The Evidence Base for Diabetes Care

SECOND EDITION

The Evidence Base for Diabetes Care

SECOND EDITION

EDITED BY

William H. Herman
Department of Internal Medicine and Epidemiology, University of Michigan, Ann Arbor, MI, USA

Ann Louise Kinmonth
Department of Public Health and Primary Care, Institute of Public Health, Cambridge, UK

Nicholas J. Wareham
MRC Epidemiology Unit, Institute of Metabolic Science, Addenbrooke's Hospital, Cambridge, UK

Rhys Williams
School of Medicine, Swansea University, Swansea, UK

WILEY-BLACKWELL
A John Wiley & Sons, Ltd., Publication

Registered office: John Wiley & Sons Ltd, The Atrium, Southern Gate, Chichester, West Sussex, PO19 8SQ, UK

Other Editorial Offices:
9600 Garsington Road, Oxford, OX4 2DQ, UK
111 River Street, Hoboken, NJ 07030-5774, USA

For details of our global editorial offices, for customer services and for information about how to apply for permission to reuse the copyright material in this book please see our website at www.wiley.com/wiley-blackwell

Library of Congress Cataloging-in-Publication Data

The evidence base for diabetes care / edited by W. Herman ... [et al.]. – 2nd ed.
     p. ; cm.
   Includes bibliographical references and index.
   ISBN 978-0-470-03274-9 (hb)
  1. Diabetes–Treatment. 2. Evidence-based medicine. I. Herman, William
   [DNLM: 1. Diabetes Mellitus–therapy. 2. Diabetes
Complications–prevention & control. 3. Diabetes Complications–therapy. 4.
Diabetes Mellitus–prevention & control. 5. Evidence-Based Medicine. WK 815
E929 2010]
   RC660.E925 2010
   616.4′62–dc22   2009031441

ISBN: 9780470032749 (HB)

A catalogue record for this book is available from the British Library.

Set in 9.5/12 Pt Palatino by Thomson Digital, Noida, India.

Printed in Singapore by Fabulous Printers Pte Ltd.

First Impression   2010

Contents

v

Contents

Part 5: Self-management, healthcare organization and public policy

List of Contributors

Amanda I. Adler
MRC Epidemiology Unit
    Institute of Metabolic Science
    Addenbrooke's Hospital
    Cambridge, UK

Ayad Al-Bemani
Department of Opthamology
Royal Victoria Infirmary
Newcastle upon Tyne, UK

Elizabeth Barrett-Connor
Department of Family and Preventive
    Medicine
University of California, San Diego
La Jolla, CA, USA

Wenche S. Borgnakke
Department of Cariology, Restorative
    Sciences and Endodontics
University of Michigan School of
    Dentistry
Ann Arbor, MI, USA

Devin L. Brown
St Joseph Mercy Hospital
Ann Arbor, MI, USA

Helen M. Colhoun
Department of Genetic Epidemiology
University College Dublin
Belfield, Dublin, Ireland

Tonya L. Corbin
Division of Cardiovascular Medicine
Department of Internal Medicine
    University of Michigan
Ann Arbor, MI, USA

Maximilian de Courten
School of Exercise and Nutrition Sciences
Faculty of Health and Behavioural Sciences
Monash University
Burwood, Victoria, Australia

Julia Critchley
Institute of Health and Society
Newcastle University
Newcastle upon Tyne, UK

Dana Dabelea
Department of Preventive Medicine and
    Biometrics
University of Colorado Health Sciences
    Center
Denver, CO, USA

Michael M. Engelgau
Division of Diabetes Translation
Center for Disease Control and
    Prevention
Atlanta, GA, USA

Eva L. Feldman
University of Michigan
Ann Arbor, MI, USA

Nita Gandhi Forouhi
Elsie Widdowson Laboratory
MRC Epidemiology Unit
Cambridge, UK

Hertzel C. Gerstein
Department of Medicine and the
    Population Health Research
    Institute
McMaster University and Hamilton
    Health Sciences
Hamilton, ON, Canada

Geoffrey Hackett
Good Hope Hospital
Sutton Coldfield
    West Midlands, UK

Richard F. Hamman
Department of Preventive Medicine and
    Biometrics
University of Colorado Health Sciences
    Center
Denver, CO, USA

William H. Herman
Department of Internal Medicine and
    Epidemiology
University of Michigan
Ann Arbor
    MI, USA

Susan L. Hickenbottom
St Joseph Mercy Hospital
Ann Arbor
    MI, USA

Teresa L. Jacobs
Departments of Neurosurgery and
    Neurology
University of Michigan
Ann Arbor
    MI, USA

Ann John
The School of Medicine
University of Wales Swansea
Swansea, UK

Ann Louise Kinmonth
General Practice and Primary Care
    Research Unit
Department of Public Health and
    Primary Care
University of Cambridge
Cambridge, UK

William R. Ledoux
VA Rehabilitation Research and
    Development Center for Excellence in
    Limb Loss
Prevention and Prosthetic
    Engineering
VA Puget Sound, and
Department of Orthopaedics and Sports
    Medicine
University of Washington
Seattle, WA, USA

Rui Li
Centers for Disease Control and
    Prevention
Atlanta, GA, USA

David R. McCance
Regional Centre for Endocrinology and
    Diabetes
Belfast, UK

Carl Erik Mogensen
Department of Internal Medicine M
    (Diabetes and Endocrinology)
Aarhus University Hospital
Aarhus, Denmark

K.M. Venkat Narayan
Division of Diabetes Translation
Center for Disease Control and
    Prevention
Atlanta, GA, USA

Stephen O'Rahilly
Department of Clinical Biochemistry
School of Clinical Medicine
Cambridge University
Addenbrooke's Hospital
Cambridge, UK

Pasquale J. Palumbo
Department of Medicine
Mayo Clinic
Scottsdale, AZ, USA

Rodica Pop-Busui
Department of Internal Medicine
Division of Metabolism, Endocrinology
    and Diabetes
University of Michigan Medical Center
Ann Arbor, MI, USA

David E. Price
ABM University Trust
Morriston Hospital
Swansea, UK

Ambady Ramachandran
India Diabetes Research Foundation and
    Dr A Ramachandran's Diabetes
    Hospitals
Egmore
Chennai, India

Simon R. Redwood
Department of Cardiology
Guy's and St Thomas' Hospitals
London, UK

Gayle E. Reiber
VA Health Services Research and
    Development and VA Rehabilitation
    Research and Development Center for
    Excellence in Limb Loss Prevention
    and Prosthetic Engineering
VA Puget Sound, and
Department of Health Services and
    Epidemiology
University of Washington
Seattle, WA, USA

Debra L. Roter
Department of Health Policy and Management
Johns Hopkins School of Public Health
Baltimore, MD, USA

Zachary Simmons
Pennsylvania State University College of
    Medicine
Hershey, PA, USA

Jay S. Skyler
Division of Endocrinology, Diabetes and
    Metabolism
University of Miami
Miami, FL, USA

Chamukuttan Snehalatha
India Diabetes Research Foundation and
    Dr A Ramachandran's Diabetes
    Hospitals
Egmore
Chennai, India

George W. Taylor
Department of Cariology, Restorative
    Sciences and Endodontics
University of Michigan School of
    Dentistry
Ann Arbor, MI, USA

Roy Taylor
School of Clinical Medical Sciences
    Medical School
Newcastle University
Newcastle upon Tyne, UK

Stephen Thomas
Diabetes Centre
St Thomas' Hospital
London, UK

Nigel Unwin
Institute of Health and Society
Newcastle University
Newcastle upon Tyne, UK

GianCarlo Viberti
Department of Diabetes and
    Endocrinology
KCL Guy's Hospital
London, UK

Nicholas J. Wareham
MRC Epidemiology Unit, Institute of
    Metabolic Science, Addenbrooke's
    Hospital, Cambridge, UK

Alan B. Weder
Division of Cardiovascular Medicine
Department of Internal Medicine
University of Michigan
Ann Arbor, MI, USA

Nicole M. Wedick
Department of Family and Preventive
    Medicine
University of California, San Diego
La Jolla, CA, USA

Sydney A. Westphal
Department of Medicine
Maricopa Medical Center
Phoenix, AZ, USA

Anthony S. Wierzbicki
Department of Chemical Pathology
Guy's and St Thomas' Hospitals
London, UK

Rhys Williams
School of Medicine
Swansea University
Swansea, UK

Deborah L. Wingard
Department of Family and Preventive
    Medicine
University of California, San Diego
La Jolla, CA, USA

Ping Zhang
Centers for Disease Control and
    Prevention
Atlanta, CA, USA

1 The evidence base for diabetes care

William H. Herman[1], Ann Louise Kinmonth[2],
Nicholas J. Wareham[3], Rhys Williams[4]

[1]*Department of Internal Medicine and Epidemiology, University of Michigan, Ann Arbor, MI, USA*
[2]*General Practice and Primary Care Research Unit, Department of Public Health and Primary Care,*
University of Cambridge, Cambridge, UK
[3]*MRC Epidemiology Unit, Institute of Metabolic Science, Addenbrooke's Hospital, Cambridge, UK*
[4]*School of Medicine, Swansea University, Swansea, UK*

Evidence-based medicine

A complex set of decisions by individuals and organizations determine how health care is delivered to people with diabetes. Historically, such decisions have been made in the absence of evidence or without strict regard to it. This has led to the persistence of practices for which there is little evidence, the slow adoption of new practices that have been demonstrated to be effective and wide variation in clinical practice and the quality of care. In recent years, there has been increasing appreciation that treatment decisions should be based on sound evidence. For patients, care providers and health systems alike, this awareness represents an opportunity to shape the delivery of care on the basis of evidence of effectiveness. This book is devoted to providing the evidence base on which treatment decisions in diabetes care may be made.

Sackett *et al.* defined evidence-based medicine as 'the conscientious, explicit and judicious use of clinically relevant research in making decisions about the care of individual patients'.[1] The strength of evidence-based medicine is that it moves clinical practice from anecdotal experience and expert opinion to a refutable scientific foundation of basic and clinical research from which we can systematically progress. Evidence-based medicine advocates that experimental methods, especially randomized, controlled clinical trials (RCTs), provide the basis for clinical practice. The strength of RCTs lies in their internal validity. The use of randomization is the strongest insurance that treatment groups will differ only in their exposure to the intervention and, hence, differences in observed outcomes can be attributed to differences in the intervention.

Perhaps not surprisingly, the major limitation of RCTs lies in their external validity, that is, the extent to which they are generalizable to particular population groups, individuals, practitioners and settings. 'Efficacy' is defined by Last as the extent to which a specific intervention produces a beneficial result under ideal conditions.[2] 'Effectiveness', on the other hand, is the extent to which the intervention does what it is intended to do 'in the real world'.[2] When individuals who participate in RCTs are atypical, the health care professionals who participate are unrepresentative or the settings deviate from a usual clinical environment, the external validity or generalizability of the results of the RCT may be low. Indeed, in most instances, an RCT offers an indication of the efficacy of an intervention, what can be achieved in the most favourable circumstances, rather than its effectiveness, what can be achieved in every day clinical practice.

Another limitation of evidence-based medicine is that the evidence that we need is not always available. In some instances, lack of evidence is a result of the necessary studies not having been carried out or not having been carried out for long enough to evaluate health endpoints. The task of conducting all of the required RCTs is overwhelming. There are a huge number of health care interventions which, when added together, have many components. It is simply impossible to subject all of these interventions and their components to experimental evaluation.

The Evidence Base for Diabetes Care, Second Edition, Edited by William H. Herman, Ann Louise Kinmonth, Nicholas J. Wareham and Rhys Williams.
© 2010 John Wiley & Sons, Ltd

Some interventions are studied and some are not. Indeed, some types of interventions are more likely to be studied than others. For example, pharmacological interventions are studied more extensively than non-pharmacological interventions, because of regulatory requirements and industry support and because of the technical and methodological difficulties in designing RCTs to evaluate non-drug interventions. As a result, the literature often fails to provide convincing evidence for complex behavioural interventions such as education, diet and lifestyle modification. In other instances, RCTs may be impossible to conduct if, for example, there are ethical or legal obstacles, if some interventions cannot be allocated on a random basis or if potential participants, practitioners or investigators refuse to take part.

Another limitation of evidence-based medicine derives from an understanding of the limits of the scientific method in clinical practice. Clinical decisions involve people and the application of results from research to clinical practice must take account of people in their social context.[3] Clinical judgement is central to clinical practice and involves weighing the benefits and risks of any medical choice in consultation with individual patients. Clinical trials explicitly focus on hard endpoints such as physiological measures and disease incidence or mortality. They often fail to focus on soft endpoints such as patient preferences or quality of life. To the extent that the latter influence clinical decision making, non-scientific mechanisms may guide decisions.[3] Indeed, as stated by Sackett *et al.*, 'External clinical evidence can inform, but can never replace, individual clinical expertise. It is this expertise that decides whether the external evidence applies to the individual patient at all and, if so, how it should be integrated into a clinical decision. Any external guideline must be integrated with individual clinical expertise in deciding whether and how it matches the patient's clinical state, predicament and preferences and thus whether it should be applied.'[1]

One of the 'credibility gaps' developing between the advocates of evidence-based medicine and the practitioners engaged in day-to-day patient care is that studies which faithfully reflect the clinical and behavioural complexities of individual patients not only have not yet been done but are unlikely ever to be done. Many clinicians 'struggle to apply the results of studies that do not seem that relevant to their daily practice'.[4] RCTs have a number of strong points but the ready generalization of their results to 'real life' clinical situations is not one of them. Too strong an emphasis on the need for evidence to support practice can easily be translated into an unwillingness to do anything which is not based on evidence. Thus the positive message of evidence-based medicine can, if taken to extremes, become a form of 'evidence-based paralysis', which acts to the detriment of the patient and the population.

Evidence-based practice

For these reasons, we prefer the term 'evidence-based practice' to the narrower, but more widely used term, 'evidence-based medicine'. Evidence-based practice emphasizes the importance of practitioners other than doctors and the importance of health-related activities other than those most obviously associated with physicians. In defining evidence-based practice, three components are essential:

• the determination, whenever possible, to base decisions on evidence accumulated through research
• use of the best possible evidence available at the time the decision needs to be made and
• use of the evidence most appropriate to a particular patient or population.

We would widen that definition of evidence-based practice to include people who are not yet patients and may never become patients, that is, to include prevention as well as care, cure and rehabilitation. In addition, although evidence-based practice uses the evidence from RCTs to provide evidence for clinical practice, it does not diminish the importance of human relationships or ignore the fact that clinical decisions in primary care involve consideration of the unique problems and concerns of individual patients.

We have chosen to call this book 'The Evidence Base for Diabetes Care' to emphasize, from the outset, that our focus is on the extent to which diabetes prevention and treatment can be based on high-quality evidence. It is not intended to be a comprehensive text book on how to care for people with diabetes. Although it refers to clinical guidelines, it is not a collection of evidence-based guidelines. This book sets out to examine critically the best evidence that is currently available in the field of diabetes prevention and care and to present it in an accessible form. The enormous potential of evidence-based practice to prevent illness, identify it early, treat it, reduce suffering and rehabilitate people to normal life presents a challenge which cannot be ignored.

Evidence-based diabetes practice

Diabetes is a particularly good example of the potential for evidence-based practice. There are at least four

1	The person with diabetes is central to the management of the condition
2	Diabetes care is multidisciplinary – evidence-based practice is important
3	The worldwide impact of diabetes is increasing at a dramatic rate
4	There is a considerable quantity of high-quality evidence available

Figure 1.1 The potential of diabetes for evidence-based practice

reasons for this (Figure 1.1). First, most diabetes care is based on long-term behavioural change. Such change will not take place unless the affected person is willing to make these changes and is assisted in making these changes. What better way is there of encouraging evidence-based practice than to make both patients and practitioners aware of the evidence that exists and the benefits (and harms) of implementing it? Second, diabetes care is multidisciplinary. The person with diabetes and, in most instances, the family, are at the centre of all diabetes health care activities. To be successful, diabetes care needs to involve the cooperation and collaboration of many practitioners – nurses, dieticians, podiatrists, psychologists and doctors. Thus diabetes care is a particularly striking example of evidence-based practice as opposed to evidence-based medicine. Third, the increasing prevalence of diabetes and its public health importance, particularly in developing countries, are a major impetus for this book. Finally, there is a considerable quantity of high-quality evidence relevant to diabetes prevention and care that needs to be translated into practice. As with other fields, there is also evidence which is not of such high quality and areas for which little evidence exists at all.

A brief explanation of terms

Throughout this book, various epidemiological terms have been used to describe risk in the context of clinical trials. These can be summarized as follows in relation to a trial which randomizes participants to two groups – an intervention group and a control group. Imagine, for the sake of simplicity, two dichotomous outcomes – prevention and non-prevention, for example:

	Outcome		
	Prevention	Non-prevention	
Intervention group	A	B	A + B
Control group	C	D	C + D

The following rates can be defined:

Experimental event rate (EER) = A/(A + B)
Control event rate (CER) = C/(C + D)
Absolute risk reduction (ARR) = CER − EER
Relative risk reduction (RRR) = (CER − EER)/CER
Number needed to treat (NNT) = 1/ARR

Analogous calculations can be performed in relation to adverse events:

	Adverse event		
	Present	Not present	
Intervention group	A	B	A + B
Control group	C	D	C + D

Experimental (adverse) event rate (E(A)ER) = A/(A + B)
Control (adverse) event rate (C(A)ER) = C/(C + D)
Absolute risk of adverse events = E(A)ER − C(A)ER
Relative risk of adverse events = (E(A)ER − C(A)ER)/C(A)ER
Number treated for one adverse event = 1/absolute risk of adverse event

Both absolute and relative risk measures have their place in evidence-based practice, but in order to understand relative risk measures, knowledge of what they are relative to is needed. For example, a relative risk reduction of 50% could mean going from an absolute risk of 1% to 0.5% or from an absolute risk of 20% to 10%. However, the absolute risk reductions, which in this case would be 0.5% and 10%, respectively, demonstrate markedly different benefits. When available, authors have been encouraged to include absolute measures, with or without their relative equivalents.

The hierarchy of evidence

There are several suggested hierarchies for grading evidence. Examples of two of these are that used by the United States Preventive Services Task Force

3

Strength of the recommendation:

A   There is good evidence to support the use of the procedure

B   There is fair evidence to support the use of the procedure

C   There is poor evidence to support the use of the procedure

D   There is fair evidence to reject the procedure

E   There is good evidence to support the rejection of the procedure

Quality of the evidence:

(I)   Evidence obtained from at least one properly randomized controlled trial

(II-1)   Evidence obtained from well-designed controlled trials without randomization

(II-2)   Evidence obtained from well-designed cohort or case–control analytical studies, preferably from more than one centre or research group

(II-3)   Evidence obtained from multiple timed series with or without the intervention or from dramatic results in uncontrolled experiments

(III)   Opinions of respected authorities based on clinical experience, descriptive studies or reports of expert committees

Figure 1.2 USPSTF template for assessing recommendations and evidence[5]

(USPSTF)[5] and that suggested by Chalmers *et al.*[6] The USPSTF template distinguishes between strength of a recommendation and the quality of the evidence (Figure 1.2). Chalmers *et al.*'s hierarchy ranks the source of evidence in a similar fashion to the second component of the USPSTF's template (Figure 1.3).

In this book, the frameworks used to review the evidence change from time to time. We have been flexible if authors have chosen different ways to summarize the existing evidence.

This book and how to use it

Systematic reviews of the literature are a necessary component of evidence-based practice. Inaccessible evidence, even of the highest quality, is of no use to a practitioner. There are several current resources which make evidence more accessible and provide assessments of its quality. These include the Cochrane Collaboration, which prepares and maintains rigorous, systematic and up-to-date reviews and meta-analyses of the benefits and risks of health care interventions,[7,8]

'Effective Healthcare Bulletins'[9] and a clutch of new journals and evidence-based medicine reviews that enable searches of databases to be made for articles that meet criteria for evidence-based decision-making.[10]

In this book, we summarize these reviews. The chapters are arranged to reflect the chronology of diabetes. They start with considerations of definition and classification, proceed through prevention of the condition itself, the prevention of complications and then the organization of care. When necessary, there are separate chapters for type 1 diabetes and type 2 diabetes – the chapters on prevention, for example. When the same principles apply to both, as for the treatment of established complications, they are combined in a single chapter.

We have brought together potentially contrasting views of the evidence – those of clinicians on the one hand, and epidemiologists on the other. This is intended to bring out the different perspectives and requirements of these two areas of practice. In many cases, the authors have been able to organize their

Highest	–	Meta-analysis of randomized controlled trials
	–	Randomized controlled trials
	–	Non-randomized controlled trials
	–	Cohort studies
	–	Case–control studies
	–	Case series
Lowest	-	Case reports

Figure 1.3 Hierarchy of evidence advocated by Chalmers *et al.*[6]

literature searches according to Cochrane Collaboration principles[7] and the results of these searches, for RCTs, are systematically presented in tables. In the chapters dealing with the prevention and treatment of established complications, we have asked teams to contribute since the span of topics is so wide. Throughout this book, authors have been asked to clarify and comment upon the evidence in each of their topic areas and to highlight what remains to be resolved by future research. We hope, therefore, that this book will be useful to patients and their representatives to allow them to establish whether their care includes all interventions known to be effective, to policy makers as a guide to what is already known and to those responsible for planning future research to identify major areas of uncertainty.

References

1 Sackett DI, Rosenberg WMC, Gray JAM, Haynes RB, Richardson WS. Evidence based medicine: what it is and what it isn't. It's about integrating individual clinical expertise and the best external evidence. *BMJ* 1996;**312**:71–72.

2 Last JM. *A Dictionary of Epidemiology*, Oxford Medical Publications, Oxford University Press, Oxford, 1983.

3 Kenny NP. Does good science make good medicine? Incorporating evidence into practice is complicated by the fact that clinical practice is as much art as science. *Can Med Assoc J* 1997;**157**:33–36.

4 Knottnerus JA, Dinant GJ. Medicine based evidence, a prerequisite for evidence based practice. *BMJ* 1997;**315**: 1109–1110.

5 US Preventive Service Task Force. *Report of the US Preventive Service Task Force. Guide to Clinical Preventive Services. An Assessment of the Effectiveness of 169 Interventions*, Williams and Wilkins, Baltimore, 1989.

6 Chalmers TC, Celano P, Sacks HS, Smith H Jr. Bias in treatment assignment in controlled clinical trials. *N Engl J Med* 1983;**309**:1358–1361.

7 Chalmers I, Sackett D, Silagy C, The Cochrane Collaboration. In: *Non-random Reflections on Health Services Research: on the 25th Anniversary of Archie Cochrane's 'Effectiveness and Efficiency'* (eds A Maynard, I Chalmers,), BMJ Publishing Group, London, 1997.

8 *The Cochrane Library*. BMJ Publishing Group, London. 1997, Issue 4.

9 Department of Health. *Effective Health Care: the Treatment of Depression in Primary Care*. Effective Health Care Bulletin No. 5, University of Leeds, Leeds, 1993.

10 Jadad AR, Haynes RB, Hunt D, Browman GP. The Internet and evidence-based decision-making: a needed synergy for efficient knowledge management in health care. *Can Med Assoc J* 2000;**162**:362–365.

Part 1: Evidence-based definition and classification

2 Classification of diabetes

Maximilian de Courten

School of Exercise and Nutrition Sciences, Faculty of Health and Behavioural Sciences, Monash University, Burwood, Victoria, Australia

Diabetes mellitus is defined as a metabolic disorder of multiple aetiologies – a syndrome or a collection of disorders, characterized by chronic hyperglycaemia with disturbances of carbohydrate, fat and protein metabolism resulting from defects in insulin secretion, insulin action or both. Given that a collection of disorders with a spectrum of aetiologies are put together under one clinical term, it is not surprising that the effects of diabetes mellitus are also diverse, with a range of possible long-term damages, dysfunctions and failures of various organs. The symptoms that diabetes mellitus may present, such as thirst, polyuria, blurring of vision and weight loss, are various and neither obligatory nor specific. In its most severe forms, ketoacidosis or a non-ketotic hyperosmolar state may develop, but often symptoms are not severe or may even be absent, and consequently hyperglycaemia sufficient to cause pathological and functional changes may be present for a long time before the diagnosis is made. The long-term effects of diabetes mellitus again include a variety of complications that progressively develop, such as retinopathy (the most specific diabetes complication), nephropathy, neuropathy and features of autonomic dysfunction, including sexual dysfunction. In addition, people with diabetes are at increased risk of cardiovascular, peripheral vascular and cerebrovascular disease. This variation in possible causes and consequences characterized the quest to define diagnostic thresholds for diabetes.

Evolution of the classification and terminology of diabetes

Brief history of the classification of diabetes

The term 'diabetes' was first used by Aretaeus of Cappadocia in the second century AD as a generic description for conditions causing increased urine output. Aretaeus wrote an accurate description of the condition that is instantly recognisable today as type 1 diabetes and concluded that it was due to a fault of the kidneys. The Indian physician Sushruta in the 6th century BC is thought to have been the first to describe what we now term type 2 diabetes, as a condition primarily affecting people who are obese with exercise as a key factor in its treatment.[1] Throughout history, such renowned scientists and physicians as Galen, Avicenna, Paracelsus and Maimonides have made reference to diabetes.[2] The sweet taste of the urine from patients with diabetes had been noticed by the ancient Greeks, Chinese, Egyptians, Indians and Persians, and in 1776, Matthew Dobson confirmed that it was due to an excess of a kind of sugar in the blood of people with diabetes.[3]

It took until the end of the 19th century for another huge step forward in the understanding of the aetiology of diabetes to be achieved. The experiments by Josef von Mering and Oskar Minkowski proved that removal of the pancreas produced severe and fatal diabetes in dogs and were published as 'Diabetes mellitus after extirpation of the pancreas' in 1889. The dogs began urinating large quantities and Minkowski tested the urine for glucose, as he did with clinic patients with polyuria, and found a similarly high glucose content. This discovery inspired the work which led to the isolation of insulin from the pancreas for use in the therapy of diabetes, for which Banting and Macleod won the Nobel Prize in 1923.

In 1936, Harold Himsworth[4] proposed that there were at least two clinical types of diabetes, insulin-sensitive and insulin-insensitive types. He suggested that patients with insulin-sensitive diabetes were insulin deficient and required exogenous insulin to

The Evidence Base for Diabetes Care, Second Edition, Edited by William H. Herman, Ann Louise Kinmonth, Nicholas J. Wareham and Rhys Williams.
© 2010 John Wiley & Sons, Ltd

survive, whereas the other group did not. This observation was based on clinical evidence, as at that time no assays were available for the measurement of insulin. The Australian scientist Joseph Bornstein developed the first bioassay for insulin and his measurements of insulin in individuals with diabetes made it increasingly apparent that there were at least two major distinct forms of the disease.[5] With the help of the assay, these were now separable not only on the basis of age at diabetes onset, but also on the basis of the level of endogenous insulin. The difference in age on onset led to the use of the terms 'juvenile-onset' and 'maturity-onset' diabetes. This was thought to be largely consistent with the later nomenclature based on observed treatment differences described as insulin-dependent diabetes mellitus (IDDM) and non-insulin-dependent diabetes mellitus (NIDDM) and subsequently type 1 and type 2 diabetes.

The debate concerning the classification of diabetes has not abated, with recent discussions focusing on the diabetes risk category of impaired fasting glucose with proposed changes to the threshold of diagnosis. In general, the need for disease classifications to be of therapeutic value to the patient is paramount and correct risk category identification is critical for prevention programmes. However, the expectations of what a classification should deliver might differ for a clinician whose concern is with diagnosis and treatment from the needs of a research scientist.[6] The classification of diabetes and its risk categories is therefore an example of a debate in which there is an uneasy compromise with a nomenclature influenced by scientific discoveries and therapeutic possibility and science-driven cut-off levels conflicting with clinical practice.[7]

Evolution of the diagnostic criteria for diabetes

Historically there was little debate about the diagnostic criteria for type 1 diabetes because of its acute onset and the logical link between aetiology and treatment, with insulin replacement being used to treat insulin deficiency. However, the recognition of a non-insulin-dependent form of diabetes, in which there was a much less clear distinction between normality and disease, created the need for diagnostic criteria. Classification of disease sub-types solely on the basis of symptoms and clinical signs was evidently unsatisfactory and the search for the development of diagnostic criteria was further promoted by the recognition that the absence of standardization was an obstacle to epidemiological and clinical research.[8]

In 1964, the World Health Organization (WHO) convened an Expert Committee on Diabetes Mellitus that attempted to provide a universal classification and diagnostic criteria for the diabetes syndrome.[9] However, it was not until 1980 that an internationally accepted classification was established.

Two international working groups, the National Diabetes Data Group (NDDG) of the National Institutes of Health, USA, in 1979[10] and the WHO Expert Committee on Diabetes in 1980[11] proposed and published similar criteria for diagnosis and classification. They both recognized that diabetes was an aetiologically and clinically heterogeneous group of disorders with hyperglycaemia shared in common. The NDDG/WHO classification system incorporated data from research conducted during the previous decades and set the path for a unified nomenclature and diagnostic criteria including the amount of oral glucose load to be used in the oral glucose tolerance test (OGTT). The inclusion of impaired glucose tolerance (IGT) in the diabetes classification followed the recognition that a zone of diagnostic uncertainty existed in the OGTT between normal glucose tolerance and diabetes.

However, controversy continued around the specific criteria and minor changes to the classification took place in 1985, letting the WHO slightly modify their criteria to coincide more with the NDDG values. The NDDG later modified the diagnostic requirements by dropping the intermediate sample during the OGTT to become identical with the WHO recommendations. With the 1985 WHO Study Group classification,[12] a number of clinical classes of diabetes were agreed upon, including the two major groups: *insulin-dependent diabetes mellitus (IDDM)* and *non-insulin-dependent diabetes mellitus (NIDDM)*. The terms type 1 and type 2 diabetes were omitted in the 1985 revision and *malnutrition-related diabetes mellitus (MRDM)* was introduced as a new class. The other important classes were retained from the 1980 document as *other types* and *impaired glucose tolerance (IGT)* as well as *gestational diabetes mellitus (GDM)*. These classifications were widely accepted for the next decade and represented a compromise between a clinical- and an aetiological-based system. This had the advantage that cases where the specific cause or aetiology was unknown could still be classified according to their clinical presentation.

Recent changes to the classification of diabetes

Data from genetic, epidemiological and aetiological studies continued to accumulate throughout the 1980s and 1990s and the understanding of the aetiology and pathogenesis of diabetes improved. With the application of universal criteria for diagnosis and standardized testing procedures, estimation of the global burden of diabetes became possible.[13,14]

Nevertheless, calls continued for revisiting the NDDG and WHO recommendations[6] to fulfil further the aims set out by the NDDG in 1979 in order to take into account the dynamic phasic nature of diabetes.[15] Advances such as the use of immunological markers of the type 1 diabetes process suggested that the clinical classification of diabetes into IDDM and NIDDM was unsatisfactory. Age of onset of diabetes was increasingly regarded as a confounding factor in the classification rather than its basis. Frequently clinicians observed autoimmune forms of diabetes amongst adults and diabetes with features of NIDDM in adolescents. In addition, many adult patients with NIDDM were well controlled for several years with diet and oral hypoglycaemic agents but needed insulin later in the course of their disease. At a time when autoantibody measurement was not available, it would have remained uncertain if these patients had type 2 with a progressive insulin insufficiency or if they had slowly progressing type 1 diabetes. With the help of the immune markers, many patients previously classified as type 2 were then reclassified as having type 1 diabetes,[16] type 1 1/2 or latent autoimmune diabetes mellitus in adults (LADA)[17]

A thought-provoking attempt at separating staging of glucose intolerance from sub-classification according to aetiological type was proposed by Kuzuya and Matsuda,[18] but harks back at least to a proposal by Harry Keen in 1985.[6] This concept seeks to separate the criteria related to aetiology and those related to the degree of deficiency of insulin or insulin action and to define each patient on the basis of these two criteria. This concept was adopted by the American Diabetes Association's Expert Committee, which convened in 1995 to review the literature and determine what changes to the classification were necessary, finally reporting in 1997.[19] The WHO also convened a consultation in December 1996 to consider the issues and examine the available data, and a provisional report was published in 1998,[20] which was adopted with minor modifications in 1999.[21]

This latest major revision of the classification is now based on stages of glucose tolerance with a complimentary sub-classification according to the aetiological type. Diabetes mellitus is defined as a group of metabolic diseases characterized by hyperglycaemia resulting from defects in insulin secretion, insulin action or both. Common to all types of diabetes mellitus is chronic hyperglycaemia, which is associated with long-term damage, dysfunction

and failure of various organs, especially the eyes, kidneys, nerves, heart and blood vessels.

Hyperglycaemia can be sub-categorized regardless of the underlying cause by staging into:

• *Insulin requiring for survival* (includes the former IDDM).
• *Insulin requiring for control*, that is, for metabolic control, not for survival (includes the former insulin-treated NIDDM).
• *Not insulin requiring*, that is, treatment by non-pharmacological methods or drugs other than insulin (includes NIDDM on diet alone or combined with oral agents).
• *Impaired glucose tolerance (IGT) and/or impaired fasting glycaemia (IFG)*.
• *Normal glucose tolerance*.

which can be summarized as follows:

Normoglycaemia	Hyperglycaemia			
Normal glucose tolerance	IGT or IFG	Diabetes mellitus		
		Not insulin requiring	Insulin requiring for control	Insulin requiring for survival

In this classification, stages reflecting the various degrees of hyperglycaemia are set across the disease processes which may lead to diabetes mellitus in an individual (Figure 2.1). In all circumstances it should now be possible to categorize each individual with diabetes mellitus according to clinical stage. The stage of glycaemia may change over time depending on the extent of the underlying disease process and impact of therapeutic glucose control. The presence of hyperglycaemia is not an essential consequence of the underlying disease process because in certain situations this may not have progressed far enough to cause high levels of blood glucose.

The possibility that the glycaemic stage in an individual may change over time in both directions reflects the observation that in some individuals with diabetes, adequate glycaemic control can be achieved with weight reduction, exercise and/or oral agents. These individuals, therefore, do not require insulin and may even revert from having diabetic glucose values to IGT or normoglycaemia. Other individuals require insulin for adequate glycaemic control but can survive without it. These individuals, by definition, have some residual insulin secretion. Individuals with extensive beta-cell destruction, and therefore no residual insulin secretion, require insulin for survival. This could result from any type of diabetes (Figure 2.1).

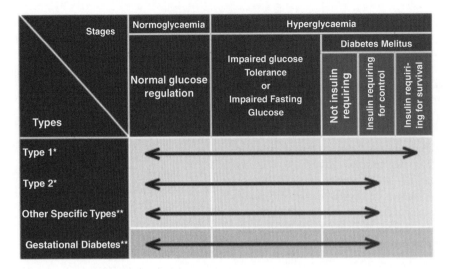

Figure 2.1 Disorders of glycaemia: aetiological types and stages. *Even after presenting in ketoacidosis, these patients can briefly return to normoglycaemia without requiring continuous therapy. **in rare instances, patients in these categories may require insulin for survival. Reproduced by permission of WHO, Ref. 32

Table 2.1 shows the classification of glycaemic disorders. As additional subtypes are discovered, it is anticipated that they will be reclassified within their own specific category.

Determining the classification in terms of aetiology allows the identification of the defect or process that leads to diabetes. For instance, the presence of islet cell antibodies makes it likely that a person has the type 1 autoimmune process even at a time when they are normoglycaemic. In contrast to type 1 and other specific types of diabetes, there are still few sensitive or highly specific indicators of the type 2 process at present, although these are likely to become apparent as aetiological research progresses.

Table 2.1 Aetiological classification of disorders of glycaemia

---

Type 1 (beta-cell destruction, usually leading to absolute insulin deficiency)
- Autoimmune
- Idiopathic

Type 2 (ranging from predominantly insulin resistance with relative insulin deficiency to a predominantly secretory defect with or without insulin resistance)

Other specific types
- Genetic defects of beta-cell function
- Genetic defects in insulin action
- Diseases of the exocrine pancreas
- Endocrinopathies
- Drug- or chemical-induced
- Infection-caused diabetes, e.g. congenital rubella
- Uncommon forms of immune-mediated diabetes
- Other genetic syndromes sometimes associated with diabetes

Gestational diabetes
- Includes the former categories of gestational impaired glucose tolerance and gestational diabetes

---

In this revision, both the ADA[19] and WHO[21] recommended the following changes to the criteria which had been used since 1985 (see Table 2.5):

- The fasting plasma glucose (FPG) threshold for the diabetes category was lowered from 7.8 to 7.0 mmol l^{-1}.
- Impaired fasting glycaemia (FPG 6.1–6.9 mmol l^{-1}) was introduced as a new category of intermediate glucose metabolism (named impaired fasting glucose by the ADA). The term IFG was originally coined by Charles et al.[22] with a fasting plasma glucose level between 6.1 and <7.8 mmol l^{-1}. The ADA and subsequently the WHO altered the upper end to correspond to the new lower diagnostic criteria for diabetes. The fasting glucose concentration of 6.1 mmol l^{-1} has been chosen as the upper limit of 'normal'.

Other revisions included changes to the nomenclature. The terms 'insulin-dependent diabetes mellitus' and 'non-insulin-dependent diabetes mellitus' and their acronyms 'IDDM' and 'NIDDM' were eliminated and type 1 and type 2 reintroduced into the nomenclature with an emphasis on using Arabic rather than Roman numerals.

The former class of 'malnutrition-related diabetes' (MRDM) was deleted, because the evidence that diabetes can be caused by malnutrition or protein deficiency *per se* was not convincing. Its subtype, protein-deficient pancreatic diabetes (PDPD or PDDM) was considered as malnutrition modulated or modified form of diabetes mellitus. The other former subtype of MRDM, fibrocalculous pancreatic diabetes (FCPD), was classified as a disease of the exocrine pancreas, which may lead to diabetes mellitus and assigned to 'other specific types'.

Gestational diabetes mellitus

Gestational diabetes mellitus (GDM) was defined as carbohydrate intolerance of variable severity with onset or first recognition during pregnancy. The definition applies irrespective of whether or not insulin is used for treatment or whether the condition persists after pregnancy. It does not exclude the possibility that unrecognized glucose intolerance may have antedated or begun concomitantly with the pregnancy. After pregnancy ends, the woman has to be reclassified, either into diabetes mellitus, IGT, IFG or normal glucose tolerance. Unfortunately, the question of the best diagnostic criteria for GDM is the major area where the ADA and WHO have not been able to come to a consensus. The WHO recommendations for diagnosing GDM have remained essentially the same since 1985. Formal testing for gestational diabetes is recommended between 24 and 28 weeks of gestation. The WHO suggests that an OGTT should be performed after overnight fasting (8–14 h) using a 75 g glucose load, with plasma glucose measured at 2 h. Pregnant women who meet WHO criteria for diabetes or IGT should be classified as having GDM. They suggest that at least 6 weeks post-pregnancy, a woman should be reclassified based on the results of 75 g load OGTT. For the WHO, the significance of IFG in pregnancy remains to be established and therefore any woman with IFG should have the 75 g OGTT.

In the 2003 ADA document,[23] the class 'gestational diabetes mellitus' is also retained as defined by the WHO and NDDG previously. However, selective rather than universal screening for glucose intolerance in pregnancy is recommended. Glucose levels meeting the threshold for the diagnosis of diabetes, a fasting plasma glucose level ≥ 126 mg dl^{-1} (7.0 mmol l^{-1}) or a casual plasma glucose ≥ 200 mg dl^{-1} (11.1 mmol l^{-1}). if confirmed on a subsequent day, preclude the need for any glucose challenge. Also, in the absence of this degree of hyperglycaemia, ADA recommends the evaluation for GDM in women with average or high-risk characteristics to follow one of two approaches:

1 One-step approach: a diagnostic OGTT without prior plasma or serum glucose screening is done. The one-step approach may be cost-effective in women at high risk.
2 Two-step approach: an initial screening is undertaken by measuring the plasma or serum glucose concentration 1 h after a 50 g oral glucose load glucose challenge test (GCT), and a diagnostic OGTT is

Table 2.2 Diagnosis of GDM with a 100 or 75 g glucose load

	mg dl^{-1}	mmol l^{-1}
100 g glucose load		
Fasting	95	5.3
1 h	180	10.0
2 h	155	8.6
3 h	140	7.8
75 g glucose load		
Fasting	95	5.3
1 h	180	10.0
2 h	155	8.6

performed only on that subset of women who exceed the glucose threshold value on the GCT.

With either approach, the diagnosis of GDM is based on an OGTT using either a 75 or 100 g glucose load. Diagnostic criteria for the 100 g OGTT are derived from the original work of O'Sullivan and Mahan, modified by Carpenter and Coustan.[24] The criteria for using the 75 g glucose load and the glucose threshold values for fasting, 1 and 2 h. are listed also in Table 2.2. The ADA maintains, however, that the 75 g test is not as well validated as the 100 g OGTT.

The test should be done in the morning after an overnight fast of between 8 and 14 h and after at least 3 days of unrestricted diet (150 g carbohydrate per day) and unlimited physical activity. Two or more of the venous plasma concentrations must be met or exceeded for a positive diagnosis.

The controversies concerning the definition of gestational diabetes are discussed in full in Chapter 11 by David McCance.

Risk categories for developing diabetes: impaired glucose tolerance and impaired fasting glycaemia/glucose

The class *Impaired Glucose Tolerance* (IGT) was defined as a stage of impaired glucose regulation diagnosed on basis of the 2 h glucose value from an OGTT. In the 1985 WHO classification of diabetes, IGT was included as a separate class of diabetes. This meant that until 1980, people with a 2 h post-glucose load plasma glucose between 7.8 and 11 mmol l^{-1} were diagnosed with diabetes. It is now categorized together with impaired fasting glycaemia (IFG) (see below) as a stage in the natural history of disordered carbohydrate metabolism with higher than normal fasting (IFG) or 2 h post-oral glucose load (IGT) glucose levels not reaching diabetic thresholds (see Table 2.5). As such, IGT and IFG were regarded, in the absence of pregnancy in which they contribute to the class of gestational diabetes, not as clinical entities in their own right but as risk factors for future diabetes and cardiovascular disease.[25] This new categorization stopped people with these risk factors from being defined as having a disease which could restrict life insurance and certain jobs and be associated with other social penalties in some countries. There are, however, calls to reinstate IGT as a disease.[26] IGT or IFG can be observed as intermediate stages in any of the disease processes listed in Figure 2.1 under the assumption that persons within this stage are at higher risk for developing diabetes than the general population. Individuals with IGT have a raised risk of macrovascular disease[27] as IGT is associated with other known CVD risk factors including hypertension, dyslipidaemia and central obesity. The diagnosis of these risk categories, therefore, may have important prognostic implications, particularly in otherwise healthy and ambulatory individuals.

A new stage of *impaired fasting glycaemia or glucose* (IFG) was also introduced to classify individuals who have fasting glucose values above the normal range, but below those diagnostic of diabetes. Although this is conceptually similar to the definition of IGT based on intermediate 2 h PG values, the thresholds chosen for IFG were not selected to be comparable to the considerations underlying the agreement on the diagnostic FPG threshold for diabetes.

The rationale for adding the category of IFG as a second diabetes risk group was to identify a risk state for diabetes and/or future cardiovascular disease and premature mortality which can be assessed more easily and reliably than IGT. Individuals with IFG, like those with IGT, have increased risks of progressing to diabetes, although the risk of progression may be lower than IGT.[27,28] There is also the suggestion that people with IFG have a lower CVD risk factor profile than those with IGT[29] and some, but not all, studies suggest that IFG is not associated with elevated cardiovascular risk.[30,31]

Current criteria for the diagnosis of diabetes mellitus

The *clinical diagnosis* of diabetes is often prompted by the classical signs and symptoms of diabetes. A single random or casual blood glucose estimation in excess of the diagnostic values indicated in Figure 2.2 (black zone) establishes the diagnosis of diabetes in such cases.

Figure 2.2 also defines levels of blood glucose below which a diagnosis of diabetes is unlikely in non-pregnant individuals. These criteria go back to the 1985 WHO report. If an OGTT is performed, blood glucose values should be measured while fasting and at 2 h after the 75 g oral glucose load.

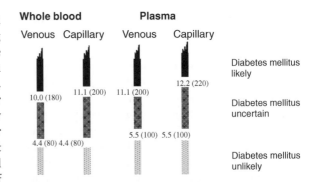

Figure 2.2 Unstandardized (casual, random) blood glucose values in the diagnosis of diabetes in mmol l^{-1} (mg dl^{-1}). Reproduced by permission of WHO, Ref. 21

Table 2.3 summarizes the current WHO and ADA recommendations for the diagnostic criteria for diabetes and intermediate hyperglycaemia. The WHO suggests that if 2 h plasma glucose is not measured when determining IFG, the status remains uncertain as diabetes or IGT based on the 2 h value cannot be excluded.

Evidence base for diagnostic thresholds

Bimodal glucose distribution as determinant of diagnostic threshold

One of the early contributions of epidemiological studies in the Pima Indians was the observation in 1971 that the population distribution of glucose values follows a bimodal shape: two separate but overlapping curves.[34] This bimodality suggested that there was, at least on the 2 h PG values, a cut-point originating from the shape of the distribution of glucose levels that could determine the difference between individuals with and without diabetes. In certain high-risk populations, bimodal distributions were confirmed and various points separating the two components of the bimodal population distribution of 2 h PG values were estimated to lie around 11.1 mmol l^{-1} and on the fasting glucose distribution at 7.8 mmol l^{-1}.[35–37]

The 2 h PG thresholds of 11.1 and 7.8 mmol l^{-1} FPG formed the basis of the 1980 diabetes classification[11] and spurred an enormous body of clinical and epidemiological data collection worldwide. However, newer data and those from lower risk populations did not demonstrate bimodality. In these populations, glucose values were more normally distributed, making it difficult to identify a threshold.[38,39] It has also been suggested that the phenomenon of bimodality is only apparent in certain high-prevalence populations because of statistical power.[40,41]

A more critical analysis of the few population data with blood glucose values following a bimodal

Table 2.3 Values for diagnosis[a] of diabetes and other categories of hyperglycaemia

	Venous plasma glucose concentration			
	WHO 2006[32]		**ADA 2003**[33]	
	mmol l^{-1}	**mg dl^{-1}**	**mmol l^{-1}**	**mg dl^{-1}**
Diabetes mellitus:				
Fasting	$\geq$7.0	$\geq$126	$\geq$7.0	$\geq$126
	or	*or*	*or*	*or*
2 h post-glucose load	$\geq$11.1	$\geq$200	$\geq$11.1	$\geq$200
Impaired glucose tolerance:				
Fasting concentration	<7.0	<126	Not required	
	and	*and*		
2 h post-glucose load	$\geq$7.8 and <11.1	$\geq$140 and < 200	$\geq$7.8 and <11.1	$\geq$140 and <200
Impaired fasting glucose:			**Impaired fasting glycaemia:**	
Fasting	$\geq$6.1 and <7.0	$\geq$110 and <126	$\geq$5.6 and <7.0	$\geq$100 and <126
	and	*and*		
2 h post-glucose load	*if measured*	*if measured*	Measurement not recommended (but <11.1 if measured)	Measurement not recommended (but <200 if measured)
	<7.8	<140		

[a]Note that both organizations (ADA and WHO) state that diabetes can only be diagnosed in an individual when these diagnostic values on confirmed on another day.

distribution and the definition of the anti-modal cut-points within those populations[32] show that the cut-points vary considerably by age, sex and ethnic group, highlighting the difficulty of selecting a single diagnostic value to be used internationally from such data. Nevertheless, the 2 h plasma glucose value derived from the OGTT was retained at 11.1 mmol l^{-1}.

Long-term diabetes complications used for defining diabetes thresholds

Microvascular changes in the kidney and retina are specific complications of diabetes which have been used to derive diagnostic cut-points for the condition. The rationale is that there is a threshold separating those individuals who are at substantially increased risk of microvascular complications from those who are not. Initially, data from epidemiological studies which have examined prevalent micro- and macrovascular complications such as retinopathy, neuropathy, nephropathy and cardiovascular disease across a range of plasma glucose levels[42–44] confirmed relationships between hyperglycaemia and the risk of developing such complications. However, many studies have compared the rates of each condition in individuals already classified according to the diagnostic criteria as having diabetes or not. Few studies considered whether the current diagnostic glucose levels represent the best level for predicting an increased risk of such complications and no formal statistical threshold for any complication has been consistently demonstrated. It is obvious that such an analysis requires large population-based cohort studies with sufficient follow-up having enough cases with diabetes-specific complications in each glycaemic interval around the thresholds tested. In the Pima Indian study of a well-characterized population with an extremely high prevalence of diabetes, the prevalence of diabetes-related microvascular disease increased sharply at 2 h PG levels of around 14 mmol l^{-1} and at fasting plasma glucose levels of 7.5 mmol l^{-1}.[44] Nevertheless, in 1997 the ADA Expert Committee confirmed the 2 h PG criterion at 11.1 mmol l^{-1} based on the relationship between glucose values and diabetes-specific complications based on data from the Pima Indians, Egypt and unpublished NHANES III analyses.[19]

The same Expert Committee compared the relationship of FPG with the development of retinopathy with that of the 2 h PG in several studies to consider a revision of the FPG diabetes criterion. In a new analysis undertaken in the Pima Indian population over a wide range of plasma glucose cut-points, both FPG and 2 h PG were similarly associated with retinopathy, indicating that by this criterion, each could work equally well for diagnosing diabetes.[45] The authors concluded that both measures were equivalent in terms of the properties previously used to justify diagnostic criteria. These findings were confirmed in a similar study in Egypt, in which the FPG and 2 h PG were each strongly and equally well associated with retinopathy.[46] For both the FPG and the 2 h PG, the prevalence of retinopathy was somewhat higher above the point of intersection of the two components of the bimodal frequency distribution ($7.2 \, \text{mmol} \, l^{-1}$ and 2 h PG $11.5 \, \text{mmol} \, l^{-1}$). The decision by the ADA Expert Committee to lower the FPG criterion was then based on equivalence to the 2 h PG relation with diabetes-specific complications and to approximate the prevalence yield for diabetes in comparison with the 2 h test.[19]

Another statistical approach to determine the value of a diagnostic test which provides the maximum sensitivity and specificity for predicting the occurrence of a given complication associated with diabetes is through the use of receiver operating characteristic (ROC) curves.[47] In the Pima Indian population, the optimum cut-off values for predicting future retinopathy were $7.2 \, \text{mmol} \, l^{-1}$ for a fasting plasma glucose test and $13.0 \, \text{mmol} \, l^{-1}$ for the 2 h PG. These values differ from the cut-off values suggested as diagnostic of diabetes from the bimodal distribution of blood glucose results in this population. The use of ROC analyses for predicting nephropathy among the Pima population indicated that the various measures of hyperglycaemia were poor at predicting renal complications of diabetes.

In summary, few studies have been ideal for the purpose of determining diagnostic glucose thresholds on the basis of the relationship to diabetes-specific complications. Most have limited statistical power either due to small sample size or limited follow-up. Different methods are used to diagnose the outcome of interest and critically studies vary as to whether or not people with previously diagnosed diabetes are included, which may introduce bias. Excluding people with diabetes can reduce this bias but reduces variation in glucose levels and excludes the participants with the highest risk of developing complications.[46] Furthermore, the specific statistical method used to derive cut-points may influence the result.

Evidence for matching the FPG threshold with the 2 h PG threshold

The 1985 WHO criteria selected the fasting and 2 h cut-offs on estimates of the bimodal glucose distribution. After reviewing the statistical relationship between the FPG distribution and 2 h PG distribution, it became evident that these criteria effectively defined diabetes by the 2 h PG alone because the fasting and 2 h cut point values were not equivalent at those levels. Almost all individuals with FPG $\geq 7.8 \, \text{mmol} \, l^{-1}$ have 2 h PG levels of $11.1 \, \text{mmol} \, l^{-1}$ or above when given an OGTT. On the other hand, only about one-quarter of those with 2 h PG exceeding $11.1 \, \text{mmol} \, l^{-1}$ without previously known diabetes have FPG greater than $7.8 \, \text{mmol} \, l^{-1}$.[48] Thus, the cut-point of FPG $7.8 \, \text{mmol} \, l^{-1}$ defined a greater degree of hyperglycae-

mia in comparison with the cut-point of 2 h PG $11.1 \, \text{mmol} \, l^{-1}$. This discrepancy was thought to be undesirable and therefore the ADA Expert Committee investigated cut-point values for both tests which reflected a similar degree of hyperglycaemia and risk of adverse outcomes. The decision to lower the diagnostic cut-point for the FPG to $7.0 \, \text{mmol} \, l^{-1}$, also adopted by the WHO,[21] was based on the belief that the cut-points for the FPG and 2 h PG should diagnose similar conditions, given the equivalence of the FPG and the 2 h PG in their association with microvascular complications. Although the overall prevalence defined by these two measures may be similar, the two tests clearly identify different individuals.[49,50]

The argument for lowering the fasting glucose diagnostic threshold in 1997 was to enable the fasting test to identify the same percentage of the population as are identified by the 2 h cut-point, an implicit assumption being that the 2 h cut-point is the optimal criterion.

In conclusion, the history of changes in diagnostic criteria and the evidence base that has led to changes in the diagnostic criteria over time highlights the tension between the need for international harmonization of criteria and possible heterogeneity between populations. There is still a need for large population-based studies preferably naïve to glucose lowering treatment. Being a multifactorial disease, it is not surprising that there are large differences in the prevalence of diabetes, their determinants and the associated complications among various ethnic groups around the world. Therefore, the development of international diagnostic criteria based on evidence from studies conducted in only a few ethnic groups is problematic.

Diagnostic thresholds for impaired glucose tolerance (IGT) and impaired fasting glycaemia (IFG)

Numerous population-based studies have calculated the risk of progression from IGT to diabetes. Two reviews[51,52] including 15 different populations from Europe, the United States, India, Africa and the Pacific island of Nauru reported an annual rate of development of diabetes varying from 2 to 14%. Risk was highest in those populations with a high background prevalence of diabetes. Data on IFG are less frequent, but in two studies there was an annual conversion rate to diabetes of 1% in middle-aged French civil servants[22] and 6% in a high-prevalence population in Mauritius.[53]

Underlying this concept of progression from an intermediate risk state is the assumption that there are three separate glycaemic states: normoglycaemia, diabetic hyperglycaemia and a non-diabetic state of hyperglycaemia in-between the two which confers a different level of risk for developing diabetes-related complications. However, across the glucose spectrum in the few longitudinal studies of the natural history of increasing glucose intolerance and development of diabetes-related complications, no clear or common threshold is observed. Indeed, the relationships are curvilinear. In addition, the development of diabetes complications seems to be related to both the duration and degree of glycaemic exposure. However, little attention has been paid to the relationship between these two variables, mainly because determination of exposure duration requires sophisticated metabolic surveillance systems or clinical datasets.[54] Comparisons are rarely made between individuals with moderate levels of hyperglycaemia for extended periods and individuals with high levels over short time frames.

The current diagnostic criteria used for the diagnosis of these two intermediate hyperglycaemic states have recently been adjusted from those in place since 1997. In 2003, the ADA issued a new expert report[23,33] recommending lowering the threshold for IFG from 6.1 mmol l^{-1} (110 mg dl^{-1}) to 5.6 mmol l^{-1} (100 mg dl^{-1}),[33] a move highly criticized by other groups led by the European Diabetes Epidemiology Group.[55] The WHO convened a Technical Guideline Development Group which published its report in 2006[32] recommending retaining the lower threshold for IFG at 6.1 mmol l^{-1} (110 mg dl^{-1}). This lack of concordance has the potential to create confusion among researchers and clinicians.[56,57] As a consequence of using different diagnostic criteria, studies and trials may no longer be directly comparable if 'diabetes', 'IGT' and 'IFG' do not mean the same thing in different studies.

A recent review investigating the reproducibility of glucose testing showed that up to 53% of dysglycaemic individuals may revert to 'normoglycaemia' within 1 year.[28] Any discussion of cut-off levels needs to be informed by knowledge of this natural variability.

What is the best diagnostic test?

Importance of reliable diabetes tests

The impact of a diagnosis of diabetes on an individual can be dramatic. Once this chronic disease is diagnosed, significant behavioural changes are often recommended which can impact not only on the people with diabetes but also on those who live with them. The ability to get health insurance and even employment may also be affected. The psychological burden associated with the diagnosis of a chronic disease for which a cure has not yet been satisfactorily developed may be significant. Given the implications of diagnosis, the diagnostic cut-off values should be highly specific or identify as few false positives as possible. The difficulty is that among those individuals who are more vulnerable to complications, the criteria would have low sensitivity and would identify fewer true cases and therefore may be unacceptable for clinical care. An ideal diagnostic test would be both highly sensitive and specific, but in the case of diabetes this is currently unattainable.

Urine glucose measurement

The first diagnostic test for diabetes was described in ancient China, with the observation that ants were attracted to the urine of persons with diabetes. The London physician Thomas Willis (1621–1675) noted that diabetic urine tasted 'wondrous sweet' and in 1776 another Englishman, Matthew Dobson, demonstrated the chemical presence of sugar in diabetic urine. By the 1840s, such chemical tests as Fehling's test were developed for sugar in the urine. Benedict's urine test was described in 1911 and remained the mainstay for assessing control of diabetes for many decades.

Urine glucose measurement, although cheap and convenient, has inadequate sensitivity[59,60] and therefore is not recommended for diagnosis,[61] although the data for these studies used high-quality blood tests as comparator and the recommendation for resource-poor settings might differ.[62]

Blood-based assessment of hyperglycaemia

Random blood glucose
Random blood glucose measured with a reflectance meter could theoretically be used as a diagnostic test but by comparison with an OGTT (Table 2.4) has low sensitivity and specificity. The issue of random glucose as a screening rather than a diagnostic measure is described in Chapter 6 by Engelgau and Narayan.

Blood glucose meters and whole blood glucose determination
Most portable devices measure the glucose concentration directly in the plasma component of the blood by filtering out the red blood cells. The reading is then calibrated to produce a result either as blood or as plasma glucose. Laboratory measures normally use plasma separated from blood cells, with determination of the concentration of glucose in a fixed

Table 2.4 The performance of a random whole blood glucose determination in comparison to an OGTT

Engelgau et al.[63]	
At sensitivity of 90%[a]	Median specificity 48–52% (according to age group)
At specificity of 90%	Median sensitivity 49–52%
Optimal	Median sensitivity 73–76%
	Median specificity 76–78%
Qiao et al.[64]	
Cut-off 5.8 mmol l^{-1}	Sensitivity 63%, specificity 85%[b]
Cut-off 5.2 mmol l^{-1}	Sensitivity 78%, specificity 62%[b]
Rolka et al.[65]	
Cut-off 7.8 mmol l^{-1}	Sensitivity 56%, specificity 96%
Cut-off 6.7 mmol l^{-1}	Sensitivity 75%, specificity 88%

[a]The cut-off value of random whole blood glucose for a sensitivity of 90% was 4.4–6.7, depending on age and post-prandial period.
[b]Sensitivities and specificities were worse in women than men at all thresholds.

volume. As glycolysis inhibitors take time to penetrate into red blood cells, only immediate separation of plasma will avoid some lowering of glucose levels in the sample, although rapid cooling can reduce this loss.

The precision of glucose meters is limited and the diagnosis of diabetes should be made on laboratory measurements of glucose.[66] The accuracy of glucose results measured by glucose meters may be low, with only 35–83% of readings being within ±10% of the adjusted laboratory plasma glucose values.[67,68] There seems to have been little improvement in accuracy over the past decade.[69,70]

Comparability of venous and capillary blood glucose measurements

Differences in glucose results could also be partially due to different sites of blood collection. Venous and capillary samples give the same result in the fasting state but in the non-fasting state capillary blood gives higher results than venous samples.[33]

Glucose measured in plasma was previously thought to be approximately 10% higher than glucose measured in whole blood.[21] However, this difference is dependent on the haematocrit of the blood, increasing to 15% at a high haematocrit of 0.55 from 8% at a low haematocrit of about 0.30,[71] and seems also to differ across the glycaemic range.[72] Hence the simple conversion of whole blood glucose to plasma glucose by adding 10% to the value is problematic and the previously published WHO conversion tables have not been repeated in the organization's latest publication and no recommendations regarding whole blood glucose-based cut-offs are given.[32]

Oral glucose tolerance test

The oral glucose tolerance test (OGTT) is the accepted standard for the diagnosis of diabetes. It is, however, time consuming and inconvenient, requiring often overlooked preparation of the patient. As recent dietary intake and the duration of the pre-test fast can affect the results,[73,74] the OGTT should be administered in the morning after at least 3 days of unrestricted diet (greater than 150 g of carbohydrate daily) and usual physical activity. A reasonable carbohydrate-containing meal (30–50 g) should be consumed on the evening before the test. The test should be preceded by an overnight fast of 8–14 h, during which period water may be drunk. Smoking should not be permitted during the test. The presence of factors that influence interpretation of the results of the test should be recorded (e.g. medications, inactivity and infection). Many would therefore regard this test as unsuitable for widespread use among people with risk factors for diabetes, let alone in a busy primary health care practice – an argument consistently brought forward in the USA.[19,23,75]

Paired OGTTs performed 2–6 weeks apart have shown that amongst people who are diagnosed as having diabetes on an initial OGTT, 95% of values in the second OGTT lie within ±20% of the initial fasting glucose and ±36% of the initial 2 h glucose.[76] At lower glucose cut-off values, the reproducibility of OGTT test results is even more uncertain. When retesting study participants with IGT within 6 weeks, the proportion of people classified with IGT on the first OGTT and on retesting was found to range from 33 to 48% with 39–61% being reclassified as normal and 6–13% as having diabetes on the second test.[28] Some of this variability might be explained by differing gastric emptying times.[77] This poor reproducibility led the American Association for Clinical Chemistry in their 2002 *Guidelines and Recommendations for Laboratory Analysis in the Diagnosis and Management of Diabetes Mellitus* to recommend not using the OGTT for diabetes diagnosis.[66]

Blood glucose measurements show considerable day-to-day variability and therefore it is recommended that diabetes only be diagnosed when two abnormal values have been found for tests conducted on separate days. This recommendation is based on concerns about the potential implications of the disease label to an individual. Duplicate testing reduces the probability of attributing the label in error. However, the evidence base for determining the diagnostic threshold as discussed below is based on studies using data from single, that is, once only, OGTTs. The requirement for duplicate testing as required for the clinical diagnosis in ambiguous cases is, however, in effect equivalent to raising the diagnostic threshold for a single test.

There is also little recent published evidence supporting the appropriate glucose amount. Early comparisons of various glucose loads (50, 75 and 100 g) led to the recommendation for the highest amount resulting in the lowest coefficient of variation of the blood glucose measurement.[78] Currently 75 g anhydrose glucose for adults and 1.75 g of glucose per kilogram body weight up to a total of 75 g of glucose for children is recommended in 250–300 ml of water drunk over the course of 5 min. The origin of these recommendations is a mid-Atlantic compromise between the 50 and 100 g used in Europe and the United States before international standardization. When glucose monohydrate is used, the corresponding amount is 82.5 g, which may give rise to confusion and another potential source of measurement error.

Fasting blood glucose measurement

The ADA Expert Committee recommended using fasting glucose alone as a diagnostic criterion, thus simplifying fieldwork and reducing the burden on participants. The WHO, by contrast, recommended retention of the OGTT.[32]

The processing of the blood sample after collection is important to ensure accurate measurement of plasma glucose. This requires rapid separation of the plasma after blood collection. Blood collection into a tube containing a glycolytic inhibitors (e.g. sodium fluoride) is only partially effective. A minimum requirement is that the sample should be placed immediately in ice–water after collection and before separating, and separation should occur within 30 min.[79]

Fasting versus oral glucose tolerance testing

The ADA classification document from 1997 received a lot of attention with the recommendations to perform diabetes diagnosis generally with fasting plasma glucose alone. This was a deviation from the 1985 WHO recommendations and not completely followed by the 1999 or 2006 WHO statements, which supported the retention of the OGTT unless circumstances would prevent it from being performed. Furthermore, the WHO retained in 1999 the recommendation for epidemiological studies to restrict diabetes screening to the 2 h post-OGTT value in situations where the fasting state of the participants cannot be assured.

In a situation of partial overlap of the distributions of fasting and 2 h diabetes values in a population, any algorithm utilizing several tests in parallel (such as scoring individuals using their fasting and their 2 h glucose value for classification by whichever meets the diabetes criterion) will yield increased numbers. Table 2.5 shows how the different criteria used over the history of diabetes classifications would classify patients with different blood glucose levels and how changing thresholds affect glucose intolerance groups. When both tests, FPG and 2 h PG, are applied

Table 2.5 Diagnostic category of individuals with different glucose cut-off levels according to various classification criteria

		2 h plasma glucose (mmol l^{-1})			Classification
		<7.8	7.8–11.1	≥11.1	
Fasting plasma glucose (mmol/l)	<5.6	N	IGT	D	WHO 1985[12]
		N	IGT	D	ADA 1997[19]
		N	IGT	D	ADA 2003[23]
		N	IGT	D	WHO 1999[21]/2006[33]
	5.6–6.0	N	IGT	D	WHO 1985
		N	IGT	D	ADA 1997
		IFG	IGT	D	ADA 2003
		N	IGT	D	WHO 1999/2006
	6.1–6.9	N	IGT	D	WHO 1985
		IFG	IFG + IGT	D	ADA 1997
		IFG	IFG + IGT	D	ADA 2003
		IFG	IFG + IGT	D	WHO 1999/2006
	7.0–7.8	N	IGT	D	WHO 1985
		D	D	D	ADA 1997
		D	D	D	ADA 2003
		D	D	D	WHO 1999/2006
	≥7.8	D	D	D	WHO 1985
		D	D	D	ADA 1997
		D	D	D	ADA 2003
		D	D	D	WHO 1999/2006

N = normal glucose tolerance, IFG = impaired fasting glycaemia, IGT = impaired glucose tolerance, D = diabetes mellitus on the same individual a whole 3×4 table emerges to classify their glucose intolerance status.

There is complete agreement in classifying individuals at either extreme of the glucose distribution (the grey shaded areas in Table 2.5). However, for individuals with an FPG between 5.6 and 7.8 mmol l^{-1} and a 2 h glucose between 7.8 and 11.1 mmol l^{-1}, how they are classified depends on the criteria that are used. This discordance between the classification systems means that if either criterion were used alone, they would inevitably identify different groups of individuals. This will also impact on incidence and prevalence rates. A number of recent studies have shown that using FPG would result in the misclassification of a significant proportion of people with diabetes, defined according to the 2 h level.[27,50,80]. It is likely that all of these people are at risk of diabetes-related complications and therefore the OGTT may be necessary to exclude diabetes in anyone with a positive screening blood test. However, approximately 35% of all people with newly diagnosed diabetes still have a normal fasting glucose, whereas 15–20% have a normal 2 h value.[28,32] This distribution differs between men and women, with women being more commonly diagnosed on the basis of the 2 h glucose.[81] This is also reflected in the observation that IGT seems to occur more often in women than elevated but not yet diabetic fasting glucose levels (IFG).[82]

HbA$_{1c}$ as a diagnostic test

Glycosylated haemoglobin (HbA$_{1c}$) is attractive as a diagnostic test, because it is simple, requires no preparation of the patient and directly relates to treatment targets. However, the 2003 and 2006 expert groups suggested that it should not yet be used for the diagnosis of diabetes, although they conceded that HbA$_{1c}$ predicted retinopathy as well as FPG and 2 h PG.[45] Data from prospective population studies identified HbA$_{1c}$ as a continuously distributed risk factor which has a linear association with all-cause mortality and CHD incidence and mortality.[83] Furthermore, in type 2 diabetes HbA$_{1c}$ is increasingly the measurement of choice in monitoring treatment and deciding when and how to implement therapy.

In the past, the utility of HbA$_{1c}$ testing was limited in part by relatively poor reproducibility and lack of standardization across laboratories. More recently, widespread adoption of standardized HbA$_{1c}$ measurements was achieved and the newer laboratory techniques are highly reproducible.[84] Measurement errors caused by non-glycaemic factors affecting HbA$_{1c}$ such as the occurrence of haemoglobinopathies are infrequent and can be minimized by confirming the diagnosis of diabetes with a plasma glucose specific test in such situations. A systematic review in 1996 found that a HbA$_{1c}$ cutoff value of 6.4% was 66% sensitive and 98% specific and was associated with a positive predictive value of 63% in a population with a diabetes prevalence of 6%.[85] Increasing the cut-off value to 7.0% increased the positive predictive value to 90%. HbA$_{1c}$ values in the high-normal range (5.6–6.0%) seem to predict a higher incidence of future diabetes[86] and could obliterate the need of an OGTT.[87] These observations have led some to recommend HbA$_{1c}$ measurement for diabetes screening[75] and even as diagnostic test[88] and the Japanese Diabetes Association has already included HbA$_{1c}$ into their diagnostic classification.

Non-invasive tests to diagnose diabetes

There is increasing evidence that advanced glycation end products (AGEs) play a crucial role in the development of atherosclerosis in diabetes.[89] AGE accumulation is seen not only to reflect the mid-term level of hyperglycaemia, but also to represent the cumulative metabolic burden due to hyperglycaemia and hyperlipidaemia, oxidative stress and inflammation.[90] AGEs accumulate not only on haemoglobin but also on other long-lived proteins such as skin collagen, lens crystallins and cartilage proteins. Importantly, the sites where chronic complications develop in diabetes are also those where long-lived proteins are present (e.g. glomerular basement membrane). It may be preferable to use assays of tissue AGE accumulation rather than only blood samples.

Several studies have now demonstrated that elevated skin AGEs are good biomarkers of diabetes, highly correlated with its complications and are predictive of future diabetic retinopathy and nephropathy.[91–93] Thus, skin AGEs could constitute a sensitive summary metric for the integrated glycaemic exposure that the body has endured. Recently, skin AGEs have been assessed non-invasively through autofluorescence.[89]

The performances of a non-invasive device determining skin AGEs compared with FPG and HbA$_{1c}$ were evaluated for sensitivity and specificity against OGTT-based classification for detecting undiagnosed diabetes and impaired glucose tolerance. The non-invasive technology showed clinical performance advantages over both FPG and HbA$_{1c}$ testing. The authors concluded that the combination of higher sensitivity and greater convenience – rapid results with no fasting or blood draws – makes the non-invasive skin AGE testing suitable for diabetes diagnosis.[94]

Conclusions

Diabetes mellitus is a complex of diseases sharing in common raised blood glucose levels that lead to short and long-term complications. The causative factors for diabetes are diverse and range from infections to single gene defects with complex environmental and biological interactions probably predominant.

Scientific progress and better understanding of diabetes had led to a classification expanding from describing a single disease state to distinguishing at least four different types of diabetes mellitus. This number of overall sub-types may not be expanded in the future because the classification allows newly described specific types of diabetes with a distinct aetiology to be moved out of the type 2 class to the class labelled 'other specific types'.

The classification of diabetes into different types is driven by differing needs, including aetiological research and clinical practice. The old descriptive age-of-onset classes gave way to a treatment-related classification, which has in turn been superseded by a system based on aetiology. Gestational diabetes mellitus as a class is still the exception as the basis for the classification is the common context rather than the aetiology.

The diagnostic criteria for diabetes are based on the common characteristic of hyperglycaemia. Achievements in accuracy and methodological standardization of internationally accepted testing procedures resulted in the widespread application of two diagnostic tests: fasting blood glucose determination and measurement of blood glucose 2 h after an oral glucose tolerance test. In the near future, a third marker of hyperglycaemia, HbA_{1c}, is likely to be added to this list. However, using several tests in parallel for the classification of glucose-intolerant states is undesirable as it creates confusion for clinicians.

The acceptance of a diagnostic standard across the various aetiological sub-types of diabetes has resulted in considerable progress in describing its epidemiology and pathogenesis. With improved characterizations of diabetic phenotypes across many populations and sub-groups (such as the elderly), it is apparent that the threshold distinguishing normal and abnormal blood glucose levels may not be universal. If this observation is correct, it would be a major challenge to diagnostic uniformity, especially as national groups increasingly seem prone to applying their own classification criteria in parallel to standard international ones.

References

1 Dwivedi G, Dwivedi S. Sushruta – the clinician – teacher par excellence. *Indian J Chest Dis Allied Sci* 2007;**49**:243–244.

2 Major R (ed.) *A History of Medicine*. Blackwell, Oxford, 1954, p. 67.

3 Dobson M. Experiments and observations on the urine in diabetes. *Medical Observations and Inquiries* 1776;**5**:298–316.

4 Himsworth H. Diabetes mellitus: its differentiation into insulin-sensitive and insulin insensitive types. *Lancet* 1936; **i**:117–120.

5 Bornstein J, Lawrence R. Plasma insulin in human diabetes mellitus. *BMJ* 1951;**ii**:1541–1542.

6 Keen H. Limitations and problems of diabetes classification from an epidemiological point of view. *Adv Exp Med Biol* 1985;**189**:31–46.

7 Abourick NN. Dialogue between clinicians and researchers will lead to a better diabetes classification. *Diabetes Care* 1996;**19**(3):270–271.

8 Danowski TS, Tinsman CA. Diabetes mellitus: still an inadequately recorded disease. *Diabetes* 1962;**11**:239–240.

9 World Health Organization. *World Health Organization Expert Committee on Diabetes Mellitus: First Report*. WHO, Geneva, 1965.

10 National Diabetes Data Group. National Diabetes Data Group classification and diagnosis of diabetes mellitus and other categories of glucose intolerance. *Diabetes* 1979;**28**: 1039–1057.

11 World Health Organization. *World Health Organization Expert Committee on Diabetes Mellitus Second Report*. WHO, Geneva, 1980.

12 World Health Organization. *Diabetes Mellitus: Report of a WHO Study Group*. WHO, Geneva, 1985.

13 King H, Aubert RE, Herman W. Global burden of diabetes 1995–2025. Prevalence numerical estimates and projections. *Diabetes Care* 1998;**21**:1414–1431.

14 King H, Rewers M. Global estimates for prevalence of diabetes mellitus and impaired glucose tolerance in adults. *Diabetes Care* 1993;**16**(1):157–177.

15 Abourizk N, Dunn J. Types of diabetes according to National Diabetes Data Group classification. Limited applicability and need to revisit. *Diabetes Care* 1990;**13**(11): 1120–1123.

16 Turner R *et al.* UKPDS 25: autoantibodies to islet-cell cytoplasm and glutamic acid decarboxylase for prediction of insulin requirement in type 2 diabetes. UK Prospective Diabetes Study Group. *Lancet* 1997;**350**(9087): 1288–1293.

17 Zimmet PZ *et al.* Latent autoimmune diabetes mellitus in adults (LADA): the role of antibodies to glutamic acid decarboxylase in diagnosis and prediction of insulin dependency. *Diabet Med* 1994;**11**(3):299–303.

18 Kuzuya T, Matsuda A. Classification of diabetes on the basis of etiologies versus degree of insulin deficiency. *Diabetes Care* 1997;**20**(2):219–220.

19 Expert Committee on the Diagnosis and Classification of Diabetes Mellitus. Report of the Expert Committee on the Diagnosis and Classification of Diabetes Mellitus. *Diabetes Care* 1997;**20**(7):1183–1197.

20 Alberti KG, Zimmet PZ. Definition, diagnosis and classification of diabetes mellitus and its complications. Part 1: Diagnosis and classification of diabetes mellitus provisional report of a WHO consultation. *Diabetic Med* 1998;**15**(7): p. 539–53.

21 World Health, Organization. *Definition Diagnosis and Classification of Diabetes Mellitus and its Complications. Part 1: Diagnosis and Classification of Diabetes Mellitus. Report of a WHO Consultation.* WHO, Geneva, 1999.

22 Charles MA *et al*. Risk factors for NIDDM in white population. Paris prospective study. *Diabetes* 1991;**40**(7):796–799.

23 Expert Committee on the Diagnosis and Classification of Diabetes Mellitus. Report of the Expert Committee on the Diagnosis and Classification of Diabetes Mellitus. *Diabetes Care* 2003;**26**(Suppl 1): S5–S20.

24 Carpenter MW, Coustan DR. Criteria for screening tests for gestational diabetes. *Am J Obstet Gynecol* 1982;**144**(7):768–773.

25 Fuller JH *et al*. Coronary-heart-disease risk and impaired glucose tolerance. The Whitehall study. *Lancet* 1980; **i**(8183):1373–1376.

26 Perry RC, Baron AD. Impaired glucose tolerance. Why is it not a disease?. *Diabetes Care* 1999;**22**(6):883–885.

27 Unwin N *et al*. Impaired glucose tolerance and impaired fasting glycaemia: the current status on definition and intervention. *Diabet Med* 2002;**19**(9):708–723.

28 Santaguida P *et al*. Diagnosis prognosis and treatment of impaired glucose tolerance and impaired fasting glucose. Evidence Report/Technology Assessment 2005;AHRQ Pub. No. 05-E026-2(128).

29 Blake DR *et al*. Impaired glucose tolerance but not impaired fasting glucose is associated with increased levels of coronary heart disease risk factors: results from the Baltimore Longitudinal Study on Aging. *Diabetes* 2004;**53** (8):2095–2100.

30 Pankow JS *et al*. Cardiometabolic risk in impaired fasting glucose and impaired glucose tolerance: the Atherosclerosis Risk in Communities Study. *Diabetes Care* 2007;**30**(2):325–331.

31 Levitzky YS *et al*. Impact of impaired fasting glucose on cardiovascular disease: the Framingham Heart Study. *J Am Coll Cardiol* 2008;**51**(3):264–270.

32 World Health Organization. *Definition and Diagnosis of Diabetes Mellitus and Intermediate Hyperglycemia: Report of a WHO/IDF Consultation.* WHO, Geneva, 2006.

33 Genuth S *et al*. Follow-up report on the diagnosis of diabetes mellitus. *Diabetes Care* 2003;**26**(11):3160–3167.

34 Rushforth NB *et al*. Diabetes in the Pima Indians. Evidence of bimodality in glucose tolerance distributions. *Diabetes* 1971;**20**(11):756–765.

35 Raper LR *et al*. Plasma glucose distributions in two pacific populations: the bimodality phenomenon. *Tohoku J Exp Med* 1983;**141**(Suppl): 199–206.

36 Flock EV *et al*. Bimodality of glycosylated hemoglobin distribution in Pima Indians: relationship to fasting hyperglycemia. *Diabetes* 1979;**28**(11):984–989.

37 Zimmet P, Whitehouse S. Bimodality of fasting and two-hour glucose tolerance distributions in a Micronesian population. *Diabetes* 1978;**27**(8):793–800.

38 Friedlander Y *et al*. Univariate and bivariate admixture analyses of serum glucose and glycated hemoglobin distributions in a Jerusalem population sample. *Hum Biol* 1995;**67**(1):151–170.

39 Cohen P, Dix D. The oral glucose tolerance test: an objective method of interpretation. *Acta Diabetol Lat* 1984;**21**(2):181–189.

40 Spielman RS *et al*. Glucose tolerance in two unacculturated Indian tribes of Brazil. *Diabetologia* 1982;**23**(2):90–93.

41 Omar MA *et al*. South African Indians show a high prevalence of NIDDM and bimodality in plasma glucose distribution patterns. *Diabetes Care* 1994;**17**(1):70–73.

42 Collins VR *et al*. Prevalence and risk factors for micro- and macroalbuminuria in diabetic subjects and entire population of Nauru. *Diabetes* 1989;**38**(12):1602–1610.

43 Collins VR *et al*. High prevalence of diabetic retinopathy and nephropathy in Polynesians of Western Samoa. *Diabetes Care* 1995;**18**(8):1140–1149.

44 Rushforth NB, Miller M, Bennett PH. Fasting and two-hour post-load glucose levels for the diagnosis of diabetes. The relationship between glucose levels and complications of diabetes in the Pima Indians. *Diabetologia* 1979; **16**(6):373–379.

45 McCance DR *et al*. Comparison of tests for glycated haemoglobin and fasting and two hour plasma glucose concentrations as diagnostic methods for diabetes. *BMJ* 1994;**308** (6940):1323–1328.

46 Engelgau MM *et al*. Comparison of fasting and 2-hour glucose and HbA1c levels for diagnosing diabetes. Diagnostic criteria and performance revisited. *Diabetes Care* 1997; **20**(5):785–791.

47 Smith PJ *et al*. A generalized linear model for analysing receiver operating characteristic curves. *Stat Med* 1996; **15**(3):323–333.

48 Harris MI *et al*. Prevalence of diabetes and impaired glucose tolerance and plasma glucose levels in U S. population aged 20–74 yr. *Diabetes* 1987;**36**(4):523–534.

49 DECODE Study Group. Will new diagnostic criteria for diabetes mellitus change phenotype of patients with diabetes? Reanalysis of European epidemiological data. DECODE Study Group on behalf of the European Diabetes Epidemiology Study Group. *BMJ* 1998;**317**(7155):371–375.

50 DECODE Study Group. Consequences of the new diagnostic criteria for diabetes in older men and women. DECODE Study (Diabetes Epidemiology: Collaborative Analysis of Diagnostic Criteria in Europe). *Diabetes Care* 1999;**22**(10): 1667–1671.

51 Edelstein SL *et al*. Predictors of progression from impaired glucose tolerance to NIDDM: an analysis of six prospective studies. *Diabetes* 1997;**46**(4):701–710.

52 Alberti KG. Impaired glucose tolerance – fact or fiction? *Diabet Med* 1996;**13**(3 Suppl 2):S6–S8.

53 Soderberg S *et al*. High incidence of type 2 diabetes and increasing conversion rates from impaired fasting glucose and impaired glucose tolerance to diabetes in Mauritius. *J Intern Med* 2004;**256**(1):37–47.

54 Orchard TJ *et al*. Cumulative glycemic exposure and microvascular complications in insulin-dependent diabetes mellitus. The glycemic threshold revisited. *Arch Intern Med* 1997;**157**(16):1851–1856.

55 Forouhi NG *et al*. The threshold for diagnosing impaired fasting glucose: a position statement by the European Diabetes Epidemiology Group. *Diabetologia* 2006;**49**:822–827.

56 Harris MI *et al*. Comparison of diabetes diagnostic categories in the U.S. population according to the 1997 American Diabetes Association and 1980–1985 World Health

Organization diagnostic criteria. *Diabetes Care* 1997;**20**(12): 1859–1862.

57 Borch-Johnsen K *et al.* Creating a pandemic of prediabetes: the proposed new diagnostic criteria for impaired fasting glycaemia. *Diabetologia* 2004;**47**(8):1396–1402.

58 Welborn TA, Reid CM, Marriott G. Australian Diabetes Screening Study: impaired glucose tolerance and non-insulin-dependent diabetes mellitus. *Metabolism* 1997; **46**(12 Suppl 1):35–39.

59 Davies MJ *et al.* Community screening for non-insulin-dependent diabetes mellitus: self-testing for post-prandial glycosuria. *Q J Med* 1993;**86**(10):677–684.

60 Bitzen PO, Schersten B. Assessment of laboratory methods for detection of unsuspected diabetes in primary health care. *Scand J Prim Health Care* 1986;**4**(2):85–95.

61 Friderichsen B, Maunsbach M. Glycosuric tests should not be employed in population screenings for NIDDM. *J Public Health Med* 1997;**19**(1):55–60.

62 van der Sande MA *et al.* Is there a role for glycosuria testing in sub-Saharan Africa? *Trop Med Int Health* 1999;**4**(7): 506–513.

63 Engelgau MM *et al.* Screening for diabetes mellitus in adults. The utility of random capillary blood glucose measurements. *Diabetes Care* 1995;**18**(4):463–466.

64 Qiao Q *et al.* Random capillary whole blood glucose test as a screening test for diabetes mellitus in a middle-aged population. *Scand J Clin Lab Invest* 1995;**55**(1):3–8.

65 Rolka DB *et al.* Performance of recommended screening tests for undiagnosed diabetes and dysglycemia. *Diabetes Care* 2001;**24**(11):1899–1903.

66 Sacks DB *et al.* Guidelines and recommendations for laboratory analysis in the diagnosis and management of diabetes mellitus. *Clin Chem* 2002;**48**(3):436–472.

67 Chan JC *et al.* Accuracy precision and user-acceptability of self blood glucose monitoring machines. *Diabetes Res Clin Pract* 1997;**36**(2):91–104.

68 Poirier JY *et al.* Clinical and statistical evaluation of self-monitoring blood glucose meters. *Diabetes Care* 1998;**21** (11):1919–1924.

69 Bohme P *et al.* Evolution of analytical performance in portable glucose meters in the last decade. *Diabetes Care* 2003; **26**(4):1170–1175.

70 Chen ET *et al.* Performance evaluation of blood glucose monitoring devices. *Diabetes Technol Ther* 2003;**5**(5):749–768.

71 Fogh-Andersen N *et al.* Direct reading glucose electrodes detect the molality of glucose in plasma and whole blood. *Clin Chim Acta* 1990;**189**(1):33–38.

72 Colagiuri S *et al.* Comparability of venous and capillary glucose measurements in blood. *Diabet Med* 2003;**20**(11): 953–956.

73 Kanan W *et al.* Glycaemic and insulinaemic responses to natural foods frozen foods and their laboratory equivalents. *Indian J Physiol Pharmacol* 1998;**42**(1):81–89.

74 Sermer M *et al.* Impact of time since last meal on the gestational glucose challenge test. The Toronto Tri-Hospital Gestational Diabetes Project. *Am J Obstet Gynecol* 1994; **171**(3):607–616.

75 US Preventive Services Task Force. Screening for type 2 diabetes mellitus in adults: US Preventive Services Task Force recommendation statement. *Ann Intern Med* 2008; **148**(11):846–854.

76 Mooy JM *et al.* Intra-individual variation of glucose specific insulin and proinsulin concentrations measured by two oral glucose tolerance tests in a general Caucasian population: the Hoorn Study. *Diabetologia* 1996;**39**(3):298–305.

77 Horowitz M *et al.* Relationship between oral glucose tolerance and gastric emptying in normal healthy subjects. *Diabetologia* 1993;**36**(9):857–862.

78 Toeller M, Knussmann R. Reproducibility of oral glucose tolerance tests with three different loads. *Diabetologia* 1973; **9**(2):102–107.

79 Burrin JM, Alberti KG. What is blood glucose: can it be measured? *Diabet Med* 1990;**7**(3):199–206.

80 DECODE Study Group. Is fasting glucose sufficient to define diabetes? Epidemiological data from 20 European studies. The DECODE Study Group: European Diabetes Epidemiology Group: Diabetes Epidemiology: Collaborative Analysis of Diagnostic Criteria in Europe. *Diabetologia* 1999; **42**(6): 647–654.

81 Williams JW *et al.* Gender differences in the prevalence of impaired fasting glycaemia and impaired glucose tolerance in Mauritius. Does sex matter? *Diabet Med* 2003; **20**(11): 915–920.

82 Tripathy D *et al.* Insulin secretion and insulin sensitivity in relation to glucose tolerance: lessons from the Botnia Study. *Diabetes* 2000;**49**(6):975–980.

83 Khaw KT, Wareham N, Bingham S, Luben R, Welch A, Day N. Association of glycated hemoglobin with cardiovascular disease and mortality in adults: the EPIC–Norfolk prospective study. *Ann Intern Med* 2004;**141**:413–420.

84 Little RR *et al.* The national glycohemoglobin standardization program: a five-year progress report. *Clin Chem* 2001; **47**(11):1985–1992.

85 Peters AL *et al.* A clinical approach for the diagnosis of diabetes mellitus: an analysis using glycosylated hemoglobin levels. Meta-analysis Research Group on the Diagnosis of Diabetes Using Glycated Hemoglobin Levels. *JAMA* 1996;**276**(15):1246–52.

86 Edelman D *et al.* Utility of hemoglobin A1c in predicting diabetes risk. *J Gen Intern Med* 2004;**19**(12):1175–1180.

87 Norberg M *et al.* A combination of HbA1c fasting glucose and BMI is effective in screening for individuals at risk of future type 2 diabetes: OGTT is not needed. *J Intern Med* 2006; **260**(3): 263–271.

88 Saudek CD *et al.* A new look at screening and diagnosing diabetes mellitus. *J Clin Endocrinol Metab* 2008;**93**(7): 2447–2453.

89 Meerwaldt R *et al.* The clinical relevance of assessing advanced glycation endproducts accumulation in diabetes. *Cardiovasc Diabetol* 2008;**7**:29.

90 Baynes JW, Thorpe SR. Glycoxidation and lipoxidation in atherogenesis. *Free Radic Biol Med* 2000;**28**(12):1708–1716.

91 Genuth S *et al.* Glycation and carboxymethyllysine levels in skin collagen predict the risk of future 10-year progression of diabetic retinopathy and nephropathy in the diabetes control and complications trial and epidemiology of diabetes interventions and complications participants with type 1 diabetes. *Diabetes* 2005;**54**(11):3103–3111.

92 Meerwaldt R *et al.* Increased accumulation of skin advanced glycation end-products precedes and correlates with clinical manifestation of diabetic neuropathy. *Diabetologia* 2005; **48**(8):1637–1644.

93 Monnier VM *et al.* Skin collagen glycation glycoxidation and crosslinking are lower in subjects with long-term intensive versus conventional therapy of type 1 diabetes: relevance of glycated collagen products versus HbA1c as markers of diabetic complications. DCCT Skin Collagen Ancillary Study Group. Diabetes Control and Complications Trial. *Diabetes* 1999;**48**(4):870–880.

94 Maynard JD *et al.* Noninvasive type 2 diabetes screening: superior sensitivity to fasting plasma glucose and A1C. *Diabetes Care* 2007;**30**(5):1120–1124.

3 Commentary on the classification and diagnosis of diabetes

Stephen O'Rahilly[1], Nicholas J. Wareham[2]

[1]Department of Clinical Biochemistry, School of Clinical Medicine, Cambridge University, Addenbrooke's Hospital, Cambridge, UK
[2]MRC Epidemiology Unit, Institute of Metabolic Science, Addenbrooke's Hospital, Cambridge, UK

Max de Courten has provided an elegant historical account of concepts regarding the taxonomy of diabetes and their evolution over time. In his chapter, he considers three related but essentially different questions concerning diagnosis, aetiology and prognosis. An alternative way of framing these questions is to imagine issues that a patient with newly diagnosed hyperglycaemia might raise with their primary care physician. In this framework, these questions become: 'Doctor, are you sure I have diabetes?', 'Why did this happen?' and 'How bad is it, Doctor?'.

• *Doctor, are you sure I have diabetes?*

How we best define and explain diabetes, normoglycaemia and the hinterland between the two comes down to a debate about the practical utility of creating categorical states from continuously distributed phenomena. This debate is not particular to diabetes and is something that is widespread throughout medicine. It is perhaps illuminating that there is no WHO definition of disease, whereas there is one for health. Although we do not wish to delve too much into an epistemological discourse in this commentary, it is impossible to address the patient's perfectly reasonable question about whether or not they have diabetes without reflecting on the definition of normality and abnormality in medicine.

• *Why did this happen?*

Most people given a disease label are not only seeking clarity about whether or not they truly have the condition but also some idea of the underlying cause that led them to become diseased in the first place. In the case of diabetes, the reductionist challenge is to produce meaningful and useful aetiological subtypes. In this commentary, we consider the current status and likelihood of future progress in defining these sub-groups and the related issue of the development of therapeutic interventions that are specific to those sub-groups.

• *How bad is it, Doctor?*

The final question that most people with a disease label wish to address is one that can be characterized as being about the related issues of staging (how far has my disease progressed?) or about prognosis (what does the future hold?). In part, these questions are linked to the issue of aetiological sub-typing as this may, at least in theory, allow more individualized prognostic information to be provided. All forms of human diabetes are ultimately due to an absolute or relative incapacity of the pancreatic beta-cell to cope with the demands put on it. In the course of diabetes therapy, there is a point at which beta-cell function becomes so impaired that exogenous insulin treatment is required. There is, of course, marked heterogeneity between people in the timing of this transition. Even though the timing of this transition point may not be associated with clinical outcomes, it is perceived by patients and doctors alike as a seminal 'crisis point' in the trajectory of their disease. In some ways, the undoubted major personal and clinical impact of a decision to initiate insulin therapy has rather muddied the waters when it comes to a rational and scientific approach to the issues of diabetes diagnosis and classification. If one uses the analogy of

The Evidence Base for Diabetes Care, Second Edition, Edited by William H. Herman, Ann Louise Kinmonth, Nicholas J. Wareham and Rhys Williams.
© 2010 John Wiley & Sons, Ltd

cancer, questions relating to the need for insulin therapy are more akin to those of 'disease staging' rather than to the issues of diagnosis (do I have cancer or not?) or classification (what sort of cancer is it?).

Max de Courten has carefully dissected and précised the current consensus views emanating from major international organizations regarding the diagnosis, classification and staging of diabetes. This commentary tries to look beyond the current common consensus to predict how the key issues of diabetes diagnosis, classification and staging are likely to evolve over the next decade and how such an evolution will aid both the biological understanding of the variety of diabetes syndromes and the quality of health care delivered to individual people and populations.

Diagnosis

As de Courten outlines, the means by which we define the boundary between normal and abnormal glucose levels has undergone transition over time and mirrors the possible approaches summarized by David Sackett and colleagues in their textbook on clinical epidemiology.[1] The early statistical definitions which placed cut-points at a particular place on the normal distribution of glucose levels in the population fall into Sackett's 'percentile' approach to defining normality. The approach for at least the last 40 years or so has been one dominated by assessment of risk with the cut-points for defining the boundary between normality and abnormality being determined by the shape of the risk curve relating levels of glycaemia to future risk of the specific microvascular complications of diabetes. The demonstration of a curvilinear risk relationship and an apparent threshold has been the cornerstone of the justification for the current cut-points. More recent studies have questioned whether this relationship is or is not curvilinear, with some suggestion that the risk is in fact linear without an obvious threshold.[2,3] Part of the problem is that in contemporary cohorts the risk of microvascular disease in the population is low once people with prevalent diabetes are removed. The task of identification of risk thresholds in epidemiology is always extremely taxing when risk is low and it may be that this is an unresolvable issue.

The question of non-linearity in risk has only ever applied to the microvascular complications of diabetes as it is generally accepted that the association between glycaemia and cardiovascular risk is linear. Although this linearity of risk for cardiovascular disease may not have direct relevance to the decision about the cut-point for defining diabetes, it does have major implications for defining the point at which to determine intermediate states of hyperglycaemia

such as IFG and IGT. For some, the existence of a definable state of 'prediabetes' and trial evidence showing that intervention can reduce progression to diabetes is sufficient justification for the use of these categories not only in research but also in routine clinical practice. For others, the lack of evidence of impact on the long-term complications of diabetes rather than just glucose levels is a barrier to clinical adoption. The central issue underlying this debate is a tension between a risk-based definition of normality and abnormality and one that goes further to adopt an approach based on capacity to benefit which Sackett refers to as the therapeutic paradigm. In this way of thinking, the boundary between normality and abnormality would be determined by evidence of treatment effectiveness. As this evidence emerges over time, it follows that the threshold would also change but that change would be based on evidence from clinical trials rather than historical observational studies of risk. The problem in the diabetes field is that, unlike blood pressure or hyperlipidaemia, there is a dearth of long-term clinical trials of glucose lowering in people with non-diabetic hyperglycaemia. Future expert committees defining where to draw the line for defining diabetes and non-diabetic hyperglycaemia need to be informed by trials, but for that to happen there needs to be a considerable increase in clinical trial activity in people at risk of diabetes.

Another issue taxing groups responsible for recommending approaches to the diagnosis of diabetes is the gulf between what is possible in research settings and in the real life situation of busy clinical practice. Although the oral glucose tolerance test has been the basis for defining type 2 diabetes, it is, in truth, only used to define the condition in a minority of cases. In an effort to try to diminish the gap between the epidemiological and pathophysiological communities and clinical practice, a recent ADA/IDF/EASD-convened expert group discussed moving to an HbA_{1c}-based definition of diabetes since this would be much more practical for many in clinical practice.[4] To date, however, the issues of test availability in developing countries are restricting the potential to make this a global recommendation. However, the central problem of the practicality of the diagnostic test for diabetes will not go away and the need for this to be harmonized with the clinical measures for defining therapeutic strategies and for monitoring treatment response will only increase as the prevalence of the condition rises.

Classification

Classification of natural phenomena into aetiological subgroups appears to be a strong human instinct. We probably do it for two reasons. First, being intrinsically curious, we like to understand the natural world and sub-categorization of observable phenomena into more manageable subtypes has been a powerful drive to taxonomy for millennia. Second, we are a practical species and like to use such knowledge for tangible human benefit. In his review, Max de Courten presents the currently accepted WHO classification whereby diabetes is split into four main classes, namely type 1, type 2, 'other specific types' and gestational diabetes, purportedly on the basis of aetiology. While this classification is undoubtedly an improvement on the old 'IDDM and NIDDM' categorization, its imperfections are readily revealed under the most superficial scrutiny. These imperfections are not the fault of the classifiers but simply reflect the relatively primitive state of our knowledge of aetiology. Thus, the term 'type 1' covers not only people whose pancreatic beta-cell destruction is clearly due to an auto-immune insulitis, but also that sizeable group of people who present with insulinopaenic, insulin-requiring diabetes with no markers of auto-immunity. The term 'type 2' is really little better than a portmanteau term to catch any form of diabetes that does not fall clearly into the other three categories.

Much of the most exciting contemporary diabetes research both in terms of understanding of aetiology and using that information to improve treatment is in the 'other specific type' category. Over the last 20 years, the genes responsible for more than 80% of Maturity Onset Diabetes of the Young (MODY) type diabetes have been identified, bringing fresh insights into the biology of the human beta-cell.[5] Importantly, defining the precise molecular subtype does have clinical relevance. Patients with glucokinase mutations have stable modest hyperglycaemia whereas those with mutations in one or other of the Hepatocyte Nuclear Factors (HNFs) tend to show deteriorating beta-cell function with time. Patients with MODY 5 have a high prevalence of renal impairment and have particular problems with achieving good glycaemic control because of the coexistence of beta-cell dysfunction and hepatic, but not muscle, insulin resistance. A critical therapeutic observation is that patients with MODY 3 due to HNF1 alpha mutations show extreme sensitivity to sulfonylureas. This is a double-edged sword for these patients. On the positive side, many patients previously on insulin can transition to sulfonylureas once the diagnosis has been made. The downside is that the administration of full doses of sulfonylureas to such patients can inadvertently lead to severe hypoglycaemia. Identifying people whose diabetes is due to lipodystrophy is clinically important as these patients are particularly prone to severe dyslipidaemia and can show a beneficial therapeutic response to leptin

therapy.[6] However, in the case of partial lipodystrophy, making the diagnosis, particularly in males, is not as straightforward as it may seem.

Perhaps the most striking example of the clinical importance of establishing the precise diagnosis of diabetes comes from patients who present with diabetes in the neonatal period. Andrew Hattersley and colleagues have recently found that a substantial fraction of these patients have activating mutations affecting the KIR6.2 potassium channel in the pancreatic beta-cell.[7] Thus those patients have beta-cells but they are electrically silenced. Remarkably, administration of sulfonylureas can reverse the defect, even in patients who have been insulin treated for decades. Not only does the transition make these patients insulin-free but it also improves glycaemic control. These 'other specific types' add up to an appreciable fraction of the burden of diabetes and are clear models of sub-groups where appropriate diagnosis and management can radically alter patient outcomes. It is likely that increased molecular understanding will result in further sub-categorization of diabetes and an increase in the number of people for whom the specific aetiology and pathogenesis of their disease is known. There is an increasing and understandable pressure to deliver the bulk of diabetes care outside the hospital setting and to have that care delivered by non-specialist staff following proforma guidelines. The high and growing prevalence of obesity-associated type 2 diabetes makes such a policy almost inevitable. However, this approach could impact negatively on a substantial fraction of people with diabetes whose disease does not conform to the 'typical' model. The maintenance of a cadre of clinicians expert in the diagnosis, classification and management of different sub-categories of diabetes is a key part of the process of avoiding this pitfall.

What is the future for aetiological classification? Will we be able to use biochemical or genetic biomarkers to further subdivide usefully patients with either type 1 or type 2 diabetes into sub-groups of different prognostic or therapeutic relevance? It is, in fact, rather too early to say. The fruits of genome-wide approaches to diabetes genetics are only beginning to emerge and as yet explain only a small proportion of the heritability of diabetes. Perhaps more will come from study of copy number variation and low-frequency variants. The understanding of the precise autoimmune mechanism in type 1 diabetes could conceivably lead to a 'magic bullet', if not for those whose beta-cells have already been destroyed then perhaps for those at risk of the disease. The behemoth of type 2 diabetes is so large and multifaceted that the victories we will achieve in the battle to understand and treat patients better are likely to occur in a piecemeal fashion. We should not, however, underestimate the importance of such patient, quiet, grinding work. Eventually we can look to a time when the accrual of information can help us towards, if not 'individualized medicine', then at least a better ability to classify our patients meaningfully in ways that allows us to target and optimize their therapy better.

Staging

The concept of staging and its orthogonal relationship to aetiological classification as presented in Max de Courten's chapter is largely uncontroversial. Although it is not biologically based, it appears to be helpful to clinicians in thinking about the practical management of patients. For people with a typical presentation of type 1 diabetes at an early age, the question of staging has not historically been an issue as the assumption of insulin requirement was a safe bet. However, the changing epidemiology of type 2 diabetes with an ever younger age of diagnosis is definitely clouding the picture, and a better system of diagnostic classification and staging is required. In older people with more typical type 2 diabetes, the point of transition between stages has been determined on the basis of the degree of glycaemic control on medication. It has not been necessary to determine formally the degree of endogenous beta-cell function in order stage the disease and tailor therapy. Even if it had been necessary, the existing measures of insulin secretory capacity and function are relatively poor and difficult to interpret without reference to a synchronous assessment of the degree of insulin resistance. However, therapies are beginning to emerge for which knowledge of the capacity of the beta-cell to respond is a prerequisite to determining whether therapy should be commenced. We would anticipate that there will be an increasing need in the future to develop, validate and apply new methods for clinical assessment of the underlying disease processes in diabetes in order to tailor therapy to the appropriate pathophysiological defect at the right stage in the disease trajectory.

References

1 Sackett DL, Haynes RB, Guyatt GH, Tugwell P. *Clinical Epidemiology: a Basic Science for Clinical Medicine*, Lippincott, Williams and Wilkins, Baltimore, 1991.

2 Wong TY, Liew G, Tapp RJ, Schmidt MI, Wang JJ, Mitchell P, Klein R, Klein BE, Zimmet P, Shaw J. Relation between fasting glucose and retinopathy for diagnosis of diabetes: three population-based cross-sectional studies. *Lancet* 2008; **371** (9614):736–743.

3 Sabanayagam C, Liew G, Tai ES, Shankar A, Lim SC, Subramaniam T, Wong TY. Relationship between glycated hemoglobin and microvascular complications: is there a natural cut-off point for the diagnosis of diabetes. *Diabetologia* 2009; **52**:1279–1289.

4 International Expert Committee. International Expert Committee report on the role of the A1C assay in the diagnosis of diabetes. *Diabetes Care* 2009; **32**(7):1327–1334.

5 Hattersley AT, Pearson ER. Minireview: pharmacogenetics and beyond: the interaction of therapeutic response, beta-cell physiology and genetics in diabetes. *Endocrinology* 2006; **147**(6):2657–2663.

6 Oral EA, Simha V, Ruiz E, Andewelt A, Premkumar A, Snell P, Wagner AJ, DePaoli AM, Reitman ML, Taylor SI, Gorden P, Garg A. Leptin-replacement therapy for lipodystrophy. *N Engl J Med* 2002; **346**(8):570–578.

7 Pearson ER, Flechtner I, Njlstad PR, Malecki MT, Flanagan SE, Larkin B, Ashcroft FM, Klimes I, Codner E, Iotova V, Slingerland AS, Shield J, Robert JJ, Holst JJ, Clark PM, Ellard S, Svik O, Polak M, Hattersley AT and the Neonatal Diabetes International Collaborative Group. Switching from insulin to oral sulfonylureas in patients with diabetes due to Kir6.2 mutations. *N Engl J Med* 2006; **355**(5):467–477.

Part 2: Primary and primordial prevention and early detection

4 Prevention of type 1 diabetes

Jay S. Skyler

Division of Endocrinology, Diabetes and Metabolism, University of Miami, Miami, FL, USA

Type 1 diabetes is characterized by immune-mediated pancreatic islet β-cell destruction, absolute insulin deficiency and thus dependence on insulin therapy for the preservation of life.[1] The type 1 diabetes disease process is thought to involve (1) a genetic predisposition, conferred principally by 'diabetogenic' genes, principally ones in the major histocompatibility complex (MHC) on the short arm of chromosome 6, (2) non-genetic (environmental) factors that appear to act as triggers in genetically susceptible people and (3) activation of immune mechanisms targeted against pancreatic islet β-cells. The process may be a relapsing and remitting disease, similar to other autoimmune diseases.[2] The initial immune response engenders secondary and tertiary responses which collectively result in impairment of β-cell function, progressive destruction of β-cells and consequent development of type 1 diabetes. The process is insidious and may evolve over many years, with the overt expression of clinical symptoms becoming apparent only when most β-cells have been destroyed. Yet, even at disease onset, 10–20% of β-cells remain. Improvement in their function accounts for the 'honeymoon' period often seen during the first years after onset of type 1 diabetes.

Over the last quarter of a century, much investigation has been directed at interdicting the type 1 diabetes disease process, both during the stage of evolution of the disease and at the time of disease onset.[3–11] The goal of intervention prior to disease onset is to arrest the immune destruction and thus delay or prevent clinical disease. The goal of intervention at disease onset is to halt the destruction of β-cells, perhaps allowing residual β-cells to recover function, thus modifying the severity of clinical manifestations.

Studies aimed at delay or prevention of clinical type 1 diabetes are critically dependent on the ability to identify individuals at risk of the disease. Although family members of patients with type 1 diabetes have a 10–20-fold increased risk compared with the general population, amongst newly diagnosed patients with type 1 diabetes only 10–15% have a relative known to have the disease.[12] Therefore, efforts have been directed at identifying potential risk markers both in relatives and, to a lesser extent, in the general population. Because case finding is easier amongst relatives (due to their 10–20-fold increased risk), most intervention studies aimed at disease prevention have focused on relatives. All evidence suggests that the type 1 disease process is the same in sporadic non-familial cases[13,14] as it is in relatives.[15–17]

Although studies in animal models have used degree of insulitis as a histopathological indicator of the type 1 diabetes disease process, histological studies in human beings are very limited.[18,19]. Thus, β-cell function (insulin secretion), measured by assessing C-peptide response (either basal or, more likely, in response to a provocative challenge) has been used to evaluate interventions in new-onset type 1 diabetes,[20,21] while the evolution from prediabetes to overt hyperglycaemia has been used in trials prior to disease onset.

This chapter will review the evidence concerning interventions designed to interdict the type 1 diabetes disease process. To facilitate the discussion, the evolution of the disease can be divided into a number of stages, depicted in Figure 4.1, through which individuals progress. Interruption of the sequence at any stage is likely to be important[22] The stages are (1) genetic susceptibility, modulated by genetic protection, identified by finding of susceptibility genes without

The Evidence Base for Diabetes Care, Second Edition, Edited by William H. Herman, Ann Louise Kinmonth, Nicholas J. Wareham and Rhys Williams.

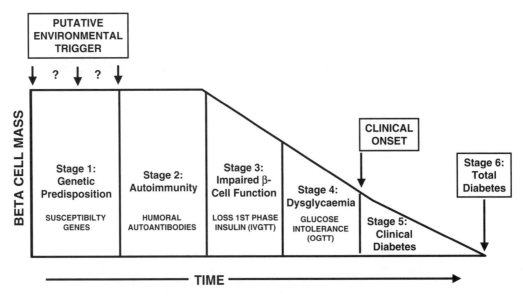

Figure 4.1 Schematic depiction of the progressive stages of development of type 1 diabetes

dominant protective genes; (2) initiation of autoimmunity, presumably by an environmental trigger, with a cellular immune response leading to immune mediated islet infiltration (insulitis), with the stage identified by the presence of circulating autoantibodies; (3) impairment of β-cell function resulting in loss of first-phase insulin response (FPIR) during an intravenous glucose tolerance test (IVGTT); (4) dysglycaemia, manifested by impaired glucose tolerance (IGT), 'indeterminate' glycaemia and/or impaired fasting glucose (IFG), but without overt diabetes; (5) clinical onset of type 1 diabetes; and (6) 'total' diabetes with loss of all β-cell function and mass (evidenced by lack of any C-peptide response to provocative challenge).

Risk identification

The identification of individuals at risk of the type 1 diabetes, and the ability to predict disease development, are crucial for studies of disease prevention. In family members, testing for autoantibodies (i.e. identification at stage 2) is usually used and in this circumstance genetic testing is of limited value. On the other hand, genetic testing may be useful in identifying individuals in the general population or in infant relatives for prospective follow-up for the appearance of autoantibodies or for recruitment into trials aimed at prevention of initiation of autoimmunity. Indeed, there are several studies underway involving screening of newborns or infants for genetic markers[23–26] with the goal of following these participants (with or without intervention) for the appearance of autoimmunity. In addition, there are studies following

offspring of parents with diabetes for the appearance of autoimmunity.[27,28]

Genetics

About 40–50% of the genetic predisposition to type 1 diabetes is conferred by genes on the short arm of chromosome 6, either within or in close proximity to the class II human leukocyte antigen (HLA) region of the MHC.[29–32] At least 16 other loci have been suggested to be involved, with the largest contribution (about 10% of the genetic predisposition) being accounted for by the flanking region of the insulin gene on chromosome 11.[30]

The relationship between type 1 diabetes and specific HLA region alleles is complex. There is a strong positive relationship with HLA-DR3 and DR4 and a strong negative relationship with DR2. Indeed, more than 90% of Caucasians with type 1 diabetes are HLA-DR3 and/or DR4. There is an even stronger relationship of type 1 diabetes when DQ loci (DQα and DQβ) are considered together with DR loci so that the predisposition to type 1 diabetes in Caucasians is with DR3,DQB1*0201 and DR4,DQB1*0302, with the strongest association being the DQαDQβ combination DQA1*0501–DQB1*0302. Other DQ alleles confer protection from type 1 diabetes; DQA1*0201–DQB1*0602 provides protection even in the presence of DQ susceptibility alleles.[33] suggesting that protection is dominant over susceptibility.

To date, for the purposes of most studies of type 1 diabetes prevention, genetic attention has focused solely on the HLA region genes. The other loci have been ignored. Studies of infants have screened for high-risk alleles and some intervention studies have excluded individuals with protective HLA alleles.[34]

Autoantibodies

A number of circulating autoantibodies to islet cell markers may be detected at diagnosis of type 1 diabetes. Indeed, current classification of diabetes uses the presence of autoantibodies to define type 1 diabetes or autoimmune diabetes (the exception being those individuals prone to ketoacidosis but without antibodies, classified as type 1 idiopathic).[35] The autoantibodies include cytoplasmic islet cell antibodies (ICAs), insulin autoantibodies (IAAs) and antibodies to directed against glutamic acid decarboxylase (GAD) and islet tyrosine phosphatases IA-2 and IA-2β.[36] [The antibodies to IA-2 include the antibody ICA-512 directed at a component of IA-2, while the antibodies to IA-2β include one directed against an insulin granule membrane protein, phogrin (phosphatase homologue of granules from rat insulinoma)]. More recently, an additional antigen, the zinc transporter ZnT8 (Slc30A8), has been identified.[37]

The first antibody to be identified was ICA, using a classical immunofluorescence assay.[38] Although the presence of ICA has been shown to be predictive of type 1 diabetes[13–16] and although the addition of IAA can improve prediction,[39] it has become clear that ICA alone is not a reliable predictor of diabetes.[40] Moreover, it has been demonstrated that prediction is greatly improved by using a combination of autoantibodies to ICA, insulin, GAD, IA-2 and perhaps IA-2β.[27,36,41–43] Nonetheless, accurate assessment of the risk of type 1 diabetes in siblings is complicated, as not all those with four autoantibodies progress.[44] In the circumstance of infants of mothers with diabetes, one needs to be cautious during the first year of life that transient maternally acquired antibodies are not present.[45] A strategy has been proposed for distinguishing these as maternal in nature.[45]

Metabolic changes

In people destined to have type 1 diabetes, a progressive metabolic defect can be demonstrated, measured as decline in β-cell function detected by a decrease in early first-phase insulin release (FPIR) during an intravenous glucose tolerance test (IVGTT).[46–48] Standardized procedures have been agreed upon, so that the test is done uniformly throughout the world.[49] The decrease in FPIR correlates strongly with other risk factors, such as autoantibodies, and the combined use of autoantibodies and FPIR response permits more accurate risk quantification.[50,51] For example, the Childhood Diabetes in Finland Study assessed

whether it is clinically relevant to classify siblings of children with recent-onset type 1 diabetes mellitus into various stages of preclinical diabetes.[52] A total of 758 siblings were graded using two classification systems, based on number of autoantibodies and FPIR. There was a greater risk of progression and a shorter time to diagnosis of diabetes in those with more antibodies and particularly with loss of FPIR.[52] In the Diabetes Prevention Trial – Type 1 (DPT-1), low FPIR in ICA-positive relatives was projected to be indicative of a risk of type 1 diabetes of 50% over 5 years and 60% of people who were identified in this way progressed to diabetes.[53]

Metabolic testing with evaluation of FPIR can be used to identify the sub-group of individuals with elevated levels of autoantibodies who are at the high risk of relatively rapid progression to diabetes. Nonetheless, individuals with multiple islet autoantibodies in whom FPIR is intact have an increased risk for development of diabetes, although this may be delayed for years after first detection of autoantibodies.

The highest risk for development of diabetes is in those relatives who already have dysglycaemia – defined as impaired glucose tolerance, indeterminate glucose tolerance and/or impaired fasting glucose[54,55] – and it is possible to calculate a risk score for progression.[56] In this circumstance, 'indeterminate glucose tolerance' is defined as a glucose level above 11.1 mmol l^{-1} (200 mg dl^{-1}) at 30, 60 or 90 min during a standard oral glucose tolerance test, performed in antibody-positive relatives of patients with type 1 diabetes. These individuals, together with those who have 'impaired glucose tolerance', have an 80–90% projected 5 year risk of developing diabetes.

Summary

In summary, risk identification for prediction of type 1 diabetes is possible. Such risk assessment may be accomplished by using a combination of genetic, immunological (autoantibodies) and metabolic (FPIR, dysglycaemia) parameters both in relatives of patients with type 1 diabetes and in the general population.

Interruption of the type 1 diabetes disease process

Given that type 1 diabetes is an immunologically mediated disease, a number of immune intervention strategies have been proposed to interdict the disease process. The scientific basis for all of the intervention strategies tested in human beings has been well established in animal models. In particular, there have been extensive studies in the NOD (non-obese diabetic) mouse and the BB (BioBreeding) rat, two models of spontaneous type 1 diabetes.[6,57,58] Although the NOD mouse has been championed as the best model[59] and studied with at least 463 interventions,[60] it has been noted that there are many pitfalls in attempting to translate success in animals into human interventions.[58,61–63] Most of the animal studies have been aimed at disease prevention. In contrast, the first human studies were initiated at the time of clinical diagnosis.[3–11] This was done to ensure that the patients participating in clinical investigations clearly had disease. Yet, the trade-off is that by the time of disease onset, most β-cell function has been lost, making the demonstration of successful intervention more difficult. In fact, it is possible that interventions that might be successful if applied early in the disease process would fail to show effectiveness when tested so late in the course of the disease. Appreciation of this dilemma, coupled with better predictors of disease development, has led to some controlled trials designed to test interventions that might delay or prevent the development of clinical hyperglycaemia. However, interventions used in these otherwise healthy individuals have been confined to ones with a very favourable safety profile.

Studies in newly diagnosed diabetes

Several interventions have been evaluated in individuals with newly diagnosed type 1 diabetes, in an attempt to interdict the disease process and preserve β-cell function. Interpretation of these has been complicated by a number of factors. Early studies often used 'remission' as an outcome, based on cessation of insulin therapy or very low dose of insulin. In fact, there even was a recommended definition of remission promulgated.[64] However, most recent investigations have focused more on preservation of C-peptide, as a biochemical marker of β-cell function.[65] Moreover, it has come to be appreciated that more intensive insulin therapy and/or better maintenance of glycaemic control results in better preservation of β-cell function.[65–70] Of these, probably the best data come from the Diabetes Control and Complications Trial (DCCT).[65,69,70] Individuals who entered the DCCT with high residual β-cell function (stimulated C-peptide levels of 0.2–0.5 pmol ml^{-1}) ($n = 303$) and who were randomized to intensive therapy to maintain normoglycaemia showed a significantly slower decline in stimulated C-peptide levels than did those randomized to conventional therapy.[69] As a consequence of these observations, aggressive glycaemic control with intensive insulin therapy is important for preservation of

endogenous β-cell function in patients with type 1 diabetes. Current strategy involves maintaining insulin therapy at the highest dose that does not induce hypoglycaemia. Moreover, this precludes the use of remission characterized by cessation of insulin therapy or reduction of insulin dose as an endpoint in clinical trials. The current approach, used by most investigators in the field and consistent with the recommendations of the American Diabetes Association[65] and the Immunology of Diabetes Society,[71] is to use C-peptide response to evaluate β-cell function.

A wide variety of interventions have been considered and many have been tested in small pilot studies or in small clinical trials.[3–11] In this chapter, discussion generally will be confined to those interventions that have been tested in randomized, controlled clinical trials.

Cyclosporin

Cyclosporin has been studied in new-onset diabetes in several randomized trials, and also a number of open trials.[72–80] Two of these – the Canadian/European Study[73] and the French Cyclosporin Study[72] – were large. multicentre. randomized controlled trials with sufficient participants (188 and 122, respectively) to draw meaningful conclusions. These (and also the other smaller studies) have demonstrated that cyclosporin results in either better preservation of β-cell function and/or a greater likelihood of remission than that seen in placebo or historical control patients. Most studies suggested that the early beneficial effects were not sustained,[74,78] although at least one study suggested that there was a sustained beneficial effect after discontinuation of cyclosporin.[79] Nonetheless, even in that study, the authors concluded that the magnitude and duration of that benefit do not appear sufficient to justify cyclosporin treatment in clinical practice.[79] This is particularly the case given the potential of nephrotoxicity with cyclosporin usage.[81,82] The toxicity of cyclosporin is such that it cannot safely be considered in new-onset type 1 diabetes. The cyclosporin studies included the first two large-scale randomized controlled trials of immune intervention in type 1 diabetes. Moreover, they were important in that they convincingly demonstrated that the type 1 diabetes disease process could be impacted by immune intervention, thus fulfilling the criteria that human type 1 diabetes is an immune-mediated disease.

Azathioprine

Azathioprine has been studied in several small randomized trials in new-onset diabetes, either alone or in combination with glucocorticoids.[83–85] As with cyclosporin, in some[83,84] – but not all – of the studies, patients treated with azathioprine had more insulin-free 'remissions', lower insulin requirement and higher glucagon-stimulated C-peptide levels. One exception was a study in children aged 2–20 years.[85] Azathioprine may result in severe leukopenia (but this can be avoided with careful monitoring and dose titration) and there is an unquantified concern about oncogenic potential. As a consequence of fears about potential toxicity, there were no further studies of azathioprine in type 1 diabetes.

Nicotinamide

Nicotinamide has been used in many studies in new-onset diabetes.[86–102] The results of the individual studies have been mixed, with some showing marginal beneficial effects of nicotinamide and others being negative. A meta-analysis of the first 10 of these studies has been reported.[103] The 10 randomized controlled trials (five of which involved placebo) conducted in recent-onset diabetes and included in the meta-analysis involved a total of 211 nicotinamide-treated patients. One year after diagnosis, baseline C-peptide was significantly higher in nicotinamide-treated patients compared with control patients $(0.73 \pm 0.65$ vs $0.32 \pm 0.56\,\text{ng ml}^{-1}$, $p < 0.005)$. Moreover, the statistical difference remained when the analysis was confined to the five placebo-controlled trials. This combined analysis suggests a therapeutic effect of nicotinamide in preserving residual β-cell function when given at diabetes diagnosis in addition to insulin. Adverse effects of nicotinamide were minimal. Hence it is surprising that there has not been much apparent use of nicotinamide in new-onset diabetes, although it has been studied in a large prevention trial, as discussed below.

BCG vaccine

Vaccination with BCG (bacillus Calmette–Guerin strain of *Mycobacterium bovis*) has been studied in new-onset diabetes. A pilot trial in 17 patients appeared promising, in that it led to transient 'clinical remission'.[104] However, three randomized controlled trials (involving a total of 192 participants) of BCG in new-onset diabetes failed to demonstrate a beneficial effect after 1–2 years.[105–107] Although this apparently would put to rest the notion of using BCG vaccine, unfortunately these studies may suffer from each being too small and thus too under-powered to allow the firm conclusion that there was not an effect.

Linomide

Linomide (quinoline-3-carboxamide) is a synthetic immunomodulator which results in complete protection from insulitis and diabetes in NOD mice.[108] The effects of linomide on insulin needs and β-cell function were evaluated in a 1 year study in 63 patients (randomized 2:1 linomide:placebo) with recent-onset diabetes.[109] In the linomide group, both insulin dose and HbA$_{1c}$ were lower and there was a trend for higher C peptide values. In a *post hoc* subgroup analysis performed in 40 patients (25 from the linomide group and 15 from the placebo group) who still had detectable residual β-cell function at entry, linomide was associated with higher C-peptide values. The authors felt that these results support further studies to define the effects of linomide in type 1 diabetes. Unfortunately, the manufacturer withdrew linomide from further study due to side-effects in other (non-diabetes) trials. A similar drug, leflunomide, has been marketed for the treatment of rheumatoid arthritis, but has not been evaluated for potential effects in type 1 diabetes.

Insulin

As noted previously, several studies have suggested that early and more aggressive insulin treatment may result in preservation of β-cell function, better metabolic control and/or a prolonged honeymoon period.[66–69] As a consequence, at least two studies were specifically designed to evaluate the effects of vigorous insulin therapy on preservation of β-cell function in recent-onset diabetes. In a study in Tampa, 26 adolescents were randomized either to conventional insulin therapy or to a 2 week course of intravenous insulin delivered via an artificial pancreas to maintain blood glucose levels in the low normal range.[110] During the 2 week intervention, the experimental therapy group received four times more insulin than the conventionally treated group. Subsequently, both groups were treated similarly. The experimental group had better preservation of β-cell function (meal-stimulated C-peptide levels) and lower HbA$_{1c}$ levels for at least 1 year after randomization. A study in Munich sought to clarify whether the beneficial effect seen in the Tampa study was a consequence of the intensification of therapy or the route of insulin administration (intravenous).[111] To that end, 10 patients with newly diagnosed diabetes were randomized to either a 2 week high-dose intravenous insulin infusion or intensive insulin therapy with four injections per day. By week 3, both groups were treated similarly with intensive insulin therapy and were followed for 1 year. Changes in stimulated

C-peptide concentrations between months 0 and 12 were not significant in either group, suggesting that both therapies were effective in preserving β-cell function.

Oral insulin

Oral administration of insulin to young NOD mice decreases insulitis and delays onset of diabetes.[112–114] This is consistent with the immunological concept of 'oral (or mucosal) tolerance',[115–117] which suggests that antigens administered by the oral route (or across another mucosal surface) favour the generation of the T-helper-2 (Th2) and T-helper-3 (Th3) subsets of CD4$^+$ T-cells and the 'type 2' and 'type 3' cytokines they respectively produce, cytokines which inhibit the T-helper-1 (Th1), and 'type 1' cytokine-mediated β-cell destruction which leads to type 1 diabetes. That these regulatory cells have been generated was shown by the fact that co-transfer of spleen cells from animals treated with oral insulin prevents adoptive transfer of diabetes.[112] The idea of using oral insulin to slow the destructive processes in human type 1 diabetes is appealing, since oral insulin does not have metabolic effects and since the safety of the insulin molecule in humans is well established. Three randomized controlled trials (involving a total of 418 patients) evaluated oral insulin in new-onset diabetes.[118–120] Unfortunately, oral insulin did not modify the rate of decline of β-cell function, although one study claimed potential beneficial effects using *post hoc* analyses.

Heat-shock protein peptide

The 60 kDa heat-shock protein (hsp60) is thought to be one of the target self-antigens involved in the β-cell destruction which leads to type 1 diabetes.[121] An immunomodulatory peptide from hsp60, p277, arrests β-cell destruction and maintains insulin production in newly diabetic NOD mice.[122,123] In a small randomized controlled trial in 35 patients with diabetes diagnosed within 6 months, the treated group showed better preservation of C-peptide at 10 months,[124] continuing to 18 months,[125] suggesting a potential beneficial effect. Additional studies in both adults[126,127] and children[127,128] with type 1 diabetes failed to show similar effects, although the therapy was not associated with any significant side-effects.

Anti-CD3 monoclonal antibody

Studies in mouse models of type 1 diabetes have shown that non-FcR-binding anti-CD3 monoclonal antibody can prevent the development of insulitis and hyperglycaemia and can even reverse diabetes and appear to induce a state of tolerance to diabetes.[129–131] Two humanized, non-mitogenic, Fc-mutated CD3 monoclonal antibodies are available – hOKT3g1(Ala–Ala) and ChAglyCD3. The hOKT3g1 (Ala–Ala) antibody was studied in a randomized controlled Phase I/II trial in 24 patients with new-onset type 1 diabetes.[132,133] Treatment involved a 14 day course of the antibody in escalating doses for 4 days followed by full dose (45 µg kg^{-1} day^{-1}) for 10 days, whereas the control group did not receive any infusion. The treated group showed improved glycaemic control and better preservation of C-peptide (in response to a mixed meal) at 12 months,[132] with the treatment effect maintained at 24 months also.[133] In another randomized controlled Phase I/II trial, the ChAglyCD3 antibody was studied in 80 patients with new-onset type 1 diabetes who were randomly assigned to receive infusions of placebo or ChAglyCD3 for six consecutive days at a dose of 8 g day^{-1}.[134] At 6, 12 and 18 months, residual β-cell function was better maintained with ChAglyCD3 than with placebo. The insulin dose increased in the placebo group but not in the ChAglyCD3 group. The effect of ChAglyCD3 was most pronounced among patients with initial residual β-cell function at or above the 50th percentile of the 80 patients.[134] Thus, these small studies suggested beneficial effects and indicated that anti-CD3 therapy warrants further evaluation in larger randomized controlled trials. With hOKT3g1(Ala-Ala), the most common side-effects were fever, rash and anaemia.[132] Administration of ChAglyCD3 was associated with a moderate 'flu-like' syndrome and transient symptoms of Epstein–Barr viral mononucleosis.[134]

GAD-alum vaccination

Preclinical studies in the NOD mouse have demonstrated that the administration of small quantities of GAD65 effectively prevents autoimmune β-cell destruction and reduces or delays the development of spontaneous diabetes.[135–139] A Phase II study was conducted to evaluate whether alum-formulated human recombinant GAD65 is safe and does not compromise β-cell function in patients with latent autoimmune diabetes in adults (LADA).[140] That study was conducted as a randomized, double-blind, placebo-controlled, dose-escalation clinical trial in a total of 47 patients. There were no safety issues and, although three of the doses studied showed no effects, there was the suggestion of minor benefit at 24 weeks from the 20 µg dose, which was administered at weeks 1 and 4. A subsequent Phase II randomized, double-blind and placebo-controlled trial has been conducted in 70 patients with type 1 diabetes between the ages of 10 and 18 years.[141] Patients received either placebo or 20 µg of GAD-alum at day 1 and day 28. Stimulated C-peptide levels were better sustained in the treatment than control group over 30 months of observation. Additional analyses demonstrated that the effect was confined to individuals treated within 6 months of diagnosis, with the effect not seen in those treated between 6 and 18 months after diagnosis. In the group treated with GAD-alum, GAD autoantibody levels increased rapidly, reached a maximum at 3 months and then decreased but remained significantly higher than in the placebo group. Increased GAD-induced expression of FOXP3 and TGF-β was found at month 15 in cells from the GAD-alum group, compared with the placebo group. The suggestion of potential beneficial effects, without adverse effects, indicates that GAD-alum warrants further investigation.

Mycophenolate mofetil (MMF) with or without initial treatment with antiCD25 (daclizumab)

This study, conducted by Type 1 Diabetes TrialNet,[142] was designed to determine the ability of two immunosuppressive therapies (MMF alone or in combination with DZB, both compared with placebo) to arrest the ongoing β-cell destruction in recently diagnosed type 1 diabetes. A total of 126 patients were randomized. The original plan was to follow them for 2 years. However, the study was halted prior to completion because the Data Safety and Monitoring Board (DSMB) determined that the C-peptide results were no different between each intervention and the control group and that it was futile to expect a difference to emerge.[143] It should be noted, however, that there also was no difference between groups in A_{1c} or insulin dose.

Anti-CD20 monoclonal antibody (rituximab)

There has been growing evidence that many T-lymphocyte-mediated diseases may depend on the contribution of B-lymphocytes. Success with the use of the anti-CD20 monoclonal antibody rituximab in other human immune-mediated diseases, such as rheumatoid arthritis and systemic lupus erythematosus, led to consideration of this therapy in new-onset type 1 diabetes by Type 1 Diabetes TrialNet.[144] Rituximab selectively depletes the majority of B-lymphocytes. It was studied in a randomized, double-masked, placebo-controlled trial in 87 patients with new-onset type 1 diabetes who were randomly assigned to receive infusions of rituximab or placebo weekly for 4 weeks at a dose of 375 mg m^{-2}. C-peptide

was significantly higher at 1 year in those assigned to rituximab as compared with placebo. This was accompanied by lower HbA_{1c} and less insulin use. Adverse events were minimal. Thus, this study suggested beneficial effects and indicated that anti-CD20 therapy warrants further evaluation in larger randomized controlled trials.

Studies in individuals at high risk of type 1 diabetes

In addition to attempts to interdict the disease process and preserve β-cell function in newly diagnosed type 1 diabetes, studies have been initiated to try actually to delay or prevent the clinical onset of type 1 diabetes. Although a number of immunosuppressive drugs (e.g. azathioprine and cyclosporin) have been considered and some even given to a few individuals,[145–148] these were not really evaluated in a disciplined way. More recently, large-scale multicentre randomized controlled clinical trials have been initiated to evaluate nicotinamide, parenteral insulin, oral insulin, nasal insulin and the elimination of cow's milk from infant feeding.

Nicotinamide

Nicotinamide has been used in prediabetes. Several very small pilot studies were inconclusive. In the first, no effect was seen.[149] In two others, treated participants appeared to fare better than untreated historical controls.[150] In a fourth, insulin secretion seemed better preserved in six treated individuals than seven controls.[151]

A very large nicotinamide study, with an unusual design, emanates from Auckland, New Zealand.[152] In this study, during the period 1988–1991, school children aged 5–8 years (with no immediate family history of diabetes) were randomized *by the school* to receive ICA testing. A total of 33 658 children were offered testing; 20 195 accepted and 13 463 declined. Of those tested, 185 were ICA positive. Of these, 173 were treated with nicotinamide (maximum dose 1.5 g day^{-1}) on the basis of either ICA levels of ≥ 10 JDF units and first phase insulin release <25th percentile of normal or those with ICA > 20 JDF units. Another 48 335 children were neither screened nor treated and served as controls. They were followed for 7.1 years. The rate of development of diabetes was $7.14/10^5$ per year in the nicotinamide-treated group versus $16.07/10^5$ per year in the comparison group. The rate in those who refused testing was $18.48/10^5$ per year. After age adjustment, the tested group had a rate of diabetes of 41% (95% CI 20 to 85%) of the other groups combined, which is significant ($p = 0.008$). When an intention-to-treat analysis was performed by combining the treated group with those who refused testing, the rate of diabetes was less than in the comparison group, but the difference did not reach statistical significance. No adverse effects were seen in treated children.

Two large, multicentre, randomized, double-masked, controlled clinical trials have evaluated the effects of nicotinamide in high-risk relatives of individuals with type 1 diabetes. These are the German (Deutsch) Nicotinamide Diabetes Intervention Study (DENIS) and the European Nicotinamide Diabetes Intervention Trial (ENDIT).

In DENIS, individuals at high risk for developing type 1 diabetes within 3 years were identified by screening siblings (age 3–12 years) of patients with diabetes for the presence of high-titre ICA.[153] Participants ($n = 55$) were randomized into placebo and high-dose nicotinamide slow release ($1.2\,g\,m^{-2}$ day^{-1}) groups and followed prospectively in a controlled clinical trial using a sequential design. Rates of diabetes onset were similar in both groups throughout the observation period (maximum 3.8 years, median 2.1 years). The authors asserted that the sequential design provides a 10% probability of a type II error against a reduction in the cumulative diabetes incidence at 3 years from 30 to 6% by nicotinamide. The trial was terminated when the second sequential interim analysis after the 11th case of diabetes showed that the trial had failed to detect a reduction of the cumulative diabetes incidence at 3 years from 30 to 6% ($p = 0.97$). The data do not exclude the possibility of a less strong, but potentially meaningful, risk reduction in this cohort or a major clinical effect of nicotinamide in individuals with less risk of progression to type 1 diabetes than those studied.

ENDIT was a prospective, placebo-controlled double-blind international trial conducted in 20 countries.[154] The participants recruited were ICA-positive, first-degree relatives, aged 5–40 years, of individuals who developed type 1 diabetes under the age of 20 years and who were themselves positive for ICA.[155] These enrolment criteria were projected to yield a risk of type 1 diabetes of 40% over a 5 year period. Participants ($n = 552$) were randomized into placebo and high-dose nicotinamide ($1.2\,g\,m^{-2}\,day^{-1}$) groups to determine if a 35% reduction in incidence of type 1 diabetes can be achieved during 5 years of treatment. More than 35 000 first-degree relatives were screened. Of 159 participants who developed diabetes in the course of the trial, 82 were taking nicotinamide and 77 were on placebo.[156] The unadjusted hazard ratio for development of diabetes was 1.07 (95% CI 0.78 to 1.45; $p = 0.69$) and the hazard ratio adjusted for age-at

entry, baseline glucose tolerance and number of islet autoantibodies detected was 1.01 (95% CI 0.73 to 1.38; $p = 0.97$). Thus, unfortunately, nicotinamide had no effect on the development of diabetes.[156]

Insulin

Insulin has been shown to delay the development of diabetes and of insulitis in animal models of spontaneous diabetes (BB rats and NOD mice).[157–163] In humans, several pilot studies of insulin use in high-risk relatives of individuals with type 1 diabetes were conducted. In one pilot study, in Boston, insulin was offered to 12 participants, five of whom accepted and seven declined and served as a comparison group.[164] In this study, insulin therapy consisted of 5 days of continuous intravenous insulin every 9 months coupled with twice daily subcutaneous insulin. Although life table analysis suggested that this treatment may delay the appearance of diabetes, there were only a small number of patients.

In another pilot study, in Munich – the Schwabing Insulin Prophylaxis Trial – there were 14 high-risk firs-degree relatives of people with type 1 diabetes randomized to either experimental treatment or a control group.[165,166] In the experimental treatment group, intravenous insulin was given by continuous infusion for 7 days, followed by daily injections for 6 months. Intravenous insulin infusions were repeated every 12 months. In the treatment group, three of the seven individuals (follow-up from time of eligibility: 2.3–7.1 years) and in the control group six of the seven untreated individuals (1.7–7.1 years) developed clinical diabetes. Life table analysis showed that clinical onset of type 1 diabetes appeared to be delayed in experimental compared with control patients (diabetes-free survival: 5.0 ± 0.9 versus 2.3 ± 0.7 years, $p < 0.03$).

A third non-randomized, observational pilot study, in Gainesville, recruited 26 participants (12 with impaired glucose tolerance), aged 3–60 years, who were ICA positive and had a first-phase insulin response (FPIR) <5th percentile ($<75\,mU\,ml^{-1}$) on two occasions.[167] They were treated with NPH insulin twice daily at a 'maximum tolerable dose' (reduced for any hypoglycaemia) (mean dose 0.33 ± 0.15; range 0.09–$0.66\,U\,kg^{-1}\,day^{-1}$). The median duration of follow-up was 5.5 years. Diabetes occurred in 10 of 12 people with IGT and five of 14 with normal glucose tolerance. In non-progressors, as opposed to progressors, there was no fall in C-peptide.

The preliminary results from these pilot studies suggested that in high-risk relatives insulin has the potential to delay or prevent the development of overt diabetes. It also was appreciated that insulin is β-cell specific, does not have generalized effects on the immune system, has well-understood effects on people and has known side-effects that are controllable. This led to the Diabetes Prevention Trial of Type 1 Diabetes (DPT-1), a randomized, controlled, multicentre clinical trial, conducted throughout the United States and Canada to test whether intervention with insulin can delay the appearance of overt clinical diabetes.[53] For the insulin injection study, DPT-1 screened and analysed 84 228 samples from relatives of patients with type 1 diabetes for islet cell antibodies (ICA) and found 3152 (3.73%) relatives who were ICA positive on initial testing. Of these, 2103 (67%) underwent staging to quantify the risk of type 1 diabetes and 372 relatives progressed in their staging evaluations to be classified as having a risk projection for type 1 diabetes of >50%. A total of 339 participants were randomized either to the intervention group or to the close observation group. The experimental intervention group received parenteral insulin – both annual intravenous insulin infusions and twice daily low-dose subcutaneous insulin injections (0.25 U kg^{-1} day^{-1} of human ultralente insulin). An oral glucose tolerance test was performed every 6 months; the diagnosis of diabetes was confirmed by a second test. The median duration of follow-up was 3.7 years. Diabetes was diagnosed in 139 participants – 69 in the intervention group and 70 in the close observation group. The average proportion of participants who progressed to diabetes was 15.1% per year in the intervention group and 14.6% per year in the close observation group. There was a higher rate of progression to diabetes among those with abnormal baseline glucose tolerance (22% per year) than among those with normal baseline glucose tolerance (10% per year, $p < 0.001$). The hazard ratio for development of diabetes was 0.96 (95% CI 0.69 to 1.34; $p = 0.80$). Thus, the cumulative incidence of diabetes in the intervention group was virtually the same as that in the observation group. Consequently, insulin in the dose and regimen used did not delay or prevent the development of type 1 diabetes. However, most participants diagnosed with diabetes were asymptomatic at the time of diagnosis.

Oral insulin

As noted earlier, oral administration of insulin[112,113] or insulin B-chain[114] to young NOD mice decreases insulitis and delays the onset of diabetes. Moreover, spleen cells from animals treated with oral insulin prevent adoptive transfer of diabetes.[112] Therefore, DPT-1 also included a protocol testing whether oral insulin (7.5 mg day^{-1}) can delay the appearance of overt clinical diabetes.[168] In this randomized, placebo-controlled, double-masked, multicentre clinical trial, 103 391 relatives of patients with type 1 diabetes were screened and 97 273 samples were analysed for islet cell antibodies (ICA), with 3483 (3.58%) ICA positive on initial testing. Of 2523 who underwent staging to quantify risk of type 1 diabetes, 388 relatives were classified as having a risk projection for type 1 diabetes of 26–50% over 5 years. They had insulin autoantibodies, intact first-phase insulin response to intravenous glucose and normal oral glucose tolerance. A total of 372 participants were randomized either to oral insulin or to placebo. The median duration of follow-up was 4.3 years. Diabetes was diagnosed in 97 participants – 44 in the oral insulin group and 53 in the placebo group. The average proportion of participants who progressed to diabetes was 6.4% per year in the oral insulin group and 8.2% per year in the placebo group. The hazard ratio for development of diabetes was 0.764 (95% CI 0.511 to 1.142; $p = 0.189$). Thus, overall there was no benefit of oral insulin. However, among participants with confirmed insulin autoantibodies (IAA) ≥ 80 nU ml^{-1} ($n = 263$), the proportion who developed diabetes was 6.2% per year in the oral insulin group and 10.4% per year in the placebo group (hazard ratio 0.566, 95% CI 0.361 to 0.888; $p = 0.015$). In this sub-group, unfortunately not pre-specified, there was a delay in diabetes, calculated from median survival times, projected as 4.5 years.[168] This led to the development of another large oral insulin prevention study, conducted by Type 1 Diabetes TrialNet, in relatives with characteristics similar to those of the DPT-1 sub-group with apparent benefit.[169]

Nasal insulin

In addition to oral insulin, since it is also given across a mucosal barrier, nasal insulin may also lead to tolerance.[115] As a consequence, three studies have been developed to examine the effects of nasal insulin on diabetes prevention. The first to be reported was a double-blind, placebo-controlled, pilot crossover study in Melbourne, Australia – the Intranasal Insulin Trial (INIT).[170] In that study, a total of 38 antibody-positive individuals, median age 10.8 years, were randomized to treatment with intranasal insulin (1.6 mg) or a carrier solution, daily for 10 days and then 2 days per week for 6 months, before crossover. Diabetes developed in 12 participants with negligible β-cell function at entry, after a median of 1.1 year. Of the remaining 26, β-cell function generally remained stable over a median follow-up of 3.0 years. Intranasal insulin was associated with an increase in antibody and a decrease in T-cell responses to insulin. The authors concluded that these findings justified a formal trial to determine whether intranasal insulin is immunotherapeutic and retards progression to clinical diabetes. They now have initiated such a study as a randomized, double-blind, placebo-controlled trial, in relatives of patients with type 1 diabetes, evaluating two doses of nasal insulin (40 and 440 U) in which there will be 12 months of treatment and a further 4 years of follow-up.

The other, the Diabetes Prediction and Prevention (DIPP) Study, is a study that was conducted in Finland amongst newborns from the general population (i.e. without relatives) with high-risk genotypes for type 1 diabetes[171] and a parallel study amongst siblings of infants identified as high risk.[172] In the birth cohort, the DIPP Study screened 116 720 consecutively born Finnish infants and identified 17 397 (~15%) with high or moderate genetic risk, of whom 10 577 participated in a prospective study in which there was serial analysis for diabetes autoantibodies.[173] Of these, 328 were found to meet the enrolment criteria of two or more antibodies in at least two consecutive samples, and 224 of these children were then randomized to receive intranasal insulin ($1\,U\,kg^{-1}$ body weight daily) or placebo. They were followed for up to 10 years, with a median follow-up of 2 years. Diabetes was diagnosed in 42 treated and 38 control individuals (hazard ratio 1.14, 95% CI 0.73 to 1.77; $p = 0.55$). In the sibling cohort, the DIPP Study screened 3430 siblings and identified 1613 (~47%) with high or moderate risk genes, of whom 1423 participated in prospective follow-up.[173] Of these, 52 met the enrolment criteria and 40 were randomized to receive nasal insulin or placebo. Diabetes was diagnosed in seven treated and four control individuals (hazard ratio 1.93, 95% CI 0.56 to 2.68; $p = 0.30$). Thus, in both cohorts the cumulative incidence of diabetes in the nasal insulin group was virtually the same as that in the placebo group. Consequently, nasal insulin did not delay or prevent the development of type 1 diabetes. However, again, most participants diagnosed with diabetes were asymptomatic at the time of diagnosis.

Milk proteins

In some epidemiological and case–control studies, it has been suggested that there is a reciprocal relationship between infant breast feeding and subsequent development of type 1 diabetes.[174,175] It has been proposed that breast feeding may be a surrogate for the absence of consumption of cow milk proteins (CMP).[175] These highly controversial hypotheses are supported by one meta-analysis,[175] but challenged in another as being confounded by bias.[176] In Finland, a small prospective study suggested that exclusive

breast feeding reduces the risk of diabetes development.[177] On the other hand, a prospective study in the United States, using appearance of antibodies as the endpoint, failed to find a relationship.[178] Another Finnish study of a cohort of high-risk newborns found that short duration of breast feeding, together with early introduction of cow milk proteins, led to increased appearance of islet autoantibodies.[179]

In spite of the controversy, the notion has been developed that consumption of CMP, particularly during a 'critical window of vulnerability' early in life, may lead to the initiation of the immunological attack against pancreatic islet β-cells and increase susceptibility to type 1 diabetes.[180] Others argue that the issue really relates to the immune function of the mucosal barrier.[181] The champions of the cow milk hypothesis cite an array of evidence in support of the CMP hypothesis – epidemiological data, disease rates in animal models, humoral and cellular immune markers directed against CMP in patients with new-onset type 1 diabetes and identification of a peptide sequence on bovine serum albumin (BSA) with homology to sequence on the islet cell protein ICA-69 (or p69) ('molecular mimicry').[180]

To test the hypothesis, a multi-national randomized prospective trial, TRIGR (Trial to Reduce Incidence of Diabetes in Genetically at Risk), has been initiated to determine whether the frequency of type 1 diabetes can be reduced by preventing exposure to CMP during early life.[182] In fact, a small pilot study was conducted in Finland that included 242 newborn infants who had a first-degree relative with type 1 diabetes and carried risk-associated HLA-DQB1 alleles.[183] After exclusive breast feeding, the infants underwent a double-blind, randomized trial of either a casein hydrolysate formula or a conventional cow milk-based formula until the age of 6–8 months. During a mean observation period of 4.7 years, after adjustment for duration of study formula feeding, life-table analysis showed a significant protection by the intervention from positivity for ICA ($p = 0.02$) and at least one autoantibody ($p = 0.03$).[183]

The full-scale TRIGR Study[182] involves 77 centres in 15 countries and registered approximately 5000 newborns and randomized a total of 2160 newborns over a 4.7 year period, completing enrolment at the end of 2006.[184] Only subjects with the risk HLA genotypes (approximately 45%) were included in the nutritional prevention trial, which involves randomization to either a casein hydrolysate formula or a conventional cow's milk-based formula. The planned duration of the intervention is until at least 6 months of age with the goal of a minimum of 2 months of daily exposure to the study formula. For 8 months they will receive either a casein hydrolysate formula or a conventional cow milk-based formula. These children will be followed for 10 years for the development of type 1 diabetes. Hence this is a 'true' primary prevention strategy.

Conclusion

In individuals with new-onset type 1 diabetes mellitus, two large, randomized controlled trials with adequate power to answer the question of preservation of β-cell function have been conducted, both with cyclosporin, and both demonstrating positive effect (Evidence Level I). Unfortunately, the side-effects result in a risk:benefit ratio that precludes the use of this intervention. Also, in new-onset type 1 diabetes, a meta-analysis has been performed that demonstrates a small beneficial effect of nicotinamide on C-peptide (Evidence Level I). Unfortunately, because of the relatively small magnitude of the effect, this intervention has not been widely used. A subset analysis from the Diabetes Control and Complications Trial – of individuals who entered the with high residual β-cell function and were randomized to intensive therapy – showed a slower decline in stimulated C-peptide than those randomized to conventional therapy (Evidence Level I). Although this demonstrated that aggressive glycaemic control can preserve β-cell function (in addition to many other beneficial effects), this approach is not as widely used as it should be. None of the other studies described above – completed or under way – will be able to provide Level I or Level II evidence.

In prevention of diabetes, four large, randomized controlled trials have been completed – the DPT-1 parenteral insulin study,[53] the ENDIT nicotinamide study,[156] the DPT-1 oral insulin study[168] and the DIPP nasal insulin study.[173] All four studies were carefully conducted and confirmed the ability to predict the development of type 1 diabetes. Unfortunately, in the doses and in the manner used in these studies, all were without beneficial effect in delaying or preventing type 1 diabetes (Evidence Level I). Of the ongoing studies, the TrialNet Oral Insulin Trial[169] and the TRIGR study,[182] also have the potential to provide Level I Evidence.

References

1 Atkinson M, Eisenbarth G. Type 1 diabetes: new perspectives on disease pathogenesis and treatment. *Lancet* 2001;**358**:221–229.

2 von Herrath M, Sanda S, Herold K. Type 1 diabetes as a relapsing-remitting disease?. *Nature Reviews Immunology* 2007;**7**:988–994.

3 Skyler JS. Immune intervention studies in insulin-dependent diabetes mellitus. *Diabetes Metabolism Reviews* 1987;**3**:1017–1035.

4 Andreani D, DiMario U, Pozzilli P. Prediction, prevention and early intervention in insulin dependent diabetes. *Diabetes Metabolism Reviews* 1991;**7**:61–77.

5 Skyler JS, Marks JB. Immune intervention in type 1 diabetes mellitus. *Diabetes Reviews* 1993;**1**:15–42.

6 Bach JF. Insulin-dependent diabetes mellitus as an autoimmune disease. *Endocrine Reviews* 1994;**15**:516–542.

7 Slover RH, Eisenbarth GS. Prevention of type I diabetes and recurrent-cell destruction of transplanted islets. *Endocrine Reviews* 1997;**18**:241–258.

8 Rabinovitch A, Skyler JS. Prevention of type 1 diabetes. *Medical Clinics of North America* 1998;**82**:739–755.

9 Eldor R, Cohen IR, Raz I. Innovative immune-based therapeutic approaches for the treatment of type 1 diabetes mellitus. *International Reviews of Immunology* 2005;**24**:327–339.

10 Aly T, Devendra D, Eisenbarth GS. Immunotherapeutic approaches to prevent, ameliorate and cure type 1 diabetes. *American Journal of Therapeutics* 2005;**12**:481–490.

11 Staeva-Vieira T, Peakman M, von Herrath M. Translational mini-review series on type 1 diabetes: immune-based therapeutic approaches for type 1 diabetes. *Clinical and Experimental Immunology* 2007;**148**:17–31.

12 Gardner SG, Bingley PJ, Sawtell PA, Weeks S, Gale EAM. Rising incidence of insulin dependent diabetes in children aged under 5 years in the Oxford region: time trend analysis. *BMJ* 1997;**315**:713–717.

13 Schatz D, Krischer J, Horne G, Riley W, Spillar R, Silverstein J, Winter W, Muir A, Derovanesian D, Shah S, Vadheim CM, Rotter JI, Maclaren NK. Islet cell antibodies predict insulin-dependent diabetes in United States school age children as powerfully as in unaffected relatives. *Journal of Clinical Investigation* 1994;**93**:2403–2407.

14 Bingley PJ, Bonifacio E, Williams AJK, Genovese S, Bottazzo GF, Gale EAM. Prediction of IDDM in the general population: strategies based on combinations of autoantibody markers. *Diabetes* 1997;**46**:1701–1710.

15 Riley WJ, Maclaren NK, Krischer J, Spillar RP, Silverstein JH, Schatz DA, Schwartz S, Malone J, Shah S, Vadheim C, *et al.* A prospective study of the development of diabetes in relatives of patients with insulin-dependent diabetes. *New England Journal of Medicine* 1990;**323**:1167–1172.

16 Bingley PJ, Christie MR, Bonifacio E, Bonfanti R, Shattock M, Fonte MT, Bottazzo GF, Gale EA. Combined analysis of autoantibodies improves prediction of IDDM in islet cell antibody-positive relatives. *Diabetes* 1994;**43**(11):1304–1310.

17 Kockum I, Wassmuth R, Holmberg E, Michelsen B, Lernmark Å. Inheritance of MHC class II genes in IDDM studied in population-based affected and control families. *Diabetologia* 1994;**37**:1105–1112.

18 Foulis AK. The pathogenesis of beta cell destruction in type I (insulin-dependent) diabetes mellitus. *Journal of Pathology* **152**:1987;141–148.

19 Imagawa A, Hanafusa T, Tamura S, Moriwaki M, Itoh N, Yamamoto K, Iwahashi H, Yamagata K, Waguri M, Nanmo T, Uno S, Nakajima H, Namba M, Kawata S, Miyagawa JI,

Matsuzawa Y. Pancreatic biopsy as a procedure for detecting in situ autoimmune phenomena in type 1 diabetes: close correlation between serological markers and histological evidence of cellular autoimmunity. *Diabetes* 2001;**50**: 1269–1273.

20 Kolb H, Gale EA. Does partial preservation of residual beta-cell function justify immune intervention in recent onset Type I diabetes? *Diabetologia* 2001;**44**:1349–1353.

21 Palmer JP, Fleming GA, Greenbaum CJ, Herold KC, Jansa LD, Kolb H, Lachin JM, Polonsky KS, Pozzilli P, Skyler JS, Steffes MW. C-peptide is the appropriate outcome measure for type 1 diabetes clinical trials to preserve beta cell function: report of an ADA Workshop, 21–22 October 2001. *Diabetes* **53**:2004;250–264.

22 Schatz DA, Krischer JP, Skyler JS. Now is the time to prevent type 1 diabetes. *Journal of Clinical Endocrinology and Metabolism* 1999;**85**:495–498.

23 Rewers M, Bugawan TL, Norris JM, Blair A, Beaty B, Hoffman M, McDuffie RS, Hamman RF, Klingensmith G, Eisenbarth GS, Erlich HA. Newborn screening for HLA markers associated with IDDM: Diabetes Autoimmunity Study in the Young (DAISY). *Diabetologia* 1996;**39**: 807–812.

24 Barker JM, Barriga KJ, Yu L, Miao D, Erlich HA, Norris JM, Eisenbarth GS, Rewers M. Diabetes Autoimmunity Study in the Young. Prediction of autoantibody positivity and progression to type 1 diabetes: Diabetes Autoimmunity Study in the Young (DAISY). *Journal of Clinical Endocrinology and Metabolism* 2004;**89**:3896–3902.

25 Nejentsev S, Sjoroos M, Soukka T, Knip M, Simell O, Lovgren T, Ilonen J. Population-based genetic screening for the estimation of Type 1 diabetes mellitus risk in Finland: selective genotyping of markers in the HLA-DQB1, HLA-DQA1 and HLA-DRB1 loci. *Diabetic Medicine* 1999;**16**:985–992.

26 Kupila A, Muona P, Simell T, Arvilommi P, Savolainen H, Hamalainen AM, Korhonen S, Kimpimaki T, Sjoroos M, Ilonen J, Knip M, Simell O. Juvenile Diabetes Research Foundation Centre for the Prevention of Type I Diabetes in Finland. Feasibility of genetic and immunological prediction of type I diabetes in a population-based birth cohort. *Diabetologia* 2001;**44**:290–297.

27 Ziegler AG, Hummel M, Schenker M, Bonifacio E. Autoantibody appearance and risk for development of childhood diabetes in offspring of parents with type 1 diabetes: the 2-year analysis of the German BABYDIAB Study. *Diabetes* 1999;**48**:460–468.

28 TEDDY Study Group. The Environmental Determinants of Diabetes in the Young (TEDDY) study: study design. *Pediatric Diabetes* **8**:2007;286–298.

29 Todd JA, Farrall M. Panning for gold: genomewide scanning in type 1 diabetes. *Diabetes Reviews* 1997;**5**:284–291.

30 Pugliese A. Unraveling the genetics of insulin-dependent type 1A diabetes: the search must go on. *Diabetes Reviews* 1999;**7**:39–54.

31 Barker JM. Clinical review: Type 1 diabetes-associated autoimmunity: natural history, genetic associations and screening. *Journal of Clinical Endocrinology and Metabolism* 2006;**91**:1210–1217.

32 Steenkiste A, Valdes AM, Feolo M, Hoffman D, Concannon P, Noble J, Schoch G, Hansen J, Helmberg W, Dorman JS, Thomson G, Pugliese A, and 13th IHWS 1 Diabetes Component participating investigators. 14th International HLA and Immunogenetics Workshop: report on the HLA component of type 1 diabetes. *Tissue Antigens* 2007;**69**(Suppl 1): 214–225.

33 Pugliese A, Gianani R, Moromisato R, Awdeh ZL, Alper CA, Erlich HA, Jackson RA, Eisenbarth GS. HLA DQB1*0602 is associated with dominant protection from diabetes even among islet cell antibody positive first degree relatives of patients with insulin-dependent diabetes. *Diabetes*. 1995;**44**:608–613.

34 Greenbaum CJ, Schatz DA, Cuthbertson D, Zeidler A, Eisenbarth GS, Krischer JP, for the DPT-1 Study Group. Islet cell antibody positive relatives with human leukocyte antigen DQA1*0102, DQB1*0602: identification by the Diabetes Prevention Trial-1. *Journal of Clinical Endocrinology and Metabolism* 2000;**85**:1255–1260.

35 American Diabetes Association Expert Committee on the Diagnosis and Classification of Diabetes Mellitus. Follow-up report on the diagnosis of diabetes mellitus. *Diabetes Care* 2003;**26**:3160–3167.

36 Verge CF, Stenger D, Bonifacio E, Colman PG, Pilcher C, Bingley PJ, Eisenbarth GS. Combined use of autoantibodies (IA-2ab, Gadab, IAA, ICA) in type 1 diabetes: Combinatorial Islet Autoantibody Workshop. *Diabetes* **47**:1998; 1857–1866.

37 Wenzlau JM, Juhl K, Yu L, Moua O, Sarkar SA, Gottlieb P, Rewers M, Eisenbarth GS, Jensen J, Davidson HW, Hutton JC. The cation efflux transporter ZnT8 (Slc30A8) is a major autoantigen in human type 1 diabetes. *Proceedings of the National Academy of Sciences of the USA* 2007;**104**: 17040–17045.

38 Bottazzo GF, Florin-Christensen A, Doniach D. Islet-cell antibodies in diabetes mellitus with autoimmune polyendocrine deficiencies. *Lancet* 1974;**ii**:1279–1283.

39 Krischer JP, Schatz D, Riley WJ, Spillar RP, Silverstein JH, Schwartz S, Malone J, Shah S, Vadheim CM, Rotter JI, Maclaren NK. Insulin and islet cell autoantibodies as time-dependent covariates in the development of insulin-dependent diabetes: a prospective study in relatives. *Journal of Clinical Endocrinology and Metabolism* 1993;**77**:743–749.

40 Gardner SG, Gale EA, Williams AJ, Gillespie KM, Lawrence KE, Bottazzo GF, Bingley PJ. Progression to diabetes in relatives with islet autoantibodies. Is it inevitable? *Diabetes Care* 1999;**22**:2049–2054.

41 Verge CF, Gianani R, Kawasaki E, Yu L, Pietropaolo M, Jackson RA, Chase HP, Eisenbarth GS. Prediction of type I diabetes in first-degree relatives using a combination of insulin, GAD and ICA512bdc/IA-2 autoantibodies. *Diabetes* 1996;**45**:926–933.

42 Maclaren N, Lan M, Coutant R, Schatz D, Silverstein J, Muir A, Clare-Salzer M, She JX, Malone J, Crockett S, Schwartz S, Quattrin T, DeSilva M, Vander Vegt P, Notkins A, Krischer J. Only multiple autoantibodies to islet cells (ICA), insulin, GAD65, IA-2 and IA-2beta predict immune-mediated (Type 1) diabetes in relatives. *Journal of Autoimmunity* 1999;**12**:279–287.

43 Krischer JP, Cuthbertson D, Yu L, Orban T, Maclaren NK, Jackson R, Winter WE, Schatz DA, Palmer JP, Eisenbarth GS,and the DPT-1 Study Group. Screening strategies for the identification of multiple antibody positive individuals. *Journal of Clinical Endocrinology and Metabolism* 2003;**88**:103–108.

44 Kulmala P, Savola K, Petersen JS, Vahasalo P, Karjalainen J, Lopponen T, Dyrberg T, Akerblom HK, Knip M. Prediction of insulin-dependent diabetes mellitus in siblings of children with diabetes. A population-based study. The Childhood Diabetes in Finland Study Group *Journal of Clinical Investigation* 1998;**101**:327–336.

45 Naserke HE, Bonifacio E, Ziegler AG. Prevalence, characteristics and diabetes risk associated with transient maternally acquired islet antibodies and persistent islet antibodies in offspring of parents with type 1 diabetes. *Journal of Clinical Endocrinology and Metabolism* 2001;**86**: 4826–4833.

46 Srikanta S, Ganda OP, Gleason RE, Jackson RA, Soeldner JS, Eisenbarth GS. Pre-type 1 diabetes. Linear loss of beta cell response to intravenous glucose. *Diabetes* 1984;**33**:717–20.

47 Chase HP, Garg SK, Butler-Simon N, Klingensmith G, Norris L, Ruskey CT, O'Brien D. Prediction of the course of pre-type 1 diabetes. *Journal of Pediatrics* 1991;**118**:838–841.

48 Bohmer KP, Kolb H, Kuglin B, Zielasek J, Hubinger A, Lampeter EF, Weber B, Kolb-Bachofen V, Jastram HU, Bertrams J, Gries FA. Linear loss of insulin secretory capacity during the last six months preceding IDDM. *Diabetes Care* 1994;**17**:138–141.

49 Bingley PJ, Colman P, Eisenbarth GS, Jackson RA, McCulloch DK, Riley WJ, Gale EA. Standardization of IVGTT to predict IDDM. *Diabetes Care* 1992;**15**:1313–1316.

50 Bingley PJ. Interactions of age, islet cell antibodies, insulin autoantibodies and first-phase insulin response in predicting risk of progression to IDDM in ICA+ relatives: the ICARUS data set. Islet Cell Antibody Register Users Study. *Diabetes* 1996;**45**:1720–1728.

51 Chase HP, Cuthbertson D, Dolan LM, Kaufman F, Krischer JP, Schatz DA, White N, Wilson DM, Wolfsdorf J. The DPT-1 Study Group: first-phase insulin release during the intravenous glucose tolerance as a risk factor for type 1 diabetes. *Journal of Pediatrics* **138**:2001;244–249.

52 Mrena S, Savola K, Kulmala P, Akerblom HK, Knip M, and the Childhood Diabetes in Finland Study Group. Staging of preclinical type 1 diabetes in siblings of affected children. *Pediatrics* 1999;**104**:925–930.

53 Diabetes Prevention Trial – Type 1 Study Group. Effects of insulin in relatives of patients with type 1 diabetes mellitus. *New England Journal of Medicine* 2002;**346**:1685–1691.

54 Sosenko JM, Palmer JP, Greenbaum CJ, Mahon J, Cowie C, Krischer JP, Chase HP, White NH, Buckingham B, Herold KC, Cuthbertson D, Skyler JS, and the Diabetes Prevention Trial – Type 1 Study Group. Patterns of metabolic progression to type 1 diabetes in the Diabetes Prevention Trial – Type 1. *Diabetes Care* 2006;**29**:643–649.

55 Sosenko JM, Palmer JP, Greenbaum CJ, Mahon J, Cowie C, Krischer JP, Chase HP, White NH, Buckingham B, Herold KC, Cuthbertson D, Skyler JS, and the Diabetes Prevention Trial – Type 1 Study Group. Increasing the accuracy of oral glucose tolerance testing and extending its application to individuals with normal glucose tolerance for the prediction of type 1 diabetes: the Diabetes Prevention Trial – Type 1. *Diabetes Care* 2007;**30**:38–42.

56 Sosenko JM, Krischer JP, Palmer JP, Mahon J, Cowie C, Greenbaum CJ, Cuthbertson D, Lachin JM, Skyler JS, and the Diabetes Prevention Trial – Type 1 Study Group. A risk score for type 1 diabetes derived from autoantibody positive participants in the Diabetes Prevention Trial – Type 1 Study Group. *Diabetes Care* 2008;**31**:528–533.

57 Atkinson MA, Leiter EH. The NOD mouse model of type 1 diabetes: as good as it gets? *Nature Medicine* 1999;**5**:601–604.

58 Greiner DL, Rossini AA, Mordes JP. Translating data from animal models into methods for preventing human autoimmune diabetes mellitus: *caveat emptor* and *primum non nocere*. *Clinical Immunology* 2001;**100**:134–143.

59 Anderson MS, Bluestone JA. The NOD mouse: a model of immune dysregulation. *Annual Review of Immunology* 2005;**23**:447–485.

60 Shoda LK, Young DL, Ramanujan S, Whiting CC, Atkinson MA, Bluestone JA, Eisenbarth GS, Mathis D, Rossini AA, Campbell SE, Kahn R, Kreuwel HT. A comprehensive review of interventions in the NOD mouse and implications for translation. *Immunity* 2005;**23**:115–126.

61 Roep BO. Are insights gained from NOD mice sufficient to guide clinical translation? Another inconvenient truth. *Annals of the New York Academy of Sciences* 2007;**1103**:1–10.

62 Roep BO, Atkinson M. Animal models have little to teach us about type 1 diabetes: 1. In support of this proposal. *Diabetologia* 2004;**47**:1650–1656.

63 Leiter EH, von Herrath M. Animal models have little to teach us about type 1 diabetes: 2. In opposition to this proposal. *Diabetologia* 2004;**47**:1657–1660.

64 Kolb H, Bach JF, Eisenbarth GS, Harrison LC, Maclaren NK, Pozzilli P, Skyler J, Stiller CR. Criteria for immune trials in type 1 diabetes. *Lancet* 1989;**ii**:686.

65 Palmer JP, Fleming GA, Greenbaum CJ, Herold KC, Jansa LD, Kolb H, Lachin JM, Polonsky KS, Pozzilli P, Skyler JS, Steffes MW. C-peptide is the appropriate outcome measure for type 1 diabetes clinical trials to preserve beta cell function: report of an ADA Workshop, 21–22 October 2001. *Diabetes* 2004;**53**:250–264.

66 Mirouze J, Selam JL, Pham TC, Mendoza E, Orsetti A. Sustained insulin induced remissions of juvenile diabetes by means of an external artificial pancreas. *Diabetologia* 1978;**14**:223–227.

67 Madsbad S, Krarup T, Faber OK, Binder C, Regeur L. The transient effect of strict glycemic control on B cell function in newly diagnosed type 1 (insulin-dependent) diabetic patients. *Diabetologia* 1982;**22**:16–20.

68 Perlman K, Ehrlich RM, Filler RM, Albisser AM. Sustained normoglycemia in newly diagnosed type I diabetic subjects: short term effects and one year follow-up. *Diabetes* 1984;**33**:995–1001.

69 Effect of intensive therapy on residual β-cell function in patients with type 1 diabetes in the diabetes control and complications trial: a randomized, controlled trial. The Diabetes Control and Complications Trial Research Group. *Annals of Internal Medicine* 1998;**128**:517–523.

70 Steffes MW, Sibley S, Jackson M, Thomas W. Beta-cell function and the development of diabetes-related complications in the diabetes control and complications trial. *Diabetes Care* 2003;**26**:832–836.

71 Greenbaum CJ, Harrison LC.,and Immunology of Diabetes Society. Guidelines for intervention trials in subjects with newly diagnosed type 1 diabetes. *Diabetes* 2003;**52**: 1059–1065.

72 Feutren G, Papoz L, Assan R, Vialettes B, Karsenty G, Vexiau P, DuRostu H, Rodier M, Sirmai J, Lallemand A, Bach JF, for the Cyclosporin/Diabetes French Study Group. Cyclosporin increases the rate and length of remissions in insulin dependent diabetes of recent onset: results of a multicentre double-blind trial. *Lancet* 1986;**ii**:119–124.

73 The Canadian–European Randomized Control Trial Group. Cyclosporin-induced remission of IDDM after early intervention: association of 1 year of cyclosporin treatment with enhanced insulin secretion. *Diabetes* 1988; **37**:1574–1582.

74 Martin S, Schernthaner G, Nerup J, Gries FA, Koivisto VA, Dupre J, Standl E, Hamet P, McArthur R, Tan MH, Dawson K, Mehta AE, Van Vliet S, von Graffenried B, Stiller C, Kolb H. Follow-up of cyclosporin A treatment in type 1 (insulin dependent) diabetes mellitus: lack of long-term effects. *Diabetologia* 1991;**34**:429–434.

75 Chase HP, Butler-Simon N, Garg SK, Hayward A, Klingensmith GJ, Hamman RF, O'Brien D. Cyclosporin A for the treatment of new-onset insulin-dependent diabetes mellitus. *Pediatrics* 1990;**85**:241–45.

76 Skyler JS, Rabinovitch A, and the Miami Cyclosporine Diabetes Study Group. Cyclosporine in recent onset type 1 diabetes mellitus: effects on islet beta cell function. *Journal of Diabetes and Its Complications* 1992;**6**:77–88.

77 Bougneres PF, Carel JC, Castano L, Boitard C, Gardin JP, Landais P, Hors J, Mihatsch MJ, Paillard M, Chaussain JL, Bach JF. Factors associated with early remission of type 1 diabetes in children treated with cyclosporine. *New England Journal of Medicine* 1988;**318**:663–670.

78 Bougneres PF, Landais P, Boisson C, Carel JC, Frament N, Boitard C, Chaussain JL, Bach JF. Limited duration of remission of insulin dependency in children with recent overt type 1 diabetes treated with low-dose cyclosporine. *Diabetes* 1990;**39**:1264–1272.

79 De Filippo G, Carel JC, Boitard C, Bougnères PF. Long-term results of early cyclosporin therapy in juvenile IDDM. *Diabetes* 1996;**45**:101–104.

80 Jenner M, Bradish G, Stiller C, Atkison P, for the London Diabetes Study Group. Cyclosporine A treatment of young children with newly-diagnosed type 1 (insulin dependent) diabetes mellitus. *Diabetologia* 1992;**35**:884–888.

81 Parving HH, Tarnow L, Nielsen FS, Rossing P, Mandrup-Poulsen T, Osterby R, Nerup J. Cyclosporine nephrotoxicity in type 1 diabetic patients. A 7-year follow-up study. *Diabetes Care* 1999;**22**:478–483.

82 Assan R, Timsit J, Feutren G, Bougneres P, Czernichow P, Hannedouche T, Boitard C, Noel LH, Mihatsch MJ, Bach JF. The kidney in cyclosporin A-treated diabetic patients: a long-term clinicopathological study. *Clinical Nephrology* 1994;**41**:41–49.

83 Harrison LC, Colman PG, Dean B, Baxter R, Martin FIR. Increase in remission rate in newly diagnosed type 1 diabetic subjects treated with azathioprine. *Diabetes* 1985;**34**:1306–1308.

84 Silverstein J, Maclaren N, Riley W, Spillar R, Radjenovic D, Johnson S. Immunosuppression with azathioprine and prednisone in recent onset insulin-dependent diabetes mellitus. *New England Journal of Medicine* 1988;**319**:599–604.

85 Cook JJ, Hudson I, Harrison LC, Dean B, Colman PG, Werther GA, Warne GL, Court JM. A double-blind controled trial of azathioprine in children with newly-diagnosed type 1 diabetes. *Diabetes* 1989;**38**:779–783.

86 Vague P, Viallettes B, Lassman-Vague V, Vallo JJ. Nicotinamide may extend remission phase in insulin dependent diabetes. *Lancet* **i**:1987;619–620.

87 Mendola G, Casamitgana R, Gomis R. Effects of nicotinamide therapy upon B-cell function in newly diagnosed type 1 (insulin-dependent) diabetes mellitus patients. *Diabetologia* 1989;**32**:160–162.

88 Pozilli P, Visalli N, Ghirlanda G, Manna R, Andreani D. Nicotinamide increases C-peptide secretion in patients with recent onset type 1 diabetes. *Diabetic Medicine* 1989;**6**: 568–572.

89 Chase HP, Butler-Simon N, Garg S, McDuffie M, Hoops SL, O'Brien D. A trial of nicotinamide in newly diagnosed patients with type 1 (insulin-dependent) diabetes mellitus. *Diabetologia* 1990;**33**:444–446.

90 Viallettes B, Picq R, du Rostu M, Charbonnel B, Rodier M, Mirouze J, Vexiau P, Passa Ph, Pehuet M, Elgrably F, Vague Ph. A preliminary multicentre study of the treatment of recently diagnosed type 1 diabetes by combination nicotinamide–cyclosporin therapy. *Diabetic Medicine* 1990;**7**: 731–35.

91 Lewis MC, Canafx DM, Sprafka JM, Barbosa JJ. Double-blind randomized trial of nicotinasmide on early onset diabetes. *Diabetes Care* 1992;**15**:121–123.

92 Ilkova H, Gorpe U, Kadioglu P, Ozyazar M, Bagriacik N. Nicotinamide in type 1 diabetes of recent onset: a double-blind placebo controlled trial. *Diabetologia* 1991;**34**(Suppl 2): A179.

93 Guastamacchia E, Ciampolillo A, Lollino G, Caragiulo L, De Robertis O, Lattanzi V, Giorgino R. Effetto della terapia con nicotinamide sull'induzione della durata della remissione clinica in diabetici tipo 1 all'esordio sottoposti a terapia insulinica ottimizzata mediante microinfusore. *Il Diabete* 1992;**4**(Suppl 1): 210.

94 Gonzalez-Clemente JM, Munoz A, Fernandez-Usac E. Desferrioxamine and nicotinamide in newly diagnosed type 1 diabetes: a randomized double-blind placebo controlled trial. *Diabetologia* 1992;**35**(Suppl 1):A202.

95 Paskova M, Ikao I, Trozova D, Bono P. Nicotinamide in children with newly diagnosed type 1 diabetes mellitus. *Diabetologia* 1992;**35**:(Suppl 1):A203.

96 Pozzilli P, Visalli N, Boccuni ML, Baroni MG, Buzzetti R, Fioriti E, Signore A, Cavallo MG, Andreani D, Lucentini L, Crino A, Cicconetti CA, Teodonio C, Amoretti R, Pisano L, Pennafina MG, Santopadre G, Marozzi G, Multari G, Campea L, Suppa MA, De Mattia GC, Cassone-Faldetta M, Perrone F, Greco A, Ghirlanda G,and The IMDIAB Study

Group. Randomized trial comparing nicotinamide and nicotinamide plus cyclosporin in recent onset insulin-dependent diabetes (IMDIAB 1). The IMDIAB Study Group. *Diabetic Medicine* 1994;**11**:98–104.

97 Pozzilli P, Visalli N, Boccuni ML, Baroni MG, Buzzetti R, Fioriti E, Signore A, Cavallo MG, Andreani D, Lucentini L, Matteoli MC, Crino A, Cicconetti CA, Teodonio C, Amoretti R, Pisano L, Pennafina MG, Santopadre G, Marozzi G, Multari G, Campea L, Suppa MA, De Mattia GC, Cassone-Faldetta M, Marietta G, Perrone F, Greco A, Ghirlanda G. Combination of nicotinamide and steroid versus nicotinamide in recent-onset IDDM. The IMDIAB II Study. *Diabetes Care* 1994;**17**:897–900.

98 Taboga C, Tonutti L, Noacco C. Residual B cell activity and insulin requirements in insulin-dependent diabetic patients treated from the beginning with high doses of nicotinamide. A two-year follow-up. *Recenti Progressi in Medicina* 1994;**85**:513–516.

99 Pozzilli P, Visalli N, Signore A, Baroni MG, Buzzetti R, Cavallo MG, Boccuni ML, Fava D, Gragnoli C, Andreani D, Lucentini L, Matteoli MC, Crino A, Cicconetti CA, Teodonio C, Paci F, Amoretti R, Pisano L, Pennafina MG, Santopadre G, Marozzi G, Multari G, Suppa MA, Campea L, De Mattia GC, Cassone-Faldetta M, Marietta G, Perrone F, Greco AV, Ghirlanda G,and The IMDIAB Study Group. Double blind trial of nicotinamide in recent-onset IDDM (the IMDIAB III study). *Diabetologia* 1995;**38**: 848–852.

100 Satman I, Dinccag N, Karsidag K, Ozer E, Altuntas Y, Yilmaz MT. The effect of nicotinamide in recent-onset type 1 diabetes regarding the level of beta cell reserve. *Klinik Gelisim* 1995;**8**:3882–3886.

101 Visalli N, Cavallo MG, Signore A, Baroni MG, Buzzetti R, Fioriti E, Mesturino C, Fiori R, Lucentini L, Matteoli MC, Crino A, Corbi S, Spera S, Teodonio C, Paci F, Amoretti R, Pisano L, Suraci C, Multari G, Sulli N, Cervoni M, De Mattia G, Faldetta MR, Boscherini B, Bitti MLM, Marietta G, Ferrazzoli F, Bizzarri C, Pitocco D, Ghirlanda G, Pozzilli P, and The IMDIAB Study Group. A multi-centre randomized trial of two different doses of nicotinamide in patients with recent-onset type 1 diabetes (the IMDIAB VI). *Diabetes Metabolism Research and Reviews* 1999;**15**:181–185.

102 Vidal J, Fernandez-Balsells M, Sesmilo G, Aguilera E, Casamitjana R, Gomis R, Conget I. Effects of nicotinamide and intravenous insulin therapy in newly diagnosed type 1 diabetes. *Diabetes Care* 2000;**23**:360–364.

103 Pozzilli P, Browne PD, Kolb H. Meta-analysis of nicotinamide treatment in patients with recent-onset IDDM. The Nicotinamide Trialists. *Diabetes Care* 1996;**19**:1357–1363.

104 Shehadeh N, Calcinaro F, Bradley BJ, Bruchlim I, Vardi P, Lafferty K. Effects of adjuvant therapy on development of diabetes in mouse and man. *Lancet* 1994;**343**:706–707.

105 Pozzilli P, on behalf of the IMDIAB Group. BCG vaccine in insulin-dependent diabetes mellitus. IMDIAB Group. *Lancet* 1997;**349**:1520–1521.

106 Elliott JF, Marlin KL, Couch RM. Effect of Bacille Calmette–Guérin vaccination on C-peptide secretion in children newly diagnosed with IDDM. *Diabetes Care* 1998;**21**:1691–1693.

107 Allen HF, Klingensmith GJ, Jensen P, Simoes E, Hayward A, Chase HP. Effect of Bacillus Calmette–Guerin vaccination on new-onset type 1 diabetes. A randomized clinical study. *Diabetes Care* 1999;**22**:1703–1707.

108 Gross D, Sidi H, Weiss L, Kalland T, Rosenmann E, Slavin S. Prevention of diabetes mellitus in non-obese diabetic mice by linomide, a novel immunomodulating drug. *Diabetologia* 1994;**37**:1195–1201.

109 Coutant R, Landais P, Rosilio M, Johnsen C, Lahlou N, Chatelain P, Carel JC, Ludvigsson J, Boitard C, Bougneres PF. Low dose linomide in Type I juvenile diabetes of recent onset: a randomised placebo-controlled double blind trial. *Diabetologia* 1998;**41**:1040–1046.

110 Shah SC, Malone JI, Simpson NE. A randomized trial of intensive insulin therapy in newly diagnosed type 1 insulin-dependent diabetes mellitus. *New England Journal of Medicine* 1989;**320**:550–554.

111 Schnell O, Eisfelder B, Standl E, Ziegler AG. High-dose intravenous insulin infusion versus intensive insulin treatment in newly diagnosed IDDM. *Diabetes* 1997;**46**: 1607–1611.

112 Zhang ZJ, Davidson LE, Eisenbarth G, Weiner HL, Suppression of diabetes in NOD mice by oral administration of porcine insulin. *Proceedings of the National Academy of Sciences of the USA* 1991;**88**:10252–10256.

113 Bergerot I, Fabien N, Maguer V, Thivolet C. Oral administration of human insulin to NOD mice generates CD4$^+$ T cells that suppress adoptive transfer of diabetes. *Journal of Autoimmunity* 1994;**7**:655–663.

114 Polanski M, Melican NS, Zhang J, Weiner HL. Oral administration of the immunodominant B-chain of insulin reduces diabetes in a co-transfer model of diabetes in the NOD mouse and is associated with a switch from Th1 to Th2 cytokines. *Journal of Autoimmunity* 1997;**10**:339–346.

115 Mayer L, Shao L. Therapeutic potential of oral tolerance. *Nature Reviews Immunology* 2004;**4**:407–419.

116 Faria AM, Weiner HL. Oral tolerance. *Immunological Reviews* 2005;**206**:232–259.

117 Faria AM, Weiner HL. Oral tolerance: therapeutic implications for autoimmune diseases. *Clinical and Developmental Immunology* 2006;**13**:143–157.

118 Pozzilli P, Pitocco D, Visalli N, Cavallo MG, Buzzetti R, Crino A, Spera S, Suraci C, Multari G, Cervoni M, Manca Bitti ML, Matteoli MC, Marietti G, Ferrazzoli F, Cassone Faldetta MR, Giordano C, Sbriglia M, Sarugeri E, Ghirlanda G. No effect of oral insulin on residual beta-cell function in recent-onset type I diabetes (the IMDIAB VII). IMDIAB Group. *Diabetologia* 2000;**43**:1000–1004.

119 Chaillous L, Lefevre H, Thivolet C, Boitard C, Lahlou N, Atlan-Gepner C, Bouhanick B, Mogenet A, Nicolino M, Carel JC, Lecomte P, Marechaud R, Bougneres P, Charbonnel B, Sai P. Oral insulin administration and residual beta-cell function in recent-onset type 1 diabetes: a multicentre randomised controlled trial. Diabete Insuline Orale group. *Lancet* 2000;**356**:545–549.

120 Ergun-Longmire B, Marker J, Zeidler A, Rapaport R, Raskin P, Bode B, Schatz D, Vargas A, Rogers D, Schwartz S, Malone J, Krischer J, Maclaren NK. Oral insulin therapy to prevent progression of immune-mediated (type 1)

diabetes. *Annals of the New York Academy of Sciences* 2004;**1029**:260–277.

121 Cohen IR. Peptide therapy for Type I diabetes: the immunological homunculus and the rationale for vaccination. *Diabetologia* 2002;**45**:1468–1474.

122 Elias D, Markovits D, Reshef T, Van der Zee R, Cohen IR, Induction and therapy of autoimmune diabetes in the nonobese diabetic (NOD/LT) mouse by a 65-kDa heat shock protein. *Proceedings of the National Academy of Sciences of the USA* 1990;**87**:1576–1580.

123 Elias D, Reshef T, Birk OS, Van der Zee R, Walker MD, Cohen IR, Vaccination against autoimmune mouse diabetes with a T-cell epitope of the human 65 kDa heat shock protein. *Proceedings of the National Academy of Sciences of the USA* 1991;**88**:3088–3091.

124 Raz I, Elias D, Avron A, Tamir M, Metzger M, Cohen IR. β-cell function in new-onset type 1 diabetes and immunomodulation with a heat-shock protein peptide (DiaPep277): a randomised, double-blind, phase II trial. *Lancet* 2001;**358**: 1749–1753.

125 Raz I, Avron A, Tamir M, Metzger M, Symer L, Eldor R, Cohen IR, Elias D. Treatment of new-onset type 1 diabetes with peptide DiaPep277 is safe and associated with preserved beta-cell function: extension of a randomised, doubleblind, phase II trial. *Diabetes/Metabolism Research and Reviews* 2007;**23**:292–298.

126 Huurman VA, Decochez K, Mathieu C, Cohen IR, Roep BO. Therapy with the hsp60 peptide DiaPep277 in C-peptide positive type 1 diabetes patients. *Diabetes/Metabolism Research and Reviews* 2007;**23**:269–275.

127 Schloot NC, Meierhoff G, Lengyel C, Vándorfi G, Takács J, Pánczél P, Barkai L, Madácsy L, Oroszlán T, Kovács P, Sütö G, Battelino T, Hosszufalusi N, Jermendy G. Effect of heat shock protein peptide DiaPep277 on beta-cell function in paediatric and adult patients with recent-onset diabetes mellitus type 1: two prospective, randomized, double-blind phase II trials. *Diabetes/Metabolism Research and Reviews* 2007;**23**:276–285.

128 Lazar L, Ofan R, Weintrob N, Avron A, Tamir M, Elias D, Phillip M, Josefsberg Z. Heat-shock protein peptide DiaPep277 treatment in children with newly diagnosed type 1 diabetes: a randomised, double-blind phase II study. *Diabetes/Metabolism Research and Reviews* 2007;**23**:286–291.

129 Herold KC, Bluestone JA, Montag AG, Parihar A, Wiegner A, Gress RE, Hirsch R. Prevention of autoimmune diabetes with nonactivating anti-CD3 monoclonal antibody. *Diabetes* 1992;**41**:385–391.

130 Chatenoud L, Thevet E, Primo J, Bach J-F, Anti-CD3 antibody induces long-term remission of overt autoimmunity in nonobese diabetic mice. *Proceedings of the National Academy of Sciences of the USA* 1994;**91**:123–127.

131 Chatenoud L, Primo J, Bach J-F. CD3 antibody-induced self tolerance in overtly diabetic NOD mice. *Journal of Immunology* 1997;**158**:2947–2954.

132 Herold KC, Hagopian W, Auger J, Poumain-Ruiz E, Taylor L, Donaldson D, Gitelman SE, Harlan D, Xu D, Zivin RA, Bluestone JA. Anti-CD3 monoclonal antibody in new-onset type 1 diabetes mellitus. *New England Journal of Medicine* 2002;**346**:1692–1698.

133 Herold KC, Gitelman SE, Masharani U, Hagopian W, Bisikirska B, Donaldson D, Rother K, Diamond B, Harlan DM, Bluestone JA. A single course of anti-CD3 monoclonal antibody hOKT3gamma1(Ala-Ala) results in improvement in C-peptide responses and clinical parameters for at least 2 years after onset of type 1 diabetes. *Diabetes* 2005;**54**: 1763–1769.

134 Keymeulen B, Vandemeulebroucke E, Ziegler AG, Mathieu C, Kaufman L, Hale G, Gorus F, Goldman M, Walter M, Candon S, Schandene L, Crenier L, De Block C, Seigneurin JM, De Pauw P, Pierard D, Weets I, Rebello P, Bird P, Berrie E, Frewin M, Waldmann H, Bach JF, Pipeleers D, Chatenoud L. Insulin needs after CD3-antibody therapy in new-onset type 1 diabetes. *New England Journal of Medicine* 2005;**352**:2598–2608.

135 Kaufman DL, Clare-Salzler M, Tian J, Forsthuber T, Ting GS, Robinson P, Atkinson MA, Sercarz EE, Tobin AJ, Lehman PV. Spontaneous loss of T-cell tolerance to glutamic acid decarboxylase in murine insulin-dependent diabetes. *Nature* 1993;**366**:69–72.

136 Tisch R, Yang XD, Singer SM, Liblau RS, Fugger L, McDevitt HO. Immune response to glutamic acid decarboxylase correlates with insulitis in non-obese diabetic mice. *Nature* 1993;**366**:72–75.

137 Tian J, Atkinson MA, Clare-Salzler M, Herschenfeld A, Forsthuber T, Lehmann PV, Kaufman DL. Nasal administration of glutamate decarboxylase (GAD65) peptides induces Th2 responses and prevents murine insulin-dependent diabetes. *Journal of Experimental Medicine* 1996;**183**:1–7.

138 Petersen JS, Karlsen AE, Markholst H, Worsaae A, Dyrberg T, Michelsen B. Neonatal tolerization with glutamic acid decarboxylase but not with bovine serum albumin delays the onset of diabetes in NOD mice. *Diabetes* 1994;**43**: 1478–1484.

139 Pleau JM, Fernandez-Saravia F, Esling A, Homo-Delarche F, Dardenne M. Prevention of autoimmune diabetes in nonobese diabetic female mice by treatment with recombinant glutamic acid decarboxylase (GAD65). *Clinical Immunology and Immunopathology* 1995;**76**:90–95.

140 Agardh CD, Cilio CM, Lethagen A, Lynch K, Leslie RD, Palmér M, Harris RA, Robertson JA, Lernmark A. Clinical evidence for the safety of GAD65 immunomodulation in adult-onset autoimmune diabetes. *Journal of Diabetes and Its Complications* 2005;**19**:238–246.

141 Ludvigsson J, Faresjö M, Hjorth M, Axelsson S, Chéramy M, Pihl M, Vaarala O, Forsander G, Ivarsson S, Johansson C, Lindh A, Nilsson NO, Aman J, Ortqvist E, Zerhouni P, Casas R. GAD treatment and insulin secretion in recent-onset type 1 diabetes. *New England Journal of Medicine* 2008;**359**:1909–1920.

142 Skyler JS, Greenbaum CJ, Lachin JM, Leschek E, Rafkin-Mervis L, Savage P, Spain L,and the Type 1 Diabetes TrialNet Study Group. Type 1 Diabetes TrialNet – an international collaborative clinical trials network. *Annals of the New York Academy of Sciences* 2008;**1150**:14–24.

143 Gottlieb P. The Mycophenolate Mofetil/Daclizumab Trial in Recent-Onset Type 1 Diabetes. Presented at American Diabetes Association 68th Annual Meeting, June 2008.

Available at: http://webcasts.prous.com/netadmin/webcast_viewer/Preview.aspx?type=0andlid=3948.

144 Pescovitz MD, Greenbaum CJ, Krause-Steinrauf H, Becker DJ, Gitelman SE, Goland R, Gottlieb PA, Marks JB, McGee PF, Moran AM, Raskin P, Rodriguez H, Schatz D, Wherrett D, Wilson DM, Lachin JM, Skyler JS, and The Type 1 Diabetes TrialNet Anti-CD20 Study Group. Preservation of beta-cell function by B-lymphocyte depletion with rituximab Submitted for publication.

145 Riley WJ, Maclaren NK, Spillar R. Reversal of deteriorating glucose tolerance with azathioprine in prediabetes. *Transplantation Proceedings* 1986;**18**:819–822.

146 Levy-Marchal C, Czernichow P, Quiniou MC, Sachs M, Bach JF. Cyclosporin administration reversed abnormalities in a prediabetic child. *Diabetes* 1984;**33**(Suppl 1): 183A.

147 Rakotoambinina B, Timsit J, Deschamps I, Laborde K, Jos J, Boitard C, Assan R, Robert JJ. Cyclosporin A does not delay insulin dependency in asymptomatic IDDM patients. *Diabetes Care* 1995;**18**:1487–1490.

148 Carel JC, Boitard C, Eisenbarth G, Bach JF, Bougnères PF. Cyclosporine delays but does not prevent clinical onset in glucose intolerant pre-type 1 diabetic children. *Journal of Autoimmunity* 1996;**9**:739–745.

149 Dumont-Herskowitz R, Jackson RA, Soeldner JS, Eisenbarth GS. Pilot trial to prevent type 1 diabetes: progression to overt IDDM despite oral nicotinamide. *Journal of Autoimmunity* 1989;**2**:733–737.

150 Elliott RB, Chase HP. Prevention or delay of type 1 (insulin-dependent) diabetes mellitus in children using nicotinamide. *Diabetologia* 1991;**34**:362–365.

151 Manna R, Migliore A, Martin LS, Ferrara E, Ponte E, Marietti G, Scuderi F, Cristiano G, Ghirlanda G, Gambassi G. Nicotinamide treatment in subjects at high risk of developing IDDM improves insulin secretion. *British Journal of Clinical Practice* 1992;**46**:177–179.

152 Elliott RB, Pilcher CC, Fergusson DM, Stewart AW. A population based strategy to prevent insulin-dependent diabetes using nicotinamide. *Journal of Pediatric Endocrinology and Metabolism* 1996;**9**:501–509.

153 Lampeter EF, Klinghammer A, Scherbaum WA, Heinze E, Haastert B, Giani G, Kolb H. The Deutsche Nicotinamide Intervention Study: an attempt to prevent type 1 diabetes. DENIS Group. *Diabetes* 1998;**47**:980–984.

154 Williams AJK, Bingley PJ, Moore WPM, Gale EAM and the ENDIT Screening Group. Islet autoantibodies, nationality and gender: a multinational screening study in first-degree relatives of patients with Type I diabetes. *Diabetologia* 2002;**45**:217–223.

155 European Nicotinamide Diabetes Intervention Trial (ENDIT) Group. Gale EAM. Intervening before the onset of Type 1 diabetes: baseline data from the European Nicotinamide Diabetes Intervention Trial (ENDIT). *Diabetologia* 2003;**46**:339–346.

156 European Nicotinamide Diabetes Intervention Trial (ENDIT) Group. European Nicotinamide Diabetes Intervention Trial (ENDIT): a randomized controlled trial of intervention before the onset of type 1 diabetes. *Lancet* 2004;**363**:925–931.

157 Gotfredsen GF, Buschard K, Frandsen EK. Reduction of diabetes incidence of BB Wistar rats by early prophylactic

insulin treatment of diabetes-prone animals. *Diabetologia* 1985;**28**:933–935.

158 Like AA, Morphology and mechanisms of autoimmune diabetes as revealed by studies of the BB/Wor rat. In: Perspectives on the Molecular Biology and Immunology of the Pancreatic Beta Cell, (eds Hanahan D, McDevitt HO, Cahill GJ), Current Communications in Molecular Biology, Cold Spring Harbor Laboratory Press, Cold Spring Harbor, NY, 1989;pp. 81–91.

159 Like AA. Insulin injections prevent diabetes (DB) in BioBreeding/Worcester (BB/W) rats. *Diabetes* 1986;**136**:3254–3258.

160 Vlahos WD, Seemayer TA, Yale JF. Diabetes prevention in BB rats by inhibition of endogenous insulin secretion. *Metabolism* 1991;**40**:825–829.

161 Gottlieb PA, Handler ES, Appel MC, Greiner DL, Mordes JP, Rossini AA. Insulin treatment prevents diabetes mellitus but not thyroiditis in RT6-depleted diabetes resistant BB/Wor rats. *Diabetologia* 1991;**34**:296–300.

162 Atkinson MA, Maclaren NK, Luchetta R. Insulitis and insulin dependent diabetes in NOD mice reduced by prophylactic insulin therapy. *Diabetes* 1990;**39**:933–937.

163 Bowman MA, Campbell L, Darrow BL, Ellis TM, Suresh A, Atkinson MA. Immunological and metabolic effects of prophylactic insulin therapy in the NOD-scid/scid adoptive transfer model of IDDM. *Diabetes* 1996;**45**:205–208.

164 Keller RJ, Eisenbarth GS, Jackson RA. Insulin prophylaxis in individuals at high risk of type 1 diabetes. *Lancet* 1993;**341**:927–928.

165 Ziegler A, Bachmann W, Rabl W. Prophylactic insulin treatment in relatives at high risk for type 1 diabetes. *Diabetes Metabolism Reviews* 1993;**9**:289–293.

166 Füchtenbusch M, Rabl W, Grassl B, Bachmann W, Standl E, Ziegler AG. Delay of type I diabetes in high risk, first degree relatives by parenteral antigen administration: the Schwabing Insulin Prophylaxis Pilot Trial. *Diabetologia* 1998;**41**:536–541.

167 Schatz D, Cuthbertson D, Atkinson M, Salzler MC, Winter W, Muir A, Silverstein J, Cook R, Maclaren N, She JX, Greenbaum C, Krischer J. Preservation of C-peptide secretion in subjects at high risk of developing type 1 diabetes mellitus – a new surrogate measure of non-progression? *Pediatric Diabetes* 2004;**5**:72–79.

168 Diabetes Prevention Trial – Type 1 Diabetes Study Group. Effects of oral insulin in relatives of patients with type 1 diabetes mellitus. *Diabetes Care* 2005;**28**:1068–1076.

169 Type 1 Diabetes TrialNet Oral Insulin Study. http://www2. diabetestrialnet.org/oins.

170 Harrison LC, Honeyman MC, Steele CE, Stone NL, Sarugeri E, Bonifacio E, Couper JJ, Colman PG. Pancreatic beta-cell function and immune responses to insulin after administration of intranasal insulin to humans at risk for type 1 diabetes. *Diabetes Care* 2004;**27**:2348–2355.

171 Kimpimaki T, Kupila A, Hamalainen AM, Kukko M, Kulmala P, Savola K, Simell T, Keskinen P, Ilonen J, Simell O, Knip M. The first signs of beta-cell autoimmunity appear in infancy in genetically susceptible children from the general population: the Finnish Type 1 Diabetes Prediction and Prevention Study. *Journal of Clinical Endocrinology and Metabolism* 2001;**86**:4782–4788.

172 Kukko M, Kimpimäki T, Kupila A, Korhonen S, Kulmala P, Savola K, Simell T, Keskinen P, Ilonen J, Simell O, Knip M. Signs of beta-cell autoimmunity and HLA-defined diabetes susceptibility in the Finnish population: the sib cohort from the Type 1 Diabetes Prediction and Prevention Study. *Diabetologia* 2003;**46**:65–70.

173 Näntö-Salonen K, Kupila A, Simell S, Siljander H, Salonsaari T, Hekkala A, Korhonen S, Erkkola R, Sipilä JI, Haavisto L, Siltala M, Tuominen J, Hakalax J, Hyöty H, Ilonen J, Veijola R, Simell T, Knip M, Simell O. Nasal insulin to prevent type 1 diabetes in children with HLA genotypes and autoantibodies conferring increased risk of disease: a double-blind, randomised controlled trial. *Lancet* 2008;**372**:1746–1755.

174 Borch-Johnsen K, Joner G, Mandrup-Paulsen T, Christy M, Zachan-Christiansen B, Kastrup K, Nerup J. Relationship between breastfeeding and incidence rates of insulin dependent diabetes mellitus. *Lancet* 1984;**ii**:1083–1086.

175 Gerstein H. Cow's milk exposure and type 1 diabetes mellitus. *Diabetes Care* 1994;**17**:13–19.

176 Norris JM, Scott FW. A meta-analysis of infant diet and insulin-dependent diabetes mellitus: do biases play a role? *Epidemiology* 1996;**7**:87–92.

177 Virtanen SM, Rasanen L, Aro A, Lindstrom J, Sippola H, Lounamaa R, Toivanen L, Tuomilehto J, Akerblom HK, Childhood Diabetes in Finland Study Group Infant feeding in Finnish children <7yr of age with newly diagnosed IDDM. *Diabetes Care* 1991;**14**:415–417.

178 Norris JM, Beaty B, Klingensmith G, Yu L.-P., Hoffman M, Chase HP, Erlich HA, Hamman RF, Eisenbarth GS, Rewers M. Lack of association between early exposure to cow's milk protein and beta-cell autoimmunity. Diabetes Autoimmunity Study in the Young (DAISY). *JAMA* 1996;**276**:609–614.

179 Kimpimaki T, Erkkola M, Korhonen S, Kupila A, Virtanen SM, Ilonen J, Simell O, Knip M. Short-term exclusive breast-feeding predisposes young children with increased genetic risk of Type I diabetes to progressive beta-cell autoimmunity. *Diabetologia* 2001;**44**:63–69.

180 Akerblom HK, Savilahti E, Saukkonen TT, Paganus A, Virtanen SM, Teramo K, Knip M, Ilonen J, Reijonen H, Karjalainen J, Vaarala O, Reunanen A. The case for elimination of cow's milk in early infancy in prevention of type 1 diabetes: the Finnish experience. *Diabetes Metabolism Reviews* 1993;**9**:269–278.

181 Harrison LC, Honeyman MC. Cow's milk and type 1 diabetes: the real debate is about mucosal immune function. *Diabetes* 1999;**48**:1501–1507.

182 TRIGR Study Group. Study design of the Trial to Reduce IDDM in the Genetically at Risk (TRIGR). *Pediatric Diabetes* 2007;**8**:117–137.

183 Akerblom HK, Virtanen SM, Ilonen J, Savilahti E, Vaarala O, Reunanen A, Teramo K, Hämäläinen AM, Paronen J, Riikjärv MA, Ormisson A, Ludvigsson J, Dosch HM, Hakulinen T, Knip M, and the National TRIGR Study Groups. Dietary manipulation of beta cell autoimmunity in infants at increased risk of type 1 diabetes: a pilot study. *Diabetologia* 2005;**48**:829–837.

184 TRIGR Study. http://trigr.epi.usf.edu/news.html.

5 Prevention of type 2 and gestational diabetes

Richard F. Hamman, Dana Dabelea

Department of Preventive Medicine and Biometrics, University of Colorado Health Sciences Center, Denver, CO, USA

Introduction

Eliot P. Joslin, founder of the Joslin Clinic, was the first to propose primary prevention of what is now classified as type 2 diabetes, when in 1921 he wrote:[1]

> A real headway against the ravages of a disease begins with its prevention rather than its treatment. Prevention implies a knowledge of the predisposing agency. Overweight is a predisposition to diabetes. The individual overweight is at least twice, and at some ages forty times, as liable to the disease. For the prevention of more than half of the cases of diabetes in this country, no radical undernutrition is necessary; the individual is simply asked to maintain the weight of his average fellow man. Diabetes, therefore, is largely a penalty of obesity and the greater the obesity, the more likely is Nature to enforce it. Granted there is one person in a thousand who has some inherent peculiarity of the metabolism which has led to obesity, there are 999 for whom being fat implies too much food or too little exercise or both combined.

Since that time, substantial research has confirmed and extended these observations. In addition to the role of obesity as a major risk factor, studies aimed at understanding the basic pathogenesis and physiology have led us closer to an understanding of the interacting pathways leading to type 2 and gestational diabetes mellitus. It has become clearer in the past 5 years that interventions aimed at reversing these steps can succeed in optimal circumstances (efficacious interventions) due to the completion of several randomized controlled trials (RCTs) of diabetes prevention. However, much work remains to understand

how to intervene in an effective and efficient way in large numbers of people to prevent diabetes. Most of the work reviewed here focuses on interventions aimed at individuals, to alter lifestyle and to reduce the metabolic derangements now known to be part of the pathways to disease. Less work has been done on broader social and psychological determinants (primordial prevention – preventing the appearance of mediating risk factors in the population), yet it is likely that diabetes prevention will require a combination of both individual and societal approaches to be successful. In a later section, the limited attempts to change the environment of schools, churches and communities as approaches to primordial prevention are reviewed.

There have been a number of summaries of the primary prevention of type 2 diabetes, previously called non-insulin-dependent diabetes mellitus (NIDDM), which serve as background for this review,[2–13] including a previous edition of this chapter.[14] Here, the focus is on studies that attempt to prevent the onset of type 2 diabetes or gestational diabetes through lifestyle modification, reduction in obesity or through pharmacological means. Studies that attempt to understand the subsequent development of complications of diabetes after onset, even if detected during an asymptomatic stage, are not included but are dealt with in a later chapter. The next chapter deals with the evidence surrounding the early detection of type 2 diabetes through screening.

Rationale and requirements for the prevention of type 2 diabetes

Several observations align to indicate the increasing need to prevent type 2 diabetes, rather than simply

The Evidence Base for Diabetes Care, Second Edition, Edited by William H. Herman, Ann Louise Kinmonth, Nicholas J. Wareham and Rhys Williams.
© 2010 John Wiley & Sons, Ltd

treat it, once established. Chapter 1 described the increasing prevalence and incidence, excess mortality and limited effectiveness of interventions once diabetes is manifest. In addition to these, diabetes, and particularly type 2 diabetes, incurs high health care costs.[15] It is the purpose of this chapter to review relevant research to determine if preventive interventions are effective. Chapter 27 reviews the evidence on their potential cost-effectiveness.

As is further developed in the next chapter in relation to screening, several pieces of knowledge must be available in order to know if it is possible to prevent any chronic disorder, including diabetes. These include knowledge of the natural history of diabetes (with a reasonably long pre-clinical phase of the natural history), an effective and simple screening test or tests for a high-risk state and effective interventions that, if applied earlier in the pre-clinical phase, would prevent or delay the onset of the disease.

The pre-clinical stages of the development of type 2 diabetes are well known. For many years it has been shown that glucose levels become elevated prior to the development of diabetes. This stage of the natural history has been called 'chemical diabetes', IGT,[16] or most recently IFG.[17] Impairment of glucose regulation at levels which are lower than used for diagnosis increases the risk of subsequent diabetes 5–8-fold.[18] Thus, there is at least one pre-clinical stage for intervention prior to the development of diabetes. Two major questions need to be answered: (1) are there efficacious and effective interventions to prevent (or delay) the onset of diabetes and (2) does treatment at the time of early diagnosis reduce complications as much or perhaps more than waiting until the time of usual clinical intervention? This chapter will summarize the available clinical trials and selected observational studies relevant to the first question. The second question is dealt with in the next chapter.

Selection criteria for studies

Studies are included if they were either RCTs or community-based trials or if they were large, prospective epidemiological studies of sufficient rigor and generalizability to be useful. The numerous clinical, ecological, cross-sectional and retrospective studies that have been conducted were largely omitted, unless they provide the only evidence bearing on an issue. The previous edition of this chapter summarized much of the observational data on diet and activity as risk factors for diabetes. Although substantial new work has occurred, it is not included here in the interest of focusing on the RCT evidence at hand.

Studies exploring the prevention of gestational diabetes have been added, largely from an observational perspective as RCTs have not yet been conducted.

Studies were identified through computerized searches of several databases, including MEDLINE, Cochrane Collaboration, Clinical Trials Registry and Best Evidence, and a thorough search of cited references in published papers. Unpublished prevention trials were sought through contacts with researchers, although none were found that had been completed but not published, at least in abstract form. Trials in progress are included in a later section of this chapter.

Definition of type 2 diabetes mellitus

The studies reviewed here use a variety of criteria to define type 2 diabetes. This is inevitable, given the long time period included. It was not possible to identify consistent criteria for all studies. However, the 1985 WHO criteria[16] or the more current American Diabetes Association criteria[19] were used as a reference when possible. In prevention trials, the development of any clinical diagnosis of diabetes or measured hyperglycaemia meeting defined criteria was usually the outcome of the trial.

Only one prevention study published to date has tested for autoimmune markers that would identify individuals developing autoimmune diabetes.[20] Since well over 90% of people developing diabetes over the age of 50 years will have type 2 diabetes,[21] this is a minor limitation. However, proper diagnosis of the etiological type of diabetes as an outcome will become increasingly important in trials in the future, since specific interventions aimed at defined metabolic and immunological pathways will increasingly be tested.

Screening and diagnosis of gestational diabetes mellitus

Health care providers disagree about several aspects of GDM, including criteria for diagnosis, associated perinatal and maternal morbidity and optimal therapeutic strategies.[22–27] The current approach in the United States consists of a non-fasting 50 g oral glucose challenge test (GCT) at 24–28 weeks' gestation with determination of plasma glucose levels 1 h after the load, followed by a diagnostic 3 h, 100 g oral glucose tolerance test (OGTT) *only* in women with an abnormal screening test. The GCT is positive in 14–18% of women using a cut-off value of $\geq$140 mg day^{-1} (7.8 mmol l^{-1}) and in 20–25% using a cut-off value of $\geq 130\,\mathrm{mg\,dl^{-1}}$ ($7.2\,\mathrm{mmol\,l^{-1}}$), with respective sensitivities for the diagnosis of GDM of approximately 80 and 90%.[28]

The American College of Obstetricians and Gynecologists[29] suggests that although universal screening for GDM is the most sensitive approach, there may be pregnant women at low risk who are less likely to benefit from the screening, such as women aged <25 years, of an ethnic group other than Hispanic, African-American, American Indian or Asian, with a body mass index (BMI) <25, without a prior history of abnormal glucose tolerance or GDM and with no known diabetes in a first-degree relative.

The final diagnosis of GDM is based on results from the OGTT. There is no agreement on the performance or interpretation of OGTT in pregnant women, but two or more pathological glucose values are required for a diagnosis of GDM. The National Diabetes Data Group criteria[30] (Table 5.1) are based on quantifying the risk of subsequent DM in the mother.[31] More recently, Carpenter and Coustan[32] derived new cut-points (Table 5.1) based on the associated risk of fetal macrosomia and Caesarean delivery in the absence of treatment.[33,34] However, women with lesser degrees of glucose intolerance, who exhibit an abnormal glucose screening test but do not meet diagnostic criteria for GDM, may also be at risk for delivering a macrosomic infant.[35,36] Furthermore, the reproducibility of the 100 g OGTT used to diagnose GDM is imperfect, with ~25% of patients exhibiting disparate results when given two tests 1 week apart.[37] These differences make direct comparison of the prevalence of GDM difficult, although risk factor relationships across studies are likely to be valid.

Natural history and risk factors for type 2 diabetes

Primary prevention of diabetes is based on knowledge of the natural history of the development of glucose intolerance and risk factors. Once these have been established from observational studies, it is at least theoretically possible that interventions aimed at any of the factors could reduce diabetes risk. A number of recent reviews of risk factors exist.[4,7,38–45] and are summarized in Table 5.2 for individual level risk factors, that is, those that operate on or within a person. This table does not include the more antecedent group-, societal- or population-level risk factors such as westernization, commercialization of the food supply, increased motorized transport,

Table 5.1 Screening and diagnostic criteria for gestational diabetes mellitus[a]

Time (h)	Glucose cut-point (mg dl^{-1})		
	Screening test 50 g OGTT	Diagnostic test 100 g OGTT	
		NDDG	Carpenter and Coustan[32]
Fasting	–	105	95
1	130 or 140	190	180
2	–	165	155
3	–	145	140

[a]Values are cut-points (mg dl^{-1}). A dash (–) indicates glucose levels not used for the test indicated. For the 100 g test, any two values over these cut-points represent a positive test.[32]

Table 5.2 Summary of established and *possible*[a] individual level risk factors for type 2 diabetes mellitus

Demographic variables	Obesity-related variables
Older age	Higher total adiposity
Male gender	Central fat distributions
Minority racial/ethnic group	Intra-abdominal fat
Family history of diabetes	Longer duration of obesity
Maternal history of diabetes	Weight gain
	Short stature
Physiological variables	
High glucose level (fasting and post-challenge)	**Reproductive variables**
Low insulin secretion	Diabetes during pregnancy
Insulin resistance syndrome: low HDL-C, high triglycerides, hypertension, fibrinolytic defects, glucose intolerance	Polycystic ovary syndrome
	Higher parity
	Lack of breast feeding
	Low birth weight
Low magnesium level	*High birth weigh*
Low chromium level	*Catch-up growth*
High plasma non-esterified fatty acids	**Dietary and nutritional variables**
Low sex hormone binding globulin	High caloric intake
	High total and saturated fat intake
Behavioural variables	*Low alcohol intake*
Low physical activity	*Low fibre intake*
Cigarette smoking	*High glycaemic index foods*
	Low vitamin D intake
	Low magnesium intake
	Low potassium intake
	Low polyunsaturated fatty acid intake
	Low vegetable fat intake
	Low whole grain intake
	Low caffeine (coffee) intake

[a]Variables in *italics* are not firmly established – differing amounts of evidence exist to support them, although the balance of observational data favours them at this time.

television and computer time replacing group and individual activity and interaction and changes in social morays which alter individual factors over large numbers of people simultaneously.

Risk factors for GDM

Given the controversies around screening and diagnosis, systematic investigation of the epidemiology of GDM has been difficult. The most often reported risk factors for GDM are older age, minority racial/ethnic background, family history of diabetes, obesity and parity. Not surprisingly, they are virtually identical with those reported for type 2 diabetes itself. Table 5.3 summarizes factors that could identify groups at high risk for the development of GDM (left) and factors that could be targeted and modified by preventive interventions (right).

Prevention of type 2 diabetes

Interventions have been targeted at altering a number of behavioural factors including obesity, dietary intake and physical activity. Obesity, of course, is the result of behavioural, genetic and physiological factors and is not simply behavioural. Pharmacological interventions have used hypoglycaemic or anti-hyperglycaemic medication to reverse insulin resistance (biguanides, thiazolidinediones), failure of insulin secretion (sulfonylureas) or glycaemic excursions (α-glucosidase inhibitors). Trials have attempted to alter glucose metabolism using metal supplementation (magnesium, chromium) or antioxidants (β-carotene, vitamin E). In addition, several recent trials have explored the use of angiotensin-converting enzyme inhibitors (ACE-I), angiotensin receptor blockers (ARB) and statin therapy on diabetes incidence.

1 Combined lifestyle interventions

Table 5.4 summarizes the intervention studies that have attempted to prevent type 2 diabetes using a combination of lifestyle interventions. These typically include a dietary intervention of various types together with increased physical activity. The intensity of the intervention for either component has often varied substantially. Inclusion criteria have also been variable, with most studies including people without diabetes.

Some studies have used diabetes related endpoints as the main outcome rather than the incidence of diabetes itself. These have included glucose tolerance testing with various criteria, infusion tests and fasting glucose levels. Such studies were included in the previous edition[14] since they might inform future trial designs. However, they have not been included in this edition because accumulating evidence from larger primary prevention trials with diabetes as the primary or secondary endpoint is now available. Non-randomized interventions (e.g.[46,47]) and a summary of observational prospective studies of physical activity and diet were also not included.

Whitehall study, London, UK

In one of the earliest attempted lifestyle interventions, Jarrett and co-workers identified Whitehall civil service workers with borderline glucose tolerance from a large ($N = 20\,000$) survey.[48–50] Men aged 40–64 years were asked to participate in an RCT of dietary carbohydrate restriction and the biguanide phenformin ($50\,\text{mg}\,\text{day}^{-1}$) for 5 years. Dietary carbohydrate was limited to $120\,\text{g}\,\text{day}^{-1}$. Progression to diabetes was confirmed by OGTT or development of intercurrent symptoms and elevated glucose levels. There were no significant differences between the diet and control groups in this small study ($N = 99$) in the incidence of diabetes. Weight change, which was not a primary goal of the trial, did not predict incidence.

Table 5.3 Risk factors for gestational diabetes mellitus

Factors that can identify high-risk populations	Factors that can be targeted by preventive interventions
Demographic variables Older age Minority racial/ethnic group Family history of diabetes	**Obesity-related variables** High pre-pregnancy BMI High pre-pregnancy waist circumference High pregnancy weight gain Low physical activity before and during pregnancy
Reproductive variables Previous GDM History of GDM in women's mother High parity Previous obstetric outcomes: macrosomia, congenital malformations, stillbirth, Caesarean section Polycystic ovary syndrome	**Dietary variables** High saturated fat intake Low alcohol intake Low vitamin C intake
Anthropometric variables Low birth weight Short stature	**Physiological variables** High screening glucose challenge test (GCT) Insulin resistance-related factors: hypertension

Uppsala, Sweden

Following a community screening programme in Uppsala, Sweden, Cederholm[51] identified 51 people with glucose intolerance classified by 1980 WHO criteria.[52] He was able to sequentially randomize 43

of these to a diet and physical activity regimen for six months ($N = 25$) or to no advice or treatment ($N = 18$). After 6 months, the intervention group was 2.2 times (95% CI 0.8 to 5.6) more likely to have normal glucose tolerance than the controls. Inverting this relative risk

Table 5.4 Combined lifestyle interventions in the primary prevention of type 2 diabetes mellitus[a]

Reference	Population	Intervention	Results	Comments
Jarrett et al., 1979[48,49]	**Whitehall, London, UK** 204 men with borderline glucose tolerance aged 40–64 years ($x = 57$); follow-up 5 years. Outcome: diabetes	**Diet** ($N = 44$) limit to 120 g day^{-1} carbohydrate **Placebo** ($N = 45$)	*Diet*: 18.2/100 worsened to diabetes *Placebo*: 13.3/100 ($p = $ NS; rate higher in intervention group)	Most men would have IGT by current criteria. 23/204 men dropped out (11.3%). No relation of weight change to diabetes incidence; diet intervention very limited in scope and impact. Diabetes required ≥ 2 positive tests. Randomization method not specified. Multiple logistic regression used to account for minor imbalances at entry
Cederholm, 1985[51]	**Uppsala, Sweden** 53 people aged 47–54 years with glucose intolerance by 1980 WHO criteria;. follow-up 6 months Outcome: diabetes	**Diet + exercise**: ($N = 25$) lower sugar, fat, calories; at 6 months with abnormal OGTT, given glipizide: ($N = 10$) **Control**: ($N = 18$); no advice or therapy	*Diet + exercise*: RR = 0.67 (95% CI 0.43–1.05), ARR = 25.8/100 PY to remain glucose intolerant on OGTT at 6 months vs *control*. Decrease in glucose AUC, relative BMI, cholesterol, TGs and SBP ($p < 0.01$). *Glipizide*: 4/10 became normal in additional 4–6 months; no control data	Glipizide given to 10/13 persons who did not normalize OGTT at 6 months, but no controls were followed so these data are not interpretable. Unmasked sequential randomization; no multivariate analysis
Pan et al., 1997[62]	**Da Qing IGT and Diabetes Study**, China 577 25 + − year-olds with IGT by WHO criteria, randomized by clinic, followed for 6 years. Outcome: diabetes	**Diet** ($N = 130$): lower fat, alcohol, higher vegetables; weight loss in those with BMI >25 **Exercise** ($N = 141$): increase by 1 U day^{-1} (local scales) **Diet + exercise** ($N = 126$) **Control** ($N = 133$): information only	*Diet*: 10.0/1000 PY, RR^b = 0.69 ($p = 0.028$), ARR = 5.7/1000 PY *Exercise*: 8.3/1000 PY, RR^b = 0.54 ($p = 0.000$), ARR = 7.4/1000 PY *Diet + exercise*: 9.6/1000 PY, RR^b = 0.58 ($p = 0.001$), ARR = 6.1/1000 PY *Control*: 15.7/1000 PY, RR^b = 1.0	Randomized by clinic; 8.1% dropout in 6 years. Similar results in lean and obese individuals. No blinding; allocation not masked, since by clinic
Dyson et al., 1997[64,65]	**Fasting Hyperglycaemia Study (FHS)** (Lifestyle) UK and France; 227 persons aged 30–65 years ($x = 50$ years); factorial design with sulfonylurea; follow-up 1 year Outcome: diabetes	**Basic lifestyle** ($N = 116$); **Reinforced lifestyle** ($N = 111$); low-fat diet, increased fibre, hypocaloric if BMI >22; aerobic physical activity given 1 × year in basic group, every 3 months in reinforced group	*Basic*: 1.5 kg weight loss at 3 months, no change at 1 year; no changes in percentage with diabetes, glucose intolerance or high BP *Reinforced*: weight loss similar to basic group; no changes in percentage with diabetes, glucose intolerance or high BP; fitness, insulin sensitivity, TGs improved significantly	Dropouts 18% in reinforced advice, 7% in basic advice at 1 year. Randomization schedule not masked

(continued)

Table 5.4 *(Continued)*

Reference	Population	Intervention	Results	Comments
Wing *et al.*, 1998[66]	**Pittsburgh, PA, USA** 154 overweight non-diabetic patients, aged 40–55 years ($x = 46$) with 1 + diabetic parent; follow-up up to 2 years. 72/154 with IGT at baseline. Outcome: diabetes	**Diet** ($N = 37$): low fat, low calorie **Exercise** ($N = 37$): 1500 kcal per week moderate exercise **Diet + exercise** ($N = 40$): combination of other interventions **Control** ($N = 40$): written material	*6 months*: decreases in F glucose, F insulin in D and D + E groups; also in lipids, BP *12 months:* no change in F glucose between groups, although weight loss maintained in D, D + E at 60% and 72% of 6 month levels *24 months: Control*: 7% with diabetes; D 30.3%; E 14%; D + E 15.6%. FPG, OGTT, weight loss did not differ between groups. 4.5 kg weight loss (4.5% of initial weight) predicted RR of 0.696 (95% CI 0.526 to 0.865) for type 2 DM among NGT; RR = 0.744 (95% CI 0.592 to 0.897) among IGT participants. No differences in type 2 DM between intervention groups, once weight loss accounted for	Groups similar at baseline. Dropouts: 6 months 15%, 12 months 22%, 24 months 16%. Class attendance averaged only 27% in last 18 months. Little change in diet or exercise at 24 months between groups. Much of the cohort not exposed to intervention during the last 18 months. Not blinded, allocation not said to be masked. ITT analysis used on persons attending follow-up
Bergenstal *et al.*, 1998[70]	**Community Diabetes Prevention Project (CDPP)**, Minnesota, USA 418 community dwelling non-diabetic persons aged $x = 46$ years; follow-up 2 years. Outcome: diabetes	**Intervention** ($N = 209$) diet, exercise, stress management yearly **Standard** ($N = 209$) no intervention	RR = 1.0 (95% CI 0.38 to 2.80) for diabetes progression (3.5% in each group); no changes in risk factors for insulin resistance at 2 years between groups	Low-intensity intervention with two meetings per year, monthly telephone calls, newsletters. Details of randomization and blinding not given
Wein *et al.*, 1999[71]	**Melbourne, Australia** 200 women with prior GDM and IGT; aged $x = 38$ years; BMI = 25; follow-up $x = 51$ months. Outcome: diabetes by WHO criteria	**Intervention** ($N = 100$) 3 monthly dietician telephone contact; primarily healthy eating; brisk walking encouraged, not reinforced **Control** ($N - 100$) baseline healthy eating, brisk walking, no reinforcement	*Intervention*: annual incidence rate = 6.1/100 PY *Control* = 7.3/100 PY RR = 0.83 (95% CI 0.47 to 1.48, $p = 0.5$) ARR = 1.2/100 PY; 17% reduction	Low-intensity telephone intervention; both groups gained weight; no difference in diet or activity scores. Adjustment for baseline differences in risk and weight change showed Cox HR = 0.63 (95% CI 0.35 to 1.14, $p = 0.12$). Lost to follow-up = 3% (intervention), 4% (control)
Eriksson *et al.*, 1999[72]; Tuomilehto, 2001[73]	**Diabetes Prevention Study (DPS)** Finland: 5 centres 522 men and women; aged $x = 55$ years, BMI = 31, WHO IGT × 2; follow-up 3.2 years. Outcome: diabetes by WHO criteria	**Intervention** ($N = 265$) diet, exercise, weight loss in 7 sessions in year 1, then 4 times per year **Control** ($N = 257$) annual information	*Lifestyle*: incidence rate = 3.2/100 PY vs *Control* = 7.8/100; HR = 0.4 (95% CI 0.3 to 0.7) for incident diabetes; ARR = 4.6/100 PY; 58% reduction	Achieved 4.2 kg weight loss in intervention group. Persons with best compliance to lifestyle change had greatest reduction in incidence

Table 5.4 *(Continued)*

Reference	Population	Intervention	Results	Comments
DPP Research Group, 2002[78–80]	**Diabetes Prevention Program (DPP)** 27 US centres, 3234 men and women; IGT with elevated FPG; 45% non-Caucasian; aged $x = 51$ years, BMI = 34; follow-up 2.8 years. Outcome: diabetes by ADA criteria	**Intensive Lifestyle (ILS)** ($N = 1079$) 16-session curriculum on diet, activity, weight loss; at least monthly contact with coach **Placebo** ($N = 1082$) annual meeting with written material on lifestyle	*ILS*: incidence rate = 4.8/100 PY vs *Placebo* = 11.0/100 PY; 58% reduction in incidence; similar in both genders, all ethnic groups, all ages; ARR = 6.2/100 PY	Achieved 5.6 kg weight loss in lifestyle vs 0.1 kg in placebo groups. Suggestion of greater reduction in persons aged >60 years (71%); NNT = 6.9 to prevent one case
Ramachandran *et al.*, 2005[87]	**Indian Diabetes Prevention Program (IDPP)** 531 men and women; IGT × 2; aged $x = 46$ years; BMI = 25.8; follow-up 3 years. Outcome: diabetes by WHO criteria	**Lifestyle modification (LSM)** ($N = 133$) diet, activity; monthly telephone; 6-monthly in person **Metformin (MET)** ($N = 133$); 250 mg bid **LSM + MET** ($N = 129$) **Control** ($N = 136$) limited reinforcement	*LSM* cumulative 3 year incidence = 39.3% (annual incidence rate (AIR) = 16.6/100 PY; ARR = 10.0/100 PY) vs *Control* = 55.0% (AIR = 26.6/100 PY) vs *MET* = 40.5% (AIR = 17.3/100 PY; ARR = 9.3/100 PY) vs *LSM + MET* 39.5% (AIR = 16.8/100 PY; ARR = 9.9/100 PY).	Weight increase in controls (~0.8 kg) with about 0.3–0.4 kg lower weight in intervention groups (similar) and significant weight gain in LSM groups at 24 months. No blinding or placebo used; 36 month follow-up for 213 persons, 30 month close-out for 132. 5.8% lost to follow-up, slightly higher in LSM groups. Consecutive allocation
Kosaka *et al.*, 2005[89]	**Tokyo, Japan** 458 Japanese males; aged 30–60s; BMI = 24; follow-up = 4 years. Outcome: diabetes by 100 g OGTT	**Intensive lifestyle (ILS)** ($N = 102$) visits every 2–3 months on diet, weight loss, increased activity **Standard (STD) Intervention** ($N = 356$) baseline session on weight loss or maintenance, smaller dietary portion size; reinforced every 6 months	*ILS*: 4 year cumulative incidence = 3.0% (0.76/100 PY) vs *STD* = 9.3% (2.44/100 PY); 67% reduction in incidence; ACRR = 6.3/100 (ARR = 1.68/100 PY); returned to NGT: ILS = 53.8% vs STD = 33.9%	ILS lost 2.18 kg at 4 years vs 0.39 kg in STD. STD group that lost most weight had lowest incidence. 9.0% of STD, 6.9% of ILS lost to follow-up after year 1. No mention of allocation method or number lost to follow-up from baseline to year 1. NNT = 60 to prevent one case over 4 years
Davey-Smith *et al.*, 2005[93]	**MRFIT, USA, 1973–76** Subset of 11 287 non-diabetic men; aged 35–57 years, $x = 46$ years; BMI ≈ 27; follow-up = 6 years. Outcome: diabetes by fasting ADA criteria, single test	**Special intervention** ($N = 5934$) 10 initial intensive sessions followed by counselling sessions approx. every 4 months; lower dietary fat, weight loss, increased activity, smoking cessation, BP control **Usual care** ($N = 5893$) 3 screenings, annual risk factor measurement	*Special intervention* (non-smokers): cumulative 6 year incidence = 10.0% (1.76/100 PY) vs *Usual care* (non-smokers) = 12% (2.13/100 PY); HR = 0.82 (95% CI 0.68 to 0.98) (ARR = 0.37/100 PY)	*Post-hoc* sub-group analysis of lower risk men in MRFIT trial. Significant interaction by smoking; smokers had higher diabetes risk among intervention group (HR = 1.26, 95% CI 1.10 to 1.45). CVD risk factors, glucose and BMI higher in non-smokers by design. 41% of all men had fasting glucose between 100 and 125 mg dl^{-1} at baseline. Increased risk for diabetes among men taking antihypertensive medications

(continued)

Table 5.4 *(Continued)*

Reference	Population	Intervention	Results	Comments
Oldroyd *et al.*, 2006[94]	**Newcastle-upon-Tyne, UK, 1994–98** 78 men and women; aged 24–75 years; weight = 85 kg; follow-up = 2 years. Outcome: glucose and diabetes by OGTT	**Lifestyle intervention** (*N* = 39) 12 routine visits with dietician and physiotherapist over 24 months on diet, physical activity **Control** (*N* = 39) no intervention; 6, 12, 24 month assessments	*Lifestyle*: group 2 year cumulative incidence = 17.9% (9.9/100 PY) vs *Control* = 20.5% (11.5/100 PY); ARR = 1.6/100 PY (NS). Lifestyle lost 1.8 kg vs 1.5 kg gain in controls. No change in mean glucose levels; significant improvement in whole body insulin sensitivity. Non-significant improvement in reversion to NGT among lifestyle group (20%) vs control (13%) at 24 months.	Underpowered trial; not masked; modest improvement in weight with low-intensity intervention. Self-reported improvements in diet and activity, but no change in fitness test or CVD risk factors. 31% dropouts, higher among controls

[a]ARR = absolute risk reduction (if not present, data were insufficient to calculate); ITT = intention-to-treat; NNT = number needed to treat.
[b]Adjusted for FPG, BMI at baseline.

for consistency with other prevention studies, participants were 0.67 times (95% CI 0.43 to 1.05) times as likely to remain abnormal, given the intervention. The absolute risk reduction (ARR) was 25.8/100 or a 33.2% risk reduction (%RR). There were significant, although small, decreases in glucose area under the OGTT curve, systolic BP, BMI, cholesterol and triglycerides compared with the controls. This important work, together with other pilot RCTs of glycaemic and insulinaemic endpoints[53–61] and non-randomized studies, set the stage for the larger trials to follow.

Da Qing IGT and diabetes study, China

The first large RCT among high-risk persons with IGT using diabetes as the endpoint was conducted in China in collaboration with the NIDDK Phoenix Epidemiology group. Pan *et al.* identified 577 people with IGT from among 110,660 men and women screened in Da Qing, in northern China.[62] Subjects were randomized using their primary care clinic (i.e. all people in a clinic received the same intervention) to a factorial design of diet, physical activity, diet plus physical activity or control given only limited written advice about diabetes and IGT. The intervention encouraged fewer simple sugars and less alcohol consumption, more vegetable intake and, if BMI was ≥25, weight loss to ≤23 kg m^{-2}. Physical activity advice was aimed at increasing walking or running at least 1 unit on a simple scale of activities and both interventions were conducted through individual and group sessions at a frequency starting weekly and decreasing to quarterly over the 6 year follow-up period. Glucose tolerance was systematically tested every 2 years and people with interim symptoms or elevations of fasting

glucose were tested as required. Repeat testing by OGTT confirmed diabetes.

Compared with the control group, all intervention groups significantly decreased the incidence of diabetes over the 6 years. Reductions in diabetes incidence ranged from 31 to 46% across the groups in adjusted models to account for baseline BMI and fasting glucose. The absolute risk reduction (ARR) ranged from 5.7 to 6.1/100 person-years (PY) across the intervention groups. Analysis by clinic, which was the original unit of randomization, showed similar results and reductions in incidence rates were also comparable in both lean and overweight groups. Of interest, in the intention-to-treat (ITT) analysis, the diet plus physical activity group appeared to be no more effective than either diet or physical activity alone, although crossover effects (e.g. changes in diet in the physical activity group) would have been difficult to detect given the simple assessment tools used.

A subsequent analysis of this study stratified 284 of the 577 participants with fasting insulin measurements into higher and lower estimated insulin sensitivity at trial baseline.[63] This analysis suggested that persons who were more insulin sensitive had a greater impact of the interventions and that the combined intervention (diet plus increased activity) had a somewhat greater impact than diet or exercise alone, when stratified in this manner. Since this is a *post hoc* sub-group analysis, it was exploratory and should be replicated. It implies that attempts to prevent diabetes maybe more effective before severe insulin resistance has developed.

These results suggest that a lifestyle intervention can delay or prevent diabetes. The study does have limitations, due largely to the limited resources available. It was difficult to determine the size of, and compliance with, the actual lifestyle changes made by individuals. No blinding was used in the evaluation of diet or physical activity, so some amount of reporting bias is likely in the assessment of lifestyle change, though the primary endpoint is unlikely to be biased by the lack of blinding. Group-based randomization, necessary due to logistical constraints in performing the intervention, although susceptible to imbalance at study entry, resulted in good balance at baseline and a reasonably consistent intervention effect was seen across clinics. Several strengths of the study should be noted.

The dropout (8.6% in 6 years) and mortality (1.9% in 6 years) rates were low. Follow-up was consistent across all groups and the intervention was developed to be applied in a country with limited resources. The authors estimated that 980 000 new cases of diabetes per year will occur in China in the next century, so feasible and effective interventions such as this are crucial to reduce the burden of disease.

Fasting hyperglycaemia study, UK and France

The Fasting Hyperglycaemia Study (FHS) was designed to identify high-risk participants for lifestyle and sulfonylurea (gliclazide) prevention therapy.[64,65] Two elevated fasting glucose levels (5.5–<7.8 mmol l^{-1}) 2 weeks apart, in people aged 30–65 years (mean = 50 years) were used to define people with IFG. People with a history of GDM, a first-degree relative with NIDDM, moderate obesity or a history of hyperglycaemia or glycosuria were identified via general practitioners in three English and two French centres. There were 227 participants with IFG, of whom 223 had an OGTT [37% were normal, 37% had IGT (by WHO criteria) and 26% had NIDDM (by WHO criteria)]. These 227 participants were randomized to a factorial lifestyle or sulfonylurea (gliclazide) intervention. In the lifestyle portion of the FHS, participants were randomly allocated to basic (N = 116) or reinforced healthy living advice (N = 111). Basic advice included weight loss (if BMI ≥ 25) and increased physical activity, which was not reinforced. In the reinforced lifestyle group, a low-fat, higher fibre diet was individually prescribed. Participants with a BMI ≥ 22 were given a detailed calorie-restricted diet for weight loss and increased activity in the form of swimming, cycling, brisk walking and so on was recommended, with increasing frequency to 5–6 times per week.

There was an average 1.5 kg weight loss in *both* groups, with maximum weight loss at 3 months and return to near baseline at 1 year. There were no differences at 1 year in the proportion with diabetes, in the mean fasting or 2 h glucose levels or BP between the groups, or any changes within group from baseline. There was a significant small increase in insulin

sensitivity by CIGMA assessment in the reinforced group, with no changes in the basic advice group. Small changes in total and LDL-cholesterol occurred similarly in both groups. Relatively small lifestyle changes were induced in this group of volunteers over 1 year which were not sufficient to alter glucose tolerance, given the small sample size studied. This is not an adequate test of alterations in lifestyle from an efficacy point of view. However, it does represent a level of intervention that can be accomplished within constraints of most health care systems. Unfortunately, at this level of lifestyle change, no improvements were realized. The heterogeneous eligibility criterion with a range of risk from NGT through diabetes on OGTT at baseline complicates the interpretation.

Pittsburgh, PA, USA

Wing *et al.* conducted a 2 year randomized intervention among overweight non-diabetic participants with a family history of diabetes.[66] Of these 154, 72 had IGT at baseline. They were randomized to one of four interventions: control (literature only), diet (low calorie, low fat), physical activity (moderate walking to 1500 kcal per week) or both diet and physical activity. The intervention groups received intensive group sessions early and refresher sessions throughout the period, although participation dropped to only 27% in the last 18 months and weight regain occurred.

Maximum weight loss occurred at 6 months and decreases in fasting glucose and insulin levels were seen in the diet and diet plus physical activity groups. By 12 months, there were no changes in fasting glucose levels between groups, although weight loss was maintained in 60% of diet intervention participants and 72% of diet plus physical activity participants. At 2 years there were no significant differences between groups, with the control group having the lowest overall incidence of diabetes (7%). When the groups were pooled, modest weight loss (−4.5 kg, which equalled 4.5% of initial weight) predicted a reduction in diabetes incidence. The relative risk (RR) was 0.696 (95% CI 0.526 to 0.865) among people with normal glucose tolerance at entry and 0.744 (95% CI 0.592 to 0.897) among those with IGT. Similar reductions were seen in all groups, with the primary predictors of diabetes incidence being IGT at baseline (higher risk) and weight loss (lower risk). No additional effect of improvement in VO_{2max} was seen.

The authors concluded that the three lifestyle approaches differed in their initial effectiveness but not in their long-term impact, such that baseline glucose and weight had returned to or exceeded baseline levels. However, the finding that modest weight loss in the entire group reduced the incidence of diabetes is very important. It is consistent with the findings from Malmö[67] and other studies[54,59] that weight loss, although perhaps not physical activity alone,[68] can reduce the development of diabetes and that the degree of weight loss does not have to be large. However, weight loss has not been found consistently to be associated with improvements in glucose levels or diabetes incidence.[53,55,69] The reasons for these discrepancies remain uncertain but may be related to the magnitude of the initial weight loss, the failure to maintain weight loss or the degree of initial hyperglycaemia.

Community diabetes prevention project (CDPP), Minnesota, USA

Bergenstal *et al.* took a lower intensity approach to preventing glucose intolerance in Minnesota.[70] They randomly allocated 418 patients to standard and intervention groups. Intervention participants received two meetings per year focusing on nutrition, physical activity and stress, with monthly calls from nutrition students for encouragement, along with a quarterly newsletter and annual individual counselling. The 418 participants at entry included 3% with diabetes and 4% with IGT. The remainder had normal glucose tolerance. After 2 years of follow-up, there were no differences in progression to diabetes or changes in fasting glucose levels between the groups.[70] No further follow-up has been published. While the low-intensity community-based intervention was designed to be of low cost, it appears that it was not effective in reducing glucose intolerance or making important changes in cardiovascular risk parameters, at least over 2 years in low-risk individuals. Given the relatively small changes seen in more intensive interventions, this result may not be surprising.

Melbourne, Australia

A small intervention was conducted by Wein *et al.* among women with prior gestational diabetes and IGT on repeat OGTT.[71] They randomized 100 women to each group and gave both healthy diet and brisk walking advice, having them return annually for testing. In the intervention group, they reinforced the dietary advice via telephone contact with a dietician every 3 months over the course of an average of 51 months of follow-up. Both groups gained weight ($\sim$1 BMI unit) and had no differences in diet or activity scores. There was a non-significant reduction in diabetes incidence in the intervention group [annual incidence rate $= 6.1/100$ PY; control $= 7.3/100$ PY; RR $= 0.83$ (95% CI 0.47 to 1.48, $p = 0.5$; ARR $= 1.2/100$ PY; 17% reduction]. Adjusting for baseline differences in risk and for weight change resulted in an unchanged hazard ratio (HR $= 0.63$ (95% CI 0.35 to 1.14, $p = 0.12$). This trial was a very low-intensity

intervention which was also underpowered. The small reduction in diabetes risk may have been due to chance, although it is consistent with the later trials reviewed below, given the intensity of the intervention. Overall, this young cohort of post-GDM women with little overweight had about a 30% cumulative risk of diabetes at 5 years, indicating that a history of GDM is a potent risk factor.

Diabetes prevention study (DPS), Finland

The aim of the DPS was to determine if an intensive diet and physical activity intervention could delay or prevent type 2 diabetes and worsening of cardiovascular risk factors among people with IGT.[72] A total of 522 overweight people at five centres with IGT on two OGTTs were randomized to either a control or an unmasked intervention group. The mean age was 55 years, BMI was 31 and 67% were women. Seven sessions were held with a nutritionist in the first year, followed with quarterly visits thereafter. The aim of the intervention was to reduce weight by 5% or more and reduce saturated fat intake to less than 30% of energy consumed, while increasing dietary fibre and physical activity. Supervised circuit resistance training sessions were available and group walking and other activities were organized. The control group received limited annual diet and physical activity advice.

One year results were reported for the first 212 participants who were randomized[72] and the primary results were published in 2001.[73] During the average follow-up period of 3.2 years, 86 participants developed diabetes: 27 in the intervention group (incidence rate 3.2/100 PY) and 59 in the control group (7.8/100 PY). The lifestyle intervention reduced the incidence of diabetes by 58% (Cox adjusted hazard ratio $= 0.4$, 95% CI 0.3 to 0.7, ARR $= 4.6/100$ PY). Persons who were more successful in achieving the lifestyle goals had a lower incidence of diabetes than persons who were less successful. On average, the intervention group lost 4.2 kg of weight and the control group lost 0.8 kg. The authors noted that this modest level of weight loss led to substantial reductions in diabetes incidence and that among individuals who lost at least 5% of their initial weight, the risk reduction was even greater. Diabetes risk was reduced in a dose-dependent fashion with weight loss.[74] Hence the overall results are somewhat conservative as an estimate of the relationship between weight loss and reduction of diabetes incidence. Among participants who did not meet the weight loss goal, but did meet the exercise goal (>4 h per week), diabetes was also reduced significantly, even after adjustment for baseline BMI (adjusted hazard ratio $= 0.3$, 95% CI 0.1 to 0.7). Over a longer follow-up period (4.1 years) Laaksonen and DPS colleagues showed that participants reporting physical activity in the upper one-third of the total leisure-time physical activity (LTPA) distribution were 80% less likely to develop diabetes than those in the lower third (RR = 0.2, 95% CI 0.10 to 0.41) adjusted for multiple baseline risk factors and weight change.[75] Reported dietary changes are summarized later in this chapter.

The diet and activity changes also resulted in improvements in insulin sensitivity in a sample of DPS participants, strongly correlated with weight change.[76] Insulin secretion remained stable among persons able to lose weight, but deteriorated in those who did not. Plasminogen activator inhibitor (PAI-1) also decreased in the intervention group by 31% with no change in the control group, again correlated with weight change.[77] Hence the benefits of lifestyle change were seen in metabolic parameters related to diabetes risk, body weight and fat distribution and ultimately on diabetes risk itself in this well-conducted trial.

Diabetes prevention program (DPP), USA

The Diabetes Prevention Program (DPP) was a multi-centre primary prevention study among people with IGT.[78] The 27 clinical centres screened over 158 000 people and conducted over 30 000 OGTTs to identify people with IGT and a fasting glucose level from 95 to 125 mg dl^{-1} (5.3–6.9 mmol l^{-1}). The trial included 3234 people randomized to three intervention groups, each with slightly over 1000 individuals per group. There was an unmasked intensive lifestyle group, aimed at reduction of body weight by 7% or more and increased moderate physical activity (usually brisk walking) to at least 150 min per week. This was accomplished using an intensive 16-session curriculum, followed by weekly or biweekly contact and reinforcement, with a toolbox of retention and relapse approaches. The pharmacological arms (metformin, troglitazone and placebo) are discussed later. The primary endpoint was clinical or OGTT diabetes, confirmed on at least two tests, using ADA criteria. Intervention groups were well balanced at baseline with respect to a number of risk factors. The average age of participants was 50.6 years, 68% were women, average BMI was 34.0 and 69% of participants reported a first-degree family history of diabetes.[79] In May 2002, after an average of 2.8 years of follow-up, the data monitoring board found evidence of significant and substantial effectiveness of both interventions and terminated the DPP 1 year early.[80] The intensive lifestyle intervention reduced the incidence of diabetes by 58%, from an average annual incidence of 11/100 PY in the placebo group to 4.8/100 PY in the lifestyle group (ARR = 6.2/100 PY). This effect was consistent across all sub-groups

examined, including persons of all racial/ethnic groups, both genders and all ages, including individuals over 60 years of age, where the estimated reduction was 71%. Persons in the lifestyle group lost an average of 5.6 kg of weight compared with 0.1 kg in the placebo group and 74% met self-reported physical activity goals at the end of the core curriculum.

Dietary self-monitoring was positively related to meeting both the activity and dietary goals and those who met initial goals (at the end of the 16 week core curriculum) were significantly more likely to continue to meet goals at study end.[81] The total incidence of diabetes was lower the more goals were met. If all three goals (dietary fat ≤25% of calories, weight loss of ≥7%, increased physical activity ≥150 min per week) were met, the risk of developing diabetes was reduced by 89%.[82] Weight loss was the dominant factor in predicting lower diabetes incidence. For every 1 kg of weight loss over the study, there was a 16% reduction in incidence (adjusted for multiple baseline and follow-up risk factors). Not surprisingly, both decreased intake of dietary fat and increased physical activity significantly predicted weight loss. Subsequent reports have shown that the lifestyle intervention not only reduced diabetes incidence, but also significantly improved cardiovascular risk factors,[83] reduced markers of inflammation (fibrinogen, CRP)[84] and the incidence of the metabolic syndrome[85] and improved markers of autonomic function.[86]

Diabetes prevention program (IDPP), India

Ramachandran *et al.* conducted a community-based randomized trial in urban Asian Indian participants with persistent IGT (on two tests within a week).[87] They randomized consecutively into four groups: standard health care advice (control), lifestyle modification (LSM), metformin (MET) and, unique among trials to date, a lifestyle plus metformin (LSM + MET) group. Overall, 531 individuals were included and followed every 6 months with capillary tests, confirmed by OGTT. The LSM intervention consisted of walking or cycling ≥30 min per day and dietary advice to include reduced caloric intake, reduced refined sugars and fats and increased fibre-rich foods. Little emphasis appeared to be placed on weight loss, since the average BMI at study entry was about 26 kg m^{-2} The MET group ultimately received 250 mg of drug twice per day. At study end, 345 individuals had either 36 months of follow-up ($N = 213$) or 30 months ($N = 132$) and 44% had developed diabetes. The 3 year cumulative incidence of diabetes was significantly reduced to similar levels in all intervention groups (control = 55% vs LSM = 39%; MET = 40.5%) and there was no additional effect of combining lifestyle and metformin (LSM + MET = 39.5%). The number needed to treat (NNT) over 3 years was 6.4–6.9 across the groups with an ARR of 9.3–10/100 PY.

Several results from this trial are noteworthy, some surprising. The overall cumulative incidence of 55% in 3 years among persons with a baseline BMI of 26.3 confirms the high-risk nature of Asian Indian populations.[88] The risk was probably enhanced by the requirement for 'stable IGT' – that is, two OGTTs in the IGT range at baseline, which identified an especially high-risk group. However, the risk in this study (18.3% per year) was even higher than in DPS (6% per year) and Da Qing (11.3% per year) which also required 'stable IGT'. The reduction in incidence of diabetes (of 26–28%) was achieved in the LSM groups with little if any weight loss, although the control group gained approximately 0.8 kg on average and was heavier than any of the intervention groups over the course of the trial. This suggests that improvement in diet and increased activity resulted in the majority of the effect; however, no details of sub-group analyses are yet available. A 1 kg weight loss in the DPP study resulted in a 16% reduction in risk,[82] so perhaps the weight differential in the IDPP also accounts for a portion of the findings. Surprising to the authors was the lack of added benefit from combining lifestyle and metformin. The risk reduction was nearly identical with either lifestyle of metformin alone.

Diabetes prevention trial, Tokyo, Japan

Kosaka *et al.* conducted a hospital-based diabetes screening programme among Japanese government employees.[89] Using a 100 g OGTT, they identified males with hyperglycaemia said to be equivalent to IGT (using 1980 WHO criteria) and randomized one of five to an intensive lifestyle intervention ($N = 102$) or standard treatment ($N = 356$). The lifestyle intervention consisted of weight loss advice (for participants with a BMI ≥ 22), weekly body weight, a dietary intervention including smaller portion size, lower fat intake, increased fruits and vegetables and increased physical activity (equivalent to 30–40 min of walking per day). Participants were seen every 2–3 months during the 4 year follow-up period. The standard intervention consisted of 6 monthly advice (at regular glucose testing visits) to lose weight (if BMI ≥ 24) using smaller meal portion size and increased physical activity. No adherence to specific components of the interventions were measured; however, the ILS group lost 2.18 kg over 4 years, compared to the standard group (0.39 kg). The baseline BMI in both groups was approximately 24, one of the lowest of any trial conducted to date. The incidence of diabetes (based on 6 monthly OGTTs) was reduced by 67% through the intervention (3.0% 4 year cumulative incidence in lifestyle; 9.3% in standard group; NNT = 16 over

4 years). This translates into an annual incidence rate of 0.76/100 PY in lifestyle compared with 2.44/100 PY in control. The absolute risk reduction (ARR) was 1.68/100 PY. The authors also noted a higher reversion from IGT to non-IGT over time in the lifestyle group (53.8 vs 33.9% in standard intervention) and a graded lower incidence of diabetes with greater reduction in weight over the trial. Among control participants, the greater the weight loss, the lower was the incidence of diabetes, even though the baseline BMI of these groups did not differ. This small trial had relatively low loss to follow-up after the first year (6.9% in lifestyle; 9.0% in control), but no data were reported on losses from randomization to year 1, nor were methods for allocation noted. At baseline (among individuals who were present at year 1) there were no significant differences in important risk factors between intervention groups.

Multiple risk factor intervention trial (MRFIT), USA, 1973–1982

There are no large diabetes-specific RCTs that have targeted lower risk individuals for intervention. However, several cardiovascular risk reduction trials have explored diabetes as a secondary outcome or conducted sub-group analyses,[90–92] with mixed results. The largest of these was the MRFIT trial, conducted in the United States in the 1970s and 1980s.[93] There were almost 13 000 men randomized in the trial, of whom 11 827 were at risk for developing diabetes (after *post hoc* exclusions). Of these, approximately 41% had a fasting glucose between 100 and 125 mg dl^{-1} at baseline (now called IFG) and the mean BMI was about 27 kg m^{-2} at entry. The special intervention was aimed at reducing multiple cardiovascular risk factors and included advice on lowering saturated fat and cholesterol intake, weight reduction, increased physical activity, smoking cessation and blood pressure control (mostly with thiazide diuretics). There were ten initial intensive sessions followed by counselling sessions approximately every 4 months. The usual care group received no intervention. Among non-smoking participants there was an 18% reduction in diabetes risk over 6 years in the intervention group compared with usual care (HR = 0.82, 95% CI 0.68 to 0.98; ARR = 0.37/100 PY). Unexpectedly, there was a 26% *increase* in diabetes among smokers exposed to the special intervention. Several exploratory analyses adjusting for baseline risk factors and subsequent treatment were similar; however, individuals who lost weight had lower diabetes risk and individuals taking antihypertensive medications had increased risk. Accounting for these factors among smokers reduced the hazard ratio to from 1.26 to 1.13 (95% CI 0.97 to 1.31). In both groups, weight loss was associated with lower diabetes incidence; for every 1 unit decrease in BMI $(kg\,m^{-2})$ there was a significant 19–25% decrease in diabetes incidence over 6 years. Among non-smokers, accounting for weight loss during the trial increased the hazard ratio from 0.82 to 0.97, suggesting that weight loss was largely responsible for the improvements seen. Because of the unexpected opposite results by smoking status, the results must be interpreted with some caution. However, the authors believe that it is likely that this intervention in lower risk non-smokers reduced the incidence of diabetes significantly.

Newcastle-upon-Tyne, UK

A small randomized intervention was conducted in Newcastle-upon-Tyne, UK, from 1994 to 1998 among 78 persons with stable IGT using a less intensive lifestyle intervention, but was only recently published.[94] Participants were given 12 appointments over 24 months of follow-up with a clinic dietician and physiotherapist for counselling about diet change and increased physical activity. Lifestyle participants lost 1.8 kg at 24 months compared with controls who gained 1.5 kg. The 2 year cumulative incidence was 17.9% (9.9/100 PY) in the lifestyle group versus 20.5% (11.5/100 PY) in the control (ARR = 1.6/100 PY), a non-significant difference but of the magnitude seen in some larger studies.[89] Surprisingly, there were no significant differences in fasting or post-load glucose levels. The study was underpowered and might not have been able to detect improvements in glucose tolerance, since a higher proportion of intervention individuals returned to NGT, but this was also not statistically significant. Modest improvement in whole body insulin sensitivity was noted, without important changes in cardiovascular disease risk factors. This study and others[71] suggest that less intense interventions may produce small changes in risk factors for diabetes but may be less able to reduce diabetes incidence. An important challenge is to understand whether less intensive interventions such as this one are actually cost-effective, since they utilize resources at a lower level, but may not impact outcomes as favourably as more intensive, albeit more expensive, interventions.

At least one other trial has been conducted that is not available in the English literature, suggesting that a lifestyle intervention reduces diabetes onset by 43% over 3 years in 321 individuals with IGT in China.[95]

RCTs using glucose or weight change as outcomes

Several RCTs have been conducted using primarily changes in weight and fasting or post-load glucose as the outcomes. An RCT requiring participants to live for a month at a wellness centre for supervised low-fat diets, weight loss and 2.5 h of physical activity per day showed significant reductions in body weight in the intervention compared with the control (−5.4 kg vs −0.5 kg), and also lower fasting glucose (intervention −0.5 mmol l^{-1}, control = −0.31 mmol l^{-1}, $p = 0.01$) and improved parameters of fibrinolysis.[96] Diabetes outcomes were not reported.

A combined diet and physical activity study in The Netherlands [Study on Lifestyle Intervention and Impaired Glucose Tolerance Maastricht (SLIM)] followed 88 individuals for 2 years (from the original 114 individuals randomized).[97,98] Significant decreases in body weight ($\Delta - 2.3$ kg) and 2 h glucose levels ($\Delta - 1.4$ mmol l^{-1}) between intervention and control groups were seen, greatest in those adherent to the combined diet and activity regimen. Insulin sensitivity also improved at 1 year.[99] These reductions in glucose levels were consistent with a recent meta-analysis[100] of eight trials (including this one) that reported a reduced mean 2 h plasma glucose of 0.84 mmol l^{-1} (95% CI 0.58 to 1.29) with lifestyle interventions.

The Women's Healthy Lifestyle Project attempted to prevent weight gain and increased cholesterol levels among 489 healthy women who experienced the menopause through dietary changes and increased physical activity (walking, aerobics, dancing, etc.).[101,102] After 18 months of follow-up there were significant decreases in weight (−3.0 kg), waist:hip ratio, blood pressure, lipids and fasting glucose levels.[101] By 54 months,[102,103] weight returned to baseline levels for the lifestyle group, but controls had gained 2.4 kg. Fasting glucose was statistically significantly lower in the lifestyle than control group, although both had small elevations [lifestyle, +1.6 mg dl^{-1} (0.09 mmol l^{-1}) from baseline; control, +3.3 mg dl^{-1} (0.18 mmol l^{-1})]. No OGTT was conducted and no comments were made about the incidence of clinical diabetes, which would be unlikely given the age and good health of participants. This intervention suggests that weight gain can be minimized through middle age with positive effects on cardiovascular risk factors common to the insulin resistance syndrome. However, the impact on glucose levels *per se* among participants was very small.

Swinburn and colleagues conducted a 1 year education program in New Zealand aimed at reduction in dietary fat[104] with a 5 year follow-up of 103 of the original 176 randomized participants at baseline.[105] Subjects were screened for glucose intolerance during a work-site programme, selected for the study, but not entered into the study until ~2 years later. A repeat OGTT was done prior to randomization and showed that ~30% of individuals at entry had diabetes in both groups. Participants with diabetes were included in the intervention, which makes it impossible to calculate diabetes incidence rates over time. The intervention was delivered in small groups monthly over the first year, without later reinforcement. The authors noted that a lower proportion of the intervention group had type 2 diabetes or impaired glucose tolerance at 1 year (47 vs 67%, $p < 0.015$). Differences in the prevalence of abnormal glucose tolerance were not maintained in later years. There were significant reductions in 2 h glucose levels over time in the intervention group. While accomplishing a dietary fat reduction, the authors noted that there were concomitant increases in physical activity, greater in the intervention group during most of the study. Weight loss was greater in the intervention group (-3.32 kg vs $+0.59$ kg in the control group at 1 year); however, by year 5 the intervention group was 1 kg heavier than at baseline, whereas controls were 1.26 kg heavier. Given the decline in follow-up (only 76% of those available at 1 year, 59% of those from baseline), some of these changes may have been due to differential dropout. Greater compliance with the education programme (and likely greater changes in *both* diet and activity) resulted in the greatest weight loss and changes in fasting and 2 h glucose, consistent with both the DPS and DPP. There appear to have been reasonable long-term impacts of this relatively modest intervention on dietary fat (and by focus on healthy lifestyle – increased activity) that resulted in improvement in weight, although inclusion of persons with diabetes at baseline and relatively high losses to follow-up make it difficult to ascertain any improvement in diabetes risk.

Watanabe *et al.* conducted a trial of 'new dietary education' (without recommended changes in physical activity) among 173 high-risk men over 1 year in Tokyo.[106] They found that on reducing total energy intake and improving meal portion size, and increasing whole grains, fruits and vegetables, among other changes, participants in the intervention group had an 8.2% lower 2 h plasma glucose compared with controls (an increase of 11.2%). The intervention was conducted with only two sessions, the first in person and the second by mail. No measurement of physical activity was conducted so concomitant changes cannot be ruled out.

Fujimoto and colleagues conducted an RCT of the American Heart Association Step 2 diet plus endurance training compared with a Step 1 diet and stretching exercise among 74 Japanese-Americans living in Seattle.[107,108] Subjects had IGT on two occasions at entry. The intervention included supervised endurance training over 6 months and diet prescriptions. From 6 to 24 months, diet and activity were home-based and unsupervised. Of the randomized group, 58 completed a 2 year follow-up. The authors reported higher reversion to NGT during follow-up among the intervention group (67 vs 30% in control), although the study was designed primarily to look at changes in adiposity and insulin sensitivity rather than diabetes. Significant and sustained weight loss was seen in the intervention group (-2.7 kg at 6 months, -1.8 kg at 24 months) than control (-0.9, $+0.7$ at 6 and 24 months respectively); intra-abdominal fat area was also lower in the intervention group and insulin sensitivity improved more in the intervention group than control.[108] No change in β-cell function was noted, suggesting that this modest lifestyle change may not protect against long-term deterioration of β-cell decline, known to predict the development of diabetes.

Brekke *et al.* allocated 77 first-degree relatives of persons with type 2 diabetes to a diet intervention (D), diet plus exercise (DE) or control.[109] This small study had few persons with IFG/IGT (9/77) and used telephone contact on average every 10 days for 4 months, then less frequently for 2 years. The DE group lost -2.16 kg at 1 year vs C ($+0.52$ kg, $p = 0.029$) and the D group lost -0.45 kg ($p = $ ns). No significant differences in fasting or 2 h glucose were seen in this largely NGT group and diabetes outcomes were not reported. In addition to self-reported changes in diet for most variables, erythrocyte fatty acid composition also improved in the D and DE groups. This is one of the few studies reporting an objective measure of dietary change. The intervention was relatively low intensity and did accomplish longer term dietary changes, although no changes in activity were found at 1 or 2 years. It is not surprising that among this small group with NGT no important changes in glycaemia were noted.

A recent meta-analysis of RCTs of lifestyle modification or education alone included many of the studies reviewed here.[100] Overall, the authors reported that lifestyle education (based on eight trials) reduced the 2 h post-load glucose level by 0.84 mmol l^{-1} (95% CI 0.39 to 1.29) compared with controls. They also reported that the overall relative risk for diabetes (from five studies) was 0.55 (95% CI 0.44 to 0.69) in lifestyle intervention groups compared with controls. These pooled estimates were relatively free from selection bias and robust to the method of pooling. Other recent comprehensive reviews have come to similar conclusions.[39,110,111]

Cost-effectiveness of lifestyle interventions

Following the publication of the primary results of the DPP in the United States, reports of the costs[112] and within trial cost-effectiveness[113] of the interventions have been published. Over 3 years, the lifestyle and metformin interventions cost US $16 000 and $31 000 (year 2000 dollars), respectively, per case of diabetes delayed or prevented and $32 000 and $100 000 per quality-adjusted life-year (QALY) gained, as implemented in the DPP and from a health system perspective. If implemented in routine clinical practice, using a group format for lifestyle and with generic medication pricing, the lifestyle and metformin interventions cost $4500 and $11 100, respectively, per case of diabetes delayed or prevented and $9000 and $35 000 per QALY gained.[113] Both of these are well within the range suggested for implementation for other diabetes interventions[114] and are likely to be affordable in routine clinical practice. Using similar modelling techniques, Palmer *et al.* estimated the likely impact of implementing the DPP style interventions in five European countries from a single-payers perspective.[115] They noted that there are estimated improvements in life expectancy, diabetes-free years of life and either cost savings or minor increases in costs (in the UK) when compared with standard (control) lifestyle recommendations. The costs per life-year gained versus standard lifestyle advice would generally be considered to fall within the ranges considered attractive or very attractive by international standards. Thus, they concluded that in persons with IGT, implementation of such programmes should not be constrained by finances.

The DPP research group has recently estimated the *lifetime* impact (as compared with the within-trial 3 year impact) of interventions and the cost of implementation using Markov modelling.[116] The absolute incidence of diabetes was estimated to be reduced by 20 and 8% using lifestyle and metformin, respectively, and there was important impact on micro- and macrovascular outcomes. In all models, the lifestyle intervention was superior to metformin. Using a health system perspective (including only direct medical costs), metformin was estimated to cost approximately US $31 300 and lifestyle cost $1100 per QALY gained over a lifetime. There were important effects of age in the models, with lifestyle being cost-saving under age 45 years and cost-effective even in the oldest groups; metformin was not cost-effective on individuals aged ≥65 years. The authors suggested that health systems should choose to reimburse a lifestyle intervention and that such intervention might begin to 'stem the tide' of the current diabetes epidemic. Using results from the Finnish DPS and a Markov model, Avenell and colleagues modelled UK data and suggested that the incremental cost per QALY over 6 years was £13 389 for a lifestyle intervention,[110] only slightly higher than the US results.

These conclusions have recently been challenged by Eddy *et al.*[117] using a different modelling approach and assumptions. While similarly estimating lifetime improvements in outcomes, they concluded that 'the program used in the DPP study may be too expensive for health plans or a national program to implement'. At present, it is not clear why this different conclusion about cost-effectiveness was reached, but it is probably due to differences in assumptions about perspective, rates of disease progression and length of programme implementation, among others.[118]

The Indian Diabetes Prevention Program recently published their within-trial estimated costs to prevent a case of diabetes for lifestyle modification, metformin or a combination.[478] The bulk of the evidence to date suggests that lifestyle interventions in high-risk persons are not only effective, but are also likely to be either cost-effective or cost-saving over a lifetime, depending on when they are initiated.

Summary

Table 5.4 shows that there are now 13 RCTs testing combined lifestyle interventions that used diabetes as an endpoint. Seven studies[51,62,73,80,87,89,93] now provide strong evidence that lifestyle changes significantly reduce diabetes risk by up to 58%; two showed positive but non-significant results;[71,94] one showed neutral findings for diabetes but a strong effect of weight loss on diabetes;[66] and three were negative.[48,65,70] These last three studies had the least intensive interventions. In addition, there are at least eight additional RCTs[100] that used glucose levels with or without measurements of insulin or insulin resistance syndrome (IRS) components (e.g. blood pressure, triglycerides, HDL cholesterol) showing important reductions in glucose levels, body weight and cardiovascular risk factors. It now appears established from well-conducted RCTs that lifestyle changes resulting in modest weight loss (5–7% of body weight) through dietary change and modestly increased physical activity result in a substantial delay or prevention of diabetes over relatively short periods (3–6 years) of intervention. Since both the Finnish and US prevention trials were of relatively short duration, it remains uncertain how long the reduced incidence of diabetes can be maintained. Lifetime modelling of the DPP results suggests that benefits may extend substantially longer;[116] however, longer term follow-up is required to determine if these projections will occur. Both the DPS and the DPP are conducting longer term surveillance for diabetes. Results from the DPS have been published suggesting that the lifestyle risk reduction for diabetes seen at 3 years continues at least until 6 years and the rates continue to diverge.[479] The Da Qing study also suggests that delay of diabetes up to 6 years is possible. Hence important longer term delay or prevention is very likely using a lifestyle intervention aimed at weight loss and improved physical activity.

A recent publication from the Nurse's Health Study combined several of the lifestyle factors reviewed in other sections of this chapter in an analysis of diabetes incidence over 16 years of follow-up.[119] Almost 85 000 nurses who did not have diagnosed diabetes or heart disease at baseline were followed from 1980 to 1996. Clinically diagnosed diabetes was the outcome and no OGTTs were conducted. A low-risk group was defined as: (1) BMI <25; (2) no current smoking; (3) drinking one-half or more glasses of alcoholic beverage per day; (4) diet high in cereal fibre and polyunsaturated fat and low in *trans* fat and glycaemic load; and (5) at least one half hour of moderate-to-vigorous activity per day. Only 3.4% of the nurses were in this low-risk group. Each of the low-risk factors were significantly related to diabetes. The relative risk of developing diabetes decreased as the number of protective factors increased. Women with three factors in the low-risk group (diet, BMI and exercise as above) had RR = 0.12 (95% CI 0.08 to 0.16) and a population attributable risk (PAR%) of 87%. This suggests that 87% of incident diabetes cases could be prevented if all women had these three factors present, other things being equal. The PAR% rose to 91% among women with all five factors present (RR = 0.09, 95% CI 0.05 to 0.17). This analysis of a large observational cohort suggests that findings from RCTs such as the DPS and DPP are likely to apply to a less selected group of women, at least, and that the average reductions in incidence seen in the RCTs could be even greater among persons adopting from three to five lifestyle changes. Persons who met all five of the goals in the DPS had an estimated 3 year diabetes incidence rate of 1 vs 35% in persons not meeting any of the goals. In the DPP, meeting the three goals of the lifestyle programme resulted in HR = 0.11 (95% CI 0.05 to 0.24, $p < 0.0001$)[82] and an 89% reduction in risk.

2 Physical activity

Physical activity is one of the primary determinants of energy balance and obesity. It is also one of the factors that has undergone recent decreases in developing countries around the world. The potential for the prevention of diabetes by increases in physical activity has been attractive for many years.[1] Physiological studies have shown that physical activity increases insulin sensitivity and reduces insulin secretion, which may be the primary conduit through which most behavioural risk factors travel to decrease diabetes risk.

Physical activity has been shown to reduce obesity and central fat distribution in short-term clinical studies.[120] As physical activity patterns in free living populations are complex, so is the assessment of physical activity in epidemiological studies.[120] Many have used questionnaires to assess leisure time physical activity, which in many urban populations is the primary determinant of differences in energy expenditure between individuals. This is not the case in rural populations, where a more comprehensive evaluation of work activities is required.[121,122] More exact measures are needed to account for all components of total energy expenditure (including resting metabolic rate and the thermic effect of food), but these are not feasible in large populations over extended periods of time. Even the gold standard method of doubly labelled water to estimate energy expenditure can only be utilized on limited numbers of participants. A number of review papers[120,122–126] and an NIH consensus statement[127] have summarized earlier work on physical activity. The previous edition of this chapter reviewed the prospective observational evidence exploring diabetes and related endpoints, which have not been updated here, but are reviewed elsewhere.[4,40,128,129] This prospective observational evidence is consistent in showing that higher levels of physical activity are associated with lower risk of type 2 diabetes. The protective effect appears to exist in people across the age span[130] and is similar in men and women.[128]

RCTs including physical activity

There is only one RCT that used increased physical activity alone as one of the interventions to prevent diabetes.[62] Combination interventions of dietary change and increased activity have become the standard approach since caloric restriction more rapidly induces weight loss and weight loss can be more easily maintained with increases in activity.[81] There are also two RCTs that have analysed patterns of activity within the trial and have diabetes incidence as the outcome.[73,82] The Da Qing study[62] found that the physical activity intervention alone reduced diabetes risk by 47% (Table 5.4) which was similar in lean and obese participants. Participants in the exercise-only group increased their activity level from baseline to 6 years by 0.6 units. However, the measure of activity in this study is difficult to compare with other metrics. The reports do not provide sufficient details of the computation of activity score to allow understanding of the amount or intensity of activity achieved.

The DPS study analyses provide much more information on the level and type of activity undertaken.[75] Laaksonen *et al.*[75] explored changes in types of activities reported by the lifestyle intervention group compared with control participants. During the 4.1 years of follow-up, moderate to vigorous leisure time physical activity (LTPA) increased by a mean of 0.8 h per week in the lifestyle group, with little change overall in the control group. The clearest difference was in structured strenuous activities, since these were offered uniquely to the intervention participants. They then combined the groups for an epidemiological analysis and explored the influence of multiple types of LTPA (structured, strenuous; moderate to vigorous; walking; commuting). Perhaps most important from a public health standpoint, even low-intensity LTPA ($\leq$3.5 METS) conferred benefits on diabetes risk. Persons in the highest tertile of increase in low intensity LTPA ($\sim +3$ h per week) had approximately 60% lower diabetes risk (HR = 0.36, 95% CI 0.19 to 0.67) than the lowest tertile (~ -3 h per week), which was not influenced by multiple baseline risk factors or by the addition of changes in weight over time. Since persons in the lowest tertile actually decreased their LPTA, it may be more correct to compare the upper (improvement) and lower (worsening) tertiles to the middle tertile (no change). This calculation (not reported by the authors) suggests that reducing low-intensity LTPA increases diabetes risk by about 60% compared with persons with stable patterns (HR = 1.59) and improving activity reduces risk by about 40% (HR = 0.57). Regardless of how results are presented, they suggest important, independent effects of physical activity to reduce diabetes incidence, at least in high-risk persons with IGT.

In the DPP there was also no independent randomization of lifestyle components. An analysis of the lifestyle sub-group showed that over the first year of the intervention, participants increased their self-reported activity levels by approximately 7–8 MET-hours per week, which was largely sustained for the duration of the trial.[82] While weight loss was the dominant factor resulting in lower diabetes incidence, there was a 46% reduction in risk (HR = 0.54, 95% CI 0.34 to 0.84, $p = 0.007$; adjusted for baseline variables only) for participants who met the physical activity goal (i.e. 150 min of moderate-intensity activity per week). Additional adjustment for weight change over follow-up (average of -2.6 kg) did not change the impact of physical activity (HR = 0.56, 0.36–0.89, $p = 0.012$). The -2.6 kg of weight loss in this sub-group was also significantly ($p < 0.0001$) and independently related to lower diabetes risk, suggesting that even small amounts of weight loss decrease risk. The DPP investigators have also shown that participants reported somewhat higher levels of baseline activity than a nationally representative sample of the United States using the NHANESIII population and methods.[131] This probably indicates that participants were more motivated and already somewhat more active than non-participants and has important implications for translation of findings to even more sedentary and potentially less motivated populations.

These results from *post hoc* analyses of the two largest RCTs yet conducted are consistent with the large body of observational evidence (e.g.[128]) of the importance of increased physical activity of multiple types in reducing diabetes incidence. Although there is ongoing debate about the amount of activity needed to produce improvements in insulin sensitivity[132] and weight loss[128] or prevention of weight gain,[40] it appears that relatively low levels of increased activity (30 min of brisk walking per day for 5–7 days per week), coupled with small amounts of weight loss (2–3 kg), can significantly lower diabetes risk.

3 Diet composition

Composition of the diet has been explored as an aetiological factor in the risk of type 2 diabetes for many years. Because of major recent changes in 'western' diets (including increases in simple refined carbohydrates and in dietary fat from animal sources, with decreased complex carbohydrate and fibre intake), dietary constituents have received significant attention. An early hypothesis was that refined and simple sugars played a major role. This early debate has been summarized by Mann and Houston,[133] who noted that a number of studies both supported and did not support the hypothesis. It is important to note that the majority of those early studies were methodologically weak and few were prospective in design. West also provided a review of nutrition in the aetiology and prevention of type 2 diabetes with published evidence from before 1975.[134,135] His conclusion was that total calories and obesity seem to be of primary importance and that there was little support for specific diet constituents, including dietary fat, simple carbohydrates and fibre.[136]

Dietary fat intake has been explored in numerous studies, since it might play a role in the development of obesity, alterations of insulin action or in diabetes incidence itself. Willett reviewed the evidence relating dietary fat to the development of obesity and concluded that 'Diets high in fat do not appear to be the primary cause of the high prevalence of excess body fat in our society and reductions in fat will not be a solution'.[137] Hannah and Howard came to a similar conclusion about glucose tolerance and the role of dietary fats,[138] although Virtanen and Aro's review did suggest a role for high dietary fats based on their synthesis of the literature.[139] A more recent review by Hu *et al.* updates this literature and notes that quality of dietary fat and carbohydrate, rather than just quantity, may be the important variables.[140]

Hence there are conflicting opinions about the role of dietary fats in the aetiology of type 2 diabetes. Based on a synthesis of animal and human studies, it appears likely that high saturated fat diets do play a role in increasing insulin resistance,[141] although the type of fat and fatty acid composition of the diet play a major role.[142] The following section reviews the current evidence on dietary constituents in diabetes prevention.

RCTs including diet

There have been no RCTs of specific dietary constituents on the incidence of diabetes in humans. Such trials would require the identification and follow-up of large numbers of high-risk people, with modification of carbohydrate, fat type or content or protein with maintenance of energy balance, to be independent of weight change. Consequently, the only RCTs are those that have explored effects of dietary composition on defined changes in intermediate endpoints such as insulin levels or action, glucose levels and lipids over short time periods (e.g.[143–145]). While providing important physiological insight, such studies beg the question of the influence of long-term dietary intake in free-living populations. Some of the strongest evidence that changes in dietary intake (coupled with increased activity and weight loss) can reduce diabetes incidence come from *post hoc* analyses from both the DPS[146] and DPP[147] RCTs. Although not able to isolate compositional changes directly due to lack of specific randomization, these analyses have explored the variations in dietary intake among persons in these trials.

In the DPS, diet was measured annually using a 3 day food diary. Lindstrom *et al.*[146] found that weight loss was greater in those with higher fibre intake and less fat and energy density, adjusted for sex and baseline physical activity, very low calorie diet use, weight and nutrient intake. Reduced diabetes risk at 4.1 years was associated with higher fibre and lower fat intake, adjusted for intervention group, age, sex and baseline weight, 2 h glucose, activity and nutrient intake. Adjustment for weight change during the trial did not change the findings importantly. In the highest quartile of fibre intake (>15.55 g per 100 kcal), diabetes risk was reduced (adjusted HR = 0.38, 95% CI 0.19 to 0.77) compared with the lowest quartile. In the highest quartile of fat intake, risk was increased (HR = 2.14, 95% CI 1.16 to 3.92). Due to multicollinearity, neither fibre nor fat was significant in the same model. However, when four sub-groups were formed by median splits in fibre and fat intake, the group with high fibre/low fat intake lost the most

weight (−3.1 kg) and had the lowest diabetes risk [HR = 0.53 vs low fibre/high fat (p = 0.024) and HR 0.37 vs high fibre/high fat (p = 0.003)]. Although it is possible that some reporting bias may exist, the association of these patterns with both weight loss and reduced diabetes risk in this clinical trial is consistent with the body of observational evidence.

DPP authors have also reported dietary changes that occurred over the first year of the trial.[147] Measurements were not made at study end due to the premature termination of the trial. Dietary improvements at 1 year in the lifestyle group were seen for each of the seven nutrient groups (including lower percent of calories from fat, energy and higher fibre), for six of the eight targeted food groups (including increases in fruits, vegetables and poultry and decreases in red meat, diary and sweets) and for the two targeted fat-related behaviours (increased use of low-fat foods and less fat/oil in cooking). There were no changes between the metformin and placebo groups over the first year. There was a stepwise reduction in diabetes risk with meeting more of the goals of the trial, including the dietary fat goal (≤25% of calories from fat).[82]

Prospective epidemiological studies

Much of the detailed evidence for dietary intake has come from prospective epidemiological studies of populations. Earlier evidence was summarized in the previous edition of this chapter[14] and has recently been updated in published reviews.[41,148] Over many years, studies have shown no important association of simple dietary carbohydrates with diabetes risk. Numerous studies have explored the ability of foods to raise blood glucose [the 'glycaemic index' (GI) of foods] and have explored the total glycaemic load of the diet as a risk factor.[149] Glycaemia improves with lower GI foods and there appears to be a higher risk of diabetes with a higher glycaemic load diet, especially in combination with lower dietary fibre intake. Most epidemiological studies are consistent in showing lower diabetes risk with higher cereal fibre intake, together with higher fruit and vegetable intake.[41,148] Several prospective studies have found higher DM risk with higher intake of total and saturated (animal) fat.[150–154] or with lower levels of polyunsaturated fats.[155–157] Intake of *trans*-fats has been shown in some studies to also increase risk.[155] The evidence from observational studies indicates that changing to a diet in which vegetable fat is more often consumed is likely to be beneficial for the prevention of type 2 diabetes. An exception to this may be fish consumption, since in some studies it is associated with a lower risk of diabetes.[152] Consistent with this, recent observational results suggest that 'prudent' diets, that is, those with lower saturated fats, higher fruit, vegetable and fibre intake and less red meat and processed meats, reduce the risk of diabetes by 30–40%,[158–160] and if combined with lower weight and increased activity, may reduce it substantially more.[119] Although there are no long-term clinical trials of diet composition and incident diabetes, the *post hoc* analyses of the DPS and DPP and the body of observational data briefly summarized here strongly suggest that a diet aimed at weight maintenance (if not overweight) or weight reduction, including lower total and saturated fat, more fruits, vegetables and fibre in a balanced fashion as currently recommended,[161–164] will reduce diabetes risk.

4 Weight change and diabetes

Several types of studies have explored weight change and subsequent diabetes. These include RCTs aimed at weight loss or obesity prevention with diabetes as the outcome, reviewed above. It also includes observational studies that explore the influence of weight change prospectively over much longer periods of time and in more representative populations than has been achieved in RCTs to date. In addition, animal studies allow unique observations not possible in humans.

Animal studies

Animal studies are mentioned briefly since two models of type 2 diabetes are relevant to the human condition and have allowed caloric restriction over much of the lifespan, which is difficult to achieve in humans. In the first model, using Israeli sand rats (*Psammomys obesus*), Walder *et al.* showed that restriction of food intake to 75% of *ad libitum* levels post-weaning led to complete restriction of the hyperglycaemia that develops in this animal in laboratory settings.[165]

The second model is the primate rhesus monkey (*Macaca mulatta*). Hansen and colleagues, in a series of elegant prospective studies, studied the development of obesity, hyperinsulinaemia, β-cell responsiveness and other parameters in male adult monkeys who are prone to the development of obesity and diabetes with characteristics similar to type 2 in humans.[166,167] They identified sequential stages of development of diabetes which began with obesity, followed by elevations in fasting insulin and decreases in insulin-stimulated glucose disposal. Acute insulin secretion then rose to compensate and later declined as hyperglycaemia developed.[168] Some monkeys went on to develop diabetic retinopathy with characteristics very similar to those in humans.[169]

These studies were followed by a prevention trial in which eight male monkeys were fed three meals per day (13% fat, 17% protein, 70% carbohydrate as monkey chow) and calories were titrated to maintain stable young adult body weight (diet restricted, DR).[167] Age-matched control monkeys ($N = 19$) were fed *ad libitum* (AL) on the same diet and both groups were followed for 5–9 years. Four (21%) of the AL-fed monkeys developed diabetes by human OGTT criteria and six (32%) had IGT, compared with no glucose intolerance among weight-stable monkeys. Fasting and glucose-stimulated insulin levels were also significantly lower among weight-stable monkeys and β-cell responsiveness was maintained. Body fat also remained at young adult levels. A 10 year follow-up of these monkeys showed a significant and sustained long-term reduction in energy expenditure from the caloric restriction.[170] Later follow-up has recently been reported.[171,172] The AL fed monkeys had a 2.6-fold increased risk of death compared with the DR monkeys and hyperinsulinaemia led to a 3.7-fold increased risk of death ($p < 0.05$). This prevention study in monkeys strongly suggests that preventing the development of obesity can delay, if not completely prevent, type 2 diabetes over the lifespan.

Human studies

Most of the over 600 human weight loss studies prior to 1998 have been critically reviewed using standardized criteria[173] and recently compiled for older adults.[174] Estimates of cost-effectiveness have also recently been published.[110] Most of the large number of studies were of relatively short duration and were not large enough to test directly whether a categorical endpoint such as diabetes was avoided, but rather focused on weight change and often glucose changes. There is substantial evidence from these studies that weight loss produced by lifestyle modifications reduced blood glucose levels in overweight and obese people without type 2 diabetes.

In larger observational prospective studies, weight loss is followed by an improvement of glucose tolerance and a reduced risk of type 2 diabetes in both women and men across the age span, in several race/ethnic groups and in several countries.[175–186] Weight gain from age 20 years to middle age has also been reported to increase the risk of the insulin resistance syndrome,[187] although no data on weight loss were presented. In many of these studies, it is often not possible to determine whether the weight loss was intentional and this may dilute the effects seen, since weight loss may be a sign of incipient disease or the effect of developing diabetes itself. For example, in the British Regional Heart Study,[180] exclusion of people developing diabetes within the first 4 years after baseline increased the risk of weight gain for diabetes in the subsequent 8 years.

A recent longitudinal study by Black *et al.* followed Danish draft board examinees from age 20 years to a mean age of 51 years.[186] At the final examination, participants were tested with an OGTT which was compared with their baseline weight and weight trajectory. Of the almost 600 men available at the final examination, persons who gained the greatest weight from age 20 years had the highest risk of IGT, even higher than men who had been obese at age 20 years but were weight stable. Importantly, persons who were overweight at age 20 years and lost weight were estimated to have substantially lower risk of IGT and elevated fasting glucose. For example, among men with a BMI of $30\,\mathrm{kg\,m^{-2}}$ at age 20 years, the estimated probability of having IGT at age 52 years was 0.2 among weight-stable men, but was reduced to 0.08 for men with a BMI of 25 and to 0.03 if the later BMI was 20. Conversely, men who gained weight from age 20 years (BMI from 20 to 30 by age 51 years) had a probability of IGT of 0.37 at the examination. Although losses to follow-up and failure to test participants on intermediate visits temper the conclusions, these results add to the understanding of the timing of weight change throughout early adult life and suggest that weight loss during adulthood is protective and that early adult weight gain substantially increases risk for glucose intolerance.

There is now substantial RCT and observational study evidence that intentional weight loss improves glycaemic outcomes and reduces the risk of IGT and diabetes.

5 Pharmacological studies

Pharmacological interventions to prevent diabetes or its complications early in the natural history have been published since the 1960s.[188] The rationale for drug intervention includes the following: (1) the drug may reverse one or more specific pathophysiological defects; (2) changes in lifestyle for otherwise healthy people are difficult to make even though they have demonstrated efficacy; (3) some people are unable to change lifestyle due to disability or other disease; and (4) it may be easier to take a drug over longer periods than it is to make significant behavioural changes. Although each of these issues has some validity, it is also important to show, through well-designed clinical trials, that pharmacological interventions are efficacious before they enter widespread use, especially if they are to be given to otherwise healthy, non-diseased persons as preventive agents.[189]

Reviews of the use of such agents have been published.[2,188,190–196] Early trials were often aimed at individuals with 'chemical diabetes', considered being 'early diabetes' by older criteria. Such studies often included a majority of people with what would now be considered IGT and thus are relevant to a review of primary prevention. Agents available in the 1960s included first-generation sulfonylureas and biguanides. Similarly to lifestyle studies, criteria for outcomes varied and were a mixture of glucose tolerance, fasting glucose and other endpoints. These early studies were summarized in detail in the previous edition of this chapter.[14] Table 5.5 summarizes the more recent RCTs using pharmacological agents. None of the licensed agents is currently licensed for prevention of diabetes in people who do not have diabetes when receiving therapy.

Sulfonylureas

Studies using the first-generation sulfonylurea tolbutamide began in the 1960s[197–207] and were published through the 1980s,[208] with newer generation sulfonylureas being reported through the late 1990s.[53,65,209,210] Details of these trials were reported in detail previously,[14] but were essentially negative. Many of them suffered from a number of methodological weaknesses, including small samples size, limited follow-up, poor compliance, inadequate or inappropriate analysis, lack of randomization or lack of concealment of method of allocation. However, there are four studies which randomized reasonably large number of individuals who were followed over several years and used ITT analysis or reported data that could be calculated in this way *post hoc*. The study by Feldman and colleagues[187,188,200,201] reported a low but not significant risk [RR = 0.16 (95% CI 0.02 to 1.54)]. The other widely quoted study by Sartor *et al.*[208] also had non-significant risk reductions when analysed by ITT (RR = 0.82, 95% CI 0.27 to 2.50, vs placebo, RR = 0.73, 95% CI 0.25 to 2.14, vs diet, *post hoc* analyses). The 10 year Bedford study[205] found no decrease in risk (OR = 1.04), consistent with previous studies. The 6 year follow-up of the Fasting Hyperglycemia Study.[53,65,209,210] did not support an effect on diabetes incidence. The remaining studies were essentially negative or uninformative. Thus, the current evidence does not support a consistent role for sulfonylurea derivatives in the prevention of type 2 diabetes.

Biguanides (metformin)

Trials using first-generation biguanides (dimethylbiguanide,[211] phenformin[48,49,212]) were discussed in the previous edition, but since they are no longer on the market, they have been omitted here. This section reviews trials using metformin alone or in combination.

Table 5.5 Pharmacological interventions (including mixed interventions) – randomized controlled trials[a]

Study, reference	Population	Intervention	Results	Comments
Biguanides (metformin) BIGPRO 1[213,214]	France; 457 participants with high waist:hip ratio, aged 35–60 years; follow-up 1 year. Outcome: OGTT	**Metformin** ($N = 164$) 850 mg bid **Placebo** ($N = 160$) Both groups given diet and exercise	*Metformin*: 2.0 kg weight loss; less rise in F glucose and insulin; lower LDL cholesterol; tPA antigen, von Willebrand factor; no change in 2 h glucose or insulin, BP, triglycerides, HDL cholesterol. No diabetes developed. Fasting glucose improved only in those with IGT at baseline. *Placebo*: 5 persons developed diabetes. Increase in fasting glucose.	28–30% dropout at 1 year. 21.5% had abnormal OGTT at entry. Assuming all persons with diabetes were detected, absence of cases in metformin group and 5 in placebo group give exact $p = 0.06$. Double blind, randomization not said to be masked
BIGPRO 1.2[216,217]	France; 168 men with high waist-hip ratio, mild hypertension, fasting glucose <7.8 mmol l^{-1}; follow-up 3 months. Outcome: fasting glucose, lipids	**Metformin** ($N = 83$) 850 mg bid **Placebo** ($N = 83$) No lifestyle changes	*Metformin*: -0.5 kg weight loss (ns), decreases in fasting glucose, insulin, LDL cholesterol, Apo B, tPA as in BIGPRO 1. No change in BP or triglycerides. No diabetes developed in either group	Double blind, randomization not said to be masked. Short follow-up. Dropouts only 3%.
Indian Diabetes Prevention Program (IDPP)[87]	India; 531 men and women; IGT × 2; mean age = 46 years; BMI = 25.8; follow-up 3 years. Outcome: diabetes by WHO criteria	**Lifestyle modification** (LSM) ($N = 133$), diet, activity; monthly telephone; 6 monthly in person **Metformin** (MET) ($N = 133$); 250 mg bid **LSM + MET** ($N = 129$) **Control** ($N = 136$) Limited reinforcement	*LSM* cumulative 3 year incidence = 39.3% [annual incidence rate (AIR) = 16.6/100 PY; ARR = 10.0/100 PY] vs **Control** = 55.0% (AIR = 26.6/100 PY) vs *MET* = 40.5% (AIR = 17.3/100 PY; ARR = 9.3/100 PY) vs *LSM + MET* 39.5% (AIR = 16.8/100 PY; ARR = 9.9/100 PY)	Weight increase in controls (~0.8 kg) with about 0.3–0.4 kg lower weight in intervention groups (similar) and significant weight gain in LSM groups at 24 months. No blinding or placebo used; 36 month follow-up for 213 persons, 30 month close-out for 132. 5.8% lost to follow-up, slightly higher in LSM groups. Consecutive allocation
Thiazolidinediones Multicentre study of troglitazone in IGT[232]	USA; 51 people aged 24–77 years (mean 47 years) with IGT; follow-up 3 months. Outcome: OGTT	**Troglitazone** ($N = 25$) 400 mg qd **Placebo** ($N = 26$)	*Troglitazone*: RR = 0.38 (95% CI 0.15 to 1.00) to remain IGT vs placebo; lower glucose and insulin AUC, triglyceride levels; no change in fasting glucose, insulin or C-peptide, LDL or HDL-C, BP, weight, HbA$_{1c}$ in either group	80% of troglitazone participants returned to normal OGTT vs 48% of placebo group. Dropouts 20%, similar in each group. Said to be lower, but text disagrees with tables. Allocation was masked, double blind
TRIPOD;[235,236] PIPOD[237]	Los Angeles, CA; 235 Latina women, history of GDM; follow-up 30 months. Outcome: diabetes	**Troglitazone** 400 mg day^{-1} ($N = 114$) **Placebo** ($N = 121$) **Pioglitazone** 45 mg day^{-1} open label to all women non-diabetic at end of TRIPOD ($N = 89$)	*Placebo*: 12.3/100 PY *Troglitazone*: 5.4/100 PY RR = 0.44, ARR = 6.9/100 PY, $p = 0.001$, NNT = 14.5 *Pioglitazone*: 5.2/100 PY No control	Largest reduction in diabetes incidence seen in women with most improvement in insulin sensitivity in sub-set analysis. Effects appear to continue for up to 8 months off drug. Dropouts = 11.3%, balanced between groups

(continued)

Table 5.5 *(Continued)*

Study, reference	Population	Intervention	Results	Comments
TZD in private practice[239]	Denver, CO; 172 men and women, mean age 57 years; follow-up 36 months. Outcome: diabetes by fasting glucose and HbA$_{1c}$	**Troglitazone** 400 mg day^{-1} for 10 months, switched to **pioglitazone** 30 mg day^{-1} or **rosiglitazone** 4 mg day^{-1} (or more) (N = 101) **Control** (N = 71)	*TZD:* 2.97% (3 year cumulative incidence); 1.4/100 PY. *Control:* 26.8% (3 year); 9.4/100 PY. RR = 0.11 (95% CI 0.021 to 0.377); ARR = 23.8% (3 years), 8.0/100 PY. NNT (3 years) = 4.2	Selected for therapy based on which MD seen in practice; no masking; no dropouts; diabetes outcome by fasting or HbA$_{1c}$: criteria not specified. Fasting C-peptide, HbA$_{1c}$ significantly lower in treated participants. Weight gain of 5.4 lb (2.4 kg) in pioglitazone group, 0.7 lb (0.32 kg) in rosiglitazone group and 4.5 lb (2.0 kg) in control
Diabetes Prevention Program (DPP)[240]	USA; men and women; IGT with elevated FPG; 45% non-Caucasian; mean age 51 years, BMI = 34; follow-up 0.9 years. Outcome: diabetes by ADA criteria	**Troglitazone** 400 mg day^{-1} (N = 585) **Placebo** (N = 582)	*Troglitazone:* 3.0/100 PY. *Placebo:* 12.0/100 PY. HR = 0.25, p < 0.001, ARR = 9.0/100 PY, NNT = 11 over 0.9 years	Includes participants randomized prior to June 1998; same period as those on troglitazone. Rates not different between troglitazone and placebo after 1 year off drug. 4 Native American centres excluded
DREAM[242,243]	21 countries, 191 centres; 5269 men and women; mean age 55 years; BMI = 30; IGT or IFG at baseline; follow-up 3 years. Outcome: OGTT diabetes or death	**Rosiglitazone** 8 mg day^{-1} (N = 2635) vs **Placebo** (N = 2634)	*Rosiglitazone:* 11.6% *Placebo:* 26.0% 3 year cumulative incidence; HR = 0.40, 95% CI 0.35 to 0.46, p < 0.0001; ARR = 15.6%; NNT = 6.4 over 3 years	OGTT diabetes had similar HR = 0.38; 6% loss-to-follow-up for glucose outcomes; 80% on active drug at 3 years; elevated CVD outcomes (NS) except CHF (p = 0.01)
α-Glucosidase inhibitors				
STOP-NIDDM[246,247]	Canada, Europe, 1368 men and women, mean age 54.5 years, WHO IGT × 1; follow-up 3.3 years. Outcome: diabetes	**Acarbose** 100 mg tid (N = 682) or **Placebo** (N = 686)	*Acarbose:* 10.1/100 PY; HR = 0.75 (95% CI 0.63 to 0.90; ARR = 9.1/100 PY) vs *Placebo:* 12.1/100 PY. Higher reversion to normal glucose tolerance (p < 0.0001). HR = 0.64 (95% CI 0.498 to 0.813) using 2 positive OGTT as endpoint	NNT = 11 persons with IGT to prevent 1 case; dropouts 23.9%, higher in acarbose (221) than placebo (130)
Anti-obesity agents				
XENDOS[263]	Sweden; 3277 non-diabetic men and women; 694 with IGT; mean age 43 years; BMI x = 37; follow-up 4 years. Outcome: diabetes	**Orlistat** (N = 1290 NGT; 350 IGT) **Placebo** (N = 1292 NGT; 344 IGT)	*Orlistat:* 4 year cumulative incidence 6.2%; HR = 0.63 (95% CI 0.46 to 0.86); ARR = 2.8/100 vs *Placebo:* 9.0%, p = 0.0032; among IGT only, HR = 0.55, p = 0.0024	NNT = 36 (all patients), 10 (IGT over 4 years.); 48% dropouts in orlistat group; 66% in placebo group. No significant effect in NGT participants; no difference in progression from NGT to IGT
Antihypertensive agents				
EWPHE[283]	Europe; men and women 60 + years; follow-up 3 years. Outcome: clinical diabetes (ICD8)	**Triamterene hydrochlorothiazide + methyldopa** (N = 416) vs **Placebo** (N = 424)	*Active:* 22.4/1000 PY vs *Placebo:* 16.2/1000 PY; RR = 1.4 (95% CI 0.8 to 2.6)	Methyldopa (up to 2 g, daily) was added in 35% of patients; on-treatment analysis; excess of prescriptions for hypoglycaemic drugs and abnormal OGTT, neither significant

Table 5.5 (Continued)

Study, reference	Population	Intervention	Results	Comments
SHEP[284]	USA; 3680 men and women aged 60+ years without diabetes at entry; follow-up: 4.5 years. Outcome: WHO diabetes or medication	**Chlorthalidone + atenolol** (N = 1870 without DM) vs **Placebo** (N = 1810 without DM)	*Active*: 8.6% at 3 years vs *Placebo*: 7.5%; RR = 1.15 (95% CI 0.91 to 1.45, p = 0.25)	Fasting glucose levels slightly higher at 3 years among persons without diabetes (p = 0.005)
HOPE;[286] HOPE-TOO[287]	Canada, North and South America and Europe; 9297 people aged 55 years and older (mean 66 years); follow-up 4.5 years; extended in 174 centres for 7.2 years, N = 4528. Outcome: self-reported diabetes	**Ramipril** (N = 2837 non-diabetic); 10 mg qd **Placebo**: (N = 2883 non-diabetic) in 2 × 2 factorial with vitamin E	*Ramipril*: RR = 0.66 (95% CI 0.51 to 0.85) vs *Placebo* for incidence of new diabetes. No interaction with vitamin E noted. *HOPE-TOO*: *Ramipril*: 7.3% vs *Placebo*: 10.3%; RR = 0.69 (95% CI 0.56 to 0.85, p = 0.0006) over entire trial period. ARR = 3%; NNT = 33 over 7 years	Ramipril discontinued in 29%, placebo in 27%; 18% of placebo group used any ACE inhibitor. Dropouts not stated. Side-effects. primarily cough that differed from placebo. HOPE-TOO had further reduction in diabetes incidence among those not diabetic at extension start. Open-label extension had similar rates of ACE use in both groups
SOLVD[288]	Montreal Center; 291 non-diabetic at baseline with LV dysfunction; follow-up 2.9 years. Outcome: FPG × 2 >126 mg dl^{-1} chart review	**Enalapril** (5–20 mg day^{-1}) (N = 153) vs **Placebo** (N = 138)	*Enalapril*: 5.9%, multivariate HR = 0.22, (95% CI 0.10 to 0.46, p < 0.0001) vs *Placebo*: 22.4%, ARR = 16.5%; NNT = 6 over 2.9 years	Not ITT; chart review for FPG; participants randomized to treatments comparable at baseline, although persons with DM removed; strongest effect in person with IFG. Other medication use similar in groups
PEACE[293]	187 sites, USA, Canada, Italy; 6896 men and women; mean age 64 years; follow-up 4.8 years; prior CHD and no CHF; no known DM. Outcome: clinical diabetes	**Trandolapril** (4 mg day^{-1}) (N = 3424) or **Placebo** (N = 3472) in addition to usual CVD therapy	*Trandolapril*: 9.8%, HR = 0.83 (95% CI 0.72 to 0.96, p = 0.01) vs *Placebo*: 11.5%, ARR = 1.7%, NNT = 59 over ~5years	Secondary analysis, not pre-specified; 70% on lipid lowering medication; 60% on beta-blockers; 35% on CCB; no definition of diabetes; no systematic DM testing; overall trial negative for mortality or CHD outcomes
CHARM[290,291]	26 countries; 5486 non-diabetic men and women aged 18+ years with LV failure; mean age = 66 years; follow-up, median 3.1 years. Outcome: clinical diabetes	**Candesartan** (4–32 mg qd) (N = 2715) vs **Placebo** (N = 2721)	*Candesartan*: 6% vs *Placebo*: 7.4%, HR = 0·78 (95% CI 0·64 to 0·96, p = 0·020); ARR = 1.4% (95% CI −2.8 to −0.05); NNT = 71 (95% CI 36 to 1613) over 3 years Composite of new DM or death: HR = 0.86 (95% CI 0.78 to 0.95, p = 0.004)	Planned sub-group analysis; various clinical criteria for DM used; dropout <1%
SCOPE[292]	15 countries; 4943 patients aged 70–89 years, with mildly elevated BP and decreased cognition; follow-up, mean 3.7 years.	**Candesartan** (8–16 mg qd) (N = 2477) vs **Placebo** (N = 2466)	*Candesartan*: 4.3% vs *Placebo*: 5.3%, RR = 0.81 (95% CI 0.63 to 1.04, p = 0.09); ARR = 1.0% (95% CI −2.2 to +0.2%); NNT = 100 over 3.7 years	84% of placebo group treated with multiple anti-hypertensive agents including diuretics and beta-blockers; DM criteria not specified; dropouts <1%

(continued)

Table 5.5 *(Continued)*

Study, reference	Population	Intervention	Results	Comments
	Outcome: clinical diabetes			
DREAM[242,289]	21 countries, 191 centres; 5269 men and women; mean age 55 years; BMI = 30; IGT or IFG at baseline; follow-up 3 years. Outcome: OGTT diabetes or mortality	**Ramipril** (15 mg qd) ($N = 2623$) vs **Placebo** ($N = 2646$)	*Ramipril*: 18.1% vs *Placebo*: 19.5%; HR = 0.91 (95% CI 0.81 to 1.03; $p = 0.15$), ARR = 1.4%; NNT = 71 over 3 years. Regression to NGT higher with Ramipril [HR = 1.16 (95% CI 1.07 to 1.27. $p = 0.001$]	OGTT diabetes similar HR = 0.91; 6% loss-to-follow-up for glucose outcomes; 80% on active drug at 3 years; no effect on mortality or CVD events
Lipid-lowering agents				
WOSCOPS[295]	Scotland, primary care practices; 5974 men ($x = 55$ years), non-diabetic, elevated cholesterol; follow-up 4.9 years. Outcome: diabetes by modified ADA criteria $\times$ 2	**Pravastatin** (40 mg qd) vs **Placebo**	*Pravastatin*: multivariate HR = 0.7 (95% CI 0.50 to 0.99, $p = 0.042$) vs *Placebo*	Sub-group *post hoc* analysis; absolute incidence rates not given by group; side-effects minimal. Approximately 30% withdrawals at 5 years in primary study
LIPID[296]	Australia, New Zealand; 7937 patients without diabetes mellitus, age 31–75 years, with prior MI or unstable angina; follow-up 6 years. Outcome: diabetes by FPG >7 mmol l^{-1} or medication	**Pravastatin** (40 mg qd) ($N = 3970$) vs **Placebo** ($N = 3967$)	*Pravastatin*: 4.5%, RR = 0.89 (95% CI 0.70 to 1.13, $p = 0.32$) vs *Placebo*: 4.0%, ARR = 0.5% (95% CI −1.5 to +0.5%) IFG: pravastatin 9.7%, placebo 9.2%	Limited results for diabetes presented; dropouts not specified for DM analyses
Heart Protection Study[477]	UK general practice;14 573 men and women without diabetes; mean age = 64.7 years; follow-up 5 years. Outcome: clinical diabetes	**Simvistatin** (40 mg qd) vs **Placebo**	*Simvistatin*: 4.6% vs *Placebo*: 4.0%, RR = 1.14 (95% CI 0.98 to 1.33; $p = 0.1$)	Development of diabetes pre-specified. No details about number randomized among those without diabetes; no information on dropouts
ASCOT-LLA[297]	UK, Scandinavia primary care; 7773 men and women; mean age 63 years, with high BP and 3 RF for CHD, cholesterol <6.5 mmol l^{-1}, no diabetes; follow-up 3.3 years. Outcome: clinical diabetes	**Atorvastatin** (10 mg) plus antihypertensives ($N = 3910$) vs **Placebo** plus antihypertensives ($N = 3863$)	*Atorvastatin*: 9.4/1000 PY vs *Placebo*: 8·2/1000 PY, HR = 1·15 (95% CI 0·91 to 1·44, $p = 0·25$)	No details on confounding treatment or dropouts among non-diabetic participants. Overall, dropouts only 1.2%
BIP[298]	303 men and women with CHD and IFG; mean age = 61 years; follow-up 6.2 years.	**Bezafibrate** (400 mg) ($N = 156$) vs **Placebo** ($N = 147$)	*Bezafibrate*: 42.3% cumulative incidence vs	Pan-PPAR activator; *post hoc* sub-group analysis; no differences in diuretics

Table 5.5 (Continued)

Study, reference	Population	Intervention	Results	Comments
	Outcome: diabetes by FPG >126 mg dl^{-1}		*Placebo*: 54.4%; HR = 0.70 (95% CI 0.49 to 0.99, $p = 0.04$, adjusted for multiple confounders); RRR = 30% (95% CI 0.1 to 51%); ARR = 12.1%, NNT = 8 over 6 years.	between groups. No data on losses to follow-up
BIP[299]	339 men and women with CHD and BMI >30; non-diabetic, 85% with NGT; mean age = 61 years; follow-up 6.2 years. Outcome: diabetes by FPG >126 mg dl^{-1}	**Bezafibrate** (400 mg) (*N* = 178) vs **Placebo** (*N* = 161)	*Bezafibrate*: 27.1% cumulative incidence vs *Placebo*: 37.0%; HR = 0.59 (95% CI 0.39 to 0.91, $p = 0.01$, adjusted for multiple confounders); RRR = 41%; ARR = 9.9%, NNT = 10 over 6 years	*Post hoc* analysis of same study as above, but looking at obese participants largely with NGT
Hormone replacement therapy				
HERS[301]	20 US centres; 2029 women with CHD, without diabetes; mean age = 67 years; follow-up 4.1 years. Outcome: clinical diabetes or FPG > 126 mg dl^{-1}	**Estrogen** (0.625 mg) + **progesterone** (2.5 mg) (*N* = 999) vs **Placebo** (*N* = 1030)	*E + P*: 6.2% over 4 years vs *Placebo*: 9.5%, HR = 0.65 (95% CI 0.48 to 0.89, $p = 0.006$); RRR = 35%; ARR = 3.3% over 4 years; NNT = 30	Multiple adjustments for BMI, drugs and changes did not impact HR. Dropouts ~10% and balanced. Compliance 43% in hormone group, 56% in placebo group; no OGTT, single FPG for Dx
WHI[302]	40 US centres; 15 641 post-menopausal women with uterus; mean age = 63 years; follow-up 5.6 years. Outcome: clinical diabetes requiring therapy	**Estrogen** (0.625 mg) + **progesterone** (2.5 mg) (*N* = 8014) vs **Placebo** (*N* = 7627)	*E + P*: 3.5% over 5.6 years vs *Placebo*: 4.2%; HR = 0.79 (95% CI 0.67 to 0.93, $p = 0.004$); RRR = 21%; ARR = 0.7%, NNT = 143 over 6 years	Primary outcome not sensitive; 3% of women had FPG >7 mmol l^{-1} or higher at baseline. Insulin resistance improved in sample on treatment vs placebo. HR adjusted for change in weight and waist circumference similar
WHI[303]	40 US centres; 9712 post-menopausal women without uterus; mean age = 64 years; follow-up 7.1 years. Outcome: clinical diabetes requiring therapy	**Estrogen** (0.625 mg) (*N* = 4806) vs **Placebo** (*N* = 4906)	*Estrogen*: 8.3% over 7.1 years vs *Placebo*: 9.3%; HR = 0.88 (95% CI 0.77 to 1.01, $p = 0.072$); RRR = 12%, ARR = 1.0%, NNT = 100	54% stopped estrogen by study end. Among users, HR = 0.73 (95% CI 0.60 to 0.88). Significant improvement in glucose and insulin at 1 year, but not at 3 or 6 years

[a]HR = hazard ratio; RR = relative risk or risk ratio; RRR = relative risk reduction; ARR = absolute risk reduction; ITT = intention-to-treat; NNT = number needed to treat (if not present, data were not available to calculate).

French investigators conducted two studies using the second-generation biguanide metformin, to determine the impact of this agent on components of the insulin resistance syndrome. In the first study, BIguanides and Prevention of Risks of Obesity (BIGPRO 1),[213,214] they selected 457 people with high waist:hip ratio (men ≥0.95, women ≥0.80) aged 35–60 years, randomly allocated them to 850 mg of metformin twice daily or placebo and followed them every 3 months for 1 year. Both groups were given diet and physical activity instruction. The metformin group showed small (−2 kg) but significant weight loss, less rise in fasting glucose and marginally greater fall in fasting insulin, without change in 2 h glucose or insulin. Lower LDL cholesterol but no changes in BP, triglycerides or HDL cholesterol were found. Of a number of haemostatic factors explored, the metformin group showed decreases in tissue plasminogen activator (tPA) antigen and von Willebrand factor,[215] but no change in plasminogen activator inhibitor-1 (PAI-1) activity or antigen not accounted for by weight loss. Five individuals in the placebo group developed diabetes, versus none in the metformin group (exact $p = 0.06$, *post hoc* analysis). The results are difficult to interpret since there was a 28 and 30% dropout rate in the two groups at 1 year. While people who dropped out were similar to those remaining in the trial, unexplained bias could have accounted for the results.

The investigators undertook a confirmatory study (BIGPRO 1.2) among 168 men who had slightly higher BP and triglyceride levels.[216,217] A similar randomization procedure and dose of metformin were used, although men were followed only for 3 months. Results were consistent with BIGPRO 1, in that fasting glucose, insulin, LDL cholesterol, ApoB and tPA antigen declined, without change in BP or triglycerides. No diabetes occurred in either group and weight loss was only 0.5 kg. In both studies, metformin produced more diarrhoea, nausea and vomiting, but no hypoglycaemic episodes.[214] The authors concluded that metformin would be an acceptable intervention in a type 2 diabetes prevention trial.

In a study in China, Li *et al.* evaluated the use of low-dose metformin (250 mg three times per day) compared with placebo to prevent the development of diabetes.[218] People with IGT were identified during screening of a large workforce in Beijing, and 90 were randomly assigned to metformin or placebo. After 1 year of follow-up, three people on metformin developed diabetes (7.1%), compared with six on placebo (14.0%) (RR = 0.51, 95% CI 0.02 to 1.91, ARR = 6.9/100 PY) (*post hoc* ITT analysis). There were also fewer people remaining with IGT and more reverting to normal glucose tolerance ($p = 0.091$). Using an efficacy analysis (including only the 70 persons who were compliant and continued in follow-up), the reduction in risk was naturally greater (RR = 0.19, 95% CI 0.02 to 1.47), but it was not statistically significant unless the lower frequency of people with IGT were also included ($p = 0.011$).

The Diabetes Prevention Program (DPP) also included metformin (850 twice daily) or placebo with simple annual lifestyle advice, in a double-blind design.[80] The design and intensive lifestyle results were discussed previously. The primary endpoint was clinical or OGTT diabetes, confirmed on at least two tests. Randomization procedures and drug assignments were carefully masked to investigators and the metformin and placebo groups were similar at baseline on all risk factors measured.[79] Metformin significantly reduced the incidence of diabetes by 31% compared with placebo (95% CI 17 to 43%) (average annual incidence of 7.8/100 PY vs 11.0/100 PY in placebo; ARR = 3.2/100 PY).[72] About 72% of participants reported ≥80% adherence to the drug. In contrast to consistent results in sub-groups for the DPP lifestyle intervention, metformin was less effective in persons with lower BMI and in persons aged 60 years or greater. The lifestyle intervention was 39% more effective than metformin ($p < 0.001$). The NNT over 3 years was 13.9 for metformin. Interestingly, fasting plasma glucose levels were reduced similarly in the metformin and lifestyle groups, although 2 hour glucose levels were reduced much more by the lifestyle intervention, consistent with metformin's action on hepatic glucose production. There were no differences in the rates of serious adverse events (hospitalizations, mortality) between groups, although mild gastrointestinal symptoms were significantly more common in the metformin group.[80]

Understanding whether the reduction in incidence is due to an acute effect of treatment of hyperglycaemia or a more fundamental change in glucose homeostasis was the goal of the DPP washout study.[219] There were 1274 participants who were asked to stop either metformin or placebo prior to unmasking of the drug assignment (79% of those eligible, excluding persons who previously developed diabetes). After a mean of 11 days off drug, a repeat OGTT was conducted. A non-significant excess of the metformin participants had a diabetic OGTT than persons on placebo (OR = 1.49, 95% CI 0.93 to 2.38, $p = 0.098$). Adding the persons with diabetes during the washout to those developing diabetes prior to the washout lowered the overall effectiveness of metformin from 34% ($p < 0.001$) to 25% ($p = 0.005$), still highly significant. The authors concluded that there remained an important effect of metformin on delaying or preventing diabetes beyond its acute metabolic effect. While the long-term duration of the metformin effect is not known, the lifetime modelling of the development of diabetes suggests that the median time to onset may be delayed by at least 3.4 years and that overall, at least 8% fewer high-risk persons using metformin would not develop diabetes in their lifetime, compared with persons on placebo.[116]

In addition to delay or prevention of diabetes, metformin in the DPP has also been shown to reduce the incidence of the metabolic syndrome by 17% compared with placebo and partially to reverse abnormalities in persons with the syndrome at trial entry.[85] Cardiovascular risk factors were also improved in persons taking metformin compared with placebo, with reductions in hypertension, LDL phenotype B, overall dyslipidaemia and increased HDL levels.[83] Metformin reduced CRP in women by 14% compared with the placebo group but by only 7% in men.[84] These cardiovascular risk improvements were always less marked with metformin than in persons in the intensive lifestyle group. The roles of insulin sensitivity and secretion were also explored.[220] Among metformin users, both insulin sensitivity and markers of secretion improved over 1 year, but to levels intermediate between the lifestyle and placebo group, consistent with the intermediate lowering of diabetes risk in the metformin group. The DPP was the first large, carefully randomized study to show that metformin will delay or prevent diabetes in high-risk IGT individuals.

The Indian Diabetes Prevention Program (IDPP) was the second large trial to include metformin, but uniquely also combined with lifestyle in one of the four arms.[87] As noted above, the 3 year cumulative incidence of diabetes was significantly reduced to similar levels in all intervention groups (control = 55% vs LSM = 39%; MET = 40.5%) and there was no additional effect of combining lifestyle and metformin (LSM + MET = 39.5%). The NNT over 3 years was 6.4–6.9 across the groups with an ARR of 9.3–10/100 PY.

Several recent studies have used metformin in obese adolescents[221] or adults with insulin resistance[222–224] or polycystic ovary syndrome.[225–228] Most, although not all,[223] have shown improvement in markers of insulin resistance or resumption of menses, although none were powered to explore diabetes incidence. At present, metformin is not licensed for prevention of diabetes or treatment of insulin resistance in the United States.

Thiazolidinediones

A class of insulin sensitizing agents has become available in the past few years, the thiazolidinediones (TZDs).[229] TZDs are peroxisomal proliferator-activated receptor (PPAR)-γ agonists, increasing insulin action by stimulation of the expression of genes that increase fat oxidation and lower plasma free fatty acid levels; increasing expression, synthesis and release of adiponectin; and stimulating adipocyte differentiation, leading to larger numbers of smaller fat cells. The first-generation agent troglitazone has been taken off the market and replaced with pioglitazone and rosiglitazone, second-generation drugs with a safer adverse event profile.

The first study to explore this class of agents used the drug troglitazone in 18 non-diabetic obese (BMI > 27) individuals, of whom 50% had IGT.[230,231] Nolan and colleagues randomly allocated 12 people to 200 mg twice daily troglitazone and six to placebo in a double-blind fashion. They were given a weight maintenance diet and activity instructions and followed weekly for 12 weeks. At study end, those taking troglitazone had lower fasting and OGTT glucose and insulin levels and higher insulin sensitivity by glucose clamp. Six out of seven people with IGT on active drug had reverted to normal glucose tolerance, however. There were only two people with IGT on placebo, so no comparison was given. Side-effects were mild and well tolerated. The authors suggested that this drug might have a role in prevention of diabetes. A second study of troglitazone was conducted by Antonucci et al. in six sites[232] and included only people with IGT by WHO criteria, in contrast to the previous study (Table 5.5). They randomized 51 participants with IGT on a single OGTT to either 400 mg of troglitazone per day (N = 25) or placebo (N = 26). After 12 weeks of follow-up, 80% of people on troglitazone had reverted to normal glucose tolerance compared with 48% of those in the placebo group (p = 0.016). The RR for remaining IGT was 0.38 (95% CI 0.15 to 1.00, unadjusted, ARR = 32/100 persons) for those receiving troglitazone. Glucose and insulin areas under the OGTT curve were significantly improved. However, there were no changes in fasting glucose, insulin or C-peptide levels. Triglycerides decreased significantly on active drug, but there were no changes in other lipids, blood pressure, weight or HbA$_{1c}$. No-one in this short study developed diabetes. Drop-out was approximately 20% in each group and no details of adverse events were given.

Change in insulin sensitivity using troglitazone was the primary outcome in a study of 42 women with prior gestational diabetes and current IGT carried by Berkowitz et al.[233] Women were randomized to placebo, 200 mg or 400 mg of troglitazone and studied before treatment and after 12 weeks using the frequently sampled intravenous glucose tolerance test (FSIGT) with minimal model assessment to determine changes in insulin sensitivity (S$_I$). There was a dose-dependent improvement in S$_I$ to a maximum of 88% in the 400 mg group. Interestingly, there were no significant changes in fasting or post-challenge glucose levels, in contrast to the study by Nolan et al.,[230] but consistent with others.[232,234] for glucose. Although not statistically significant, there were declines in AUC glucose on the 400 mg dose among women with prior GDM, which is also consistent with people with IGT and no prior GDM.[232] This study served as the pilot study for the larger TRIPOD study.

The TRoglitazone In the Prevention Of Diabetes (TRIPOD) trial was a single-centre, randomized, placebo-controlled, double-blind 5 year study to determine if troglitazone prevented or delayed the onset of type 2 diabetes in high-risk Latina women with a history of GDM.[235,236] A total of 266 women with confirmed GDM were randomized to placebo or 400 mg of troglitazone per day and 235 had at least one follow-up visit. The primary endpoint was the development of OGTT diabetes (single 2 h glucose $\geq$200 mg dl^{-1} (11.1 mmol l^{-1}) or single fasting glucose $\geq$140 mg dl^{-1} (7.8 mmol l^{-1}). After a median of 30 months of follow-up, the incidence rate in the placebo group was 12.3/100 PY and in the troglitazone group 5.4/100 PY (HR = 0.45, 95% CI 0.25 to 0.83; ARR = 6.9/100 PY, p = 0.001, NNT = 14.5). The HR did not change with adjustment for small differences in baseline characteristics. Troglitazone was discontinued in the study on removal from the market in 2000. Sub-group analysis showed that the majority of the effect was in women who improved their insulin sensitivity and reduced β-cell workload. In the sub-group considered, non-responders to treatment (lowest tertile of S_I change) diabetes developed at 9.8% per year, whereas in the responders (upper two tertiles) it was 3.0% per year. During a post-trial washout period of $\sim$8 months, the risk of developing diabetes since stopping the drug or placebo was also reduced among women who took troglitazone (HR = 0.13, 95% CI 0.02 to 1.14). The authors concluded that troglitazone has persistent effects beyond the acute pharmacological effects, although the sample size resulted in a non-significant result.

Buchanan and colleagues extended the TRIPOD study after switching women to pioglitazone (45 mg day^{-1}) (PIPOD) from troglitazone after it was removed from the market.[237] Women (N = 89/95 eligible) without diabetes at the end of TRIPOD and whose HbA$_{1c}$ was <7% were provided open-label pioglitazone in an observational study, with regular OGTT and IVGTT testing. The average annual incidence of diabetes from the start of PIPOD to the end of drug washout was 5.2%, similar to the rate in TRIPOD of 5.4% and lower than the rates during the placebo period in TRIPOD of 12.3%. Understanding of these rate differences is complicated by the lack of a comparable untreated control during PIPOD and the relatively high dropout rates (26% over 3 years). Exploration of insulin sensitivity and secretion from both studies suggests that women with the best response to the drugs (greatest reduction in insulin output during IVGTT) had the lowest risk of diabetes,

also consistent with a small mechanistic study.[238] Thus, improvement in insulin sensitivity during active treatment, which reduces the need for β-cell secretory response, appears to reduce diabetes risk over a period extending at least 6–8 months beyond active therapy (end of the drug washout). Taken together, TRIPOD and PIPOD also argue for a drug class effect.

Durbin conducted a private practice-based trial of thiazolidinediones versus watchful waiting (control) in 172 adults with a mean age of $\sim$57 years.[239] Persons had IGT at baseline with elevated C-peptide levels and were placed on 400 mg day^{-1} of troglitazone (N = 101) or watchful waiting (N = 71) based on which physician was seen in the practice. After a mean of 10 months (when troglitazone was taken off the market), persons on active treatment were assigned either rosiglitazone or pioglitazone depending on which informational session they attended. People were followed for an average of 3 years. In those treated with TZDs, the 3 year cumulative incidence was 2.97% (1.4/100 PY) compared with controls (26.8% 3 years; RR = 0.11, 95% CI 0.021 to 0.377; ARR = 23.8% 3 years), leading to a 3 year NNT of 4.2. There were no dropouts in this practice-based study. However, the randomization method was weak and no data were shown about the comparability of groups on diabetes risk factors. Criteria for diabetes were not specified and masking was not noted. Nonetheless, the significant reduction in treated persons was of the magnitude seen in other TZD studies such as the DPP.

The DPP originally included troglitazone as one of the agents to be tested. After 585 people were randomized to troglitazone, one participant experienced hepatic failure and death, causing the investigators and NIH to stop its use in the trial. Troglitazone was subsequently withdrawn from the market. The troglitazone-treated participants were given group lifestyle classes and followed off drug,[240] having been treated for a mean of 0.9 months (range 0.5–1.5 years). The diabetes incidence rate was 3.0/100 PY, compared with 12.0, 6.7 and 5.1 cases/100 PY in the placebo, metformin and ILS participants randomized during the same interval (HR = 0.25 vs placebo, p < 0.001; ARR = 9.0/100 PR, NNT = 11). The effect of troglitazone was shown to be due to improved insulin sensitivity with no worsening of insulin secretion. During the 3 years after troglitazone withdrawal, the diabetes incidence density rate was almost identical with that of the placebo group, suggesting that after the drug was stopped, risk returned to that of untreated participants.

One other small RCT of troglitazone was conducted in high-risk African-American individuals with NGT.[241] Using only 200 mg day^{-1} of drug in

49 individuals (81 on placebo), after 24 months there were no significant improvements in glucose or insulin levels or area under the curve, although trends to lower levels were seen in treated people. There was improvement in the disposition index and the insulin: glucose ratio and no people in this low-risk (NGT) group converted to diabetes in either group. Whether the small changes seen are clinically relevant is not clear, but the results suggest that a lower dose of TZD among NGT persons may have limited effects. It also highlights the utility of conducting prevention trials in higher risk individuals (such as IGT) in order to detect treatment effects.

A large trial of the TZD rosiglitazone for diabetes prevention has been reported [Diabetes REduction Assessment with ramipril and rosiglitazone Medication (DREAM)].[242,243] DREAM was a 2×2 factorial, double-blind RCT comparing rosiglitazone (8 mg day^{-1}) with placebo and ramipril/placebo (see below) in 5269 men and women aged ≥ 30 years (mean 55 years) from 21 countries, with 3 years of follow-up. Persons had IGT or isolated IFG at baseline, were at relatively low risk for CVD events and had diabetes on OGTT or death as the primary composite outcome. There was a 60% reduction in the composite endpoint (HR = 0.40, 95% CI 0.35 to 0.46, $p < 0.0001$) and a nearly identical reduction in diabetes alone (HR = 0.38, 95% CI 0.33 to 0.44, $p < 0.0001$; ARR = 15.6%, NNT = 6.4 over 3 years), indicating that there was little mortality and no major effect. In addition to reducing the risk of diabetes, rosiglitazone also improved the transition to NGT by approximately 70%, modestly lowered blood pressure and reduced serum ALT enzyme levels, suggesting an improvement in hepatic fatty acid deposition. There was no interaction with ramipril for any endpoint. However, these benefits came with small amounts of weight gain on active drug ($\sim$3%) and a 37% non-significant increase in composite cardiovascular outcomes (MI, stroke, CVD death, CHF, new angina and revascularization). Congestive heart failure was significantly increased, although the numbers were relatively small (14 vs 2 on placebo) and none were fatal. The authors noted that for every 1000 people treated with rosiglitazone for $\sim$3 years, 144 cases of diabetes would be prevented with an excess of about four cases of CHF. Nonetheless, excess weight gain and a trend towards increased, rather than decreased, CVD events and CHF raise important cautions about the widespread use of this drug, even with its potent lowering of diabetes risk. A recent meta-analysis[480] and an editorial summarizing cardiovascular risk concerns with rosiglitazone taking a number of recent trials together[481] suggest that rosiglitazone may

significantly increase myocardial infarction rates (odds ratio 1.36, 95% CI 1.04 to 1.78). Given the balance of costs and potential side-effects, lifestyle modification should remain the first-line preventive therapy.[244]

The ACT NOW (*Actos Now for Prevention of Diabetes*) trial (NCT00220961, www.clinicaltrials.gov) was conducted at eight US centres among 602 persons with IGT, with random allocation to either pioglitazone (ACTOS®) or placebo,[467] and a 2.9 year median follow-up. The primary outcome was diabetes incidence using repeated OGTTs and follow-up was a minimum of 24 months post-randomization. Participants had insulin sensitivity measured using a frequently sampled intravenous glucose tolerance test (FSIGT) in addition to carotid intimal media thickness measures using carotid B-mode ultrasound at baseline and 45 months post-drug washout. The study began in 2004 and finished in late 2007 but results were available only as presented orally in June 2008. Participants taking pioglitazone had 81% lower diabetes risk (HR = 0.19) and 42% of the pioglitazone participants but only 28% of placebo participants returned to normal glucose tolerance at the end of the study. The 1 year NNT was 3.5. A washout phase was due to be completed late in 2008. Further details await publication of complete results. Whether pioglitazone has excess CVD events is not known at present in persons with prediabetes, although a recent report from a large trial of persons with diabetes (PROactive 10)[482] and a recent meta-analysis[483] found reductions in most major classes of CVD endpoints, with the exception of congestive heart failure. Hence it is possible that excess CVD risk is not a thiazolidinedione class effect.

α-Glucosidase inhibitors

α-Glucosidase inhibitors cause dose-dependent inhibition of α-glucosidase enzymes located in the brush border of enterocytes throughout the small intestine that hydrolyse oligo- and polysaccharides into absorbable monosaccharides. These agents induce a significant decrease in the post-prandial rise in glucose and insulin. Three α-glucosidase inhibitor molecules have been developed: acarbose, miglitol and voglibose. No prevention trials with the last two agents have been reported. Chiasson *et al.* in Montreal conducted a small pilot study ($N = 18$) of acarbose in people with IGT.[245] After 4 months, those on acarbose showed lower post-meal and 12 h glucose and insulin profiles with no change among those on placebo. Results in this short-term study suggested the potential utility of acarbose to improve glucose tolerance and insulin sensitivity and led the authors to begin a larger multicentre trial in Canada and Europe.

The Study to Prevent NIDDM (STOP-NIDDM)[246,247] was designed to test whether acarbose would delay or prevent type 2 diabetes among people with IGT. A total of 1429 participants were recruited with IGT and other eligibility criteria and were followed for an average of 3.3 years. Randomization was to acarbose (titrated to 100 mg three times daily) or placebo. Mean age at baseline was 54.5 years, with a mean BMI of 30.9. The outcome was diabetes diagnosed annually on OGTT. After exclusions, there were 1368 persons in the ITT analysis, of whom 341 (23.9%) discontinued prematurely, 211 in the acarbose group and 130 in the placebo group. Acarbose treatment reduced overall risk of diabetes by 25% using proportional hazards (hazard ratio = 0.75, 95% CI 0.63 to 0.90; ARR = 9.1/100 PY over 3.3 years). It also resulted in a significant increase in conversion from IGT to normal glucose tolerance ($p < 0.0001$). Acarbose was equally effective across the age span and across BMI levels. A small amount of weight loss occurred in the acarbose group (0.5 kg) with weight gain in the placebo (0.3 kg). Accounting for weight change over time did not alter the efficacy of the drug.[247] If the same endpoint criteria as used in the DPP are applied to this trial (two positive OGTTs rather than one), the acarbose HR = 0.64 (95% CI 0.498 to 0.813) and a relative reduction in diabetes risk of 36% were similar to that produced by metformin.[80] There was a higher dropout rate in the active treatment group, due in part to the higher rate of gastrointestinal side-effects and a relatively high dropout rate over-all.

Over the 3.3 year follow-up period, acarbose was also shown to reduce major CVD endpoints by 49% (HR = 0.51, 95% CI 0.28 to 0.95) and hypertension development (HR = 0.66, 95% CI 0.49 to 0.89), largely unaffected by adjustment for CVD risk factors.[248] In a sub-group of 132 individuals, subclinical atherosclerosis, as measured using carotid intimal–medial thickness (IMT), was also slowed by ~50% ($p = 0.027$). One of the possible hypothesized mechanisms for the action of α-glucosidase inhibitors is reduction of post-prandial hyperglycaemia and hypertriglyceridaemia, both of which can induce oxidative stress, leading to endothelial dysfunction.[249]

The STOP-NIDDM trial has been criticized for irregularities in the definition of study groups, inadequate blinding, multiple *post hoc* cardiovascular endpoints, inclusion of persons with endpoints at baseline (diabetes, hypertension) and potential sponsor bias.[250,251] These criticisms have been rebutted by the investigators and additional results were provided.[252] The primary results on the prevention or delay of diabetes appear robust, with or without the inclusion of the persons 'developing' diabetes during the 3 month washout period.[252] As the authors noted, it appears from this study, as from the washout studies of metformin and troglitazone in the DPP,[219,240] that it is very likely that any medication needs to be taken continuously to maintain a longer term benefit.[252]

There have been few other trials of acarbose reported to date. A 3 year primary prevention study has been completed in Hoorn, The Netherlands, also using acarbose among 150 people with IGT (DAISI). Participants with a mean of two fasting plasma glucose levels $< 7.8 \text{ mmol l}^{-1}$ (140 mg dl^{-1}) and the mean of two 2 h post-load glucoses $> 8.6 - < 11.1 \text{ mmol l}^{-1}$ ($> 155.0 - < 200 \text{ mg dl}^{-1}$) have been randomized to either 50 mg of acarbose three times per day or placebo. Participants in the trial had 3 monthly fasting glucose levels and an OGTT at 1.5 and 3 years for the primary endpoint of type 2 diabetes. A useful addition to this small trial is the performance of a hyperglycaemic clamp at randomization and at 3 years to assess insulin resistance. The trial is completed and manuscripts are being prepared, although no results are available as yet (Prof. G. Nijpels, personal communication).

The Early Diabetes Intervention Trial (EDIT) was a 6 year, prospective, randomized, placebo-controlled study in individuals with a mean of two consecutive fasting plasma glucose levels in the range 5.5–7.7 mmol l^{-1} (100–139 mg dl^{-1}). Nine UK clinical centres recruited 631 people. The primary aim of the trial was to determine whether deterioration in glucose tolerance could be delayed or prevented using acarbose or metformin in a 2×2 factorial design. Three year interim[253] and 6 year final results[254] have only been presented in abstract form, now several years ago. No significant effect was seen at 3 years. At 6 years, there was no reduction overall in diabetes risk among those on acarbose (RR = 1.04, $p = 0.81$), on metformin (RR = 0.99, $p = 0.94$) or on combination therapy (RR = 1.02, $p = -0.91$). However, among those with IGT at baseline, acarbose reduced the risk (RR = 0.66, $p = 0.046$), although metformin (RR = 1.09, $p = 0.70$) or combination therapy (RR = 0.72, $p = 0.27$) did not. Further details have not been published. These results provide limited support for the use of acarbose among persons with IGT, but given the heterogeneous nature of glucose intolerance at baseline (17% had diabetes by 2 h glucose $\geq 11.0 \text{ mmol l}^{-1}$; 37% IGT, 21% IFG and 46% NGT) the overall the results are negative. The authors suggest that the interventions may differ in their efficacy depending on the type and level of initial glucose abnormality. It appears that compliance was poor, with only 37% taking acarbose at study end (versus 46% taking placebo, with similar results for metformin), so these results may reflect not a lack of efficacy of either drug, but the failure to take them.

A 3 year trial in China included lifestyle, acarbose, metformin or placebo.[255] The authors noted that the annual diabetes incidence was 11.6% in the control group, which was lower with diet and exercise (8.2%) and even lower with metformin (4.1%) or acarbose (2%) treatment. Using a proportional hazard regression model, risk reductions for the onset of type 2 diabetes were reported to be 87.8% for acarbose (HR = 0.20, 95% CI 0.05–0.89), 76.8% for metformin (HR = 0.31, 95% CI 0.09–1.1) and 8.2% for diet and exercise intervention. Methodological details of this trial are not easily accessible, so these results, together with a shorter trial by Pan *et al.*,[256] can be taken only as weakly suggestive of additional evidence that acarbose delays or prevents diabetes.

At present, there is only one published trial confirming the effect of acarbose,[247] with suggestive evidence from three other RCTS.[254–256] No studies other than STOP-NIDDM have reported cardiovascular endpoint reduction. Whether drugs which reduce post-prandial or post-load hyperglycaemia can reduce cardiovascular disease awaits the results of larger trials, such as NAVIGATOR, described later.

Newer agents may be useful for diabetes prevention. One new class of agents are the dipeptidyl peptidase-IV (DPP-4) inhibitors.[257] These agents lower glucose levels through inhibition of the DPP-4-mediated degradation of the active form of incretins, particularly glucagon-like peptide-1 (GLP-1). At present, there are no trials focused on diabetes prevention, but early studies in non-diabetic volunteers suggest that this may occur.[258,484] Whether incretin pathways are central to the development of type 2 diabetes also remains to be firmly established.[257] Another new class of agents are the selective cannabinoid CB1 receptor antagonists, such as rimonabant.[259] The endocannabinoid system is thought to influence food intake via the mesolimbic dopaminergic system. In 1 year studies of non-diabetic individuals, rimonabant (20 mg day^{-1}) decreased body weight (by a mean of 6–7 kg) and visceral obesity (waist circumference) compared with placebo.[260,261] In addition, lipid profiles were shifted towards a less atherogenic pattern and glucose levels were lower on treatment. A diabetes prevention trial with this agent is under way (RAPOSDI; see below).

Anti-obesity agents

Given the efficacy of weight loss to delay or prevent diabetes, the use of weight loss agents to accomplish this has been evaluated in a limited way. A meta-analysis.[262] of three smaller weight loss trials with orlistat (a lipase inhibitor that reduces dietary fat absorption) found that the pooled reduction in diabetes incidence over ~2 years was 3.0% in the treated groups versus 7.6% (RR = 0.39). However, there were only six cases of diabetes in total. There was a shift in the glucose tolerance distribution such that more individuals abnormal at baseline became NGT at follow-up. High dropout rates and small sample size limit the usefulness of this meta-analysis.

A much larger RCT used orlistat together with lifestyle advice versus placebo plus advice for weight loss: the XENDOS study.[263] There were 3277 obese individuals with a non-diabetic OGTT randomized to 120 mg tid of drug or placebo, together with a weight-reducing diet and increased physical activity. After 4 years, the cumulative incidence of diabetes was 6.2% on orlistat and 9.0% on placebo (HR = 0.63, 95% CI 0.46 to 0.86; ARR = 2.8/100, p = 0.0032). Analysis of planned sub-groups found that the effect was seen primarily in those with IGT at baseline (HR = 0.55, p = 0.0024) and the reduction seen among those with NGT was not significant. Weight loss was significantly greater on drug (10.6 vs 6.2 kg on placebo; p = 0.001), using the last observation carried forward (LOCF) method, necessary due to high dropout rates (48% in the drug group, 66% in the placebo group) that characterize weight loss studies. The primary limitation of this trial is the high dropout rates, which make significant bias possible and interpretation difficult. Nonetheless, the apparent greater weight loss on drug and subsequent lower incidence of diabetes among persons with IGT is consistent with other studies. Several other RCTs using orlistat have been conducted in groups including both persons with and without diabetes, making interpretation of the prevention effect impossible to determine given pooled analyses (e.g.[264,265]). Gastrointestinal side-effects and multiple dosing per day (with each meal) make the use of orlistat difficult, but if taken, together with an effective lifestyle programme, it appears likely to result in greater weight loss than with lifestyle alone and should lead to improved delay/prevention of diabetes.

No studies of the primary prevention of diabetes through weight loss using sibutramine, a norepinephrine and serotonin reuptake inhibitor, were identified. However, this agent has been shown to be effective in producing weight loss[266,267] and often in reducing insulin resistance and cardiovascular risk, especially when combined with a lifestyle programme,[268] and thus may be a useful adjunct to weight loss in high-risk individuals. Without formal trials with diabetes as an endpoint, it is not possible to determine whether unanticipated side-effects could result in higher diabetes development, although this appears unlikely given the multiple risk factors that are improved.

Antihypertensive agents

There are multiple RCTs of various antihypertensive agents that have examined diabetes outcomes, usually as *post hoc* analyses, although some have defined diabetes as a planned secondary endpoint among persons without diabetes at trial entry. The trials that explored specific agents versus placebo with at least 1 year of follow-up are included in Table 5.5.

The trials comparing two or more active agents without a placebo are numerous;[192,193,196,269,270] most have reported differences between agents, but the interpretation of whether the primary agent(s) lowered diabetes risk or the comparison agent(s) increased risk is not possible to ascertain. These trials include studies of angiotensin-converting enzyme inhibitors (ACEs) (CAPPP,[271] STOP-2,[272] ALLHAT[273] and ANBP2[274]), angiotensin II receptor blockers (ARBs) (LIFE,[275] ALPINE[276] and VALUE[277,278]), calcium channel blockers (NORDIL,[279] ALLHAT,[273] INSIGHT[280] and INVEST[281]) and beta blockers (HAPPHY[282]), often compared against diuretics or other combinations. Readers are referred to review articles on these agents for further details of these studies.[192,193,196,269,270] Chapter 12 also includes information on many of these RCTs from the antihypertensive perspective.

Diuretics

In one of the earliest RCTs to explore the incidence of diabetes among persons taking antihypertensive agents, the European Working Party on Hypertension in the Elderly randomized 840 persons older than 60 years to placebo or combination diuretics plus methyldopa (35%) in a stepped fashion.[283] A non-significant excess incidence of clinically diagnosed diabetes was seen (RR = 1.4, 95% CI 0.8 to 2.6). The Systolic Hypertension in the Elderly Trial (SHEP) randomized over 4700 elderly individuals with isolated systolic hypertension to diuretics and beta-blockers versus placebo over an average of 4.5 years. In a *post hoc* analysis among the 3680 without known diabetes at entry, the incidence of diabetes by fasting glucose, history or medication was 8.6% versus 7.5% in the actively treated group versus placebo, respectively (RR = 1.15, 95% CI 0.91 to 1.45, $p = 0.25$).[284] Both trials suggest non-significant increases in diabetes incidence with the use of diuretics and/or beta-blockers, similar to other cohort studies.[269,285] Since this drug combination is often used as the referent therapy for trials of newer agents, it is difficult to determine whether the newer agents reduce diabetes incidence or the active control increases it.

Angiotensin-converting enzyme (ACE) inhibitors and receptor blockers (ARBS)

There are now six RCTs of ACE[286–289] or ARB therapy[290–292] versus placebo that provide information about the possible prevention of diabetes. While the potential mechanism of action is not clear, several studies suggest both ACE and ARB act through multiple pathways to enhance insulin sensitivity.[291] Ramipril, one of the newer ACE inhibitors, has been studied in a cardiovascular prevention trial among high-risk individuals, including people both with diabetes and at risk for it. The Heart Outcomes Prevention Evaluation (HOPE) Study[286] found, in a subset analysis, that people at risk for type 2 diabetes who were randomized to ramipril had a lower incidence of diabetes than those on placebo (RR = 0.66, 95% CI 0.51 to 0.85, ARR = 1.8/100 PY) over an average of 4.5 years of follow-up. There was no effect or interaction with the factorial vitamin E arm of the trial for diabetes incidence. The HOPE-TOO extension included 174 of the original 276 centres and 67% of the originally randomized participants.[287] In analyses over the entire 7.2 years of follow-up, people randomized to ramipril had a 31% lower diabetes risk compared with placebo. Interestingly, the proportion taking an ACE inhibitor in the open-label extension period was almost identical in both groups. The investigators suggested that this meant that early versus later initiation of therapy was more effective. However, since diabetes was self-reported and not systematically tested, they initiated the DREAM trial with OGTT outcomes to test whether ACE inhibition prevented diabetes.

A *post hoc* analysis of the Studies Of Left Ventricular Dysfunction (SOLVD) trial at the Montreal centre compared the ACE inhibitor enalapril versus placebo.[288] There were 291 persons without diabetes but with low cardiac ejection fraction at baseline who had available fasting glucose levels measured prospectively and retrieved from chart review. Adjustment for multiple risk factors found that after 2.9 years, persons randomized to enalapril had a multivariate HR = 0.22 (95% CI 0.10 to 0.46, $p < 0.0001$, ARR = 16.5%) versus placebo. The effect was larger among persons with IFG at baseline. This small cohort was not analysed as ITT, although baseline characteristics were well balanced and accounted for in adjusted analyses.

The PEACE Trial studied whether addition of an ACE (trandolapril, 4 mg day^{-1} or placebo) to standard antihypertensive and lipid-lowering therapy among

6896 lower risk individuals with previous CHD but without CHF or diabetes reduced diabetes incidence.[293] After almost 5 years of follow-up, people on trandolapril had a diabetes HR = 0.83 (95% CI 0.72 to 0.96, p = 0.01) versus placebo. However, 70% were on lipid-lowering medication, 60% were on beta-blockers, 35% were on calcium channel blockers and the trial suffered from a lack of systematic diabetes testing. Overall, the trial was negative for improvement in mortality or CHD outcomes, probably due to the lower risk of the participants.

Two RCTs of candesartan, an angiotensin II type 1 receptor blocker (ARB), have been conducted versus placebo. In the CHARM study,[290,291] three predefined sub-group trials among persons with varying degrees of heart failure and exposure to prior treatment were pooled for the analysis of diabetes incidence. Among the 5486 persons without diabetes at baseline, new diabetes was significantly less likely in the candesartan group (6% over 3.1 years) than placebo (7.4%; HR = 0.78, 95% CI 0.64 to 0.96, p = 0.02; ARR = 1.4%, 95% CI −2.8 to −0.05). Sub-group analyses showed no evidence of heterogeneity, as did comparison of the three subtrials, although there was a suggestion that the drug did not reduce diabetes when candesartan was added to prior ACE therapy.

The SCOPE trial[292] was conducted in multiple centres internationally and originally designed to evaluate candesartan versus placebo in elderly people with mildly elevated blood pressure and mild cognitive deficit. However, due to ethical concerns, 84% of the placebo group was treated with multiple anti-hypertensive agents including diuretics, beta-blockers and ACE inhibitors. Overall, diabetes incidence was 4.3% in the candesartan group versus 5.3% in the 'placebo' group (RR = 0.81, p = 0.09). This trial suffers from two major problems, an apparent placebo group that was actually an actively treated control with agents which may increase the rate of diabetes and, like the CHARM trial,[291] reliance on clinical identification of diabetes, without systematic glucose testing. Hence SCOPE, although consistent with other studies, provides little evidence that candesartan reduces diabetes risk.

While most of the *post hoc* analyses of ACE and ARB trials that have been published suggest lower diabetes incidence on active treatment,[269,294] most trials suffer from weak diabetes endpoint definition and lack of systematic testing, opening up the possibility that detection bias or elevation in risk among actively treated 'placebo' patients play a role in the findings. In addition, most have been conducted in patients with multiple risk factors for diabetes, but especially among heart failure patients, who may reflect very different risk for diabetes compared with individuals who have been included in primary prevention trials such as DPP and DPS. Both the HOPE[286,287] and CHARM[291] trials have presented more thorough analyses of diabetes which suggest that competing mortality, use of other agents and differential hospitalization between groups which could lead to altered rates of diabetes detection, seem not to play a role. Nonetheless, the evidence from these trials is inconclusive that these drugs reduce diabetes incidence.

The DREAM trial was designed to directly test whether ramipril (15 mg day^{-1}) versus placebo would decrease the risk of OGTT diabetes and/or mortality as the primary composite outcome.[242] Among the 5269 participants in 191 centres and 21 countries who were followed for a mean of 3 years, there was a non-significant 9% reduction of diabetes incidence (HR = 0.91, 95% CI 0.81 to 1.03; p = 0.15; ARR = 1.4%) and regression to NGT was significantly higher on active drug (HR = 1.16, 95% CI 1.07 to .27; p = 0.001).[289] Adherence to ramipril was 87% at 1 year and 75% at 3 years, with a similar side-effect profile except for increased cough, as expected. The 9% reduction in diabetes risk is smaller than estimated in HOPE and other ACE studies and may reflect differences in study population (lower CVD risk, no diabetes at baseline, younger age), endpoint definitions (use of OGTT testing at entry and follow-up) or shorter duration of follow-up (3 years versus an average of 4.5 years). There is a suggestion of lowering of diabetes risk after 3 years in persons taking ramipril who were followed longer. Taken together with the higher reversion rate to NGT, this suggests that a small benefit may exist.[289]

Overall, ACE inhibitors cannot currently be recommended for diabetes prevention. It is likely that they do not increase diabetes risk, however, and therefore may be preferred agents for blood pressure reduction in complex patients, especially those with heart failure. The small positive effects on glucose metabolism may be of some benefit in such patients.

Lipid-lowering agents

Freeman *et al.* reported a sub-group analysis of the West of Scotland Coronary Prevention Study (WOSCOPS)[295] using pravastatin, one of a number of HMG-CoA reductase inhibitors. There were 5974 men aged 45–64 years (x = 55 years) without diabetes at baseline among the 6595 persons randomized to either pravastatin (40 mg day^{-1}) or placebo. Participants at entry had normal fasting glucose levels, elevated LDL cholesterol and no history of diabetes, myocardial infarction or unstable angina or coronary revascularization at entry. Diabetes was defined by modified ADA criteria, requiring two fasting glucose levels ≥7.0 mmol l^{-1} (126 mg dl^{-1}) and an increment from baseline of ≥ 2.0 mmol l^{-1} (36 mg dl^{-1}) or treatment with diabetes medications. After 4.9 years of follow-up, men randomized to pravastatin had a 30% lower incidence of diabetes ($p = 0.042$) (multivariate hazard ratio = 0.7, 95% CI 0.50 to 0.99). The authors noted that the risk reduction could be due to effects of triglycerides and insulin resistance or perhaps through anti-inflammatory mechanisms of the statins. No information was reported on the use of antihypertensive or other agents in either group.

A second pravastatin trial, the LIPID Trial,[296] randomized slightly more than 6800 persons without diabetes at entry to placebo or pravastatin (40 mg day^{-1}). The limited results presented for diabetes prevention indicated no significant benefit of the statin (RR = 0.89, 95% CI 0.70 to 1.13, $p = 0.32$) and no information on potential confounding drug therapy.

The Heart Protection Study randomized 14 573 men and women from general practices throughout the UK, with low to moderate risk of CHD but without clinical diabetes, to simvastatin (40 mg day^{-1}) or placebo. After a mean of 5 years of follow-up, there was no significant difference in diabetes incidence (simvastatin = 4.6% versus placebo = 4.0%; RR = 1.14, 95% CI 0.98 to 1.33; $p = 0.1$). The 95% CI excluded results seen in both the previous trials.

The Anglo Scandinavian Cardiac Outcomes Trial – Lipid Lowering Arm (ASCOT-LLA)[297] used atorvastatin (10 mg) or placebo together with antihypertensive agents in men and women aged 40–79 years from UK and Scandinavian primary care practices. Participants were hypertensive and had at least three risk factors for CHD and, in this subset of the trial, had total cholesterol levels ≤ 6.5 mmol l^{-1} (250 mg dl^{-1}) and no previous diagnosis of diabetes. The trial was stopped early after 3.3 years due to beneficial effects of the statin on CHD endpoints. However, as in the Heart Protection Study, there was no benefit of atorvastatin on diabetes development (HR = 1.15, 95% CI 0.91 to 1.44; $p = 0.25$). No details on confounding medications, cross-overs or testing for diabetes were given. Taking these studies together, there is only one positive study of a statin and three of reasonable size that were negative. The evidence to date does not indicate that statins lower diabetes risk, although they clearly reduce CHD risk in persons with and without diabetes.

Two *post hoc* sub-group analyses of the Bezafibrate Infarction Prevention Study (BIP) conducted in the early 1990s have recently been published, examining the effect of this pan-PPAR activator versus placebo on diabetes development. In a high-risk sub-group of 303 men and women with prior CHD and IFG (fasting plasma glucose 110–125 mg dl^{-1}) at baseline, bezafi-brate reduced the incidence of diabetes over 6.2 years from 54.4% in the placebo group to 42.3% (adjusted HR = 0.70, 95% CI 0.49 to 0.99, $p = 0.04$; ARR = 12.1%, NNT = 8).[298] In a second sub-group of 339 men and women defined by a BMI ≥ 30 and non-diabetic (85% had NGT, 15% IFG), a similar reduction in diabetes incidence was seen (HR = 0.59, 95% CI 0.39 to 0.91, $p = 0.01$ adjusted; ARR = 9.9%, NNT = 10 over 6 years).[299] Both analyses accounted for increasing use of ACE and adjusted for slight imbalances at baseline. Even though diabetes was defined both as clinically diagnosed/treated and as FPG ≥ 126 mg dl^{-1} on follow-up testing, no OGTTs were used and no data were presented on losses to follow-up. Although the results are interesting in the light of the mechanism of action of insulin sensitization and lipid-lowering effects (predominant PPAR-α action, but also -γ and -δ activity), the practical utility of this drug seems limited, given that it had a limited effect on CVD endpoints in the BIP trial[300] and that more potent PPAR-γ insulin sensitizers are now available. Newer agents with dual PPAR-α and -γ activity (the glitazars, e.g. muraglitazar, tesaglitazar) are under regulatory review,[259] although none have entered longer term prevention trials at present.

Estrogen/progestin

Two large clinical trials (HERS, WHI) reported on the effects of hormone replacement therapy (HRT) on diabetes risk. The Heart and Estrogen/Progestin Replacement Study (HERS) examined diabetes development in *post hoc* analyses of 2029 women with CHD but without diagnosed diabetes at baseline in 20 US centres.[301] Women were randomly assigned to 0.625 mg of conjugated estrogen plus 2.5 mg of medroxyprogesterone acetate versus placebo and followed for a mean of 4.1 years. Women on HRT had significantly lower diabetes incidence at 4 years (HR = 0.65, 95% CI 0.48 to 0.89, $p = 0.006$; RRR = 35%; ARR = 3.3% over 4 years; NNT = 30). Adjustment for multiple potential mediators for this effect (e.g. BMI and change in weight, waist, lipids, antihypertensive drug therapy) had no appreciable effect on the HR. Smaller HRT trials summarized by Kanaya *et al.*[301] have mostly found consistent reductions in glucose levels on HRT, although none reported diabetes incidence outcomes.

The Women's Health Initiative (WHI) has recently published results for estrogen plus progesterone[302] and for estrogen alone[303] versus placebo. In the analysis of conjugated equine estrogen (0.625 mg) plus medroxyprogesterone acetate (2.5 mg) versus placebo, 15 641 post-menopausal women with an intact uterus and without clinical diabetes were followed for 5.6 years, when the trial was stopped due to increased breast cancer and overall harm. Diabetes, defined as self-reported and on-treatment, occurred in 4.2% of the placebo group (annualized rate = 0.76%) compared with 3.5% in women treated with HRT (annualized rate = 0.61%). The HR was 0.79 (95% CI 0.67 to 0.93, $p = 0.004$), with RRR = 21%, ARR 0.7% and NNT = 143 over 5.6 years. In a sample of women, improvements in glucose levels and estimated insulin resistance were seen at 1 year, which diminished somewhat by 3 years. Adjustment for changes in weight or waist circumference did not impact the overall results.

In the analysis of the WHI estrogen-only trial among post-menopausal women without a uterus, similar definitions of outcome were used.[303] After 7.1 years of follow-up, 8.3% of women (annualized rate = 1.16%) in the estrogen-alone group developed diabetes compared with 9.3% (annualized rate 1.3%) in the placebo group (HR = 0.88, 95% CI 0.77 to 1.01; RRR = 12%, ARR = 1.0%, NNT = 100 over 7 years). As the authors of both studies noted, however, any potential benefit on diabetes outcomes must be weighed against increases in venous thromboembolic events and increased risk for breast cancer with long-term use for estrogen plus progesterone and the lack of protection for CVD and breast cancer in the estrogen-only trial. For these reasons, hormone therapy cannot be recommended as a viable approach to diabetes prevention in post-menopausal women at this time. Further study of mechanisms may be useful to explore the role of hormonal factors in diabetes prevention, including studies of alternative post-menopausal hormone therapy regimens and selective estrogen agonists or antagonists on insulin resistance and diabetes.

Other interventions

Chromium Chromium (Cr) has been shown to play an important role in the regulation of glucose, insulin and lipid metabolism, as reviewed by Anderson[304] and Mertz.[305] It is likely that the response to chromium depends on the chromium nutritional status of the individual, so that heterogeneous results may have occurred due to inclusion of people in various nutritional states at entry. Methods for the evaluation of chromium status or diagnosis of chromium deficiency are not clinically established.[304] These facts present difficult obstacles in defining risk groups or clinical responders.

Based on recent reviews[306,307] and a meta-analysis,[308] there appear to be at least 10 small RCTs of short duration among people without diabetes.[309–318] None of these were long or large enough to evaluate the effects of chromium on diabetes outcomes. These short-term trials give little evidence that

larger studies of chromium supplementation should be mounted, though one longer-term epidemiological study has suggested lower levels of chromium in persons with diabetes and/or heart disease than controls.[319] At present there is no evidence that supplementation with chromium in any form can reduce diabetes incidence.

Antioxidants and other vitamins Several observational studies have explored the role of antioxidants in diabetes and on related variables such as glucose levels, HbA_{1c}, etc. Feskens *et al.*[152] found that intake of vitamin C at baseline was inversely related to 2 h glucose level 20 years later, independent of dietary fat intake, BMI and energy expenditure in the prospective follow-up of the Finnish and Dutch cohorts of the Seven Countries Study. Various other studies have shown cross-sectional associations between vitamin C and measures of hyperglycaemia.[320,321]

After 4 years of prospective follow-up of 944 men in eastern Finland, Salonen *et al.*[322] found that low plasma vitamin E was independently associated with a 3.9-fold (95% CI 1.8 to 8.6) increase in diabetes incidence. The IRAS investigators showed a statistically significant protective association of increasing concentration of plasma α-tocopherol with reduced risk of diabetes incidence over 5 years; however, this effect was limited to individuals who did not take vitamin E supplements.[323]

The HOPE multi-centre RCT included vitamin E supplementation (400 IU) and ACE among high-risk people for cardiovascular disease and diabetes in a factorial design.[286] They found no effect of vitamin E supplementation on diabetes incidence among the 5720 participants followed 4.5 years. A second RCT was recently reported from the Women's Health Study among 38 716 apparently healthy female health professionals followed over 10 years and given either 600 IU of vitamin E (α-tocopherol) every other day or matching placebo.[324] No effect of vitamin E on self-reported diabetes incidence was seen (RR = 0.95, 95% CI 0.87 to 1.05, $p = 0.31$), nor were there important interactions with diabetes risk factors, except for women with a negative family history, where there was a suggestion of a slight protective effect (RR = 0.88, 95% CI 0.78 to 1.00). These two RCTs together suggest no important effect of vitamin E on diabetes incidence.

One RCT explored β-carotene supplements alone. Liu *et al.* gave 50 mg of β-carotene every other day or placebo to over 22 000 US male physicians.[325] After a median of 12 years of follow-up, there was no difference in diabetes incidence rates (RR = 0.98, 95% CI 0.85 to 1.12) adjusted for other risk factors.

In the observational follow-up of the National Health and Nutrition Examination Survey – I Epidemiological Follow-up Survey,[326] Ford found that persons who developed diabetes over approximately 20 years were significantly less likely to report baseline use of multivitamins (21.4%) during the previous month than persons who did not develop diabetes (33.5% use). After multiple adjustment, the hazard ratio for the use of multivitamins was 0.76 (95% CI 0.63 to 0.93; ARR $\approx$ 1.6/1000 PY). Persons reporting more sustained use had greater reductions and persons starting vitamin intake after baseline had no reduction in risk. Whether this finding is due to the vitamin use itself or to other aspects of lifestyle clustering in persons who use multivitamins, remains unclear.

A recent French trial (SU.VI.MAX)[327] has directly explored the use of a multiple antioxidant pill (120 mg vitamin C, 30 mg vitamin E, 6 mg β-carotene, 100 μg selenium and 20 mg zinc) in a *post hoc* analysis of persons with available fasting plasma glucose (FPG) and other data. No effect was seen on FPG after 7.5 years. An inverse association with baseline β-carotene dietary intake and plasma concentrations was found in mixed models using both baseline and 7.5 year values and lower plasma concentrations of vitamin C were also related to higher FPG. Given that a number of observational cohort studies have found lower incidences of diabetes with higher fruit and vegetable intake,[152,328,329] the authors believe that the lack of evidence of multivitamin supplementation on FPG, plus the finding that β-carotene intake and plasma levels were related to FPG, suggests that β-carotene is simply an indirect marker of fruit and vegetable intake.

There is no current RCT evidence that supplementation with β-carotene or other antioxidants alters diabetes risk. However, it is possible that longer term studies of antioxidants may be required to understand their effects, since they may act at an earlier stage in disease,[330] requiring a cohort at lower risk at entry. They may also require intake of multiple antioxidants and other cofactors to be effective, as would occur in a diet higher in combinations of fruits and vegetables rather than single vitamin supplements.[331]

There have been reports of other potential risk factors for type 2 diabetes noted in observational studies which could hold some potential for preventive interventions, including magnesium, calcium and vitamin D. Observational data for these substances are reviewed briefly below. However, few RCTs have been conducted to determine the role that supplementation might play in reducing diabetes incidence.

Magnesium Among nurses[329,332] and other health professionals,[333] lower magnesium intake was found to be associated with an increased risk of diabetes in a dose–response fashion, with the relative risk steadily dropping as intake increased to the highest quartile (nurses RR = 0.62, 95% CI 0.50 to 0.78); male health professionals RR = 0.72, 95% CI 0.54 to 0.96). A recent extension of these studies with longer follow-up and adjustment for a wide variety of dietary, medication and behavioural factors found even stronger results.[334] Similar findings for magnesium have also been reported from the Iowa Women's Health Study.[335] While lower serum Mg^{2+} levels were associated with higher diabetes incidence in ARIC, low dietary intake was not.[336] A recent meta-analysis of prospective studies (including those noted above) found that the overall relative risk for a 100 mg per day increase in magnesium intake was 0.85 (95% CI 0.79 to 0.92), which was similar for intake of dietary magnesium (RR = 0.86, 95% CI 0.77 to 0.95) and total magnesium (RR = 0.83, 95% CI 0.77 to 0.89). A single small ($N = 63$) RCT of oral magnesium supplementation (2.5 g day^{-1} MgCl$_2$) among Mexican non-diabetic participants with insulin resistance (HOMA-IR $\geq$ 3) and low serum magnesium levels $\leq$0.74 mmol l^{-1}) found that insulin resistance significantly improved over 3 months (without concomitant weight change) and with no change in the placebo group.[485] Longer term clinical implications for diabetes prevention remain unclear.

Vitamin D, calcium There is a growing body of observational data that low intake of vitamin D, low calcium intake and combinations are associated in cohort studies with higher risk of type 2 diabetes.[329,337] For example, in the Nurses Health Study, a daily intake of >1200 mg calcium and >800 IU vitamin D was associated with a lower risk of type 2 diabetes (RR = 0.67, 95% CI 0.49 to 0.90) compared with an intake of <600 mg calcium and 400 IU vitamin D.[338] Lower circulating levels of vitamin D (usually 25-hydroxy-vitamin D) have been shown to be associated with higher prevalence of diabetes, glucose concentrations and insulin resistance and the prevalence of the metabolic syndrome.[339] These observations were tested in the Women's Health Initiative Calcium/Vitamin D randomized trial, which has been recently published.[486] Post-menopausal women aged 50–79 years received 1000 mg of elemental calcium plus 400 IU of vitamin D$_3$ daily, or placebo, in a double-blind fashion. There were 33 951 participants without self-reported diabetes at baseline and outcome was the new diagnosis of treated diabetes. Over 7 years of follow-up, the hazard ratio for incident diabetes associated with calcium/vitamin D treatment was 1.01 (95% CI 0.94 to 1.10) and was robust in sub-group analyses, efficacy analyses accounting for non-adherence and analyses examining change in laboratory measurements (fasting glucose, insulin or HOMA-IR). Thus, there was no evidence that this combination was associated with reduced clinical diabetes incidence. The authors noted that 'higher doses of vitamin D may be required, and/or associations of calcium and vitamin D intake with improved glucose metabolism observed in non-randomized studies may be the result of confounding or of other components of foods containing these nutrients'.

Smoking Observational results increasingly support the role of cigarette smoking as a reversible risk factor for diabetes. Manson *et al.* reported results from the Physician's Health Study[340] that found a dose-dependent increased risk for development of type 2 diabetes among smokers compared with never smokers. After adjustment for BMI, activity and alcohol consumption (but not dietary factors), the RR for smoking were 1.0 (95% CI 0.8 to 1.3) for 1–19.9 pack-years; 1.3 (95% CI 1.0 to 1.6) for 20–39.9 pack-years and 1.6 (95% CI 1.3 to 2.1) for 40 + pack-years ($p < 0.001$ for trend). The other Health Professional follow-up studies showed consistent elevations in diabetes risk,[341,342] as did the Zutphen Study,[343] a Japanese worker cohort,[344] the Osaka Health Survey,[345] the cohort of the MONICA/KORA Augsburg Study,[346] a large elderly Japanese cohort of men and women,[347] a Finnish cohort (independent of BMI and levels of physical activity)[348] and the large US Cancer Prevention Study.[349] Three other older prospective studies found no associations.[205,350,351] Each of these negative studies had fewer cases of incident diabetes than seen in the positive studies. Smoking cessation for diabetes prevention has not been evaluated in randomized studies. However, two observational reports suggest that risk falls after smoking cessation,[349,352] although weight gain following quitting increased the risk for diabetes within 5 years and risk returned to baseline only after 10–20 years. Smoking is now a well-established independent risk factor for diabetes, based on observational studies.[340]

Alcohol Elective alcohol consumption has also been studied in several observational prospective studies[342,353–358] and moderate intake appears to reduce risk for diabetes, as it does for cardiovascular disease.[359] Recent systematic reviews have shown that the risk of diabetes has a U-shaped relationship with consumption;[360–362] risk is reduced compared with non-drinkers by 30–60%, regardless of BMI or other risk factors. Heavy consumption (more than

three drinks per day) appears to be associated with increased risk of diabetes. Cardiovascular risk among persons with diabetes appears also to be reduced.[363] No RCTs have yet examined the use of moderate alcohol intake as a possible prevention for diabetes.

Bariatric surgery Use of surgery to limit food intake and induce long-term weight loss is one of the most radical and costly approaches to induce weight loss and treat obesity. The most common approaches include vertical banded gastroplasty or gastric bypass. There is reasonably convincing evidence that the significant weight loss induced by surgery can markedly reduce obesity, diabetes incidence, hypertension, hyperinsulinaemia and hypertriglyceridaemia.[364,365] In one of the largest studies reporting 10 year outcomes,[366] the Swedish Obese Subjects (SOS) study showed that diabetes incidence was reduced 75% at 10 years (OR = 0.25, 95% CI 0.17 to 0.38, $p < 0.001$) compared with matched (non-randomized) controls, as was development of hypertriglyceridaemia and hyperuricaemia. Recovery from diabetes to normal glucose tolerance also occurred 3.5 times more frequently among persons undergoing surgery. Although some evaluations suggest that obesity surgery can be cost-effective,[367] Segal *et al.* found that gastric surgery was less cost-effective per life-year saved compared with lifestyle modification to prevent diabetes.[368]

Prevention of gestational diabetes (GDM)

Gestational diabetes (GDM) is defined as glucose intolerance with onset or first recognition during pregnancy.[369,370] Approximately 135 000 cases of GDM, representing on average 3–8% of all pregnancies,[369] are diagnosed annually in the United States.[29] Marked variation in GDM prevalence among different racial/ethnic groups has been documented, with higher prevalence among American-Indian, Asian, African-American and Hispanic populations than among non-Hispanic whites.[371–375] Several factors contribute to this variation: differences in diagnostic criteria and screening methods and differences in the underlying population incidence and prevalence of type 2 diabetes.[376] In addition, the current definition of GDM precludes the distinction between GDM and pre-existing undiagnosed diabetes mellitus, which makes the degree of surveillance in a given population have an important impact on the estimated prevalence of GDM. This is especially the case for high-risk populations in which type 2 diabetes occurs at an early age, such as American-Indians.[376]

In general, the prevalence of GDM varies in direct proportion to the prevalence of type 2 diabetes in a given population or ethnic group. Recent data suggest that GDM prevalence has been increasing over the last decade, in parallel with the increase in the prevalence of obesity and type 2 diabetes. Two studies by Kaiser Permanente Health plan members showed significant increases in the cumulative incidence of GDM: ~3.5% per year in Northern California[377] and 11% annually (1994 to 2002) in Colorado.[378] Disturbingly, both studies showed increasing rates of GDM among all racial/ethnic groups. As many as 50% of women with GDM may develop type 2 diabetes within 5 years of the index pregnancy.[379] Further, increasing exposure to diabetes during pregnancy may be an important determinant of the increasing prevalence of obesity and type 2 diabetes in youth.[380,381] This creates a postulated cross-generational vicious cycle of diabetes in pregnancy, by which maternal diabetes pro-duces more diabetes in the offspring.[382,383] In addi-tion, as recently shown by the Australian Carbohy-drate Intolerance Study,[384] close monitoring and treatment of GDM women with diet and insulin (compared with usual care for women without GDM) results in significantly lower risk (RR = 0.33, 95% CI 0.14 to 0.75) of serious perinatal complications. GDM screening, diagnosis, treatment and, possibly, preven-tion warrants further attention.

There are no current randomized clinical trials spe-cifically designed to prevent GDM. Most data suggest-ing that prevention of GDM may be achievable through lifestyle interventions are provided by observational epidemiological studies (summarized in Table 5.6).

Diet and prevention of GDM

It is likely that the most important dietary factor in the development of insulin resistance and type 2 diabetes

Table 5.6 Observational studies of diet, physical activity and gestational diabetes

Reference	Population (no. of participants), study type	Instrument/ measurement	Comparison	Results (OR or RR, 95% CI)
Dietary macronutrients and antioxidants				
Moses, 1997[386]	Australia (N = 36), case–control	Food diaries	Total fat intake before or during pregnancy (% of total calories)	Higher total fat intake associated with GDM recurrence (41.4 vs 33.1%, $p < 0.001$)
Wang, 2000[387]	China (N = 133), case–control	24 h food diaries (3rd trimester)	Total fat intake (% of total calories) Polyunsaturated/saturated fat ratio (24 h recall; % of total calories)	Lower total fat intake associated with GDM [29.1% in GDM vs 33.2% in BMI-matched NGT women ($p < 0.05$)]. Low polyunsaturated/ saturated fat ratio associated with GDM, independent of BMI ($p < 0.0014$)
Saldana, 2004[388]	Chapel Hill, NC (N = 1698), historical prospective	Food frequency questionnaires (3rd trimester)	Isocaloric diets, replacing 1% calories from fat with 1% calories from carbohydrates	RR = 1.1 (95% CI 1.02 to 1.1), adjusted for pre-pregnancy age, BMI, race, physical activity
Zhang, 2004[392]	Seattle, WA (N = 327), case–control	Food frequency questionnaire (1st trimester) Plasma ascorbic acid	Low periconceptional vitamin C intake ($<70\,mg\,day^{-1}$) vs other Lowest vs highest plasma ascorbic acid quartile (<42.6 vs $>63.3\,\mu mol\,l^{-1}$)	OR = 3.7 (95% CI 1.7 to 8.2), adjusted for pre-pregnancy age, BMI, race, energy intake, family history of DM OR = 12.8 (95% CI 3.5 to 46.2), adjusted as above
Zhang, 2004[393]	Seattle, WA (N = 755), prospective	Food frequency questionnaire (1st trimester) Plasma ascorbic acid	Low periconceptional vitamin C intake ($<70\,mg\,day^{-1}$) vs other Lowest vs highest plasma ascorbic acid quartile (<55.9 vs $>74.6\,\mu mol\,l^{-1}$)	RR = 1.8 (95% CI 0.8 to 4.4), adjusted as above RR = 3.1 (95% CI 1.0 to 9.7), adjusted as above

Table 5.6 *(Continued)*

Reference	Population (no. of participants), study type	Instrument/ measurement	Comparison	Results (OR or RR, 95% CI)
Recreational physical activity				
Dye, 1997[402]	New York State, cross-sectional, population-based birth registry	Questionnaire	Inactive vs active during pregnancy	OR = 1.9 (95% CI 1.2 to 3.1), only when BMI >33
Dempsey, 2004[403]	Seattle WA (N = 541), case–control	Minnesota Leisure-time Physical Activity Questionnaire (1st trimester)	Any vs no activity before and during pregnancy	OR = 0.40 (95% CI 0.23 to 0.68), adjusted for covariates, including pre-pregnancy BMI
Dempsey, 2004[404]	Seattle, WA (N = 909), prospective	Minnesota Leisure-time Physical Activity Questionnaire (1st trimester: type, frequency, time spent in recreational activities)	Any vs no activity before and during pregnancy Time spent (≥4.2 h per week vs inactive) Energy spent (≥21.1 MET-h per week vs inactive)	RR = 0.31 (95% CI 0.12 to 0.79), adjusted for maternal age, race, parity and pre-pregnancy RR = 0.24 (95% CI 0.10 to 0.64), adjusted as above RR = 0.26 (95% CI 0.10 to 0.65), adjusted as above
Solomon, 1997[405]	Nurses Health Study II, Boston (N = 14 613), prospective	Validated questionnaire (time spent per week in specific activities) administered in 1989	Vigorous vs less vigorous activity	NS, before or after BMI adjustment
Zhang, 2006[406]	Nurses Health Study II, Boston (N = 21 765), prospective	Validated questionnaire (time spent per week in specific activities) administered in 1989	Vigorous vs less vigorous activity Brisk walking vs easy walking TV watching and no vigorous activity vs less TV watching and vigorous activity	RR = 0.77 (95% CI 0.69 to 0.94), adjusted for covariates, including pre-pregnancy BMI RR = 0.66 (95% CI 0.46 to 0.95), adjusted as above RR = 2.3 (95% CI 1.06 to 4.97), adjusted as above

is excess caloric intake relative to caloric expenditure.[385] However, several hypotheses regarding specific nutrients that have been evaluated in adults related to either diabetes risk or insulin resistance, independent of total calories, have also been studied in relation to GDM risk. These include fat, carbohydrate and vitamin C intake.

Fat and carbohydrates

In 1997, Moses *et al.*[386] found that high-fat diets were associated with an increased risk for GDM recurrence in future pregnancies. Women who developed GDM in a follow up pregnancy consumed 41.1% of their diet from fat compared with 33.1% for women who did not develop GDM ($p < 0.001$). However, Wang *et al.*[387] found that women with GDM consumed a lower percentage of their total calories from fat than did age- and BMI-matched women with normal glucose tolerance. However, a lower polyunsaturated/saturated fat ratio had a strong protective effect on GDM

development, independent of pre-pregnancy BMI ($p = 0.0014$).

An observational study of 1698 women enrolled in the Pregnancy, Infection and Nutrition Study in North Carolina, Saldana *et al.*[388] suggested that adding 100 kcal from carbohydrates to the diet was associated with a 9% lower likelihood of developing GDM (as compared with normal glucose tolerance), based on regression modelling including calorie intake constant. Substituting fat for carbohydrates significantly increased the likelihood of developing GDM (as compared with normal glucose tolerance: RR = 1.1, 95% CI 1.02 to 1.10). The predicted probability of GDM was reduced by half with a 10% decrease in dietary fat and a 10% increase in carbohydrate.

Although weight gain has been shown to increase the risk of GDM, there was no effect of diet on weight gain during pregnancy in this population. These data suggest that pregnant women who maintain a diet with a similar macronutrient distribution to that recommended outside the pregnancy (<30% fat and >50% carbohydrate) will reduce their GDM risk. However, more studies are needed to try to identify the composition of carbohydrate and fat that may be associated with a decreased risk, since this was not a randomized intervention.

Vitamin C

Lower maternal plasma ascorbic acid concentrations in early pregnancy were associated with a subsequent increased risk of GDM in a prospective cohort study of women initiating prenatal care before 16 weeks gestation.[393] After adjustment for confounding, women with plasma ascorbic acid <55.9 μmol l^{-1}, the lowest quartile, had a 3.1-fold increased risk of GDM (95% CI 1.0 to 9.7) compared with women whose concentrations were in the upper quartile. Women who consumed <70 mg vitamin C daily experienced a 1.8-fold increased risk of GDM compared with women who consumed higher amounts (95% CI 0.8 to 4.4). These findings suggest the need for RCTs of vitamin C during pregnancy as a possible way to reduce GDM.

Physical activity and prevention of GDM

Epidemiological studies

Several studies suggest that engaging in recreational physical activity before and/or during pregnancy could reduce the risk of GDM. Dye et al.[402] reported that maternal inactivity during pregnancy was associated with a 1.9-fold increased risk of GDM (OR = 1.9, 95% CI 1.2 to 3.1) compared with women who did exercise during this period. However, this association was limited to women with a pre-pregnancy BMI of >33 kg m^{-2}. Thus, obese women who exercised during this period experienced a 47% lower risk (OR = 0.53, 95% CI 0.32 to 0.83).

In a case–control study of 155 women with GDM and 386 controls, Dempsey et al.[403] showed that women who engaged in any physical activity during the year before pregnancy or during the first 20 weeks of pregnancy experienced a halving of the risk of GDM compared with those who did not exercise. Moreover, the greatest benefit was noted in women who engaged in any recreational physical activity both before and during pregnancy in whom there was 60% reduction in GDM. These associations were independent of pre-pregnancy BMI. Even physically inactive women who reported climbing as few as 1–4 flights of stairs per day experienced significant reductions in GDM prevalence, independent of their pre-pregnancy BMI. In addition, the number of hours spent performing recreational activities and the energy expended were also related to a decrease in GDM prevalence.

The same investigators further explored the relationship between recreational physical activity before and during pregnancy and GDM risk in a prospective study.[404] In 1996–2000, 909 normotensive, non-diabetic women in Washington State were questioned during early gestation about physical activity performed during the previous year and 7 days prior to the interview during early pregnancy. Compared with inactive women, those who participated in any physical activity *during the previous year* experienced a 66% risk reduction (RR = 0.34, 95% CI 0.17 to 0.70). This association was attenuated after adjusting for maternal age, race, parity and pre-pregnancy BMI (RR = 0.44, 95% CI 0.21 to 0.91), suggesting that part of the association between physical activity and GDM risk reduction is mediated through changes in BMI. However, as with the previous case–control study, the greatest reduction in GDM risk was seen among women who exercised both before and during pregnancy (adjusted RR = 0.31, 95% CI 0.12 to 0.79).

Solomon et al.[405] queried participants in the Nurses Health Study II at least 1 year prior to a completed singleton pregnancy about their physical activity level (MET score), frequency of vigorous activity (times per week) and walking pace. Women engaged in vigorous activity (four or more times per week versus less than one time per week) or brisk walking (versus casual walking) were less likely to develop GDM, but these associations did not reach statistical significance. This analysis was subsequently extended with more years of follow-up and more detailed measures of physical activity status.[406] This report included 21 765 women in the Nurses Health Study II with at least one singleton pregnancy between 1990 and 1998. Both total and vigorous activity scores were significantly and inversely associated with GDM risk. The inverse associations remained significant (although were attenuated) after controlling for pre-pregnancy BMI. Among women who did not perform vigorous physical activity, brisk walking was associated with a significantly lower GDM risk (RR = 0.66, 95% CI 0.46 to 0.95). This association was attenuated after further adjustment for total physical activity and dietary factors, but was no longer significant after controlling for BMI. Greater time spent watching television was also associated with higher GDM risk.

Clinical studies

Human pregnancy is an insulin-resistant condition,[407] which facilitates the transfer of nutrients from mother to fetus.[408] The insulin resistance of normal pregnancy that occurs in the second and third trimesters is a physiological adaptation that ensures that maternal glucose is adequately delivered to the fetus.[409] Moderate and vigorous physical activity (aerobic dance and walking) are associated with reduced insulin resistance and fat mass during pregnancy.[410] Importantly, Clapp and Capeless reported that the typical acute exercise-induced hyperglycaemia observed outside pregnancy is reversed in healthy pregnant women who exercise regularly,[411] thus supporting the biological plausibility of using physical activity as a disease prevention strategy in pregnant women. Other studies suggest that habitual physical activity may reduce the pregnancy-induced dyslipidaemia common in GDM pregnancies,[412] and it may also be associated with lower plasma leptin concentrations.[399] In addition, Clapp and Kiess demonstrated that the magnitude of pregnancy-associated changes in TNF-α is altered by regular sustained weight-bearing activity during early, mid and late pregnancy[410] TNF-α is a pro-inflammatory cytokine which likely has regulatory influences on insulin resistance and other cytokine levels and has been shown to be related to insulin resistance in pregnancy.[413]

Conclusions

These results from observational and clinical studies are likely to have practical significance in guiding primary prevention efforts for GDM. They also support the concept of adoption by reproductive-aged women of lifestyle changes for which there is already evidence of their effectiveness in preventing type 2 diabetes. GDM (or gestational hyperglycaemia) is an important risk factor for the development of type 2 diabetes over the life course of a woman and it is also the main initiator of an inter-generational vicious cycle by which diabetes begets diabetes. RCTs aimed at preventing GDM are urgently needed to provide further conceptual and practical support for the prevention of diabetes.

Primordial prevention

Primary prevention is directed at reducing the incidence of diabetes at a time when an individual has demonstrable risk factors (such as IGT or obesity), a high-risk strategy. A broader concept is that of 'primordial' prevention, first introduced in the field of cardiovascular disease prevention in the 1980s[426] and conceptualized to be 'upstream' from the individual and aimed at preventing or delaying the emergence of the risk factors altogether as a population strategy. Examples could include social, cultural and market forces that impact on the individual, family and community to alter the occurrence of obesity,

physical activity and dietary patterns that lead to IGT.[427] A related approach is to focus on healthy lifestyles in youth rather than adults, directed at slowing the rate of change of risk factors in addition to lowering the risk of developing 'treatable' risk factors,[428] an approach consistent with the results of numerous life-course studies.[429–436] Even though type 2 diabetes is now more frequent in youth than recognized previously and occurs in all racial/ethnic groups in the United States, it is still relatively uncommon.[437] Thus, intervention studies have not yet been able to explore the primordial modification of the group or individual environment using diabetes as the primary study endpoint. Rather, they have examined the development of the major risk factors for diabetes, including diet and physical activity knowledge and behaviour, obesity (BMI and skinfolds) and occasionally elevated glucose levels, by changing individual, school, worksite or community environments.[438–443]

An early review of community-based interventions from 1990 to 2001 identified six studies in youth and nine in adults, with one study conducted in both.[438] Studies conducted during this time period often focused on process and knowledge outcomes, with limited exploration of obesity and often without control groups.[444] Other common study limitations included short intervention durations, high dropout rates, lack of matching of pre- and post-test data or linking of self-reported lifestyle changes to health outcomes (e.g. BMI, prevalence of IGT).[438] Overall, only two of these 16 studies showed positive effects in the intervention groups.[445,446] A similar review by The Task Force on Community Preventive Services conducted in the published literature from 1986 to 2001 agreed with the conclusion that there was insufficient evidence of effectiveness of combination nutrition and physical activity interventions to prevent or reduce overweight and obesity in school-based interventions to recommend them.[447]

Since this time, a number of additional studies have been reported addressing some of these methodological shortcomings. In three recent systematic reviews,[439,440,487] 49 newer studies were identified that attempted interventions among youth in school settings and included measures of obesity, weight, BMI or skinfolds. Many additional studies have also been published exploring other outcomes.[440] The approaches used usually targeted most or all youth in a grade level regardless of risk and varied from highly focused interventions, such as reduction of carbonated beverage intake[448] or decreased TV watching,[449] to more comprehensive school curriculum, after-school, cafeteria and physical education programme alterations (e.g. [450,451]). Many were aimed at increasing knowledge of nutrition and activity, in addition to behaviour change, and some included secondary interventions of youth found to be at high individual risk. Of the 28 studies included until late 2005, 17 (61%) were found to be effective using the criteria of reduced obesity or less obesity increase among youth in the intervention arm. Virtually all of these studies had concurrent control groups rather than pre–post designs. Similar conclusions were noted by Flodmark *et al.* in an additional recent review.[441] In contrast, two recent reviews of dietary interventions in children and youth to prevent obesity concluded that there was currently lack of sufficient evidence for the use of diet change alone,[442,443] although in a subset of RCTs meeting strict methodological criteria for pooling there was evidence of some benefit of dietary interventions.[443]

One additional large ($N = 1419$) school-based study did not appear in the reviews noted above, though it is useful, since it used capillary glucose levels as a primary outcome measure. The Bienestar Health Program was conducted in 13 San Antonio, Texas, elementary schools (with 14 randomly allocated control schools) and consisted of a health class and physical education curriculum, a family programme, a school cafeteria programme and an after-school health club.[452] The programme was aimed at decreasing dietary saturated fat intake, increasing dietary fibre intake and physical activity. After 7 months of intervention (i.e. one school year), fasting capillary glucose levels decreased in intervention schools and increased in control schools after adjusting for covariates [-2.24 mg dl^{-1} (0.12 mmol l^{-1}); $p = 0.03$]. Self-reported dietary fibre intake ($p = .009$) and fitness scores ($p = .04$) also increased in intervention children and decreased in control children. Percentage of body fat and dietary saturated fat intake did not differ significantly between intervention and control children and weight change was not reported. Follow-up was reasonably complete (85%) and baseline differences were adjusted in the analyses. This programme would have been considered not effective by the reviews since it did not report weight change. However, there was a significant improvement in glucose levels. Whether this was the result of the intervention is not certain, although increases in fitness also occurred and would be consistent with some improvement in glucose metabolism. Further follow-up is planned.

Worksites can provide access to over 60% of the adult population, which makes them potentially important settings in which to implement strategies for reducing the prevalence and burden of overweight and obesity. Worksites allow access to employees in a relatively controlled setting through established channels of communication and social support networks. Incentives for ongoing support of health promoting activities in worksites may be important since such programmes might translate into cost savings for employers, although the evidence on this point is not well established. A systematic review of published studies, conducted on behalf of the Task Force on Community Preventive Services in 2004, found that interventions in the worksite that combined nutrition and physical activity are effective in helping employees lose weight [at least 4 lb (1.8 kg)] and keep it off, at least over the short term (minimum of 6 months). Single-component interventions were less effective. The Task Force recommended use of worksite interventions to help employees control overweight and obesity.[447]

Jenum *et al.* conducted a public health-oriented intervention in one of two low-income health districts in Oslo, Norway.[454] They provided health-related information on increasing physical activity, weight reduction and nutrition change, implemented through the use of low-cost leaflets, reminders of the health benefits of using stairs, local meetings, display stands and mass media communication activities, coordinated by a community organizing committee. Individual counselling during the biannual fitness tests was provided to increase perceived behavioural control for physical activity. Organized walking groups and group sessions for indoor activity were provided at no cost for participants during the entire intervention period. Of the 6140 invited by letter in both districts (22% of whom were migrants to Norway), 48% participated in the baseline measurement survey for CVD and diabetes risk and 67% attended the follow-up survey 3 years later. Overall, there was significantly less weight gain among men and persons >50 years of age in the intervention district compared with control and there were improvements in reported physical activity (9%), triglyceride and cholesterol/HDL ratio, systolic blood pressure, smoking and for men in glucose levels (-0.35 mmol l^{-1}, $p = 0.03$). Further studies are needed to determine if rates of diabetes would be altered by the changes seen, but risk factor changes are in a favourable direction and suggest that this low-cost community intervention was at least partially successful.

A second large community-based study of 3114 individuals aged 31–70 years was conducted over 5 years in the Maastricht region (population 185 000) of The Netherlands as a prospective intervention with a concurrent reference population comparison.[455] Hartslag Limburg was comprised of two strategies: a population-wide strategy aimed at all inhabitants and specifically at low SES groups and a sub-group strategy focused on individuals diagnosed with CVD or multiple physical risk factors for CVD. The intervention, not unlike that in Oslo,[454] integrated collaborating community and health organizations using local health committees. Multiple 'interventions' were implemented, of which almost 600 were 'major' (193 diet, 361 physical activity and nine antismoking), including such things as computer-assisted nutrition education, nutrition education tours in supermarkets, television programmes, food labelling, smoke-free areas, walking and bicycling clubs and campaigns and a stop-smoking campaign, in addition to commercials on local television and radio, newspaper articles and pamphlet distribution. Over the 5 year follow-up, during which over 80% of participants returned, risk factors changed unfavourably in the reference group, whereas changes were less pronounced or absent in the intervention group. The adjusted difference in mean change in risk factors between intervention and reference group was significant ($p < 0.05$) for BMI, $-0.36\,\mathrm{kg\,m^{-2}}$ in men and $-0.25\,\mathrm{kg\,m^{-2}}$ in women, and for waist circumference, $-2.9\,\mathrm{cm}$ in men and $-2.1\,\mathrm{cm}$ in women, and also for systolic blood pressure, serum glucose and total cholesterol in women. The authors acknowledge that participants may have been more motivated than non-participants, but it appears that this broad-based community and high-risk strategy had favourable outcomes over moderately long follow-up periods. Whether these last two studies (Oslo and Maastricht) represent successful community interventions, in part because they involved activated community members (participatory research), also remains unclear, but they seemed to achieve greater results than some of the previous large-scale US studies of community intervention that have been deemed largely unsuccessful (e.g. Stanford Five Cities[456] and the Minnesota Heart Health Program[457,458]).

The evidence available to date suggests that some school, worksite and community-based lifestyle approaches may be effective in changing behaviour at different times in the life course. They may require substantial resources to implement and are often difficult to evaluate. Of interest are the observations that reduced television watching, at least in the United States, may be an important pathway to reduced obesity rates in both youth and adults. Future studies should be done on larger populations over longer periods with careful measurement of outcomes and attention to adherence and intervention modifiers,[459] to ensure that such interventions are effective over longer periods. Such studies should receive high priority given the rapid increases in diabetes and obesity risks that are occurring across the age span. Multifaceted interventions aimed at individuals, communities, advertising and social policy are likely to be required to reverse the obesity trends among youth, analogous to methods used to reverse the smoking

trends of the past three decades.[441,460] Whether a typical RCT will be the best method to evaluate such studies has been questioned and a broader framework for such evaluation has been proposed.[461] Colagiuri *et al.* summarized the broad approaches to prevention of diabetes and concluded that social policy is the key to achieving and sustaining social and physical environments required to achieve widespread reductions in the incidence of diabetes, given the likelihood that such policy will impact large numbers of persons and achieve primordial prevention in many.[460]

Type 2 diabetes prevention studies currently under way

There are several pharmacological primary prevention trials under way that should report results in the near future. These are summarized in Table 5.7 and briefly below. In addition, a number of school-, church- and worksite-based trials have been registered at www.clinicaltrials.gov, but will not be discussed here.

NAVIGATOR (nateglinide and valsartan in impaired glucose tolerance outcomes research)

The Navigator Trial (NCT00097786; www.clinicaltrials.gov) will test the prevention of type 2 diabetes using two novel agents in a 2×2 factorial design with placebo.[463] Nateglinide is an amino acid derivative that reduces post-prandial glycaemia when taken immediately before meals.[464] Valsartan is an angiotensin II receptor blocker, indicated for high blood pressure and heart failure.[465] The goal is to determine whether restoration of early-phase insulin secretion and improvements in insulin sensitivity can arrest decline to type 2 diabetes and prevent cardiovascular disease. The study is being conducted in ~800 centres in 39 countries and has recruited over 9300 people who have IGT and either a history of cardiovascular disease (if aged 50 years or older) or one or more cardiovascular risk factors (if aged 55 years or older). Diabetes incidence will be examined at 3 years (phase 1) and CVD prevention at 5–6 years (phase 2). More than 43 000 patients were screened for enrolment using an OGTT. Of the patients screened, 12% had isolated IFG, 30% had IGT and 28% had undiagnosed diabetes.[466] Recruitment began in 2002 and the trial is expected to continue until 2009.

CANOE (Canadian normoglycaemia outcomes study)

CANOE is a small ($N = 200$) RCT in two Ontario centres including persons with IGT who are receiving

Table 5.7 Primary prevention trials for type 2 diabetes mellitus under way as of 2006

Study, reference, clinical trial registration number	Population	Intervention	Study start	Study end	Comments
DAISI – Dutch Acarbose Trial	Hoorn, The Netherlands; 150 men and women, age 45–70 years, IGT × 2 Outcome: diabetes	Acarbose 50 mg tid or placebo	1998	2003	Papers being prepared?
NAVIGATOR[463] NCT00097786	800 centres in 40 countries; 9300 participants with IGT; age 50 + years with at least one CV disease or 55 + years with at least one CV risk factor Outcomes: diabetes (phase 1); CVD (phase 2)	Nateglinide (60 mg before meals), Valsartan (160 mg daily), both or placebo. 2 × 2 factorial design	2002	2008	Enrolment completed
ACT NOW NCT00220961	600 participants; 8 US sites; IGT by OGTT with 1 other risk factor, follow-up 37 months, with FSIVGTT and Carotid IMT at 45 months Outcome: diabetes by OGTT	Pioglitazone vs placebo	2004	2007	Enrolment completed
CANOE[468] NCT00116922	200 participants; 2 Canadian sites; IGT with 4 year follow-up Outcome: diabetes by OGTT	Lifestyle plus: rosiglitazone 2 mg/metformin 500 mg bid vs placebo	2004	2010	Recruiting
ONTARGET[469,470] NCT00153101	25 620 participants; 730 centres in 40 countries; age 55 + years, prior CVD or diabetes with end organ damage; sub-set without diabetes with OGTT at entry, 2 years, study end; outcome: diabetes	Telmisartan (80 mg day^{-1}) plus ramipril (10 mg day^{-1}) vs ramipril alone	2000–1	2008	Enrolment completed
TRANSCEND[469,470] NCT00153101	6000 participants; 730 centres in 40 countries; age 55 + years, prior CVD or diabetes with end organ damage; sub-set without diabetes with OGTT at entry, 2 years, study end Outcome: diabetes	Telmisartan (80 mg day^{-1}) vs placebo, in ACE-intolerant participants	2000–1	2008–09	Enrolment completed; participants not eligible for ONTARGET due to ACE intolerance are enrolled in TRANSCEND
ŁODZ post GDM NCT00265746	300 women aged 18–50 years with prior GDM in Poland Outcome: diabetes	Lifestyle vs lifestyle plus metformin			2005
Taiwan Lifestyle Trial NCT00257218	600 participants aged 40–60 years with IFG in Taiwan Outcome: diabetes 150 participants with NGT as comparison	Lifestyle vs control	2006		
J-PREDICT NCT00301392	1240 IGT participants aged 30–74 years in Tokyo Outcome: diabetes	Pitavastatin vs placebo	2006	2013	Recruiting

Table 5.7 *(Continued)*

Study, reference, clinical trial registration number	Population	Intervention	Study start	Study end	Comments
Role of Pioglitazone in Preventing Diabetes NCT00276497	6643 people screened, 406 with IGT aged 35–55 years randomized in Chennai India Outcome: diabetes	Pioglitazone vs placebo	2003	2008	Follow-up
RAPSODI NCT00325650	2100 subjects aged 35–75 years with IGT, IFG or both; outcome: diabetes Outcome: diabetes	Rimonabant vs. placebo	2006	2008	Study terminated by company in 2009

a lifestyle intervention plus randomly allocated insulin sensitizing medication (Avandamet®: rosiglitazone 2 mg/metformin 500 mg bid) or placebo.[468] The primary outcome is diabetes occurrence by fasting or OGTT. Average follow-up will be 4 years, with a planned 45% lowering of diabetes risk. Trial results are expected in 2010.

ONTARGET (ongoing telmisartan alone and in combination with ramipril global endpoint trial) and TRANSCEND (telmisartan randomized assessment study in ACE intolerant subjects with cardiovascular disease)

The primary objectives of the ONTARGET trial (NCT00153101; *www.clinicaltrials.gov*) are to determine if the combination of the ARB telmisartan (80 mg day^{-1}) and the ACE inhibitor ramipril (10 mg day^{-1}) is more effective than ramipril alone and if telmisartan is at least as effective as ramipril. The TRANSCEND study will determine if telmisartan is superior to placebo in patients who are intolerant of ACE inhibitors.[469,470] High-risk patients with CVD or diabetes with end-organ damage are being recruited and followed for 3.5–5.5 years in these two parallel RCTs. The primary outcome for both trials is a CVD composite. At baseline, approximately 35–37% of individuals had pre-existing diabetes. The remaining persons without diabetes comprise a pre-specified substudy that underwent an OGTT at 2 years and study end to determine if either drug combination reduces diabetes incidence. Recruitment from 730 centres in 40 countries for ONTARGET ($n = 25\ 620$) was completed in July 2003. Results were recently published for ONTARGET and showed no significant difference between the two drugs in the CVD composite endpoint and no difference in new diabetes risk among those without

diabetes at baseline. Diabetes incidence rates were lowest for combination therapy (6.1/100 person-years) compared with ramipril alone (6.7/100) and telmisartan (7.5/100), although these small differences were not statistically significant. For TRANSCEND, 5776 patients (out of a projected total of 6000) have been recruited (by 10 May 2004). Results were expected in 2008–2009 after 3.5–5.5 years of follow-up.

Lifestyle trials (Łodz, Taiwan)

Two lifestyle trials have been initiated, one in Łodz, Poland, among 300 women with a history of GDM and the other in Taiwan among 600 individuals aged 40–60 years. In the post-GDM trial, metformin or placebo will be added to lifestyle.

J-predict (pitavastatin)

A primary prevention trial of the lipid-lowering stain pitavastatin was started in Tokyo in 2006. Estimated recruitment will be 1240 participants aged 30–74 years with IGT who will be followed for OGTT diabetes and changes in lipid and CVD endpoints. Limited details of the protocol are available. The trial is scheduled to end in 2013.

Role of pioglitazone in preventing diabetes (Chennai, India)

A double-blind randomized prospective study of pioglitazone was begun in 2003 (enrolment completed in May 2005) to determine if the drug (versus placebo) would delay the onset of OGTT diabetes over 3 years among non-obese participants with IGT (NCT00276497; www.clinicaltrials.gov). A total of 6643 individuals were screened and 406 participants of both sexes aged 35–55 years were randomized either to pioglitazone or placebo. All participants were given advice on diet, exercise and benefits of lifestyle modification. The authors have recently reported the three year results of this trial.[488] The cumulative incidence of diabetes was not significantly different in the pioglitazone treated group compared with placebo (unadjusted HR 1.084 [95% CI 0.75–1.56], p = 0.665). These results are at odds with those seen in the other trials that have reported use of thiazolidediones (DPP, DREAM).

RAPSODI (rimonabant in prediabetic subjects to delay onset of type 2 diabetes)

Sanofi-Aventis has undertaken a weight loss, primary diabetes prevention trial of the selective cannabinoid CB1 receptor antagonist rimonabant (NCT00325650; www.clinicaltrials.gov). The trial, started in 2006, recruited 2100 people aged 35–75 years with IFG, IGT or both and is following individuals for OGTT diabetes, among other outcomes.

Prevention strategies

Type 2 diabetes has multiple risk factors and, at the current state of knowledge, is regarded as a heterogeneous disorder. Interventions can be targeted at the multiple risk factors, either in the entire population or in high-risk individuals, perhaps using both approaches.[11] Given the widespread and increasing prevalence of obesity in the United States and other countries,[471,472] a population-based strategy to reduce obesity is likely to lead to widespread benefits for diabetes and related disorders.

The evidence to date suggests that obesity prevention or reduction may be effective in school and worksite locations, with emerging evidence from a handful of community studies. Unfortunately, the longer term impact on obesity is an area that needs further work, especially given the strong environmental components working to reduce physical activity and increase energy intake in Western societies.[473] The studies of obesity prevention in children must be confirmed and expanded. Public policy must be addressed and changes made in order to increase activity, maintain weight for adults at near-normal levels and induce weight loss for overweight and obese people.[474] Such strategies echo the recommendations of Joslin nearly 90 years ago.[1]

A high-risk strategy involves the identification of persons with levels of pre-diabetic risk factors that place them at high risk of developing diabetes in the near future.[11] This is the approach that was taken in all of the larger clinical trials recently completed. These approaches have now been shown to work for

lifestyle change, which has been replicated in four studies in very different populations (China,[62] Finland,[73] United States,[78–80] India[87] and Japan[89]). Results for metformin have been significant in two[80,87] of three trials, with consistent but non-significant results in one smaller study.[218] Further details are required to understand more fully the acarbose results, which were positive in two studies.[247,254]

With efficacy of lifestyle changes established, it remains to be determined what the most efficient, cost-effective strategies are to identify and intervene in such high-risk individuals. Longer term follow-up is needed to determine the duration of the effects of lifestyle change, before beginning to understand the impacts on chronic complications and mortality. Pharmacological treatment approaches in high-risk individuals who are otherwise well must be carefully considered from a side-effect and cost standpoint, and also for their efficacy. High-risk approaches must complement a wider public health approach aimed at general reduction of obesity and physical inactivity, since it is not possible to medically treat all high-risk individuals.

A number of questions in the high-risk strategy remain unanswered. Although it is now known that diabetes incidence can be reduced among persons with IFG or IGT, it is not clear whether there are additional subsets of high-risk individuals among those with IFG or IGT who can be identified. Such people might include those with altered insulin sensitivity[63] or higher levels of obesity, who may respond to specific subinterventions. The evidence available suggests that weight loss is important if glucose levels are to be lowered; however, physical activity improves insulin action, even in the absence of weight loss. The effect of these different components of risk over the longer term remains largely unknown. Will it be useful to identify high-risk patterns of genes in individuals to target for intervention? With evolving technology, it might be cost-effective to identify genetically high-risk people for intervention in the near future.

Because of the success of studies aimed at lifestyle change, plans have been developed to promote diabetes prevention in health systems and populations. In Finland, a comprehensive three part strategy has been developed.[475] A *population strategy* promotes the health of the entire population by means of nutritional interventions and increased physical activity so that the risk factors for type 2 diabetes, such as obesity and metabolic syndrome, are reduced in all age groups, including both society-oriented measures and measures targeting individuals with the aim of preventing obesity. A high-risk strategy targets individuals with a particularly high risk of developing type 2 diabetes.

This strategy provides a systematic model for the screening, education and monitoring of people at risk. A strategy for early diagnosis and management is directed at individuals with newly diagnosed type 2 diabetes, to help provide systematic treatment to prevent diabetic complications. This comprehensive approach requires cooperation between many players to promote healthy nutrition and physical activity, and also to improve the Finnish health-care system and restructure health-promotion activities. All current health policy strategies, programmes and projects will be used in implementation, in addition to the services of non-governmental organizations involved in public health, nutrition and physical education.

Conclusion

The available data now provide a firm answer that type 2 diabetes can be delayed or prevented in high-risk individuals using lifestyle change and selected pharmacological agents.

With the current level of information, it is reasonable to recommend a programme of regular moderate physical activity, weight maintenance or modest weight loss for overweight people and a low-fat, calorie-moderated diet, with smoking cessation. In addition, people at high risk should have specific risk factors for cardiovascular disease treated (e.g. lipids, blood pressure).

GDM (or gestational hyperglycaemia) is an important risk factor for the development of type 2 diabetes over the life course of a woman and it is also the main initiator of an inter-generational vicious cycle by which diabetes becomes self-perpetuating in populations. Among women of reproductive age, lifestyle changes for which there is already evidence of their effectiveness in preventing type 2 diabetes should be adopted, which may also reduce the risk of GDM during pregnancy, though clinical trial evidence is not available to support this recommendation and RCTs aimed at preventing GDM are urgently needed.

References

1 Joslin EP. The prevention of diabetes mellitus. *JAMA* 1921;**76**:79–84.

2 Liberopoulos EN, Tsouli S, Mikhailidis DP, Elisaf MS. Preventing type 2 diabetes in high risk patients: an overview of lifestyle and pharmacological measures. *Curr Drug Targets* 2006;**7**(2):211–228.

3 Inzucchi SE, Sherwin RS. The prevention of type 2 diabetes mellitus. *Endocrinol Metab Clin North Am* 2005;**34**(1):199.

4 LaMonte MJ, Blair SN, Church TS. Physical activity and diabetes prevention. *J Appl Physiol* 2005;**99**(3):1205–1213.

5 Chiasson JL, Rabasa-Lhoret R. Prevention of type 2 diabetes: insulin resistance and beta-cell function. *Diabetes* 2004;**53**(Suppl 3): S34–S38.

6 Davies MJ, Tringham JR, Troughton J, Khunti KK. Prevention of Type 2 diabetes mellitus. A review of the evidence and its application in a UK setting. *Diabet Med* 2004; **21**(5):403–414.

7 Costacou T, Mayer-Davis EJ. Nutrition and prevention of type 2 diabetes. *Annu Rev Nutr* 2003;**23**:147–170.

8 Kanaya AM, Narayan KM. Prevention of type 2 diabetes: data from recent trials. *Primary Care Clin Office Pract* 2003; **30**(3):511–526.

9 Paffenbarger RS Jr, Lee IM, Kampert JB. Physical activity in the prevention of non-insulin-dependent diabetes mellitus. *World Rev Nutr Diet* 1997;**82**:210–218.

10 Helmrich SP, Ragland DR, Paffenbarger RS Jr. Prevention of non-insulin-dependent diabetes mellitus with physical activity. *Med Sci Sports Exerc* 1994;**26**(7):824–830.

11 Tuomilehto J, Knowler WC, Zimmet P. Primary prevention of non-insulin-dependent diabetes mellitus. *Diabetes Metab Rev* 1992;**8**:339–353.

12 King H, Dowd JE. Primary prevention of type 2 (non-insulin-dependent) diabetes mellitus. *Diabetologia* 1990; **33**(1):3–8.

13 Zimmet P. The prevention and control of diabetes: An epidemiological perspective. *J Med Assoc Thai* 1987; **70**(Suppl 2): 30–35.

14 Hamman RF. Prevention of type 2 diabetes mellitus. In: *The Evidence Base for Diabetes Care* (eds Williams RL, Tuomilehto J, Herman WH,), John Wiley and Sons, Ltd, Chichester, 2002.

15 American Diabetes Association. Economic costs of diabetes in the U.S. in Diabetes Care 2002. 2003;**26**(3):917–932.

16 WHO Study Group. *Diabetes Mellitus – Technical Report Series 727*, World Health Organization, Geneva, 1985.

17 American Diabetes Association. Report of the Expert Committee on the Diagnosis and Classification of Diabetes Mellitus. *Diabetes Care* **20**(7):1997;1183–1197.

18 Edelstein SL, Knowler WC, Bain RP *et al.* Predictors of progression from impaired glucose tolerance to non-insulin-dependent diabetes mellitus: an analysis of six prospective studies. *Diabetes* **46**:1997;701–710.

19 Expert Committee on the Diagnosis, Classification of Diabetes Mellitus. Report of the Expert Committee on the Diagnosis and Classification of Diabetes Mellitus. *Diabetes Care* 2003;**26**(90001):5S–20S.

20 Dabelea D, Ma Y, Knowler WC, *et al.* Autoimmunity and prevention of type 2 diabetes: The Diabetes Prevention Program (DPP). *Diabetes* 2006;**55**(Suppl 1): LB–20.

21 Harris MI., Classification, diagnostic criteria and screening for diabetes. In: *Diabetes in America*, 2nd edn; (ed. National Diabetes Data Group), NIDDK No. 95-1468, National Institutes of Health, Bethesda, MD, 1995, pp. 15–35.

22 Ratner RE. Clinical review 47. Gestational diabetes mellitus: after three international workshops do we know how to diagnose and manage it yet? *J Clin Endocrinol Metab* 1993; **77**(1):1–4.

23 Jarrett RJ. Gestational diabetes: a non-entity? *BMJ* 1993; **306**(6869):37–38.

24 Buchanan TA, Kjos, SL. Gestational diabetes: risk or myth? *J Clin Endocrinol Metab* 1999;**84**(6):1854–1857.

25 Kjos SL, Buchanan TA. Gestational diabetes mellitus. *N Engl J Med* 1999;**341**(23):1749–1756.

26 Dornhorst A, Chan, SP. The elusive diagnosis of gestational diabetes. *Diabet Med* 1998;**15**(1):7–10.

27 Ferrara A, Hedderson MM, Quesenberry CP, Selby JV. Prevalence of gestational diabetes mellitus detected by the national diabetes data group or the Carpenter and Coustan plasma glucose thresholds. *Diabetes Care* 2002;**25**(9): 1625–1630.

28 Hanna FW, Peters, JR. Screening for gestational diabetes; past, present and future. *Diabet Med* 2002;**19**(5):351–358.

29 American College of Obstetricians and Gynecologists. ACOG Practice Bulletin. Assessment of risk factors for preterm birth. Clinical management guidelines for obstetrician-gynecologists. Number 31, October 2001. (Replaces Technical Bulletin number 206, June 1995; Committee Opinion number 172, May 1996; Committee Opinion number 187, September 1997; Committee Opinion number 198, February 1998; and Committee Opinion number 251, January 2001). *Obstet Gynecol* 2001; **98** (4): 709–716.

30 National Diabetes Data Group. Classification and diagnosis of diabetes mellitus and other categories of glucose intolerance. *Diabetes* 1979;**28**:1039–1057.

31 O'Sullivan JB, Mahan CM. Criteria for the oral glucose tolerance test in pregnancy. *Diabetes* 1964;**13**:278–285.

32 Carpenter MW, Coustan DR. Criteria for screening tests for gestational diabetes. *Am J Obstet Gynecol* 1982;**144**(7):768–773.

33 Magee MS, Walden CE, Benedetti TJ, Knopp RH. Influence of diagnostic criteria on the incidence of gestational diabetes and perinatal morbidity. *JAMA* 1993;**269**(5):609–615.

34 Sacks DA, Abu-Fadil S, Greenspoon JS, Fotheringham N. Do the current standards for glucose tolerance testing in pregnancy represent a valid conversion of O'Sullivan's original criteria? *Am J Obstet Gynecol* 1989;**161**(3):638–641.

35 Sermer M, Naylor CD, Gare DJ *et al.* Impact of increasing carbohydrate intolerance on maternal–fetal outcomes in 3637 women without gestational diabetes. The Toronto Tri-Hospital Gestational Diabetes Project. *Am J Obstet Gynecol* 1995;**173**(1):146–156.

36 Leikin EL, Jenkins JH, Pomerantz GA, Klein L. Abnormal glucose screening tests in pregnancy: a risk factor for fetal macrosomia. *Obstet Gynecol* 1987;**69**(4):570–573.

37 Harlass FE, McClure GB, Read JA, Brady K. Use of a standard preparatory diet for the oral glucose tolerance test. Is it necessary? *J Reprod Med* 1991;**36**(2):147–150.

38 Murakami K, Okubo H, Sasaki S. Effect of dietary factors on incidence of type 2 diabetes: a systematic review of cohort studies. *J Nutr Sci Vitaminol* 2005;**51**(4):292–310.

39 Schulze M, Hu F. Primary prevention of diabetes: what can be done and how much can be prevented? *Annu Rev Public Health* 2005;**26**:445–467.

40 Wareham NJ, van Sluijs EM, Ekelund U. Physical activity and obesity prevention: a review of the current evidence. *Proc Nutr Soc* 2005;**64**(2):229–247.

41 Parillo M, Riccardi G. Diet composition and the risk of type 2 diabetes: epidemiological and clinical evidence. *Br J Nutr* 2004;**92**(1):7–19.

42 Swinburn BA, Caterson I, Seidell JC, James WPT. Diet, nutrition and the prevention of excess weight gain and obesity; review. *Public Health Nutr* 2004;**7**(1A):123–146.

43 van Dam RM. The epidemiology of lifestyle and risk for type 2 diabetes. *Eur J Epidemiol* 2003;**18**(12):1115–1125.

44 Rewers M, Hamman RF. Risk factors for Non-insulin-dependent diabetes. In: *Diabetes in America – 1995*; (ed. Harris MI) US Government Printing Office, Washington, DC, 1995.

45 Hamman RF. Genetic and environmental determinants of non-insulin-dependent diabetes mellitus (NIDDM). *Diabetes Metab Rev* 1992;**8**:287–338.

46 Eriksson KF, Lindgarde F. Poor physical fitness and impaired early insulin response but late hyperinsulinaemia, as predictors of NIDDM in middle-aged Swedish men. *Diabetologia* 1996;**39**(5):573–579.

47 Eriksson KF, Lindgarde F. No excess 12-year mortality in men with impaired glucose tolerance who participated in the Malmo Preventive Trial with diet and exercise. *Diabetologia* 1998;**41**(9):1010–1016.

48 Jarrett RJ, Keen H, Fuller JH, McCartney M. Treatment of borderline diabetes: controlled trial using carbohydrate restriction and phenformin. *BMJ* 1977;**ii**:861–865.

49 Jarrett RJ, Keen H, Fuller JH, McCartney M. Worsening to diabetes in men with impaired glucose intolerance ('borderline diabetes'). *Diabetologia* 1979;**16**:25–30.

50 Jarrett RJ, Keen H, McCartney P. The Whitehall Study: ten year follow-up report on men with impaired glucose tolerance with reference to worsening to diabetes and predictors of death. *Diabetic Med* 1984;**1**:279–283.

51 Cederholm J. Short-term treatment of glucose intolerance in middle-aged subjects by diet, exercise and sulfonylurea. *Uppsala J Med Sci* 1985;**90**:229–242.

52 WHO Expert Committee on Diabetes Mellitus. *WHO Expert Committee on Diabetes Mellitus Second Report.* World Health Organization, Geneva, 1980.

53 Page RCL, Harnden KE, Cook JTE, Turner RC. Can life-styles of subjects with impaired glucose tolerance be changed? A feasibility study. *Diabetic Med* 1992;**9**:562–566.

54 Singh RB, Singh NK, Rastogi SS, Mani UV, Niaz MA. Effects of diet and lifestyle changes on atherosclerotic risk factors after 24 weeks on the Indian Diet Heart Study. *Am J Cardiol* 1993;**71**(15):1283–1288.

55 Hellenius ML, Brismar KE, Berglund BH, de Faire UH. Effects on glucose tolerance, insulin secretion, insulin-like growth factor 1 and its binding protein, IGFBP-1, in a randomized controlled diet and exercise study in healthy, middle-aged men. *J Intern Med* 1995;**238**(2):121–130.

56 Hellenius ML, de Faire U, Berglund B, Hamsten A, Krakau I. Diet and exercise are equally effective in reducing risk for cardiovascular disease. Results of a randomized controlled study in men with slightly to moderately raised cardiovascular risk factors. *Atherosclerosis* 1993;**103**(1):81–91.

57 Colman E, Katzel LI, Rogus E, Coon P, Muller D, Goldberg AP. Weight loss reduces abdominal fat and improves insulin action in middle- aged and older men with impaired glucose tolerance. *Metabolism* 1995;**44**(11):1502–1508.

58 Holme I. The Oslo Diet and Exercise Study (ODES): design and objectives. *Control Clin Trials* 1993;**14**:229–243.

59 Anderssen SA, Hjermann I, Urdal P, Torjesen PA, Holme I. Improved carbohydrate metabolism after physical training and dietary intervention in individuals with the 'atherothrombogenic syndrome'. Oslo Diet and Exercise Study (ODES). A randomized trial. *J Intern Med* 1996;**240**(4): 203–209.

60 Anderssen SA, Holme I, Urdal P, Hjermann I. Associations between central obesity and indexes of hemostatic, carbohydrate and lipid metabolism. Results of a 1-year intervention from the Oslo Diet and Exercise Study. *Scand J Med Sci Sports* 1998;**8**(2):109–115.

61 Torjesen PA, Birkeland KI, Anderssen SA, Hjermann I, Holme I, Urdal P. Lifestyle changes may reverse development of the insulin resistance syndrome. The Oslo Diet and Exercise Study: a randomized trial. *Diabetes Care* 1997;**20**(1): 26–31.

62 Pan XR, Li GW, Hu YH et al. Effects of diet and exercise in preventing NIDDM in people with impaired glucose tolerance. The Da Qing IGT and Diabetes Study. *Diabetes Care* 1997;**20**(4):537–544.

63 Li G, Hu Y, Yang W, et al. Effects of insulin resistance and insulin secretion on the efficacy of interventions to retard development of type 2 diabetes mellitus: the DA Qing IGT and Diabetes Study. *Diabetes Res Clin Pract* 2002;**58**(3): 193–200.

64 Dyson PA, Hammersley MS, Morris RJ, Holman RR, Turner RC. The Fasting Hyperglycaemia Study: II. Randomized controlled trial of reinforced healthy-living advice in subjects with increased but not diabetic fasting plasma glucose. *Metabolism* 1997;**46**(12 Suppl 1): 50–55.

65 Hammersley MS, Meyer LC, Morris RJ, Manley SE, Turner RC, Holman RR. The Fasting Hyperglycaemia Study: I. Subject identification and recruitment for a non-insulin-dependent diabetes prevention trial. *Metabolism* 1997;**46** (12 Suppl 1): 44–49.

66 Wing RR, Venditti E, Jakicic JM, Polley BA, Lang W. Lifestyle intervention in overweight individuals with a family history of diabetes. *Diabetes Care* 1998;**21**(3):350–359.

67 Eriksson KF, Lindgarde F. Prevention of type 2 (non-insulin-dependent) diabetes mellitus by diet and physical exercise. The 6-year Malmo feasibility study. *Diabetologia* 1991;**34**:891–898.

68 Katzel LI, Bleecker ER, Colman EG, Rogus EM, Sorkin JD, Goldberg AP. Effects of weight loss vs aerobic exercise training on risk factors for coronary disease in health, obese, middle-aged and older men: a randomized controlled trial. *JAMA* 1995;**274**(24):1915–1921.

69 Nilsson PM, Lindholm LH, Schersten BF. Life style changes improve insulin resistance in hyperinsulinaemic subjects: a one-year intervention study of hypertensives and normotensives in Dalby. *J Hypertens* 1992;**10**:1071–1078.

70 Bergenstal R, Monk A, Upham P, Nelson JB, List S. The Community Diabetes Prevention Project (CDPP): identification of the natural history of the insulin resistance syndrome (IRS) and whether progression to Type 2 diabetes can be altered – year 2 data. *Diabetes* 1998;**47**(Suppl 1): abstracts.

71 Wein P, Beischer N, Harris C, Permezel M. A trial of simple versus intensified dietary modification for prevention of progression to diabetes mellitus in women with impaired glucose tolerance. *Aust N Z J Obstet Gynaecol* 1999;**39**(2): 162–166.

72 Eriksson J, Lindstrom J, Valle T, et al. Prevention of Type II diabetes in subjects with impaired glucose tolerance: the Diabetes Prevention Study (DPS) in Finland – study design and 1-year interim report on the feasibility of the lifestyle intervention programme. *Diabetologia* 1999;**42**(7):793–801.

73 Tuomilehto J, Lindstrom J, Eriksson JG et al. Prevention of type 2 diabetes mellitus by changes in lifestyle among subjects with impaired glucose tolerance. *N Engl J Med* 2001;**344**(18):1343–1350.

74 Lindstrom J, Peltonen M, Tuomilehto J. Lifestyle strategies for weight control: Experience from the Finnish Diabetes Prevention Study. *Proc Nutr Soc* 2005;**64**(1):81–88.

75 Laaksonen DE, Lindstrom J, Lakka TA, et al. Physical activity in the prevention of type 2 diabetes: The Finnish *Diabetes* Prevention Study. *Diabetes* 2005;**54**(1):158–165.

76 Uusitupa M, Lindi V, Louheranta A, Salopuro T, Lindstrom J, Tuomilehto J. Long-term improvement in insulin sensitivity by changing lifestyles of people with impaired glucose tolerance: 4-year results from the Finnish Diabetes Prevention Study. *Diabetes* 2003;**52**(10):2532–2538.

77 Hamalainen H, Ronnemaa T, Virtanen A, et al. Improved fibrinolysis by an intensive lifestyle intervention in subjects with impaired glucose tolerance. The Finnish Diabetes Prevention Study. *Diabetologia* 2005;**48**(11):2248–2253.

78 The Diabetes Prevention Program Research Group. The Diabetes Prevention Program. Design and methods for a clinical trial in the prevention of type 2 diabetes. *Diabetes Care* 1999;**22**(4):623–634.

79 The Diabetes Prevention Program Research Group. The Diabetes Prevention Program. Baseline characteristics of the randomized cohort. *Diabetes Care* 2000;**23**(11):1619–1629.

80 The Diabetes Prevention Program Research Group. Reduction in the incidence of type 2 diabetes with lifestyle intervention or metformin. *N Engl J Med* 2002;**346**(6):393–403.

81 Wing RR, Hamman RF, Bray GA, et al. Achieving weight and activity goals among diabetes prevention program lifestyle participants. *Obes Res* 2004;**12**(9):1426–1434.

82 Hamman RF, Wing RR, Edelstein SL, et al. Effect of weight loss with lifestyle intervention on risk of diabetes. *Diabetes Care* 2006;**29**(9):2102–2107.

83 The Diabetes Prevention Program Research Group. Impact of intensive lifestyle and metformin therapy on cardiovascular disease risk factors in the Diabetes Prevention Program. *Diabetes Care* 2005;**28**(4):888–894.

84 Haffner S, Temprosa M, Crandall J, et al. Intensive lifestyle intervention or metformin on inflammation and coagulation in participants with impaired glucose tolerance. *Diabetes* 2005;**54**(5):1566–1572.

85 Orchard TJ, Temprosa M, Goldberg R, et al. The effect of metformin and intensive lifestyle intervention on the metabolic syndrome: the Diabetes Prevention Program randomized trial. *Ann Intern Med* 2005;**142**(8):611–619.

86 Carnethon MR, Prineas RJ, Temprosa M, Zhang ZM, Uwaifo G, Molitch ME. The association among autonomic nervous system function, incident diabetes and intervention arm in the diabetes prevention program. *Diabetes Care* 2006;**29**(4):914–919.

87 Ramachandran A, Snehalatha C, Mary S, et al. The Indian Diabetes Prevention Programme shows that lifestyle modification and metformin prevent type 2 diabetes in Asian Indian subjects with impaired glucose tolerance (IDPP-1). *Diabetologia* 2006;**49**(2):289–297.

88 Ramachandran A, Snehalatha C, Vijay V. Low risk threshold for acquired diabetogenic factors in Asian Indians. *Diabetes Res Clin Pract* 2004;**65**(3):189–195.

89 Kosaka K, Noda M, Kuzuya T. Prevention of type 2 diabetes by lifestyle intervention: a Japanese trial in IGT males. *Diabetes Res Clin Pract* 2005;**67**(2):152–162.

90 Hjermann I, Leren P, Norman N, Helgeland A, Holme I. Serum insulin response to oral glucose load during a dietary intervention trial in healthy coronary high risk men: the Oslo study. *Scand J Clin Lab Invest* 1980;**40**(1):89–94.

91 Wood DA, Kinmonth AL, Davies GA, et al Randomised controlled trial evaluating cardiovascular screening and intervention in general practice: principal results of British family heart study. *BMJ* 1994;**308**(6924):313–320.

92 Miettinen TA, Huttunen JK, Naukkarinen V, *et al*. Multifactorial primary prevention of cardiovascular diseases in middle-aged men. Risk factor changes, incidence and mortality. *JAMA* 1985;**254**(15):2097–2102.

93 Davey Smith G, Bracha Y, Svendsen KH, *et al*. Incidence of type 2 diabetes in the Randomized Multiple Risk Factor Intervention Trial. *Ann Intern Med* 2005;**142**(5):313–322.

94 Oldroyd JC, Unwin NC, White M, Mathers JC, Alberti KG. Randomised controlled trial evaluating lifestyle interventions in people with impaired glucose tolerance. *Diabetes Res Clin Pract* 2006;**72**:117–127.

95 Wenying L, Lixiang L, Jinwu Q, *et al*. The preventive effect of acarbose and metformin on the progression to diabetes mellitus in the IGT population: a 3 year multicenter prospective study. *Chin J Endocrinol Metab* 2001;**17**:131–136.

96 Lindahl B, Nilsson TK, Jansson JH, Asplund K, Hallmans G. Improved fibrinolysis by intense lifestyle intervention. A randomized trial in subjects with impaired glucose tolerance. *J Intern Med* 1999;**246**(1):105–112.

97 Mensink M, Feskens EJ, Saris WH, De Bruin TW, Blaak EE. Study on Lifestyle Intervention and Impaired Glucose Tolerance Maastricht (SLIM): preliminary results after one year. *Int J Obesity Relat Metab Disorders: J Int Assoc Study Obesity* 2003;**27**(3):377–384.

98 Mensink M, Blaak EE, Corpeleijn E, Saris WH, De Bruin TW, Feskens EJ. Lifestyle intervention according to general recommendations improves glucose tolerance. *Obesity Res* 2003;**11**(12):1588–1596.

99 Corpeleijn E, Feskens JM, Jansen EHJM, *et al*. Improvements in glucose tolerance and insulin sensitivity after lifestyle intervention are related to changes in serum fatty acid profile and desaturase activities: the SLIM study. *Diabetologia* 2006;**49**(10):2392–2401.

100 Yamaoka K, Tango T. Efficacy of lifestyle education to prevent type 2 diabetes: a meta-analysis of randomized controlled trials. *Diabetes Care* 2005;**28**(11):2780–2786.

101 Simkin-Silverman LR, Wing RR, Boraz MA, Meilahn EN, Kuller LH. Maintenance of cardiovascular risk factor changes among middle-aged women in a lifestyle intervention trial. *Womens Health* 1998;**4**(3):255–271.

102 Kuller LH, Simkin-Silverman LR, Wing RR, Meilahn EN, Ives DG. Women's Healthy Lifestyle Project: a randomized clinical trial: results at 54 months. *Circulation* 2001;**103**(1):32–37.

103 Simkin-Silverman LR, Wing RR, Boraz MA, Kuller LH. Lifestyle intervention can prevent weight gain during menopause: results from a 5-year randomized clinical trial. *Ann Behav Med* 2003;**26**(3):212–220.

104 Swinburn BA, Woollard GA, Chang EC, Wilson MR. Effects of reduced-fat diets consumed *ad libitum* on intake of nutrients, particularly antioxidant vitamins. *J Am Diet Assoc* 1999;**99**(11):1400–1405.

105 Swinburn BA, Metcalf PA, Ley SJ. Long-term (5-year) effects of a reduced-fat diet intervention in individuals with glucose intolerance. *Diabetes Care* 2001;**24**(4):619–624.

106 Watanabe M, Yamaoka K, Yokotsuka M, Tango T. Randomized controlled trial of a new dietary education program to prevent type 2 diabetes in a high-risk group of Japanese male workers. *Diabetes Care* 2003;**26**(12):3209–3214.

107 Liao D, Asberry PJ, Shofer JB, *et al*. Improvement of BMI, body composition and body fat distribution with lifestyle modification in Japanese Americans with impaired glucose tolerance. *Diabetes Care* 2002;**25**(9):1504–1510.

108 Carr DB, Utzschneider KM, Boyko EJ *et al*. A reduced-fat diet and aerobic exercise in Japanese Americans with impaired glucose tolerance decreases intra-abdominal fat and improves insulin sensitivity but not beta-cell function. *Diabetes* 2005;**54**(2):340–347.

109 Brekke HK, Jansson PA, Lenner RA. Long-term (1- and 2-year) effects of lifestyle intervention in type 2 diabetes relatives. *Diabetes Res Clin Pract* 2005;**70**(3):225–234.

110 Avenell A, Broom J, Brown TJ, *et al*. Systematic review of the long-term effects and economic consequences of treatments for obesity and implications for health improvement. *Health Technol Assess* 2004;**8**(21):1–182.

111 Norris SL, Zhang X, Avenell A, Gregg E, Schmid CH, Lau J. Long-term non-pharmacological weight loss interventions for adults with prediabetes. *Cochrane Database Syst Rev* 2005;(2):CD005270.

112 Herman WH, Brandle M, Zhang P, *et al*. Costs associated with the primary prevention of type 2 diabetes mellitus in the diabetes prevention program. *Diabetes Care* 2003;**26**(1):36–47.

113 Diabetes Prevention Program Research Group. Within-trial cost-effectiveness of lifestyle intervention or metformin for the primary prevention of type 2 diabetes. *Diabetes Care* 2003;**26**(9):2518–2523.

114 Klonoff DC, Schwartz DM. An economic analysis of interventions for diabetes. *Diabetes Care* 2000;**23**(3):390–404.

115 Palmer AJ, Roze S, Valentine WJ, Spinas GA, Shaw JE, Zimmet PZ. Intensive lifestyle changes or metformin in patients with impaired glucose tolerance: modeling the long-term health economic implications of the diabetes prevention program in Australia, France, Germany. Switzerland and the United Kingdom. *Clin Ther* 2004;**26**(2): 304–321.

116 Herman WH, Hoerger TJ, Brandle M, *et al*. The cost-effectiveness of lifestyle modification or metformin in preventing type 2 diabetes in adults with impaired glucose tolerance. *Ann Intern Med* 2005;**142**(5):323–332.

117 Eddy DM, Schlessinger L, Kahn R. Clinical outcomes and cost-effectiveness of strategies for managing people at high risk for diabetes. *Ann Intern Med* 2005;**143**(4):251–264.

118 Engelgau MM. Trying to predict the future for people with diabetes: a tough but important task. *Ann Intern Med* 2005;**143**(4):301–302.

119 Hu FB, Manson JE, Stampfer MJ, *et al*. Diet, lifestyle and the risk of type 2 diabetes mellitus in women. *N Engl J Med* 2001;**345**(11):790–797.

120 Kriska AM, Blair SN, Pereira MA. The potential role of physical activity in the prevention of non-insulin-dependent

diabetes mellitus: the epidemiological evidence. *Exerc Sport Sci Rev* 1994;**22**:121–143.

121 Mayer EJ, Alderman BW, Regensteiner JG et al. Physical-activity-assessment measures compared in a biethnic rural population: the San Luis Valley *Diabetes* Study. *Am J Clin Nutr* 1991;**53**:812–820.

122 Kriska AM, Bennett PH. An epidemiological perspective of the relationship between physical activity and NIDDM: from activity assessment to intervention. *Diabetes Metab Rev* 1992;**8**:355–372.

123 Pate RR, Pratt M, Blair SN, *et al.* Physical activity and public health. A recommendation from the Centers for Disease Control and Prevention and the American College of Sports Medicine. *JAMA* 1995;**273**(5):402–407.

124 Spelsberg A, Manson JE. Physical activity in the treatment and prevention of diabetes. *Compr Ther* 1995;**21**(10):559–562.

125 Blair SN, Kohl HW, Gordon NF, Paffenbarger RS Jr. How much physical activity is good for health? *Annu Rev Public Health* 1992;**13**:99–126.

126 Blair SN, Horton E, Leon AS, *et al.* Physical activity, nutrition and chronic disease. *Med Sci Sports Exerc* 1996;**28**(3): 335–349.

127 NIH Consensus Development Panel on Physical Activity, Cardiovascular Health. Physical activity and cardiovascular health. *NIH Consensus Statement* 1995;**13**(3):1–33.

128 Bassuk SS, Manson JE. Epidemiological evidence for the role of physical activity in reducing risk of type 2 diabetes and cardiovascular disease. *J Appl Physiol* 2005;**99**(3): 1193–1204.

129 Kriska A, Can a physically active lifestyle prevent type 2 diabetes? *Exerc Sport Sci Rev* 2003;**31**(3):132–137.

130 Gurwitz JH, Field TS, Glynn RJ, *et al.* Risk factors for non-insulin-dependent diabetes mellitus requiring treatment in the elderly. *J Am Geriatr Soc* 1994;**42**(12):1235–1240.

131 Kriska AM, Edelstein SL, Hamman RF, *et al.* Physical activity in individuals at risk for diabetes: Diabetes Prevention Program. *Med Sci Sports Exerc* 2006;**38**(5):826–832.

132 McAuley KA, Williams SM, Mann JI, *et al.* Intensive lifestyle changes are necessary to improve insulin sensitivity: a randomized controlled trial. *Diabetes Care* 2002;**25**(3): 445–452.

133 Mann JI, Houston A. The aetiology of non-insulin dependent diabetes mellitus. In: *Diabetes in Epidemiological Perspective* (eds Mann JI, Pyorala K, Teuscher A,) Churchill Livingstone, Edinburgh, 1983;pp. 122–164.

134 West KM. *Epidemiology of Diabetes and its Vascular Lesions*, Elsevier Biomedical Press, New York, 1978.

135 West KM. Prevention and therapy of diabetes mellitus. *Nutr Rev* 1975;**33**(7):193–198.

136 West KM. Diet and diabetes. *Postgrad Med* 1976;**60**(9): 209–216.

137 Willett WC. Is dietary fat a major determinant of body fat? *Am J Clin Nutr* 1998;**67**(3 Suppl): 556S–562S.

138 Hannah JS, Howard BV. Dietary fats, insulin resistance and diabetes. *J Cardiovasc Risk* 1994;**1**(1):31–37.

139 Virtanen SM, Aro A. Dietary factors in the aetiology of diabetes. *Ann Med* 1994;**26**(6):469–478.

140 Hu FB, vanDam RM, Liu S. Diet and risk of Type II diabetes: the role of types of fat and carbohydrate. *Diabetologia* 2001;**44**(7):805–817.

141 Storlien LH, Baur LA, Kriketos AD, *et al.* Dietary fats and insulin action. *Diabetologia* 1996;**39**(6):621–631.

142 Storlien LH, Kriketos AD, Jenkins AB, *et al.* Does dietary fat influence insulin action? *Ann N Y Acad Sci* 1997;**827**:287–301.

143 Sarkkinen E, Schwab U, Niskanen L, *et al.* The effects of monounsaturated-fat enriched diet and polyunsaturated-fat enriched diet on lipid and glucose metabolism in subjects with impaired glucose tolerance. *Eur J Clin Nutr* 1996;**50**(9):592–598.

144 Howard BV, Abbott WG, Swinburn BA. Evaluation of metabolic effects of substitution of complex carbohydrates for saturated fat in individuals with obesity and NIDDM. *Diabetes Care* 1991;**14**:786–795.

145 Vessby B, Unsitupa M, Hermansen K, *et al.* Substituting dietary saturated for monounsaturated fat impairs insulin sensitivity in healthy men and women: The KANWU Study. *Diabetologia* 2001;**44**(3):312–319.

146 Lindstrom J, Peltonen M, Eriksson JG, *et al.* High-fibre, low-fat diet predicts long-term weight loss and decreased type 2 diabetes risk: the Finnish Diabetes Prevention Study. *Diabetologia* 2006;**49**(5):912–920.

147 Mayer-Davis EJ, Sparks KC, Hirst K, *et al.* Dietary intake in the diabetes prevention program cohort: baseline and 1-year post randomization. *Ann Epidemiol* 2004;**14**(10): 763–772.

148 Steyn NP, Mann J, Bennett PH, *et al.* Diet, nutrition and the prevention of type 2 diabetes. *Public Health Nutr* 2004;**7**(1A): 147–165.

149 Willett W, Manson J, Liu S. Glycemic index, glycemic load and risk of type 2 diabetes. *Am J Clin Nutr* 2002;**76**(1): 274S–280S.

150 Marshall JA, Hoag S, Shetterly SM, Hamman RF. Dietary fat predicts conversion from impaired glucose tolerance to NIDDM: The San Luis Valley Diabetes Study. *Diabetes Care* 1994;**17**(1):50–56.

151 van Dam RM, Willett WC, Rimm EB, Stampfer MJ, Hu FB. Dietary fat and meat intake in relation to risk of type 2 diabetes in men. *Diabetes Care* 2002;**25**(3):417–424.

152 Feskens EJ, Virtanen SM, Rasanen L, *et al.* Dietary factors determining diabetes and impaired glucose tolerance. A 20-year follow-up of the Finnish and Dutch cohorts of the Seven Countries Study. *Diabetes Care* 1995;**18**(8): 1104–1112.

153 Wang L, Folsom AR, Zheng ZJ, Pankow JS, Eckfeldt JH, for the ARIC Study Investigators. Plasma fatty acid composition and incidence of diabetes in middle-aged adults: the Atherosclerosis Risk in Communities (ARIC) Study. *Am J Clin Nutr* 2003;**78**(1):91–98.

154 Meyer KA, Kushi LH, Jacobs DR Jr, Folsom AR. Dietary fat and incidence of type 2 diabetes in older Iowa women. *Diabetes Care* 2001;**24**(9):1528–1535.

155 Salmeron J, Hu FB, Manson JE, *et al.* Dietary fat intake and risk of type 2 diabetes in women. *Am J Clin Nutr* 2001;**73**(6): 1019–1026.

156 Laaksonen DE, Lakka TA, Lakka HM, *et al.* Serum fatty acid composition predicts development of impaired fasting glycaemia and diabetes in middle-aged men. *Diabet Med* 2002;**19**(6):456–464.

157 Harding AH, Day NE, Khaw KT, *et al.* Dietary fat and the risk of clinical type 2 diabetes: the European prospective investigation of Cancer – Norfolk study. *Am J Epidemiol* 2004;**159**(1):73–82.

158 Fung TT, Schulze M, Manson JE, Willett WC, Hu FB. Dietary patterns, meat intake and the risk of type 2 diabetes in women. *Arch Int Med* 2004;**164**(20):2235–2240.

159 Montonen J, Knekt P, Harkanen T, *et al*. Dietary patterns and the incidence of type 2 diabetes. *Am J Epidemiol* 2005;**161**(3):219–227.

160 Montonen J, Jarvinen R, Heliovaara M, Reunanen A, Aromaa A, Knekt P. Food consumption and the incidence of type II diabetes mellitus. *Eur J Clin Nutr* 2005;**59**(3): 441–448.

161 Lichtenstein AH, Appel LJ, Brands M, *et al*. Diet and Lifestyle Recommendations Revision 2006: a scientific statement from the American Heart Association Nutrition Committee. *Circulation* 2006;**114**(1):82–96.

162 American Dietetic Association. Position of the American Dietetic Association: dietary guidance for healthy children ages 2 to 11 years. *J Am Diet Assoc* 2004;**104**(4):660–677.

163 Mann JI, De Leeuw I, Hermansen K, *et al*. Evidence-based nutritional approaches to the treatment and prevention of diabetes mellitus. *Nutr Metab Cardiovasc Dis* 2004;**14**(6):373–394.

164 Klein S, Sheard NF, Pi-Sunyer X, *et al*. Weight management through lifestyle modification for the prevention and management of type 2 diabetes: rationale and strategies. A statement of the American Diabetes Association, the North American Association for the Study of Obesity and the American Society for Clinical Nutrition. *Am J Clin Nutr* 2004;**80**(2):257–263.

165 Walder K, Dascaliuc CR, Lewandowski PA, Sanigorski AJ, Zimmet P, Collier GR. The effect of dietary energy restriction on body weight gain and the development of noninsulin-dependent diabetes mellitus (NIDDM) in *Psammomys obesus*. *Obes Res* 1997;**5**(3):193–200.

166 Hansen BC, Bodkin NL. Beta-cell hyperresponsiveness: earliest event in development of diabetes in monkeys. *Am J Physiol* 1990;**259**(3 Pt 2): R612–R617.

167 Hansen BC, Bodkin NL. Primary prevention of diabetes mellitus by prevention of obesity in monkeys. *Diabetes* 1993;**42**(12):1809–1814.

168 Bodkin NL, Ortmeyer HK, Hansen BC. Longitudinal study of the insulin resistance trajectory preceding non-insulin-dependent diabetes mellitus in Rhesus monkeys. *Diabetes* 1994. **43**(Suppl 1): abstracts.

169 Kim SY, Johnson MA, McLeod DS, *et al*. Retinopathy in monkeys with spontaneous type 2 diabetes. *Invest Ophthalmol Vis Sci* 2004;**45**(12):4543–4553.

170 DeLany JP, Hansen BC, Bodkin NL, Hannah J, Bray GA. Long-term calorie restriction reduces energy expenditure in aging monkeys. *J Gerontol A Biol Sci Med Sci* 1999;**54**(1):B5–B11.

171 Bodkin NL, Alexander TM, Ortmeyer HK, Johnson E, Hansen BC. Mortality and morbidity in laboratory-maintained Rhesus monkeys and effects of long-term dietary restriction. *J Gerontol A Biol Sci Med Sci* 2003;**58**(3):212–219.

172 Tigno XT, Gerzanich G, Hansen BC. Age-related changes in metabolic parameters of nonhuman primates. *J Gerontol A Biol Sci Med Sci* 2004;**59**(11):1081–1088.

173 National Institutes of Health. *Clinical Guidelines on the Identification, Evaluation and Treatment of Overweight and Obesity in Adults*, NIH, NHLBI, Bethesda, MD, 1998.

174 Villareal DT, Apovian CM, Kushner RF, Klein S. Obesity in older adults: technical review and position statement of the American Society for Nutrition and NAASO. The Obesity Society. *Am J Clin Nutr* 2005;**82**(5):923–934.

175 Holbrook TL, Barrett-Connor E, Wingard DL. The association of lifetime weight and weight control patterns with diabetes among men and women in an adult community. *Int J Obes* 1989;**13**:723–729.

176 Chan JM, Rimm EB, Colditz GA, Stampfer MJ, Willett WC. Obesity, fat distribution and weight gain as risk factors for clinical diabetes in men. *Diabetes Care* 1994;**17**(9):961–969.

177 Colditz GA, Willett WC, Rotnitzky A, Manson JE. Weight gain as a risk factor for clinical diabetes mellitus in women. *Ann Intern Med* 1995;**122**(7):481–486.

178 Hanson RL, Jacobsson LT, McCance DR, *et al*. Weight fluctuation, mortality and vascular disease in Pima Indians. *Int J Obes Relat Metab Disord* 1996;**20**(5):463–471.

179 Viswanathan M, Snehalatha C, Viswanathan V, Vidyavathi P, Indu J, Ramachandran A. Reduction in body weight helps to delay the onset of diabetes even in non-obese with strong family history of the disease. *Diabetes Res Clin Pract* 1997;**35**(2–3):107–112.

180 Wannamethee SG, Shaper AG. Weight change and duration of overweight and obesity in the incidence of type 2 diabetes. *Diabetes Care* 1999;**22**(8):1266.

181 French SA, Jeffery RW, Folsom AR, McGovern P, Williamson DF. Weight loss maintenance in young adulthood: prevalence and correlations with health behavior and disease in a population-based sample of women aged 55–69 years. *Int J Obes Relat Metab Disord* 1996;**20**(4):303–310.

182 Ford ES, Williamson DF, Liu SM. Weight change and diabetes incidence – findings from a national cohort of US adults. *Am J Epidemiol* 1997;**146**(3):214–222.

183 Sakurai Y, Teruya K, Shimada N, *et al*. Relationship between weight change in young adulthood and the risk of NIDDM. The Sotetsu Study. *Diabetes Care* 1997;**20**(6):978–982.

184 Moore LL, Visioni AJ, Wilson PW, *et al*. Can sustained weight loss in overweight individuals reduce the risk of diabetes mellitus? *Epidemiology* 2000;**11**(3):269–273.

185 Resnick HE, Valsania P, Halter JB, Lin X. Relation of weight gain and weight loss on subsequent diabetes risk in overweight adults. *J Epidemiol Community Health* 2000; **54**(8):596–602.

186 Black E, Holst C, Astrup A, *et al*. Long-term influences of body-weight changes, independent of the attained weight, on risk of impaired glucose tolerance and Type 2 diabetes. *Diabetic Med* 2005;**22**(9):1199–1205.

187 Everson SA, Goldberg DE, Helmrich SP, *et al*. Weight gain and the risk of developing insulin resistance syndrome. *Diabetes Care* 1998;**21**:(10):1637–1643.

188 Fuller JH. Clinical trials in diabetes mellitus. In: *Diabetes in Epidemiological Perspective* (eds Mann JI, Pyorala K, Teuscher A,), Churchill Livingstone, Edinburgh, 1983, pp. 265–285.

189 Stern MP. Kelly West Lecture. Primary prevention of type II diabetes mellitus. *Diabetes Care* 1991;**14**:399–410.

190 Melander A. Oral antidiabetic drugs: an overview. *Diabetic Med* 1996;**13**(9 Suppl 6): S143–S147.

191 Melander A, Bitzen PO, Sartor G, Schersten B, Wahlin-Boll E. Will sulfonylurea treatment of impaired glucose tolerance delay development and complications of NIDDM? *Diabetes Care* 1990;**13**(Suppl 3): 53–58.

192 Padwal R, Majumdar SR, Johnson JA, Varney J, McAlister FA. A systematic review of drug therapy to delay or prevent type 2 diabetes. *Diabetes Care* 2005;**28**(3):736–744.

193 Prisant LM. Preventing type II diabetes mellitus. *J Clin Pharmacol* 2004;**44**(4):406–413.

194 Li ZP, Maglione M, Tu WL, *et al.* Meta-analysis: pharmacologic treatment of obesity. *Ann Intern Med* 2005;**142**(7): 532–546.

195 Anderson DC Jr. Pharmacologic prevention or delay of type 2 diabetes mellitus. *Ann Pharmacother* 2005;**39**(1):102–109.

196 Jermendy G. Can type 2 diabetes mellitus be considered preventable? *Diabetes Res Clin Pract* 2005;**68**(1):S73–S81.

197 Engelhardt HT, Vecchio TJ. The long-term effect of tolbutamide on glucose tolerance in adults, asyptomatic, latent diabetes. *Metabolism* 1965;**14**:885–890.

198 Belknap BH, Bagdade JD, Amaral JAP, Bierman EL. Plasma lipids and mild glucose tolerance. A double blind study of the effect of tolbutamide and placebo in mild adult diabetic outpatients. *Excerpta Med Int Congr Ser* 1967;**149**:171–176.

199 Camerini-Davalos RA. Treatment of 'chemical' diabetes. *Excerpta Med Int Congr Ser* 1967;**149**:228–242.

200 Feldman R, Fitterer D. The prophylactic use of oral hypoglycemic drugs in asymptomatic diabetes. *Excerpta Med Int Congr Ser* 1967;**149**:243.

201 Feldman R, Crawford D, Elashoff R, Glass A. Progress report on the prophylatic use of oral hypoglycemic drugs in asymptomatic diabetes: neurovascular studies. *Adv Metab Dis* 1973;**2**(Suppl 2): 557–567.

202 Keen H, Jarrett RJ, Fuller JH. Tolbutamide and arterial disease in borderline diabetics. *Excerpta Med Int Congr Ser* 1973;**312**:588–602.

203 Keen H, Jarrett RJ, Chlouverakis C, Boyns DR. The effect of treatment of moderate hyperglycemia on the incidence of arterial disease. *Postgrad Med J* 1968;**44**:960–965.

204 Keen H, Jarrett RJ, Ward JD, Fuller JH. Borderline diabetics and their response to Tolbutamide. *Adv Metab Dis* 1973; **2** (Suppl2): 521–531.

205 Keen H, Jarrett RJ, McCartney P. The ten-year follow-up of the Bedford Survey (1962–1972): Glucose tolerance and diabetes. *Diabetologia* 1982;**2**:73–78.

206 Paasikivi J. Long-term tolbutamide treatment after myocardial infarction. *Acta Med Scand* 1970;**507**(Suppl): 1–82.

207 Tan MH, Graham CA, Bradley RF, Gleason RE, Soeldner JS. The effects of long-term therapy with oral hypoglycemic agents on the oral glucose tolerance test dynamics in male chemical diabetics. *Diabetes* 1977;**26**:561–570.

208 Sartor G, Schersten B, Carlstrom S, Melander A, Norden A, Persson G. Ten-year follow-up of subjects with impaired glucose tolerance. Prevention of diabetes by tolbutamide and diet regulation. *Diabetes* 1980;**29**:41–49.

209 Karunakaran S, Hammersley MS, Morris RJ, Turner RC, Holman RR. The Fasting Hyperglycaemia Study: III. Randomized controlled trial of sulfonylurea therapy in subjects with increased but not diabetic fasting plasma glucose. *Metabolism* 1997;**46**(12 Suppl 1): 56–60.

210 Herlihy OM, Morris RJ, Karunakaran S, Holman RR. Sulphonylurea therapy over six years does not delay progression to diabetes. *Diabetologia* 2000;**43**(Suppl 1): A73.

211 Papoz L, Job D, Eschwege E, *et al.* Effect of oral hypoglycemic drugs on glucose tolerance and insulin secretion in borderline diabetic patients. *Diabetologia* 1978;**15**: 373–380.

212 Kasperska-Czyzykowa T, Jaskolska K, Galecki A, Trzcaski M, Woy-Wojciechowski J. Effect of biguanide derivatives (phenformin) on carbohydrate tolerance in 'borderline' and asymptomatic ('chemical') diabetes. Results of a 5-year prospective study. *Acta Med Pol* 1986;**27**:141–152.

213 Fontbonne A, Andre P, Eschwege E. BIGPRO (Biguanides and the Prevention of the Risk of Obesity): study design. A randomized trial of metformin versus placebo in the correction of the metabolic abnormalities associated with insulin resistance. *Diabete Metab* 1991;**17**:249–254.

214 Fontbonne A, Charles MA, Juhanvague I, *et al.* The effect of metformin on the metabolic abnormalities associated with upper-body fat distribution. *Diabetes Care* 1996;**19**(9): 920–926.

215 Charles MA, Morange P, Eschwege E, Andre P, Vague P, Juhan-Vague I. Effect of weight change and metformin on fibrinolysis and the von Willebrand factor in obese non-diabetic subjects: the BIGPRO1 Study. Biguanides and the Prevention of the Risk of Obesity. *Diabetes Care* 1998;**21**(11): 1967–1972.

216 Crepaldi G, Tiengo A, DelPrato S (eds). *Metformin and the Treatment of the Insulin Resistance Syndrome. The BIGPRO Studies*, Elsevier, Amsterdam, 1999.

217 Charles MA, Eschwege E, Grandmottet P, *et al.* Treatment with metformin of non-diabetic men with hypertension and hypertriglyceridaemia and central fat distribution. The BIGPRO 1. 2 Trial. *Diabetes Metab Res. Rev* 2000;**16**(1):2–7.

218 Li CL, Pan CY, Lu JM, *et al.* Effect of metformin on patients with impaired glucose tolerance. *Diabetic Med* 1999;**16**(6): 477–481.

219 The *Diabetes* Prevention Program Research Group. Effects of withdrawal from metformin on the development of diabetes in the Diabetes Prevention Program. *Diabetes Care* 2003;**26**(4):977.

220 The *Diabetes* Prevention Program Research Group. Role of insulin secretion and sensitivity in the evolution of type 2 diabetes in the Diabetes Prevention Program: effects of lifestyle intervention and metformin. *Diabetes* 2005;**54**(8): 2404–2414.

221 Srinivasan S, Ambler GR, Baur LA, *et al.* Randomized, controlled trial of metformin for obesity and insulin resistance in children and adolescents: improvement in body composition and fasting insulin. *J Clin Endocrinol Metab* 2006;**91**(6):2074–2080.

222 Rodriguez Y, Giri M, Feyen E, Christophe AB. Effect of metformin vs placebo treatment on serum fatty acids in non-diabetic obese insulin resistant individuals. *Prostaglandins Leukot Essent Fatty Acids* 2004;**71**(6):391–397.

223 Rodriguez-Moctezuma JR, Robles-Lopez G, Lopez-Carmona JM, Gutierrez-Rosas MJ. Effects of metformin on the body composition in subjects with risk factors for type 2 diabetes. *Diabetes Obes Metab* 2005;**7**(2):189–192.

224 Schuster D, Gaillard T, Rhinesmith S, Habash D, Osei K. Impact of metformin on glucose metabolism in non-diabetic, obese African Americans: a placebo-controlled, 24-month randomized study. *Diabetes Care* 2004;**27**(11): 2768–2769.

225 Bridger T, MacDonald S, Baltzer F, Rodd C. Randomized placebo-controlled trial of metformin for adolescents with polycystic ovary syndrome. *Arch Pediatr Adolesc Med* 2006; **160**(3):241–246.

226 Eisenhardt S, Schwarzmann N, Henschel V, *et al.* Early effects of metformin in women with polycystic ovary

syndrome: a prospective randomized, double-blind, placebo-controlled trial. *J Clin Endocrinol Metab* 2006;**91**(3):946–952.

227 Tang T, Glanville J, Hayden CJ, White D, Barth JH, Balen AH. Combined lifestyle modification and metformin in obese patients with polycystic ovary syndrome. A randomized, placebo-controlled, double-blind multicentre study. *Hum Reprod* 2006;**21**(1):80–89.

228 James AP, Watts GF, Mamo JC. The effect of metformin and rosiglitazone on post-prandial lipid metabolism in obese insulin-resistant subjects. *Diabetes Obes Metab* 2005;**7**(4): 381–389.

229 Boden G, Zhang M. Recent findings concerning thiazolidinediones in the treatment of diabetes. *Expert Opin Invest Drugs* 2006;**15**(3):243–250.

230 Nolan JJ, Ludvik B, Beerdsen P, Joyce M, Olefsky J. Improvement in glucose tolerance and insulin resistance in obese subjects treated with troglitazone. *N Engl J Med* 1994;**331**:1188–1193.

231 Iwamoto Y, Kosaka K, Kuzuya T, Akanuma Y, Shigeta Y, Kaneko T. Effects of troglitazone – a new hypoglycemic agents in patients with niddm poorly controlled by diet therapy. *Diabetes Care* 1996;**19**(2):151–156.

232 Antonucci T, Whitcomb R, Norris RM, McLain R, Lockwood D. Impaired glucose tolerance is normalized by treatment with the thiazolidinedione troglitazone. *Diabetes Care* 1997;**20**(2):188–193.

233 Berkowitz K, Peters R, Kjos SL, *et al.* Effect of troglitazone on insulin sensitivity and pancreatic beta-cell function in women at high risk for NIDDM. *Diabetes* 1996;**45**(11): 1572–1579.

234 Levin K, Hother-Nielsen O, Henriksen JE, Beck-Nielsen H. Effects of troglitazone in young first-degree relatives of patients with type 2 diabetes. *Diabetes Care* 2004;**27**(1): 148–154.

235 Azen SP, Peters RK, Berkowitz K, Kjos S, Xiang A, Buchanan TA. TRIPOD (TRoglitazone In the Prevention Of Diabetes): a randomized, placebo-controlled trial of troglitazone in women with prior gestational diabetes mellitus. *Control Clin Trials* 1998;**19**(2):217–231.

236 Buchanan TA, Xiang AH, Peters RK, *et al.* Preservation of pancreatic beta-cell function and prevention of type 2 diabetes by pharmacological treatment of insulin resistance in high-risk hispanic women. *Diabetes* 2002;**51**(9):2796–2803.

237 Xiang AH, Peters RK, Kjos SL, *et al.* Effect of pioglitazone on pancreatic beta-cell function and diabetes risk in Hispanic women with prior gestational diabetes. *Diabetes* 2006;**55**(2): 517–522.

238 Cavaghan MK, Ehrmann DA, Byrne MM, Polonsky KS. Treatment with the oral antidiabetic agent troglitazone improves beta cell responses to glucose in subjects with impaired glucose tolerance. *J Clin Invest* 1997;**100**(3): 530–537.

239 Durbin RJ. Thiazolidinedione therapy in the prevention/delay of type 2 diabetes in patients with impaired glucose tolerance and insulin resistance. *Diabetes Obes Metab* 2004; **6**(4):280–285.

240 The Diabetes Prevention Program Research Group. Prevention of type 2 diabetes with troglitazone in the *Diabetes Prevention Program*. *Diabetes* 2005;**54**(4):1150–1156.

241 Schuster D, Gaillard T, Rhinesmith S, Habash D, Osei K. The impact of an insulin sensitizer, troglitazone, on glucose metabolism in African Americans at risk for type 2 diabetes mellitus: a placebo-controlled, 24-month randomized study. *Metabolism* 2003;**52**(9):1211–1217.

242 Gerstein HC, Yusuf S, Holman R, Bosch J, Pogue J. Rationale, design and recruitment characteristics of a large, simple international trial of diabetes prevention: the DREAM trial. *Diabetologia* 2004;**47**(9):1519–1527.

243 The DREAM (Diabetes REduction Assessment with ramipril, rosiglitazone Medication) Trial Investigators. Effect of rosiglitazone on the frequency of diabetes in patients with impaired glucose tolerance or impaired fasting glucose: a randomised controlled trial. *Lancet* 2006;**368**(9541):1096–1105.

244 Tuomilehto J, Wareham N. Glucose lowering and diabetes prevention: are they the same? *Lancet* 2006;**368**(9543): 1218–1219.

245 Chiasson JL, Josse RG, Leiter LA, *et al.* The effect of acarbose on insulin sensitivity in subjects with impaired glucose tolerance. *Diabetes Care* 1996;**19**(11):1190–1193.

246 Chiasson JL, Gomis R, Hanefeld M, Josse RG, Karasik A, Laakso M. The STOP-NIDDM Trial: an international study on the efficacy of an alpha-glucosidase inhibitor to prevent type 2 diabetes in a population with impaired glucose tolerance: rationale, design and preliminary screening data. Study to Prevent Non-Insulin-Dependent Diabetes Mellitus. *Diabetes Care* 1998;**21**(10):1720–1725.

247 Chiasson JL, Josse RG, Gomis R, *et al.* Acarbose for prevention of type 2 diabetes mellitus: the STOP-NIDDM randomised trial. *Lancet* 2002;**359**(9323):2072–2077.

248 Chiasson JL, Josse RG, Gomis R, Hanefeld M, Karasik A, Laakso M. Acarbose treatment and the risk of cardiovascular disease and hypertension in patients with impaired glucose tolerance: the STOP-NIDDM trial. *JAMA* 2003; **290**(4):486–494.

249 Delorme S, Chiasson JL. Acarbose in the prevention of cardiovascular disease in subjects with impaired glucose tolerance and type 2 diabetes mellitus. *Curr Opin Pharmacol* 2005;**5**(2):184–189.

250 Kaiser T, Sawicki PT. Acarbose for prevention of diabetes, hypertension and cardiovascular events? A critical analysis of the STOP-NIDDM data. *Diabetologia* 2004;**47**(3):575–580.

251 Sawicki PT, Kaiser T. Response to Chiasson *et al.*: acarbose for the prevention of Type 2 diabetes, hypertension and cardiovascular disease in subjects with impaired glucose tolerance: facts and interpretations concerning the critical analysis of the STOP-NIDDM Trial data. *Diabetologia* 2004;**47**(6):976–977.

252 Chiasson JL, Josse RG, Gomis R, Hanefeld M, Karasik A, Laakso M. Acarbose for the prevention of Type 2 diabetes, hypertension and cardiovascular disease in subjects with impaired glucose tolerance: facts and interpretations concerning the critical analysis of the STOP-NIDDM Trial data. *Diabetologia* 2004;**47**(6):969–975.

253 Citroen HA, Tunbridge FKE, Holman RR. Possible prevention of type 2 diabetes with acarbose or metformin over three years. *Diabetologia* 2000;**43**(Suppl 1): A73–279.

254 Holman RR, Blackwell H, Stratton IM, Manley SE, Tucker L, Frighi V. Six-year results from the Early Diabetes Intervention Trial. *Diabet Med* 2003;**20**(Suppl 2): 15.

255 Yang W, Lin L, Qi J, *et al.* The preventive effect of acarbose and metformin on the progression to diabetes mellitus in

the IGT population: a 3-year multicentre prospective study. *Chin J Endocrinol Metab* 2001;**17**:131–136.

256 Pan CY, Gao Y, Chen JW, *et al.* Efficacy of acarbose in Chinese subjects with impaired glucose tolerance. *Diabetes Res Clin Pract* 2003;**61**(3):183–190.

257 Meier JJ, Nauck MA. Incretins and the development of type 2 diabetes. *Curr Diab Rep* 2006;**3**(194):201.

258 Herman GA, Bergman A, Liu F, *et al.* Pharmacokinetics and pharmacodynamic effects of the oral DPP-4 inhibitor sitagliptin in middle-aged obese subjects. *J Clin Pharmacol* 2006;**46**(8):876–886.

259 Lebovitz H. Diabetes: assessing the pipeline. *Atherosclerosis Suppl* 2006;**7**(1):43–49.

260 Despres JP, Golay A, Sjostrom L,and the Rimonabant in Obesity – Lipids Study Group. Effects of rimonabant on metabolic risk factors in overweight patients with dyslipidemia. *N Engl J Med* 2005;**353**(20):2121–2134.

261 Van Gaal LF, Rissanen AM, Scheen AJ, Ziegler O, Rossner S. Effects of the cannabinoid-1 receptor blocker rimonabant on weight reduction and cardiovascular risk factors in overweight patients: 1-year experience from the RIO-Europe study. *Lancet* 2005;**365**(9468):1389–1397.

262 Heymsfield SB, Segal KR, Hauptman J, *et al.* Effects of weight loss with orlistat on glucose tolerance and progression to type 2 diabetes in obese adults. *Arch Intern Med* 2000;**160**(9):1321–1326.

263 Torgerson JS, Hauptman J, Boldrin MN, Sjostrom L. XENical in the Prevention of *Diabetes* in Obese Subjects (XENDOS) Study: a randomized study of orlistat as an adjunct to lifestyle changes for the prevention of type 2 diabetes in obese patients. *Diabetes Care* 2004;**27**(1):155–161.

264 Lindgarde F. The effect of orlistat on body weight and coronary heart disease risk profile in obese patients: the Swedish Multimorbidity Study. *J Intern Med* 2000;**248**(3):245–254.

265 Broom I, Wilding J, Stott P, Myers N. Randomised trial of the effect of orlistat on body weight and cardiovascular disease risk profile in obese patients: UK Multimorbidity Study. *Int J Clin Pract* 2002;**56**(7):494–499.

266 Arterburn DE, Crane PK, Veenstra DL. The efficacy and safety of sibutramine for weight loss: a systematic review. *Arch Intern Med* 2004;**164**(9):994–1003.

267 Kim SH, Lee YM, Jee SH, Nam CM. Effect of sibutramine on weight loss and blood pressure: a meta-analysis of controlled trials. *Obes Res* 2003;**11**(9):1116–1123.

268 Wadden TA, Berkowitz RI, Womble LG, *et al.* Randomized trial of lifestyle modification and pharmacotherapy for obesity. *N Engl J Med* 2005;**353**(20):2111–2120.

269 Padwal R, Laupacis A. Antihypertensive therapy and incidence of type 2 diabetes: a systematic review. *Diabetes Care* 2004;**27**(1):247–255.

270 Pepine CJ, Cooper-Dehoff RM. Cardiovascular therapies and risk for development of diabetes. *J Am Coll Cardiol* 2004;**44**(3):509–512.

271 Hansson L, Lindholm LH, Niskanen L, *et al.* Effect of angiotensin-converting-enzyme inhibition compared with conventional therapy on cardiovascular morbidity and mortality in hypertension: the Captopril Prevention Project (CAPPP) randomized trial. *Lancet* 1999;**353**(9153): 611–616.

272 Hansson L, Lindholm LH, Ekbom T, *et al.* Randomised trial of old and new antihypertensive drugs in elderly patients: cardiovascular mortality and morbidity: The Swedish Trial in Old Patients with Hypertension-2 study. *Lancet* 1999;**354** (9192):1751–1756.

273 The ALLHAT Officers and Coordinators for the ALLHAT Collaborative Research Group. The Antihypertensive and Lipid-Lowering Treatment to Prevent Heart Attack Trial. Major outcomes in high-risk hypertensive patients randomized to angiotensin-converting enzyme inhibitor or calcium channel blocker vs diuretic: The Antihypertensive and Lipid-Lowering Treatment to Prevent Heart Attack Trial (ALLHAT). *JAMA* 2002;**288**(23):2981–2997.

274 Reid CM, Johnston CI, Ryan P, Willson K, Wing LM. Diabetes and cardiovascular outcomes in elderly subjects treated with ACE inhibitors or diuretics: findings from the 2nd Australian National Blood Pressure Study. *Am J Hypertens* 2003;**16**:11A.

275 Dahlof B, Devereux RB, Kjeldsen SE, *et al.* Cardiovascular morbidity and mortality in the Losartan Intervention For Endpoint reduction in hypertension study (LIFE): a randomised trial against atenolol. *Lancet* 2002;**359**(9311):995–1003.

276 Lindholm LH, Persson M, Alaupovic P, Carlberg B, Svensson A, Samuelsson O. Metabolic outcome during 1 year in newly detected hypertensives: results of the Antihypertensive Treatment and Lipid Profile in a North of Sweden Efficacy Evaluation (ALPINE study). *J Hypertens* 2003;**21**(8): 1563–1574.

277 Julius S, Kjeldsen SE, Weber M, *et al.* Outcomes in hypertensive patients at high cardiovascular risk treated with regimens based on valsartan or amlodipine: the VALUE randomised trial. *Lancet* 2004;**363**(9426):2022–2031.

278 Kjeldsen SE, Julius S, Mancia G, *et al.* Effects of valsartan compared to amlodipine on preventing type 2 diabetes in high-risk hypertensive patients: the VALUE trial. *J Hypertens* 2006;**24**(7):1405–1412.

279 Hansson L, Hedner T, Lund-Johansen P, *et al.* Randomised trial of effects of calcium antagonists compared with diuretics and beta-blockers on cardiovascular morbidity and mortality in hypertension: the Nordic Diltiazem (NORDIL) study. *Lancet* 2000;**356**(9227):359–365.

280 Mancia G, Brown M, Castaigne A, *et al.* Outcomes with nifedipine GITS or Co-amilozide in hypertensive diabetics and non-diabetics in Intervention as a Goal in Hypertension (INSIGHT). *Hypertension* 2003;**41**(3):431–436.

281 Pepine CJ, Handberg EM, Cooper-Dehoff RM, *et al.* A calcium antagonist vs a non-calcium antagonist hypertension treatment strategy for patients with coronary artery disease. The International Verapamil–Trandolapril Study (INVEST): a randomized controlled trial. *JAMA* 2003;**290**(21): 2805–2816.

282 Wilhelmsen L, Berglund G, Elmfeldt D, *et al.* Beta-blockers versus diuretics in hypertensive men: main results from the HAPPHY trial. *J Hypertens* 1987;**5**(5):561–572.

283 Fletcher A, Amery A, Birkenhager W, *et al.* Risks and benefits in the trial of the European Working Party on High Blood Pressure in the Elderly. *J Hypertens* 1991;**9**(3):225–230.

284 Savage PJ, Pressel SL, Curb JD, *et al.* Influence of long-term, low-dose, diuretic-based, antihypertensive therapy on glucose, lipid, uric acid and potassium levels in older men and women with isolated systolic hypertension: The

Systolic Hypertension in the Elderly Program. SHEP Cooperative Research Group. *Arch Intern Med* 1998;**158**(7):741–751.

285 Gress TW, Nieto FJ, Shahar E, Wofford MR, Brancati FL. Hypertension and antihypertensive therapy as risk factors for type 2 diabetes mellitus. Atherosclerosis Risk in Communities Study. *N Engl J Med* 2000;**342**(13):905–912.

286 Yusuf S, Gerstein H, Hoogwerf B, *et al*. Ramipril and the development of diabetes. *JAMA* 2001;**286**(15):1882–1885.

287 Bosch J, Lonn E, Pogue J, Arnold JM, Dagenais GR, Yusuf S. Long-term effects of ramipril on cardiovascular events and on diabetes: results of the HOPE study extension. *Circulation* 2005;**112**(9):1339–1346.

288 Vermes E, Ducharme A, Bourassa MG, *et al*. Enalapril reduces the incidence of diabetes in patients with chronic heart failure: insight from the Studies Of Left Ventricular Dysfunction (SOLVD). *Circulation* 2003;**107**(9):1291–1296.

289 The DREAM Trial Investigators. Effect of ramipril on the incidence of diabetes. *N Engl J Med* 2006;**355**:1551–1562.

290 Pfeffer MA, Swedberg K, Granger CB, *et al*. Effects of candesartan on mortality and morbidity in patients with chronic heart failure: the CHARM-Overall programme. *Lancet* 2003;**362**(9386):759–766.

291 Yusuf S, Ostergren JB, Gerstein HC, *et al*. Effects of candesartan on the development of a new diagnosis of diabetes mellitus in patients with heart failure. *Circulation* 2005; **112**(1):48–53.

292 Lithell H, Hansson L, Skoog I, *et al*. The Study on Cognition and Prognosis in the Elderly (SCOPE): principal results of a randomized double-blind intervention trial. *J Hypertens* 2003;**21**(5):875–886.

293 The PEACE Trial Investigators. Angiotensin-converting-enzyme inhibition in stable coronary artery disease. *N Engl J Med* 2004;**351**(20):2058–2068.

294 Abuissa H, Jones PG, Marso SP, O'Keefe JH Jr. Angiotensin-converting enzyme inhibitors or angiotensin receptor blockers for prevention of type 2 diabetes: a meta-analysis of randomized clinical trials. *J Am Coll Cardiol* 2005;**46**(5): 821–826.

295 Freeman DJ, Norrie J, Sattar N, *et al*. Pravastatin and the development of diabetes mellitus: evidence for a protective treatment effect in the West of Scotland Coronary Prevention Study. *Circulation* 2001;**103**(3):357–362.

296 Keech A, Colquhoun D, Best J, *et al*. Secondary prevention of cardiovascular events with long-term pravastatin in patients with diabetes or impaired fasting glucose: results from the LIPID trial. *Diabetes Care* 2003;**26**(10):2713–2721.

297 Sever PS, Dahlof B, Poulter NR, *et al*. Prevention of coronary and stroke events with atorvastatin in hypertensive patients who have average or lower-than-average cholesterol concentrations, in the Anglo-Scandinavian Cardiac Outcomes Trial – Lipid Lowering Arm (ASCOT-LLA): a multicentre randomised controlled trial. *Lancet* 2003;**361**(9364): 1149–1158.

298 Tenenbaum A, Motro M, Fisman EZ, *et al*. Peroxisome proliferator-activated receptor ligand bezafibrate for prevention of type 2 diabetes mellitus in patients with coronary artery disease. *Circulation* 2004;**109**(18):2197–2202.

299 Tenenbaum A, Motro M, Fisman EZ, *et al*. Effect of bezafibrate on incidence of type 2 diabetes mellitus in obese patients. *Eur Heart J* 2005;**26**(19):2032–2038.

300 Secondary prevention by raising HDL cholesterol and reducing triglycerides in patients with coronary artery disease: the Bezafibrate Infarction Prevention (BIP) study. *Circulation* 2000;**102**(1):21–27.

301 Kanaya AM, Herrington D, Vittinghoff E, *et al*. Glycemic effects of post-menopausal hormone therapy: the Heart and Estrogen/progestin Replacement Study. A randomized, double-blind, placebo-controlled trial. *Ann Intern Med* 2003;**138**(1):1–9.

302 Margolis KL, Bonds DE, Rodabough RJ, *et al*. Effect of oestrogen plus progestin on the incidence of diabetes in post-menopausal women: results from the Women's Health Initiative Hormone Trial. *Diabetologia* 2004;**47**(7): 1175–1187.

303 Bonds DE, Lasser N, Qi L, *et al*. The effect of conjugated equine oestrogen on diabetes incidence: the Women's Health Initiative randomised trial. *Diabetologia* 2006; **49**:1–10.

304 Anderson RA. Nutritional factors influencing the glucose/insulin system: chromium. *J Am Coll Nutr* 1997;**16**(5): 404–410.

305 Mertz W. Chromium in human nutrition: a review. *J Nutr* 1993;**123**:626–633.

306 Guerrero-Romero F, Rodriguez-Moran M. Complementary therapies for diabetes: the case for chromium, magnesium and antioxidants. *Arch Med Res* 2005;**36**(3):250–257.

307 Cefalu WT, Hu FB. Role of chromium in human health and in diabetes. *Diabetes Care* 2004;**27**(11):2741–2751.

308 Althuis MD, Jordan NE, Ludington EA, Wittes JT. Glucose and insulin responses to dietary chromium supplements: a meta-analysis. *Am J Clin Nutr* 2002;**76**(1):148–155.

309 Uusitupa MI, Mykkanen L, Siitonen O, *et al*. Chromium supplementation in impaired glucose tolerance of elderly: effects on blood glucose, plasma insulin, C-peptide and lipid levels. *Br J Nutr* 1992;**68**:209–216.

310 Abraham AS, Brooks BA, Eylath U. The effects of chromium supplementation on serum glucose and lipids in patients with and without non-insulin-dependent diabetes. *Metabolism* 1992;**41**(7):768–771.

311 Thomas VL, Gropper SS. Effect of chromium nicotinic acid supplementation on selected cardiovascular disease risk factors. *Biol Trace Elem Res* 1996;**55**(3):297–305.

312 Anderson RA, Polansky MM, Bryden NA, Canary JJ. Supplemental-chromium effects on glucose, insulin, glucagon and urinary chromium losses in subjects consuming controlled low-chromium diets. *Am J Clin Nutr* 1991;**54** (5):909–916.

313 Wilson BE, Gondy A. Effects of chromium supplementation on fasting insulin levels and lipid parameters in healthy, non-obese young subjects. *Diabetes Res Clin Pract* 1995;**28** (3):179–184.

314 Volpe SL, Huang HW, Larpadisorn K, Lesser II. Effect of chromium supplementation and exercise on body composition, resting metabolic rate and selected biochemical parameters in moderately obese women following an exercise program. *J Am Coll Nutr* 2001;**20**(4):293–306.

315 Amato P, Morales AJ, Yen SSC. Effects of chromium picolinate supplementation on insulin sensitivity, serum lipids and body composition in healthy, nonobese, older men and women. *J Gerontol A Biol Sci Med Sci* 2000;**55**(5): M260–M263.

316 Gunton JE, Cheung NW, Hitchman R, *et al.* Chromium supplementation does not improve glucose tolerance, insulin sensitivity or lipid profile: a randomized, placebo-controlled, double-blind trial of supplementation in subjects with impaired glucose tolerance. *Diabetes Care* 2005;**28**(3):712–713.

317 Joseph LJ, Farrell PA, Davey SL, Evans WJ, Campbell WW. Effect of resistance training with or without chromium picolinate supplementation on glucose metabolism in older men and women. *Metabolism* 1999;**48**(5):546–553.

318 Cefalu WT, Bell-Farrow AD, Stegner J, *et al.* Effect of chromium picolinate on insulin sensitivity in vivo. *J Trace Elem Exp Med* 1999;**12**:71–83.

319 Rajpathak S, Rimm EB, Li T, *et al.* Lower toenail chromium in men with diabetes and cardiovascular disease compared with healthy men. *Diabetes Care* 2004;**27**(9):2211–2216.

320 Shoff SM, Mares-Perlman JA, Cruickshanks KJ, Klein R, Klein BE, Ritter LL. Glycosylated hemoglobin concentrations and vitamin E, vitamin C and beta-carotene intake in diabetic and non-diabetic older adults. *Am J Clin Nutr* 1993;**58**(3):412–416.

321 Sargeant LA, Wareham NJ, Bingham S, *et al.* Vitamin C and hyperglycemia in the European Prospective Investigation into Cancer – Norfolk (EPIC-Norfolk) study: a population-based study. *Diabetes Care* 2000;**23**(6):726–732.

322 Salonen JT, Nyyssonen K, Tuomainen TP, *et al.* Increased risk of non-insulin dependent diabetes mellitus at low plasma vitamin E concentrations: a four year follow up study in men. *BMJ* 1995;**311**(7013):1124–1127.

323 Mayer-Davis EJ, Costacou T, King I, Zaccaro DJ, Bell RA. Plasma and dietary vitamin E in relation to incidence of type 2 diabetes: The Insulin Resistance and Atherosclerosis Study (IRAS). *Diabetes Care* 2002;**25**(12):2172–2177.

324 Liu S, Lee IM, Song Y, *et al.* Vitamin E and risk of type 2 diabetes in the Women's Health Study randomized controlled trial. *Diabetes* 2006;**55**(10):2856–2862.

325 Liu S, Ajani U, Chae C, Hennekens C, Buring JE, Manson JE. Long-term β-carotene supplementation and risk of type 2 diabetes mellitus. *JAMA* 1999;**282**(11):1073–1075.

326 Ford ES. Vitamin supplement use and diabetes mellitus incidence among adults in the United States. *Am J Epidemiol* 2001;**153**(9):892–897.

327 Czernichow S, Couthouis A, Bertrais S, *et al.* Antioxidant supplementation does not affect fasting plasma glucose in the Supplementation with Antioxidant Vitamins and Minerals (SU.VI. MAX) study in France: association with dietary intake and plasma concentrations. *Am J Clin Nutr* 2006;**84**(2):395–399.

328 Montonen J, Knekt P, Jarvinen R, Reunanen A. Dietary antioxidant intake and risk of type 2 diabetes. *Diabetes Care* 2004;**27**(2):362–366.

329 Colditz GA, Manson JE, Stampfer MJ, Rosner B, Willett WC, Speizer FE. Diet and risk of clinical diabetes in women. *Am J Clin Nutr* 1992;**55**:1018–1023.

330 Steinberg D. Clinical trials of antioxidants in atherosclerosis: are we doing the right thing? *Lancet* 1995;**346**:36–38.

331 Yusuf S, Dagenais G, Pogue J, Bosch J, Sleight P. Vitamin E supplementation and cardiovascular events in high-risk patients. The Heart Outcomes Prevention Evaluation Study Investigators. *N Engl J Med* 2000;**342**(3):154–160.

332 Salmeron J, Manson JE, Stampfer MJ, Colditz GA, Wing AL, Willett WC. Dietary fiber, glycemic load and risk of non-insulin-dependent diabetes mellitus in women. *JAMA* 1997;**277**(6):472–477.

333 Salmeron J, Ascherio A, Rimm EB, *et al.* Dietary fiber, glycemic load and risk of NIDDM in men. *Diabetes Care* 1997;**20**(4):545–550.

334 Lopez-Ridaura R, Willett WC, Rimm EB, *et al.* Magnesium intake and risk of type 2 diabetes in men and women. *Diabetes Care* 2004;**27**(1):134–140.

335 Meyer KA, Kushi LH, Jacobs DR Jr, Slavin J, Sellers TA, Folsom AR. Carbohydrates, dietary fiber and incident type 2 diabetes in older women. *Am J Clin Nutr* 2000;**71**(4):921–930.

336 Kao WH, Folsom AR, Nieto FJ, Mo JP, Watson RL, Brancati FL. Serum and dietary magnesium and the risk for type 2 diabetes mellitus: the Atherosclerosis Risk in Communities Study. *Arch Intern Med* 1999;**159**(18):2151–2159.

337 Boucher BJ. Inadequate vitamin D status: does it contribute to the disorders comprising syndrome 'X'? *Br J Nutr* 1998;**79**(4):315–327.

338 Pittas AG, wson-Hughes B, Li T, *et al.* Vitamin D and calcium intake in relation to type 2 diabetes in women. *Diabetes Care* 2006;**29**(3):650–656.

339 Ford ES, Ajani UA, McGuire LC, Liu S. Concentrations of serum vitamin D and the metabolic syndrome among U.S. adults. *Diabetes Care* 2005;**28**(5):1228–1230.

340 Manson JE, Ajani UA, Liu S, Nathan DM, Hennekens CH. A prospective study of cigarette smoking and the incidence of diabetes mellitus among US male physicians. *Am J Med* 2000;**109**(7):538–542.

341 Rimm EB, Manson JE, Stampfer MJ, *et al.* Cigarette smoking and the risk of diabetes in women. *Am J Public Health* 1993;**83**(2):211–214.

342 Rimm EB, Chan J, Stampfer MJ, Colditz GA, Willett WC. Prospective study of cigarette smoking, alcohol use and the risk of diabetes in men. *BMJ* 1995;**310**(6979):555–559.

343 Feskens EJM, Kromhout D. Cardiovascular risk factors and the 25-year incidence of diabetes mellitus in middle-aged men. *Am J Epidemiol* 1989;**130**:1101–1108.

344 Kawakami N, Takatsuka N, Shimizu H, Ishibashi H. Effects of smoking on the incidence of non-insulin-dependent diabetes mellitus – replication and extension in a Japanese cohort of male employees. *Am J Epidemiol* 1997;**145**(2):103–109.

345 Uchimoto S, Tsumura K, Hayashi T, *et al.* Impact of cigarette smoking on the incidence of Type 2 diabetes mellitus in middle-aged Japanese men: the Osaka Health Survey. *Diabet Med* 1999;**16**(11):951–955.

346 Meisinger C, Doring A, Thorand B, Lowel H. Association of cigarette smoking and tar and nicotine intake with development of type 2 diabetes mellitus in men and women from the general population: the MONICA/KORA Augsburg Cohort Study. *Diabetologia* 2006;**49**(8):1770–1776.

347 Sairenchi T, Iso H, Nishimura A, *et al.* Cigarette smoking and risk of type 2 diabetes mellitus among middle-aged and elderly Japanese men and women. *Am J Epidemiol* 2004;**160**(2):158–162.

348 Patja K, Jousilahti P, Hu G, Valle T, Qiao Q, Tuomilehto J. Effects of smoking, obesity and physical activity on the risk

of type 2 diabetes in middle-aged Finnish men and women. *J Intern Med* 2005;**258**(4):356–362.

349 Will JC, Galuska DA, Ford ES, Mokdad A, Calle EE. Cigarette smoking and diabetes mellitus: evidence of a positive association from a large prospective cohort study. *Int J Epidemiol* 2001;**30**(3):540–546.

350 Medalie JH, Papier CM, Goldbourt U, Herman JB. Major factors in the development of diabetes mellitus in 10,000 men. *Arch Intern Med* 1975;**135**:811–817.

351 Wilson PW, Anderson KM, Kannel WB. Epidemiology of diabetes mellitus in the elderly. The Framingham Study. *Am J Med* 1986;**80**:3–9.

352 Wannamethee SG, Shaper AG, Perry IJ. Smoking as a modifiable risk factor for type 2 diabetes in middle-aged men. *Diabetes Care* 2001;**24**(9):1590–1595.

353 Ajani UA, Hennekens CH, Spelsberg A, Manson JE. Alcohol consumption and risk of type 2 diabetes mellitus among US male physicians. *Arch Intern Med* 2000;**160**(7):1025–1030.

354 Perry IJ, Wannamethee SG, Walker MK, Thomson AG, Whincup PH, Shaper AG. Prospective study of risk factors for development of non-insulin dependent diabetes in middle aged British men. *BMJ* 1995;**310**(6979):560–564.

355 Stampfer MJ, Colditz GA, Willett WC, *et al.* A prospective study of moderate alcohol drinking and risk of diabetes in women. *Am J Epidemiol* 1988;**128**:549–558.

356 Balkau B, Eschwege E, Ducimetiere P, Richard JL, Warnet JM. The high risk of death by alcohol related diseases in subjects diagnosed as diabetic and impaired glucose tolerant: the Paris Prospective Study after 15 years of follow-up. *J Clin Epidemiol* 1991;**44**:465–474.

357 Holbrook TL, Barrett-Connor E, Wingard DL. A prospective population-based study of alcohol use and non-insulin-dependent diabetes mellitus. *Am J Epidemiol* 1990;**132**: 902–909.

358 Kao WH, Puddey IB, Boland LL, Watson RL, Brancati FL. Alcohol consumption and the risk of type 2 diabetes mellitus: atherosclerosis risk in communities study. *Am J Epidemiol* 2001;**154**(8):748–757.

359 Colsher PL, Wallace RB. Is modest alcohol consumption better than none at all? An epidemiologic assessment. *Annu Rev Public Health* 1989;**10**:203–219.

360 Carlsson S, Hammar N, Grill V. Alcohol consumption and type 2 diabetes. Meta-analysis of epidemiological studies indicates a U-shaped relationship. *Diabetologia* 2006;**48**(6): 1051–1054.

361 Koppes LL, Dekker JM, Hendriks HF, Bouter LM, Heine RJ. Moderate alcohol consumption lowers the risk of type 2 diabetes: a meta-analysis of prospective observational studies. *Diabetes Care* 2005;**28**(3):719–725.

362 Howard AA, Arnsten JH, Gourevitch MN. Effect of alcohol consumption on diabetes mellitus: a systematic review. *Ann Intern Med* 2004;**140**(3):211–219.

363 Tanasescu M, Hu FB. Alcohol consumption and risk of coronary heart disease among individuals with type 2 diabetes. *Curr Diabet Rep* 2001;**1**(2):187–191.

364 Maggard MA, Shugarman LR, Suttorp M, *et al.* Meta-analysis: surgical treatment of obesity. *Ann Intern Med* 2005;**142** (7):547–559.

365 Buchwald H, Avidor Y, Braunwald E, *et al.* Bariatric surgery: a systematic review and meta-analysis. *JAMA* 2004; **292**(14):1724–1737.

366 Sjostrom CD. Systematic review of bariatric surgery. *JAMA* 2005;**293**(14):1726–1737.

367 Sjostrom L, Narbro K, Sjostrom D. Costs and benefits when treating obesity. *Int J Obes Relat Metab Disord* 1995; **19**(Suppl 6): S9–S12.

368 Segal L, Dalton AC, Richardson J. Cost-effectiveness of the primary prevention of non-insulin dependent diabetes mellitus. *Health Promotion Int* 1998;**13**(3):197–209.

369 Metzger BE, Coustan DR. Summary and recommendations of the Fourth International Workshop – Conference on Gestational Diabetes Mellitus. The Organizing Committee. *Diabetes Care* 1998;**21**(Suppl 2): B161–B167.

370 WHO Study Group. *Prevention of Diabetes Mellitus,* WHO Technical Report Series No. 844, World Health Organization, Geneva, 1994.

371 Green JR, Pawson IG, Schumacher LB, Perry J, Kretchmer N. Glucose tolerance in pregnancy: ethnic variation and influence of body habitus. *Am J Obstet Gynecol* 1990;**163**(1 Pt 1): 86–92.

372 Beischer NA, Oats JN, Henry OA, Sheedy MT, Walstab JE. Incidence and severity of gestational diabetes mellitus according to country of birth in women living in Australia. *Diabetes* 1991;**40**(Suppl 2): 35–38.

373 Dooley SL, Metzger BE, Cho NH. Gestational diabetes mellitus. Influence of race on disease prevalence and perinatal outcome in a U. S. population. *Diabetes* 1991;**40** (Suppl 2): 25–29.

374 Berkowitz GS, Lapinski RH, Wein R, Lee D. Race/ethnicity and other risk factors for gestational diabetes. *Am J Epidemiol* 1992;**135**(9):965–973.

375 Murphy NJ, Bulkow LR, Schraer CD, Lanier AP. Prevalence of diabetes mellitus in pregnancy among Yup'ik Eskimos, 1987–1988. *Diabetes Care* 1993;**16**(1):315–317.

376 King H. Epidemiology of glucose intolerance and gestational diabetes in women of childbearing age. *Diabetes Care* 1998;**21**(Suppl 2): B9–B13.

377 Ferrarra A, Kahn HS, Quesenberry CP, Riley C, Hedderson MM. An increase in the incidence of gestational diabetes mellitus: Northern California, 1991–2000. *Obstet Gynecol* 2004;**103**:526–533.

378 Dabelea D, Snell-Bergeon JK, Hartsfield CL, Bischoff KJ, Hamman RF, McDuffie RS. Increasing prevalence of gestational diabetes mellitus (GDM) over time and by birth cohort: Kaiser Permanente of Colorado GDM Screening Program. *Diabetes Care* 2005;**28**(3):579–584.

379 Kim C, Newton KM, Knopp RH. Gestational diabetes and the incidence of type 2 diabetes: a systematic review. *Diabetes Care* 2002;**25**(10):1862–1868.

380 Dabelea D, Hanson RL, Bennett PH, Roumain J, Knowler WC, Pettitt DJ. Increasing prevalence of Type II diabetes in American Indian children. *Diabetologia* 1998;**41**(8):904–910.

381 Dabelea D, Hanson RL, Lindsay RS, *et al.* Intrauterine exposure to diabetes conveys risks for type 2 diabetes and obesity: a study of discordant sibships. *Diabetes* 2000;**49** (12):2208–2211.

382 Freinkel N. Banting Lecture 1980. Of pregnancy and progeny (review). *Diabetes* 1980;**29**:1023–1035.

383 Pettitt DJ, Knowler WC. Diabetes and obesity in the Pima Indians: a crossgenerational vicious cycle. *J Obesity Weight Regul* 1988;**7**:61–65.

384 Crowther CA, Hiller JE, Moss JR, McPhee AJ, Jeffries WS, Robinson JS. Effect of treatment of gestational diabetes mellitus on pregnancy outcomes. *N Engl J Med* 2005;**352**(24):2477–2486.

385 Carlsson A, Sundkvist G, Groop L, Tuomi T. Insulin and glucagon secretion in patients with slowly progressing autoimmune diabetes (LADA). *J Clin Endocrinol Metab* 2000;**85**(1):76–80.

386 Moses RG, Shand JL, Tapsell LC. The recurrence of gestational diabetes: could dietary differences in fat intake be an explanation? *Diabetes Care* 1997;**20**(11):1647–1650.

387 Wang Y, Storlien LH, Jenkins AB, *et al.* Dietary variables and glucose tolerance in pregnancy. *Diabetes Care* 2000;**23**(4):460–464.

388 Saldana TM, Siega-Riz AM, Adair LS. Effect of macronutrient intake on the development of glucose intolerance during pregnancy. *Am J Clin Nutr* 2004;**79**(3):479–486.

389 Will JC, Byers T. Does diabetes mellitus increase the requirement for vitamin C? *Nutr Rev* 1996;**54**(7):193–202.

390 Colditz GA, Manson JE, Stampfer MJ, Rosner B, Willett WC, Speizer FE. Diet and risk of clinical diabetes in women. *Am J Clin Nutr* 1992;**55**(5):1018–1023.

391 Feskens EJ, Virtanen SM, Rasanen L, *et al.* Dietary factors determining diabetes and impaired glucose tolerance. A 20-year follow-up of the Finnish and Dutch cohorts of the Seven Countries Study. *Diabetes Care* 1995;**18**(8):1104–1112.

392 Zhang C, Williams MA, Frederick IO, *et al.* Vitamin C and the risk of gestational diabetes mellitus: a case–control study. *J Reprod Med* 2004;**49**(4):257–266.

393 Zhang C, Williams MA, Sorensen TK, *et al.* Maternal plasma ascorbic acid (vitamin C) and risk of gestational diabetes mellitus. *Epidemiology* 2004;**15**(5):597–604.

394 Borghouts LB, Keizer HA. Exercise and insulin sensitivity: a review. *Int J Sports Med* 2000;**21**(1):1–12.

395 Kriska AM, Saremi A, Hanson RL, *et al.* Physical activity, obesity and the incidence of type 2 diabetes in a high-risk population. *Am J Epidemiol* 2003;**158**(7):669–675.

396 Helmrich SP, Ragland DR, Leung RW, Paffenbarger RS Jr. Physical activity and reduced occurrence of non-insulin-dependent diabetes mellitus. *N Engl J Med* 1991;**325**(3):147–152.

397 Manson JE, Rimm EB, Stampfer MJ, *et al.* Physical activity and incidence of non-insulin-dependent diabetes mellitus in women. *Lancet* 1991;**338**(8770):774–778.

398 Hinton PS, Olson CM. Predictors of pregnancy-associated change in physical activity in a rural white population. *Matern Child Health J* 2001;**5**(1):7–14.

399 Ning Y, Williams MA, Dempsey JC, Sorensen TK, Frederick IO, Luthy DA. Correlates of recreational physical activity in early pregnancy. *J Matern Fetal Neonatal Med* 2003;**13**(6):385–393.

400 Kirwan JP, Varastehpour A, Jing M, *et al.* Reversal of insulin resistance postpartum is linked to enhanced skeletal muscle insulin signaling. *J Clin Endocrinol Metab* 2004;**89**(9):4678–4684.

401 Harding AH, Williams DE, Hennings SH, Mitchell J, Wareham NJ. Is the association between dietary fat intake and insulin resistance modified by physical activity? *Metabolism* 2001;**50**(10):1186–1192.

402 Dye TD, Knox KL, Artal R, Aubry RH, Wojtowycz MA. Physical activity, obesity and diabetes in pregnancy. *Am J Epidemiol* 1997;**146**(11):961–965.

403 Dempsey JC, Butler CL, Sorensen TK, *et al.* A case–control study of maternal recreational physical activity and risk of gestational diabetes mellitus. *Diabetes Res Clin Pract* 2004;**66**(2):203–215.

404 Dempsey JC, Sorensen TK, Williams MA, *et al.* Prospective study of gestational diabetes mellitus risk in relation to maternal recreational physical activity before and during pregnancy. *Am J Epidemiol* 2004;**159**(7):663–670.

405 Solomon CG, Willett WC, Carey VJ, *et al.* A prospective study of pregravid determinants of gestational diabetes mellitus. *JAMA* 1997;**278**(13):1078–1083.

406 Zhang C, Solomon CG, Manson JE, Hu FB. A prospective study of pregravid physical activity and sedentary behaviors in relation to the risk for gestational diabetes mellitus. *Arch Intern Med* 2006;**166**(5):543–548.

407 Catalano PM, Vargo KM, Bernstein IM, Amini SB. Incidence and risk factors associated with abnormal postpartum glucose tolerance in women with gestational diabetes. *Am J Obstet Gynecol* 1991;**165**(4 Pt 1): 914–919.

408 Cousins L. Insulin sensitivity in pregnancy. *Diabetes* 1991;**40** (Suppl2): 39–43.

409 Barbour LA. New concepts in insulin resistance of pregnancy and gestational diabetes: long-term implications for mother and offspring. *J Obstet Gynaecol* 2003;**23**(5):545–549.

410 Clapp JF III, Kiess W. Effects of pregnancy and exercise on concentrations of the metabolic markers tumor necrosis factor alpha and leptin. *Am J Obstet Gynecol* 2000;**182**(2): 300–306.

411 Clapp JF III, Capeless EL. The changing glycemic response to exercise during pregnancy. *Am J Obstet Gynecol* 1991;**165**: (6 Pt 1): 1678–1683.

412 Butler CL, Williams MA, Sorensen TK, Frederick IO, Leisenring WM. Relation between maternal recreational physical activity and plasma lipids in early pregnancy. *Am J Epidemiol* 2004;**160**(4):350–359.

413 Kirwan JP, Hauguel-De Mouzon S, Lepercq J, *et al.* TNF-alpha is a predictor of insulin resistance in human pregnancy. *Diabetes* 2002;**51**(7):2207–2213.

414 Broussard BA, Sugarman JR, Bachman-Carter K, *et al.* Toward comprehensive obesity prevention programs in Native American communities. *Obes Res* 1995;**3**(Suppl 2): 289s–297s.

415 Maggio CA, Pi-Sunyer FX. The prevention and treatment of obesity. Application to type 2 diabetes. *Diabetes Care* 1997;**20**(11):1744–1766.

416 Williamson DF. The prevention of obesity. *N Engl J Med* 1999;**341**(15):1140–1141.

417 Campbell K, Waters E, O'Meara S, Kelly S, Summerbell C. Interventions for preventing obesity in children. *Cochrane Database Syst Rev* 2002;(2):CD001871.

418 Wadden TA, Butryn ML, Byrne KJ. Efficacy of lifestyle modification for long-term weight control. *Obes Res* 2004. **12**:(Suppl): 151S–162S.

419 Douketis JD, Macie C, Thabane L, Williamson DF. Systematic review of long-term weight loss studies in obese adults: clinical significance and applicability to clinical practice. *Int J Obes* 2005;**29**(10):1153–1167.

420 Taylor CB, Fortmann SP, Flora J, *et al.* Effect of long-term community health education on body mass index. The Stanford Five-City Project. *Am J Epidemiol* 1991;**134**: 235–249.

421 Jeffery RW. Community programs for obesity prevention: the Minnesota Heart Health Program. *Obes Res* 1995;**3** (Suppl 2): 283s–288s.

422 Cambien F, Richard JL, Ducimetiere P, Warnet JM, Kahn J. The Paris Cardiovascular Risk Factor Prevention Trial. Effects of two years of intervention in a population of young men. *J Epidemiol Community Health* 1981;**35**(2):91–97.

423 Stevens VJ, Corrigan SA, Obarzanek E, *et al.* Weight loss intervention in phase 1 of the Trials of Hypertension Prevention. The TOHP Collaborative Research Group. *Arch Intern Med* 1993;**153**(7):849–858.

424 Cutler JA. Randomized clinical trials of weight reduction in nonhypertensive persons. *Ann Epidemiol* 1991;**1**(4):363–370.

425 Elmer PJ, Grimm R Jr, Laing B, *et al.* Lifestyle intervention: results of the Treatment of Mild Hypertension Study (TOMHS). *Prev Med* 1995;**24**(4):378–388.

426 Farquhar JW. Primordial prevention: the path from Victoria to Catalonia. *Prev Med* 1999;**29**:(6 Pt 2): S3–S8.

427 Liburd LC, Jack L Jr, Williams S, Tucker P. Intervening on the social determinants of cardiovascular disease and diabetes. *Am J Prev Med* 2005;**29**:(5 Suppl 1): 18–24.

428 Labarthe DR. Prevention of cardiovascular risk factors in the first place. *Prev Med* 1999;**29**:(6 Pt 2): S72–S78.

429 Raitakari OT, Juonala M, Viikari JS. Obesity in childhood and vascular changes in adulthood: insights into the Cardiovascular Risk in Young Finns Study. *Int J Obes (Lond)* 2005;**29**(Suppl 2): S101–S104.

430 shmukh-Taskar P, Nicklas TA, Morales M, Yang SJ, Zakeri I, Berenson GS. Tracking of overweight status from childhood to young adulthood: the Bogalusa Heart Study. *Eur J Clin Nutr* 2006;**60**(1):48–57.

431 Berenson GS, Srnivasan SR. Cardiovascular risk factors in youth with implications for aging: the Bogalusa Heart Study. *Neurobiol Aging* 2005;**26**(3):303–307.

432 Freedman DS, Khan LK, Serdula MK, Dietz WH, Srinivasan SR, Berenson GS. The relation of childhood BMI to adult adiposity: the Bogalusa Heart Study. *Pediatrics* 2005;**115**(1): 22–27.

433 Lynch J, Smith GD. A life course approach to chronic disease epidemiology. *Annu Rev Public Health* 2005;**26**:1–35.

434 Darnton-Hill I, Nishida C, James WP. A life course approach to diet, nutrition and the prevention of chronic diseases. *Public Health Nutr* 2004;**7**(1A):101–121.

435 Kuh D, Ben Shlomo Y, Lynch J, Hallqvist J, Power C. Life course epidemiology. *J Epidemiol Community Health* 2003; **57**(10): 778–783.

436 Lamont D, Parker L, White M, *et al.* Risk of cardiovascular disease measured by carotid intima-media thickness at age 49–51: lifecourse study. *BMJ* 2000;**320**(7230):273–278.

437 The SEARCH for *Diabetes* in Youth Study Group. The burden of diabetes among U.S. youth: prevalence estimates from the SEARCH for Diabetes in Youth Study. *Pediatrics* 2006;**118**:1510–1518.

438 Satterfield DW, Volansky M, Caspersen CJ, *et al.* Community-based lifestyle interventions to prevent type 2 diabetes. *Diabetes Care* 2003;**26**(9):2643–2652.

439 Sharma M. School-based interventions for childhood and adolescent obesity. *Obes Rev* 2006;**7**(3):261–269.

440 Doak CM, Visscher TL, Renders CM, Seidell JC. The prevention of overweight and obesity in children and adolescents: a review of interventions and programmes. *Obes Rev* 2006;**7**(1):111–136.

441 Flodmark CE, Marcus C, Britton M. Interventions to prevent obesity in children and adolescents: a systematic literature review. *Int J Obes* 2006;**30**(4):579–589.

442 Gibson LJ, Peto J, Warren JM, dos Santos Silva I. Lack of evidence on diets for obesity for children: a systematic review. *Int J Epidemiol* 2006;**35**:1544–1552.

443 Collins CE, Warren J, Neve M, McCoy P, Stokes BJ. Measuring effectiveness of dietetic interventions in child obesity: a systematic review of randomized trials. *Arch Pediatr Adolesc Med* 2006;**160**(9):906–922.

444 Simmons D, Voyle J, Swinburn B, O'Dea K. Community-based approaches for the primary prevention of non-insulin-dependent diabetes mellitus. *Diabet Med* 1997;**14**(7): 519–526.

445 Simmons D, Fleming C, Cameron M, Leakehe L. A pilot diabetes awareness and exercise programme in a multi-ethnic workforce. *N Z Med J* 1996;**109**(1031):373–376.

446 Simmons D, Fleming C, Voyle J, Fou F, Feo S, Gatland B. A pilot urban church-based programme to reduce risk factors for diabetes among Western Samoans in New Zealand. *Diabet Med* 1998;**15**(2):136–142.

447 Katz DL, O'Connell M, Yeh MC, *et al.* Public health strategies for preventing and controlling overweight and obesity in school and worksite settings: a report on recommendations of the Task Force on Community Preventive Services. *MMWR Recomm Rep* 2005;**54**(RR-10):1–12.

448 James J, Thomas P, Cavan D, Kerr D. Preventing childhood obesity by reducing consumption of carbonated drinks: cluster randomised controlled trial. *BMJ* 2004;**328**(7450): 1237–1239.

449 Robinson TN. Reducing children's television viewing to prevent obesity. *JAMA* 1999;**282**(16):1561–1567.

450 Gortmaker SL, Peterson K, Wiecha J, *et al.* Reducing obesity via a school-based interdisciplinary intervention among youth: Planet Health. *Arch Pediatr Adolesc Med* 1999; **153**(4):409–418.

451 Muller MJ, Asbeck I, Mast M, Langnase K, Grund A. Prevention of obesity – more than an intention. Concept and first results of the Kiel Obesity Prevention Study (KOPS). *Int J Obes Relat Metab Disord* 2001;**25**(Suppl 1): S66–S74.

452 Trevino RP, Yin Z, Hernandez A, Hale DE, Garcia OA, Mobley C. Impact of the Bienestar school-based diabetes mellitus prevention program on fasting capillary glucose levels: a randomized controlled trial. *Arch Pediatr Adolesc Med* 2004;**158**(9):911–917.

453 Ramaiya KL, Swai ABM, Alberti KGMM, McLarty D. Lifestyle changes decrease rates of glucose intolerance and cardiovascular (CVD) risk factors: a six-year intervention study in a high risk Hindu Indian sub-community. *Diabetologia* 1992;**35**(Suppl 1): A60.

454 Jenum AK, Anderssen SA, Birkeland KI, *et al.* Promoting physical activity in a low-income multiethnic district: effects of a community intervention study to reduce risk

factors for type 2 diabetes and cardiovascular disease: a community intervention reducing inactivity. *Diabetes Care* 2006;**29**(7):1605–1612.

455 Schuit AJ, Wendel-Vos GC, Verschuren WM, *et al.* Effect of 5-year community intervention Hartslag Limburg on cardiovascular risk factors. *Am J Prev Med* 2006;**30**(3): 237–242.

456 Winkleby MA, Taylor CB, Jatulis D, Fortmann SP. The long-term effects of a cardiovascular disease prevention trial: the Stanford Five-City Project. *Am J Public Health* 1996;**86**(12): 1773–1779.

457 Luepker RV, Murray DM, Jacobs DR Jr, *et al.* Community education for cardiovascular disease prevention: risk factor changes in the Minnesota Heart Health Program. *Am J Public Health* 1994;**84**(9):1383–1393.

458 Luepker RV, Rastam L, Hannan PJ, *et al.* Community education for cardiovascular disease prevention. Morbidity and mortality results from the Minnesota Heart Health Program. *Am J Epidemiol* 1996;**144**(4):351–362.

459 Gross D, Fogg L. A critical analysis of the intent-to-treat principle in prevention research. *J Primary Prev* 2004;**25**(4): 475–489.

460 Colagiuri R, Colagiuri S, Yach D, Pramming S. The answer to diabetes prevention: science, surgery, service delivery or social policy? *Am J Public Health* 2006;**96**(9): 1562–1569.

461 Swinburn B, Gill T, Kumanyika S. Obesity prevention: a proposed framework for translating evidence into action. *Obes Rev* 2005;**6**(1):23–33.

462 Oxford Health Alliance. http://www.oxha.org/: (last accessed June 2009).

463 The NAVIGATOR Trial Steering Committee. Nateglinide and valsartan in impaired glucose tolerance outcomes research: rationale and design of the NAVIGATOR trial. *Diabetes* (Suppl 2): 2002;**51**:A116.

464 Dunn CJ, Faulds D. *Nateglinide*. *Drugs* 2000;**60**(3):607–615.

465 Thurmann PA. Valsartan: a novel angiotensin type 1 receptor antagonist. *Expert Opin Pharmacother* 2000;**1**(2): 337–350.

466 The NAVIGATOR Trial Steering Committee. NAVIGATOR Trial Screening Suggests that Abnormal Glucose Tolerance Is Common in People at Risk for Cardiovascular Disease (CVD). *Diabetes* 2003.

467 National Institutes of Health. http://wwwclinicaltrialsgov: identifier NCT00220961 (last accessed June 2009).

468 Zinman B, Harris SB, Gerstein HC, *et al.* Preventing type 2 diabetes using combination therapy: design and methods of the CAnadian Normoglycaemia Outcomes Evaluation (CANOE) trial. *Diabetes Obes Metab* 2006;**8**(5):531–537.

469 Teo K, Yusuf S, Sleight P, *et al.* Rationale, design and baseline characteristics of 2 large, simple, randomized trials evaluating telmisartan, ramipril and their combination in high-risk patients: the Ongoing Telmisartan Alone and in Combination with Ramipril Global Endpoint Trial/Telmisartan Randomized Assessment Study in ACE Intolerant Subjects with Cardiovascular Disease (ONTARGET/TRANSCEND) trials. *Am Heart J* 2004;**148**(1):52–61.

470 Sleight P. The ONTARGET/TRANSCEND Trial Programme: baseline data. *Acta Diabetol* 2005;**42**(Suppl 1): S50–S56.

471 Blanck HM, Dietz WH, Galuska DA, *et al.* State-specific prevalence of obesity among adults – United States, 2005. *MMWR* 2006;**55**(36):985–988.

472 James PT, Rigby N, Leach R and the International Obesity Task Force. The obesity epidemic, metabolic syndrome and future prevention strategies. *Eur J Cardiovasc Prev Rehabil* 2004;**11**(1):3–8.

473 Hill JO, Peters JC. Environmental contributions to the obesity epidemic. *Science* 1998;**280**:1371–1374.

474 Koplan JP, Dietz WH. Caloric imbalance and public health policy. *JAMA* 1999;**282**(16):1579–1581.

475 Finnish *Diabetes* Association. *Program for the Prevention of Type 2 Diabetes in Finland 2003–2010*, Finnish Diabetes Association, Tampere, 2003.

476 Andersson CM, Bjaras GE, Ostenson CG. A stage model for assessing a community-based diabetes prevention program in Sweden. *Health Promotion Int* 2002;**17**(4):317–327.

477 Collins R, Armitage J, Parish S, Sleigh P, Peto R and the Heart Protection Study Collaborative Group. MRC/BHF Heart Protection Study of cholesterol-lowering with simvastatin in 5963 people with diabetes: a randomised placebo-controlled trial. *Lancet* 2003;**361**(9374):2005–2016.

478 Ramachandran A, Snehalatha C, Yamuna A, Mary S, Ping Z. Cost-effectiveness of the interventions in the primary prevention of diabetes among Asian Indians: within-trial results of the Indian Diabetes Prevention Programme (IDPP). *Diabetes Care* 2007;**30**(10):2548–2552.

479 Lindstrom J, Ilanne-Parikka P, Peltonen M, Aunola S, Eriksson JG, Hemio K, Hamalainen H, Harkonen P, Keinanen-Kiukaanniemi S, Laakso M. Sustained reduction in the incidence of type 2 diabetes by lifestyle intervention: follow-up of the Finnish Diabetes Prevention Study. *Lancet* 2006;**368**(9548):1673–1679.

480 Nissen SE, Wolski K. Effect of rosiglitazone on the risk of myocardial infarction and death from cardiovascular causes. *N Engl J Med* 2007;**356**(24):2457–2471.

481 Psaty BM, Furberg CD. The record on rosiglitazone and the risk of myocardial infarction. *N Engl J Med* 2007; **357**(1):2025–2027.

482 Wilcox R, Kupfer S, Erdmann E. Effects of pioglitazone on major adverse cardiovascular events in high-risk patients with type 2 diabetes: results from PROspective pioglitAzone Clinical Trial In macro Vascular Events (PROactive 10). *Am Heart J* 2008;**155**(4):712–717.

483 Lincoff AM, Wolski K, Nicholls SJ, Nissen SE. Pioglitazone and risk of cardiovascular events in patients with type 2 diabetes mellitus: a meta-analysis of randomized trials. *JAMA* 2007;**298**(10):1180–1188.

484 Utzschneider KM, Tong J, Montgomery B, Udayasankar J, Gerchman F, Marcovina SM, Watson CE, Ligueros-Saylan MA, Foley JE, Holst JJ, Deacon CF, Kahn SE. The dipeptidyl peptidase-4 inhibitor vildagliptin improves cell function and insulin sensitivity in subjects with impaired fasting glucose. *Diabetes Care* 2008;**31**(1):108–113.

485 Guerrero-Romero F, Tamez-Perez HE, Gonzales-Gonzales G, Salinas-Martinez AM, Montes-Villarreal J, Trevino-Ortiz JH, Rodriguez-Moran M. Oral magnesium supplementation improves insulin sensitivity in non-diabetic subjects with insulin resistance. A double-blind placebo-controlled randomized trial. *Diabetes Metab* 2004;**30**(3): 253–258.

486 de Boer I, Tinker LF, Connelly S, Curb JD, Howard BV, Kestenbaum B, Larson JC, Manson JE, Margolis KL, Siscovick DS, Weiss NS. Calcium plus vitamin D supplementation and the risk of incident diabetes in the Women's Health Initiative. *Diabetes Care* 2008;**31**(4):701–707.

487 Sharma M. International school-based interventions for preventing obesity in children. *Obes Rev* 2007;**8**(2): 155–167.

488 Ramachandran A, Snehalatha C, Mary S, Selvam S, Kumar C, Seeli A, Shetty A: Pioglitazone does not enhance the effectiveness of lifestyle modification in preventing conversion of impaired glucose tolerance to diabetes in Asian Indians: results of the Indian Diabetes Prevention Programme-2 (IDPP-2). *Diabetologia* **52**: 1019–1026, 2009.

6

The evidence to screen for type 2 diabetes

Michael M. Engelgau, K.M. Venkat Narayan

Division of Diabetes Translation, Center for Disease Control and Prevention, Atlanta, GA, USA

Introduction

In 2000, an estimated 171 million people worldwide had diabetes and by 2030 this number may more than double, perhaps to 366 million or even more.[1] A complex disease that frequently has devastating consequences, diabetes is also an economic scourge around the world.[2,3] Clearly a pandemic at this point, diabetes is a major public health problem.

What role should screening for undiagnosed type 2 diabetes play in combating the pandemic? Because type 2 diabetes accounts for 90–95% of all diabetes cases, it represents the majority of the public health burden and is the form of the disease considered in this chapter. At present, even though improved levels of care can clearly help delay the development of complications and prevent disability,[4] the benefits of early detection of type 2 diabetes through screening have not been empirically established.[5,6] Despite the scant evidence for diabetes screening, several health organizations have already decided to recommend it. Why might screening be recommended?

First, the fact that undiagnosed diabetes is common and widespread has been demonstrated repeatedly. Population-based surveys have found one-third to half of the total cases to be undiagnosed.[7–10] Second, numerous studies[11–17] have found diabetic complications to be common at clinical diagnosis. Existing recommendations, primarily based on expert opinion, perhaps in part reflect the clinical experience and frustration of health care providers at seeing newly diagnosed persons with established complications. Finally, even without data to support their arguments,

some have contended that treatment of early disease improves health outcomes and saves resources.[18]

Although detecting type 2 diabetes early might intuitively be expected to yield health benefits, the decision to screen should be based on the best available quantitative evidence.[5,6] Perhaps screening for diabetes and providing earlier exposure to treatment may potentially reduce the incidence of complications, require fewer resources and improve quality of life. However, we must also consider pitfalls in assessing the benefits of screening, such as biases in evaluation, side-effects of treatment and other adverse consequences. The purpose of this chapter is to examine the evidence for type 2 diabetes screening.

Historical perspective

Some of the first organized diabetes screening activities were conducted in the United States among insurance applicants during the early 1900s.[19] Later, large-scale diabetes screening was conducted among inductees into the armed services during World Wars I and II. The advent of automated glucose measurement techniques in the latter half of the twentieth century led to even more widespread screening activity in many communities, in workplaces and at health fairs. Still, despite rather broad implementation, at that time little was known or understood about what these efforts accomplished.

Although initial qualitative assessments of diabetes screening tests in the United States during the 1950s found high false-positive and false-negative rates and

The Evidence Base for Diabetes Care, Second Edition, Edited by William H. Herman, Ann Louise Kinmonth, Nicholas J. Wareham and Rhys Williams.

overall poor performance,[19] not until the 1970s was formal evaluation of diabetes screening efforts considered. In both that decade and in the 1980s, problems were noted with mass indiscriminate screening and the value of such initiatives was questioned.[20–25] Major issues raised were that the criteria for a positive screening test and standardized diagnostic criteria for diabetes were not established and that long-term benefits of screening had not been evaluated. Diagnostic criteria were more firmly established in the early and mid 1980s. In the late 1980s and early 1990s, following widespread implementation of diagnostic criteria and also reports from population-based studies that nearly half of all diabetes cases were undiagnosed, some organizations began to recommend screening.

Principles of screening for type 2 diabetes

There are important distinctions between screening and diagnostic tests. First, screening involves attempts to detect asymptomatic disease and screening tests differentiate those at high risk from those at low risk using a variety of methods that are typically rapid, simple and safe.[26–28] By contrast, when individuals encountered in the clinic exhibit symptoms or signs of disease and diabetes is suspected, the tests undertaken do not represent screening, but rather diagnosis. Second, diagnostic tests using standard criteria[29a] are required after screening tests to establish a diagnosis.

From a public health perspective, is screening for type 2 diabetes appropriate? A good way to answer this question is to consider responses to seven queries:[26–37] (1) does diabetes represent an important health problem imposing a significant burden from losses in quality and quantity of life?; (2) does it have a natural history that is understood?; (3) is there a preclinical or asymptomatic state during which the disease can be diagnosed?; (4) are treatments available following early detection that yield benefits superior to those obtained by delayed treatment?; (5) are there tests that can detect the preclinical state that are reliable and have acceptable risks?; (6) are the costs of case finding and treatment reasonable and balanced in relationship to health expenditures as a whole and are there resources available to treat detected cases?; and (7) will screening be a continuing systematic process incorporated into routine health care, rather than a single effort? Below we critically review the available evidence for each of these issues. As issues 4 and 5 are critical to this evaluation, we will devote most of this chapter to these two.

Issue 1: Does diabetes represent an important health problem that imposes a significant burden from losses in quantity and quality of life?

The global burden of diabetes is large and increasing, with an estimated worldwide prevalence of 2.8% in 2000 and a predicted 4.4% in 2030.[1] The three countries with the largest burdens – India, China and the United States – were estimated in 2000 to have 31.7 million, 20.8 million and 17.7 million affected persons, respectively.

Diabetes is a complex disease that damages nearly every organ in the body. It is a major cause of visual impairment and blindness, end-stage renal disease (ESRD) and lower extremity amputations.[38] It is also a significant cause of cardiovascular disease, stroke, peripheral vascular disease, congenital malformations, perinatal mortality, disability and premature mortality.[38] Currently, diabetes is the sixth leading cause of death in the United States, but it ranks even higher among some minority populations there.[39]

Diabetes consumes an extraordinary amount of resources and places a heavy economic burden on societies. The annual cost of the disease worldwide was estimated to be between US$153 and 286 billion.[2] Diabetic populations tend to consume health care resources at a rate 2–3 times that of unaffected populations.[3] Indirect costs from losses in productivity, although poorly characterized, are significant in both developed and developing countries.

Issue 2: Does type 2 diabetes have a natural history that is understood?

A chronic degenerative condition, diabetes progresses through several identifiable states. The true onset is followed by a period during which the disease remains undiagnosed. After a person develops typical symptoms or following incidental tests, a diagnostic test is typically performed. Diabetic microvascular complications (retinopathy, nephropathy and neuropathy) and macrovascular disease (cardiovascular, cerebrovascular and peripheral vascular disease) eventually develop in most patients and can result in major disability and, ultimately, death. Major risk factors for microvascular complications include poor glycaemic control and hypertension. For macrovascular disease they include hypertension, smoking, dyslipidaemia and possibly glycaemic control.

Understanding the natural history of diabetes within and between populations requires standard diagnostic criteria. In 1979–1980, the National Diabetes Data Group (NDDG) in the United States and the World Health Organization (WHO), in parallel, reviewed the available scientific knowledge and developed and widely disseminated recommendations for diagnosing diabetes.[40,41] In 1995–1997, the ADA Expert Committee on the Diagnosis and Classification of Diabetes Mellitus proposed a revision of these recommendations and in 1999 a WHO Committee completed a similar review.[29a,42] Both reached similar conclusions for diagnostic criteria. When typical symptoms (polyuria, polydipsia or unexplained weight loss) are present, a casual (i.e. any time during the day without regard to the last meal) plasma glucose concentration of $11.1\,mmol\,l^{-1}$ (≥ 200 $mg\,dl^{-1}$) confirms the diagnosis. Alternatively, the diagnosis can be made with fasting glucose or oral glucose tolerance test (OGTT). The ADA Expert Committee suggested lowering the previous fasting diagnostic criterion of a plasma glucose of 7.7–$7.0\,mmol\,l^{-1}$.[29a] The one difference between the two groups was that although the ADA Committee retained the 2 h OGTT value of $11.1\,mmol\,l^{-1}$, it eliminated routine use of this test, whereas the WHO Committee proposed retention of both tests. Both groups recommended that persons with only one positive test have a repeat test on a different day to confirm the diagnosis.

Thus, the natural history of diabetes has been described in several populations and diagnostic criteria are well established. While variations exist in diabetes risk factor profiles, the magnitude of risk associated with each factor and the progression rates across different populations, the diabetes-related clinical states are common to all.

Issue 3: Does diabetes have a recognizable and diagnosable preclinical state?

Using the same diagnostic criteria as for symptomatic cases,[29a,42] diabetes can be detected in the preclinical state. Population-based prevalence studies designed to identify all cases (diagnosed and undiagnosed) involve testing many asymptomatic persons and commonly detect large numbers of undiagnosed cases.

Definitely establishing the duration of the preclinical state is not possible directly.[43] Attempts using currently available data have required major assumptions. One study estimated the duration of preclinical diabetes as 9–12 years before clinical diagnosis when assuming that the prevalence of retinopathy is linear with the duration of diabetes and the prevalence is zero in non-diabetic persons.[15] Another study, which used a non-linear regression model, estimated the preclinical duration as between 7 and 8 years.[44] Thus, depending on the investigators' assumptions and the populations studied, the preclinical phase may vary widely but may last for several years.

Complications are by no means uncommon during the early stages of disease. Among people with either undiagnosed or newly diagnosed type 2 diabetes detected during population studies or in clinical trials, 2–39% have retinopathy,[11–15] 8–18% nephropathy,[16,45,46] 5–13% neuropathy[11,47] and 8% cardiovascular disease. In addition, the prevalence of cardiovascular disease, peripheral vascular disease and premature death, are at the same level in persons with undiagnosed diabetes as they are in those with diagnosed diabetes.[17,48,49]

Issue 4: Does treatment following early detection of type 2 diabetes yield benefits superior to those obtained when treatment is delayed?

The issue of treatment is of major importance to consideration of the evidence base for screening. In this section, we discuss methods to assess benefits from screening, review studies that help determine the potential benefits, examine the issue of improved glycaemic control in detail, briefly address the issue of complications and conclude by examining the potential risks of early treatment.

Assessing benefit

Four measures can be used to assess the benefits of screening and early treatment:[29b,50–52] (1) the relative reduction in morbidity or mortality rates, (2) the absolute reduction in morbidity and mortality rates, (3) the number of patients needed to treat (NNT) to prevent one adverse event in a given time period and (4) the total mortality rate of a cohort (from all-cause mortality, not just diabetes-related). Absolute differences are preferred because they measure the actual units of benefit, whereas relative differences do not. For example, a reduction in relative risk reduction of 50% could mean going from 1.0 to 0.5% or from 20 to 10%. However, the absolute reductions in risk of 0.5 and 10 percentage points are markedly different. The NNT is the inverse of the absolute reduction in risk. For example, if the absolute reduction in risk is from 20 to 10% over 5 years, the NNT to prevent one event over 5 years would be $100/10 = 10$. However, in the lower risk scenario, the risk reduction from 1.0 to 0.5% would produce an NNT of $100/0.5 = 200$ people treated for 5 years to prevent one event. The total mortality rate accounts for competing mortality risks from chronic diseases (e.g. cardiovascular diseases and cancer) and other causes (e.g. infectious diseases, injury) and can be used to determine additional life-years and quality-adjusted life-years (QALYs). QALYs take into account whether years are lived

Table 6.1 Criteria for the diagnosis[a] of diabetes mellitus[29a]. Reproduced by permission of the American Diabetes Association

---

1. Symptoms of diabetes[b] and a casual[c] plasma glucose $\geq$200 mg dl^{-1} (11.1 mmol l^{-1})

2. Fasting plasma glucose $\geq$126 mg dl^{-1} (7.0 mmol l^{-1})

3. 2 h plasma glucose on an oral glucose tolerance test $\geq$200 mg dl^{-1}

---

[a]Need meet only one criterion. Test must be repeated and remain positive on a separate day except when symptoms of unequivocal hyperglycaemia with acute metabolic decompensation are present.
[b]Polyuria, polydipsia and unexplained weight loss.
[c]Any time during day without regard to the time since the last meal.

with disabilities such as blindness, amputation or ESRD.[50,53]

In assessing the net benefit of screening, one must consider four types of bias that may lead to spurious conclusions: selection, lead time, length time and over-diagnosis (Table 6.1).[27,30] Selection bias occurs if screen-detected persons are more likely than the general population to have good health outcomes. For example, if those who have interest and participate in screening programs are more likely to follow health recommendations than those diagnosed through standard procedures, they may prevent or delay the complications of diabetes for reasons other than early detection.

Lead time is the period between detection of disease by screening and diagnosis through standard procedures. If early treatment of screening-detected diabetes during the lead time is ineffective compared with persons diagnosed through standard procedures, then those detected through screening would appear to have a longer interval before diabetes complications develop simply because of their earlier diagnosis rather than because of a positive impact of the treatment on prognosis. Length time bias occurs if people with screening-detected disease have a slower natural progression of disease than those diagnosed through standard practice, resulting in lower morbidity and mortality. The chance that diabetes is detected through screening depends on the duration of the preclinical disease state.[27] Thus, a person who has a short preclinical state has little chance for detection before becoming symptomatic. On the other hand, those with long preclinical states are more likely to be detected in a screening programme. Thus screening would tend to detect disease with a slower progression. Finally, overdiagnosis bias can occur when vigorous screening efforts result in diagnoses being made among those who do not have true disease.

Although conditions or behaviours that accelerate diabetic complications (such as hypertension, hyperlipidaemia or smoking) might also be detected at diagnosis,[36] these conditions can be detected without

diabetes screening and their presence does not specifically warrant screening for type 2 diabetes. However, screening, identification and treatment of these other conditions in the population directly may be more efficient.[5] Thus, examination of studies that might support diabetes screening should consider the specific benefit gained from improved glycaemic control alone.

Randomized controlled trials (RCTs) would be the best design to evaluate the benefits and risks of early diabetes treatment and are superior to case–control designs or observational studies because they measure the effect of the screening procedure alone and not other health behaviours that relate to whether an individual agrees to screening.[54] In an RCT, an unscreened control group who would receive routine care for diabetes only after clinical diagnosis would be compared with an intervention group diagnosed earlier before symptomatic hyperglycaemia by active screening.

RCTs of diabetes screening have not been conducted and may be difficult to conduct in the future because of ethical concerns and costs. Random assignment to the no screening control group might be seen as unethical because several organizations have already recommended it. The benefits may be small and accrue over many years. Thus, large numbers of participants and long-term follow-up would require substantial resources. These issues may be part of the reason that diabetes screening has been on few research agendas.[55,56], However, one such study examining the benefits of intensive interventions for glycaemic control and cardiovascular risk factors reduction *after* screening for diabetes compared with standard care is the Anglo–Danish–Dutch Study of Intensive Treatment in People with Screen Detected Diabetes in Primary Care (ADDITION).[57]

ADDITION is a population-based screening programme among persons aged 40–69 years in three European countries followed by an open RCT of conventional treatment from current national guidelines and contrasted with a group that receives intensive multifactorial treatments, including lifestyle advice, aspirin, ACE inhibitors and protocol-driven tight control of blood glucose, blood pressure and cholesterol. Endpoints include mortality, macrovascular and microvascular complications, patient health status and satisfaction, processes of care and costs.

Other forms of evidence of the effectiveness of screening may be derived from observational data by either comparison of outcomes before and after commencement of screening or by comparison of similar geographically defined communities that adopt different screening policies. Future observational studies may characterize some of the benefits because screening recommendations are at various levels of implementation and may create screened and not-screened groups for systematic comparisons.

Potential benefits of screening

Few empirical data exist about the benefits of screening for diabetes. However, two small observational studies from the 1960s are available. The first, conducted in the former German Democratic Republic, was a follow-up study of 250 patients detected by glycosuria who were compared with patients matched by age, sex and weight diagnosed through standard clinical practice.[58] No difference between the groups was noted in survival times or risk of vascular complications at 10 or 20 years. A second study conducted in Italy compared 105 patients with diabetes detected through screening to 104 patients matched by age, sex, weight, family history, therapy and smoking, diagnosed through standard clinical practice.[59] After 6 years of follow-up the average glycaemia was significantly less in the screening-detected group, although there was no difference between the groups with regard to development of retinopathy, cataracts or neuropathy, lipid levels or cardiovascular or peripheral vascular disease. These older studies provide only weak evidence. Neither was a RCT, and the understanding of the benefits of glycaemic control and clinical practice patterns during this era were very different from our current understanding and practices. The ADDITION study should help answer some of these questions.[57]

Potential benefits of glycaemic control

In the face of limited direct data on the benefits of screening, we are forced to examine less direct evidence of the benefit of glucose control for preventing microvascular and macrovascular complications by the combination of reviewing RCTs and disease modelling (Table 6.2) We have good evidence that persons with new clinically diagnosed diabetes typically have glucose levels that warrant treatment. For example, in the United Kingdom Prospective Diabetes Study (UKPDS), the average HbA_{1c} among persons with newly diagnosed type 2 diabetes at recruitment was 9.0%.[45] In a more recent study in the United States, persons with newly diagnosed diabetes had an average HbA_{1c} of 8.8%.[60] Therefore, it is relevant to consider the benefits (i.e. microvascular and macrovascular and mortality outcomes) and the risks (i.e. hypoglycaemia, weight gain, quality of life) associated with improved glycaemic control in type 2 diabetes. However, these benefits may not translate to persons diagnosed through screening.

The landmark UKPDS directly examined the relationship between improved glycaemic control and

Table 6.2 Types of bias and their effect on evaluations of screening

Bias	Effect
Selection	Having healthy participants leads to better outcomes in screening-detected persons
Lead time	Earlier diagnosis results in screening-detected persons living longer with disease than persons diagnosed through standard procedures
Length time	Persons detected through screening have a slower natural progression of disease and a better prognosis than those detected through standard procedures
Overdiagnosis	Enthusiasm for screening leads to erroneous diagnosis among persons who do not have true disease

complications.[61–63] In this large study ($n = 5102$) of persons with newly diagnosed type 2 diabetes who were followed for an average of 10 years, the intensive treatment group using oral hypoglycaemic agents and insulin achieved an average HbA_{1c} of 7.0%; the conventional therapy group averaged 7.9%. Overall the intensive group had a 25% lower rate of aggregate microvascular endpoints and there was a 16% statistically non-significant decrease ($p = 0.52$) in the risk of non-fatal and fatal cardiovascular endpoints. By contrast, the observational Epidemiology of Diabetes Interventions and Complications study (the follow-up to the type 1 Diabetes Control and Complications Trial cohort), found that after 17 years of follow-up, the risk of any cardiovascular disease event was reduced by 42% (95% CI 9 to 63%; $p = 0.02$), of a non-fatal myocardial infarction, stroke or death from cardiovascular disease by 57% (95% CI 12 to 79%; $p = 0.02$).[64] Whether or not this will hold in persons with type 2 is unclear.

A Markov simulation model of diabetes was used to examine the cost-effectiveness of improved glycaemic control and cardiovascular risk reduction in screen-detected diabetes.[50] The benefits of early detection resulted from delivering hyperglycaemic and hypertension control to a screen-detected cohort of persons with diabetes over their lifetime. The benefits applied were those found in the UKPDS[61] and Hypertension Optimal Treatment (HOT)[65] studies. This model estimated the lifetime benefits and costs associated with early detection and treatment of one-time opportunistic clinic-based screening for type 2 diabetes and compared them with the benefits and costs for persons diagnosed by current clinical practice. The results are summarized in Table 6.3. Data for the model were obtained from clinical trials, epidemiological studies and population surveys. In brief, a

Table 6.3 Effectiveness of targeted screening for type 2 diabetes for people with hypertension[a,b]

	Lifetime cumulative incidence				Results per person screened[c]		
	ESRD	Blindness	LEA	CHD	LYs gained	QALYs gained	Cost per QALY (US$)
Age 35 years							
Without screening (%)	25.3	12.3	40.2	21			
With screening (%)	24.7	12.4	40.3	21			
Change in absolute risk (%)	−0.6	+0.1	−0.1	−0.4			
Number needed to treat	166			250			
					0.18	0.08	87.096
Age 55 years							
Without screening (%)	6.5	5.2	15.1	29.9			
With screening (%)	6.4	5.3	15.4	27.4			
Change in absolute risk (%)	−0.1	+0.1	+0.3	−2.5			
Number needed to treat	1000			40			
					0.35	0.22	34.375
Age 75 years							
Without screening (%)	0.23	0.84	1.69	24.4			
With screening (%)	0.22	0.88	1.72	21.1			
Change in absolute risk (%)	−0.01	+0.04	+0.03	−3.3			
Number needed to treat	10000			30			
					0.23	0.18	32.106

[a]Data are from a lifetime simulation model and are per true case of diabetes.

[b]See reference 50. Intensive glycaemic control and intensive hypertension control given after diagnosis regardless of screening status. ESRD, end-stage renal disease; LEA, lower extremity amputation; CHD, coronary heart disease; LY, life-year; QALY, quality-adjusted life-year; NA, not applicable because denominator is zero. Number needed to treat is over the lifetime.

[c]Cost-effectiveness ratios are results per person screened.

hypothetical cohort of persons from the general United States population aged ≥35 years who had newly diagnosed diabetes were followed from onset of disease, which was assumed to be 10 years before clinical diagnosis and 5 years before screening diagnosis until death. The outcomes were dependent on age. However, in general, the lifetime incidences of ESRD, blindness and lower extremity amputation were reduced in the screened group and both life-years and quality-adjusted life-years were gained. The benefits of early detection and treatment were found to accrue more from postponement of complications such as end-stage renal disease and coronary heart disease. The impact of blindness and amputations was less than from the resulting improvement in the quality of life than from additional years of life gained. Cost-effectiveness ratios were more favourable in middle age and the elderly than in younger persons.

Potential benefit from detecting and treating complications

Early diagnosis following screening may also provide an opportunity to prevent morbidity from major microvascular complications. Such complications are common at diagnosis; but timely laser therapy for retinopathy may prevent or delay loss of vision,[66–68] instituting treatment with angiotensin-converting-enzyme inhibitor therapy may prevent or delay nephropathy[69,70] and initiating comprehensive foot care may prevent lower extremity amputations. Evidence from epidemiological studies suggests that hyperglycaemia increases cardiovascular risk,[73] and follow-up studies of the Diabetes Control and Complications Trial suggest that better glycaemic control lowers such risk.[64]

Within the UKPDS cohort, those who entered the study with lower glycaemic levels had significantly reduced risks for most of the outcomes.[74] Another potential benefit is that once diabetes is diagnosed, control of glycaemia and cardiovascular risk factors may improve in primary care.[60]

Potential risks of early detection and treatment

To make a good policy decision about screening, any potential treatment benefits should be examined against possible adverse effects of screening or of subsequent diagnostic tests. At present, such negative effects are poorly understood, but may include physical, psychological and social harm.[29b,32]

In terms of physical effects, one might consider the possibility that hyperinsulinaemia, which has been associated with atherosclerosis in prospective epidemiological studies,[75–77] might result from intensified glycaemic control by insulin treatment. However, the UKPDS and two other studies (the University Group Diabetes Study and the Kumomoto Study in Japan) provide supportive evidence that the risk of cardiovascular events does not increase and actually may reduce with improved glycaemic control.

The risks associated with drugs or insulin therapy in screen-detected populations are not known.[78] However, in all the RCTs reviewed here. hypoglycaemia occurred more frequently in the intensive treatment groups than among the conventional treatment groups. The UKPDS noted hypoglycaemic episodes in both groups, but the rate was higher in the intensive group (1.0–1.8% annual rate in oral- and insulin-treated intensive groups versus 0.7% in the conventional group, $p < 0.001$).[62]

Improved glycaemic control in persons with diagnosed diabetes may result in weight gain. Over the 6 years of the Kumomoto Study, there was a slight increase in body mass index in both treatment groups that was not statistically significant.[79] However, in the UKPDS, there was a significantly greater increase in weight in the intensive treatment group compared with the conventional treatment group (2.9 kg, $p < 0.001$).[62]

Very little is known about how well asymptomatic persons who have been diagnosed following screening will comply with advice about diet and exercise and little is known about the long-term safety and effectiveness of pharmacological therapy in this population. However, some evidence suggests that risk factor levels do improve.[60] Improved glycaemic control may require more intensive self-care and substantial lifestyle change which may affect quality of life (QOL). Among participants in the UKPDS with diagnosed diabetes who were participating in the UKPDS, there was neither improvement nor decline in QOL assessments of mood, cognitive function, symptoms or general health between the two groups.[80] However, QOL was lowered by the occurrence of hypoglycaemia.

If patients largely ignore advice about diet and exercise and if pharmacological therapy is associated with substantial side-effects, any benefits of early detection through screening may be diminished. Finally, if a large percentage of those detected through screening are elderly, the benefits may be limited because of a shortened life expectancy,[50,81] and the risk of morbidity associated with workup and treatment may outweigh the relatively modest benefits.[34,82]

In terms of psychological and social effects, patients may become overly frightened about where their 'disease' will lead them. In addition, after being told they have diabetes, they may have difficulty obtaining health insurance or employment even though they are apparently healthy. However, one study found that screening for diabetes does not induce significant anxiety,[83] nor was health-related QOL reduced 1 year after screen diagnosis, compared with people who were screen-negative.[84]

Conclusions

In summary, RCTs and disease models provide evidence for a potential benefit from treating glycaemic levels in newly diagnosed persons and one disease model suggests that screening and early treatment decrease some microvascular complications and have substantial benefit in reducing macrovascular disease. Screening may prevent disability from microvascular complications that are already present at clinical diagnosis. On the other hand, the potential harm from early treatment is poorly understood. Using data from observational and clinical trials and disease modelling there would appear to be modest evidence for benefit from early improved glycaemic control in type 2 diabetes.

Issue 5: Are there tests that can detect preclinical diabetes that are reliable and have acceptable risks?

This issue has been extensively studied and a vast literature exists. Here we review the characteristics of screening tests, discuss the methodological issues for evaluating screening tests, examine the performance of both questionnaire and biochemical screening tests and discuss risks that can be associated with applying screening tests.

Characteristics of screening tests

Ideally, a diabetes screening test should be both sensitive, that is, have a high probability of being positive when the person truly has diabetes, and specific, that is, have a high probability of being negative when the person does not have diabetes. Generally, a tradeoff must be made between sensitivity and specificity. When considering a test or evaluating studies, one will frequently examine the positive predictive value (PPV), which is the probability of having diabetes when the screening test is positive.[85–87] The determinants of the PPV are the sensitivity and specificity of the screening test and the prevalence of disease in the population. When sensitivity and specificity are constant, the PPV increases with the prevalence of disease. Because an increase in PPV translates into more cases detected for each diagnostic test, it has significant implications for resources use. Information about the type of population, for example, volunteers, community based or clinic based, and the distribution of risk factors, such as age, race or ethnicity, family history, obesity and physical activity, can be used to target groups with a higher prevalence of diabetes and thereby enhance the efficiency.

Screening tests should also be reliable. Consistent results should be obtained when the test is performed more than once on the same person under the same conditions.[85] Uniform procedures and methods, standardized techniques, properly functioning equipment and quality control are necessary to ensure reliability.

Methodological issues for evaluation studies of screening tests

When evaluating studies of the performance of type 2 diabetes screening tests, four issues must be considered: the characteristics of the study population, the referral policies for positive tests, the validity of the diagnostic test and the selection of cutpoints. The population's characteristics are important because they affect sensitivity and specificity. For example, both of these values will be higher in populations that include persons with severe hyperglycaemia, as is the case when persons with diagnosed diabetes are included, because it is easier to distinguish between those with frank diabetes and those without disease than between those with asymptomatic undiagnosed diabetes and those without disease. Hence studies including persons with diagnosed diabetes should be interpreted cautiously. Referral policies are important because if participants with positive screening tests are preferentially referred to receive verification by the gold standard test, work-up bias may occur that substantially distorts sensitivity and specificity. The validity of the diagnostic test is important because some studies have not performed definitive testing with a diagnostic gold standard.

Finally, the issue of cutpoints and their tradeoffs is important, particularly in relation to sensitivity and specificity.[85] For example, selection of a high blood glucose test cutpoint results in low sensitivity and high specificity, whereas selection of a low cutpoint results in high sensitivity and low specificity. The choice of a cutpoint will be influenced by policy, priorities and costs. Ideally, receiver operating characteristic (ROC) curve analyses, which can evaluate performance over the entire range of cutpoints, should be used to compare different types of tests (e.g. fasting glucose to HbA_{1c}).[86,89–93] Unfortunately, few studies have performed such analyses. However, ROC curves are not always useful in selecting the 'best' cutpoint. While the cutpoint that optimizes both

sensitivity and specificity can be determined in an ROC plot, this is not necessarily the best cutpoint for a screening programme. Other factors, such as the number of people referred for diagnostic tests, the resources available and health care system capacity, need to be considered.

Types of screening tests and their performance

The two major types of screening tests for type 2 diabetes are questionnaires and biochemical tests.

Questionnaires With questionnaires, self-reported demographic, behavioural and medical information is used to assign a person to a high- or low-risk group. Community-based diabetes prevention programmes may use questionnaires to assess diabetes symptoms and risk factors and refer those at risk for a medical evaluation.[94] Questionnaires are popular and less expensive than biochemical tests but when used alone they generally perform poorly.

In 1989, the American Diabetes Association (ADA) published a questionnaire in which participants were asked about various diabetes risk factors: family history, obesity, at-risk race/ethnicity, history of impaired glucose tolerance, hypertension or hyperlipidaemia and history of gestational diabetes or delivery of a baby weighing >4 kg. The expected results were that persons with one or more risk factors would be more likely than those with none to have abnormal capillary glucose values. However, there was actually no difference in that 8% of those with no risk factors and 9% of those with one or more factors had elevated capillary glucose measurements.[95] The sensitivity was 69% and the specificity was 34%. Significant increases in the likelihood of an elevated capillary measurement were found if a history of impaired glucose tolerance was reported or if there were three or more diabetes risk factors.

In 1993, the ADA disseminated a second questionnaire, 'Take the Test. Know the Score', which was designed to increase public awareness in addition to assessing risk.[96] Points were given for positive responses with scores of 5 and >5 points termed low risk and high risk, respectively. Subsequent use among populations in both United States[97] and United Kingdom[98] populations showed that the test performed rather poorly. For example, in the United Kingdom, when a score of >5 was used to predict persons with random capillary glucose >6.5 mmol l^{-1}, the sensitivity was 46% and the specificity was 59%. In addition, participants commonly reported symptoms of diabetes regardless of capillary glucose measurement. Overall, approximately one-third of participants reported frequent urination, extreme fatigue and blurred vision, and nearly 20% reported excessive thirst.

A third risk assessment questionnaire was developed in the United States, using data from the US National Health and Nutritional Examination Survey II (NHANES II).[99] A test of the questionnaire in the population from which it was developed found a sensitivity of 79% and a specificity of 65% for detection of undiagnosed diabetes using WHO criteria.[40] By ROC curve comparisons, it performed better than the ADA's 'Take the Test. Know the Score'. High-risk groups were identified through only five risk factors; older age, obesity, sedentary lifestyle, family history of diabetes and delivering a baby weighing more than 4 kg. Participants were considered high risk if they had one or more of these factors. The questionnaire did not depend on prior medical evaluations or care to ensure its applicability to all populations, including the medically underserved.[100] The ADA has incorporated an adaptation of this instrument in its current diabetes screening position statement as a risk test for use in community-based programmes.[94] Subsequently, this adapted risk test was used in a community screening programme in Onondaga County, New York, where it had an overall sensitivity of 80% but a specificity of only 35% and a very low yield (PVP <10%).[100]

A questionnaire developed in The Netherlands' Hoorn Study population incorporated symptoms such as thirst, pain or shortness of breath during walking, plus demographic and clinical characteristics including age, sex, obesity, family history of diabetes, hypertension and preferences such as reluctance to use a bicycle for transportation.[101] This questionnaire was subsequently evaluated in a separate sub-group of the Hoorn Study population and found to have a sensitivity of 56% and a specificity of 72% and a performance better than the ADA questionnaires (as judged by ROC analyses).

In summary, in the light of the rather poor performance of risk assessment questionnaires as a stand-alone test, they might best be limited to education and awareness efforts.[102–104]

More recently, there have been screening tests that have developed risk 'scores'. This approach uses regression models that include a range of information from demographic (e.g. age, sex), self-report histories (e.g. family history of diabetes, lifestyle), clinical information (e.g. BMI, waist circumference, hypertension, hyperlipidaemia, steroid use) and in some cases laboratory information (Table 6.4). Risk scores, which are continuous values across the population, are used to identify a group at higher risk for having undiagnosed diabetes. An arbitrary threshold score can be determined, depending on the programme's goals and the performance characteristics, in terms of sensitivity, specificity and predictive values, number of diagnostic tests required and other logistics.

An emerging issue with questionnaires and risk scores is their utility across different populations other than the one in which they were developed. One study found that a risk score screening tool developed in a Danish population performed similarly among an Australian population.[105] However, other researchers have found different results. Using four screening tests (the Rotterdam Diabetes Study, the Cambridge Risk Score, the San Antonio Health Study and the Finnish Diabetes Risk Score) and applying them to a German population, it was found that the sensitivity, specificity and predictive values were substantially worse than originally described.[106] In part this result was due to differences in the population characteristics. It was suggested that risk scores are probably only of value in the population in which they were developed and that risk score tools should be assessed in the population being targeted. Others have suggested that the value of using risk factors adds little when an actual measure of blood glucose is planned.[107]

Biochemical tests Measurements of glucose and highly correlated metabolites (e.g. HbA_{1c} and fructosamine) have been used extensively for diabetes screening (Table 6.3). Urine glucose or venous and capillary blood glucose is measured under various conditions – fasting, at random, post-prandial or after glucose loading – to represent different metabolic states. Characteristics of several biochemical screening tests can be found in Table 6.3.

Use of trace glycosuria as a positive test tends to have low sensitivity and high specificity. Performance is usually better with random, post-prandial or glucose-loaded measurements than with fasting measurements, probably because the renal threshold for glucose is reached more often in the non-fasting state.

Studies of fasting venous blood screening test have often used measurements collected as part of diagnostic testing with the 2 h glucose concentration serves as the gold-standard test In populations where persons with previously diagnosed diabetes have been excluded or the population has not been enriched with high-risk persons,[25,116,117,128,129] sensitivity has ranged from 40 to 65% at a specificity of >90%. Other studies have reported higher sensitivity (up to 95%),[109,115,118,130–132] but some included persons with diagnosed diabetes or populations with an increased proportion of persons with abnormal glucose tolerance. Studies of fasting capillary glucose tests have had ranges in performance similar to that for fasting venous tests.

In some cases, random and post-prandial venous and capillary glucose tests perform better than fasting tests. This happens because persons without diabetes,

Table 6.4 Sensitivity and specificity of various biochemical tests and combinations of tests for detecting undiagnosed type 2 diabetes

Test	Metabolic state	Cutpoint	Sensitivity (%)	Specificity (%)	Ref.
Urine glucose[a]	Fasting	≥Trace	16	98	110
	Fasting	≥Trace	35	100	25
	Random	≥Trace	18	99	108
	Random	≥Trace	64	99	109
	1 h pp[d]	≥Trace	43	98	111, 114
	2 h OGTT[e]	≥Trace	48	96	25
	2–4 h pp	≥Trace	39	98	25
Venous glucose[b]	Fasting	≥5.8	85	84	132
	Fasting	≥6.1	65	93	117
	Fasting	≥6.1	80	96	118
	Fasting	≥6.1	95	90	109
	Fasting	≥6.1	66	96	130
	Fasting	≥6.5	74	93	115
	Fasting	≥6.7	44	98	25
	Fasting	≥6.7	32	97	123
	Fasting	≥6.9	48	97	138
	Fasting	≥7.0	56	98	128
	Fasting	≥7.0	40	99	129
	Fasting	≥7.0	59	96	131
	Fasting	≥7.8	52	99	116
	Fasting	≥5.8	28	87	148
	Fasting	≥6.1	92	68	149
	1 h OGTT	≥11.1	87–93	89–90	118
	2 h OGTT	≥11.1	90–93	100	118
	2–4 h pp	≥7.2	50	99	25
Capillary glucose[b]	Fasting	≥5.5	90	94	110
	Fasting	≥6.7	65	94	133
	Fasting	≥6.7	90	90	134
	Random	Age, pp time specific	50–60	90	150
	Random	≥7.2	80	80	134
	Random	≥8.0	69	95	108
	Random	≥6.7	75	88	151
	2 h OGTT	≥11.1	69	98	119
	2 h OGTT	≥8.6	90	93	110
	2 h OGTT	≥9.7	98	98	135
Glycosylated haemoglobin[c]	–	≥5.6	35	100	138
	–	≥5.6	83	84	152
	–	≥5.8	92	89	109
	–	≥6.0	60	91	116
	–	≥6.03	85	91	139
	–	≥6.1	78	79	132
	–	>6.3	48	100	137
	–	≥8.0	87	87	134
	–	≥8.1	37	96	140
	–	≥8.3	48	100	137
	–	≥8.3	43	96	144
	–	>8.42	27	88	141
	–	≥8.5	15	100	143
	–	≥8.6	67	97	147
	6.1–6.9	Annual incidence of diabetes 7.8%			153
Fructosamine[b]	–	≥1.18	19	99	123
	–	≥1.78	19	97	143

Table 6.4 (Continued)

Test	Metabolic state	Cutpoint	Sensitivity (%)	Specificity (%)	Ref.
	–	≥1.92	74	95	154
	–	≥2.50	67	96	147
	–	≥2.90	23	98	138
Combination tests	Fasting glucose and HbA$_{1c}$	≥7.8 mmol l^{-1} ≥6.0%	40	99	116
	Fasting glucose and HbA$_{1c}$	≥5.6 mmol l^{-1} ≥5.5%	83	83	132
	Fasting glucose and fructosamine	≥5.4 mmol l^{-1} ≥235 mol l^{-1}	82	83	132
	Fasting glucose and HbA$_{1c}$	≥6.1 mmol l^{-1} ≥6.1%	69	96	136
	Risk questions and capillary glucose	≥6.7	58	94	151
	Risk score and fasting glucose		56	71	148
	Risk score and fasting glucose	≥9 ≥6.1	83	59	149
	Risk factors and fasting glucose	≥5.5	80	80	155
	Risk factors and fasting glucose and A$_{1c}$	≥5.5 ≥5.3	74	89	155
Risk scores[f]	Multiple factors	≥11 points	66 men; 70 women		156
	Age, sex, BMI, HTN, PA, FH	≥31 points	76	72	157
	Multiple factors	≥4 points	57	65	148
	Multiple factors	South Asians >0.127	63	63	158
		Caribbean >0.236	69	64	
	Multiple factors	≥0.11	85	51	159
	Multiple factors	>9	86	41	149
Risk equations[f]	Age, BMI, waist circumference, HTN, PA, diet Age, sex, BMI, capillary glucose, post-prandial time	None	62	96	160
	Age, sex, ethnicity, SBP, HDL, BMI, FH (predicting 10 year risk of developing diabetes)	None	65	78	161
	Age, sex, ethnicity, SBP, HDL, BMI, FH (predicting 7.5 year risk of developing diabetes)	None	Range	Range	162

[a]Cutpoint expressed as qualitative dipstick determination.
[b]Cutpoint expressed as mmol l^{-1}.
[c]Cutpoint expressed as % haemoglobin A$_{1c}$.
[d]pp, Postprandial.
[e]OGTT, oral glucose tolerance test.
[f]SBP, systolic blood pressure; HDL, high-density lipid; BMI, body mass index; FH, family history; HTN, hypertension.

compared with those with undiagnosed diabetes, are more likely to have post-prandial rather than fasting hyperglycaemia.[150] Higher cutpoints are needed to account for the post-prandial state to obtain optimal performance from random and post-prandial tests.[150,163]

Glycated haemoglobin measurement, which is now widely available,[164] has a moderate to low sensitivity and moderate to high specificity at the cutpoints generally reported. Sensitivities of 15–67% have been reported at a specificity of >90% (Table 6.3). Higher sensitivity at high specificity has been reported, but this was in populations that included persons with diagnosed diabetes or a high level of glucose intolerance.[109,139]

HbA_{1c} may be considered unsuited for diabetes screening if the comparison is with current diagnostic criteria. A study in a small number of persons with normoglycaemia failed to find a relationship between fasting venous glucose and A_{1c} values.[165] Others have found that only 2–30% of the non-diabetic variance in glycosylated haemoglobin can be explained by fasting or post-load blood glucose, the remainder presumably being related to other factors independent of glycaemia, such as the rate of glycation and differences in red cell survival.[166,167]

Screening tests using anhydroglucitol, a polyol sugar alcohol fund in reduced serum concentrations in persons with diabetes,[115] and serum fructosamine, a measure of glycosylated total serum proteins,[120,123,138,143,147,154] are independent of fasting status, but neither has performed better than other available tests.

Combinations of biochemical tests have also been evaluated.[116,132,136] Using multiple tests in a series when second and subsequent screening tests are performed only when the preceding test is positive can enhance the yield from certain screening. For example, a second screening test performed only in the population of persons who had positive initial screening test yields a 'double positive' population that will have a higher prevalence of disease than if either test was administered alone. Screening programmes can use a less expensive test first such as a questionnaire, followed by the more complicated or expensive test such as capillary glucose measurement. Strategies that use multiple screening tests will not detect more undiagnosed cases (i.e. they will not improve sensitivity), but will be more efficient.

The risks of screening tests

There are several risks associated with screening tests. Exposure to additional diabetes and other comorbidity may convey harmful risks[5,168] and may increase worry and reduce health-related QOL. In addition, persons without diabetes who have positive screening tests are subject to the costs of unnecessary evaluations in addition to the hazards they present. Furthermore, the inconvenience of screening and such adverse effects as 'labelling' of false-positive persons must be considered.[78] On the other hand, persons with dia-

betes who have negative screening tests will not receive appropriate diagnostic testing and will be falsely reassured that they are disease free. Finally, among persons who do not have diabetes and have negative screening tests, accurate interpretation and communication of their diabetes risk may be challenging.

Although community-level screening interventions may be more effective than those in clinical practice,[78,169] it may be difficult to ensure proper referral for screen-positive persons and appropriate repeated testing in screen-negative individuals.[170] Furthermore, screening outside clinical settings may mean that abnormal tests are never discussed with the primary health care provider, that compliance with recommendations is low and that a positive long-term impact on health is unlikely.[168]

The issue of informed consent for screening is complex, as failure to obtain truly informed consent for screening is unethical.[31] Before conducting screening, health care providers and public health workers need to be aware of complex information about risks and benefits so that they can fully inform their patients. There is rarely sufficient time for providers to provide this information and patients may have trouble assimilating the important details.

Conclusions

Our review of various screening methods for detecting undiagnosed type 2 diabetes shows that questionnaires tend to perform poorly and are inconsistent across populations, and biochemical tests may be a better alternative. Because test performance typically depends on the populations being evaluated and the cutpoint reported, interpretation can be difficult and comparisons with other studies challenging. Finally, the risks associated with screening tests remain poorly understood.

Issue 6: Are the costs of case finding and treatment balanced in relationship to health expenditures as a whole and are there resources available to treat detected cases?

Diabetes screening programmes include screening tests in populations, diagnostic tests in those with positive screening tests and the initiation of lifelong care for those confirmed to have diabetes. Information on the cost per case detected can be very useful for programme planning and can guide the selection of cutpoints for various screening tests. A cost evaluation of using fasting glucose, random glucose or HbA_{1c} was conducted recently.[171] When the test's cost, performance characteristics (sensitivity, specificity, PPV, PPN) and the number and cost of referrals for diagnostic testing are all considered, a profile of

Table 6.5 Population-based, selective and opportunistic screening programme strategies and yields[a]

Type	Setting	Target population	Total tests	Screening test used	Total No. positive screening tests	Total No. new cases detected	Yield (%)[d]	Ref.
Population	Community	Volunteers, awareness campaign	NR	Self-referral after advertising campaign	41	7	17	187
	Community sample for diabetes study	Volunteers responding to invitation	320	Risk score	21	4	19	195
	Community education and outreach	Volunteers	320	Risk score	18	3	17	195
		Volunteers	3031	CG	72	52	72	191
	Community screening	Volunteers	2016	CG	148	6	4	97
	Community health fair	Volunteers	3212	VG	120	25	21	196
	Community outreach	Volunteers	253 190	VG	9682	5370	55	197
	Community diabetes detection drive	Volunteers	559	VG, CG, urine	164	42	26	198
	Community diabetes promotion	Volunteers	23 228	CG	860	64	7	199
	Community outreach	Volunteers	396	Risk score	264	28	11	103
	Clinic	≥40 years	9042	CG, VG	–	–	2.2	200
	Community study	55–74 years	1353	OGTT	–	–	7–10	201
	Community	All	3506	Risk score, CG	153	–	1	202
	Hospital waiting room	Volunteers	548	CG	NR	5	–	189
	Dental clinic	All patients	119	VG	24	6	25	21
	Pharmacy (distributed 35000 urine kits)	Volunteers (preference to high risk: >40 years, obese, FH, large baby)	3409	Urine	164	22	13	197
Selective	Community outreach (mailed 7426 risk questionnaires to households)	Volunteers (>60 years)	349	Risk score	181	11	6	102
	Community physician's patients	20% sample of patients >40 years	1767	BG	48	19	40	172
	Clinic population (mailed urine glucose kits)	Volunteers 45–70 years	2984	Urine	73	17	23	22

(continued)

Table 6.5 (Continued)

Type	Setting	Target population	Total tests	Screening test used	Total No. positive screening tests	Total No. new cases detected	Yield (%)[a]	Ref.
Selective	Clinic population (mailed urine glucose kits)	Volunteers 45–70 years	3231	Urine	52	10	19	181
	Clinic population (mailed urine glucose kits)	Volunteers 45–70 years	13 795	Urine	343	99	29	114
	Motor vehicle license renewal department	Volunteers >70 years	410	CG	11	NR	–	92
	Industry workers	Volunteers 18–74 years	4048	CG	267	13	5	203
	Clinic registries	Volunteers 50–69 years	367	CG	28	5	18	188
	School	6–18 years	250	CG, VG	0	0	0	204
	Community	Volunteers all ages	704	VG, A$_{1c}$	–	–	3.4	205
	Community	Volunteers all ages	32 954	Risk score, CG	1564	354	22	206
Opportunistic	Clinic population	Volunteers	3268	CG, urine	234	66	28	108
	Health insurance beneficiaries	Volunteers >25 years	8818	VG	176	30	17	168
	Clinic population	Volunteers ≥45 years	5752	PG, A$_{1c}$, OGTT	202	35	17	207
	Emergency room	All	500	CG	36	13	30	208
	Medicare	NR	826	NR	NR	32	4	209

[a]CG, capillary glucose; VG, venous glucose; NR, not reported; risk score, use of questionnaire or risk classification scheme.
[b]Positive predictive value (PPV).

Table 6.6 Screening recommendations for type 2 diabetes by health agencies, professional organizations and associations and health task forces

Agency, organization, task force[a]	Strategy	Recommended test	Repeat interval (years)	Year published	Ref.
WHO	Country specific	Locally determined	Not stated	2003	212
DUK	Selective, target high-risk group	Fasting, random, urine glucose	3	2006	213
USPSTF[b]	Selective, persons with hyperlipidaemia or hypertension	Not stated	Not stated	2003	214, 215
CTFPHE	Selective, persons with hyperlipidaemia or hypertension	Fasting glucose	Not stated	2005	216
CDA	Selective, risk factors	Fasting glucose	3	2003	217
ADA	Selective, risk factors	Risk questionnaire	3	2006	210

[a]WHO, World Health Organization; DUK, Diabetes United Kingdom; USPSTF, United States Preventive Services Task Force; CTFPHE, Canadian Task Force on the Periodic Health Examination; CDA, Canadian Diabetes Association; ADA, American Diabetes Association.
[b]The American College of Physicians and the American Academy of Family Physicians have adopted the USPSTF recommendations.

the cost per case identified can provide the best value for different screening tests. From a single-payer perspective, if the purpose of screening was to identify both pre-diabetes and undiagnosed diabetes, the costs per case ranged from US$125 to $321 for the capillary blood glucose test, from $114 to $476 for the fasting blood glucose test and from $153 to $536 for the HbA$_{1c}$ test.

Determining programme costs and additional burden on the health care system requires an understanding of the prevalence of undiagnosed diabetes, the method of case finding and the operation of the health care delivery system. As each of these three factors may vary widely by setting, making general statements about the costs and burden of screening is fraught with difficulty. One safe generalization is that for early detection to provide benefits, access to diabetes treatment is essential.[5,36] For countries with publicly funded national health care and universal access to services, where most patients see a physician often, screening yields may be low and not justify the effort. Within the United States, in contrast, where there may be up to 40 million persons with either no medical care coverage at all or inadequate medical coverage,[173] yields may be greater than in other countries.

In the screening simulation model discussed earlier in this chapter, an opportunistic screening programme for the United States population aged 35 years and older with hypertension was developed.[50] Diabetes was diagnosed approximately 5 years earlier with a screening programme. The estimated average annual cost for a programme per

person screened varied from $4000–5000 for a 35-year-old cohort to $200–400 for an 85-year-old cohort. With screening, there were benefits in terms of reducing the lifetime incidence of the major diabetes complications and in additional QALYs (Table 6.2). Across the age range, older persons had a more favourable cost-effectiveness. Reviews of guidelines and previous cost-effectiveness studies of interventions for diseases and conditions other than diabetes suggest that interventions whose cost-effectiveness is between $20 000 and $100 000 per QALY are often provided, but their availability may be limited.

From an economic, clinical and public health perspective, the issue of how diabetes screening complements efforts to control other diseases should be considered. The diagnosis of type 2 diabetes can be combined with detection efforts for other conditions (e.g. smoking, hypertension, hyperlipidaemia)[5,36] and the optimal mix of screening tests that produces the most benefits could then be determined.[36,53,55]

For a health care system to implement diabetes screening, either obtaining new resources or redirecting current resources away from other activities is required. Because health care budgets are finite, redirection is more common and hence there is an 'opportunity cost' in taking on a new activity (i.e. other activities may have to be reduced or eliminated altogether).[53] Competing opportunities could be improving care for those already diagnosed with diabetes or targeting persons at high risk for developing diabetes with prevention efforts. Health care policy leaders in each country will need to document their current situation and priorities and then assess where diabetes screening fits. Cost-effectiveness studies can help but the absolute cost for the entire population of the effort must be considered and the decision may be very different for developed countries as compared with developing countries.

In summary, the global impact of a screening programme on the health care system may be substantial but can vary greatly from country to country. Generally, there is limited information about the expected impact on health care systems.

Issue 7: Will screening be a continuing process, rather than a single effort?

Screening programmes inevitably miss some cases and new-onset cases continue to replenish the pool of undiagnosed cases. Therefore, to address fully the undiagnosed burden, screening programmes must be ongoing. To accomplish this, there must be a commitment to developing and sustaining screening capacity which should include programme support, coordination and evaluation. If screening is made part of routine preventive care, it could be conducted in the clinic setting at designated intervals. However, the optimal interval between screenings is not clear and few studies have examined the appropriate frequency of screening. In one United Kingdom study that conducted a repeat diabetes screening at 30 months by self-testing of post-prandial glycosuria in 3200 persons registered at a general clinic, the repeat screening response rate was slightly lower than the initial (73% versus 79%, $p < 0.0001$), but the yields were not significantly different (0.44% versus 0.72%, $p = 0.2$).[175] The optimal interval would be one where cost-effectiveness would be equal for each screening.

Another study found that after a 1 year interval, 48% of those who tested positive were disease free, whereas after a 5 year interval, 28% who tested positive were disease free.[176] A third study found that the balance of tradeoffs between false positives and negatives was optimal at an interval of approximately 3 years.[177]

The yield of programmes that screen for diabetes

Direct evaluation of the effectiveness of screening programmes has been restricted to their ability to detect undiagnosed cases. Three approaches to conducting screening programmes for diabetes have been used: universal, selective and opportunistic; results from all these types are presented in Table 6.4.[168,178,180] Classification for this chapter is based on the information

within each report and what was deemed the dominant mode of the screening effort.

Universal approaches screen every person. Costly and potentially inefficient, this method is not widely favoured except in very high prevalence populations. Selective screening, often conducted outside the health care system, targets sub-groups of the population with a high prevalence of risk factors for diabetes.[94,181,182] Opportunistic screening tests focus on persons during routine encounters with the health care system, such as primary care visits or periodic health evaluations.[178–180,183–186] Both selective and opportunistic screening can significantly reduce the resources needed to reach high-risk groups, but some important groups may be missed.[186] Opportunistic screening may often have poor coverage and a tendency to be misdirected – some persons getting too many tests too often with others getting too few.

Most screening programmes report using either universal, selective or combined strategies (Table 6.4). Some of the selective programmes, for example, have begun with universal health promotion and diabetes awareness programmes targeting entire communities, then screened volunteers with diabetes risk factors. Testing strategies have included questionnaires in addition to fasting, random, post-prandial and post-challenge biochemical measurements. Some programmes have conducted public awareness campaigns that have resulted in increased patient requests for screening when making clinic visits,[187] while others have advocated increasing professional alertness as an efficient approach.[170] The yields reported, which are highly variable and depend on the screening test cutpoint, range from 4 to 72% (Table 6.4).

Selective screening has been used in widely varied settings, including doctors' offices and medical clinics,[188] clinic and hospital waiting rooms,[189] dental clinics,[21] community pharmacies,[190] shopping and community centres,[191] drivers' license registration centres,[192] work sites and community churches.[193,194] Groups with an expected rate higher than the general population have been targeted using factors such as age and risk factors such as family history of diabetes and obesity.[82,192] Reported yields for selective screening have ranged from 5 to 40%.

Although data on the effectiveness of screening from simulation models are available only for opportunistic methods,[50] few reports have used such methods Strategies have included the sponsorship by health insurance companies of multichannel chemistry screening through widespread phlebotomy centres[168] and the use of patient clinic registries. Yields from opportunistic screening are reported to range from 4 to 30%.

Current screening policies and recommendations and practices

Several health agencies, task forces and professional organizations have provided recommendations on screening for type 2 diabetes (Table 6.5). Because definitive studies on the benefits of screening are not available, all the recommendations rely on expert opinion, consensus and extrapolation from observational studies and clinical trials. None of the recommendations encourages universal screening, but some suggest using a selective approach in populations with diabetes risk factors. The WHO suggests that national health officials determine whether screening should be pursued and that the methods used be determined at the local level. None of the strategies or recommended screening intervals has been formally evaluated.

The United States Preventive Services Task Force (USPSTF) in its current recommendations, which were published in 2003 (Table 6.6), cites insufficient evidence to recommend universal, routine screening. However, using the potential benefits from lifetime statistical models such as those in Table 6.3, persons with hypertension or hyperlipidaemia are a reasonable target group to screen.

The current ADA recommendations state that early detection and treatment may well reduce the burden of type 2 diabetes and its complications and that screening may be appropriate in certain circumstances.[210] The recommendations suggest that screening be considered at any age if risk factors for diabetes are present, that is, family history, obesity, belonging to a high-risk minority group, abnormal glucose tolerance, hypertension, hyperlipidaemia, previous gestational diabetes or history of delivery of a large baby (>4 kg). In addition, the ADA recommends screening for all persons aged ≥45 years old regardless of risk factor status and repetition of screening at 3 year intervals. Its rationale for these latter recommendations is that there is a steep rise in the incidence of diabetes after age 45 years, that there is a negligible likelihood of developing any significant complications of diabetes within 3 years of a negative test and the risk factors included in its recommendations are firmly established.

In the light of these recommendations, just how common is screening for type 2 diabetes? Limited information describing the level of screening activities is available and is restricted to the experience in the United States. A 1989 population-based survey found that approximately 40% of persons who did not have diabetes reported being checked for the disorder during the previous year by a doctor or other health professional,[182] but this report did not describe the location or the circumstances of the screening tests. In 1998, a population-based survey in Montana found that 39% of persons without diabetes had been screened during the previous year.[211] With several organizations and agencies recommending it, screening is without doubt taking place in several countries, but it seems unlikely that it is systematically applied. More probable is that it is left up to patients, health care providers and various public health and health promotion workers. In addition, there is a good deal of incidental diabetes screening in the health care setting as the widespread use of multichannel chemistry tests means that glucose values are frequently available when laboratory tests are conducted for other reasons.

Summary

We have considered the evidence to address seven key issues to determine whether diabetes screening is an appropriate clinical and public health activity. We have clearly shown that diabetes is an important public health problem, it has a well-characterized natural history and it can be diagnosed in the preclinical asymptomatic state. However, currently there is little direct evidence to support diabetes screening. The effect of early treatment on long-term health outcomes and the risks associated with it are unclear. In addition, while several screening tests and some screening strategies have been evaluated, there is no clear evidence that broad implementation of these strategies will be effective and sustainable.

Definitive studies on the effectiveness of screening may be forthcoming, however. The ADDITION study may help in understanding whether early detection and intensive glycaemic control and reduction of cardiovascular risk factors improve outcomes.

Statistical models have already helped to answer some of the key questions and may continue to do so. This approach is attractive because of their relatively low cost compared with a clinical trial, the ability to incorporate data from many clinical and epidemiological studies, to perform economic evaluations and the capability of modifying treatment algorithms relatively easily. Models will need to be refined as new clinical and epidemiological results become available. In addition, future models need to include better information on the natural history of the preclinical phase, comprehensive cardiovascular disease modules and the joint influence of glucose and cardiovascular risk factor reduction, comprehensive QOL information and economic evaluations using common outcome measures. These studies should consider all costs associated with a comprehensive screening programme including, at a minimum, the direct costs of screening, diagnostic testing and care for persons with type 2 diabetes detected through screening. However, these models require multiple assumptions which must be considered when interpreting their results. Finally, various combinations of disease screening interventions should be considered in economic studies to allow for selection of the optimal combination of interventions within the financial and resource limitations of the health care system.

Conclusions

The effectiveness of diabetes screening has not been directly demonstrated. Indirect examination of the potential benefits of screening using data from RCTs of treatment of diagnosed diabetes, observational studies and disease models lends support to the idea that early improvement in glycaemic control may help reduce the lifetime occurrence of microvascular disease. The physical, psychological and social effects of screening and early diagnosis and treatment remain unclear. Thus, on balance, there is modest evidence, at best, to support screening for type 2 diabetes.

References

1 Wild S, Roglic G, Green A, Sicree R, King H. Global prevalence of diabetes. Estimates for the years 2000 and 2030. *Diabetes Care* 2004;**27**:1047–1053.

2 www.eatlas.idf.org/Cost_of_diabetes (last accessed 2 November 2009).

3 American Diabetes Association. Economic costs of diabetes in the United States 2002. *Diabetes Care* 2003;**27**:917–932.

4 Clark CM Jr. How should we respond to the worldwide diabetes epidemic? *Diabetes Care* 1998;**21**:475–476.

5 Wareham NJ, Griffin SJ. Should we screen for type 2 diabetes? Evaluation against National Screening Committee criteria. *BMJ* 2001;**322**:986–988.

6 Engelgau MM, Narayan KM, Herman WH. Screening for type 2 diabetes. *Diabetes Care* 2000;**23**:1563–1580.

7 Cowie CC, Rust KF, Byrd-Holt DD, Eberhardt MS, Flegal KM, Engelgau MM, Saydah SH, Williams DE, Geiss LS, Gregg EW. Prevalence of diabetes and impaired fasting glucose in adults in the U.S. population: National Health and Nutrition Examination Survey 1999–2002. *Diabetes Care* 2006;**29**:1263–1268.

8 Oliveira JE, Milech A, Franco LJ. The prevalence of diabetes in Rio de Janeiro. Brazil. The Cooperative Group for the Study of Diabetes Prevalence in Rio De Janeiro. *Diabetes Care* 1996;**19**:663–666.

9 McLarty DG, Pollitt C, Swai AB. Diabetes in Africa. *Diabet Med* 1990;**7**:670–684.

10 Flegal KM, Ezzati TM, Harris MI, Haynes SG, Juarez RZ, Knowler WC, Perez-Stable EJ, Stern MP. Prevalence of diabetes in Mexican Americans, Cubans, and Puerto Ricans from the Hispanic Health and Nutritional Examination Survey, 1982–1984. *Diabetes Care* 1991;**14**:628–638.

11 Wang WQ, Ip TP, Lam KS. Changing prevalence of retinopathy in newly diagnosed non-insulin dependent diabetes mellitus patients in Hong Kong. *Diabetes Res Clin Pract* 1998;**39**:185–191.

12 Harris MI, Klein R, Cowie CC, Rowland M, Byrd-Holt DD. Is the risk of diabetic retinopathy greater in non-Hispanic blacks and Mexican Americans than in non-Hispanic whites with type 2 diabetes? A U. S. population study. *Diabetes Care* 1998;**21**:1230–1235.

13 Rajala U, Laakso M, Qiao Q, Keinanen-Kiukaanniemi S. Prevalence of retinopathy in people with diabetes, impaired glucose tolerance and normal glucose tolerance. *Diabetes Care* 1998;**21**:1664–1669.

14 Kohner EM, Aldington SJ, Stratton IM, Manley SE, Holman RR, Matthews DR, Turner RC. United Kingdom Prospective Diabetes Study, 30: diabetic retinopathy at diagnosis of non-insulin-dependent diabetes mellitus and associated risk factors. *Arch Ophthalmol* 1998;**116**:297–303.

15 Harris MI, Klein R, Welborn TA, Knuiman MW. Onset of NIDDM occurs at least 4–7 yr before clinical diagnosis. *Diabetes Care* 1992;**15**:815–819.

16 Ballard DJ, Humphrey LL, Melton LJ III, Frohnert PP, Chu PC, O'Fallon WM, Palumbo PJ. Epidemiology of persistent proteinuria in type II diabetes mellitus. Population-based study in Rochester, Minnesota. *Diabetes* 1988;**37**:405–412.

17 Harris MI. Impaired glucose tolerance in the U.S. population. *Diabetes Care* 1989;**12**:464–474.

18 Pauker SG. Deciding about screening. *Ann Intern Med* 1993;**118**:901–902.

19 Davidson JK (ed.). *Clinical Diabetes Mellitus. A Problem Oriented Approach*, 2nd edn, Thieme Medical Publishers, New York, 1991.

20 Genuth SM, Houser HB, Carter JR Jr, Merkatz IR, Price JW, Schumacher OP, Wieland RG. Observations on the value of mass indiscriminate screening for diabetes mellitus based on a five-year follow-up. *Diabetes* 1978;**27**:377–383.

21 Kupfer IJ. Diabetes screening in an outpatient oral surgery clinic. *NY State Dent J* 1970;**36**:31–32.

22 Hawthorne VM, Cowie CC. Some thoughts on early detection and intervention in diabetes mellitus. *J Chronic Dis* 1984;**37**:667–669.

23 Bennett PH, Knowler WC. Early detection and intervention in diabetes mellitus: is it effective? *J Chronic Dis* 1984;**37**: 653–666.

24 West KM. Community screening programs for diabetes? *Diabetes Care* 1979;**2**:381–384.

25 West KM, Kalbfleisch JM. Sensitivity and specificity of five screening tests for diabetes in ten countries. *Diabetes* 1971;**20**:289–296.

26 Calman K. Developing screening in the NHS. *J Med Screen* 1994;**1**:101–105.

27 Morrison AS. *Screening in Chronic Disease*, 2nd edn, Oxford University Press, New York, 1992.

28 Wilson JMG, Jungner G, *Principles and Practice of Screening for Disease*, World Health Organization, Geneva, 1968.

29 (a) The Expert Committee on the Diagnosis and Classification of Diabetes Mellitus. Report of the Expert Committee on the Diagnosis and Classification of Diabetes Mellitus. *Diabetes Care* 1997;**20**:1183–1197; (b) Marshall KG. Prevention. How much harm? How much benefit? 1. Influence of reporting methods on perception of benefits. *CMAJ* 1996;**154**:1493–1499.

30 Gordis L. The scope of screening. *J Med Screen* 1994;**1**:98–100.

31 Marshall KG. Prevention. How much harm? How much benefit? 4. The ethics of informed consent for preventive screening programs. *CMAJ* 1996;**155**:377–383.

32 Marshall KG. Prevention. How much harm? How much benefit? 3. Physical, psychological and social harm. *CMAJ* 1996;**155**:169–176.

33 Marshall KG. Prevention. How much harm? How much benefit? 2. Ten potential pitfalls in determining the clinical significance of benefits. *CMAJ* 1996;**154**:1837–1843.

34 Trilling JS. Screening for non-insulin-dependent diabetes mellitus in the elderly. *Clin Geriatr Med* 1990;**6**:839–848.

35 Browder AA. Screening for diabetes. *Prev Med* 1974;**3**: 220–224.

36 de Courten M, Zimmet P. Screening for non-insulin-dependent diabetes mellitus: where to draw the line? *Diabet Med* 1997;**14**:95–98.

37 Cadman D, Chambers L, Feldman W, Sackett D. Assessing the effectiveness of community screening programs. *JAMA* 1984;**251**:1580–1585.

38 Engelgau MM, Geiss LS, Saaddine JB, Boyle JP, Benjamin SM, Gregg EW, Tierney EF, Rios-Burrows N, Mokdad AH, Ford ES, Imperatore G, Narayan KM. The evolving diabetes burden in the United States. *Ann Intern Med* 2004;**140**: 945–950.

39 Centers for Disease Control and Prevention. *National Diabetes Fact Sheet 2005*. Centers for Disease Control and Prevention, US Department of Health and Human Services, Atlanta, GA, 2005.

40 World Health Organization Expert Committee on Diabetes Mellitus. *Second Report on Diabetes Mellitus*. Technical Report Series No. 646. World Health Organization, Geneva, 1980, pp. 8–14.

41 National Diabetes Data Group. Classification and diagnosis of diabetes mellitus and other categories of glucose intolerance. *Diabetes* 1979;**28**:1039–1057.

42 World Health Organization. *Definition Diagnosis and Classification of Diabetes Mellitus and Its Complications: Report of a WHO Consultation. Part 1: Diagnosis and Classification of Diabetes Mellitus*. World Health Organization, Geneva, 1999.

43 Brookmeyer R, Day NE, Moss S. Case–control studies for estimation of the natural history of preclinical disease from screening data. *Stat Med* 1986;**5**:127–138.

44 Thompson TJ, Engelgau MM, Hegazy M, Ali MA, Sous ES, Badran A, Herman WH. The onset of NIDDM and its relationship to clinical diagnosis in Egyptian adults. *Diabet Med* 1996;**13**:337–340.

45 Turner R, Cull C, Holman R. United Kingdom Prospective Diabetes Study 17: a 9-year update of a randomized, controlled trial on the effect of improved metabolic control on complications in non-insulin-dependent diabetes mellitus. *Ann Intern Med* 1996;**124**:136–145.

46 Klein R, Klein BE, Moss SE. Prevalence of microalbuminuria in older-onset diabetes. *Diabetes Care* 1993;**16**:1325–1330.

47 Eastman RC, Neuropathy in diabetes. In: *Diabetes in America*, 2nd edn, NIH Publication 95-1468, National Diabetes Data Group, National Institutes of Health, National Institute of Diabetes and Digestive and Kidney Diseases, Bethesda, MD, 1996.

48 Wingard D.L., Barrett-Connor E., Heart disease in diabetes. In: *Diabetes in America*, 2nd edn, NIH Publication 95-1468, National Diabetes Data Group, National Institutes of Health, National Institute of Diabetes and Digestive and Kidney Diseases, Bethesda, MD, 1996.

49 Eastman RC, Cowie CC, Harris MI. Undiagnosed diabetes or impaired glucose tolerance and cardiovascular risk. *Diabetes Care* 1997;**20**:127–128.

50 Hoerger TJ, Harris R, Hicks KA, Donahue K, Sorensen S, Engelgau M. Screening for type 2 diabetes mellitus: a cost-effectiveness analysis. *Ann Intern Med* 2004;**140**:689–699.

51 Gold MR, Siegel JE, Russell LB, Weinstein MC, *Cost-Effectiveness in Health and Medicine*, Oxford University Press, New York, 1996.

52 Rembold CM. Number needed to screen: development of a statistic for disease screening. *BMJ* 1998;**317**:307–312.

53 Donaldson C. Using economics to assess the place of screening. *J Med Screen* 1994;**1**:124–128.

54 Sasco AJ. Validity of case–control studies and randomized controlled trials of screening. *Int J Epidemiol* 1991;**20**: 1143–1144.

55 Davies M, Day J. The Cochrane Collaborative Diabetes Review Group. *Diabet Med* 1996;**13**:390–391.

56 Airey CM, Williams DRR. Cochrane Collaboration Review Group: Diabetes. *Diabet Med* 1995;**12**:375–376.

57 Lauritzen T, Griffin S, Borch-Johnsen K, Wareham NJ, Wolffenbuttel BH, Rutten G. The ADDITION study: proposed trial of the cost-effectiveness of an intensive multifactorial intervention on morbidity and mortality among people with type 2 diabetes detected by screening. *Int J Obes Relat Metab Disord* 2000;**24**(Suppl 3): S6–S11.

58 Panzram G. Mortality and survival in type 2 (non-insulin-dependent) diabetes mellitus. *Diabetologia* 1987;**30**:123–131.

59 Manservigi D, Samori G, Graziani R, Bottoni L. Impaired glucose tolerance and clinical diabetes: a 6-year follow-up of screened versus non-screened subjects. *Diabetologia* 1982;**23**:185.

60 O'Connor PJ, Gregg E, Rush WA, Cherney LM, Stiffman MN, Engelgau MM. Diabetes: how are we diagnosing and initially managing it? *Ann Fam Med* 2006;**4**:15–22.

61 UKPDS Group. Tight blood pressure control and risk of macrovascular and microvascular complications in type 2 diabetes: UKPDS 38. *BMJ* 1998;**317**:703–713.

62 UKPDS Group. Intensive blood-glucose control with sulphonylureas or insulin compared with conventional treatment and risk of complications in patients with type 2 diabetes (UKPDS 33). *Lancet* 1998;**352**:837–853.

63 UKPDS Group. Effect of intensive blood-glucose control with metformin on complications in overweight

patients with type 2 diabetes (UKPDS 34). *Lancet* 1998;**352**: 854–865.

64 The Diabetes Control and Complications Trial/Epidemiology of Diabetes Interventions and Complications Study Research Group. Intensive diabetes treatment and cardiovascular disease in patients with type 1 diabetes. *N Engl J Med* 2005;**353**:2643–2653.

65 Hansson L, Zanchetti A, Carruthers SG, Dahlof B, Elmfeldt D, Julius S, Menard J, Rahn KH, Wedel H, Westerling S. Effects of intensive blood-pressure lowering and low-dose aspirin in patients with hypertension: principal results of the Hypertension Optimal Treatment (HOT) randomised trial. HOT Study Group. *Lancet* 1998;**351**:1755–1762.

66 Ferris FL III. How effective are treatments for diabetic retinopathy? *JAMA* 1993;**269**:1290–1291.

67 Diabetic Retinopathy Study Group. Photocoagulation treatment of proliferative diabetic retinopathy: clinical application of diabetic retinopathy study (DRS) findings. *Ophthalmology* 1981;**88**:583–600.

68 ETDRS Research Group. Photocoagulation for diabetic macular edema. *Arch Ophthalmol* 1985;**103**:1796–1806.

69 Lewis EJ, Hunsicker LG, Bain RP, Rohde RD. The effect of angiotensin-converting-enzyme inhibition on diabetic nephropathy. The Collaborative Study Group. *N Engl J Med* 1993;**329**:1456–1462.

70 Kasiske BL, Kalil RS, Ma JZ, Liao M, Keane WF. Effect of antihypertensive therapy on the kidney in patients with diabetes: a meta-regression analysis. *Ann Intern Med* 1993;**118**:129–138.

71 Reiber GE, Pecoraro RE, Koepsell TD. Risk factors for amputation in patients with diabetes mellitus. A case–control study. *Ann Intern Med* 1992;**117**:97–105.

72 Bild DE, Selby JV, Sinnock P, Browner WS, Braveman P, Showstack JA. Lower-extremity amputation in people with diabetes. Epidemiology and prevention. *Diabetes Care* 1989;**12**:24–31.

73 Khaw KT, Wareham N, Bingham S, Luben R, Welch A, Day N. Association of hemoglobin A1c with cardiovascular disease and mortality in adults: the European prospective investigation into cancer in Norfolk. *Ann Intern Med* 2004;**141**:413–420.

74 Colagiuri S, Cull CA, Holman RR. Are lower fasting plasma glucose levels at diagnosis of type 2 diabetes associated with improved outcomes?: U K. prospective diabetes study 61. *Diabetes Care* 2002;**25**:1410–1417.

75 Welborn TA, Wearne K. Coronary heart disease incidence and cardiovascular mortality in Busselton with reference to glucose and insulin concentrations. *Diabetes Care* 1979;**2**: 154–160.

76 Pyorala K, Savolainen E, Kaukola S, Haapakoski J. Plasma insulin as a coronary heart disease risk factor: relationship to other risk factors and predictive value during $9^1/_2$-year follow-up of the Helsinki Policemen Study Population. *Acta Med Scand Suppl* 1985;**701**:38–52.

77 Fontbonne A, Charles MA, Thibult N, Richard JL, Claude JR, Warnet JM, Rosselin GE, Eschwege E. Hyperinsulinaemia as a predictor of coronary heart disease mortality in a healthy population: the Paris Prospective Study 15-year follow-up. *Diabetologia* 1991;**34**:356–361.

78 US Preventive Services Task, Force. *Guide to Clinical Preventive Services*, 2nd edn, International Medical Publishing, Alexandria, VA, 1996.

79 Ohkubo Y, Kishikawa H, Araki E, Miyata T, Isami S, Motoyoshi S, Kojima Y, Furuyoshi N, Shichiri M. Intensive insulin therapy prevents the progression of diabetic microvascular complications in Japanese patients with non-insulin-dependent diabetes mellitus: a randomized prospective 6-year study. *Diabetes Res Clin Pract* 1995;**28**:103–117.

80 UKPDS Group Quality of life in type 2 diabetic patients is affected by complications but not by intensive policies to improve blood glucose or blood pressure control (UKPDS 37). *Diabetes Care* 1999;**22**:1125–1136.

81 Vijan S, Hofer TP, Hayward RA. Estimating benefits of glycemic control in microvascular complications in type 2 diabetes. *Ann Intern Med* 1997;**127**:788–795.

82 Bulpitt CJ, Benos AS, Nicholl CG, Fletcher AE. Should medical screening of the elderly population be promoted? *Gerontology* 1990;**36**:230–245.

83 Skinner TC, Davies MJ, Farooqi AM, Jarvis J, Tringham JR, Khunti K. Diabetes screening anxiety and beliefs. *Diabet Med* 2005;**22**:1497–1502.

84 Edelman D, Olsen MK, Dudley TK, Harris AC, Oddone EZ. Impact of diabetes screening on quality of life. *Diabetes Care* 2002;**25**:1022–1026.

85 Mausner JS, Kramer S. *Epidemiology – An Introductory Text*. W.B. Saunders, Philadelphia, PA, 1985.

86 Fletcher RH, Fletcher SW, Wagner EH. *Clinical Epidemiology: the Essentials*. Williams and Wilkins, Baltimore, MD, 1988.

87 Hennekens CH, Buring JE. In: *Epidemiology in Medicine* (ed. In: Mayrent SL,), LittleBrown and Company, Boston, MA, 1987; pp. 336–339.

88 Reid MC, Lachs MS, Feinstein AR. Use of methodological standards in diagnostic test research Getting better but still not good. *JAMA* 1995;**274**:645–651.

89 Centor RM, Schwartz JS. An evaluation of methods for estimating the area under the receiver operating characteristic (ROC) curve. *Med Decis Making* 1985;**5**: 149–156.

90 Hanley JA, McNeil BJ. A method of comparing the areas under receiver operating characteristic curves derived from the same cases. *Radiology* 1983;**148**:839–843.

91 Bamber D. The area above the ordinal dominancy graph and the area below the receiver operating characteristic graph. *J Math Psychol* 1975;**12**:387–415.

92 Beck JR, Shultz EK. The use of relative operating characteristic (ROC) curves in test performance evaluation. *Arch Pathol Lab Med* 1986;**110**:13–20.

93 Centor RM. A Visicalc program for estimating the area under a receiver operating characteristic (ROC) curve. *Med Decis Making* 1985;**5**:139–148.

94 American Diabetes Association. Screening for type 2 diabetes. *Diabetes Care* 1999;**22**:S20–S23.

95 Duncan WE, Linville N, Clement S. Assessing risk factors when screening for diabetes mellitus. *Diabetes Care* 1993;**16**:1403–4.

96 American Diabetes Association. American diabetes alert. *Diabetes Forecast* 1993;**46**:54.

97 Newman WP, Nelson R, Scheer K. Community screening for diabetes. Low detection rate in a low-risk population. *Diabetes Care* 1994;**17**:363–365.

98 Burden ML, Burden AC. The American Diabetes Association screening questionnaire for diabetes. Is it worthwhile in the U.K.? *Diabetes Care* 1994;**17**:97.

99 Herman WH, Smith PJ, Thompson TJ, Engelgau MM, Aubert RE. A new and simple questionnaire to identify people at increased risk for undiagnosed diabetes. *Diabetes Care* 1995;**18**:382–387.

100 Herman WH, Smith PJ, Thompson TJ, Engelgau MM, Aubert RE. Response to Knudson et al. *Diabetes Care* 1998;**21**:1030–1031.

101 Ruige JB, de Neeling JN, Kostense PJ, Bouter LM, Heine RJ. Performance of an NIDDM screening questionnaire based on symptoms and risk factors. *Diabetes Care* 1997;**20**: 491–496.

102 McGregor MS, Pinkham C, Ahroni JH, Herter CD, Doctor JD. The American Diabetes Association Risk Test for diabetes. *Diabetes Care* 1995;**18**:585–586.

103 Knudson PE, Turner KJ, Sedore A, Weinstock RS. Utility of the American Diabetes Association risk test in a community screening program. *Diabetes Care* 1998;**21**:1029–1031.

104 McGregor MS, Pinkham C, Ahroni JH, Herter CD, Doctor JD. The American Diabetes Association Risk Test for diabetes. Is it a useful screening tool? *Diabetes Care* 1995;**18**: 585–586.

105 Glumer C, Borch-Johnsen K, Colagiuri S. Can a screening programme for diabetes be applied to another population? *Diabet Med* 2005;**22**:1234–1238.

106 Rathmann W, Martin S, Haastert B, Icks A, Holle R, Lowel H, Giana G. Performance of screening questionnaires and risk scores for undiagnosed diabetes: the KORA Survey 2000. *Arch Intern Med* 2005;**165**:436–441.

107 Simmons D, Thompson CF, Engelgau MM. Controlling the diabetes epidemic: how should we screen for undiagnosed diabetes and dysglycaemia? *Diabet Med* 2005;**22**:207–212.

108 Andersson DK, Lundblad E, Svardsudd K. A model for early diagnosis of type 2 diabetes mellitus in primary health care. *Diabet Med* 1993;**10**:167–173.

109 Hanson RL, Nelson RG, McCance DR, Beart JA, Charles MA, Pettitt DJ, Knowler WC. Comparison of screening tests for non-insulin-dependent diabetes mellitus. *Arch Intern Med* 1993;**153**:2133–2140.

110 Forrest RD, Jackson CA, Yudkin JS. The glycohaemoglobin assay as a screening test for diabetes mellitus: the Islington Diabetes Survey. *Diabet Med* 1987;**4**:254–259.

111 Davies M, Alban-Davies H, Cook C, Day J. Self testing for diabetes mellitus. *BMJ* 1991;**303**:696–698.

112 Anokute CC. Epidemiological studies of diabetes mellitus in Saudi Arabia – Part I – Screening of 3158 males in King Saud University. *J R Soc Health* 1990;**110**:201–203.

113 Orzeck EA, Mooney JH, Owen JA Jr. Diabetes detection with a comparison of screening methods. *Diabetes* 1971;**20**: 109–116.

114 Davies MJ, Williams DR, Metcalfe J, Day JL. Community screening for non-insulin-dependent diabetes mellitus: self-testing for post-prandial glycosuria. *Q J Med* 1993;**86**: 677–684.

115 Robertson DA, Albeti KG, Dowse GK, Zimmet P, Toumilehto J, Gareeboo H. Is serum anhydroglucitol an alternative to the oral glucose tolerance test for diabetes screening? The Mauritius Noncommunicable Diseases Study Group. *Diabet Med* 1992;**10**:56–60.

116 Simon D, Coignet MC, Thibult N, Senan C, Eschwege E. Comparison of glycosylated hemoglobin and fasting plasma glucose with two-hour post-load plasma glucose in the detection of diabetes mellitus. *Am J Epidemiol* 1985;**122**: 589–593.

117 Modan M, Harris MI. Fasting plasma glucose in screening for NIDDM in the U. S. and Israel. *Diabetes Care* 1994;**17**: 436–439.

118 Haffner SM, Rosenthal M, Hazuda HP, Stern MP, Franco LJ. Evaluation of three potential screening tests for diabetes mellitus in a biethenic population. *Diabetes Care* 1984; **7**:347–353.

119 Forrest RD, Jackson CA, Judkin JS. The abbreviated glucose tolerance test in screening for diabetes: the Islington Diabetes Study. *Diabet Med* 1988;**5**:557–561.

120 Tsuji I, Nakamoto K, Hasegawa T, Hisashige A, Inawashiro H, Fukao A, Hisamichi S. Receiver operating characteristic analysis on fasting plasma glucose. HbA1c and fructosamine on diabetes screening. *Diabetes Care* 1991;**14**:1075–1077.

121 Blunt BA, Barrett-Conner E, Wingard DL. Evaluation of fasting plasma glucose as a screening test for NIDDM in older adults. Rancho Bernardo Study. *Diabetes Care* 1991;**14**:989–993.

122 Modan M, Halkin H, Karasik A, Lusky A. Effectiveness of glycosylated hemoglobin, fasting plasma glucose and a single post load plasma glucose level in population screening for glucose intolerance. *Am J Epidemiol* 1984;**119**: 431–444.

123 Swai AB, Harrison K, Chuwa LM, Makene W, McLarty D, Alberti KG. Screening for diabetes: does measurement of serum fructosamine help? *Diabet Med* 1988;**5**:648–652.

124 Bourn D, Mann J. Screening for noninsulin dependent diabetes mellitus and impaired glucose tolerance in a Dunedin general practice – is it worth it? *N Z Med J* 1992;**105**:208–210.

125 Abernethy MH, Andre C, Beaven DW, Taylor HW, Welsh G. A random blood sugar diabetes detection survey. *N Z Med J* 1977;**86**:123–126.

126 Sigurdsson G, Gorrskalksson G, Thorsteinsson T, Davidsson D, Olafsson O, Samuelsson S, Sigfusson N. Community screening for glucose intolerance in middle-aged Icelandic men. Deterioration to diabetes over a period of $7^1/_2$ years. *Acta Med Scand* 1981;**210**:21–26.

127 Moses RG, Colagiuri S, Shannon AG. Effectiveness of mass screening for diabetes mellitus using random capillary blood glucose measurements. *Med J Aust* 1985;**143**:544–6.

128 Lee CH, Fook-Chong S. Evaluation of fasting plasma glucose as a screening test for diabetes mellitus in Singaporean adults. *Diabet Med* 1997;**14**:119–122.

129 Chang CJ, Wu JS, Lu FH, Lee HL, Yang YC, Wen MJ. Fasting plasma glucose in screening for diabetes in the Taiwanese population. *Diabetes Care* 1998;**21**:1856–1860.

130 Nitiyanant W, Ploybutr S, Sriussadaporn S, Yamwong P, Vannasaeng S. Evaluation of the new fasting plasma

glucose cutpoint of 7.0 mmol/l in detection of diabetes mellitus in the Thai population. *Diabetes Res Clin Pract* 1998;**41**:171–176.

131 Wiener K. Fasting plasma glucose as a screening test for diabetes mellitus. *Diabet Med* 1997;**14**:711–712.

132 Ko GT, Chan JC, Yeung VT, Chow CC, Tsang LW, Li JK, So WY, Wai HP, Cockram CS. Combined use of a fasting plasma glucose concentration and HbA1c or fructosamine predicts the likelihood of having diabetes in high-risk subjects. *Diabetes Care* 1998;**21**:1221–1225.

133 Bortheiry AL, Malerbi DA, Franco LJ. The ROC curve in the evaluation of fasting capillary blood glucose as a screening test for diabetes and IGT. *Diabetes Care* 1994;**17**:1269–1272.

134 Ferrell RE, Hanis CL, Aguilar L, Tulloch B, Garcia C, Schull WJ. Glycosylated hemoglobin determination from capillary blood samples. Utility in an epidemiological survey of diabetes. *Am J Epidemiol* 1984;**119**:159–166.

135 Forrest RD, Jackson CA, Yudkin JS. Screening for diabetes mellitus in general practice using a reflectance meter system. The Islington Diabetes Survey. *Diabetes Res* 1987;**6**:119–122.

136 Ko GT, Chan JC, Cockram CS. Supplement to the use of a paired value of fasting plasma glucose and glycated hemoglobin in predicting the likelihood of having diabetes. *Diabetes Care* 1998;**21**:2032–2033.

137 Santiago JV, Davis JE, Fisher F. Hemoglobin A1c levels in a diabetes detection program. *J Clin Endocrinol Metab* 1978;**47**: 578–580.

138 Sekikawa A, Tominaga M, Takahashi K, Watanabe H, Miyazawa K, Sasaki H. Is examination of fructosamine levels valuable as a diagnostic test for diabetes mellitus? *Diabetes Res Clin Pract* 1990;**8**:187–192.

139 Little RR, England JD, Wiedmeyer HM, McKenzie EM, Pettitt DJ, Knowler WC, Goldstein DE. Relationship of glycosylated hemoglobin to oral glucose tolerance. Implications for diabetes screening. *Diabetes* 1988;**37**:60–64.

140 Orchard TJ, Daneman D, Becker D, Kuller LH, LaPorte RE, Drash AL, Wagener D. Glycosylated hemoglobin: a screening test for diabetes mellitus? *Prev Med* 1982;**11**:595–601.

141 Motala AA, Omar MA. The value of glycosylated haemoglobin as a substitute for the oral glucose tolerance test in the detection of impaired glucose tolerance (IGT). *Diabetes Res Clin Pract* 1992;**17**:199–207.

142 Verrillo A, de Teresa A, Golia R, Nunziata V. The relationship between glycosylated haemoglobin levels and various degrees of glucose intolerance. *Diabetologia* 1983;**24**: 391–393.

143 Guillausseau PJ, Charles MA, Paolaggi F, Timsit J, Chanson P, Peynet J, Godard V, Eschwege E, Rousselet F, Lubetzki J. Comparison of HbA1 and fructosamine in diagnosis of glucose-tolerance abnormalities. *Diabetes Care* 1990;**13**: 898–900.

144 Kesson CM, Young RE, Talwar D, Whitelaw JW, Robb DA. Glycosylated hemoglobin in the diagnosis of non-insulin-dependent diabetes mellitus. *Diabetes Care* 1982;**5**:395–398.

145 Goldstein D.E., Little R.R., England J.D., Wiedmeyer H.M., McKenzie E., Glycated hemoglobin: is it a useful screening test for diabetes mellitus? *In: Frontiers of Diabetes Research: Current Trends in Non-insulin-dependent Diabetes Mellitus*

(eds Alberti KGMM, Mazze R,), Elsevier, Amsterdam, 1989.

146 Lester E, Frazer AD, Shepard CA, Woodroffe FJ. Glycosylated haemoglobin as an alternative to the glucose tolerance test for the diagnosis of diabetes mellitus. *Ann Clin Biochem* 1985;**22**:74–78.

147 Salemans TH, Van Dieijen–Visser MP, Brombacher PJ. The value of HbA1 and fructosamine in predicting impaired glucose tolerance – an alternative to OGTT to detect diabetes mellitus or gestational diabetes. *Ann Clin Biochem* 1987;**24**:447–452.

148 Schmidt MI, Duncan BB, Vigo A, Pankow J, Ballantyne CM, Couper D, Brancati F, Folsom AR, and the ARIC Investigators. Detection of undiagnosed diabetes and other hyperglycemia states: The Atherosclerosis Risk in Communities Study. *Diabetes Care* 2003;**16**:1338–1343.

149 Franciosi M, De Berardis G, Rossi MC, Sacco M, Belfiglio M, Pellegrini F, Tognoni G, Valentini M, Nicolucci A. Use of the diabetes risk score for opportunistic screening of undiagnosed diabetes and impaired glucose tolerance: the IGLOO (Impaired Glucose Tolerance and Long-Term Outcomes Observational) study. *Diabetes Care* 2005;**28**:1187–1194.

150 Engelgau MM, Thompson TJ, Smith PJ, Herman WH, Aubert RE, Gunter EW, Wetterhall SF, Sous ES, Ali MA. Screening for diabetes mellitus in adults. The utility of random capillary blood glucose measurements. *Diabetes Care* 1995;**18**:463–466.

151 Rolka DB, Narayan KM, Thompson TJ, Goldman D, Lindenmayer J, Alich K, Bacall D, Benjamin EM, Lamb B, Stuart DO, Engelgau MM. Performance of recommended screening tests for undiagnosed diabetes and dysglycemia. *Diabetes Care* 2001;**24**:1899–1903.

152 Rohlfing CL, Little RR, Wiedmeyer HM, England JD, Madsen R, Harris MI, Flegal KM, Eberhardt MS, Goldstein DE. Use of GHb (HbA1c) in screening for undiagnosed diabetes in the U. S. population. *Diabetes Care* 2000;**23**:187–191.

153 Edelman D, Olsen MK, Dudley TK, Harris AC, Oddone EZ. Utility of hemoglobin A1c in predicting diabetes risk. *J Gen Intern Med* 2004;**19**:1175–1180.

154 Croxson SC, Absalom S, Burden AC. Fructosamine in diabetes screening of the elderly. *Ann Clin Biochem* 1991;**28**:279–282.

155 Colagiuri S, Hussain Z, Zimmet P, Cameron A, Shaw J. AusDiab. Screening for type 2 diabetes and impaired glucose metabolism: the Australian experience. *Diabetes Care* 2004;**27**:367–371.

156 Saaristo T, Peltonen M, Lindstrom J, Saarikoski L, Sundvall J, Eriksson JG, Tuomilehto J. *Diab Vasc Dis Res* 2005;**2**:67–72.

157 Glumer C, Carstensen B, Sandbaek A, Lauritzen T, Jorgensen T, Borch-Johnsen K. Inter99 study. *Diabetes Care* 2004;**27**:727–733.

158 Spijkerman AM, Yuyun MF, Griffin SJ, Dekker JM, Nijpels G, Wareham NJ. The performance of a risk score as a screening test for undiagnosed hyperglycemia in ethic minority groups: data from the 1999 health survey for England. *Diabetes Care* 2004;**27**:116–122.

159 Park PJ, Griffin SJ, Sargeant L, Wareham NJ. The performance of a risk score in predicting undiagnosed hyperglycemia. *Diabetes Care* 2002;**25**:984–988.

160 Tabaei BP, Herman WH. A multivariate logistic regression equation to screen for diabetes: development and validation. *Diabetes Care* 2002;**25**:1999–2003.

161 McNeely MJ, Boyko EJ, Leonetti DL, Kahn SE, Fujimoto WY. Comparison of a clinical model, the oral glucose tolerance test and fasting glucose for prediction of type 2 diabetes risk in Japanese Americans. *Diabetes Care* 2003;**26**:758–763.

162 Stern MP, Williams K, Haffner SM. Identification of persons at high risk for type 2 diabetes mellitus: do we need the oral glucose tolerance test? *Ann Intern Med* 2002;**136**:575–581.

163 Blunt BA, Barrett-Connor E, Wingard DL. Evaluation of fasting plasma glucose as screening test for NIDDM in older adults. Rancho Bernardo Study. *Diabetes Care* 1991;**14**: 989–993.

164 Goldstein DE, Little RR, Wiedmeyer HM, England JD, Rohlfing CL, Wilke AL. Is glycohemoglobin testing useful in diabetes mellitus? Lessons from the diabetes control and complications trial. *Clin Chem* 1994;**40**:1637–1640.

165 Kilpatrick ES, Maylor PW, Keevil BG. Biological variation of glycated hemoglobin. Implications for diabetes screening and monitoring. *Diabetes Care* 1998;**21**:261–264.

166 Yudkin JS, Forrest RD, Jackson CA, Ryle AJ, Davie S, Gould BJ. Unexplained variability of glycated haemoglobin in non-diabetic subjects not related to glycaemia. *Diabetologia* 1990;**33**:208–215.

167 Modan M, Meytes D, Rozeman P, Yosef SB, Sehayek E, Yosef NB, Lusky A, Halkin H. Significance of high HbA1 levels in normal glucose tolerance. *Diabetes Care* 1988;**11**:422–428.

168 Mold JW, Aspy CB, Lawler FH. Outcomes of an insurance company-sponsored multichannel chemistry screening initiative. *J Fam Pract* 1998;**47**:110–117.

169 Frame PS, Berg AO, Woolf S. U. S. Preventive Services Task Force: highlights of the 1996 report. *Am Fam Physician* 1997;**55**:567–576, 581–582.

170 Home PD. Diagnosing the undiagnosed with diabetes. *BMJ* 1994;**308**:611–612.

171 Zhang P, Engelgau MM, Valdez R, Cadwell B, Benjamin SM, Narayan KM. Efficient cutoff points for three screening tests for detecting undiagnosed diabetes and pre-diabetes: an economic analysis. *Diabetes Care* 2005;**28**:1321–1325.

172 Worrall G. Screening the population for diabetes. *BMJ* 1994;**308**:1639.

173 Davidoff F, Reinecke RD. The 28th Amendment. *Ann Intern Med* 1999;**130**:692–694.

174 Laupacis A, Feeny D, Detsky AS, Tugwell PX. How attractive does a new technology have to be to warrant adoption and utilization? Tentative guidelines for using clinical and economic evaluations. *CMAJ* 1992;**146**:473–481.

175 Davies M, Day J. Screening for non-insulin-dependent diabetes mellitus (NIDDM): how often should it be performed? *J Med Screen* 1994;**1**:78–81.

176 Park PJ, Griffin SJ, Duffy SW, Wareham NJ. The effect of varying the screening interval on false positives and duration of undiagnosed diabetes in a screening program for type 2 diabetes. *J Med Screen* 2000;**7**:91–96.

177 Johnson SL, Tabaei BP, Herman WH. The efficacy and cost of alternative strategies for systematic screening for type 2 diabetes in the U. S. population 45–74 years of age. *Diabetes Care* 2005;**28**:307–311.

178 Worrall G. Screening for diabetes - an alternative view. *Br J Gen Pract* 1992;**42**:304.

179 Santrach PJ, Burritt MF. Point-of-care testing. *Mayo Clin Proc* 1995;**70**:493–449.

180 Law M. 'Opportunistic' screening. *J Med Screen* 1994;**1**:208.

181 Davies M, Day J. Screening for non-insulin-dependent diabetes mellitus (NIDDM): how often should it be performed? *J Med Screen* 1994;**1**:78–81.

182 Cowie CC, Harris MI, Eberhardt MS. Frequency and determinants of screening for diabetes in the U. S. *Diabetes Care* 1994;**17**:1158–1163.

183 Luckmann R, Melville SK. Periodic health evaluation of adults: a survey of family physicians. *J Fam Pract* 1995;**40**:547–554.

184 Herbert CP. Clinical health promotion and family physicians: a Canadian perspective. *Patient Educ Couns* 1995;**25**: 277–282.

185 Stange KC, Flocke SA, Goodwin MA. Opportunistic preventive services delivery. Are time limitations and patient satisfaction barriers? *J Fam Pract* 1998;**46**:419–424.

186 Dickey LL, Kamerow DB. Primary care physicians' use of office resources in the provision of preventive care. *Arch Fam Med* 1996;**5**:399–404.

187 Singh BM, Prescott JJ, Guy R, Walford S, Murphy M, Wise PH. Effect of advertising on awareness of symptoms of diabetes among the general public: the British Diabetic Association Study. *BMJ* 1994;**308**:632–636.

188 Bourn D, Mann J. Screening for noninsulin dependent diabetes mellitus and impaired glucose tolerance in a Dunedin general practice – is it worth it? *N Z Med J* 1992;**105**: 207–210.

189 Clement S, Duncan W, Coffey L, Dean K, Kinum N. Screening for diabetes mellitus. *Ann Intern Med* 1989; **110**:572–573.

190 Solomon AC, Hoag SG, Kloesel WA. A community pharmacist-sponsored diabetes detection program. *J Am Pharm Assoc* 1977;**17**:161–163.

191 Bernard JA. Diabetic screening program held in El Paso, Nov. 19–21, 1970. *Southwest Med* 1971;**52**:33–34.

192 Ross BC. Diabetes screening for over 70 motor drivers. *N Z Med J* 1985;**98**:1093.

193 Engelgau MM, Narayan KM, Geiss LS, Thompson TJ, Beckles GL, Lopez L, Hartwell T, Visscher W, Liburd L. A project to reduce the burden of diabetes in the African-American community: Project DIRECT. *J Natl Med Assoc* 1998;**90**:605–613.

194 Porterfield DS, Din R, Burroughs A, Burrus B, Petteway R, Treiber L, Lamb B, Engelgau M. Screening for diabetes in an African-American community: the Project DIRECT experience. *J Natl Med Assoc* 2004;**96**:1325–1331.

195 Azzopardi J, Fenech FF, Junoussov Z, Mazovetsky A, Olchanski V. A computerized health screening and follow-up system in diabetes mellitus. *Diabet Med* 1995;**12**: 271–276.

196 Abernethy MH, Andre C, Beaven DW, Taylor HW, Welsh G. A random blood sugar diabetes detection survey. *N Z Med J* 1977;**86**:123–126.

197 Kent GT, Leonards JR. Analysis of tests for diabetes in 250,000 persons screened for diabetes using finger blood after a carbohydrate load. *Diabetes* 1968;**17**:274–280.

198 Orzeck EA, Mooney JH, Owen JA Jr. Diabetes detection with a comparison of screening methods. *Diabetes* 1971;**20**: 109–116.

199 Moses RG, Colagiuri S, Shannon AG. Effectiveness of mass screening for diabetes mellitus using random capillary blood glucose measurements. *Med J Aust* 1985;**143**:544–546.

200 Leiter LA, Barr A, Belanger A, Lubin S, Ross SA, Tildesley HD, Fontaine N. Diabetes Screening in Canada (DIASCAN) Study: prevalence of undiagnosed diabetes and glucose intolerance in family physician offices. *Diabetes Care* 2001;**24**:1038–1043.

201 Rathmann W, Haastert B, Icks A, Lowel H, Meisinger C, Holle R, Giani G. High prevalence of undiagnosed diabetes mellitus in Southern Germany: target populations for efficient screening. The KORA survey 2000. *Diabetologia* 2003;**46**:182–189.

202 Tabaei BP, Burke R, Constance A, Hare J, May-Aldrich G, Parker SA, Scott A, Stys A, Chickering J, Herman WH. Community-based screening for diabetes in Michigan. *Diabetes Care* 2003;**26**:668–670.

203 Rand CG, Jackson RJ, Mackie CC. A method for the epidemiological study of early diabetes. *Can Med Assoc J* 1974;**111**:1312–1314.

204 Sellers EA, Dean HJ. Screening for type 2 diabetes in high-risk pediatric population: capillary vs. venous fasting plasma glucose. *Can J Diabet* 2005;**29**:393–396.

205 Grant T, Soriano Y, Marantz PR, Nelson I, Williams E, Ramirez D, Burg J, Nordin C. Community-based screening for cardiovascular disease and diabetes using HbA1c. *Am J Prev Med* 2004;**26**:271–275.

206 Hosler AS, Berberian EL, Spence MM, Hoffman DP. Outcome and cost of a statewide diabetes screening and awareness initiative in New York. *J Public Health Manage Pract* 2005;**11**:59–64.

207 Ealovega MW, Tabaei BP, Brandle M, Burke R, Herman WH. Opportunistic screening for diabetes in routine clinical practice. *Diabetes Care* 2004;**27**:9–12.

208 George PM, Valahhji J, Dawood M, Henry JA. Screening for type 2 diabetes in the accident and emergency departments. *Diabet Med* 2005;**22**:1766–1769.

209 Lee DS, Remington P, Madagame J, Blustein J. A cost analysis of community screening for diabetes in the central Wisconsin Medicare population (results from the MetaStar pilot project in Wausau). *WMJ* 2000;**99**:39–43.

210 American Diabetes Association. Standards of medical care for diabetes – 2006. *Diabetes Care* 2006;**29**(Suppl): S4–S42.

211 Harwell TS, Smilie JG, McDowall JM, Helgerson SD, Gohdes D. Diabetes screening practices among individual-saged 45 years and older. *Diabetes Care* 2000;**23**:125–126.

212 World Health, Organization. *Report of a World Health Organization and International Diabetes Federation Meeting: Screening for Type 2 Diabetes*, World Health Organization, Geneva, 2003.

213 Diabetes UK. Position Statement: Early identification of people with type 2 diabetes. www.diabetes.org.uk (last accessed June 2009).

214 US Preventive Services Task Force. Screening for type 2 diabetes mellitus in adults: recommendations and rational. *Ann Intern Med* 2003;**138**:212–214.

215 Harris R, Donahue K, Rathore SS, Frame P, Woolf SH, Lohr KN. Screening adults for type 2 diabetes: a review of the evidence for the U. S. Preventive Services Task Force. *Ann Intern Med* 2003;**138**:215–229.

216 Feig DS, Palda VA, Lipscombe L, and the Canadian Task Force on Preventive Health Care. Screening for type 2 diabetes to prevent vascular complications: updated recommendations from the Canadian Task Force on Preventive Health Care. *CMAJ* 2005;**172**:177–180.

217 Canadian Diabetes Association Clinical Practice Guidelines Expert Committee. Screening and Prevention. *Clin Pract Guidelines* 2003;S10–S13.

Part 3: Prevention of complications

7 The effectiveness of interventions aimed at weight loss and other effects of diet and physical activity in achieving control of diabetes and preventing its complications

Nita Gandhi Forouhi[1], Nicholas J. Wareham[2]

[1]*Elsie Widdowson Laboratory, MRC Epidemiology Unit, Cambridge, UK*
[2]*MRC Epidemiology Unit, Institute of Metabolic Science, Addenbrooke's Hospital, Cambridge, UK*

Introduction

This chapter reviews the evidence for the effectiveness of interventions aimed at altering diet, physical inactivity and obesity in managing diabetes and diminishing the risks of complications among people with diabetes. The overall effectiveness of these interventions is a product of the efficacy of interventions in supporting individual behaviour change and the impact that this behaviour change has on individual risk. An important distinction has been made between studies which have measured the effectiveness of interventions *aimed* at changing physical activity and diet on more distal clinical outcomes and those which have assessed the effectiveness on behaviour change itself. This chapter is mostly concerned with the former and therefore the interventions described are mostly 'black box'. One can state what outcomes the interventions were designed to alter, but very little inference can be made about the mechanisms by which an effect was achieved or which component of the intervention was most effective in achieving it.

When reviewing the evidence for the effectiveness of lifestyle interventions, one would like, as with pharmacological interventions, to identify randomized controlled clinical trials restricted to people with diabetes in which the primary endpoint was one of the key health outcomes related to diabetes such as mortality, incident heart disease or retinopathy. Few such studies exist. Most of the evidence available comes from prospective cohort studies and short-term randomized studies. In these studies, the endpoints are often intermediate factors such as weight, blood glucose, lipid, insulin or blood pressure, that have been demonstrated in other studies to be associated with the long-term complications of diabetes. This chapter reviews this evidence, and considers possible explanations for the absence of long-term health endpoint trials of behavioural interventions.

What is the evidence for the effectiveness of weight loss in reducing the risk of the complications of diabetes?

Some 80–90% of persons with type 2 diabetes are overweight[1] and obesity worsens abnormalities associated with diabetes, such as hyperglycaemia, hyperlipidaemia and hypertension.[2] Moderate weight loss (5% of body weight) can improve insulin action, decrease fasting blood glucose concentrations and reduce the need for diabetes medications.[3–7] Not surprisingly weight loss is considered to be one of the cornerstones of diabetic therapy. In this chapter, we focus on trials of the effectiveness of weight

The Evidence Base for Diabetes Care, Second Edition, Edited by William H. Herman, Ann Louise Kinmonth, Nicholas J. Wareham and Rhys Williams.
© 2010 John Wiley & Sons, Ltd

reduction in people with diabetes, which are designed to address several different questions:

- Is weight loss effective in reducing the risks of the complications of diabetes?
- Is weight loss effective in improving glycaemia?
- What are the most effective approaches for achieving weight loss in people with diabetes?

Is weight loss effective in reducing the risks of the complications of diabetes? The importance of intentional weight loss

There are no randomized controlled trials (RCTs) of treatments aimed at weight reduction in people with diabetes where the outcome is a health-related event. Evidence from prospective population-based studies is available but may be limited by problems of confounding and reverse causality, as it is difficult to separate intentional and disease-related unintentional weight loss.[5] Williamson *et al.* reported that intentional weight loss among 34% of a cohort of 4970 overweight individuals with diabetes was associated with a 25% reduction in total mortality and a 28% reduction in cardiovascular and diabetes mortality.[8] However, the WHO multi-national study of vascular disease in diabetes illustrates well the difficulty of determining the effectiveness of weight loss on health endpoints from observational studies.[9] In this study, baseline body mass index (BMI) was positively associated with mortality in European men, whereas there was a U-shaped relationship in Native American men and East Asians and an inverted U-shape in European women and Native American women. In general, those patients who were lean also had a longer duration of diabetes, were more likely to be receiving insulin therapy and had a higher prevalence of retinopathy. Even when adjusted for such confounding, no clear relationship between BMI and mortality was observed. Weight loss in people who had a BMI less than $29\,\text{kg}\,\text{m}^{-2}$ at baseline was associated with a 2–3-fold increase in risk of mortality compared with people who were weight stable. The complexity of these associations is further highlighted by the report among 1401 overweight diabetic adults that those trying to lose weight have a reduced risk of all-cause mortality, independent of whether they actually lose weight.[10] Weight loss seems to be associated with increased mortality only if the weight loss is unintentional.[10]

As weight loss has been associated with health hazards in addition to benefits, it is important to address the limitations of observational evidence. After considerable planning, an RCT is under way in the United States to investigate whether interventions designed to produce sustained weight loss in obese individuals with type 2 diabetes mellitus improve health. This 'Look AHEAD' (Action for Health in Diabetes), a multi-centre randomized clinical trial,[11] has now completed enrolment of 5145 obese patients with type 2 diabetes and longer term follow-up is now under way. At study entry, participants were randomly assigned to one of two interventions; standard diabetes support and education alone or with an intensive lifestyle intervention to support weight loss. The intensive intervention comprised group and individual meetings to achieve and maintain weight loss through decreases in caloric intake and increased physical activity. The 1 year results, now available, show a significantly greater weight loss (8.6% of initial weight) in the intensive lifestyle group compared with the standard care group (loss of 0.7% of initial weight).[12] A greater proportion of the intensive lifestyle group (compared with the standard care group) had reductions in medication use for diabetes, hypertension and lipid-lowering therapy. There was an impressive improvement in glycaemic control, with the mean HbA_{1c} dropping from 7.3 to 6.6% in the intensive lifestyle group, whereas in the standard care group there was no significant change in HbA_{1c} level (from 7.3 to 7.2%). Finally, cardiovascular risk factors (systolic and diastolic blood pressure, triglycerides, HDL cholesterol and urine albumin-to-creatinine ratio) improved significantly more in the intensive lifestyle intervention group than in the standard care participants.[12] These 1 year results are very promising, but continued intervention for up to 11.5 years will determine whether there are sustained benefits.

Broadly similar findings have also been reported from a small Korean intervention study among 58 people with diabetes.[13] Participants were randomly assigned to either a 16 week intensive lifestyle modification programme and subsequent monthly meetings during the 6 month study period or to a control group of basic dietary education and usual care. In the intervention group there was a significant weight loss at 6 months ($-2\,\text{kg} \pm 2.6\,\text{kg}$), but not in the control group ($+0.2\,\text{kg} \pm 1.7\,\text{kg}$). Over the same period, there were significant improvements in the intervention group in glycaemic control (mean difference in HbA_{1c} 1%) and systolic blood pressure (mean difference $-8.2\,\text{mmHg}$), but not in the control group ($+0.1\%$ difference in HbA_{1c}; $+0.4\,\text{mmHg}$ systolic blood pressure). There was also a significant attenuation of the progression of carotid intima-media thickness, a marker of early atherosclerosis in the intervention group at 6 months, but not in the control group.[13]

A small 1 year cohort study supports this result, demonstrating weight loss among volunteers to be associated with improved pulse wave velocity, a marker of arterial stiffness, which is an indicator of cardiovascular risk.[14] An intensive nutritional intervention (with or without the drug orlistat) in 38 overweight individuals with diabetes was associated with an average weight loss of 7.8%, an HbA_{1c} reduction of 1.4% (mean HbA_{1c} 6.6% at 1 year compared with 8.0% at baseline) and a reduction in arterial pulse wave velocity of $50 \, \text{cm s}^{-1}$ (from $740 \, \text{cm s}^{-1}$ at baseline to $690 \, \text{cm s}^{-1}$ at 1 year follow-up). Based on estimates from cross-sectional studies, a $50\text{--}100 \, \text{cm s}^{-1}$ increase is associated with ageing 10 years, so this is a clinically meaningful effect. These improvements are promising and taken together with the Look AHEAD trial suggest that weight loss among people with established type 2 diabetes is achievable in the short term and associated with improvements in cardiovascular risk. The long-terms effects remain to be established.

Is weight loss effective in improving glycaemia?

The absence of RCT evidence concerning the efficacy of weight loss on health events in people with diabetes leads to greater emphasis on studies where the impact of weight loss on glycaemic control is evaluated. The largest observational study is the United Kingdom Prospective Diabetes Study (UKPDS),[7] described in detail in another chapter, in which 3044 people with newly diagnosed type 2 diabetes were advised to follow the British Diabetic Association recommendation of a diet containing 50% carbohydrate, 30% fat and 20% protein. Suggested energy intake was related to the degree of overweight, such that for persons with greater than 150% ideal body weight, the recommended energy intake was 4.6 MJ per day, whereas for persons with less than 110% ideal body weight, the recommendation was 7 MJ per day. Among the 2597 participants who were allocated to dietary treatment alone for 3 months, the reduction in fasting glucose, adjusted for initial level, was significantly related to the degree of attained weight loss.[7] Average weight loss was 7% of ideal body weight. It was estimated that, on average, patients needed to lose 30% of ideal body weight to achieve a fasting glucose level of $<6 \, \text{mmol l}^{-1}$ at 3 months. Improvements in glycaemic control with caloric restriction and weight loss are attributable to improved insulin sensitivity in both obese diabetic and non-diabetic persons.[15]

Is there a group of patients with type 2 diabetes who do not respond to diet?

In the UKPDS,[7] 15% of patients were considered to have shown 'primary diet failure' at 3 months, such that despite a prescription of recommended dietary change,

their fasting glucose level remained $>15 \, \text{mmol l}^{-1}$ or they had symptoms of hyperglycaemia. This group included more of the patients who were not overweight, giving rise to speculation that the underlying pathophysiology of diabetes in these individuals may be different and may influence their response to diet therapy. Other groups have shown that the effect of dietary prescription on glycaemic control is minimal in non-obese people with poorly controlled diabetes (fasting blood glucose $>10 \, \text{mmol l}^{-1}$), but that diet-induced weight loss may lead to metabolic improvements in the obese.[16] Studies have suggested that the distribution of the glucose response to weight loss is bimodal, indicating possible separation into 'responder' and 'nonresponder' groups determined by random plasma glucose below or above $10 \, \text{mmol l}^{-1}$ after a minimum weight loss of 9 kg in each group.[17] Comparison of responders and non-responders shows no difference in age, sex, initial fasting glucose or body weight. Whether groups of responders and non-responders differ in other pathophysiological characteristics, such as preferential loss of visceral fat, insulin sensitivity or secretion, remains to be determined.[18]

Watts *et al.* suggested that the success or failure of diet therapy can be predicted from the plasma glucose response to weight loss of only 2.3–4.5 kg.[17] Mild to moderately obese patients with type 2 diabetes who remain hyperglycaemic after a weight loss of 2.3 kg or more are unlikely to improve glycaemic control with further weight loss and should be considered for treatment with hypoglycaemic agents.[17] Finally, in the UKPDS, the overall weight loss by study centre was related to the availability of dietetic advice. It should be borne in mind that one type of diet therapy is unlikely to work for all overweight or obese individuals with type 2 diabetes. Dietary guidance needs to be individualized to allow for different approaches to reducing energy intake.

What are the most effective approaches for achieving weight loss in people with diabetes?

It is usually assumed that strategies that are effective for achieving weight loss among the obese in the general population will be generalizable to the subgroup of obese people with diabetes.[19] This assumption may not, however, always be correct and people with diabetes may find it harder to lose weight[20] or maintain weight loss[21] compared with non-diabetic individuals. Furthermore, anti-diabetic medication including sulfonylureas, thiazolidinediones, meglitinides and insulin may promote weight gain and make weight maintenance harder. Where possible, therefore, studies specifically aimed at the population of people with diabetes have been described in more detail.

Weight loss interventions may be categorized as being:

- focused on diet alone
- aimed at diet and exercise
- pharmacological or
- surgical.

How effective are dietary interventions on weight loss?

Dietary interventions are considered an important strategy for weight loss in diabetes. In a meta-analysis of 89 studies (with 1800 participants) examining different strategies promoting weight loss in type 2 diabetes, Brown et al. concluded that the largest reductions in body weight occurred in persons treated through dietary means when comparing diet, exercise and behavioural therapies, reporting average weight losses of 20, 3.4 and 6.4 lb (9.1, 1.5 and 2.9 kg), respectively.[22] However, methodological limitations of this study merit consideration. The meta-analysis was not restricted to RCTs, or to studies with a particular duration of follow-up. Some 72% of the studies included used a one-group pre-test/post-test comparison and only four of the 89 studies had a double-blind design. The authors scored each study for methodological quality and the average score (out of a possible total of 21) was 10. Studies that scored poorly tended to lack key attributes such as randomization, a clear description of the intervention and direct longitudinal measures of outcome. Overall effect sizes were at least two-fold greater in the non-randomized studies. Notwithstanding these limitations, there is widespread acceptance that diet is an integral component of diabetes management. In the following subsections we consider the elements of dietary interventions that may influence weight loss.

Energy restriction versus dietary fat restriction

It has been estimated that an energy deficit of $500–1000 \, \mathrm{kcal \, day^{-1}}$ ($2100–4200 \, \mathrm{kJ \, day^{-1}}$) will result in a weight loss of approximately 1–2 lb (0.5–1 kg) per week and an average total weight loss of about 8% after 6 months.[23] However, there has been an ongoing debate about the merits of calorie restriction alone versus restriction of specific dietary components such as reducing fat intake. A variety of types of diets have been proposed to influence weight loss, with fewer studies specifically among people with diabetes than among those with obesity regardless of diabetes status. For instance, one review[24] describes 12 studies, five of which were restricted to individuals with type

2 diabetes. In one of these, Pascale et al.[25] recruited 44 obese women with type 2 diabetes and randomly assigned them either to calorie restriction or to calorie restriction combined with fat restriction. Patients in the calorie restriction group were advised to consume $1000–1500 \, \mathrm{kcal \, day^{-1}}$ ($4200–6300 \, \mathrm{kJ \, day^{-1}}$) and were given general information about healthy eating and encouraged to keep their fat intake at <30% of total energy. Those in the low-calorie/low-fat group were given similar calorie targets, but were also given specific instructions on how to reduce fat intake to 20% of total calories. Both groups also participated in a 16 week 'behavioural weight loss' programme. Weight loss was significantly greater in those in the low-calorie/low-fat group than in those in the calorie restriction only group over the 16 week programme (7.7 versus 4.6 kg) and at the 1 year follow-up (5.2 versus 1 kg). However, in this study there were no detectable differences in glucose, HbA_{1c} or lipids between treatment groups. In a Cochrane Collaboration review, Moore et al. reviewed 36 articles on 18 RCTs that included a total of 1467 participants with type 2 diabetes.[26] In five studies, a low-fat diet was compared with either a moderate-fat or a low-carbohydrate diet, with more weight loss in the low-fat group, but the trials were assessed to be at high risk for bias.[25,27–30] There were only marginal changes in glycated haemoglobin and no firm conclusions could be drawn on the effectiveness of the interventions on glycaemic control. It has been suggested that a low-fat diet (e.g. 25–30% of total energy from fat) results in decreased total energy intake and weight loss and thus forms the basis for conventional dietary advice for weight loss. Data on the long-term effect of a very low-fat diet (<15% of calories from fat) on weight loss are limited because few studies have achieved this level of intake.

An alternative approach to a continued low-calorie diet is the use of intermittent very low-calorie diets. The effectiveness of these two approaches was compared in a randomized study of 93 type 2 diabetic persons by Wing and et al.[31] At 1 year, there was greater weight loss in the intermittent very low-calorie diet group (14.2 ± 10.3 kg), but this was not significantly different from the weight loss in the low-calorie group (10.5 ± 11.6 kg, $p = 0.06$). A sub-analysis stratifying by sex showed that the between-treatment group differences were significant in women only (14.1 kg versus 8.6 kg, $p = 0.02$). Ethnic differences in responses to weight control programmes have also been observed between black and white individuals with diabetes. Wing and Anglin reported[32] that black individuals randomly assigned to either a low-calorie diet or an intermittent very low-calorie diet had a greater degree of weight regain between 6 months and

1 year than an equivalent group of white individuals. The extent to which differences in response are attributable to differences in adherence or physiology are unknown. It should be noted that the benefits of low-calorie diets in people with type 2 diabetes may extend beyond their effect on weight. Wing and colleagues have speculated that the benefits on glucose control and insulin sensitivity of calorie restriction in obese patients with type 2 diabetes are independent of the effect on weight.[33,34]

Low-carbohydrate diets

Recently, there has been an increased interest in the use of low-carbohydrate diets as a potential strategy for obesity management both in the general[35] and the diabetic populations.[36] Many types of low-carbohydrate diets have been proposed, but the most famous of these is the Atkins diet,[37] which has been embraced by an estimated 20 million people worldwide. Such diets promote restriction of carbohydrate intake to as low as 5–10% of total energy, with an unlimited intake of protein or accompanying fat. The mechanism of weight loss despite *ad libitum* intake of high-fat foods might be due to severe restriction of carbohydrate-depleting glycogen stores, leading to excretion of bound water, the ketogenic nature of the diet being appetite suppressing, the high protein content being highly satiating and reducing spontaneous food intake or limited food choices leading to decreased energy intake.[35]

A systematic review of low-carbohydrate diets that included 107 articles among 3268 participants reported that among obese individuals, weight loss was associated with duration of diet ($p = 0.002$) and restriction of calorie intake ($p = 0.03$) but not with reduced carbohydrate content ($p = 0.90$).[38] Of note, most participants were on low-carbohydrate diets that were not extreme (663 participants received diets of $<60 \, \text{g day}^{-1}$ of carbohydrates, of whom only 71 received $20 \, \text{g day}^{-1}$ or less). There was no significant adverse effect on serum lipids, glucose or insulin or on blood pressure in the short term (up to 6 months), but longer term effects are unknown. However, this review was based on studies among the generally obese and not among obese individuals with type 2 diabetes. In Samaha *et al.*'s study of a low-carbohydrate versus a low-fat diet, 25 of the 64 severely obese (mean BMI $43 \, \text{kg m}^{-2}$) study participants had type 2 diabetes.[39] Those who were on a low-carbohydrate diet lost more weight than those on the low-fat diet [mean ($\pm$ SD), $-5.8 \pm 8.6 \, \text{kg}$ versus $-1.9 \pm 4.2 \, \text{kg}$; $p = 0.002$] and had greater decreases in triglyceride levels (mean, $-20 \pm 43\%$ versus $-4 \pm 31\%$; $p = 0.001$), irrespective of the use or non-use of hypoglycaemic or lipid-lowering medications. Among those with diabetes, fasting glucose decreased from a mean value of $9.3 \, \text{mmol l}^{-1}$ ($168 \, \text{mg dl}^{-1}$) to $7.9 \, \text{mmol l}^{-1}$ ($142 \, \text{mg dl}^{-1}$) after 6 months.[39] However, this finding should be interpreted with caution, given the small magnitude of overall and between-group differences in weight loss in these markedly obese individuals and the short duration of the study.

There has been a growing literature suggesting that some form of low-carbohydrate diet is a viable option for patients with diabetes, particularly as the traditional dietary recommendation of a high-carbohydrate, low-fat diet has achieved equivocal success.[36,40] Potential support for a low-carbohydrate diet comes from a retrospective non-randomized follow-up study to 22 months of 16 obese diabetic patients previously placed on a low-carbohydrate diet (20% of total energy, with 80–90 g of carbohydrate daily) and followed up closely for 6 months.[41] This study found that the mean body weight varied from $100.6 \pm 14.7 \, \text{kg}$ at the start of the initial study to $89.2 \pm 14.3 \, \text{kg}$ at 6 months and to $92.0 \pm 14.0 \, \text{kg}$ by 22 months. Seven of the 16 patients (44%) retained the same body weight from 6 to 22 months or reduced it further; all but one had lower weight at 22 months than at the beginning. Metabolic control was also improved; for instance, mean HbA_{1c} was 8.0 ± 1.5, 6.6 ± 1.0, 7.0 ± 1.3 and $6.9 \pm 1.1\%$ at baseline and after 6, 12 and 22 months, respectively. However, this study was not randomized and did not have a control arm for the longer follow-up and results need to be interpreted with great caution. A strictly supervised inpatient study of directly observed low-carbohydrate diet ($21 \, \text{g day}^{-1}$ of carbohydrate) but unlimited access to fat or protein intake was designed to compare the effects of usual diet for 7 days versus low-carbohydrate diet for 14 days, on weight loss and glucose control among 10 obese patients with type 2 diabetes.[42] On the low-carbohydrate diet the energy intake decreased from 3111 to $2164 \, \text{kcal day}^{-1}$ and the mean energy deficit ($1027 \, \text{kcal day}^{-1}$) completely accounted for the weight loss of $1.65 \, \text{kg}$ in 14 days. Glycaemic control was improved despite no changes to anti-diabetic medication, with a decrease in HbA_{1c} from 7.3 to 6.8% and an improvement in insulin sensitivity (measured by clamp) of 75%. Lipids were favourably affected, with a decrease in plasma cholesterol and triglyceride levels. Despite the potential positive effect among patients with diabetes, however, it is premature to recommend this diet because this study had several limitations, including small size, very short duration, lack of a strict control group (patients served as their own controls when on usual diet) and the setting of intense in-hospital direct diet control and observation, which would not apply to a free-living population.

Overall, there is an increasing call from some quarters to incorporate the recommendation of low-carbohydrate diets as part of the weight loss and glycaemic control strategy for type 2 diabetes. A case has been made for considering low-carbohydrate diets as a short-term safe and effective intervention if obese diabetic patients have been unsuccessful in losing weight or improving glycaemic control by other means.[36] However, a key concern among diabetic patients on a long-term low-carbohydrate diet is the potential acceleration of decline in renal function because of high protein intake. There is currently no evidence that the low-carbohydrate diets in use have an adverse effect on renal function, but the long-term effects of protein intake >20% of calories on diabetes management and its complications are unknown.

Other theoretical concerns include increased calcium loss in the urine leading to osteoporosis and nephrolithiasis and dyslipidaemia from the associated high fat intake. Hence such diets still need further evaluation, including assessment of cardiovascular outcomes and other longer term effects, and they cannot currently be recommended for a diabetic population without further study.

Glycaemic index and glycaemic load

Since the first description in 1981, the role of the glycaemic index (GI) and later the glycaemic load of diets for diabetes and obesity management has gained increased interest. The GI of foods is concerned with the quality of the carbohydrate for a given quantity of carbohydrate. Thus the GI of a food is the increase above fasting in the blood glucose area over 2 h after ingestion of a constant amount of that food (usually a 50 g carbohydrate portion) divided by the response to a reference food (usually glucose or white bread). The glycaemic load of foods or meals is calculated by multiplying the GI of the constituent foods by the quantity of carbohydrate in each food and then totalling the values for all foods. A randomized trial compared four different diets with varying GI and load in 129 overweight persons over 12 weeks for effects on weight loss and cardiovascular risk reduction.[43] Although all groups lost a similar mean percentage of weight (varying between 4.2 and 6.2%), the proportion who lost 5% or more of body weight varied significantly by diet (31% for a high-GI, high-carbohydrate diet, 56% for a low-GI, high-carbohydrate diet, 66% for a high-protein, high-GI diet and 33% for a high-protein, low-GI diet, $p = 0.01$). Mean LDL cholesterol declined significantly in the high-carbohydrate, low-GI group, but increased in the high-protein, high-GI group. Thus, high-protein and low-GI regimens increased body fat loss, while cardiovascular risk was minimized by a high-carbohydrate, low-GI diet.[43] Low-GI foods may have a meaningful utility for persons with

diabetes, but methodological issues pose difficulties including the method of dietary assessment (type of food questionnaire), application of appropriate GI tables and correlated dietary patterns. Population-based studies should provide insights into the independent association of GI and glycaemic load with obesity and diabetes and, as for other dietary interventions, for low-GI diets there is also a need for longer term intervention studies.

Many different types of dietary modification have been studied (such as calorie restriction, low-fat, high-carbohydrate diet or low-carbohydrate diet or combinations of these), but they all suffer from the limitations of poor long-term compliance and weight regain, despite short-term weight loss. Current expert opinion, based on best evidence to date, is that overweight or obese patients with type 2 diabetes should be encouraged to adopt dietary recommendations that reduce the risk of coronary heart disease, such as those by the National Cholesterol Education Programme diet that recommends a moderate decrease in caloric intake of 500–1000 kcal day^{-1} (2100–4200 kJ day^{-1}) to help with slow but progressive weight loss.[44] This diet derives 50–60% of energy from carbohydrate, ~15% from protein and 25–35% from fat (with saturated fat of <7% of total calories).[45] These dietary recommendations should go hand-in-hand with other lifestyle recommendations that include physical activity.

How effective are combined diet and physical activity interventions on weight loss?

Overall, the combination of diet and exercise appears to be more beneficial for weight loss than simply diet by itself, as shown in the UK Effective Health Care review.[24] This identified four trials of exercise in combination with a dietary programme for weight loss,[46–49] but only one trial was specifically focused on people with diabetes.[49] The benefits of combined interventions may result from the effects of exercise in reducing the loss of lean body mass and the reduction in basal metabolic rate that may occur with weight loss.[50] King and Tribble reviewed studies of weight loss and maintenance with caloric restriction alone, exercise alone or a combination of both.[51] In studies with a follow-up of at least 6 months they found that the average weight loss was 4.0 kg in four diet-only programmes, 4.9 kg in five exercise-only programmes and 7.2 kg in three combined diet and exercise programmes.[51]

Specifically among adult type 2 diabetic patients, the long-term effectiveness (at 1–5 years) of weight-loss strategies involving dietary, physical activity or behavioural interventions has been assessed in a meta-analysis of 22 studies including 4659 participants.[52] Dietary interventions included low-calorie diets [800–155 kcal day^{-1} (3350–650 kJ day^{-1})] and very low-calorie diets [<800 kcal day^{-1} (<3350 kJ day^{-1})]; physical activity interventions included counselling, an exercise prescription or participation in a supervised or unsupervised exercise programme; behavioural interventions addressed barriers to diet or physical activity, using strategies such as stimulus control and social support. The pooled weight loss for any intervention compared with usual care ($n = 585$) was 1.7 kg (95% CI 0.3 to 3.2 kg) or 3.1% of baseline body weight. Comparison groups often achieved substantial weight loss, minimising between-group differences. However, among persons who underwent a physical activity and behavioural intervention ($n = 126$), those who also received a very low-calorie diet lost 3.0 kg (95% CI 0.5 to 6.4 kg) or 1.6% of baseline body weight, more than persons who received a low-calorie diet alone. Among persons who received identical dietary and behavioural interventions ($n = 53$), those who received a more intense physical activity intervention lost 3.9 kg (95% CI 1.9 to 9.7 kg) or 3.6% of baseline body weight, more than those who received a less intense or no physical activity intervention.[52]

Hence there is support for greater weight loss with combination of diet and physical activity than either alone, but the magnitude of the associated weight loss seems to be modest and somewhat disappointing. However, although our emphasis in this section has been on the primary outcome of weight, it is important to note that other outcomes, such as medication usage, are improved to a greater extent. For example, in the study by Wing *et al.*, the diet plus exercise group had reduced medications to a greater extent than the diet-only group at the 1 year follow-up (83% versus 38%).[49] The effects of physical activity on metabolic control are also valuable and are considered in a separate section.

Does physical activity aid in the prevention of weight gain in people with diabetes?

Diabetic patients are prone to gain weight for a variety of reasons, including pharmacotherapy, such as intensified insulin therapy in individuals with type 1 diabetes[53] and type 2 diabetes.[7] With the setting of lower HbA$_{1c}$ target levels, more aggressive management of diabetic individuals is being encouraged, with the concomitant increased use of medications that enhance anabolism and weight gain. Although it is likely that increased physical activity would attenuate such weight gain, there have been few systematic studies. Beyond the specific context of diabetes, one

systematic review identified only a handful of trials that have evaluated the effectiveness of any interventions aimed at preventing weight gain,[54] a marked difference to the number of trials of interventions aimed at treating obesity or preventing weight regain in people who have successfully lost weight.

How effective are pharmacological interventions on weight loss?

When lifestyle management has failed to achieve weight loss, drug therapy to aid weight loss has a place in patients who are at high risk of complications. Orlistat, an intestinal lipase inhibitor, and sibutramine, a serotonin and noradrenaline re-uptake inhibitor, are the most widely studied and used drugs for obesity control. In a meta-analysis of 50 studies of orlistat use, Li *et al.* reported a mean weight loss over 12 months of treatment of 2.9 kg (95% CI 2.3 to 3.5 kg).[55] Although its use is limited by gastrointestinal side-effects, it is a safe drug, with use of up to 4 years now demonstrated.[56] A similar magnitude of weight loss [mean 4.5 kg (95% CI 3.2 to 5.3 kg) at 12 months] has been reported in separate meta-analyses of the effect of sibutramine.[55,57,58] Among patients with diabetes, sibutramine use was associated with a weight loss of about 5 kg on average in clinical trials. For instance, one meta-analysis reported a weight decrease of (mean $\pm$ SD) 5.5 $\pm$ 0.23 kg in the sibutramine group compared with 0.9 $\pm$ 0.17 kg in the placebo group, and another meta-analysis reported weight loss of 5.1 kg (95% CI 3.2 to 7.0 kg) in the sibutramine group at 12–52 weeks follow-up.[59,60] The longer term results of treatment with sibutramine are not yet known, but recent case reports have implicated its use with memory impairment,[61] cardiomyopathy,[62] prolonged QT interval[63] and severe bruising,[64] warranting caution in its extended use.

New drug developments for obesity treatment are the focus of efforts of many pharmaceutical companies and researchers. One such new drug is rimonabant, which works through antagonism of the cannabinoid receptor type 1 (CB1) to decrease food intake and increase energy expenditure. The RIO-Europe (rimonabant in obesity) trial compared the effects of placebo, 5 or 20 mg daily of rimonabant among 1507 individuals with BMI above 30 kg m^{-2} or a BMI of >27 kg m^{-2} in combination with poorly controlled hypertension or dyslipidaemia. All participants received dietary advice and were asked to observe a hypocaloric diet [600 kcal day^{-1} (2510 kJ day^{-1})].[65] Recently, the 2 year results of this study have been published[66] and report a significantly greater weight loss with rimonabant 20 mg (mean $\pm$ SD, -5.5 ± 7.7 kg; $p < 0.001$) and 5 mg (-2.9 ± 6.5 kg;

$p = 0.002$) than placebo (-1.2 ± 6.8 kg). Rimonabant 20 mg also showed significantly greater improvements than placebo in waist circumference and several metabolic parameters. Rimonabant was generally well tolerated and rates of adverse events, including depressed mood disorders and disturbances, were similar to placebo during year 2. Thus, by 2 years, rimonabant appears safe and efficacious. The RIO-North America study among 3045 adults in the United States and Canada followed a similar protocol to RIO-Europe and weight loss and maintenance were compared at 1 and 2 years of follow-up.[67] Patients who were switched from the 20 mg rimonabant group to the placebo group during the second year experienced weight regain while those who continued to receive 20 mg of rimonobant maintained their weight loss and favourable cardiometabolic risk profiles. A high drop-out rate (51–55%), however, places a limitation on the interpretation of such trials. More specifically for diabetes, the RIO-diabetes study has examined the effects of rimonabant in 1047 overweight or obese type 2 diabetic patients (BMI 27–40 kg m^{-2} and HbA$_{1c}$ concentration of 6.5–10.0% at baseline) already on metformin or sulfonylurea monotherapy.[68] Patients were given a mild hypocaloric diet and advice for increased physical activity and randomly assigned placebo ($n = 348$), 5 mg day^{-1} rimonabant ($n = 360$) or 20 mg day^{-1} rimonabant ($n = 339$) for 1 year. The primary endpoint was weight change from baseline after 1 year of treatment. Weight loss was significantly greater after 1 year in both rimonabant groups than in the placebo group [placebo -1.4 kg (SD 3.6), 5 mg day^{-1} -2.3 kg (4.2), $p = 0.01$, versus placebo 20 mg day^{-1} -5.3 kg (5.2), $p < 0.0001$ versus placebo]. However, the high attrition rate (66% completed the 1 year study), with over half discontinuing the study for reasons other than adverse events (mood disorders, nausea and dizziness), leaves doubt about its effectiveness in the longer term. Although there is much interest in this new drug, its long term effectiveness and safety are yet to be determined and it is not yet widely licensed for use in diabetes.

There are also other drugs in use or in development to aid weight loss. Although the list is not exhaustive, it includes fluoxetine and sertraline (centrally acting serotonin reuptake inhibitors), bupropion (used for help with smoking cessation), topiramate and zonisamide (licensed for use in epilepsy management, but may act on adipose tissue and induce weight loss) and the centrally acting sympathomimetic agents phentermine and diethylpropion, which are not available on prescription in the UK but are widely used in other countries. Isolated studies have shown potential benefits of mazindol, phenmetrazine and amphetamine or its derivatives and other drugs. There is also much interest in the glucagon-like peptide-1 (GLP-1) analogues such as exenatide and in agents that inhibit the enzyme dipeptidylpeptidase-4 (DPP-4) prolonging the half life of incretins. Some of these may offer promising prospects for effective and sustained loss of weight among diabetic individuals, but their longer term safety, tolerability and licensing arrangements for this specific indication are not yet established.

How effective are surgical interventions on weight loss?

There are two main types of surgical intervention for bariatric surgery – malabsorptive and restrictive. With malabsorptive surgery, parts of the gastrointestinal tract are bypassed so that the absorption of food is limited (such as in gastric bypass, jejunoileal bypass and biliopancreatic diversion). With restrictive surgery, the size of the stomach is restricted so the person experiences the feeling of fullness with less food (such as with gastroplasty and gastric banding). A systematic review and meta-analysis including 22 094 persons aged 16–64 years and with BMI ranging from 32.3 to 68.8 kg m^{-2} reported effective weight loss following bariatric surgery for morbid obesity.[69] In this review, a total of 136 primary studies were included, including five randomized controlled trials, 28 non-randomized controlled trials or series and 101 uncontrolled case series. The percentage of excess weight loss was defined as (weight loss/excess weight) $\times$ 100, where excess weight is the total preoperative weight minus the ideal weight. The mean percentage of excess weight loss was 61.2% (95% CI 58.1 to 64.4%) for all patients. For different procedures the excess weight loss was as follows: 47.5% (95% CI 40.7 to 54.2%) for gastric banding, 61.6% (95% CI 56.7 to 66.5%) for gastric bypass, 68.2% (95% CI 61.5 to 74.8%) for gastroplasty and 70.1% (95% CI 66.3 to 73.9%) for biliopancreatic diversion or duodenal switch. Operative mortality within 30 days of surgery ranged from 0.1 to 1.1%, depending on the procedure performed. Notably, diabetes was resolved in 76.8% of patients, such that no further therapy was required.[69] Among the five RCTs, the outcomes were within the range of values and the trends for the overall meta-analysis.

The prospective Swedish Obese Subjects Study provides support for the long-term effectiveness of weight loss following bariatric surgery.[70] On comparing those who underwent gastric surgery with those who were treated conventionally (control group) for obesity, at 10 years of follow-up weight had increased by 1.6% in the control group and decreased by 16.1% in the surgery group ($p < 0.001$). The 2 and 10 year rates of recovery from diabetes were more favourable and incidence rates of diabetes were lower in the surgery group than in the control group. A more recent meta-analysis has also confirmed that surgery is more effective than non-surgical treatment for weight loss in patients with a BMI of $40 \, \text{kg m}^{-2}$ or greater, but concluded that more data are needed to determine the efficacy of surgery relative to non-surgical therapy for less severely obese people.[71] Finally, evidence of a beneficial effect of bariatric surgery on predicted cardiovascular risk has also recently emerged. In a historical cohort study (from 1990 to 2003) in Minnesota with persons with BMI $\geq$ $35 \, \text{kg m}^{-2}$, the estimated 10 year risk of cardiovascular disease (CVD) events for the operative group decreased from 37% at baseline to 18% at 3.3 year follow-up, but remained unchanged (30%) in the non-operative group.[72]

Although there is convincing evidence that surgical intervention results in substantial weight loss and positive effects on the health of carefully selected morbidly obese patients, costs to patient and provider are also substantial. Complications are common and can require expensive care. On the basis of data from the National Hospital Discharge Survey, rates for gastric bypass surgery (per 100 000 adults) increased significantly ($p < 0.001$) from 7.0 to 38.6 from 1998 to 2002 in the United States.[73] Encinosa *et al.* reported that among 2522 bariatric surgical procedures at 308 hospitals in the United Stares, the complications rate increased by 81% (from 22 to 40%) on comparing initial surgical stay with 6 months post-discharge from hospital.[74] A total of 18% of patients required costly re-admission or emergency room or outpatient hospital visit within 6 months, highlighting longer term post-operative complication rates as an important issue.[74]

What is the evidence for the effectiveness of physical activity in Modifying the long-Term risk of the Macrovascular complications of Diabetes?

To our knowledge, there are no RCTs of interventions to increase physical activity that assess the reduction in risk of coronary heart disease (CHD) events or other long-term complications in people with diabetes. Thus the evidence supporting physical activity as a means of reducing CHD risk in diabetic populations comes from the observational relative risk reduction in the general population and the effects of activity on known cardiovascular risk factors in people with diabetes.

The epidemiological evidence for the association between physical inactivity and CHD has previously been reviewed by Powell *et al.*[75] and Berlin and Colditz.[76] These studies indicate a relative risk (RR) of future CHD in sedentary individuals of 1.9 (95% CI 1.6 to 2.2) compared with those with active occupations and an RR of 1.6 (95% CI 1.2 to 2.2) compared with individuals who are recreationally active. Many of the studies reviewed in these meta-analyses were characterized by the use of summary indices of activity which may be prone to error and bias, the introduction of surrogate markers of activity and unresolved questions of confounding. The *type* of physical activity that is most likely to be beneficial to long-term risk and the *amount* of activity that is required to have a health benefit remain unresolved. These issues arise from the difficulty of measuring physical activity in free-living populations[77] – problems that are relevant not only to the analysis of cohort studies, but also to the evaluation of intervention programmes where the goal is to measure change in physical activity.[78]

Few studies have assessed the effect of physical activity on CHD risk specifically among persons with diabetes; they show that relative risk reduction from activity is equally, if not more, beneficial among diabetic persons. In the Health Professionals' Follow-up Study among 2803 men with diabetes, physical activity was assessed every 2 years and 266 incident cases of CVD were identified during 14 years of follow-up.[79] The multivariate analysis of incidence of CVD across quintiles of total physical activity estimated risks relative to the lowest quintile (1.0) of 0.87, 0.64, 0.72 and 0.67 and walking pace was inversely associated with non-fatal and fatal CVD independently of walking hours. Among 3316 Finnish participants with type 2 diabetes followed for a mean of 18 years and experiencing 903 CVD death events, both greater leisure time (RR 1.0, 0.83 and 0.67, p trend 0.005) and occupational (RR 1.0, 0.91, 0.60, p trend < 0.001) self-reported physical activity were associated with reduced CVD mortality across the categories low, moderate and high for activity.[80] In the 25 year follow-up in the Whitehall study of British civil servants, among 352 men with diabetes or impaired glucose tolerance (IGT) or 6056 men with normoglycaemia at baseline, both walking pace and leisure-time physical activity were inversely related to CHD and total mortality.[81] Indeed, the gradient of the activity–mortality association was steeper in individuals with diabetes/IGT in comparison with normoglycaemic persons, with the linear trend across activity levels for CHD risk differing markedly for walking pace and leisure activity (p for interaction 0.05 and 0.02, respectively).[81]

The lack of RCT level evidence for benefits of physical activity among people with diabetes is not surprising since the major question may not be whether physical activity can be beneficial to people with diabetes, but rather how individual physical activity change can be supported and maintained.

Are there any specific metabolic effects of physical activity over and Above an effect on weight control?

Physical activity has a series of direct effects that impact on metabolic control independently of weight. Exercise in people with type 2 diabetes is particularly relevant because of the central role of insulin resistance in the pathogenesis of this disorder.[82] In overweight type 2 diabetic patients, plasma glucose is lowered during activity because of increased glucose utilization and lowered hepatic glucose production.[83,84] Exercise also increases insulin sensitivity at the liver and skeletal muscle.[85] Improvements in insulin sensitivity with exercise are also demonstrable in patients with type 1 diabetes.[86,87]

Two separate meta-analyses have specifically addressed the issue of whether physical activity without weight loss has beneficial metabolic effects in diabetes. In a meta-analysis in 2001 of 14 controlled trials including 504 diabetic persons, Boule et al. found that exercise training reduced glycated haemoglobin in a clinically and statistically significant way (mean difference –0.66% HbA_{1c} units, $p < 0.001$) but did not reduce body weight.[88] Meta-regression confirmed that the beneficial effect of exercise on HbA_{1c} was independent of any effect on body weight. However, this analysis included some non-randomized trials and also trials where diet was a co-intervention with exercise in the intervention group, but the same diet was not applied to the control group. Hence it was not possible to assess the 'true' independent effect of exercise in this review.[88] More recently, in 2006, a Cochrane systematic review included 14 RCTs comparing any type of well-documented aerobic, fitness or resistance training exercise with no exercise in 377 persons with type 2 diabetes and with no documented difference between the groups except for the exercise intervention.[89] In trials with durations ranging from 8 weeks to 12 months, compared with the control group, the exercise intervention significantly improved glycaemic control as indicated by a mean difference in HbA_{1c} of 0.6% (95% CI reduction of 0.3 to 0.9%, $p < 0.05$), despite no overall weight loss, thought to be due probably to an increase in fat-free

mass (muscle) with exercise. There was a significant reduction with exercise in visceral adipose tissue ($-45.5\,cm^2$, 95% CI -63.8 to -27.3) and plasma triglycerides ($-0.25\,mmol\,l^{-1}$, 95% CI -0.48 to -0.02), but not in plasma cholesterol or blood pressure.

Furthermore, in a specifically designed study, Duncan et al. tested the effects of 6 months of exercise without weight loss on insulin sensitivity and several markers of lipid metabolism in a group of 18 sedentary type 2 diabetic persons with mean BMI $28.9 \pm 4.6\,kg\,m^{-2}$.[90] Participants were instructed not to change their diet or attempt to alter their weight and were assigned to individualized exercise consisting of walking at moderate or high intensity (45–55 or 65–75% of heart rate reserve) and a frequency of either 3–4 (low frequency) or 5–7 (high frequency) days per week, with a duration of 30 min per session. Exercise improved insulin sensitivity as measured by the frequently sampled intravenous glucose tolerance test ($2.54 \pm 2.74\,\mu U\,ml^{-1}\,min^{-1}$ at baseline versus $4.41 \pm 3.30\,\mu U\,ml^{-1}\,min^{-1}$ at 6 months, $p < 0.005$). There was also a significant improvement in plasma lipase activity (with increased lipoprotein lipase:hepatic lipase ratio), but there was no significant change in fasting lipids, BMI, waist circumference, fitness (VO_{2max}) or any dietary intake measures over 6 months, leading the authors to conclude that modest amounts of exercise, without weight loss, can positively affect markers of glucose and fat metabolism in previously sedentary adults. Lee et al. examined the effect of exercise without weight loss on body fat distribution in a 13 week supervised moderate-intensity ($\sim$60% of peak oxygen uptake) aerobic exercise intervention five times per week for 60 min among 24 lean and obese men, with and without diabetes.[91] Body weight did not change in any group, but all groups significantly reduced their total, abdominal and visceral fat as measured by magnetic resonance imaging (MRI), with a proportionately greater reduction in visceral fat area among the obese and diabetic men ($p < 0.01$). They also found that there was an increase in total skeletal muscle associated with a decrease in muscle lipid as measured by computed tomography in all groups, leading them to conclude that regular exercise without weight loss reduces total and visceral fat and muscle lipid in both obesity and diabetes, providing support and a mechanistic explanation for the observations of the two meta-analyses above.[88,89]

Evidence has also just started to emerge of improvements in markers of inflammation such as interleukin-6 (IL-6) in lean and obese people with and without diabetes who underwent 12 week aerobic exercise intervention without weight loss.[92] Consistent with the findings reported by Lee et al.,[91] although there was no change in body weight or BMI, total and visceral fat measured by MRI scan and waist circumference were reduced significantly in the exercise intervention group in this study.[92] There is mounting evidence that inflammation may be related to the risk for diabetes and its control, hence these findings of reduction in inflammatory marker concentrations with physical activity without weight loss are of potential importance.

Hence it seems that structured physical activity is beneficial with or without weight loss in persons with diabetes. The majority of patients with diabetes or at high risk of developing diabetes do not, however, engage in regular physical activity. This was confirmed in a study by Morrato et al., who found that of 23 283 adults surveyed in the Medical Expenditure Panel Survey, which is a nationally representative survey of the United States population, a total of 39% of adults with diabetes ($n = 1825$) reported being physically active (moderate or vigorous activity ≥ 30 min, three times per week) versus 58% of adults without diabetes ($n = 21\,401$).[93] After adjustment for socio-demographic and clinical factors, being physically inactive was strongly correlated with lower income level, limitations in physical function, depression and severe obesity (BMI $>40 \,\mathrm{kg\,m^{-2}}$). Hence knowing the benefits of physical activity is the starting point, but translation into action is an ongoing challenge.

Is there any evidence to indicate what type and what intensity of exercise are needed?

Epidemiological studies which have relied solely on self-reported measures of activity, with inherent biases and imprecision, are unlikely to be able to separate the aetiological effects of different types of activity, nor will they be able to quantify their importance accurately. By contrast, studies which have incorporated objective measures of activity with knowledge of measurement error can better determine the relative importance of different types of activity. These studies suggest that increasing overall energy expenditure has beneficial effects on the 2 h post-glucose load glucose concentration[94] and other features of the insulin resistance syndrome[95,96] independently of the degree of obesity and cardiorespiratory fitness. These results may be of importance in translating findings into preventive action, as they suggest that approaches aimed at increasing overall energy expenditure through whatever means will have benefits. Furthermore, interventions need not necessarily be of an intensity required to increase cardiorespiratory fitness. Some experimental support for this conclusion is derived from studies such as that by Oshida et al.,[97] who measured the effects of low-intensity activity on insulin sensitivity. An improvement in insulin sensitivity was observed at 1 year, even though there was no change in BMI or fitness.

The relationship between amounts of physical activity and short-term beneficial effects in type 2 diabetic patients has been addressed by Kang et al.[98] Among six obese men with type 2 diabetes, the authors examined the effect of 1 week of low-intensity exercise compared with shorter, more intense activity providing equivalent energy expenditure. The exercise interventions consisted of two 7 day blocks of daily sessions. In the low-intensity activity, individuals exercised at 50% of maximum oxygen uptake ($\mathrm{VO_{2max}}$), whereas for the high-intensity activity they aimed at 70% of $\mathrm{VO_{2max}}$. After 7 days of exercise the area under the plasma insulin response curve during an oral glucose tolerance test was reduced only in those exercising at the higher intensity. Neither group showed a change in plasma glucose concentration. A different conclusion was reached by Braun et al., who showed that high-intensity activity and low-intensity exercise had comparable effects on insulin sensitivity in women with type 2 diabetes.[99]

Short-term improvements in glycaemic control have been demonstrated in patients with type 1 diabetes who undergo resistance training either alone[100] or in combination with aerobic activity.[101,102] However, long-term studies are few and only recently emerging. In a paper entitled 'Make your diabetic patients walk', reflecting the authors' conclusions, Di Loreto et al. examined the 2 year impact of different increments in energy expenditure on health benefits in 179 diabetic patients.[103] Six voluntary aerobic physical activity groups were randomized to a physical activity counselling intervention, based on energy expenditure [metabolic equivalents (METS) per hour per week]. These were as follows: group 0 (no activity, $n = 28$), group 1–10 (mean $\pm$ SEM MET hours 6.8 ± 0.3, $n = 27$), group 11–20 (17.1 ± 0.4, $n = 31$), group 21–30 (27.0 ± 0.5, $n = 27$), group 31–40 (37.5 ± 0.5, $n = 32$), group >40 (58.3 ± 1.8, $n = 34$). At baseline there were no differences between the six groups for energy expenditure, diabetes duration and all parameters measured. After 2 years, in groups 0 and 1–10 no parameters changed, but in all groups >10 METS energy expenditure, $\mathrm{HbA_{1c}}$, blood pressure, total cholesterol, triglycerides and estimated 10 year CHD risk improved ($p < 0.05$). In groups with >20 METS energy expenditure there was additional improvement in body weight, waist circumference, fasting glucose, serum LDL and HDL cholesterol and heart rate ($p < 0.05$). There was also financial benefit with reduced per capita yearly costs of medications in groups with >10 METS per hour per week energy expenditure, whereas in groups 0 and 1–10 there was an increase and no change, respectively. Although this study has limitations such as the self-reported nature of type, duration and intensity of exercise, the *post hoc* analysis of long-term effects of exercise and the limited range of aerobic activities undertaken, mainly brisk walking, it is suggestive of the beneficial effects of higher intensity physical activity among type 2 diabetic individuals and opens up possibilities for further improved studies.

Finally, a meta-analysis of nine RCTs ($n = 266$ adults) of structured aerobic exercise interventions of 8 weeks or more also confirmed that higher intensity exercise has the potential to improve HbA_{1c} levels and cardiorespiratory fitness in type 2 diabetic persons.[104] Mean exercise characteristics comprised 3.4 sessions per week with 49 min per session for 20 weeks and exercise intensity ranged from 50 to 75% of VO_{2max}. There was an 11.8% increase in VO_{2max} in the exercise group and a 1.0% decrease in the control group (post-intervention standardized mean difference $= 0.53$, $p < 0.003$). Studies with higher exercise intensities tended to produce larger improvements in VO_{2max} and exercise intensity predicted post-intervention weighted mean difference in $HbA_{(1c)}$ ($r = -0.91$, $p = 0.002$) to a larger extent than did exercise volume ($r = -0.46$, $p = 0.26$).[104]

How common are the adverse effects of exercise on the complications of diabetes?

There is paucity of epidemiological evidence on the risks and benefits of activity in the presence of diabetic complications. Few diabetes-specific studies exist, particularly for mortality, and therefore most authorities generalize from studies in the general population. Although silent CHD may be more prevalent in the population of people with diabetes, the absolute risk of harm even for vigorous activity is low.[105,106] The presence of autonomic neuropathy and in particular QT interval lengthening may increase the risk of adverse effects of activity such as through decreased cardiac responsiveness to exercise, but few data are available to quantify these risks.[107–111]

Epidemiological studies of the risk of diabetic eye disease in individuals who undertake increased physical activity suggest that activity has little role in promoting the development of proliferative retinopathy.[112–115] Although it is plausible that exercise may increase the risk of vitreous haemorrhage or retinal detachment in people with pre-existing proliferative retinopathy either through the mechanical effects of movement or through rises in systolic blood pressure, systematic quantification of the magnitude of this risk has not been undertaken.[116–118]

In people with type 1 diabetes who are free of renal disease, the effects of exercise on glomerular filtration rate (GFR) and renal plasma flow (RPF) are similar to those in non-diabetic individuals in that exercise causes a reduction in both GFR and RPF.[119] However, there are no data beyond small case series to indicate whether such short-term changes are associated with long-term adverse effects on renal function. One study in type 1 diabetic children found that post-exercise albuminuria was not a useful predictor of the onset of microalbuminuria at 6 years of follow-up.[120] Physical activity can increase urinary protein excretion, but the extent of the exercise-induced albuminuria is related to the level of blood pressure increase[121] and also to the degree of glycaemic control. Although less frequently studied,[122] the effects in type 2 diabetes may be similar. There is good evidence that exercise-induced albuminuria may be reduced by intensified insulin therapy.[123–125] The American Diabetes Association does not recommend any specific exercise restrictions for people with diabetic kidney disease, but because of associations with CVD, the ADA recommends an exercise ECG stress test before beginning exercise that is significantly more intense than usual.

Is exercise associated with adverse effects on metabolic control in people with diabetes?

The only available evidence on adverse effects of exercise on metabolic control relates to persons with type 1 diabetes, where the increase in glucose release from the liver and non-esterified fatty acids (NEFA) from adipose tissue that normally occur with exercise are inhibited. Muscle glucose utilization increases with exercise and, therefore, the limitation on hepatic glucose production can lead to falls in circulating glucose. Thus in a person with well treated type 1 diabetes, the risk of hypoglycaemia during periods of exercise is significant. This is a manageable problem if the person with diabetes can adjust the dose of insulin to account for periods of activity. However, if that exercise is episodic or unpredictable, or if no adjustment to insulin dosage is made, hypoglycaemia may result. Not only is this a problem during the period of activity, but because the exercise-induced increase in insulin action persists when the exercise in terminated, the risk of hypoglycaemia may also persist for several hours.[126] The risks of hypoglycaemia are compounded by an acceleration in the absorption of insulin from subcutaneous tissues during exercise.[127] This effect is exacerbated if insulin is accidentally injected intramuscularly,[128] suggesting the need for extra caution in injection prior to exercise.

The metabolic effects of physical activity in type 1 diabetes which is poorly controlled are somewhat different. In a study comparing the effects of a 3 h moderate exercise intervention in patients with type 1 diabetes with differing degrees of baseline control, Berger *et al.* demonstrated that people with poor control showed worsening of hyperglycaemia and ketosis, in contrast to those with reasonable control, in whom glucose levels fell.[129]

Individuals with type 1 diabetes differ in their metabolic response to activity[130,131] and each individual may participate in a variety of activities of differing intensity and duration. Such variations create difficulties in making uniform recommendations for adjustment to insulin dosage or carbohydrate intake and therefore in providing a clear evidence base for management. It is probably more prudent for health care professionals to base individual recommendations on physiological knowledge of the general effects of activity on glucose control in type 1 diabetes and to advocate careful individual blood glucose monitoring.

Are there any specific effects of nutritional manipulation over and above an effect on weight?

In the same way that physical activity can play a role in the management of diabetes independently of its effect on weight, nutritional factors may impact on metabolic control through non-weight-related pathways. In considering the evidence, it should be borne in mind that manipulation of one element of the diet often affects others in addition to total energy. For example, high-fat diets are lower in carbohydrate and low-carbohydrate diets are often relatively high in protein. Also, whole foods may have effects distinct from those of their constituents, making the interpretation of dietary studies complicated. A further challenge of dietary studies is the reliance on self-report of food intake, which is subject to under- or over- reporting and measurement error, making interpretation more complex.

Altering the composition of the fat content of the diet

As in the general population, so among persons with diabetes the primary goal is to limit foods rich in saturated fats, trans-fatty acids and cholesterol intake to reduce the risk of CVD.[66] The type of fat in the diet and its effect on metabolic control in diabetes are reviewed next.

Monounsaturated fats

In a meta-analysis of the effects of prescribing diets high in monounsaturated fats to people with type 2 diabetes, Garg identified nine randomized, cross-over design trials which contrasted isoenergetic, weight-maintaining diets which were high in monounsaturated fat or high in carbohydrate.[132] The primary outcome was the mean difference in changes in blood glucose and lipids between diet periods. The overall effect of diets rich in monounsaturated fat compared with those high in carbohydrate was a significant reduction in fasting triglyceride, total cholesterol and VLDL cholesterol and an increase in HDL cholesterol. The mean difference between groups in fasting glucose was $0.23 \, \text{mmol} \, l^{-1}$ in favour of the high-fat, low-carbohydrate group, with no detectable difference in insulin concentration. Only three of the studies assessed glycated haemoglobin, which was not affected by diet group. However, all of the studies considered were probably of too short a duration to impact on long-term measures of glycaemic control.[132] The question of whether the metabolic effects were independent of weight loss was studied by Low *et al.*,[133] who investigated 17 obese patients with type 2 diabetes before and after dieting for 6 weeks with a formula diet enriched with monounsaturated fatty acids (MUFA) or carbohydrates (CHO). There was no evidence of random allocation in this trial. Weight loss was comparable in the two groups but fasting glucose decreased significantly more in the MUFA group ($-4.6 \, \text{mmol} \, l^{-1}$) compared with the CHO group ($-2.4 \, \text{mmol} \, l^{-1}$, $p < 0.05$).

Polyunsaturated fats and fish oil supplementation

Diets high in polyunsaturated fatty acids (PUFA) appear to have similar beneficial effects to monounsaturated fatty acids.[134,135] Epidemiological data suggest that fish intake is inversely associated with CHD mortality[136] and the risk for diabetes.[137] These observations have given rise to considerable interest in the possible benefits of fish-derived oils, particularly *n*-3 fatty acids. Two meta-analyses of clinical trials of fish oil supplementation in people with diabetes have reached broadly similar conclusions.[138,139] Montori *et al.*[139] in their quantitative systematic review identified 18 trials, seven with a parallel group design and 11 cross-over studies. The duration of study was from 2 to 24 weeks. Twelve of the studies reported fasting glucose results in a way that allowed pooling of the data. The pooled weighted mean difference for fasting glucose was $0.26 \, \text{mmol} \, l^{-1}$ with 95% CIs of -0.08 to 0.60, suggesting no overall significant effect on glycaemia. The equivalent figures for Hba_{1c} were 0.15% (95% CI -0.08 to 0.37). By contrast, the overall effect of fish oil on triglyceride, reported in 14 trials, was beneficial with a pooled weighted mean difference of -0.56 mmol l^{-1} (95% CI -0.71 to -0.41). From these results, the authors concluded that in people with type 2 diabetes who have normal triglyceride levels, fish oil supplementation leads to a modest lowering of triglyceride without an adverse effect on glycaemia, a conclusion similar to that reached by the authors of the previous meta-analysis.[138] A recent meta-analysis of 12 RCTs of ω-3 PUFA supplements in type 2 diabetes found that in addition to beneficial effects on dyslipidaemia, there was a significant reduction in diastolic blood pressure and an increase in coagulant factor VII level. However, the latter, which is a potential adverse effect, was based on only two studies and requires further study.[140] The same authors have now also published a Cochrane Systematic Review including 23 RCTs (1075 participants) with mean duration of 9 weeks of supplementation with ω-3 PUFA.[141] They confirmed a beneficial effect on triglyceride levels: among those taking ω-3 PUFA, triglyceride levels were significantly lowered by 0.45 mmol l^{-1} (95% CI -0.58 to -0.32, $p < 0.00001$), although LDL cholesterol levels were raised by 0.11 mmol l^{-1} (95% CI 0.00 to 0.22, $p = 0.05$). However, there was no significant change in total or HDL cholesterol, HbA$_{1c}$, fasting glucose, fasting insulin or body weight. Notably, no trials with vascular events or mortality defined endpoints were available and are needed. Collectively these findings re-endorse that PUFA may be beneficial for some intermediate outcomes such as lipids, but appear not to have a consistent direct effect on glycaemic control and their effect on long-term outcomes is unknown.

Altering the nature of the carbohydrate content of the diet

Dietary carbohydrate is the major determinant of post-prandial glucose levels, normally maintained in a narrow range by the insulin secretory response, but impaired in persons with diabetes due to defects in insulin action, insulin secretion or both. Both the amount and the type of carbohydrate consumed influence post-prandial glucose levels.[142] There are intrinsic and extrinsic variables that influence the effect of carbohydrate-containing foods on blood glucose response, such as type of starch, method of cooking, degree of processing and pre-prandial glucose levels. As regards use of sugars, evidence from clinical studies confirms that dietary sucrose (disaccharide sugar) does not increase glycaemia more than isocaloric amounts of starch (polysaccharide carbohydrate), challenging the historically held notion that added sugars should be avoided and natural sugars

restricted in diabetes *per se*. Daly *et al.* identified 12 trials in which sugars were compared with starch for effect on insulin sensitivity.[143] All of these trials were of relatively short duration (range 1 week to 3 months) and five were specifically focused on people with diabetes. Overall in these studies, there was no significant effect of type of carbohydrate on insulin sensitivity. In a review by the ADA, five studies assessed the effects of single meals containing between 12 and 25% of calories as sucrose, finding no adverse effect on glycaemic response.[144] Five longer term studies lasting from 2 days to 4 weeks with 7–38% of calories from sucrose, found no adverse effects on glycaemia. It is apparent that the glycaemic response is similar if the total amount of carbohydrate is similar. Finally, over a 3 week intervention period, an isocaloric increase in the dietary intakes of sucrose to 13% of total energy per day in nine overweight people with type 2 diabetes was not associated with a decline in glycaemic control or insulin sensitivity and weight remained stable.[145] The current ADA recommendation is that the intake of sucrose and sucrose-containing foods by people with diabetes does not need to be restricted because of concern about aggravating hyperglycaemia. However, they recommend that intake of other nutrients ingested with sucrose, such as fat, need to be taken into account and care should be taken to avoid excess energy intake.[66]

Studies of the effect of fructose (monosaccharide sugar) on glycaemic control and insulin level were reviewed by Henry and Crapo.[146] In seven studies among individuals with type 2 diabetes, there were no adverse effects of fructose on glucose and insulin levels.[146] In persons with diabetes, fructose produces a lower post-prandial glucose response when it replaces sucrose or starch in the diet, but it may adversely affect plasma lipids,[146,147] hence it is not advisable as an added sweetener. Although some conventional advice has included the avoidance of fruit and vegetables containing fructose, there is no evidence that naturally occurring fructose in fruits and vegetables is harmful, and indeed fruits and vegetables have a range of beneficial effects[148] and should be encouraged.

The differing effects of foods on glycaemic response have led to the notion of the glycaemic index, reflecting the rate at which carbohydrate is digested and absorbed, as described above in the section on the effectiveness of dietary interventions on weight loss. Although one would expect that low-GI diets should improve glycaemic control, the findings of RCTs have been mixed, leading to controversy and confusion about dietary advice on GI of diets. However, a meta-analysis of 14 studies with 356 diabetic participants by Brant-Miller *et al.* showed that low-GI diets produced a 0.43% (95% CI 0.13 to 0.72%) points reduction in HbA_{1c} compared with high-GI diets.[149] Another meta-analysis of 16 RCTs confirmed a significant decrease in HbA_{1c} by 0.27% points (95% CI 0.03 to 0.5), in fructosamine by 0.1 (95% CI 0.00 to 0.20) $mmol\,l^{-1}$ and in total cholesterol by 0.33 (95% CI 0.18 to 0.47) $mmol\,l^{-1}$ compared with high-GI diets.[150] These findings prompted the American Diabetes Association to state that for diabetes management, 'the use of glycemic index and load may provide a modest additional benefit over that observed when total carbohydrate is considered alone'.[66]

The final element of carbohydrate intake that may be modulated is fibre intake. There are epidemiological data suggesting that consuming a high-fibre diet including soluble fibre supplements ($\sim$50 g of fibre per day) reduces glycaemia in persons with type 1 diabetes and glycaemia, hyperinsulinaemia and lipaemia in persons with type 2 diabetes.[144] However, achieving such a high-fibre intake can be challenging and the emphasis should generally be on promoting high intakes as part of dietary intake rather than as a supplement. In a random order cross-over trial, Kinmonth *et al.* compared isocaloric diets based on low-fibre, refined carbohydrate foods or on complex carbohydrate foods containing three times as much dietary fibre.[151] Ten children with type 1 diabetes were assigned to eat both diets in random order for 6 weeks each. Glycaemic control significantly improved on the high-fibre diet. Similar results have been observed in trials in adults.[152,153]

Changing the protein content of the diet

For diabetic persons, there is no evidence to suggest that the usual protein intake (15–20% of total daily energy intake) should be modified if renal function is normal.[66] The major interest in protein intake in people with diabetes has been in relation to the effect of protein restriction on the progression of diabetic renal disease as discussed in more detail in another chapter. Although the Modification of Diet in Renal Disease Study (MDRD) did not show any significant effect of lowering protein intake on the rate of decline of glomerular filtration rate (GFR) in non-diabetic persons,[154] the effect may be different in people with diabetes.[155] A review for the Cochrane Collaboration by Waugh and Robertson[156] focused on trials which included at least a 4 month protein restriction diet in people with type 1 diabetes. The outcomes were expressed in terms of change in GFR rather than clinical outcome. Overall the authors concluded that protein restriction was associated with slowing of progression of diabetic nephropathy.

The subject of the role of high-protein, high-fat diets, such as the Atkins diet, among people with diabetes has been discussed above in the section on low carbohydrate diets and weight loss.

Alcohol

The specific effects of alcohol in people with diabetes include a potential increased risk of hypoglycaemia especially when alcohol is consumed without food.[157] Although epidemiological data may suggest an association between increased alcohol intake and improved glycaemic control,[158] it is difficult to separate the specific effects of alcohol from other related lifestyles, including the pattern of food intake that occurs with alcohol.[159] Excessive intake of alcohol (three or more drinks per day), on a consistent basis and particularly when combined with co-ingestion of carbohydrate, may contribute to hyperglycaemia.[160]

Other forms of dietary supplementation

The final group of dietary interventions includes vitamins, micronutrients and minerals. Observational epidemiological evidence indicates that low levels of the antioxidant vitamins C[161] and E[162] are associated with worse glucose tolerance. These observations are supported both by *in vitro* evidence of the effects of antioxidants on insulin action[163] and by associations between diabetes and consumption of diets low in fresh fruit and vegetables,[164,165] the major source of dietary vitamin C. The clinical trial evidence of the benefits of these antioxidants taken as supplements is less conclusive. In the recent French SUVIMAX primary prevention cohort, 3146 adults were randomly assigned to receive a daily capsule containing 120 mg of vitamin C in combination with 30 mg of vitamin E, 6 mg of β-carotene, 100 μg of selenium and 20 mg of zinc or a placebo for 7.5 years, after which no significant difference was observed between age-adjusted mean fasting glucose in men ($p = 0.78$) and women ($p = 0.89$) in either group.[166] The possibility of a major benefit of vitamin E seems unlikely given the results of the HOPE study, in which the benefits of vitamin E and ramipril were compared in a factorial design RCT, with no effect of vitamin E on cardiovascular outcome among 3654 persons with diabetes.[167] Furthermore, no significant overall associations were observed between risk of retinopathy and intake of dietary vitamin C or E among 1353 type 2 diabetic participants from the Atherosclerosis Risk In Communities (ARIC) cohort, although it should be noted that the study included prevalent retinopathy rather than study new-onset retinopathy following antioxidant supplementation.[168] Recent evidence also suggests that, contrary to expectation, vitamin E supplements may increase blood pressure in persons with diabetes.[169] Fifty-eight type 2 diabetic persons were randomized to a daily dose of $500\,mg\,day^{-1}$ of α-tocopherol, $500\,mg\,day^{-1}$ of mixed tocopherols (60% γ-tocopherol) or placebo for 6 weeks. Both α-tocopherol and mixed tocopherols significantly increased systolic and diastolic blood pressure, pulse pressure and heart rate versus placebo.[169]

There has been recent increased interest in the potential role of vitamin D levels, which have been reported to have effects on insulin secretion and are associated with diabetes in some[170] but not all studies.[171] There are currently no trials of supplementation in people with type 2 diabetes, but a large trial for the prevention of diabetes demonstrated no benefit of supplementation.[172] The trial used a low dose of vitamin D supplementation ($400\,IU\,day^{-1}$), which may have led to the null result. No definitive recommendations can yet be given on vitamin D supplementation in type 2 diabetes management.

Minerals such as chromium, magnesium and zinc have generated interest as potential candidates for improvements in diabetes management. Although some small chromium intervention studies have suggested that supplementation may result in improved glucose control[173] or insulin secretion,[174] others have been inconclusive.[175] A meta-analysis of 15 RCTs including 618 participants by Althuis *et al.*[176] found no association between chromium and glucose or insulin concentrations among non-diabetic individuals, but a study of 155 diabetic persons in China showed that chromium reduced glucose and insulin concentrations while the combined data from the 38 diabetic individuals in other studies did not. The study among diabetic persons in China was the only one to report that chromium significantly reduced HbA_{1c}. The authors concluded that there is no overall effect of chromium on glucose or insulin concentrations in non-diabetic persons, but the data for persons with diabetes are inconclusive and require further study in well-designed trials.[176]

Magnesium levels in people with diabetes have been investigated because of evidence that hypomagnesaemia occurs frequently in individuals with diabetes, particularly those with poor glycaemic control,[177] and that increased magnesium intake may improve insulin action and secretion.[178,179] A meta-analysis of nine RCTs of oral magnesium supplementation of duration 4–16 weeks among 370 patients with type 2 diabetes found that fasting glucose was significantly lower in the treatment groups compared with the placebo groups [$-0.56\,mmol\,l^{-1}$ (95% CI -1.10 to -0.01)], HbA_{1c} levels and blood pressure did not differ significantly between groups, whereas HDL cholesterol levels were raised in the treatment group [$0.08\,mmol\,l^{-1}$ (95% CI 0.03 to 0.14)].[180] The long-term benefits and safety of magnesium treatment on glycaemic control remain to be determined and at present no specific recommendations have been made on magnesium supplementation in diabetes. Finally, zinc has also been considered as potentially important because low levels have been found in diabetes and a recent study showed that among type 2 diabetic persons, low levels of zinc were independently associated with higher risk for CHD [hazard ratio for CHD death 1.7 (95% CI 1.21 to 2.38) and for any CHD event 1.37 (95% CI 1.03 to 1.82)].[181] However, the SUVIMAX study trial discussed above, which included zinc supplementation, did not find any beneficial effect on glycaemic control in diabetic persons,[166] nor did a trial of zinc supplementation in the primary prevention of diabetes.[182]

There has been ongoing interest in the efficacy and safety of several other herbs and minerals for glycaemic control and other outcomes, too many to review individually in this chapter. A systematic review assessed 108 trials (58 controlled trials with 42 RCTs and 16 non-randomized trials and other non-controlled trials) examining 36 herbs (single or in combination) and nine vitamin/mineral supplements, involving 4565 patients with diabetes or impaired glucose tolerance.[183] Among these 58 trials, meta-analyses could not be performed due to heterogeneity and the small number of studies per supplement, but the direction of the evidence for improved glucose control was positive in 76% (44 of 58). Very few adverse effects were reported and the authors concluded that there is insufficient evidence to draw definitive conclusions about the efficacy of individual herbs and supplements for diabetes; however, they appear to be generally safe and several supplements may warrant further study. The best evidence for efficacy from adequately designed RCTs is available for *Coccinia indica* and American ginseng, chromium has been the most widely studied supplement and other supplements with positive preliminary results include *Gymnema sylvestre*, *Aloe vera*, vanadium, *Momordica charantia* and nopal.[183] The ADA does not currently recommend supplementation with any of the above micronutrients due primarily to a lack of definitive evidence combined with lack of information on long-term safety and efficacy issues.[66]

Although various dietary manipulations may be beneficial to different extents in achieving glycaemic control, there is evidence that medical nutrition therapy provided by dietitians experienced in diabetes management can be clinically effective, as comprehensively reviewed by Pastors *et al.*[184] This review of clinical trials and outcome studies reported a decrease in HbA_{1c} of 1–2% in type 2 diabetes and of ~1% in type 1 diabetes, depending on the duration of diabetes.

Why have few long-term outcome trials of lifestyle interventions been undertaken in people with established diabetes?

As interventions aimed at altering diet and physical activity are central to diabetes care, it is perhaps surprising that long-term randomized controlled studies have not been undertaken to evaluate the impact of these interventions on delaying or preventing the complications of this disorder. One possible explanation could be that as the provision of some form of dietary and physical activity advice is so widely accepted as part of routine diabetes care, randomization is considered inappropriate. Alternatively, as these behavioural interventions are seldom sufficient to limit progression of the disorder without pharmacological therapy, some may feel that they are not worth evaluating separately. The evaluation of complex lifestyle interventions is difficult as defining the interventions, ensuring fidelity of delivery and maintaining the distinction between intervention groups in longer trials are hard. Trials of this type have also been affected by high dropout rates. The measurement of the effect of any intervention on diet and physical activity is difficult because the behaviours are not easy to measure. Intervention trials which have used subjective self-report measures are likely to be affected by recall bias in which participants randomized to the intervention arm report greater activity or dietary change solely by virtue of being allocated to that group rather than as a result of true

Table 7.1 Summary of evidence provided in this chapter

Area of interest	Strength of recommendation	Quality of the evidence
Weight reduction is effective in reducing the risks of the complications of diabetes	B	II-2
Weight loss is effective in improving glycaemia	A	I
Dietary interventions in people with diabetes are effective in producing weight loss	A	I
Combined diet and physical activity interventions are effective in people with diabetes in producing weight loss	A	I
Increasing physical activity is effective in the prevention of weight gain in people with diabetes	B	II-2
Pharmacological interventions are effective in producing weight loss in people with diabetes	A	I
Surgical interventions are effective in producing weight loss in people with diabetes	A	I
Increasing physical activity results in reduction of the long-term risks of the complications of diabetes	B	II-2
Increasing physical activity has beneficial effects on metabolic control over and above the effect on weight	A	I
Altering the composition of the fat content of the diet has beneficial effects on glycaemia	B	II-1
Fish oil supplementation has a beneficial effect on triglyceride concentrations	A	I
Altering the nature of the carbohydrate content of the diet has beneficial effects on glycaemic control	B	II-1
Calorie restriction plus reduction in fat has no detectable effect on glycaemia over and above the effect on weight loss	A	I
Protein restriction is effective in reducing the rate of progression of diabetic nephropathy	A	I
High-protein diets (>20% of calories) may be effective in short-term weight loss and improved glycaemia, but long-term effects are not known and these diets are not recommended as a method for weight loss at present	C	III
Alcohol consumption should be moderate. Even moderate alcohol consumption in combination with ingestion of carbohydrates may raise blood glucose	B	I
Antioxidant supplementation may be effective in improving glycaemia but long-term effectiveness and safety are unknown. Thus routine supplementation with vitamins E and C and carotene are not currently advised	A	I
Chromium supplementation may have beneficial effects on glycaemic control, but evidence is inconclusive and therefore not currently recommended	C	I
Magnesium supplementation is effective in improving glycaemic control but long-term effects are unknown	C	I

behaviour change.[78] Although the use of objective biomarkers of activity and diet would be preferable, these have rarely been included in such studies. Probably the most important reason for the absence of long-term studies is that the time necessary to produce an impact on health endpoints makes them expensive and consequently unattractive to potential funders.

Overall, this chapter demonstrates that interventions to alter diet and physical activity can be effective in short, explanatory trials among people with diabetes in achieving weight loss and glycaemic control. Although the lure of specific medications for weight loss is attractive, the effects of these would last as long as the therapy is continued and, indeed, long-term safety is unclear. The potential for diet and physical activity to achieve weight loss and improved glycaemic and other metabolic control in the longer term, in addition to their added contribution to medication strategies, now deserves evaluation in specifically designed pragmatic studies of cost-effectiveness.

Summary of the evidence provided in this chapter

The evidence provided in this chapter is summarized in Table 7.1.

References

1 Centers for Disease Control, Prevention (CDC). Prevalence of overweight and obesity among adults with diagnosed diabetes – United States, 1988–1994 and 1999–2002. *MMWR Morb Mortal Wkly Rep* 2004;**53**(45):1066–1068.

2 Maggio CA, Pi-Sunyer FX. The prevention and treatment of obesity. Application to type 2 diabetes. *Diabetes Care* 1997;**20** (11):1744–1766.

3 Olefsky J, Reaven GM, Farquhar JW. Effects of weight reduction on obesity. Studies of lipid and carbohydrate metabolism in normal and hyperlipoproteinemic subjects. *J Clin Invest* 1974;**53**(1):64–76.

4 Pi-Sunyer FX. Short-term medical benefits and adverse effects of weight loss. *Ann Intern Med* 1993;**119**(7 Pt 2): 722–726.

5 Pi-Sunyer FX. Weight and non-insulin-dependent diabetes mellitus. *Am J Clin Nutr* 1996;**63**:426S–429S.

6 Williams KV, Kelley DE. Metabolic consequences of weight loss on glucose metabolism and insulin action in type 2 diabetes. *Diabetes Obes Metab* 2000;**2**(3):121–129.

7 UKPDS, Group. UK Prospective Diabetes Study 7: Response of fasting plasma glucose to diet therapy in newly presenting type II diabetic patients. *Metabolism* 1990;**39**(9): 905–912.

8 Williamson DF, Thompson TJ, Thun M, Flanders D, Pamuk E, Byers T. Intentional weight loss and mortality among

overweight individuals with diabetes. *Diabetes Care* 2000; **23**(10):1499–1504.

9 Chaturvedi N, Fuller JH. The WHO Multinational Study Group. Mortality risk by body weight and weight change in people with NIDDM. *Diabetes Care* 1995;**18**(6):766–774.

10 Gregg EW, Gerzoff RB, Thompson TJ, Williamson DF. Trying to lose weight, losing weight and 9-year mortality in overweight U.S. adults with diabetes. *Diabetes Care* 2004;**27**(3):657–662.

11 Ryan DH, Espeland MA, Foster GD, Haffner SM, Hubbard VS, Johnson KC *et al*. Look AHEAD (Action for Health in Diabetes): design and methods for a clinical trial of weight loss for the prevention of cardiovascular disease in type 2 diabetes. *Control Clin Trials* 2003;**24**(5):610–628.

12 Pi-Sunyer FX, Blackburn G, Brancati FL, Bray GA, Bright R, Clark JM *et al*. Reduction in weight and cardiovascular disease risk factors in individuals with type 2 diabetes: one-year results of the look AHEAD trial. *Diabetes Care* 2007;**30**(6):1374–1383.

13 Kim SH, Lee SJ, Kang ES, Kang S, Hur KY, Lee HJ *et al*. Effects of lifestyle modification on metabolic parameters and carotid intima-media thickness in patients with type 2 diabetes mellitus. *Metabolism* 2006;**55**(8):1053–1059.

14 Barinas-Mitchell E, Kuller LH, Sutton-Tyrrell K, Hegazi R, Harper P, Mancino J *et al*. Effect of weight loss and nutritional intervention on arterial stiffness in type 2 diabetes. *Diabetes Care* 2006;**29**(10):2218–2222.

15 Escalante-Pulido M, Escalante-Herrera A, Milke-Najar ME, Alpizar-Salazar M. Effects of weight loss on insulin secretion and *in vivo* insulin sensitivity in obese diabetic and non-diabetic subjects. *Diabetes Nutr Metab* 2003;**16**(5–6):277–283.

16 Wolffenbuttel BHR, Weber RFA. Van Koestsveld PM, Verschoor L. Limitations of diet therapy in patients with non-insulin-dependent diabetes mellitus. *Int J Obes* 1989;**13**(2): 173–182.

17 Watts NB, Spanheimer RG, Digirolamo M, Gebhart SSP, Musey V, Khalid Siddiq Y *et al*. Prediction of glucose response to weight loss in patients with non-insulin-dependent diabetes mellitus. *Arch Intern Med* 1990;**150**: 803–806.

18 Bosello O, Armellini F, Zamboni M, Fitchet M. The benefits of modest weight loss in type II diabetes. *Int J Obes* 1997;**21**: S10–S13.

19 World Health Organization. *Obesity: Preventing and Managing the Global Epidemic*, World Health Organization, Geneva, 2000.

20 Pi-Sunyer FX. Weight loss in type 2 diabetic patients. *Diabetes Care* 2005;**28**(6):1526–1527.

21 Guare JC, Wing RR, Grant A. Comparison of obese NIDDM and nondiabetic women: short- and long-term weight loss. *Obes Res* 1995;**3**(4):329–335.

22 Brown SA, Upchurch S, Anding R, Winter M, Ramirez G. Promoting weight loss in type II diabetes. *Diabetes Care* 1996;**19**(6):613–624.

23 National Institutes of, Health. *Clinical Guidelines on the Identification, Evaluation and Treatment of Overweight and Obesity in Adults*, National Institutes of Health, Bethesda, MD, 1998.

24 NHS, Centre for Reviews and Dissemination. The prevention and treatment of obesity. *Effective Health Care* 1997;**3**:1–11.

25 Pascale RW, Wing RR, Butler BA, Mullen M, Bononi P. Effects of a behavioral weight loss program stressing calorie restriction versus calorie plus fat restriction in obese individuals with NIDDM or a family history of diabetes. *Diabetes Care* 1995;**18**(9):1241–1248.

26 Moore H, Summerbell C, Hooper L, Cruickshank K, Vyas A, Johnstone P *et al.* Dietary advice for treatment of type 2 diabetes mellitus in adults. *Cochrane Database Syst Rev* 2004(3):CD004097.

27 de Bont AJ, Baker IA, St Leger AS, Sweetnam PM, Wragg KG, Stephens SM *et al.* A randomised controlled trial of the effect of low fat diet advice on dietary response in insulin independent diabetic women. *Diabetologia* 1981; **21** (6):529–533.

28 Hockaday TD, Hockaday JM, Mann JI, Turner RC. Prospective comparison of modified fat–high-carbohydrate with standard low-carbohydrate dietary advice in the treatment of diabetes: one year follow-up study. *Br J Nutr* 1978;**39**(2):357–362.

29 Milne RM, Mann JI, Chisholm AW, Williams SM. Long-term comparison of three dietary prescriptions in the treatment of NIDDM. *Diabetes Care* 1994;**17**(1):74–80.

30 Tsihlias EB, Gibbs AL, McBurney MI, Wolever TM. Comparison of high- and low-glycemic-index breakfast cereals with monounsaturated fat in the long-term dietary management of type 2 diabetes. *Am J Clin Nutr* 2000;**72**(2):439–449.

31 Wing RR, Blair E, Marcus M, Epstein LH, Harvey J. Year-long weight loss treatment for obese patients with type II diabetes: does including an intermittent very-low-calorie diet improve outcome? *Am J Med* 1994;**97**:354–362.

32 Wing RR, Anglin K. Efectiveness of a behavioural weight control program for blacks and whites with NIDDM. *Diabetes Care* 1996;**19**(5):409–13.

33 Wing RR, Blair EH, Bononi P, Marcus MD, Watanabe R, Bergman RN. Calorie restriction *per se* is a significant factor in improvements in glycemic control and insulin sensitivity during weight loss in obese NIDDM patients. *Diabetes Care* 1994;**17**(1):30–36.

34 Kelley DE, Wing R, Buonocore C, Sturis J, Polonsky K, Fitzsimmons M. Relative effects of calorie restriction and weight loss in noninsulin-dependent diabetes mellitus. *J Clin Endocrinol Metab* 1993;**77**(5):1287–93.

35 Astrup A, Meinert LT, Harper A. Atkins and other low-carbohydrate diets: hoax or an effective tool for weight loss?. *Lancet* 2004;**364**(9437):897–899.

36 Kennedy RL, Chokkalingam K, Farshchi HR. Nutrition in patients with Type 2 diabetes: are low-carbohydrate diets effective, safe or desirable?. *Diabet Med* 2005;**22**(7):821–832.

37 Atkins RC, *Dr. Atkins' New Diet Revolution*, Simon & Schuster, New York, 1998.

38 Bravata DM, Sanders L, Huang J, Krumholz HM, Olkin I, Gardner CD *et al.* Efficacy and safety of low-carbohydrate diets: a systematic review. *JAMA* 2003;**289**(14):1837–1850.

39 Samaha FF, Iqbal N, Seshadri P, Chicano KL, Daily DA, McGrory J *et al.* A low-carbohydrate as compared with a low-fat diet in severe obesity. *N Engl J Med* 2003;**348** (21): 2074–2081.

40 Arora SK, McFarlane SI. The case for low carbohydrate diets in diabetes management. *Nutr Metab* 2005;**2**:16–24.

41 Nielsen JV, Joensson E. Low-carbohydrate diet in type 2 diabetes. Stable improvement of bodyweight and glycemic control during 22 months follow-up. *Nutr Metab* 2006;**3**:22–26.

42 Boden G, Sargrad K, Homko C, Mozzoli M, Stein TP. Effect of a low-carbohydrate diet on appetite, blood glucose levels and insulin resistance in obese patients with type 2 diabetes. *Ann Intern Med* 2005;**142**(6):403–411.

43 McMillan-Price J, Petocz P, Atkinson F, O'Neill K, Samman S, Steinbeck K *et al.* Comparison of 4 diets of varying glycemic load on weight loss and cardiovascular risk reduction in overweight and obese young adults: a randomized controlled trial. *Arch Intern Med* 2006;**166**(14):1466–1475.

44 Klein S, Sheard NF, Pi-Sunyer X, Daly A, Wylie-Rosett J, Kulkarni K *et al.* Weight management through lifestyle modification for the prevention and management of type 2 diabetes: rationale and strategies: a statement of the American Diabetes Association, the North American Association for the Study of Obesity and the American Society for Clinical Nutrition. *Diabetes Care* 2004;**27**(8):2067–2073.

45 Expert Panel on Detection, Evaluation, Treatment of High Blood Cholesterol in Adults (Adult Treatment Panel III). Executive Summary of the Third Report of the National Cholesterol Education Program (NCEP) Expert Panel on Detection, Evaluation, and Treatment of High Blood Cholesterol in Adults (Adult Treatment Panel III). *JAMA* 2001;**285**(19):2486–2497.

46 Bertram SR, Venter I, Stewart RI. Weight loss in obese women – exercise versus dietary education. *S Afr Med J* 1990;**78**:15–18.

47 Johnson WG, Stalonas PM, Christ MA, Pock SR. The development and evaluation of a behavioral weight-reduction program. *Int J Obes* 1979;**3**(3):229–38.

48 Pavlou KN, Krey S, Steffee WP. Exercise as an adjunct to weight loss and maintenance in moderately obese subjects. *Am J Clin Nutr* 1989;**49**:1115–1123.

49 Wing RR, Epstein LH, Paternostro-Bayles M, Kriska A, Nowalk MP, Gooding W. Exercise in a behavioral weight control programme for obese patients with type 2 (non-insulin-dependent) diabetes. *Diabetologia* 1988;**31**:902–909.

50 Bouchard C, Despres J-P,. Tremblay A. Exercise and obesity. *Obes Res* 1993;**1**:133–147.

51 King AC, Tribble DL. The role of exercise in weight regulation in nonathletes. *Sports Med* 1991;**11**(5):331–349.

52 Norris SL, Zhang X, Avenell A, Gregg E, Bowman B, Serdula M *et al.* Long-term effectiveness of lifestyle and behavioral weight loss interventions in adults with type 2 diabetes: a meta-analysis. *Am J Med* 2004;**117**(10):762–774.

53 Carlson MG, Campbell PJ. Intensive insulin therapy and weight gain in IDDM. *Diabetes* 1993;**42**:1700–1707.

54 Hardeman W, Griffin S, Johnston M, Kinmonth AL, Wareham NJ. Interventions to prevent weight gain: a systematic review of psychological models and behaviour change methods. *Int J Obes* 2000;**24**:131–143.

55 Li Z, Maglione M, Tu W, Mojica W, Arterburn D, Shugarman LR *et al.* Meta-analysis: pharmacologic treatment of obesity. *Ann Intern Med* 2005;**142**(7):532–546.

56 Torgerson JS, Hauptman J, Boldrin MN, Sjostrom L. XENical in the prevention of diabetes in obese subjects

(XENDOS) study: a randomized study of orlistat as an adjunct to lifestyle changes for the prevention of type 2 diabetes in obese patients. *Diabetes Care* 2004;**27**(1):155–161.

57 Arterburn DE, Crane PK, Veenstra DL. The efficacy and safety of sibutramine for weight loss: a systematic review. *Arch Intern Med* 2004;**164**(9):994–1003.

58 Kim SH, Lee YM, Jee SH, Nam CM. Effect of sibutramine on weight loss and blood pressure: a meta-analysis of controlled trials. *Obes Res* 2003;**11**(9):1116–1123.

59 Vettor R, Serra R, Fabris R, Pagano C, Federspil G. Effect of sibutramine on weight management and metabolic control in type 2 diabetes: a meta-analysis of clinical studies. *Diabetes Care* 2005;**28**(4):942–949.

60 Norris SL, Zhang X, Avenell A, Gregg E, Schmid CH, Lau J. Pharmacotherapy for weight loss in adults with type 2 diabetes mellitus. *Cochrane Database Syst Rev* 2005;(1): CD004096.

61 Clark DW, Harrison-Woolrych M. Sibutramine may be associated with memory impairment. *BMJ* 2004;**329** (7478):1316.

62 Sayin T, Guldal M. Sibutramine: possible cause of a reversible cardiomyopathy. *Int J Cardiol* 2005;**99**(3):481–482.

63 Harrison-Woolrych M, Clark DW, Hill GR, Rees MI, Skinner JR. QT interval prolongation associated with sibutramine treatment. *Br J Clin Pharmacol* 2006;**61**(4):464–469.

64 Harrison-Woolrych M, Hill GR, Clark DW. Bruising associated with sibutramine: results from postmarketing surveillance in New Zealand. *Int J Obes* 2006;**30**: 1315–1317.

65 Van Gaal LF, Rissanen AM, Scheen AJ, Ziegler O, Rossner S. Effects of the cannabinoid-1 receptor blocker rimonabant on weight reduction and cardiovascular risk factors in overweight patients: 1-year experience from the RIO-Europe study. *Lancet* 2005;**365**(9468):1389–1397.

66 Bantle JP, Wylie-Rosett J, Albright AL, Apovian CM, Clark NG, Franz MJ *et al*. Nutrition recommendations and interventions for diabetes: a position statement of the American Diabetes Association. *Diabetes Care* 2008;**31** (Suppl 1): S61–S78.

67 Pi-Sunyer FX, Aronne LJ, Heshmati HM, Devin J, Rosenstock J. Effect of rimonabant, a cannabinoid-1 receptor blocker, on weight and cardiometabolic risk factors in overweight or obese patients: RIO-North America: a randomized controlled trial. *JAMA* 2006;**295**(7):761–775.

68 Scheen AJ, Finer N, Hollander P, Jensen MD, Van Gaal LF. Efficacy and tolerability of rimonabant in overweight or obese patients with type 2 diabetes: a randomised controlled study. *Lancet* 2006;**368**(9548):1660–1672.

69 Buchwald H, Avidor Y, Braunwald E, Jensen MD, Pories W, Fahrbach K *et al*. Bariatric surgery: a systematic review and meta-analysis. *JAMA* 2004;**292**(14):1724–1737.

70 Sjostrom L, Lindroos AK, Peltonen M, Torgerson J, Bouchard C, Carlsson B *et al*. Lifestyle, diabetes and cardiovascular risk factors 10 years after bariatric surgery. *N Engl J Med* 2004;**351**(26):2683–2693.

71 Maggard MA, Shugarman LR, Suttorp M, Maglione M, Sugerman HJ, Livingston EH *et al*. Meta-analysis: surgical treatment of obesity. *Ann Intern Med* 2005;**142**(7): 547–559.

72 Batsis JA, Romero-Corral A, Collazo-Clavell ML, Sarr MG, Somers VK, Brekke L *et al*. Effect of weight loss on predicted cardiovascular risk: change in cardiac risk after bariatric surgery. *Obesity (Silver Spring)* 2007; **15**(3):772–784.

73 Smoot TM, Xu P, Hilsenrath P, Kuppersmith NC, Singh KP. Gastric bypass surgery in the United States, 1998–2002. *Am J Public Health* 2006;**96**(7):1187–1189.

74 Encinosa WE, Bernard DM, Chen CC, Steiner CA. Healthcare utilization and outcomes after bariatric surgery. *Med Care* 2006;**44**(8):706–712.

75 Powell KE, Thompson PD, Caspersen CJ, Kendrick JS. Physical activity and the incidence of coronary heart disease. *Annu Rev Public Health* 1987;**8**:253–287.

76 Berlin JA, Colditz GA. A meta-analysis of physical activity in the prevention of coronary heart disease. *Am J Epidemiol* 1990;**132**(4):612–628.

77 Rennie KL, Wareham NJ. The validation of physical activity instruments for measuring energy expenditure: problems and pitfalls. *Public Health Nutr* 1:1998;265–271.

78 Wareham N, Rennie K. The assessment of physical activity in individuals and populations: why try to be more precise about how physical activity is assessed?. *Int J Obes* 1998;**22**: S30–S38.

79 Tanasescu M, Leitzmann MF, Rimm EB, Hu FB. Physical activity in relation to cardiovascular disease and total mortality among men with type 2 diabetes. *Circulation* 2003;**107**(19):2435–2439.

80 Hu G, Eriksson J, Barengo NC, Lakka TA, Valle TT, Nissinen A *et al*. Occupational, commuting and leisure-time physical activity in relation to total and cardiovascular mortality among Finnish subjects with type 2 diabetes. *Circulation* 2004;**110**(6):666–673.

81 Batty GD, Shipley MJ, Marmot M, Smith GD. Physical activity and cause-specific mortality in men with Type 2 diabetes/impaired glucose tolerance: evidence from the Whitehall study. *Diabet Med* 2002;**19**(7):580–588.

82 Reaven GM. Role of insulin resistance in human disease. *Diabetes* 1988;**37**:1595–1607.

83 Minuk HL, Vranic M, Marliss EB, Hanna AK, Albisser AM, Zinman B. Glucoregulatory and metabolic response to exercise in obese noninsulin-dependent diabetes. *Am J Physiol* 1981;**240**:E458–E464.

84 Jenkins AB, Furler SM, Bruce DG, Chisholm DJ. Regulation of hepatic glucose output during moderate exercise in non-insulin-dependent diabetes. *Metabolism* 1988; **37**:966–972.

85 Devlin J, Hirshman M, Horton E, Horton E. Enhanced peripheral and splanchnic insulin sensitivity in NIDDM men after a single bout of exercise. *Diabetes* 1987; **36**:434–439.

86 Landt KW, Campaigne BN, James FW, Sperling MA. Effects of exercise training on insulin sensitivity in adolescents with type 1 diabetes. *Diabetes Care* 1985;**8**(5):461–465.

87 Wallberg-Henriksson H, Gunnarsson R, Henriksson J, Defronzo R, Felig P, Ostman J *et al*. Increased peripheral insulin sensitivity and muscle mitochondrial enzymes but unchanged blood glucose control in type 1 diabetics after physical training. *Diabetes* 1982;**31**:1044–1050.

88 Boule NG, Haddad E, Kenny GP, Wells GA, Sigal RJ. Effects of exercise on glycemic control and body mass in type 2 diabetes mellitus: a meta-analysis of controlled clinical trials. *JAMA* 2001;**286**(10):1218–1227.

89 Thomas DE, Elliott EJ, Naughton GA. Exercise for type 2 diabetes mellitus. *Cochrane Database Syst Rev* 2006;**3**: CD002968.

90 Duncan GE, Perri MG, Theriaque DW, Hutson AD, Eckel RH, Stacpoole PW. Exercise training, without weight loss, increases insulin sensitivity and postheparin plasma lipase activity in previously sedentary adults. *Diabetes Care* 2003;**263**:557–562.

91 Lee S, Kuk JL, Davidson LE, Hudson R, Kilpatrick K, Graham TE *et al.* Exercise without weight loss is an effective strategy for obesity reduction in obese individuals with and without Type 2 diabetes. *J Appl Physiol* 2005;**993**: 1220–1225.

92 Dekker MJ, Lee S, Hudson R, Kilpatrick K, Graham TE, Ross R *et al.* An exercise intervention without weight loss decreases circulating interleukin-6 in lean and obese men with and without type 2 diabetes mellitus. *Metabolism* 2007;**563**:332–338.

93 Morrato EH, Hill JO, Wyatt HR, Ghushchyan V, Sullivan PW. Physical activity in U.S. adults with diabetes and at risk for developing diabetes, 2003. *Diabetes Care* 2007;**302**:203–209.

94 Wareham NJ, Wong M-Y, Day NE. Glucose intolerance and physical inactivity: the relative importance of low habitual energy expenditure and cardiorespiratory fitness. *Am J Epidemiol* 2000;**152**:132–139.

95 Wareham NJ, Wong M-Y, Hennings S, Mitchell J, Rennie K, Cruickshank K *et al.* Quantifying the association between habitual energy expenditure and blood pressure. *Int J Epidemiol* 2000;**29**:655–660.

96 Wareham NJ, Hennings SJ, Byrne CD, Hales CN, Prentice AM, Day NE. A quantitative analysis of the relationship between habitual energy expenditure, fitness and the metabolic cardiovascular syndrome. *Br J Nutr* **80**:1998;235–241.

97 Oshida Y, Yamanouchi K, Hayamizu S, Sato Y. Long-term mild jogging increases insulin action despite no influence on body mass index or VO$_{2max}$. *J Appl Physiol* 1989;**665**: 2206–2210.

98 Kang J, Robertson RJ, Hagberg JM, Kelley DE, Goss FL, DaSilva SG *et al.* Effect of exercise intensity on glucose and insulin metabolism in obese individuals and obese NIDDM patients. *Diabetes Care* 1996;**19**(4):341–349.

99 Braun B, Zimmermann MB, Kretchmer N. Effects of exercise intensity on insulin sensitivity in women with non-insulin dependent diabetes mellitus. *J Appl Physiol* 1995;**78**(1):300–306.

100 Durak EP, Jovanovic-Peterson L, Peterson CM. Randomized crossover study of effect of resistance training on glycemic control, muscular strength and cholesterol in type 1 diabetic men. *Diabetes Care* 1990;**13**(10):1039–1043.

101 Peterson CM, Jones RL, Dupuis A, Levine BS, Bernstein R, O'Shea M. Feasibility of improved blood glucose control in patients with insulin-dependent diabetes mellitus. *Diabetes Care* 1979;**2**(4):329–335.

102 Miller WJ, Sherman WM, Ivy JL. Effect of strength training on glucose tolerance and post-glucose insulin response. *Med Sci Sports Exercise* 1984;**16**(6):539–543.

103 Di Loreto C, Fanelli C, Lucidi P, Murdolo G, De Cicco A, Parlanti N *et al.* Make your diabetic patients walk: long-term impact of different amounts of physical activity on type 2 diabetes. *Diabetes Care* 2005;**28**(6): 1295–1302.

104 Boule NG, Kenny GP, Haddad E, Wells GA, Sigal RJ. Meta-nalysis of the effect of structured exercise training on cardiorespiratory fitness in Type 2 diabetes mellitus. *Diabetologia* 2003;**46**(8):1071–1081.

105 Siscovick DS, Weiss NS, Fletcher RH, Lasky T. The incidence of primary cardiac arrest during vigorous exercise. *N Engl J Med* 1984;**311**:874–877.

106 Kohl HW III, Powell KE, Gordon NF, Blair SN, Paffenbarger RS Jr. Physical Activity, physical fitness and sudden cardiac death. *Epidemiol Rev* 1992;**14**:37–58.

107 Hilsted J, Galbo H, Christensen NJ. Impaired cardiovascular responses to graded exercise in diabetic autonomic neuropathy. *Diabetes* 1979;**28**:313–319.

108 Kahn JK, Sisson JC, Vinik A. QT Interval prolongation and sudden cardiac death in diabetic autonomic neuropathy. *J Clin Endocrinol Metab* 1987;**64**:751–754.

109 Kahn JK, Sisson JC, Vinik AI. Prediction of sudden cardiac death in diabetic autonomic neuropathy. *J Nucl Med* 1988;**29**:1605–1606.

110 Ewing DJ, Boland O, Neilson JMM, Cho CG, Clarke BF. Autonomic neuropathy, QT interval lengthening and unexpected deaths in male diabetic patients. *Diabetologia* 1991;**34**:182–185.

111 Zola BE, Vinik AI. Effects of autonomic neuropathy associated with diabetes mellitus on cardiovasular function. *Curr Sci* 1992;**3**:33–41.

112 Cruikshanks KJ, Moss SE, Klein R, Klein BEK. Physical activity and proliferate retinopathy in people diagnosed with diabetes before age 30 yr. *Diabetes Care* 1992;**15**(10): 1267–1272.

113 LaPorte RE, Dorman JS, Tajima N *et al.* Pittsburgh insulin-dependent diabetes and mortality study: physical activity and diabetic complications. *Pediatrics* 1986;**78**: 1027–1033.

114 Kriska AM, LaPorte RE, Patrick SL, Kuller LH, Orchard TJ. The association of physical activity and diabetic complications in individuals with insulin-dependent diabetes mellitus: the epidemiology of diabetes complications study – VII. *J Clin Epidemiol* 1991;**44**(11):1207–1214.

115 Orchard T, Dorman J, Maser RE, Becker DJ, Ellis D, LaPorte RE *et al.* Factors associated with avoidance of severe complications after 25 yr of IDDM. *Diabetes Care* 1990;**13**(7):741–747.

116 Anderson B. Activity and diabetic vitreous haemorrhages. *Ophthalmology* 1980;**87**:173–175.

117 Graham C, Lasko-McCarthey P. Exercise options for people with diabetic complications. *Diabetes Educator* 1990;**16**: 212–220.

118 Bernbaum M, Albert SG, Cohen JD. Exercise training in individuals with diabetic retinopathy and blindness. *Arch Phys Med Rehabil* 1989;**70**:605–611.

119 Vittinghus E, Mogensen CE. Albumin excretion and renal haemodynamic response to physical exercise in normal and diabetic man. *Scand J Clin Lab Invest* 1981;**41**:627–632.

120 Bognetti E, Meschi F, Pattarini A, Zoja A, Chiumello G. Post-exercise albuminuria does not predict microalbuminuria in type 1 diabetic patients. *Diabet Med* 1994;**11**(9): 850–855.

121 Christensen CK. Abnormal albuminuria and blood pressure rise in inicipient diabetic nephropathy induced by exercise. *Kidney Int* 1984;**25**:819–823.

122 Mohamed A, Wilkin T, Leatherdale BA, Rowe D. Response of urinary albumin to submaximal exercise in newly diagnosed non-insulin dependent diabetes. *BMJ* 1984;**288**: 1342–1343.

123 Viberti G, Pickup JC, Bilous RW, Keen H, Mackintosh D. Correction of exercise-induced microalbuminuria in insulin-dependent diabetics after 3 weeks of subcutaneous insulin infusion. *Diabetes* 1981;**30**:818–823.

124 Koivisto VA, Huttunen N-P, Vierikko P. Continuous subcutaneous insulin infusion corrects exercise-induced albuminuria in juvenile diabetes. *BMJ* 1981;**282**:778–779.

125 Vittinghus E, Mogensen CE. Graded exercise and protein excretion in diabetic man and the effect of insulin treatment. *Kidney Int* 1982;**21**:725–729.

126 MacDonald MJ. Postexercise late-onset hypoglycemia in insulin-dependent diabetic patients. *Diabetes Care* 1987; **10**(5): 584–588.

127 Zinman B, Murray FT, Vranic M, Albisser AM, Leibel BS, McClean PA *et al*. Glucoregulation during moderate exercise in insulin treated diabetics. *J Clin Endocrinol Metab* 1977;**45**:641–652.

128 Frid A, Östman J, Linde B. Hypoglycemia risk during exercise after intramuscular injection of insulin in thigh in IDDM. *Diabetes Care* 1990;**13**(5):473–477.

129 Berger M, Berchtold P, Cüppers HJ, Drost H, Kley HK, Müller WA *et al*. Metabolic and hormonal effects of muscular exercise in juvenile type diabetics. *Diabetologia* 1977;**13**:355–365.

130 Caron D, Poussier P, Marliss EB, Zinman B. The effect of postprandial exercise on meal-related glucose intolerance in insulin-dependent diabetic individuals. *Diabetes Care* 1982;**5**(4):364–369.

131 Campaigne BN, Wallberg-Henriksson H, Gunnarsson R. Glucose and insulin responses in relation to insulin dose and caloric intake 12 h after acute physical exercise in men with IDDM. *Diabetes Care* 1987;**10**(6):716–721.

132 Garg A. High monounsaturated fat diets for people with diabetes mellitus: a meta-analysis. *Am J Clin Nutr* 1998;**67**:577s–582s.

133 Low CC, Grossman EB, Gumbiner B. Potentiation of effects of weight loss by monounsaturated fatty acids in obese NIDDM patients. *Diabetes* 1996;**4**(55):569–575.

134 Hu FB, van Dam RM, Liu S. Diet and risk of Type II diabetes: the role of types of fat and carbohydrate. *Diabetologia* 2001;**4**(47):805–817.

135 Summers LK, Fielding BA, Bradshaw HA, Ilic V, Beysen C, Clark ML *et al*. Substituting dietary saturated fat with polyunsaturated fat changes abdominal fat distribution and improves insulin sensitivity. *Diabetologia* 2002;**4**(53): 369–377.

136 He K, Song Y, Daviglus ML, Liu K, Van Horn L, Dyer AR *et al*. Accumulated evidence on fish consumption and coronary heart disease mortality: a meta-analysis of cohort studies. *Circulation* 2004;**109**(22):2705–2711.

137 Feskens EJM, Bowles CH, Kromhout D. Inverse association between fish intake and risk of glucose intolerance in normoglycemic elderly men and women. *Diabetes Care* 1991;**14**:935–941.

138 Friedberg CE, Janssen MJFM, Heine RJ, Grobbee DE. Fish oil and glycemic control in diabetes. *Diabetes Care* 1998; **2**(14):494–500.

139 Montori VM, Farmer A, Wollan PC, Dinneen SF. Fish oil supplementation in type 2 diabetes. *Diabetes Care* 2000; **2**(39):1407–15.

140 Hartweg J, Farmer AJ, Holman RR, Neil HA. Meta-analysis of the effects of n-3 polyunsaturated fatty acids on haematological and thrombogenic factors in type 2 diabetes. *Diabetologia* 2007;**50**(2):250–258.

141 Hartweg J, Perera R, Montori V, Dinneen S, Neil HA, Farmer A. Omega-3 polyunsaturated fatty acids (PUFA) for type 2 diabetes mellitus. *Cochrane Database Syst Rev* 2008;**1**:CD003205.

142 Sheard NF, Clark NG, Brand-Miller JC, Franz MJ, Pi-Sunyer FX, Mayer-Davis E *et al*. Dietary carbohydrate (amount and type) in the prevention and management of diabetes: a statement by the American Diabetes Association. *Diabetes Care* 2004;**27**(9):2266–2271.

143 Daly ME, Vale C, Walker M, Alberti KG, Mathers JC. Dietary carbohydrates and insulin sensitivity: a review of the evidence and clinical implications. *Am J Clin Nutr* 1997;**66**(5):1072–1085.

144 Franz MJ, Horton ES, Bantle JP, Beebe CA, Brunzell JD, Coulston AM *et al*. Nutrition principles for the management of diabetes and related complications. *Diabetes Care* 1994;**17**(5):490–518.

145 Brynes AE, Frost GS. Increased sucrose intake is not associated with a change in glucose or insulin sensitivity in people with type 2 diabetes. *Int J Food Sci Nutr* 2007; **58**(8):644–651.

146 Henry RR, Crapo PA. Current issues in fructose metabolism. *Annu Rev Nutr* 1991;**11**:21–39.

147 Uusitupa MI. Fructose in the diabetic diet. *Am J Clin Nutr* 1994;**59**(3Suppl): 753S–757S.

148 Harding AH, Wareham NJ, Bingham SA, Khaw K, Luben R, Welch A *et al*. Plasma vitamin C level, fruit and vegetable consumption and the risk of new-onset type 2 diabetes mellitus: the European prospective investigation of cancer – Norfolk prospective study. *Arch Intern Med* 2008;**168**(14): 1493–1499.

149 Brand-Miller J, Hayne S, Petocz P, Colagiuri S. Low-glycemic index diets in the management of diabetes: a meta-analysis of randomized controlled trials. *Diabetes Care* 2003; **26**(8):2261–2267.

150 Opperman AM, Venter CS, Oosthuizen W, Thompson RL, Vorster HH. Meta-analysis of the health effects of using the glycaemic index in meal-planning. *Br J Nutr* 2004;**92**(3):367–381.

151 Kinmonth AL, Angus RM, Jenkins PA, Smith MA, Baum JD. Whole foods and increased dietary fibre improve blood

glucose control in diabetic children. *Arch Dis Child* 1982;**57**:187–194.

152 Simpson RW, Mann JI, Eaton J, Carter RD, Hockaday TDR. High-carbohydrate diets and insulin-dependent diabetics. *BMJ* 1979;**ii**:523–525.

153 Simpson HCR, Lousley S, Geekie M, Simpson RW, Carter RD, Hockaday TDR. A high-carbohydrate leguminous fibre diet improves all aspects of diabetic control. *Lancet* 1981; **i**:1–5.

154 Klahr S, Levey AS, Beck GJ, Caggiula AW, Hunsicker L, Kusek JW *et al*. The effects of dietary protein restriction and blood-pressure control on the progression of chronic renal diease. *N Engl J Med* 1994;**330**(13):877–884.

155 Friedman EA. Diabetic nephropathy: strategies in prevention and management. *Kidney Int* 1982;**21**:780–791.

156 Waugh NR, Robertson AM. Protein restriction for diabetic renal disease. *Cochrane Database Syst Rev* 2000;(2): CD002181.

157 Lieber CS. Alcohol and the liver: 1994 update. *Gastroenterology* 1994;**106**(4):1085–1105.

158 Ahmed AT, Karter AJ, Warton EM, Doan JU, Weisner CM. The relationship between alcohol consumption and glycemic control among patients with diabetes: the Kaiser Permanente Northern California Diabetes Registry. *J Gen Intern Med* 2008;**23**(3):275–282.

159 Harding AH, Sargeant LA, Khaw KT, Welch A, Oakes S, Luben RN *et al*. Cross-sectional association between total level and type of alcohol consumption and glycosylated haemoglobin level: the EPIC-Norfolk study. *Eur J Clin Nutr* 2002;**56**:882–890.

160 Howard AA, Arnsten JH, Gourevitch MN. Effect of alcohol consumption on diabetes mellitus: a systematic review. *Ann Intern Med* 2004;**140**(3):211–219.

161 Sargeant LA, Wareham NJ, Bingham S, Day NE, Luben RN, Oakes S *et al*. Vitamin C and hyperglycemia in the European Prospective Investigation Into Cancer-Norfolk (EPIC-Norfolk) Study. *Diabetes Care* 2000;**23**(6):726–732.

162 Salonen JT, Nyyssonen K, Tuomainen T-P *et al*. Increased risk of non-insulin dependent diabetes mellitus at low plasma vitamin E concentrations: a four year follow up study in men. *BMJ* 1995;**311**:1124–1127.

163 Paolisso G, D'Amore A, Giugliano D *et al*. Pharmacological doses of vitamin E improve insulin action in healthy subjects and non-insulin dependent diabetic subjects. *Am J Clin Nutr* 1993;**57**:650–656.

164 Sargeant LA, Khaw KT, Bingham S, Day NE, Luben RN, Oakes S *et al*. Fruit and vegetable intake and population glycosylated haemoglobin levels: the EPIC-Norfok Study. *Eur J Clin Nutr* 2001;**55**:342–348.

165 Williams DEM, Wareham NJ, Cox BD, Byrne CD, Hales CN, Day NE. Frequent salad vegetable consumption is associated with a reduction in the risk of diabetes mellitus. *J Clin Epidemiol* 1999;**52**(4):329–335.

166 Czernichow S, Couthouis A, Bertrais S, Vergnaud AC, Dauchet L, Galan P *et al*. Antioxidant supplementation does not affect fasting plasma glucose in the Supplementation with Antioxidant Vitamins and Minerals (SU.VI. MAX) study in France: association with dietary intake and plasma concentrations. *Am J Clin Nutr* 2006;**84**(2): 395–399.

167 Lonn E, Yusuf S, Hoogwerf B, Pogue J, Yi Q, Zinman B *et al*. Effects of vitamin E on cardiovascular and microvascular outcomes in high-risk patients with diabetes: results of the HOPE study and MICRO-HOPE substudy. *Diabetes Care* 2002;**25**(11):1919–1927.

168 Millen AE, Klein R, Folsom AR, Stevens J, Palta M, Mares JA. Relation between intake of vitamins C and E and risk of diabetic retinopathy in the Atherosclerosis Risk in Communities Study. *Am J Clin Nutr* 2004;**79**(5): 865–873.

169 Ward NC, Wu JH, Clarke MW, Puddey IB, Burke V, Croft KD *et al*. The effect of vitamin E on blood pressure in individuals with type 2 diabetes: a randomized, double-blind, placebo-controlled trial. *J Hypertens* 2007;**25** (1):227–234.

170 Boucher BJ, Mannan N, Noonan K, Hales CN Evans SJW. Glucose intolerance and impairment of insulin secretion in relation to vitamin D deficiency in East London Asians. *Diabetologia* 1995;**38**:1239–1245.

171 Wareham NJ Byrne CD Carr C, Day NE, Boucher BJ Hales CN. Glucose intolerance is associated with altered calcium homeostasis: a possible link between increased serum calcium concentrations and cardiovascular disease mortality. *Metabolism* 1997;**46**(10):1171–1177.

172 de Boer IH Tinker LF, Connelly S, Curb JD, Howard BV, Kestenbaum B *et al*. Calcium plus vitamin D supplementation and the risk of incident diabetes in the Women's Health Initiative. *Diabetes Care* 2008;**31**(4):701–707.

173 Anderson RA, Cheng N, Bryden NA *et al*. Elevated intakes of supplemental chromium improve glucose and insulin variables in individuals with type 2 diabetes. *Diabetes* 1997;**1997**(46):1786–1791.

174 Grant KE, Chandler RM, Castle AL, Ivy JL. Chromium and exercise training: effect on obese women. *Med Sci Sports Exercise* 1997;**29**(8):992–998.

175 McCarty MF. Exploiting complementary therapeutic strategies for the treatment of type II diabetes and prevention of its complications. *Med Hypotheses* 1997;**49**:143–152.

176 Althuis MD, Jordan NE, Ludington EA, Wittes JT. Glucose and insulin responses to dietary chromium supplements: a meta-analysis. *Am J Clin Nutr* 2002;**761**:148–155.

177 Tosiello L. Hypomagnesemia and diabetes mellitus. A review of clinical implications. *Arch Intern Med* 1996;**156**(11): 1143–1148.

178 Barbagallo M, Dominguez LJ. Magnesium metabolism in type 2 diabetes mellitus, metabolic syndrome and insulin resistance. *Arch Biochem Biophys* 2007;**458**(1):40–47.

179 Song Y, Manson JE, Buring JE, Liu S. Dietary magnesium intake in relation to plasma insulin levels and risk of type 2 diabetes in women. *Diabetes Care* 2004;**27**(1):59–65.

180 Song Y, He K, Levitan EB, Manson JE, Liu S. Effects of oral magnesium supplementation on glycaemic control in Type 2 diabetes: a meta-analysis of randomized double-blind controlled trials. *Diabet Med* 2006;**23**(10): 1050–1056.

181 Soinio M, Marniemi J, Laakso M, Pyorala K, Lehto S, Ronnemaa T. Serum zinc level and coronary heart disease events in patients with type 2 diabetes. *Diabetes Care* 2007;**30** (3):523–528.

182 Beletate V, El Dib R, Atallah A. Zinc supplementation for the prevention of type 2 diabetes mellitus. *Cochrane Database Syst Rev* 2007;(1):CD005525.

183 Yeh GY, Eisenberg DM, Kaptchuk TJ, Phillips RS. Systematic review of herbs and dietary supplements for glycemic control in diabetes. *Diabetes Care* 2003;**26**(4):1277–1294.

184 Pastors JG, Franz MJ, Warshaw H, Daly A, Arnold MS, How effective is medical nutrition therapy in diabetes care? *J Am Diet Assoc* 2003;**103**(7):827–831.

8 What is the evidence that changing tobacco use reduces the incidence of diabetic complications?

Deborah L. Wingard, Elizabeth Barrett-Connor, Nicole M. Wedick

Department of Family and Preventive Medicine, University of California, San Diego La Jolla, CA, USA

Introduction

Diabetes is associated with the development of numerous complications, including nephropathy, neuropathy, retinopathy and heart disease. Smoking is also associated with the development of heart disease, and also cancer, stroke and lung disease.[1,2] Smoking may be associated with the development of other complications of diabetes.[3-6] Unfortunately, the prevalence of smoking appears to be essentially the same for individuals with and without diabetes.[3,5-7] Based on this information, the American Diabetes Association issued a position statement that prevention or cessation of tobacco use is an important component of clinical diabetes care.[8] This chapter reviews current evidence that changing tobacco use could reduce the incidence of diabetic complications.

Possible mechanisms

Smoking could increase the risk of complications in individuals with diabetes, if smoking interferes with metabolic control. Several studies have demonstrated that metabolic control is worse in smoking compared with non-smoking diabetic patients, the smokers having more hyperglycaemia and increased levels of glycosylated haemoglobin.[4,9-11] Smoking has also been shown to increase the secretion of catecholamines, growth hormone and cortisol,[11-14] hormones which counteract insulin action and could lead to an increased insulin requirement in diabetic patients. Targher *et al.*[15]

found that insulin resistance was markedly worse among individuals with type 2 diabetes who smoked. However, Hleve *et al.*[16] reported that neither acute nor habitual smoking caused substantial changes in insulin sensitivity in type 1 diabetic patients.

Smoking could also increase the risk of complications in individuals with diabetes, if smoking influences other risk factors for those complications. For example, research has demonstrated that smokers have higher serum concentrations of cholesterol, triglycerides, very low-density lipoprotein (VLDL) cholesterol and low-density lipoprotein (LDL) cholesterol and lower serum concentrations of high-density lipoprotein (HDL) cholesterol and apolipoprotein A1.[17-20] These associations would be expected to increase the risk of cardiovascular disease (CVD).

In clinical trials, smoking has been shown to acutely raise blood pressure[21] and reduce retinal blood flow,[22] and the vasoconstriction caused by nicotine induces a transient rise in pulse rate,[12] effects that could potentially affect the cardiovascular circulation, impair kidney function and cause retinal disease. As reviewed by Christen *et al.*, smoking also increases carboxyhaemoglobin and platelet adhesiveness and causes vasoconstriction of peripheral arteries.[23] These changes could lead to tissue hypoxia and possibly the peripheral vascular and nerve abnormalities seen in individuals with diabetes.

Alternatively, smoking may not directly or indirectly increase the risk of complications in individuals with diabetes, but rather serve as a marker for other aspects of lifestyle that influence complication rates.

The Evidence Base for Diabetes Care, Second Edition, Edited by William H. Herman, Ann Louise Kinmonth, Nicholas J. Wareham and Rhys Williams.
© 2010 John Wiley & Sons, Ltd

For example, individuals who smoke cigarettes may be more likely to drink alcohol and eat a high-fat diet, while being less likely to exercise, behaviours shown to influence the risk of heart disease. Smoking may also serve as a marker for low socioeconomic status and limited access to medical care, which may in turn increase the risk of complications. If smoking helps the diabetic individual maintain weight control, smoking could prevent complications; however, several studies indicate that smoking is associated with increased visceral adiposity, a stronger risk factor for coronary heart disease than body mass index.[24–26]

Prevalence of smoking among adults with diabetes

Despite substantial evidence of the harmful effects of smoking, over 20% of adults in the United States continue to report smoking cigarettes (23% according to the 2001 Behavioural Risk Factor Surveillance System Survey[7] and 21% according to the 2004 National Health Interview Survey[27]). Smoking is generally reported more frequently by men (23.4%) than women (18.5%) and by native Americans (33.4%) than Caucasians (22.2%), blacks (20.2%) or Hispanics (15.0%).[27] As summarized in Table 8.1, recent studies

Table 8.1 Prevalence of smoking in diabetic compared with non-diabetic adults, United States, 2000–2006

Study	Participants	'Current smoker' prevalence (%)	
		Diabetes	**No diabetes**
Cross-sectional			
West et al.[28]	**Proyecto VER**	Total = 18.9	Total = 20.9
Arizona, USA	1022 Mexican Americans with type 2	Known = 17.7	
2002	diabetes and 3717 without diabetes for	New = 25.2	
	which smoking status could be		
	determined, aged 40–80+ years		
Ford et al.[7]	**Behavioral Risk Factor Surveillance System**	*Age-specific and age-adjusted:*	*Age-specific and age-adjusted:*
USA	14 457 with diabetes and 198 053 without	Total = 23.2	Total = 23.2
2004	diabetes in 2001, aged ≥18 years	*Age, years:*	*Age, years:*
		Age 18–44 = 28.0	Age 18–44 = 27.4
		Age 45–64 = 21.3	Age 45–64 = 22.9
		Age ≥65 = 7.7	Age ≥65 = 10.5
		Sex:	*Sex:*
		Men = 24.8	Men = 24.8
		Women = 21.9	Women = 21.5
		Race or ethnicity:	*Race or ethnicity:*
		White = 25.0	White = 24.3
		African American = 20.2	African American = 22.7
		Hispanic = 18.9	Hispanic = 18.8
		Other = 29.7	Other = 23.6
Wong et al.[29]	**Multi-ethnic Study of Atherosclerosis**	Total = 11.9	Total = 12.8
6 states, USA	778 individuals with diabetes and 5322	White = 9.9	*(data for sub-groups not shown)*
2006	without diabetes, aged 45–85 years	Black = 15.3	
		Hispanic = 11.1	
		Chinese = 6.9	
Cohort (baseline)			
Cho et al.[30]	**Health Professionals Follow-up Study**	*Age standardized to age*	*Age standardized to age*
USA	1515 male health professionals with type 2	*distribution of cohort in 1986:*	*distribution of cohort in 1986:*
2002	diabetes and 49 801 without diabetes	Without CHD = 10	Without CHD = 10
	aged 40–75 years	With CHD = 6	With CHD = 13
Lifford et al.[31]	**Nurses' Health Study**	*Age-adjusted:*	*Age-adjusted:*
USA	4277 female nurses (mean age 64 years)	Total = 11.2	Total = 12.4
2005	with type 2 diabetes and 77 568 (mean		
	age 62 years) without diabetes		
	(restricted to nurses who reported		
	information on urinary function in 1996)		

that have compared adults with and without diabetes in the United States have found few differences in the prevalence of smoking and the above-noted trends by gender and race persist in both groups.[7,28–31]

Although studies of health professionals[30] and nurses[31] found lower rates of smoking overall (10–12%) than in the general population, there were still no differences in smoking rates between those with and without diabetes.

Recent international studies, summarized in Table 8.2, indicate more variation in smoking prevalence.[32–37] In France, individuals with diabetes are less likely to smoke than those without diabetes (23.1 and 29.6%, respectively).[33] Similarly in The Netherlands, in the absence of CVD, men and women with diabetes are less likely to smoke than those without diabetes. However, among those with CVD, diabetes is associated with more smoking.[37] Smoking is very high among aboriginal Canadians without diabetes

(73–80%), but substantially lower among those with diabetes (44–54%).[32]

While most recent studies in the United States and other countries have focused primarily on type 2 diabetes, one study from Germany was restricted to those with type 1 diabetes.[34] The authors reported a smoking prevalence of 10.5% in youth aged 12–16 years and 34.8% in those aged 17–26 years. Unfortunately this study included no non-diabetic children or young adults for comparison. In older studies based on the US 1989 National Health Interview Survey[38] and the London cohort from the WHO Multinational Study of Vascular Disease in Diabetes,[39] similar rates of smoking were reported for those with type 1 and type 2 diabetes. In the US National Survey, among those with diabetes the prevalence of smoking decreased with increasing duration of disease.[38] This may reflect the increased mortality associated with the combination of smoking and diabetes.

Table 8.2 Prevalence of smoking in diabetic compared with non-diabetic adults, multinational, 2000–2006

Study	Participants	'Current smoker' prevalence (%)	
		Diabetes	**No diabetes**
Cross-sectional			
Harris et al.[32]	**Sandy Lake Diabetes Complications Study**	Men = 43.8	Men:
Canada	119 Aboriginal Canadians with type 2 diabetes	Women = 53.5	NGT = 80.4
2002	and 406 without diabetes, aged 18–74 years		IGT = 50.0
			Women:
			NGT = 73.3
			IGT = 51.9
Beziaud et al.[33]	698 individuals with type 2 diabetes and	Total = 23.1	Total = 29.6
France	27079 without diabetes, aged 20–69 years	Men = 31.0	Men = 36.4
2004		Women = 9.9	Women = 24.2
Schwab et al.[34]	**Germany diabetes documentation and**	Pre-pubertal	–
Germany	**quality management system (DPV)**	(0.25–11 years) = 0.24	
2006	19 683 patients with type 1 diabetes, age	Pubertal (12–16 years) = 10.53	
	range 3 months–26 years	Adult = (17–26 years) = 34.75	
Cohort (baseline)			
Lee et al.[35]	**WHO Multinational Study of Vascular**	Total = 28.2	–
Multinational	**Disease in Diabetes**	Men = 37.1	
2001	1188 subjects with type 1 diabetes and 3234	Women = 20.5	
	subjects with type 2 diabetes from 10 centres,		
	mean age = 55 years		
Zoppini et al.[36]	**Verona Diabetes Study**	<65 years = 36	–
Italy	3398 patients with type 2 diabetes, median	≥65 years = 13	
2003	age = 66 years		
Becker et al.[37]	**Hoorn Study**	*Men:*	*Men:*
The Netherlands	208 individuals with type 2 diabetes and 2253	Without CVD = 22.6	Without CVD = 36.9
2003	without diabetes, mean age = 62 years	With CVD = 42.3	With CVD = 35.4
		Women:	*Women:*
		Without CVD = 20.5	Without CVD = 28.9
		With CVD = 28.6	With CVD = 23.1

Since the first edition of this book,[40] smoking rates have declined for both those with and without diabetes and substantially for some ethnic groups. Based on US National Health Interview Surveys, smoking declined overall from 25.9% in 1989 to 20.9% in 2004.[27,38] Based on the Behavioral Risk Factor Surveys, smoking declined from 25.5% in 1988 to 23.2% in 2001 among those without diabetes and from 26.0 to 23.2% among those with diabetes.[26,41]

All of the above studies relied on self-reported smoking status and many also relied on self-reported diabetes status. Although these self-reports may be underestimates, the data suggest that individuals with diabetes smoke at rates equivalent to the general population.

Diabetic complications in smokers versus non-smokers

Diabetes is associated with the development of numerous complications, the primary ones being nephropathy, neuropathy, retinopathy and CVD. This section reviews prospective evidence that smoking is associated with the risk of developing each of these complications.

Nephropathy

Whereas cross-sectional studies[40] of individuals with diabetes often show an association between smoking and the prevalence of nephropathy (defined variously as microalbuminuria, albuminuria and proteinuria), results from prospective studies are less consistent. As shown in Table 8.3, only two of four cohort studies which focused on type 1 diabetes found an association between smoking and the incidence of nephropathy,[44,48] and two of two studies restricted to type 2 diabetes found positive associations.[45,50] The one study to include both type 1 and type 2 diabetes, the WHO Multinational Study of Vascular Disease in Diabetes,[49] found no association between smoking and renal failure. Prospective studies of patient series (not shown in table of cohort studies) are also inconsistent: two studies of type 1 patients found positive associations between smoking and incidence of nephropathy[52,53]. However, among three studies of type 2 patients,[52,54] only one found a positive association.[55] Overall, there is inconsistent evidence for an association between smoking and development of nephropathy, based on prospective cohort studies and patient series. If cross-sectional studies are included, the majority appear to support an increased risk of nephropathy.

All three cohort studies of progression of pre-existing nephropathy have studied individuals with type 1 diabetes: two of these found no association[42,51]

whereas the third found an association with 'development and/or progression' of nephropathy.[43] Two studies based on type 1 patient series (not shown in the table) found a positive association of smoking with progression of nephropathy,[56,57] whereas a third found no association.[58] All three studies of type 2 patient series found a positive association of smoking with progression of nephropathy.[59,60] Overall, there is no consistent evidence for an association between smoking and progression of nephropathy in those with type 1 diabetes. Given the lack of any cohort studies of type 2 diabetes, there is insufficient evidence to determine if there is an association with progression of nephropathy.

Neuropathy

Smoking was significantly associated with neuropathy incidence in three prospective studies of patients with type 1 diabetes (Table 8.4): the Sorbinil Retinopthy Trial,[23] the Epidemiology of Diabetic Complications Study[61] and the EURODIAB Prospective Complications Study.[64] Each found an increased incidence of distal symmetric polyneuropathy that persisted after multivariate adjustment [hazard ratio (HR) = 1.87, HR = 1.73, odds ratio (OR) = 1.68, respectively]. Cross-sectional data (not shown in the table) from the European IDDM Complications Study found a 2.4-fold increased prevalence of neuropathy in those with type 1 diabetes.[65] In contrast, baseline data from the DCCT failed to identify an association with mild neuropathy.[66] In the latter, those with renal impairment and severe neuropathy were excluded and only prevalence data were presented.

The only prospective study among those with type 2 diabetes, the San Luis Valley Diabetes Study,[62] identified a two-fold increased risk of neuropathy for individuals with diabetes who were followed for an average of 4.7 years. This cohort study identified a possible dose–response association, in which the incidence of distal symmetric sensory neuropathy was greater in those with more than 10 pack-years of smoking compared with those with less than 10 pack-years, and persisted after multivariate adjustment including duration of diabetes.

The only prospective study of progression of neuropathy, the Stockholm Diabetes Intervention Study, did not find an association.[42]

Retinopathy

There is consistent evidence that smoking is not associated with the incidence of retinopathy in individuals with diabetes. As shown in Table 8.5, only two out of 10 prospective studies found an association

Table 8.3 Risk of development and progression of nephropathy in diabetic smokers versus non-smokers

Study	Participants	Nephropathy[a]	
		Development	Progression
Trial participants			
Reichard et al.[42]	**Stockholm Diabetes Intervention Study**	–	Smoking not associated with progression of nephropathy
Stockholm, Sweden 1991	96 participants with type 1 diabetes and non-proliferative retinopathy, mean age = 30 years, followed 5 years		
Mühlhauser et al.[43] Germany 1995	**Trial of Intensive Insulin Therapy** 601 participants with type 1 diabetes, mean age = 27 years, followed 6 years	–	Smoking associated with 'development and/or progression' of nephropathy', OR = 1.27, $p = 0.049$ (per 10 pack-years, multivariate)
Cohort			
Microalbuminuria Collaborative Study Group[44] UK 1993	**Microalbuminuria Collaborative Study** 137 patients with type 1 diabetes and normoalbuminuria from 9 clinics, followed 4 years	Smoking associated with microalbuminuria incidence, $p < 0.05$ (ever smoking, multivariate)	–
Klein et al.[45] Wisconsin, USA 1993	**Wisconsin Epidemiology Study of Diabetic Retinopathy** 839 individuals with diabetes, onset ≥30 years, mean follow-up = 4.1 years	Smoking associated with proteinuria incidence, increased risk with increasing pack-years, OR = 3.47, 95% CI 1.95 to 6.1 (per 45 pack-years, multivariate)	–
Klein et al.[46] Wisconsin, USA 1999	**Wisconsin Epidemiology Study of Diabetic Retinopathy** 891 individuals with diabetes, onset <30 years and taking insulin, followed 10 years	Smoking not related to change in creatinine clearance or incidence of renal insufficiency	–
Microalbuminuria Collaborative Study Group[47] UK 1999	**Microalbuminuria Collaborative Study** 148 patients with type 1 diabetes and normoalbuminuria, aged 17–58 years, followed 7 years	Smoking did not predict microalbuminuria as measured by AER	–
Scott et al.[48] Boston, MA, USA 2001	**Natural History of Microalbuminuria Study** 943 individuals with type 1 diabetes and normoalbuminuria, age 15–44 years, followed 4 years	Smoking associated with increased risk of microalbuminuria, OR = 3.1, 95% CI 1.9 to 5.1 (current, multivariate)	–
Colhoun et al.[49] Multinational 2001	**WHO Multinational Study of Vascular Disease in Diabetes** 959 subjects with type 1 diabetes and 2559 with type 2 diabetes from 10 centres, mean age = 55 years, mean follow-up = 8.4 years	Smoking not associated with renal failure (past or current)	–
Rossing et al.[50] Denmark 2002	537 type 2 diabetic patients with normoalbuminuria, mean age = 41 years, follow-up = 9 years	Smoking associated with development of micro/macroalbuminuria, OR = 1.61, 95% CI 1.11 to 2.33 (≥1 cigarette per day, multivariate)	–
Giorgino et al.[51] Europe 2004	**EURODIAB Prospective Complications Study** 352 individuals with type 1 diabetes and microalbuminuria from 31 centres, mean age = 32 years, mean follow-up = 7.3 years	–	Smoking not associated with progression to macroalbuminuria as measured by AER

[a]A dash (–) indicates not reported; OR = odds ratio.

Table 8.4 Risk of development of neuropathy in diabetic smokers versus non-smokers

Study	Participants	Neuropathy[a]	
		Development	Progression
Trial participants			
Reichard et al.[42] Stockholm, Sweden 1991	**Stockholm Diabetes Intervention Study** 96 participants with type 1 diabetes and non-proliferative retinopathy, mean age = 30 years, followed 5 years	–	Smoking not associated with progression of neuropathy
Christen et al.[23] USA 1999	**Sorbinil Retinopathy Trial** 407 participants with type 1 diabetes, aged 18–56 years, median follow-up = 3.3 years	Smoking associated with definite distal symmetric polyneuropathy incidence, HR = 1.87, $p = 0.023$ (ever smoking, multivariate)	–
Cohort			
Forrest, et al.[61] Pennsylvania, USA 1997	**Epidemiology of Diabetic Complications Study** 453 individuals with type 1 diabetes from Pittsburgh IDDM Registry, mean age = 25 years. mean follow-up = 5.3 years	Smoking associated with distal symmetrical polyneuropathy incidence, HR = 1.73, $p = 0.03$ (ever smoking, multivariate)	–
Sands, et al.[62] Colorado, USA **1997**	**San Luis Valley Diabetes Study** 231 individuals with type 2 diabetes, aged 20–74 years, 71% Hispanic, mean follow-up = 4.7 years	Smoking associated with distal symmetric sensory neuropathy incidence, OR = 2.2, $p = 0.05$ (current smoking, multivariate)	–
Dyck et al.[63] Minnesota, USA 1999	**Rochester Diabetic Neuropathy Study** 264 individuals with type 1 and 2 diabetes, aged 15–89 years, followed ~7 years	Correlation observed between smoking within last year (pack-years) and composite neuropathy score ($r = 0.16$, $p = 0.017$); however smoking not associated with severity of neuropathy (multivariate)	–
Tesfaye et al.[64] Europe 2005	**EURODIAB Prospective Complications Study** 1172 individuals with type 1 diabetes from 31 centres, mean age = 31 years, mean follow-up = 7.3 years	Smoking associated with neuropathy incidence OR = 1.68, 95% CI 1.20 to 2.36 (former and current smoking, multivariate)	–

[a]A dash (–) indicates not reported; OR = odds ratio; HR = hazard ratio.

between smoking and incidence of retinopathy.[42,43,67–78] In fact, the United Kingdom Prospective Diabetes Study[68] found a significant reduction in the incidence of retinopathy among individuals with type 2 diabetes who smoked [relative risk (RR) = 0.63, $p = 0.004$, 95% confidence interval (CI) 0.48 to 0.82]. Current smoking was associated with reduced retinopathy incidence for type 1 and non-insulin-treated type 2 diabetic patients (RR = 0.79, 95% CI 0.67 to 0.94; RR = 0.75, 95% CI 0.58 to 0.95, respectively) using data routinely collected from the Nottingham Clinical Information System for Diabetes.[74]

Among seven cohort studies examining retinopathy progression, four found no association with smoking: all four included individuals with type 1 diabetes[67,71,72,76] and one also included individuals with type 2 diabetes.[72] As shown in Table 8.5, the United Kingdom Prospective Diabetes Study[68] found a significant reduction in risk among individuals

with type 2 diabetes (RR = 0.50, $p = 0.004$, 95% CI 0.36 to 0.71), while two studies of individuals with type 1 diabetes found significantly increased risk of retinopathy progression.[42,43]

In summary, the majority of prospective studies of smoking and incidence of retinopathy have found no significant evidence of a harmful effect and two large studies found a reduced incidence.[68] Similarly, the majority of prospective studies have found no association between smoking and the progression of retinopathy; two found an increased risk[42,43] and one a reduced risk.[68] This inconsistency across studies from many countries argues against an association between smoking and retinopathy incidence or progression.

Heart disease morbidity and mortality

Smoking is an established risk factor for heart disease in people without diabetes. As shown in

Table 8.5 Risk of development and progression of retinopathy in diabetic smokers versus non-smokers

Study	Participants	Retinopathy[a]	
		Development	**Progression**
Trial participants			
Reichard et al.[42] Stockholm, Sweden 1991	**Stockholm Diabetes Intervention Study** 96 participants with type 1 diabetes and non-proliferative retinopathy in RCT of intense versus regular treatment, mean age = 30 years, followed 5 years	–	Smoking associated with progression of retinopathy, OR = 3.0, $p < 0.05$ (multivariate)
Muhlhauser et al.[43] Germany 1995	**Trial of intensive insulin therapy** 613 participants with type 1 diabetes, mean age = 27 years, followed 6 years	Smoking not associated with retinopathy incidence, OR = 1.17, $p = 0.2$	Smoking associated with progression of retinopathy, OR = 1.44, $p = 0.0075$ (per 10 pack-years, multivariate)
Cohen et al.[67] USA 1999	**Sorbinil Retinopathy Trial** 485 participants with type 1 diabetes in RCT of aldose reductase inhibition, aged 18–56 years, median follow-up = 3.4 years	–	Smoking not associated with progression of retinopathy, RR = 0.8, ns (current smoking, multivariate)
Stratton et al.[68] UK 2001	**United Kingdom Prospective Diabetes Study (UKPDS)** 1919 individuals with type 2 diabetes, mean age = 52 years, followed 6 years	Smoking associated with reduced retinopathy incidence, RR = 0.63, $p = 0.0043$ (current smoking, multivariate)	Smoking associated with reduced retinopathy progression, RR = 0.50, $p = 0.0045$ (current smoking, multivariate)
Cohort			
Yanko et al.[69] Israel 1983	**Israel Ischaemic Heart Disease Project** 178 men with diabetes, aged 40–65 years, followed ~15 years	Smoking not associated with retinopathy incidence	–
Ballard et al.[70] *Rochester, MN, USA* 1986	1135 individuals with type 2 diabetes, followed 13–37 years	Smoking not associated with retinopathy incidence, $p = 0.96$ (smoking at time of diagnosis, multivariate)	–
Chase et al.[71] Colorado, USA 1991	359 patients with type 1 diabetes, mean age ≈ 20 years, mean follow-up = 2.4 years	–	Smoking not associated with retinopathy progression
Moss et al.[72] Wisconsin, USA 1996	**Wisconsin Epidemiologic Study of Diabetic Retinopathy** Incidence: 130 younger-onset and 447 older-onset Progression: 529 younger-onset and 904 older-onset Followed 10 years	Smoking not associated with retinopathy incidence (current, past, pack-years, multivariate)	Smoking not associated with retinopathy progression (current, past, pack-years, multivariate)
Tudor et al.[73] Colorado, USA 1998	**San Luis Valley Diabetes Study** 244 individuals with type 2 diabetes (65% Hispanic), median follow-up = 4.8 years	Smoking not associated with retinopathy incidence, OR = 1.23, $p = 0.63$ (ever smoking, multivariate)	–
Janghorbani et al.[74] UK 2001	1334 patients with type 1 diabetes and 2090 patients with type 2 diabetes from three outpatient clinics at University Hospital, Nottingham, mean age = 49 years, mean follow-up 4.6 years	Smoking associated with retinopathy incidence *Type 1:* Current: RR = 0.79, 95% CI 0.67 to 0.94 Ex-smoker: RR = 1.21, 95% CI = 1.03 to 1.42 *Type 2:* Current: RR = 0.75, 95% CI 0.58 to 0.95	–

(continued)

Table 8.5 *(Continued)*

Study	Participants	Retinopathy[a]	
		Development	**Progression**
Chaturvedi *et al.*[75] Europe 2001	**EURODIAB Prospective Complications Study** 764 individuals with type 1 diabetes, aged 15–60 years, followed 7.3 years	Ex-smoker: RR = 1.09, ns Smoking status was not a significant predictor among insulin-treated type 2 diabetic patients (stepwise Cox proportional hazards model) Smoking not associated with retinopathy incidence (current)	–
Porta *et al.*[76] Europe 2001	**EURODIAB Prospective Complications Study** 1249 individuals with type 1 diabetes from 31 centres (16 countries), mean age = 31 years, mean follow-up = 7.3 years	–	Smoking not associated with progression to proliferative diabetic retinopathy (current)
Keen *et al.*[77] Multinational 2001	**WHO Multinational Study of Vascular Disease in Diabetes** 2877 subjects with type 1 and type 2 diabetes from 10 centres, mean age = 55 years, mean follow-up = 8.4 years	Smoking not associated with incidence of any retinopathy or proliferative retinopathy, after adjustment for blood glucose levels	–
Janghorbani *et al.*[78] Iran 2003	549 patients with type 2 diabetes from outpatient clinics at Amin University Hospital, Iran, mean age = 45.7 years, mean follow-up = 5.1 years	Smoking not associated with incident diabetic retinopathy (stepwise Cox proportional hazards model)	–

Table 8.6, virtually all of the prospective cohort studies have also identified smoking as a risk factor for heart disease in persons with diabetes.[79–90] In these studies from multiple countries, smoking increased the risk of fatal heart disease in individuals with both type 1 and type 2 diabetes by 1.5–2-fold. In addition, data from both the Multiple Risk Factor Intervention Trial (MRFIT)[79] and the Nurses Health Study[88] identified a significant dose response. Only the Whitehall Study in England[82] failed to identify smoking as a risk factor for coronary heart disease mortality in individuals with diabetes. However, only 40 diabetic men (24%) reported never having smoked.

While the majority of the early studies in Table 8.6 report only fatal heart disease, five recent studies confirm an association with heart disease morbidity.[86–90] The WHO Multinational Study of Vascular Disease in Diabetes[87] found a significant association of smoking with fatal and non-fatal myocardial infarction (women) and stroke (men), whereas the Nurses Health Study[88] found a dose–response relationship with non-fatal myocardial infarction and total (fatal and non-fatal) coronary heart disease incidence.

Data from the National Health and Nutrition Examination Survey[85] and the Rancho Bernardo Study[81] suggest that smoking may be a stronger risk factor

for fatal heart disease among those with diabetes compared with those without diabetes (2.5-fold risk versus about 1.5-fold, age-adjusted). Suarez and Barrett-Connor[81] estimated that 65% of CVD deaths could be attributed to the interaction between diabetes and smoking. In contrast, two reports from the Nurses Health Study[84,88] found a four-fold increased heart disease incidence in non-diabetic smokers compared with a two-fold increase in diabetic smokers (age-adjusted).

All-cause mortality

As can be seen in Table 8.7, smoking is almost universally associated with an increased overall mortality among individuals with diabetes.[83,85,93–97] Only the Whitehall Study in England[82] and a community study in Maryland in the United States[92] failed to identify smoking as a risk factor for overall mortality among those with diabetes. Data from both the WHO Multinational Study of Vascular Disease in Diabetes[94] and the Nurses Health Study[95] indicated a dose–response relationship: mortality risk increased with increased number of cigarettes smoked per day. The WHO Study[94] also reported that mortality risk increased with increasing duration of smoking and decreased time since quitting.

Table 8.6 Risk of heart disease morbidity and mortality in diabetic and non-diabetic smokers versus non-smokers

Study	Participants	Heart disease morbidity and mortality[a]	
		Diabetes	**No diabetes**
Trial participants			
Stamler et al.[79] USA 1993	**Multiple Risk Factor Intervention Trial (MRFIT)** 5163 men with diabetes and 342 815 men without diabetes free of baseline myocardial infarction, aged 35–57 years, mean follow-up = 12 years	Increasing No. of cigarettes associated with increasing risk of CVD mortality, $p = 0.0024$ (multivariate)	Increasing No. of cigarettes associated with increasing risk of CVD mortality, $p = 0.0006$ (multivariate)
Alderberth et al.[80] Sweden 1998	**Multifactorial Primary Prevention Trial** 249 men with diabetes and 6851 men without diabetes, aged 51–59 years, followed 16 years	Smoking predicted CHD mortality, HR = 1.74, 95% CI 1.09 to 2.77 (current, multivariate)	Smoking predicted CHD mortality, HR = 1.95, 95% CI 1.66 to 2.28 (current, multivariate)
Cohort			
Suarez and Barrett-Connor[81] Rancho Bernardo, CA, USA 1984	**Rancho Bernardo Study** 229 individuals with type 2 diabetes and 2391 without diabetes, aged 60–79 years, followed 9 years	Smoking predicted CVD mortality Men: RR = 2.6, $p = 0.05$ Women: RR = 2.4, ns (current, age-adjusted) 65% CVD deaths attributed to interaction of diabetes and smoking	Smoking did not predict CVD mortality Men: RR = 1.1, ns Women: RR = 1.4, ns (current, age-adjusted)
Jarrett and Shipley[82] London, UK 1985	**Whitehall Study** 168 male civil servants with diabetes and 18 229 without diabetes, aged 40–64 years, followed 10 years	Smoking did not predict CHD mortality Current smoking, ns Past smoking, ns No. of cigarettes per day, ns (multivariate)	Smoking predicted CHD mortality Current smoking, $p < 0.001$ Past smoking, ns No. of cigarettes per day, $p < 0.05$ (multivariate)
Moy et al.[83] Pennsylvania, USA 1990	**IDDM Morbidity and Mortality Study** 548 patients with type 1 diabetes from Pittsburgh IDDM Registry, aged $\geq$18 years, followed 6 years	Smoking predicted CHD mortality in women, HR = 5.16, 95% CI 1.29 to 20.57, but not men, HR = 0.78, 95% CI 0.21 to 2.86 (heavy smoking, multivariate)	–
Manson et al.[84] 11 states, USA 1991	**Nurses Health Study** 1483 female nurses with type 2 diabetes and 114 694 without diabetes, aged 30–55 years, followed 8 years	Smoking predicted CHD morbidity and mortality, RR current = 2.6, RR past = 1.6, (age-adjusted)	Smoking predicted CHD morbidity and mortality, RR current = 4.6, RR past = 1.4 (age = adjusted)
Ford and DeStefano[85] USA 1991	**NHANES I Epidemiologic Follow-Up Study** 602 individuals with diabetes and 12 562 without diabetes, aged 25–74 years, followed 10 years	Smoking predicted CHD mortality, HR = 2.49, 95% CI 0.94 to 6.59 (current, multivariate)	Smoking predicted CHD mortality, HR = 1.71, 95% CI 1.19 to 2.47 (current, multivariate)
Morrish et al.[39] London, UK 1991	**London cohort of the WHO Multinational Study of Vascular Disease in Diabetics** 243 patients with type 1 diabetes and 254 patients with type 2 diabetes, mean age $\approx$ 46 years, mean follow-up = 8.3 years	Smoking associated with ECG abnormality (type 2), myocardial infarction and ischaemic heart disease (types 1 and 2), $p < 0.05$ (multivariate)	–
Fuller et al.[86] Multinational 2001	**WHO Multinational Study of Vascular Disease in Diabetes** 1260 subjects with type 1 diabetes and 3483 subjects with type 2 diabetes from 10 centres, mean age = 46 years, mean follow-up = 12 years	*MI (fatal and non-fatal):* current smoking significant for women with type 2 diabetes, RR = 1.4, 95% CI 1.1 to 2.0 (age-adjusted) *Stroke (fatal and non-fatal):* current and ex-smoking significant for men with type 2 diabetes, RR = 2.1, 95% CI 1.1 to 4.0; RR = 2.2, 95% CI 1.2 to 3.9, respectively (age-adjusted)	

(continued)

Table 8.6 *(Continued)*

Study	Participants	Heart disease morbidity and mortality[a]	
		Diabetes	**No diabetes**
Al-Delaimy *et al.*[87] USA 2002	**Nurses' Health Study** 121 700 female nurses with 6547 diagnosed with type 2 diabetes, aged 30–55 years, followed 20 years	*CVD mortality:* smoking not significant with adjustment for triglycerides in multivariate analyses *Overall:* current or ex-smoking not significant for either men or women with type 1 diabetes *Age-adjusted CHD incidence rates:* Per 10 0000 person-years Never smokers = 539 Past smokers = 623 1–14 cigarettes per day = 792 ≥15 cigarettes per day = 1114 Among 68 227 person-years, multivariate RR (95% CI): *Total CHD:* Past smokers = 1.21 (0.97 to 1.51) 1–14 cigarettes per day = 1.66 (1.10 to 2.52) ≥15 cigarettes per day = 2.68 (2.07 to 3.48) *Fatal CHD:* Past smokers = 1.24 (0.90 to 1.72) 1–14 cigarettes per day = 1.73 (0.95 to 3.15) ≥15 cigarettes per day = 2.11 (1.39 to 3.19) *Non-fatal MI:* Past smokers = 1.19 (0.88 to 1.61) 1–14 cigarettes per day = 1.56 (0.88 to 2.77) ≥15 cigarettes per day = 3.05 (2.19 to 4.26)	*Age–adjusted CHD incidence rates:* Per 10 0000 person-years Never smokers = 48 Past smokers = 68 1–14 cigarettes per day = 144 ≥15 cigarettes per day = 223
Orchard *et al.*[88] Pittsburgh, PA, USA 2003	**Pittsburgh Epidemiology of Diabetes Complications Study** 603 patients with type 1 diabetes, aged 8–47 years, followed 10 years	Ever smoking (≥100 lifetime cigarettes) predicted CAD, HR = 1.58, 95% CI 1.05 to 2.38 (multivariate)	
Soedamah-Muthu *et al.*[89] Europe 2004	**EURODIAB Prospective Complications Study** 2329 subjects with type 1 diabetes, aged 15–60 years, followed 7 years	Current smoking predicted incident CHD in men, OR = 1.62, 95% CI 1.004 to 2.62, but not in women (multivariate). Ex-smoking versus non-smoking not significant	–

[a]A dash (–) indicates not reported; OR = odds ratio; RR = relative risk; HR = hazards ratio; CHD = coronary heart disease; CVD = cardiovascular disease; ns = not significant.

For the two studies that allow a direct comparison, the risk of overall mortality associated with smoking was nearly identical among those with and without diabetes.[80,85] In the study in Sweden,[80] the relative risks were 1.95 and 1.96 for those with and without diabetes, respectively. In the study in the United States,[85] based on data from the National Health and Nutrition Examination Study, the relative risks were 1.79 and 1.60 for those with and without diabetes, respectively.

Table 8.7 Risk of all-cause mortality in diabetic and non-diabetic smokers versus non-smokers

Study	Participants	All-cause mortality[a]	
		Diabetes	**No diabetes**
Trial participants			
Alderberth et al.[80] Sweden 1998	**Multifactorial Primary Prevention Trial** 249 men with diabetes and 6851 men without diabetes, aged 51–59 years, mean follow-up = 16 years	Smoking predicted mortality, RR = 1.95; 95% CI 1.41 to 2.70 (current, multivariate)	Smoking predicted mortality, RR = 1.96; 95% CI 1.79 to 2.15 (current, multivariate)
Mühlhauser et al.[90] Germany 2000	**Trial of Intensive Insulin Therapy** 3570 participants with type 1 diabetes, mean age = 27 years, mean follow-up = 10.3 years	Smoking predicted mortality, HR = 1.92, $p = 0.0001$, (current, multivariate)	–
Cohort			
Dupree and Meyer[91] Maryland, USA 1980	371 individuals with types 1 and 2 diabetes and 742 age-, race- and sex-matched controls without diabetes from a community-wide survey, aged 20–75 years, followed 39 months	Smoking did not predict mortality, RR = 1.1, ns (ever smoking)	Smoking did not predict mortality, RR = 1.3, ns (ever smoking)
Jarrett and Shipley[82] London, UK 1985	**Whitehall Study** 168 male civil servants with diabetes and 18 229 without diabetes, aged 40–64 years, followed 10 years	Smoking did not predict mortality, ns (current/past, multivariate)	Smoking predicted all-cause mortality, $p < 0.001$ (current/past, multivariate)
Klein et al.[92] Wisconsin, USA 1989	**Wisconsin Epidemiologic Study of Diabetic Retinopathy** 2366 individuals with onset either before or after 30 years, followed 6 years	Smoking predicted mortality Younger onset: HR = 2.36, $p = 0.05$ Older onset: HR = 1.58, $p = 0.0001$ (current, multivariate)	–
Moy et al.[83] Pennsylvania, USA 1990	**IDDM Morbidity and Mortality Study** 548 patients with type 1 diabetes from Pittsburgh IDDM Registry, aged ≥18 years, followed 6 years	Smoking predicted mortality Women: HR = 2.57, 95% CI 1.04 to 6.36 Men: HR = 1.21, 95% CI 0.57 to 2.55 (heavy smoking, multivariate)	–
Ford and DeStefano[85] USA 1991	**NHANES I** 602 individuals with diabetes and 12 562 without diabetes, aged 25–74 years, followed 10 years	Smoking predicted mortality, HR = 1.79, 95% CI 1.10 to 2.91 (current, multivariate)	Smoking predicted mortality, HR = 1.60, 95% CI 1.34 to 1.90 (current, multivariate)
Chaturvedi et al.[93] Multinational 1997	**WHO Multinational Study of Vascular Disease in Diabetes** 4427 patients with type 1 and 2 diabetes from 10 centres, aged 35–55 years, followed 11 years	Smoking predicted mortality; risk increased with duration and quantity, and decreased with time since quitting RR = 1.45, $p = 0.001$ (current, age-adjusted) RR = 1.53, $p = 0.001$ (quit 1–9 years, age-adjusted) RR = 1.25, $p = 0.02$ (quit ≥10 years, age-adjusted)	–
Al-Delaimy et al.[94] 11 states, USA 2001	**Nurses' Health Study** 7401 female nurses with self-diagnosed diabetes, aged 30–55 years, followed 20 years	Among 67 420 person-years, multivariate RR(95% 95% CI): Past smokers = 1.31 (1.11, 1.55) 1–14 cig/day = 1.43 (0.96, 2.14) 15–34 cig/day = 1.64 (1.24, 2.17) ≥35 cig/day = 2.19 (1.32, 3.65)	–
Mulnier et al.[95] UK 2006	General Practice Research Database 28725 patients with type 2 diabetes, aged 35–89 years, followed 7 years	Multivariate HR (95% CI): Current smoker = 1.50 (1.41 to 1.61) Ex-smoker = 1.25 (1.15 to 1.36)	–

(continued)

Table 8.7 (Continued)

Study	Participants	All-cause mortality[a]	
		Diabetes	**No diabetes**
Intervention study Yudkin[96] USA 1993	**Multiple Risk Factor Intervention Trial (MRFIT)** 5163 men with diabetes and 342815 men without diabetes free of myocardial infarction at baseline, aged 35–57 years, followed 10 years (intervention estimates from meta-analysis of MRFIT data)	Smoking cessation would prolong life by a mean of 3 years in a 45-year-old man with diabetes	Smoking cessation would prolong life by a mean of 4 years in a 45-year-old man without diabetes

[a]A dash (–) indicates not reported; RR = relative risk; HR = hazards ratio.

Clinical trials of smoking cessation among individuals with diabetes

There is overwhelming epidemiological evidence that smoking cessation decreases the risk of coronary heart disease, cancer, stroke and lung disease.[1,2] Although no clinical trials have randomized individuals with diabetes to smoking cessation versus no intervention and then monitored for incidence or progression of complications, Yudkin[96] estimated the benefits of smoking cessation for persons with and without diabetes, using data from the Multiple Risk Factor Intervention Trial (MRFIT).[97] He estimated that smoking cessation would prolong the life of a 45-year-old man with diabetes by a mean of 3 years, compared with 4 years in a 45-year-old man without diabetes.[96] This estimate is based on a multifactorial intervention in primarily white men. Cessation benefits among those with diabetes may vary by ethnicity, gender and the presence of other complications.

Current intervention techniques generally have low success in diabetic populations[98–105] and may not be as effective for individuals with diabetes compared with those without diabetes.[98,99,102] Factors potentially inhibiting success include fear of weight gain, depression and the use of smoking to suppress stress and anxiety related to diabetes management.[98–102,106] Some of these beliefs were specifically assessed in a survey of 64 patients with type 1 diabetes (mean age 41 years).[99] Approximately 50% agreed with the statement that they were reluctant to quit smoking because they might gain weight, 46% that smoking helped them not eat sweets, 38% that when they were worried about diabetes, smoking helped calm them down, and 42% that diabetes makes them give up so many things that they like that they do not also want to give up cigarettes. These attitudes influence a diabetic smoker's desire to quit and confidence to succeed.

Data from the US National Health Interview Surveys indicate that between 1974 and 1990 the prevalence of smoking declined in individuals with diabetes (from 36 to 26%), similar to those without diabetes (from 37 to 26%).[107] Data from the 2001 Behavioral Risk Factor Surveillance System (BRFSS) indicate that smoking prevalence has continued to decline, to 23% in both those with and without diabetes.[7] While a greater proportion of smokers with diabetes compared with those without diabetes reported that they had been advised by a physician to quit or cut down smoking in 1990 (58% versus 46%), more than 40% of smokers with diabetes reported never having received advice from a physician to quit smoking.[107] In 1989, Wakefield *et al.* reported that 70% of current smokers in their survey who were diabetic had been given advice to quit smoking,[106] and in 1999, Ruggiero *et al.* reported that 85% of the diabetic smokers responding to their survey reported that they had been advised to quit:[108] an encouraging trend, but based on limited data.

Conclusion

In addition to the known benefits of smoking cessation for decreasing the risk of coronary heart disease, cancer, stroke and lung disease,[1,2] the risk of most diabetic complications may also be reduced by quitting smoking. As reviewed in this chapter and summarized in Table 8.8, there is substantial evidence from patient series, case–control and cohort studies that smoking is associated with both the development and progression of heart disease. Smoking also clearly increases the risk of overall mortality and mortality from heart disease in individuals with diabetes, with a benefit from cessation that is similar to that seen in non-diabetics. Evidence for an association between smoking and nephropathy and neuropathy

Table 8.8 Summary of evidence: benefits of not smoking or quitting smoking in type 1 or 2 diabetes

Benefit	Strength of recommendation[a]	Quality of the evidence[a]
Reduction in development of		
Nephropathy	B	II-2
Neuropathy	B	II-2
Retinopathy	D	II-2
Reduction in progression of		
Nephropathy	C	II-2
Neuropathy	C	II-2
Retinopathy	D	II-2
Reduction in morbidity or mortality from		
Heart disease	A	II-2
Reduction in mortality from		
All causes	A	I[b]

[a]A good evidence supporting quitting smoking or not smoking
B fair evidence in support of quitting smoking or not smoking
C insufficient evidence
D fair evidence in support of no association
E good evidence in support of no association
I at least one randomized controlled trial
II-1 controlled trial without randomisation
II-2 cohort or case-control studies
II-3 timed series or uncontrolled experiment
III clinical expertise or expert committee
[b]Intervention estimates from meta-analysis of MRFIT data.[96]

is inconclusive, but suggests an increased risk. However, there is consistent evidence that smoking is not associated with the development or progression of retinopathy.

There are no randomized controlled trials of smoking cessation that have examined the impact of cessation on diabetic complications, but smoking cessation studies in non-diabetic individuals have shown that smoking cessation is associated with a significant reduction in risk of CVD and death.[1,2] Because individuals with diabetes are at increased risk of CVD, the major cause of morbidity and mortality in persons with and without diabetes, even a small decrease in their risk would be clinically meaningful. Unfortunately, individuals with diabetes appear to be smoking at the same rate as non-diabetic individuals. Diabetic smokers may be good candidates for smoking cessation programmes and nicotine supplements; however; evidence for the effectiveness of these programmes for those with diabetes is inconclusive.

Acknowledgement

This work was partially supported by grant DK31801 from the National Institute of Diabetes, Digestive and Kidney Disease.

References

1 US Department of Health, Human, Services. *The Health Consequences of Smoking: a Report of the Surgeon General*, US Department of Health and Human Services, Centers for Disease Control and Prevention, National Center for Chronic Disease Prevention and Health Promotion, Office on Smoking and Health, Atlanta, GA, 2004.

2 US Department of Health, Human, Services. *The Health Benefits of Smoking Cessation: a Report of the Surgeon General*, US Department of Health and Human Services, Public Health Service, Centers for Disease Control and Prevention, National Center for Chronic Disease Prevention and Health Promotion, Office on Smoking and Health, Atlanta, GA 1990.

3 Mühlhauser I. Smoking and diabetes. *Diabet Med* 1990;**7**:10–15.

4 Mühlhauser I. Cigarette smoking and diabetes: an update. *Diabet Med* 1994;**11**:336–343.

5 Dierkx RIJ, van de Hoek W, Hoekstra JBL, Erkelens DW. Smoking and diabetes mellitus (review). *Neth J Med* 1996;**48**:150–162.

6 Haire-Joshu D, Glasgow RE, Tibbs TL. Smoking diabetes (technical review). *Diabetes Care* 1999;**22**:1887–1898.

7 Ford ES, Mokdad AH, Gregg EW. Trends in cigarette smoking among US adults with diabetes: findings from the Behavioral Risk Factor Surveillance System. *Prev Med* 2004;**39**(6):1238–1242.

8 American Diabetes Association. Smoking and diabetes (position statement). *Diabetes Care* 2004;**27**(Suppl 1): S74–S75.

9 Bott U, Jorgens V, Grusser M, Bender R, Mühlhauser I, Berger M. Predictors of glycaemic control in type 1 diabetic patients after participation in an intensified treatment and teaching programme. *Diabet Med* 1994;**11**:362–371.

10 Lundman BM, Asplund K, Norberg A. Smoking and metabolic control in patients with insulin-dependent diabetes mellitus. *J Intern Med* **227**:1990;101–106.

11 Modan M, Meytes D, Rozeman P, Yosef SB, Sehayek E, Yosef NB. Significance of high HbA1 levels in normal glucose tolerance. *Diabetes Care* 1988;**11**:422–428.

12 Cryer PE, Haymond MW, Santiago JV, Shah SD. Norepinephrine and epinephrine release and adrenergic mediation of smoking-associated hemodynamic and metabolic events. *N Engl J Med* 1976;**295**:573–577.

13 Baer L, Radichevich I. Cigarette smoking in hypertensive patients-blood pressure and endocrine responses. *Am J Med* 1985;**78**:564–568.

14 Chiodera P, Volpi R, Capretti L. Abnormal effect of cigarette smoking on pituitary hormone secretions in insulin-dependent diabetes mellitus. *Clin Endocrinol* 1997;**46**:351–357.

15 Targher G, Alberiche M, Zenere M, Bonadonna R, Muggeo M, Bonora E. Cigarette smoking and insulin resistance in patients with non-insulin-dependent diabetes mellitus. *J Clin Endocrinol Metab* 1997;**82**:3619–3624.

16 Hleve E, Yki-Jarvinen H, Koivisto VA. Smoking and insulin sensitivity in type 1 diabetic patients. *Metabolism* 1986;**35**: 874–877.

17 Ganda OMP. Pathogenesis of macrovascular disease in the human diabetic. *Diabetes* 1980;**29**:931–942.

18 Craig WY, Palomaki GE, Haddow JE. Cigarette smoking and serum lipid and lipoprotein concentrations: an analysis of published data. *BMJ* 1989;**298**:784–788.

19 The DCCT Research Group. Lipid and lipoprotein levels in patients with IDDM. *Diabetes Care* 1992;**15**:886–894.

20 Oliver MF. Cigarette smoking, polyunsaturated fats, linoleic acid and coronary heart disease. *Lancet* 1989; i:1241–1243.

21 Groppelli A, Giorgi DMA, Omboni S, Parati G, Mancia G. Persistent blood pressure increase induced by heavy smoking. *J Hypertens* 1992;**10**:495–499.

22 Morgando P, Chen H, Patel V, Herbert L, Kohner E. The acute effect of smoking on retinal blood flow in subjects with and without diabetes. *Ophthalmology* 1994;**101**: 1220–1224.

23 Christen WG, Manson JE, Bubes V, Glynn RJ. Risk factors for progression of distal symmetric polyneuropathy in type 1 diabetes mellitus. *Am J Epidemiol* 1999;**150**:1142–1151.

24 Barrett-Connor E, Khaw KT. Cigarette smoking and increased central adiposity. *Ann Intern Med* 1989;**111**:783–787.

25 Troisi RJ, Heinold JW, Vokonas PS, Weiss ST. Cigarette smoking, dietary intake and physical activity: effects on body fat distribution – the Normative Aging Study. *Am J Clin Nutr* 1991;**53**:1104–1111.

26 Randrianjohany A, Balkau B, Cubeau J, Ducimetiere P, Warnet JM, Eschwege E. The relationship between behavioral pattern, overall and central adiposity in a population of healthy French men. *Int J Obes Relat Metab Disorders* 1993;**17**:651–655.

27 National Center for Chronic Disease Prevention and Health Promotion, Centers for Disease Control and Prevention. National Health Interview Survey 2004. Cigarette smoking among adults – United States 2004. *MMWR Morb Mortal Wkly Rep* 2005;**54**(44):1121–1124.

28 West SK, Munoz B, Klein R, Broman AT, Sanchez R, Rodriguez J, Snyder R. Risk factors for Type II diabetes and diabetic retinopathy in a Mexican–American population: Proyecto VER. *Am J Ophthalmol* 2002;**134**(3):390–398.

29 Wong TY, Klein R, Islam FM, Cotch MF, Folsom AR, Klein BE, Sharrett AR, Shea S. Diabetic retinopathy in a multiethnic cohort in the United States. *Am J Ophthalmol* 2006; **141** (3):446–455.

30 Cho E, Rimm EB, Stampfer MJ, Willett WC, Hu FB. The impact of diabetes mellitus and prior myocardial infarction on mortality from all causes and from coronary heart disease in men. *J Am Coll Cardiol* 2002;**40**(5):954–960.

31 Lifford KL, Curhan GC, Hu FB, Barbieri RL, Grodstein F. Type 2 diabetes mellitus and risk of developing urinary incontinence. *J Am Geriatr Soc* 2005;**53**(11):1851–1857.

32 Harris SB, Zinman B, Hanley A, Gittelsohn J, Hegele R, Connelly PW, Shah B, Hux JE. The impact of diabetes on cardiovascular risk factors and outcomes in a native Canadian population. *Diabetes Res Clin Pract* 2002;**55**(2):165–173.

33 Beziaud F, Halimi JM, Lecomte P, Vol S, Tichet J. Cigarette smoking and diabetes mellitus. *Diabetes Metab* 2004;**30**(2): 161–166.

34 Schwab KO, Doerfer J, Hecker W, Grulich-Henn J, Wiemann D, Kordonouri O, Beyer P, Holl RW, and DPV Initiative of the German Working Group for Pediatric Diabetology. Spectrum and prevalence of atherogenic risk

factors in 27,358 children, adolescents and young adults with type 1 diabetes: cross-sectional data from the German diabetes documentation and quality management system (DPV). *Diabetes Care* 2006;**29**(2):218–225.

35 Lee ET, Keen H, Bennett PH, Fuller JH, Lu M. Follow-up of the WHO Multinational Study of Vascular Disease in Diabetes: general description and morbidity. *Diabetologia* 2001;**44**(Suppl 2):S3–13.

36 Zoppini G, Verlato G, Leuzinger C, Zamboni C, Brun E, Bonora E, Muggeo M. Body mass index and the risk of mortality in type II diabetic patients from Verona. *Int J Obes Relat Metab Disord* 2003;**27**(2):281–285.

37 Becker A, Bos G, de Vegt F, Kostense PJ, Dekker JM, Nijpels G, Heine RJ, Bouter LM, Stehouwer CD. Cardiovascular events in type 2 diabetes: comparison with nondiabetic individuals without and with prior cardiovascular disease. 10-year follow-up of the Hoorn Study. *Eur Heart J* 2003;**24** (15):1406–1413.

38 Ford ES, Malarcher AM, Herman WH, Aubert RE. Diabetes mellitus and cigarette smoking: findings from the 1989 National Health Interview Survey. *Diabetes Care* 1994;**17**:688–692.

39 Morrish NJ, Stevens LK, Fuller JH, Jarrett RJ, Keen H. Risk factors for macrovascular disease in diabetes mellitus: the London follow-up to the WHO Multinational Study of Vascular Disease in Diabetics. *Diabetologia* 1991;**34**: 590–594.

40 Wingard DL, Barrett-Connor E, Wedick N, What is the evidence that changing tobacco use reduces the incidence of diabetic complications? In: *The Evidence Base for Diabetes Care* (eds R Willliams, W Herman, AL Kinmonth, NJ Wareham), John Wiley & Sons, Ltd., Chichester, 2002, Chapter 19, pp. 449–474.

41 Ford ES, Newman J. Smoking and diabetes mellitus: findings from 1988 Behavioral Risk Factor Surveillance System. *Diabetes Care* 1991;**14**:871–874.

42 Reichard P, Berglund B, Britz A, Nilsson BY, Rosenqvist U. Intensified conventional insulin treatment retards the microvascular complications of insulin-dependent diabetes mellitus (IDDM): the Stockholm Diabetes Intervention Study (SDIS) after five years. *J Intern Med* 1991;**230**:101–108.

43 Mühlhauser I, Bender R, Bott U, Jorgens V, Grusser M, Wagener W, Overmann H, Berger M. Cigarette smoking and progression of retinopathy and nephropathy in type 1 diabetes. *Diabet Med* 1995;**13**:536–543.

44 Jyo U, Microalbuminuria Collaborative Study Group. United Kingdom. Risk factors for development of microalbuminuria in insulin dependent diabetic patients: a cohort study. *BMJ* 1993;**306**:1235–1239.

45 Klein R, Klein BE, Moss SE. Incidence of gross proteinuria in older-onset diabetes: a population-based perspective. *Diabetes* 1993;**42**:381–389.

46 Klein R, Klein BEK, Moss SE, Cruickshanks KJ, Brazy PC. The 10-year incidence of renal insufficiency in people with type 1 diabetes. *Diabetes Care* 1999;**22**:743–751.

47 The Microalbuminuria Collaborative Study Group. Predictors of the development of microalbuminuria in patients with type 1 diabetes mellitus: a seven-year prospective study. *Diabet Med.* 1999;**16**(11):918–925.

48 Scott LJ, Warram JH, Hanna LS, Laffel LM, Ryan L, Krolewski AS. A nonlinear effect of hyperglycemia and current cigarette smoking are major determinants of the onset of microalbuminuria in type 1 diabetes. *Diabetes* 2001; **50**(12):2842–2849.

49 Colhoun HM, Lee ET, Bennett PH, Lu M, Keen H, Wang SL, Stevens LK, Fuller JH. Risk factors for renal failure: the WHO Mulinational Study of Vascular Disease in Diabetes. *Diabetologia* 2001;**44**(Suppl 2):S46–S53.

50 Rossing P, Hougaard P, Parving HH. Risk factors for development of incipient and overt diabetic nephropathy in type 1 diabetic patients: a 10-year prospective observational study. *Diabetes Care* 2002;**25**(5):859–864.

51 Giorgino F, Laviola L, Cavallo Perin P, Solnica B, Fuller J, Chaturvedi N. Factors associated with progression to macroalbuminuria in microalbuminuric type 1 diabetic patients: the EURODIAB Prospective Complications Study. *Diabetologia* 2004;**47**(6):1020–1028.

52 Orth SR, Schroeder T, Ritz E, Ferrari P. Effects of smoking on renal function in patients with type 1 and type 2 diabetes mellitus. *Nephrol Dial Transplant* 2005;**20**(11):2414–2419.

53 Couper JJ, Staples AJ, Cocciolone R, Nairn J, Badcock N, Henning P. Relationship of smoking and albuminuria in children with insulin-dependent diabetes. *Diabet Med* 1994;**11**:666–669.

54 Gall MA, Hougaard P, Johnsen KB, Parving HH. Risk factors for development of incipient and overt diabetic nephropathy in patients with non-insulin dependent diabetes mellitus: prospective, observational study. *BMJ* 1997;**314**:783–799.

55 Forsblom CM, Groop PH, Ekstrand A, Totterman KJ, Sane T, Saloranta C, Groop L. Predictors of progression from normoalbuminuria to microalbuminuria in NIDDM. *Diabetes Care* 1998;**21**:1932–1938.

56 Sawicki PT, Didjurgeit U, Mühlhauser I, Bender R, Heinemann L, Berger M. Smoking is associated with progression of diabetic nephropathy. *Diabetes Care* 1994;**17**:126–131.

57 Chase HP, Garg SK, Marshall G, Berg CL, Harris S, Jackson WE, Hamman RE. Cigarette smoking increases the risk of albuminuria among subjects with type 1 diabetes. *JAMA* 1991;**265**:614–617.

58 Hovind P, Rossing P, Tarnow L, Parving HH. Smoking and progression of diabetic nephropathy in type 1 diabetes. *Diabetes Care* 2003;**26**(3):911–916.

59 Rossing K, Christensen PK, Hovind P, Tarnow L, Rossing P, Parving HH. Progression of nephropathy in type 2 diabetic patients. *Kidney Int* 2004;**66**(4):1596–1605.

60 Baggio B, Budakovic A, Dalla Vestra M, Saller A, Bruseghin M, Fioretto P. Effects of cigarette smoking on glomerular structure and function in type 2 diabetic patients. *J Am Soc Nephrol* 2002;**13**(11):2730–2736.

61 Forrest KY-Z, Maser RE, Pambianco G, Becker DJ, Orchard TJ. Hypertension as a risk factor for diabetic neuropathy. A prospective study. *Diabetes* 1997;**46**:665–670.

62 Sands ML, Shetterly SM, Franklin GM, Hamman RF. Incidence of distal symmetric (sensory) neuropathy in NIDDM. *Diabetes Care* 1997;**20**:322–329.

63 Dyck PJ, Davies JL, Wilson DM, Service FJ, Melton LJ III, O'Brien PC. Risk factors for severity of diabetic polyneuropathy: intensive longitudinal assessment of the Rochester Diabetic Neuropathy Study cohort. *Diabetes Care* 1999;**22**: 1479–1486.

64 Tesfaye S, Chaturvedi N, Eaton SE, Ward JD, Manes C, Ionescu-Tirgoviste C, Witte DR, Fuller JH, and the EURODIAB Prospective Complications Study Group. Vascular risk factors and diabetic neuropathy. *N Engl J Med* 2005;**352**:341–350.

65 Tesfaye S, Stephenson JM, Fuller JH, Plater M, Ionescu-Tirgoviste C, Nuber A, Pozza G, Ward JD, and the EURODIAB IDDM Study Group. Prevalence of diabetic peripheral neuropathy and its relation to glycaemic control and potential risk factors: the EURODIAB IDDM Complications Study. *Diabetologia* 1996;**39**:1377–1384.

66 The DCCT Research Group. Factors in development of diabetic neuropathy. Baseline analysis of neuropathy in feasibility phase of Diabetes Control and Complications Trial (DCCT). *Diabetes* 1988;**37**:476–481.

67 Cohen RA, Hennekens CH, Christen WG, Krolewski A, Nathan DM, Peterson MJ, LaMotte F, Manson JE. Determinants of retinopathy progression in type 1 diabetes mellitus. *Am J Med* 1999;**107**:45–51.

68 Stratton IM, Kohner EM, Aldington SJ, Turner RC, Holman RR, Manley SE, Matthews DR. UKPDS 50: risk factors for incidence and progression of retinopathy in Type II diabetes over 6 years from diagnosis. *Diabetologia* 2001;**44**: 156–163.

69 Yanko B, Goldbourt U, Michaelson IC, Shapiro A, Yaari S. Prevalence and 15-year incidence of retinopathy *and associated characteristics in middle-aged and elderly diabetic men.* *Br J Ophthalmol* 1983;**67**:759–765.

70 Ballard DJ, Melton LJ, Dwyer MS, Trautmann JC, Chue CP, O'Fallon WM, Palumbo PJ. Risk factors for diabetic retinopathy: a population-based study in Rochester. Minnesota. *Diabetes Care* 1986;**9**:334–342.

71 Chase HP, Garg SK, Marshall G, Berg CL, Harris S, Jackson WE, Hamman RE. Cigarette smoking increases the risk of albuminuria among subjects with type 1 diabetes. *JAMA* 1991;**265**:614–617.

72 Moss SE, Klein R, Klein BE. Cigarette smoking and ten-year progression of diabetic retinopathy. *Ophthalmology* 1996;**103**:1438–1442.

73 Tudor SM, Hamman RF, Baron A, Johnson DW, Shetterly SM. Incidence and progression of diabetic retinopathy in Hispanics and non-Hispanic whites with type 2 diabetes. San Luis Valley Diabetes Study, Colorado. *Diabetes Care* 1998;**21**:53–61.

74 Janghorbani M, Jones RB, Murray KJ, Allison SP. Incidence of and risk factors for diabetic retinopathy in diabetic clinic attenders. *Ophthalmic Epidemiol* 2001;**8** (5):309–325.

75 Chaturvedi N, Sjoelie A-K, Porta M, Aldington SJ, Fuller JH, Songini M, Kohner EM. Markers of insulin resistance are strong risk factors for retinopathy incidence in type 1 diabetes. The EURODIAB Prospective Complications Study. *Diabetes Care* 2001;**24**:284–289.

76 Porta M, Sjoelie AK, Chaturvedi N, Stevens L, Rottiers R, Veglio M, Fuller JH, and the EURODIAB Prospective Complications Study Group. Risk factors for progression to proliferative diabetic retinopathy in the EURODIAB

Prospective Complications Study. *Diabetologia* 2001; **44**(12): 2203–2209.

77 Keen H, Lee ET, Russell D, Miki E, Bennett PH, Lu M. The appearance of retinopathy and progression to proliferative retinopathy: the WHO Multinational Study of Vascular Disease in Diabetes. *Diabetologia* 2001;**44**(Suppl 2): S22–S30.

78 Janghorbani M, Amini M, Ghanbari H, Safaiee H. Incidence of and risk factors for diabetic retinopathy in Isfahan. Iran. *Ophthalmic Epidemiol* 2003;**10**(2):81–95.

79 Stamler J, Vaccaro O, Neaton JD, Wentworth D, and The Multiple Risk Factor Intervention Trial Research Group. Diabetes, other risk factors and 12-year cardiovascular mortality for men screened in the Multiple Risk Factor Intervention Trial. *Diabetes Care* 1993;**16**:434–444.

80 Alderberth AM, Rosengren A, Wilhelmsen L. Diabetes and long-term risk of mortality from coronary and other causes in middle-aged Swedish men. A general population study. *Diabetes Care* 1998;**21**:539–545.

81 Suarez L, Barrett-Connor E. Interaction between cigarette smoking and diabetes mellitus in the prediction of death attributed to cardiovascular disease. *Am J Epidemiol* 1984;**120**:670–675.

82 Jarrett RJ, Shipley MJ. Mortality and associated risk factors in diabetics. *Acta Endocrinol* 1985;**110**(Suppl. 272): 21–26.

83 Moy CS, LaPorte RE, Dorman JS, Songer TJ, Orchard TJ, Kuller LH, Becker DJ, Drash AL. Insulin-dependent diabetes mellitus mortality. *Circulation* 1990;**82**:37–43.

84 Manson JE, Colditz GA, Stampfer MJ, Willett WC, Krolewski AS, Rosner B, Arky RA, Speizer FE, Hennekens CH. A prospective study of maturity-onset diabetes mellitus and risk of coronary heart disease and stroke in women. *Arch Intern Med* 1991;**151**:1141–1147.

85 Ford ES, DeStefano F. Risk factors for mortality from all causes and from coronary heart disease among persons with diabetes. Findings from the National Health and Nutrition Examination Survey I Epidemiologic Follow-Up Study. *Am J Epidemiol* 1991;**133**:1220–1230.

86 Fuller JH, Stevens LK, Wang SL. Risk factors for cardiovascular mortality and morbidity: the WHO Mutinational Study of Vascular Disease in Diabetes. *Diabetologia* 2001;**44** (Suppl 2): S54–S64.

87 Al-Delaimy WK, Manson JE, Solomon CG, Kawachi I, Stampfer MJ, Willett WC, Hu FB. Smoking and risk of coronary heart disease among women with type 2 diabetes mellitus. *Arch Intern Med* 2002;**162**(3):273–279.

88 Orchard TJ, Olson JC, Erbey JR, Williams K, Forrest KY, Smithline Kinder L, Ellis D, Becker DJ. Insulin resistance-related factors, but not glycemia, predict coronary artery disease in type 1 diabetes: 10-year follow-up data from the Pittsburgh Epidemiology of Diabetes Complications Study. *Diabetes Care* 2003;**26**(5):1374–1379.

89 Soedamah-Muthu SS, Chaturvedi N, Toeller M, Ferriss B, Reboldi P, Michel G, Manes C, Fuller JH, and the EURODIAB Prospective Complications Study Group. Risk factors for coronary heart disease in type 1 diabetic patients in Europe: the EURODIAB Prospective Complications Study. *Diabetes Care* 2004;**27**(2):530–537.

90 Mühlhauser I, Overmann H, Bender R, Jorgens V, Berger M. Predictors of mortality and end-stage diabetic complications in patients with type 1 diabetes mellitus on intensified insulin therapy. *Diabet Med* 2000;**17**:727–734.

91 Dupree EA, Meyer MB. Role of risk factors in complications of diabetes mellitus. *Am J Epidemiol* 1980;**112**:100–112.

92 Klein R, Moss SE, Klein BEK, DeMets DL. Relation of ocular and systemic factors to survival in diabetes. *Arch Intern Med* 1989;**149**:266–272.

93 Chaturvedi N, Stevens L, Fuller JH, and The World Health Organization Multinational Study Group. Which features of smoking determine mortality risk in former cigarette smokers with diabetes? *Diabetes Care* 1997;**20**:1266–1272.

94 Al-Delaimy WK, Willett WC, Manson JE, Speizer FE, Hu FB. Smoking and mortality among women with type 2 diabetes: The Nurses' Health Study cohort. *Diabetes Care* 2001;**24**(12): 2043–2048.

95 Mulnier HE, Seaman HE, Raleigh VS, Soedamah-Muthu SS, Colhoun HM, Lawrenson RA. Mortality in people with type 2 diabetes in the UK. *Diabet Med* 2006;**23**(5):516–521.

96 Yudkin JS. How can we best prolong life? Benefits of coronary risk factor reduction in non-diabetic and diabetic subjects. *BMJ* 1993;**306**:1313–1318.

97 Ockene JK, Kuller LH, Svendsen KH, Meilahn E. The relationship of smoking cessation to coronary heart disease and lung cancer in the Multiple Risk Factor Intervention Trial. *J Public Health* 1990;**80**:954–958.

98 Microalbuminuria Collaborative Study Group. United Kingdom. Risk factors for development of microalbuminuria in insulin dependent diabetic patients: a cohort study. *BMJ* 1993;**306**:1235–1239.

99 Haire-Joshu D, Heady S, Thomas L, Schechtman K, Fisher EB. Beliefs about smoking and diabetes care. *Diabetes Educator* 1994;**20**:4510–415.

100 Kirkman MS, Weinberger M, Landsman PB, Samsa GP, Shortliffe EA, Simel DL, Feussner JR. A telephone-delivered intervention for patients with NIDDM. Effect on coronary risk factors. *Diabetes Care* 1994;**17**:840–846.

101 Sawicki PT, Didjurgeit U, Mühlhauser I, Berger M. Behavioral therapy versus doctor's anti-smoking advice in diabetic patients. *J Intern Med* 1993;**234**:407–409.

102 Fowler PM, Hoskins PL, McGill M, Dutton SP, Yue DK, Turtle JR. Anti-smoking programme for diabetic patients: the agony and the ecstasy. *Diabet Med* 1989;**6**:698–702.

103 Canga N, de Irala J, Vara E, Duaso MJ, Ferrer A, Martinez-Gonzalez MA. Intervention study for smoking cessation in diabetic patients: a randomized controlled trial in both clinical and primary settings. *Diabetes Care* 2000;**23**: 1455–1460.

104 Hokanson JM, Anderson RL, Hennrikus DJ, Lando HA, Kendall DM. Integrated tobacco cessation counseling in a diabetes self-management training program: a randomized trial of diabetes and reduction of tobacco. *Diabetes Educator* 2006;**32**(4):562–570.

105 Persson LG, Hjalmarson A. Smoking cessation in patients with diabetes mellitus: results from a controlled study of an intervention programme in primary healthcare in Sweden. *Scand J Prim Health Care* 2006;**24**(2):75–80.

106 Wakefield M, Roberts L, Rosenfeld E. Prospects for smoking cessation among people with insulin-dependent diabetes. *Patient Educ Couns* 1989;(3):257–266.

107 Malarcher AM, Ford ES, Nelson DE, Chrismon JH, Mowery P, Merritt RK, Herman WH. Trends in cigarette smoking and physicians' advice to quit smoking among people with diabetes in the U.S. *Diabetes Care* 1995;**18**:694–697.

108 Ruggiero L, Rossi JS, Prochaska JO, Glasgow RE, de Groot M, Dryfoos JM, Reed GR, Orleans CT, Prokhorov AV, Kelly K. Smoking and diabetes: readiness for change and provider advice. *Addictive Behav* 1999;**24**(4):573–578.

9

Does intensive glycaemic management reduce morbidity and mortality in type 1 diabetes?

William H. Herman

Department of Internal Medicine and Epidemiology, University of Michigan, Ann Arbor, MI, USA

Introduction

The 'glucose hypothesis' attributes the complications of diabetes to chronic hyperglycaemia. It postulates that hyperglycaemia causes complications and that correction of hyperglycaemia prevents them. In humans, numerous retrospective studies have demonstrated associations between the degree and duration of hyperglycaemia and the severity of microvascular and neuropathic complications. The strong associations between hyperglycaemia and diabetic complications set the stage for randomized prospective clinical trials, the most rigorous and least biased means to test the glucose hypothesis.

It was not until the late 1970s and early 1980s that the technologies necessary to conduct prospective clinical trials to test the glucose hypothesis were in place. The technologies necessary for the conduct of such trials included (1) valid and reproducible methods to assess objectively long-term glycaemic control, specifically haemoglobin A_{1c} (HbA$_{1c}$), (2) the means to achieve near normoglycaemia in type 1 diabetes, including self-monitoring of blood glucose and protocols for multiple daily injections and continuous subcutaneous insulin infusion, and (3) valid and reproducible methods to assess microvascular and neuropathic outcomes, including stereo fundus photography, microalbuminuria testing and standardized neurological examinations. With the availability of these technologies, it was finally possible to test the glucose hypothesis rigorously.

The benefits of intensive glycaemic management on microvascular and neuropathic complications

Early randomized prospective clinical trials designed to study the relationship between glycaemic control and microvascular and neuropathic complications demonstrated that intensive and conventional treatment protocols achieved different levels of glycaemic control and that methods to measure the development and progression of complications were practical. However, these trials involved too few participants and were too brief to determine whether the different treatments changed the rates of progression of complications. A meta-analysis of these small, short-term trials estimated the impact of intensive therapy on the progression of microvascular complications in type 1 diabetes.[1] A total of 16 reports (from 12 cohorts) were selected for the meta-analysis. Reports selected for the meta-analysis were published in English between January 1966 and December 1991 and were randomized, included only patients with insulin-dependent diabetes and presented analysable data.[2–17] The duration of follow-up ranged from 8 to 60 months. Conventional therapy was accomplished by one or two injections of insulin daily and intensive therapy was achieved, for the most part, by continuous subcutaneous insulin infusion or by multiple daily injections. In the summary estimate, glycosylated haemoglobin was significantly lower, by 1.4%, in the intensive therapy groups compared with the conventionally treated groups. With intensive therapy, the risk of retinopathy

The Evidence Base for Diabetes Care, Second Edition, Edited by William H. Herman, Ann Louise Kinmonth, Nicholas J. Wareham and Rhys Williams.
© 2010 John Wiley & Sons, Ltd

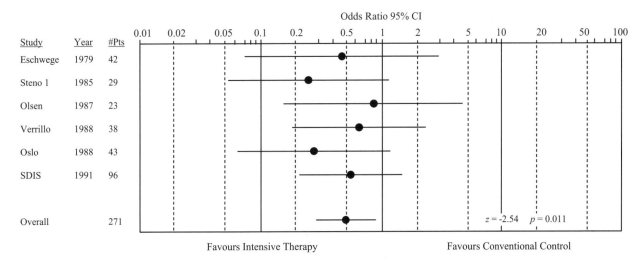

Figure 9.1 Meta-analysis of the effects of intensive glycaemic control on the progression of diabetic retinopathy. Reproduced from Ref. 1 by permission of Elsevier

progressing was slightly and non-significantly higher after 6–12 months, but significantly lower after more than 2 years [odds ratio (OR) 0.49, 95% confidence interval (CI) 0.28 to 0.85] (Figure 9.1). The risk of nephropathy progression was also significantly decreased (OR 0.34, 95% CI 0.20 to 0.58) (Figure 9.2).

Two long-term, prospective, explanatory clinical trials confirmed and extended these results. The Stockholm Diabetes Intervention Study (SDIS) compared the effects of intensified and standard treatment over 7.5 years in 102 type 1 diabetic patients (mean age 31 years, mean duration of diabetes 17 years at baseline) with non-proliferative retinopathy, normal serum creatinine concentrations and 'unsatisfactory' blood glucose control.[18] Subjects were referred to the study by their personal

physicians and 91% of patients who were asked to participate accepted. Intensified treatment consisted of individual education, three or more insulin injections per day, self-monitoring of blood glucose and increased provider contacts. Standard treatment consisted of two or three insulin injections per day and routine diabetes care with physician visits every 4 months. Self-monitoring of blood glucose was advised but test results were discussed only at routine visits. At entry, glycosylated haemoglobin was $9.5 \pm 1.3\%$ in the intensified treatment group and $9.4 \pm 1.4\%$ in the standard treatment group (normal range, 3.9–5.7%). The mean value for the whole study was $7.1 \pm 0.7\%$ in the intensified treatment group and $8.5 \pm 0.7\%$ in the standard treatment group ($p = 0.001$).

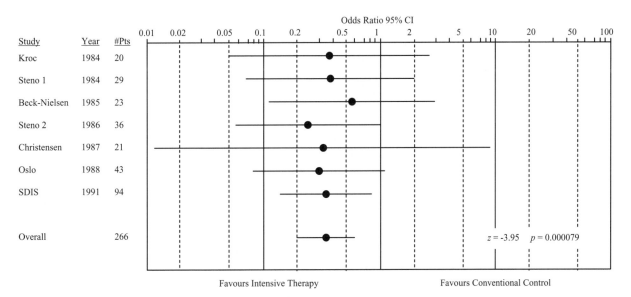

Figure 9.2 Meta-analysis of the effects of intensive glycaemic control on the progression of diabetic nephropathy. Reproduced from Ref. 1 by permission of Elsevier

Proliferative retinopathy or clinically important macular oedema requiring immediate photocoagulation developed in 27% of patients receiving intensified treatment and 52% of those receiving standard treatment ($p = 0.01$). Urinary albumin excretion >200 μg min^{-1} developed in 2% of the intensified treatment group and 18% of the standard treatment group ($p = 0.01$). None of the patients in the intensified treatment group developed a glomerular filtration rate below the normal range but 12% of those in the standard treatment group did ($p = 0.02$). During the follow-up, deterioration in nerve conduction velocities was less in the intensive than in the standard treatment group (p 0.02). This study confirmed that in type 1 diabetes, intensive therapy significantly delays progression to proliferative retinopathy or clinically important macular oedema requiring photocoagulation and to diabetic nephropathy. It also demonstrated that intensive therapy could significantly delay deterioration in nerve conduction velocities.

The Diabetes Control and Complications Trial (DCCT) confirmed and extended these findings.[19] The DCCT was a large, multi-centre, randomized controlled clinical trial that compared the impact of intensive and conventional therapy on the early microvascular and neuropathic complications of type 1 diabetes. It was designed to answer two separate but related questions: (1) could intensive therapy prevent the development of diabetic retinopathy in patients with no retinopathy (primary prevention)?; and (2) could intensive therapy slow the progression of early retinopathy (secondary intervention)? Subjects were recruited from 29 academic medical centres in the United States and Canada from 1983 through 1989. A total of 1441 patients 13–39 years of age with type 1 diabetes (726 with no retinopathy at baseline and 715 with mild retinopathy) were randomly assigned to intensive therapy administered either with external insulin pump or by three or more daily insulin injections and guided by frequent blood glucose monitoring, or to conventional therapy with one or two daily insulin injections. Subjects were followed for up to 9 years. At baseline, mean HbA$_{1c}$ was ~8.9% (normal <6.05%) and did not differ between treatment groups. HbA$_{1c}$ reached a nadir at 6 months in the patients receiving intensive therapy. Patients assigned to the intensive treatment group achieved and maintained HbA$_{1c}$ values of 7.2%. Patients randomly assigned to the conventional treatment group maintained HbA$_{1c}$ values of 9.1%.

In the primary prevention cohort, the cumulative incidence of retinopathy was similar in the two treatment groups until ~3 years, when the cumulative incidence curves began to separate. From 5 years onwards, the cumulative incidence of retinopathy was ~50% less in the intensive therapy group than in the conventional therapy group. Intensive therapy reduced the adjusted mean risk of retinopathy by 76% (95% CI 62 to 85%) and the reduction in risk became more pronounced with time. In the secondary intervention cohort, patients receiving intensive therapy had a higher cumulative incidence of retinopathy during the first year compared with those in the conventional therapy group, but a lower cumulative incidence beginning at 3 years and continuing for the rest of the study. Intensive therapy reduced the average risk of progression by 54% (95% CI 39 to 66%).

In the DCCT primary prevention cohort, intensive therapy also reduced the mean adjusted risk of microalbuminuria by 34% ($p = 0.04$). In the secondary intervention cohort, intensive therapy reduced the risk of microalbuminuria by 43% ($p = 0.001$) and the risk of albuminuria by 56% ($p = 0.01$). A *post hoc* sub-group analysis of 73 type 1 diabetic patients with microalbuminuria in the DCCT failed to find an impact of intensive therapy on progression from microalbuminuria to clinical albuminuria in patients with type 1 diabetes.[20]

These results were similar to those obtained by the Microalbuminuria Collaborative Study Group.[21] The Microalbuminuria Collaborative Study Group studied 70 type 1 diabetic patients with microalbuminuria but without arterial hypertension randomized to intensive ($n = 36$) and conventional ($n = 34$) therapy for a median of 5 years (range 2–8 years). A significant glycaemic separation between the two groups was maintained for only 3 years. Progression to clinical albuminuria occurred in six patients in each group. Intensive therapy with improved glycaemic control for 3 years had no impact on progression from microalbuminuria to albuminuria. Although both of these studies were limited by their sample size, the Microalbuminuria Collaborative Study Group concluded that the DCCT and their study together had sufficient power to detect a reduction in the risk of progression to clinical albuminuria of 33% or greater. A smaller treatment effect could not be excluded.[21]

In patients in the DCCT primary intervention cohort, intensive therapy reduced the appearance of neuropathy at 5 years by 69% ($p = 0.006$) and in the secondary intervention cohort by 57% ($p < 0.001$).

Table 9.1 summarizes the odds of development and progression of microvascular and neuropathic complications of type 1 diabetes with intensive therapy compared with conventional therapy. The results of the meta-analysis and two large, randomized prospective clinical trials conclusively demonstrate that intensive therapy slows the development and progression of retinopathy and nephropathy and the development of neuropathy in type 1 diabetes.

Table 9.1 The benefits and risks of intensive glycaemic management: risk (odds ratio) of development and progression of microvascular and neuropathic complications and hypoglycaemia with intensive versus conventional therapy[a]

Study, year, reference	Participants	Retinopathy		Nephropathy		Neuropathy	Hypoglycaemia
		Development	Progression	Development	Progression	Development	
Meta-analysis 1993[1]	12 small short-term RCTs in patients with type 1 diabetes followed for 8–60 months	–	Risk of progression halved (OR 0.5)	–	70% reduction in risk of progression (OR 0.3)	–	ns
SDIS 1993[18]	102 patients with type 1 diabetes followed for 7.5 years	–	60% reduction in risk of progression (OR 0.4)	–	90% reduction in risk of progression (OR 0.1)	–	2.8-fold increase in risk of developing severe hypoglycaemia (OR 2.8)
DCCT 1993[19]	1441 patients with type 1 diabetes followed for 6.5 years	80% reduction in risk of developing retinopathy (OR 0.2)	Risk of progression halved (OR 0.5)	30% reduction in risk of developing nephropathy (OR 0.7)	60% reduction in risk of progression (OR 0.4)	60% reduction in risk of developing neuropathy (OR 0.4)	3.3-fold increase in risk of developing severe hypoglycaemia (OR 3.3)
Meta-analysis 1997[33]	14 RCTs in patients with type 1 diabetes followed for 6–90 months	–	–	–	–	–	3.0-fold increase in risk of developing severe hypoglycaemia (OR 3.0)

[a]–, Not studied; ns, not significant.

The benefits of intensive glycaemic management: cardiovascular disease and survival

The impact of intensive therapy on cardiovascular outcomes and survival in type 1 diabetes is an important clinical question. None of the clinical trials cited was designed to assess the impact of therapy on macrovascular disease and the youth of the patients and the relative shortness of follow-up made the detection of treatment-related differences in macrovascular events unlikely. A cross-sectional analysis of the SDIS demonstrated an association between HbA_{1c}, stiffness of the carotid wall and endothelial dysfunction in type 1 diabetic individuals.[22] The effect of long-term intensive therapy on early atherosclerosis was further examined using ultrasound to assess endothelial function, carotid intima-medial thickness and arterial stiffness.[22] Fifty-nine of the 102 participants in the Stockholm Diabetes Intervention Study were studied about 12 years after randomization to intensive or conventional therapy. Endothelial function was better and arteries were less stiff in the intensive therapy group, suggesting that intensive therapy slows atherosclerosis.

At baseline, the DCCT excluded patients with hypertension, hypercholesterolaemia or clinical evidence of cardiovascular disease. When all major cardiovascular and peripheral vascular events were combined in the DCCT, intensive therapy reduced the risk of macrovascular disease by 41% (from 0.8 to 0.5 events per 100 patient-years), but the difference was not statistically significant.[19] Despite the increased incidence of overweight associated with intensive therapy, intensive therapy was associated with a small but insignificant reduction in the development of hypertension. In addition, intensive therapy was associated with small but significant reductions in the development of hypercholesterolaemia and hypertriglyceridaemia.[19] Additional follow-up of the DCCT cohort demonstrated that intensive as compared with conventional therapy reduced the progression of atherosclerosis as measured by carotid intima-media thickness[23] and reduced the prevalence of coronary artery calcification.[24]

Lawson *et al.* critically reviewed randomized controlled trials of intensive insulin therapy (IIT) in type 1 diabetes and used meta-analytical techniques to estimate the impact of IIT on the risk of developing cerebrovascular, cardiovascular and peripheral vascular complications.[25] They conducted a comprehensive literature search of articles published between January 1966 and January 1996 and selected articles if they were randomized controlled clinical trials, involved participants with type 1 diabetes and were of 2 years' duration. Early reports of studies were excluded if later reports were available. IIT was defined as a method of intensifying diabetes management with the goal of improving metabolic control over that achieved by conventional therapy (CT). IIT could be achieved through multiple daily injections or continuous subcutaneous insulin infusion pump, whereas CT was defined as one or two insulin injections per day. To be included, studies had to show a statistically significant difference in glycosylated haemoglobin between the IIT and CT groups. Studies were initially included regardless of whether data were provided on macrovascular complications and authors were contacted to confirm outcomes and/or obtain unpublished data. The primary outcome measure was the number of major cardiovascular events. These included cerebrovascular disease (cerebrovascular accident), cardiovascular disease (angina, myocardial infarction, angioplasty, coronary artery bypass), peripheral vascular disease (intermittent claudication, peripheral artery bypass) and macrovascular death (fatal cerebrovascular accident, fatal myocardial infarction, sudden death). If a patient had different types of events, they were counted separately, even if they were within the same class. In addition to abstracting data regarding the number of events, the authors contacted the study authors to obtain data on the number of individuals having one or more macrovascular events. The authors analysed separately the number of individuals having one or more macrovascular event and rates of macrovascular mortality.

The initial search identified 30 studies. Six studies met all inclusion criteria and the authors were able to obtain confirmation of macrovascular outcomes. These studies are described in Table 9.2. Subject age at entry was relatively young. Duration of diabetes ranged from 2 to 9 years. Two studies included both primary prevention and secondary intervention patients. The remaining four studies included patients with evidence of early microvascular complications. In each of the studies, the IIT and CT groups had similar baseline characteristics. All studies achieved a statistically significant difference in glycosylated haemoglobin levels.

IIT significantly reduced the total number of first major macrovascular events of each type: cerebrovascular, cardiovascular and peripheral vascular (OR 0.55, 95% CI 0.35 to 0.88, $p = 0.015$) (Figure 9.3). In three of the studies, participants had more than one event. When events within the same class (e.g. angina and myocardial infarction) were counted only once, the result became non-significant. Although there was a trend towards a decrease in the number of participants having one or more macrovascular

Table 9.2 Effect of intensive insulin treatment on number of macrovascular events: study characteristics

Study	Study duration (years)[b]	Number of patients	Age at entry (years)[b]	Type 1 diabetes duration (years)[b]	Mean study GHb percentage above normal	
					IIT (mean ± SD)	CT (mean ± SD)
Holman et al., UK, 1983	2	74	42 ± 12	18.6 ± 6.1	123 (10.5 ± 1.4)	134 (11.4 ± 1.5)
Steno 1, Denmark, 1991	8	34	34 ± 7	19.0 ± 3.0	121 (7.6 ± 0.9)	129 (8.1 ± 1.1)
Steno 2, Denmark, 1991	5	36	18–50	5 - 26	125 (7.9 ± 1.1)	140 (8.8 ± 1.0)
Oslo, Norway, 1992	7	45	26 ± 5	12.8 ± 3.6	121 (9.2 ± 1.3)	137 (10.4 ± 1.5)
DCCT, North America, 1993	6.5 (3–9)	Primary: 726	27 ± 8	2.6 ± 1.4	119 (7.2 ± 1.4)	150 (9.1 ± 1.4)
		Secondary: 715	27 ± 7	8.8 ± 3.8		
SDIS, Sweden, 1994	7.5	102	31 ± 8	17.0 ± 5.0	125 (7.1 ± 0.7)	149 (8.5 ± 0.7)

[a]Source: adapted from Ref. 25.
[b]Data for age at entry and diabetes duration are means ± SD or ranges. Study duration includes intervention and follow-up.

event with IIT, the difference between IIT and CT was not statistically significant (OR = 0.72, 95% CI 0.44 to 1.17, $p = 0.22$). Rates of macrovascular mortality were not different between IIT and CT (OR = 0.91, 95% CI 0.31 to 2.65, $p = 0.93$).

The DCCT Research Group subsequently studied whether the use of intensive therapy as compared with conventional therapy during the DCCT affected the long-term incidence of cardiovascular disease.[26] Some 93% of the 1441 patients with type 1 diabetes randomly assigned to intensive or conventional therapy in the DCCT were followed until 2005 in the observational Epidemiology of Diabetes Interventions and Complications (EDIC) Study. Cardiovascular disease, defined as confirmed angina, the need for coronary artery revascularization, non-fatal myocardial infarction or stroke or death from cardiovascular disease was assessed with standardized measures and classified by an independent committee. Over 17 years including approximately 6 years during which patients were randomized to intensive or conventional treatment, and 11 years of observational follow-up during which differences in the mean HbA$_{1c}$ values narrowed and disappeared between the treatment groups,[27] a total of 144 cardiovascular events occurred in 83 patients.[26] There were 46 events among 31 patients originally assigned to intensive treatment and 98 events among 52 patients originally assigned to conventional treatment (0.38 vs 0.80 events per 100 patient-years, $p = 0.007$). Intensive therapy was associated with a 42% (95% CI 9 to 62%, $p = 0.02$) reduction in the cumulative incidence

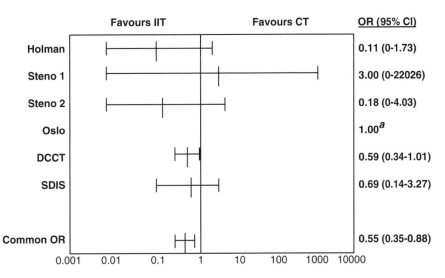

Figure 9.3 Effect of intensive insulin treatment (IIT) on the number of macrovascular events. [a]Accurate determination of CI not possible due to zero event rate in both groups. Adapted from Ref. 25

of a first cardiovascular event and a 57% (95% CI 12 to 79%, $p = 0.02$) reduction in the risk of the first occurrence of non-fatal myocardial infarction or stroke or death from cardiovascular disease. Differences in HbA_{1c} values during the DCCT explained much of the cardiovascular benefit of intensive therapy.[26] Microalbuminuria and albuminuria were also strongly associated with the risk of cardiovascular disease.[26]

Randomized, prospective clinical trials have also been too short to assess the impact of intensive therapy on survival. In the SDIS, 4/48 participants (8.3%) in the intensive therapy group died compared with 3/54 (5.6%) in the standard therapy group ($p =$ ns).[18] In the DCCT, 7/711 participants (1.0%) died in the intensive therapy group and 4/730 (0.5%) died in the conventional therapy group ($p =$ ns).[18] In the DCCT, mortality in both groups was less than expected on the basis of population-based mortality studies, perhaps suggesting that participants enrolled in the study were healthier than the general population with type 1 diabetes.[18]

Prospective observational studies have suggested an association between hyperglycaemia and mortality in type 1 diabetes. In the Wisconsin Epidemiologic Study of Diabetic Retinopathy, after a median follow-up of 10 years, the hazard ratio for mortality from ischaemic heart disease in younger-onset (<30 years of age) insulin-treated diabetic individuals for a 1% change in glycosylated haemoglobin was 1.18 and the 95% CI was 1.00 to 1.40.[28] Glycosylated haemoglobin was also significantly associated with all-cause mortality in younger-onset insulin-treated participants ($p < 0.005$).[28] Ten-year survival in the first quartile of glycosylated haemoglobin was 96.3% compared with 93.0% in the fourth quartile.[28] After correcting for age and sex, the hazard ratio of dying for the fourth relative to the first quartile was 1.9.[28] To the extent that intensive therapy prevents the development and delays the progression of diabetic nephropathy and to the extent that diabetic kidney disease is associated with excess mortality in type 1 diabetes, it is not unreasonable to hypothesize that intensive therapy might be associated with improved survival. Indeed, a computer simulation model developed by the DCCT Research Group to assess the long-term benefits and costs of intensive therapy suggested that intensive therapy might be associated with a 5.1 year increase in survival compared with conventional therapy.[29] This intriguing hypothesis must, however, be tested empirically.

In summary, data from these trials and prospective observational studies suggest that intensive therapy is associated with a reduction in adverse cardiovascular outcomes and cardiovascular mortality.

Metabolic memory

Follow-up to the DCCT has also demonstrated that the reduction in the risk of progressive retinopathy and nephropathy resulting from intensive therapy in patients with type 1 diabetes persists despite increasing hyperglycaemia.[27,30–32] At the end of the DCCT, the patients in the conventional therapy group were offered intensive therapy and the care of all patients was transferred to their own physicians. The difference in the median HbA_{1c} values between the intensive therapy and conventional therapy groups narrowed during follow-up (median during 4 years, 7.9 and 8.2%, respectively; $p < 0.001$). Four years after the DCCT ended, retinopathy was evaluated on the basis of centrally graded fundus photographs and nephropathy was evaluated on the basis of urine specimens. The proportion of patients who had worsening retinopathy, including proliferative retinopathy, macular oedema and the need for laser therapy, was lower and the proportion of patients with development of new microalbuminuria (5 vs 11%, odds reduction 26–70%, $p = 0.002$) and new albuminuria (1 vs 5%, odds reduction 60–95%, $p = 0.001$) was significantly lower in the intensive-therapy group.

After 7–8 years of EDIC follow-up, prior intensive therapy was still associated with persistent differences in retinopathy and nephropathy outcomes. At 7 years of follow-up, prior intensive therapy was associated with a 62% reduction of a further three-step progression of diabetic retinopathy (95% CI 51 to 70%, $p < 0.001$)[27] and at 10 years of follow-up, prior intensive therapy was associated with a 53% reduction of a further 3-step progression (95% CI 43 to 61%, $p < 0.001$).[32] At 8 years of follow-up, prior intensive therapy was associated with a 40% reduction in the odds of developing hypertension (95% CI 34 to 47%, $p < 0.001$),[31] a 59% reduction in the odds of developing microalbuminuria (95% CI 39 to 73%, $p < 0.001$)[31] and an 84% reduction in the odds of developing albuminuria (95% CI 67 to 92%, $p < 0.001$).[31] In addition, significantly fewer intensive-treatment patients reached a serum creatinine level 2.0 mg dl^{-1} ($p = 0.004$).[31]

These results demonstrate that the benefits of intensive therapy on the microvascular complications of type 1 diabetes, specifically retinopathy and nephropathy are long lasting and persist and even increase beyond the period of intervention. This phenomena, termed 'metabolic memory', has led the DCCT/EDIC Research Group to recommend implementation of intensive therapy as soon as possible after the onset of type 1 diabetes with a target HbA_{1c} level of 7.0% or less.

The risks of intensive glycaemic management

The benefits of intensive glycaemic management do not come without risks. Essentially all of the studies of intensive therapy for the prevention of microvascular and neuropathic complications demonstrated an increased incidence of hypoglycaemia associated with intensive therapy. In the meta-analysis by Wang et al., only six studies provided data on severe hypoglycaemia that could be analysed.[1] In intensively treated patients, there was a trend toward more frequent severe hypoglycaemic reactions but the difference was not statistically significant. In a more recent meta-analysis, Egger et al.[33] identified 14 randomized controlled trials in type 1 diabetes with at least 6 months of follow-up and the monitoring of glycaemia by glycosylated haemoglobin.[3,5,8,9,12,14,18,19,34–39] The trials contributed 1028 participants allocated to intensive therapy and 1039 participants allocated to conventional therapy. Follow-up ranged from 0.5 to 7.5 years. The median incidence of severe hypoglycaemia was 7.9 episodes per 100 person-years with intensive therapy and 4.6 episodes per 100 person-years with conventional therapy. The combined odds ratio (95% CI) for hypoglycaemia with intensive therapy was 2.99 (2.45 to 3.64) (Table 9.3). The risk of severe hypoglycaemia was determined by the degree of normalization of glycaemia achieved. In the SDIS, there were 1.1 episodes of serious hypoglycaemia

(requiring help from someone else) per patient-year in the intensified treatment group and 0.4 such episodes per patient-year in the standard treatment group.[18] In the DCCT, the corresponding rates were 0.62 episodes per patient-year in the intensive therapy group and 0.19 episodes per patient-year in the conventional therapy group.[19]

Because of concerns that recurrent severe hypoglycaemia might influence the integrity of the central nervous system and cause cognitive impairment, the SDIS and DCCT investigators performed careful measurements of neuropsychological function. Results of a 3 year analysis of the SDIS showed no consistent hypoglycaemia-associated cognitive impairment.[40] At the end of the DCCT, intensive therapy did not adversely affect neuropsychological performance[41] and patients who had repeated episodes of severe hypoglycaemia did not have any decrement in cognitive function.[42] Further testing of the DCCT cohort a mean of 18 years after randomization showed no evidence of long-term declines in cognitive function in intensively treated patients despite a relatively high rate of recurrent severe hypoglycaemia.[43]

To compare fully the benefits and personal costs of the two treatment regimens, both diabetes-specific and generic quality of life assessments were included in the DCCT along with more traditional measures of disease progression.[44] All analyses of quality of life showed no differences between intensive and conventional therapy. In the DCCT, patients undergoing

Table 9.3 Meta-analysis of the effects of intensive glycaemic control on severe hypoglycaemia, ketoacidosis, and all-cause mortality

Study[b]	Year	Ref.	No. of patients	OR (95% CI)		
				Hypoglycaemia	Ketoacidosis	All-cause mortality
Steno-1	1983	34	32	1.6 (0.2 to 11.0)	1.0 (0.1–18.0)	3.2 (0.1–84.0)
Holman	1983	3	74	1.1 (0.1 to 18.0)	–	1.1 (0.1–18.0)
Kroc	1984	5	70	7.1 (0.8 to 62.0)	22.1 (1.2–401.0)	–
Beck-Nielsen	1985	8	24	1.5 (0.3 to 8.8)	5.0 (0.8–33.0)	–
Oslo-MDI	1986	35	45	0.8 (0.2 to 3.2)	–	–
Oslo-CSII	1986	35	45	0.2 (0.1 to 1.1)	5.7 (0.3–130.0)	–
Steno-2	1986	9	36	1.0 (0.2 to 4.3)	11.5 (0.6–231.0)	1.0 (0.1–8.0)
Christensen	1987	12	24	–	3.3 (0.1–88.0)	–
Marshall	1987	36	12	2.5 (0.2 to 39.0)	–	–
Helve	1987	37	65	3.2 (0.1 to 81.0)	16.4 (0.9–305.0)	–
Verillo	1987	14	44	2.1 (0.2 to 25.0)	–	–
Bangstad	1992	38	30	1.0 (0.1 to 18.0)	5.1 (0.5–52.0)	–
SDIS	1993	18	102	2.6 (1.2 to 5.9)	1.1 (0.2–8.4)	1.6 (0.3–7.3)
DCCT-PP	1993	19	726	3.8 (2.8 to 5.2)	1.1 (0.7–1.8)	1.1 (0.2–7.8)
DCCT-SI	1993	19	715	3.1 (2.3 to 4.2)	1.5 (0.9–2.6)	2.4 (0.5–13.0)
MCSG	1995	39	70	0.9 (0.3 to 3.6)	1.5 (0.2–9.3)	0.3 (0.0–7.8)
Combined				3.0 (2.5 to 3.6)	1.7 (1.3–2.4)	1.4 (0.7–3.0)

[a]Source: adapted from Ref. 33.

[b]MDI, multiple daily injections; CSII, continuous subcutaneous insulin infusion; Pp, primary prevention; SI, secondary intervention.

intensive therapy did not face deterioration in the quality of their lives, even while the rigours of their diabetes care was increased. The occurrence of severe hypoglycaemia was not consistently associated with a subsequent increase in symptomatic distress or decline in diabetes-related quality of life. There was, however, a suggestion that in the primary prevention intensive treatment group, patients who had repeated severe hypoglycaemia (three or more events resulting in coma or seizure) tended to be at increased risk of measurable symptomatic distress.

In both the SDIS and DCCT, there was also an increase in weight associated with intensive therapy. In the SDIS, weight remained stable in the conventional therapy group but body mass index increased by 5.8% in the intensive therapy group.[17] In the DCCT, intensive therapy was associated with a 33% increase in the mean adjusted risk of becoming overweight, a condition defined as a body weight more than 120% above the ideal (12.7 cases of overweight per 100 patient-years in the intensive therapy group versus 9.3 in the conventional-therapy group).[19]

The meta-analysis by Wang et al.[1] demonstrated a significantly higher incidence of diabetic ketoacidosis (DKA) in patients treated with continuous subcutaneous insulin infusion (CSII) than in those treated conventionally.[1] Indeed, the incidence of DKA increased by 12.6 episodes per 100 person-years (95% CI 8.7 to 16.5) in patients on CSII compared to those receiving conventional therapy. This finding was not confirmed by the SDIS or the DCCT. The meta-analysis by Egger et al.[33] which included data from the SDIS and DCCT has, however, confirmed a significantly higher incidence of DKA with CSII therapy (Table 9.2). The median incidence of DKA was 0 episodes per 100 person-years with conventional therapy and 2.9 episodes per 100 person-years with intensive therapy. The combined odds ratio (95% CI) for DKA with intensive therapy was 1.74 (1.27 to 2.38). With exclusive use of CSII therapy, the odds ratio for DKA (95% CI) was 7.20 (2.95 to17.58). In contrast, with exclusive use of multiple daily injections (MDI), the odds ratio was 1.13 (0.15 to 8.35) and for trials offering a choice between CSII and MDI, the odds ratio was 1.28 (0.90 to 1.83).

The meta-analysis by Egger et al.[33] identified 26 deaths among patients with type 1 diabetes, 15 among those receiving intensive therapy and 11 among those receiving conventional therapy (OR 1.40, 95% CI 0.65 to 3.01) (Table 9.2). This analysis confirmed a non-significant reduction in cardiovascular mortality among intensively treated patients (OR 0.42, 95% CI 0.13 to 1.40). It did, however, suggest a low but increased incidence of DKA-associated mortality (5 vs 0 deaths) ($p = 0.02$).

In summary, intensive therapy in young adults with type 1 diabetes causes hypoglycaemia (Table 9.2) and weight gain but does not appear to have an adverse impact on neuropsychological function or quality of life. Intensive therapy with CSII is, however, associated with a significantly increased incidence of DKA and possibly, of death associated with DKA. What, then, should be the recommendations for glycaemic management? The answer lies in balancing the benefits and risks of intensive therapy.

The target for intensive glycaemic management

Some investigators have sought to define a glycaemic threshold for microvascular complications that might minimize the incidence of severe hypoglycaemia. Careful analysis of the DCCT demonstrated no HbA_{1c} threshold below which there was zero risk of the development or progression of complications.[45] In addition, although the absolute risk of severe hypoglycaemia in the intensive treatment group increased as the HbA_{1c} decreased, the relative risk gradient declined with decreasing HbA_{1c}.[45] Thus, in the DCCT, as HbA_{1c} was reduced, there were continuing relative reductions in the risk of complications, whereas there was a slower rate of increase in the risk of hypoglycaemia. These data would support implementation of intensive therapy with the goal of achieving normal glycaemia.

In the patient populations in whom prospective clinical trials were conducted, that is, willing, younger patients with type 1 diabetes with absent to moderate microvascular and neuropathic complications but without severe diabetic complications or other medical conditions, the goal of glycaemic management should be to achieve an HbA_{1c} as close to the non-diabetic range as possible. This is especially true as observational follow-up of the DCCT cohort has demonstrated that the benefits of prior intensive therapy may persist for at least 10 years.[26,27,30-32] Both the risks and sequelae of hypoglycaemia may be greater in children under 13 years of age, in the elderly, in patients with repeated severe hypoglycaemia or unawareness of hypoglycaemia and in patients with advanced diabetic complications. The risk–benefit ratio with intensive therapy may be less favourable in such patients. In such patients, the goal of glycaemic management must consider both the likelihood of benefit from attaining the goal and the risks associated with the therapy required to achieve the goal. Factors limiting the benefit of intensive therapy include the existence of advanced diabetes complications, major co-morbidities and limited life expectancy. Factors heightening the risk of intensive therapy include history of severe hypoglycaemia or hypoglycaemia unawareness, advanced autonomic neuropathy or cardiovascular disease and factors that might impair the detection or treatment of hypoglycaemia such as alterations in mental status, lack of mobility or lack of social support. In patients with substantial factors limiting the benefit or heightening the risk of intensive therapy, an individualized but less intensive goal for glycaemic management is probably indicated. In addition, goal setting must consider the individual's self-determined diabetes care goal and their willingness to make the necessary lifestyle modifications.

References

1 Wang PH, Lau J, Chalmers TC. Meta-analysis of effects of intensive blood glucose control on late complications of type 1 diabetes. *Lancet* 1993;**341**:1306–1309.

2 Eschwege E, Job D, Guyot-Argenton C, Aubry JP, Tchobroutsky G. Delayed progression of diabetic retinopathy by divided insulin administration: a further follow-up. *Diabetologia* 1979;**16**:13–15.

3 Holman RR, Dornan TL, Mayon-White V *et al*. Prevention of deterioration of renal and sensory-nerve function by more intensive management of insulin-dependent diabetic patients. *Lancet* 1983;**i**:204–207.

4 Deckert T, Lauritzen T, Parving HH, Christiansen JS, and the Steno Study Group. Effect of two years of strict metabolic functions in long term insulin-dependent diabetes. *Diab Nephropathy* 1984;**3**:6–10.

5 The Kroc Collaborative Study Group Blood glucose control and the evolution of diabetic retinopathy and albuminuria. *N Engl J Med* 1984;**311**:365–372.

6 Lauritzen T, Larsen KF, Larsen HW, Deckert T and the Steno Study Group. Two-year experience with continuous subcutaneous insulin infusion in relation to retinopathy and neuropathy. *Diabetes* 1985;**34**(S3):74–79.

7 Wiseman MJ Saunders AJ Keen H, Viberti G. Effect of blood glucose control on increased glomerular filtration rate and kidney size in insulin-dependent diabetes. *N Engl J Med* **312**:1985; 617–621.

8 Beck-Nielsen H, Richelsen B, Morgensen CE *et al*. Effect of insulin pump treatment for one year on renal function and retinal morphology in patients with IDDM. *Diabetes Care* 1985;**8**:585–589.

9 Feldt-Rasmussen B, Mathiesen ER Deckert T. Effect of two years of strict metabolic control on progression of incipient nephropathy in insulin-dependent diabetes. *Lancet* 1986; **ii**:1300–1304.

10 Olsen T, Richelsen B, Ehlers N, Beck-Nielsen H. Diabetic retinopathy after 3 years' treatment with continuous subcutaneous insulin infusion (CSII). *Acta Ophthalmol* 1987;**65**: 185–189.

11 Helve E, Laatikainen L, Merenmies L, Koivisto V. Continuous insulin infusion therapy and retinopathy in patients with type 1 diabetes. *Acta Endocrinol* 1987;**115**:313–319.

12 Christensen CK Christiansen JS Schmitz A *et al*. Effect of continuous subcutaneous insulin infusion on kidney function and size in IDDM patients: a 2 year controlled study. *J Diabetes Complications* 1987;**1**:91–95.

13 Dahl-Jorgensen K, Hanssen KF, Kierulf P, Bjoro T, Sandvik L, Agenaes O. Reduction of urinary albumin excretion after 4 years of continuous subcutaneous insulin infusion in insulin-dependent diabetes mellitus. *Acta Endocrinol* 1988;**117**:19–25.

14 Verrillo A, de Teresa A, Martino C, Verrillo L, di Chiara G. Long-term correction of hyperglycemia and progression of retinopathy in insulin dependent diabetes: a five-year randomized prospective study. *Diabetes Res* 1988;**8**:71–76.

15 The Kroc Collaborative Group. Diabetic retinopathy after two years of intensified insulin treatment. *JAMA* 1988;**260**: 37–41.

16 Brinchmann-Hansen O, Dahl-Jorgensen K, Hanssen KF, Sandvik L. The response of diabetic retinopathy to 41 months of multiple insulin injections, insulin pumps and conventional insulin therapy. *Arch Ophthalmol* 1988;**106**: 1242–1246.

17 Reichard P, Berglund B, Britz A, Cars I, Nilsson BY, Rosenqvist U. Intensified conventional insulin treatment retards the microvascular complications of insulin-dependent diabetes mellitus (IDDM): the Stockholm Diabetes Intervention Study (SDIS) after 5 years. *J Intern Med* 1991;**230**:101–108.

18 Reichard P, Nilsson BY, Rosenqvist U. The effect of long-term intensified insulin treatment on the development of microvascular complications of diabetes mellitus. *N Engl J Med* 1993;**329**:304–309.

19 The Diabetes Control, Complications Trial Research Group. The effect of intensive treatment of diabetes on the development and progression of long-term complications in insulin-dependent diabetes mellitus. *N Engl J Med* 1993;**329**: 977–986.

20 The Diabetes Control, Complications Trial Research Group. Effect of intensive therapy on the development and progression of diabetic nephropathy in the Diabetes Control and Complications Trial. *Kidney Int* 1995;**47**:1703–1720.

21 Microalbuminuria Collaborative Study Group, United Kingdom. Intensive therapy and progression to clinical albuminuria in patients with insulin dependent diabetes mellitus and microalbuminuria. *BMJ* 1995;**311**:973–977.

22 Jensen-Urstad KJ, Reichard PG, Rosfors JS, Lindblad LEL, Jensen-Urstad MT. Early atherosclerosis is retarded by improved long-term blood glucose control in patients with IDDM. *Diabetes* 1996;**45**:1253–1258.

23 Diabetes Control, Complications Trial/Epidemiology of Diabetes Interventions, Complications Research Group. Intensive diabetes therapy and carotid intima-media thickness in type 1 diabetes mellitus. *N Engl J Med* 2003;**348**:2294–2303.

24 Cleary P, Orchard T, Zinman B *et al*. Coronary calcification in the Diabetes Control and Complications Trial/Epidemiology of Diabetes Interventions and Complications (DCCT/EDIC) cohort. *Diabetes* 2003;**52**(Suppl 2): A152.

25 Lawson ML, Tsui E, Gerstein HC, Zinman B. Effect of intensive therapy on early macrovascular disease in young individuals with type 1 diabetes-a systematic review and meta-analysis. *Diabetes Care* 1999;**22**:(2):B35–B39.

26 The Diabetes Control, Complications Trial/Epidemiology of Diabetes Interventions, Complications (DCCT/EDIC) Study

Research Group. Intensive diabetes treatment and cardiovascular disease in patients with type 1 diabetes. *N Engl J Med* 2005;**353**:2643–2653.

27 The Writing Team for the Diabetes Control, Complications Trial/Epidemiology of Diabetes Interventions, Complications Research Group. Effect of intensive therapy on the microvascular complications of type 1 diabetes mellitus. *JAMA* 2002;**287**:2563–2569.

28 Klein R. Hyperglycemia and microvascular and macrovascular disease in diabetes. *Diabetes Care* 1995;**18**:258–268.

29 The Diabetes Control and Complications Trial (DCCT) Research Group. Lifetime benefits and costs of intensive therapy as practiced in the Diabetes Control and Complications Trial. *JAMA* 1996;**276**:1409–1415.

30 The Diabetes Control, Complications Trial/Epidemiology of Diabetes Interventions, Complications Research Group. Retinopathy and nephropathy in patients with type 1 diabetes four years after a trial of intensive therapy. *N Engl J Med* 2000;**342**:381–389.

31 The Writing Team for the Diabetes Control, Complications Trial/Epidemiology of Diabetes Interventions, Complications Research Group. Sustained effect of intensive treatment of type 1 diabetes mellitus on development and progression of diabetic nephropathy. The Epidemiology of Diabetes Interventions and Complications (EDIC) Study. *JAMA* 2003;**290**:2159–2167.

32 Diabetes Control, Complications Trial/Epidemiology of Diabetes Interventions, Complications (DCCT/EDIC) Research Group. Prolonged effect of intensive therapy on the risk of retinopathy complications in patients with type 1 diabetes mellitus. *Arch Ophthalmol* 2008;**126**:1707–1715.

33 Egger M, Smith GD, Stettler C, Diem P. Risk of adverse effects of intensified treatment in insulin-dependent diabetes mellitus: a meta-analysis. *Diabet Med* 1997;**14**:919–928.

34 Lauritzen T, Frost-Larsen, K, Larsen HW, Deckert T, and the Steno Study, Group. Effect of 1 year of near-normal blood glucose levels on retinopathy in insulin-dependent diabetics. *Lancet* 1983;**i**:200–204.

35 Dahl-Jorgensen K, Brinchmann-Hanssen O, Hanssen KF, Ganes T, Kierulf P, Smeland E, Sandvik L, Aagenaes O. Effect of near normoglycemia for two years on progression of early diabetic retinopathy, nephropathy and neuropathy: the Oslo Study. *BMJ* 1986;**293**:1195–1199.

36 Marshall SM, Home PD, Taylor R, Alberti KGMM. Continuous insulin infusion versus injection therapy: a randomized cross-over trial under usual diabetic clinic conditions. *Diabet Med* 1987;**4**:521–525.

37 Helve E, Koivisto VA, Lehtonen A, Pelkonen R, Huttunen JK, Nikkila EA. A crossover comparison of continuous insulin infusion and conventional injection treatment of type 1 diabetes. *Acta Med Scand* 1987;**221**:385–393.

38 Bangstad H-J, Kofoed-Enevoldsen A, Dahl-Jorgensen K, Hanssen KF. Glomerular charge selectivity and the influence of improved blood glucose control in type 1 (insulin-dependent) diabetic patients with microalbuminuria. *Diabetologia* 1992;**35**:1165–1169.

39 Microalbuminuria Collaborative Study Group United Kingdom. Intensive therapy and progression to clinical albuminuria in patients with insulin dependent diabetes mellitus and microalbuminuria. *BMJ* 1995;**311**:973–977.

40 Reichard P, Berglund A, Britz A, Levander S, Rosenqvist U. Hypoglycemic episodes during intensified insulin treatment: increased frequency but no effect on cognitive function. *J Intern Med* 1991;**229**:9–16.

41 The Diabetes Control, Complications Trial Research Group. Effects of intensive diabetes therapy on neuropsychological function in adults in the Diabetes Control and Complications Trial. *Ann Intern Med* 1996;**124**:379–388.

42 Austin EJ, Deary IJ. Effects of repeated hypoglycemia on cognitive function: a phychometrically validated reanalaysis of the Diabetes Control and Complications Trial data. *Diabetes Care* 1999;**22**:1273–1277.

43 The Diabetes Control, Complications Trial/Epidemiology of Diabetes Interventions, Complications (DCCT/EDIC) Study Research Group. Long-term effect of diabetes and its treatment on cognitive function. *N Engl J Med* 2007;**356**: 1842–1852.

44 The Diabetes Control, Complications Trial Research Group. Influence of intensive diabetes treatment on quality-of-life outcomes in the Diabetes Control and Complications Trial. *Diabetes Care* 1996;**19**:195–203.

45 The Diabetes Control, Complications Trial Research Group. The absence of a glycemic threshold for the development of long-term complications: The perspective of the Diabetes Control and Complications Trial. *Diabetes* 1996;**45**: 1289–1298.

10 Does intensive glycaemic management reduce morbidity and mortality in type 2 diabetes?

Amanda I. Adler

MRC Epidemiology Unit, Institute of Metabolic Science, Addenbrooke's Hospital, Cambridge, UK

Background

Observational studies have demonstrated that hyperglycaemia increases the risk of complications among individuals with type 2 diabetes.[1,2] This increase in risk is independent of risk factors with which hyperglycaemia is associated, including duration of diabetes, diabetic complications, blood pressure, blood lipids and smoking. The association between hyperglycaemia and complications spans the spectrum from microvascular complications to macrovascular complications and death. However, these observational studies do not, in general, provide sufficient evidence on which to base strategies to intensify glucose-lowering therapies given the possibility that hyperglycaemia may be linked to unmeasured or unknown risk factors for complications. These studies which document an association between blood glucose and complications, do, however, support trials of the effectiveness of lowering blood glucose.

Most trials to date have studied the effect of blood glucose lowering on coronary, cerebrovascular and peripheral arterial disease (macrovascular disease), ophthalmological, neurological and renal complications (microvascular disease) and death. Some endpoints combine macro- and microvascular disease, such as lower extremity amputation, whereas other endpoints include neither, for example, cataracts. As experiments, these trials have included an active therapeutic intervention and a comparison group. Most trials attempt to improve hyperglycaemia directly and others alter biochemical pathways downstream from hyperglycaemia.[3] Both are discussed in this chapter, as are trials which include lifestyle changes (diet and physical activity). Although observational studies inform clinical care, this chapter focuses on trials alone, and for cardiovascular disease, only on trials that address hard rather than surrogate endpoints, that is, the incidence of myocardial infarction or cardiovascular death rather than coronary angiography or estimates of cardiovascular risk. For nephropathy, given the relative rarity of end-stage renal disease, this chapter includes studies which have addressed the endpoints proteinuria and rises in plasma creatinine, and for retinopathy, retinal changes and laser photocoagulation, in addition to visual changes. Completed trials vary and test:

- the degree of blood glucose lowering testing a more aggressive versus a less aggressive strategy;
- a single blood glucose-lowering drug compared with a placebo;
- blood glucose lowering as a component of an overall approach striving for more compared with less intensive multifactorial care.

This chapter also includes a description of important ongoing studies designed to resolve outstanding questions related to glucose lowering.

Blood glucose-lowering strategies in type 2 diabetes

Interventions currently available to treat type 2 diabetes include interventions to increase physical activity and diets designed to promote weight loss (so-called 'lifestyle' changes). Oral anti-diabetic drugs include sulfonylureas, meglitinides, biguanides (metformin),

The Evidence Base for Diabetes Care, Second Edition, Edited by William H. Herman, Ann Louise Kinmonth, Nicholas J. Wareham and Rhys Williams.

α-glucosidase inhibitors (e.g. acarbose, miglitol), thiazolidinediones (pioglitazone and rosiglitazone), dipeptidylpeptidase 4 inhibitors (sitagliptin and vildagliptin) and drugs for weight loss (rimonabant, sibutramine and orlistat). Injected (subcutaneous) drugs for diabetes include glucagon-like peptide-1 mimetics (exenatide) and insulin including human insulin and analogues of insulin. Insulins include short-acting (prandial or bolus) used prior to or with meals or continuously in insulin pumps and long-acting (basal or background or intermediate acting), used once or twice daily. Patients with type 2 diabetes may use basal or bolus insulin or both, including in pre-mixed fixed combinations (biphasic insulins), used twice daily and, rarely, three times daily.

Completed clinical trials

University Group Diabetes Program (UGDP)

The UGDP started in 1960 and measured 'the efficacy of hypoglycemic treatments in the prevention of vascular complications in type 2 diabetes'.[4] The study enrolled 1027 individuals. Investigators treated patients with diet alone for 1 month and thereafter randomized them to fixed-dose insulin or variable-dose insulin, to the sulfonylurea (tolbutamide) or placebo, or (delayed randomization) to the biguanide phenformin or placebo.[5] The diet was designed to achieve and maintain a body weight within 15% of ideal weight in all patients throughout the study. Due to an apparent increase in mortality from both tolbutamide (cardiovascular deaths) and phenformin, investigators discontinued both arms and compared the placebo arms with insulin.[6]

The study showed, in the groups assigned to insulin, better blood glucose control and fewer hospitalizations for heart disease, but neither outcome differed significantly from the placebo groups. Investigators observed no differences for retinopathy, peripheral vascular disease or cardiovascular disease between the groups assigned to insulin, but the number of events was small, suggesting that the study was unlikely to find a difference even if one existed. Fewer patients randomized to insulin developed raised plasma creatinine levels relative to those assigned to placebo ($p = 0.03$).

The results of the study showed that insulin therapy neither reduced nor increased the risk of cardiovascular disease and that too few events occurred to detect a true difference.[6] The study suggested that sulfonylureas and phenformin might be harmful. Critics noted that the study's termination was premature, that death was not a pre-defined endpoint and that the placebo group to which the tolbutamide group was compared

had an implausibly low rate of death (in comparison with which the tolbutamide death rate appeared high). The study was limited by the investigators' inability to monitor glycaemia by self-monitoring of blood glucose or with haemoglobin A_{1c} (HbA_{1c}). The finding of no difference between groups was probably due to insufficient numbers of patients and events and could not be interpreted as no difference between treatments. The published writings about the UGDP are lively, if occasionally acerbic.[7–9]

Veterans Affairs Cooperative Study and Veterans Affairs Diabetes Trial (VADT)

The investigators of the Veterans Affairs Cooperative Study on Glycemic Control and Complications in Type II Diabetes performed this feasibility study in 153 men. They tested whether achieving near-normal glycaemia compared with 'standard' treatment reduced the incidence of cardiovascular events. In 27 months of follow-up, investigators observed an approximately 2.0% separation of HbA_{1c} between groups. Investigators observed no difference in rates of cardiovascular disease or death.[10] Given the small size and short duration of the study, the trial would not have been expected to detect a difference. The follow-on study, the Veterans Affairs Diabetes Trials (VADT), enrolled 1792 adults with type 2 diabetes and an $HbA_{1c} > 8.5\%$.[11] Again, the study tested the hypothesis that improved glycaemic control results in a lower incidence of major cardiovascular events. Investigators randomized subjects to either intensive or 'usual' control of blood glucose, between which the investigators hoped to achieve a difference in HbA_{1c} of at least 1.5%. Therapy in both groups included combinations of thiazolidinedione, sulfonylureas, metformin, α-glucosidase inhibitors, natiglinide and insulin and so could not test the advantages or disadvantages of any single agents.[12]

Kumamoto Study

The Japanese Kumamoto Study tested the hypothesis that intensive treatment of blood glucose prevents the development or worsening of diabetic complications in insulin-treated patients with type 2 diabetes who do not have significant complications. In this small randomized study of 110 patients, the patients were divided into those without retinopathy and those with 'simple' retinopathy. Half of each group received basal insulin only, and the other half received a regime of basal plus prandial insulin (basal-bolus). Although designed primarily to assess microvascular complications, the study included cardiovascular disease including angina pectoris, myocardial infarction, stroke, intermittent claudication, gangrene and lower extremity amputation. Retinopathy was defined as a change of at least two stages on the Early Treatment Diabetic Retinopathy Study (ETDRS) classification, nephropathy by the development of a urinary albumin excretion of >30 mg per 24 h and neuropathy by vibration perception thresholds.

Over 8 years, the group administering multiple injections achieved an HbA_{1c} of 7.2% compared with 9.4% in the group injecting basal insulin only. Despite equal insulin dosages per kilogram of body weight, randomization to a basal-bolus insulin significantly decreased the risk of retinopathy, nephropathy and neuropathy. Based on a small number of events, the investigators reported that the total cardiovascular events in the multiple injection group were 0.6% per year compared with 1.3% per year.[13]

Because of their findings, the investigators called for treatment goals of an HbA_{1c} of less than 6.5%, fasting blood glucose values less than 110 mg dl^{-1} and blood glucose values 2 h following meals of less than 180 mg dl^{-1} as a means to lower the risk of diabetic complications.[13]

United Kingdom Prospective Diabetes Sudy (UKPDS)

The UKPDS recruited 5102 patients newly diagnosed with type 2 diabetes and tested whether a policy of intensive blood glucose control striving for near-normal blood glucose levels, relative to a conventional policy, lowered the incidence of diabetic complications. The diagnostic criteria for diabetes differed from criteria of the American Diabetes Association since diabetes was diagnosed from two fasting plasma glucose values of at least 6 mmol l^{-1}, rather than 7 mmol l^{-1}. The study was powered on a composite endpoint comprising microvascular and macrovascular disease, but myocardial infarction, stroke and the combined endpoint of death from peripheral vascular disease or lower extremity amputation were pre-specified aggregate endpoints.[14]

The main study randomized 3867 patients to intensive therapy, defined as initial treatment with sulfonylurea or insulin, or to conventional therapy with diet. A subsidiary study among patients at least 120% overweight included alternate randomization to metformin. The investigators added therapies as required to maintain the goal of fasting blood glucose values of <6 mmol l^{-1} ('near normal') in the intensive group and <15 mmol l^{-1} in the conventional group. Regardless of added therapies, the investigators analysed the study on the initial randomization ('intention-to-treat').

The investigators recruited participants aged 25–65 years at study onset from centres in England, Scotland and Northern Ireland. Of these patients, 81% were white, 10% South Asian, 8% Afro-Caribbean and 1% other ethnicities. This mix over-represented non-white participants relative to the make-up of the British population. The average body mass index (BMI) was 27.5 kg m^{-2}.

Over a 10 year median follow-up, the group randomized to intensive therapy achieved a median HbA_{1c} value of 7.0% compared with 7.9% in the conventional group. The intensive therapy group experienced fewer diabetic complications but experienced more frequent hypoglycaemia and more weight gain.

Intensive treatment significantly lowered the rate of microvascular disease and was associated with a risk reduction of 25% (7–40, $p = 0.0099$). Patients randomized to the intensive treatment group were also less likely to have a myocardial infarction, with an estimated relative risk reduction of 16% (0–29).[14] The risk reduction included the possibility of no effect and was associated with a probability (p) value of 0.052, which exceeded the traditional threshold for statistical significance. There was no difference in the rates of stroke between conventional and intensive groups.[14] The results showed a highly significant reduction in risk for retinal photocoagulation. Although the association between intensive therapy and renal failure was similar in magnitude to that of retinal photocoagulation, there were too few cases of renal failure to show a significant difference. Compared with the conventional group, an intensive policy of glucose lowering reduced the risk for any diabetes-related endpoint by 12% (95% CI 1–21, $p = 0.029$). Intensive therapy was not associated with a decrease or increase in deaths. The study showed no difference in incidence of myocardial infarction between the three intensive agents (chlorpropamide, glibenclamide or insulin). There was no difference for any of the three aggregate endpoints between the three intensive agents.

For overweight patients, there was a more modest difference (−.6%) in median HbA_{1c} during follow-up between the metformin and conventional groups than between the insulin/sulfonylurea and conventional groups. Metformin-allocated patients experienced fewer diabetes-related complications (relative risk reduction 42%, 9–63, $p = 0.017$) compared with the conventional group and a rate of myocardial infarction 39% lower (11–59).[15] The magnitude of the reduction in myocardial infarction exceeded that expected from the relationship between HbA_{1c} and the incidence of myocardial infarction.[1] Metformin lowered the prevalence of retinopathy, but not of albuminuria.

Patients in whom metformin was added to sulfonylurea therapy had an increased risk of death compared with those on sulfonylureas alone. Discounting a chance finding, these results could reflect deleterious effects of combining metformin with sulfonylureas, or alternatively, could reflect a benefit of sulfonylurea therapy alone.

The UKPDS showed that lowering blood glucose lowered the risk of diabetic complications and, in overweight patients randomized to metformin, the risk of myocardial infarction and death. With the possible exception of the combination of sulfonylurea and metformin, no single randomization including sulfonylureas or insulin was associated with increased diabetic complications. No threshold in HbA_{1c} existed below which the risk of diabetes complications was absent. Therefore, choosing a level of HbA_{1c} as a goal for the treatment of type 2 diabetes is based on a balance between realistic achievement of glycaemic control, risk of hypoglycaemia and weight gain, the overall risk of diabetic complications and available resources.

Following the end of the UKPDS, investigators followed UKPDS participants, recording patient characteristics and outcomes ('post-study monitoring'), but did not encourage a difference in policies related to blood glucose lowering. Intensive control of blood glucose had proved successful in reducing microvascular disease and, accordingly, the investigators encouraged all participants to strive for a goal of an HbA_{1c} of 7.0%. Despite these efforts, the HbA_{1c} values were similar between the groups formerly randomized to intensive and to conventional control of blood glucose. In the 10 years following the end of the UKPDS, patients previously randomized to the intensive blood glucose policy were nonetheless less likely to die or have experienced a myocardial infarction than patients previously randomized to conventional control.[16] The investigators suggested a 'legacy effect', a sustained benefit from good control of blood glucose.

STENO-2

The STENO-2 investigators tested a 'targeted, intensified, multifactorial intervention' of multiple modifiable risk factors for diabetes. These included targeting of hyperglycaemia, hypertension, dyslipidaemia, microalbuminuria and existing cardiovascular disease in an effort to decrease cardiovascular disease as defined by death due to cardiovascular causes, non-fatal myocardial infarction, non-fatal stroke, revascularization and lower extremity amputation. The period of treatment was approximately 8 years. The comparison group received conventional, guideline-driven care and was adapted as guidelines changed over time. Despite its modest size (80 per group),

intensive therapy was associated with a halving of the risk of cardiovascular disease.[17]

Participants were followed after the end of the trial for another 5.5 years. Levels of HbA_{1c} in participants at the end of the observation period were not different between groups, nor were they at the level advocated by guidelines (average of 7.7 and 8.0% for the intervention and conventional therapy group, respectively).[18] Nevertheless, patients who had been randomized to intensive therapy were significantly less likely (hazard ratio 0.43, 95% CI 0.19 to 0.94) to have died.

PROactive

The prospective pioglitazone clinical trial in macrovascular events (PROactive) study tested whether pioglitazone, compared with placebo, lowered the risk of a composite endpoint of all-cause mortality, non-fatal myocardial infarction (MI) (including silent MI), stroke, acute coronary syndrome, revascularization of coronary or lower extremity arteries and lower extremity amputation. The study randomized 5238 patients with type 2 diabetes and cardiovascular disease and showed a non-significant decrease in the risk of cardiovascular disease over 2.5 years (hazard ratio 0.90, 95% CI 0.80–1.02, $p = 0.095$) at the expense of weight gain and an increased risk of congestive heart failure.[19,20] Despite more side-effects, participants randomized to pioglitazone were not more likely to discontinue their study drug. A secondary endpoint limited to death from any cause, non-fatal myocardial infarction (excluding silent MI) or stroke was associated with a hazard ratio of 0.84 (95% CI 0.72–0.98), $p = 0.027$. However, to ensure that chance did not account for these findings, many investigators would call for a more stringent probability value when considering secondary endpoints.

Action to Control Cardiovascular Risk in Diabetes (ACCORD)

The NIH-funded ACCORD Study recruited 10 251 participants with known type 2 diabetes who also had cardiovascular disease (CVD) or who were at particularly high risk of developing CVD. ACCORD tested the hypothesis that lowering glycaemia delays or prevents CVD. Investigators randomized patients to intensive control with a target HbA_{1c} level of <6.0% or to standard control with a target HbA_{1c} level of 7.0–7.9%.[21] The pre-specified primary outcome was the first occurrence of non-fatal MI or non-fatal stroke or death from cardiovascular causes. Participants randomized to intensive control started on at least two anti-diabetic drugs and therapies were added when HbA$_{1c}$ levels exceeded 6% or when blood glucose levels obtained from self-blood glucose monitoring exceeded target levels.

The study population had an average HbA$_{1c}$ of 8.3% at baseline. One year on, the median HbA$_{1c}$ was 6.4% in the intensive group and 7.5% in the standard group. Participants maintained these median values and the difference between group was sustained throughout the study. Planned to last 5.5 years, the trial was stopped after 3.5 years because of a higher rate of death in the group randomized to intensive therapy. Patients randomized to intensive therapy were 22% more likely to die (hazard ratio 1.22, 1.01–1.46, $p = 0.04$). In addition, the group randomized to intensive therapy experienced higher rates of fluid retention, hypoglycaemia and weight gain and lower rates of non-fatal MI (hazard ratio 0.76, 0.62–0.92, $p = 0.004$). The primary endpoint was not different between groups (hazard ratio 0.90, 95% CI 0.78 to 1.04, $p = 0.16$). It is uncertain whether the approach of rapid lowering of blood glucose, the levels of blood glucose achieved or an unmeasured factor was responsible for the increased risk of death.[22]

Action in Diabetes and Vascular Disease (ADVANCE)

ADVANCE addressed intensive blood glucose (and blood pressure) control, enrolling 11 140 participants with type 2 diabetes over age 55 years at otherwise high risk for CVD. The investigators randomized patients to a glucose-lowering regimen with a goal of HbA$_{1c}$ 6.5% or to one based on standard guidelines.[23] Modified-release gliclazide was the only sulfonylurea permitted in the intensive arm and the only sulfonylurea not allowed in the standard control group. Otherwise, the study permitted the addition of metformin, thiazolidinediones, acarbose and insulin. Two co-primary endpoints existed, one a composite of macrovascular disease and the other of microvascular disease. Macrovascular disease included death from CVD plus non-fatal MI or stroke; microvascular disease included nephropathy defined by end-stage renal disease and also changes in albuminuria and plasma creatinine plus retinopathy.

During the 5 years of follow-up, the difference in HbA$_{1c}$ between groups was 0.67%. Combining micro- and macrovascular disease, there were fewer events in the intensive therapy group (hazard ratio 0.90, 95% CI 0.82 to 0.98, $p = 0.01$). Broken down, intensive therapy was associated with a reduction in microvascular disease (hazard ratio 0.86, 95% CI 0.77 to 0.97, $p = 0.01$) but not macrovascular disease (hazard ratio 0.94, 95% CI 0.84 to 1.06, $p = 0.32$). The HbA$_{1c}$ target of 6.5% in the intensively-treated group did not differ

markedly from the ACCORD study but, unlike in ACCORD, the investigators observed no increase in cardiovascular deaths compared with standard therapy.

Glucose Insulin Potassium (GIK) Infusion trials

During periods of acute illness including MI, treatment of hospitalized patients with intravenous insulin, glucose and potassium (K$^+$) has been tested as a means to improve survival. The hypothesized mechanism of benefit relates to the preference of the myocardium for glucose as an energy substrate during ischaemia and reperfusion. Because insulin stimulates glucose and potassium uptake, the infused potassium replaces potassium levels in blood. Although all patients in trials of GIK have hyperglycaemia, not all have previously diagnosed diabetes; others have stress hyperglycaemia or undiagnosed diabetes.

A meta-analysis of 38 studies found no benefit for randomization to GIK. However, when trials by design also strove for normal levels of blood glucose, this approach resulted in better outcomes.[24] In analyses combining the major studies OASIS-6 and CRE-ATE-ECLA, with over 11 000 patients in each of the treatment and intervention arms, the investigators observed no differences between the groups in the rates at 1 month for death, heart failure or both. Patients with the highest levels of blood glucose had the highest mortality, regardless of allocated treatment.[25] With regard to stroke, a study that randomized patients with acute stroke and a blood glucose level of 6.0–17.0 mmol l^{-1} to GIK found no difference in outcome. However, the study recruited fewer than 1000 patients, whereas some 2300 patients would have been required to find a meaningful difference.[26] Of the studies limited to patients with diabetes, Diabetes Mellitus, Insulin Glucose Infusion in Acute Myocardial Infarction (DIGAMI) showed a increased survival beyond 3 years for patients randomized to GIK,[27] whereas DIGAMI-2 found no difference.[28] In summary, GIK is not itself associated with favourable outcomes, although attaining excellent glycaemic control during acute cardiovascular events may be.[29]

Other interventions to alter blood glucose metabolism

Interventions using inhibitors of aldose reductase to alter the polyol pathway to inhibit the metabolism of glucose to sorbitol have been tested in clinical trials. No studies with macrovascular endpoints exist. A Cochrane review reported that aldose reductase inhibitors have shown no benefit over placebo for diabetic neuropathy.[30] Aldose reductase inhibitors are not currently indicated for the prevention or treatment of diabetic complications.

Hyperglycaemia can induce an elevation in protein kinase C activity in vascular cells thought to be integral to the development of vascular complications.[31] Ruboxistaurin, an inhibitor of protein kinase C-beta, has been studied in humans with promising results for retinopathy and nephropathy.[32] Routine usage in diabetes awaits further research.

Surgical-induced weight loss improves blood glucose control in diabetes and prolongs survival. The Swedish Obesity Study tested the potential benefits and drawbacks of bariatric surgery in 4047 obese individuals (with an average BMI of approximately $40 \, kg \, m^{-2}$), 11% of whom had diabetes. Although initially designed as a randomized controlled study, the study was redesigned as an observational study because research ethics committees were unlikely to have approved a trial. Based on multivariate observational analyses, bariatric surgery was associated with a 27% reduction in the death rate. This rate was not different in individuals with diabetes.[33] No randomized trial in type 2 diabetes of surgery for obesity and cardiovascular deaths exists.

Ongoing clinical trials

Bypass angioplasty revascularization investigation in type 2 diabetes (BARI 2D)

The BARI 2D trial asks two questions of patients with type 2 diabetes and significant coronary disease: (1) is elective (non-emergent) revascularization and intensive medical therapy better than intensive medical therapy alone with respect to death rates, and (2) is an approach using insulin-sensitizing drugs better (or worse) than an approach using insulin-providing drugs with respect to death rates? Both groups have a target value for HbA_{1c} of <7.0%. Insulin 'provision' includes insulin or sulfonylureas, whereas the strategy for insulin sensitization employs treatment with thiazolidinediones and metformin.[34] BARI 2D has randomized 2800 adults.

Hyperglycaemia and its effect after acute myocardial infarction on cardiovascular outcomes in patients with type 2 diabetes (HEART 2-D)

HEART 2-D (ClinicalTrials.gov identifier NCT00191282)[35] recruited patients with type 2 diabetes admitted to cardiac care units following MI

and addressed glucose lowering via different insulin-based regimes. The study measured time to first recurrent event defined as death from CVD, non-fatal MI or stroke, hospitalization for acute coronary syndromes or coronary revascularization. The investigators randomized patients to a 'post-prandial strategy' with insulin lispro, a short-acting insulin analogue, with the possible inclusion of bedtime neutral protamine Hagedorn (NPH) insulin or to a 'basal strategy' with basal (or biphasic) insulin. This study, with follow-up to 3.5 years, aimed to achieve an HbA_{1c} of less than 7.0% in both groups. The study at the time of writing has finished, but has not been published.

Action for health in diabetes (look AHEAD)

Look AHEAD, an NIH-funded study, addresses the hypothesis that weight loss reduces the risk of CVD among 5145 adults with type 2 diabetes. While increased body weight may or may not be associated independently with an increased risk of CVD in diabetes, weight loss lowers blood glucose. The investigators encourage weight loss in the intervention group via diet and physical activity and in the control group by education alone. The composite primary endpoint of the study includes fatal and non-fatal MI, stroke and cardiovascular deaths (ClinicalTrials.gov identifier NCT00017953).[36–38] One-year results show that the group who received intensive lifestyle advice became fitter and lost more weight. HbA_{1c} also dropped by approximately 0.6% in the intervention group compared with approximately 0.1% in the control group. Whether this will result in a reduction in CVD will be determined at the study's end, estimated for 2012.

Nateglinide and Valsartan in Impaired Glucose Tolerance Outcomes Research (NAVIGATOR)

The NAVIGATOR study is a randomized controlled trial that addresses the role of glucose lowering with natiglinide [and/or randomization to the angiotensin receptor blocker (ARB) valsartan] compared with placebo treatment in individuals with impaired glucose tolerance aged over 50 years in 7500 individuals. Although not performed in individuals with type 2 diabetes, the study addresses whether either drug lowers the incidence of CVD and also diabetes.

Outcome Reduction with an Initial Glargine Intervention (ORIGIN)

The ORIGIN Study (Clinicaltrials.gov identifier NCT00069784) tests lowering blood glucose with insulin (glargine) in individuals with newly diagnosed type 2 diabetes and impaired fasting glucose and/or impaired glucose tolerance in order to lower the incidence of CVD. The rationale is based on the probable higher risk of CVD in individuals with glucose levels between 'normal' and those sufficient to meet criteria for the diagnosis of diabetes.[39,40] Of the 82% of subjects with established diabetes, the study was limited to those on at most one oral blood glucose-lowering drug. Participants randomized to insulin started at either 2, 4 or 6 units of glargine titrating to achieve fasting blood glucose levels between 4.0 and 5.3 mmol l^{-1}. The unblinded study has two co-primary composite outcomes: (3) cardiovascular death or non-fatal MI or non-fatal stroke and (4) the above-listed events plus revascularization or hospitalization for heart failure. Investigators strive for fasting plasma glucose values of 5.3 mmol l^{-1} in the group receiving insulin and for the blood glucose values thought to represent 'best practice' by the treating physician for the group not randomized to insulin. The study, which employs a factorial design, also evaluates the role of fish oil.[41]

Acarbose Cardiovascular Evaluation (ACE)

The ACE trial studies the effectiveness of acarbose to reduce the risk of recurrent cardiovascular events in Chinese patients with CVD and impaired glucose tolerance. The results of the STOP-NIDDM study showing that acarbose effectively delays or prevents diabetes, plus the knowledge that diabetes increases the risk of CVD, provides a strong rationale for this study.[42] As with the NAVIGATOR study, the study participants do not (yet) have diabetes. This randomized, placebo-controlled, outcome trial will recruit approximately 6500 individuals, with results expected in 2012.[43]

Rosiglitazone Evaluated for Cardiac Outcomes and Regulation of Glycaemia in Diabetes (RECORD)

RECORD, a non-inferiority study, assesses the combination of rosiglitazone plus either metformin or sulfonylurea compared with the combination of metformin plus sulfonylurea with respect to cardiovascular outcomes in people with type 2 diabetes. This 6 year study of 4458 patients is planned for completion in 2009.[44] An early analysis of the study precipitated by safety concerns[45,46] showed no difference in MI between the two groups. In view of insufficient power due to premature analysis and a lower than expected event rate, the analyses could neither confirm nor exclude a beneficial or harmful effect of rosiglitazone.

Safety of thiazolidinediones

Rosiglitazone and pioglitazone, PPAR-γ agonists, effectively reduce HbA$_{1c}$ and provide additional benefits in terms of glycaemic control when added to existing therapies. Rosiglitazone as monotherapy provides better sustained control of blood glucose than conventional therapies.[47]

The safety of thiazolidinediones has recently received attention. In the short term, the risks associated with rosiglitazone and pioglitazone include weight gain, fluid retention, peripheral oedema, macular oedema, expansion of plasma volume contributing to the risk of anaemia, heart failure and effects on lipid profiles. For rosiglitazone, the effects on lipids are unfavourable compared with pioglitazone.

Longer term risks associated with rosiglitazone and pioglitazone include an increased risk of bony fractures. For rosiglitazone, there is a potentially increased risk of myocardial ischaemia based on meta-analyses of interventional trials; pharmacoepidemiological studies show differing results. The available studies for pioglitazone, including published meta-analyses of trials and the completed long-term PROactive study, do not raise similar concerns about an increased risk of MI in association with pioglitazone treatment. An observational study suggests that pioglitazone users are less likely than rosiglitazone users to experience an MI or coronary revascularization.

SPREADDIMCAD

The Study on the Prognosis and Effect of Anti-Diabetic Drugs on Type 2 Diabetes Mellitus with Coronary Artery Disease (ClinicalTrials.gov identifier NCT00513630) is a double-blind, randomized trial which employs glipizide or metformin. The endpoint is recurrent cardiovascular events in patients and the study population consists of individuals with type 2 diabetes mellitus and coronary heart disease. This study is taking place in Shanghai, China, and is forecasted for completion in 2010.

Reducing weight using medications

Randomized trials have shown that the weight-loss drugs orlistat and sibutramine can achieve modest weight loss in individuals with diabetes.[48] Long-term cardiovascular benefits, if any, remain unclear. The ongoing SCOUT study addresses the effectiveness of sibutramine use (versus placebo) in patients with type 2 diabetes.[49] Rimonabant, a cannabinoid receptor antagonist, available in Europe but not the United States, reduces weight and blood glucose in patients with diabetes.[50] Currently under way is the CRES-CENDO study with the primary objective of testing whether rimonabant reduces the risk of an MI, stroke or death from MI or stroke in patients with abdominal obesity and other risks for CVD, which may include type 2 diabetes (ClinicalTrials.gov identifier NCT00263042).

Discussion

Glucose-lowering, alone or in combination with other modalities, reduces the risk of diabetic complications in type 2 diabetes. Blood glucose successfully reduces the incidence of complications, but often at the expense of increased weight gain, increased incidence of hypoglycaemia and financial costs, which vary by treatment. Investigators and clinicians, in general, consider the benefits to outweigh the risks, but acknowledge that the balance in individual patients varies.

The recent report from ACCORD of an increased risk of death in the setting of aggressive glucose lowering has raised issues of the appropriate speed and degree of glucose lowering. It also raises questions regarding the means of glucose lowering. It seems a reasonable conclusion, but remains unproved, that factors related to intensive therapy, namely hypoglycaemia, weight gain and fluid retention, were also associated with the increased risk of death. Therefore, interventions which do not cause these problems may yield more benefit and fewer concerns. Currently, these therapies include diet, metformin, acarbose, weight-loss drugs, bariatric surgery, GLP-1 mimetics and DPP-IV inhibitors. Current and as yet unplanned studies will answer some of these questions. Clinical guidelines in the future may reflect agent-specific targets for HbA_{1c}.

Authorities worldwide have addressed blood glucose-lowering goals in type 2 diabetes. Among groups who have developed guidelines following rigorous processes and with clear scope and methodology, the National Institute of Clinical Health and Excellence (NICE) has stated in guidelines that one should 'involve the person in decisions about their individual HbA_{1c} target level, which may be above that of 6.5% set for people with type 2 diabetes in general ...' and to 'avoid pursuing highly intensive management to levels of less than 6.5%'.[51] The Scottish Intercollegiate Guidelines Network (SIGN) has called for an 'HbA_{1c} ideally around 7%'.[52] The Canadian Diabetes Association, which has been noted to place greater emphasis on observational studies,[53] calls for an HA_{1c} of 7% or lower and a value of lower than 6%, if achievable safely.[54] In a review of existing guidelines, weighing those performed with appropriate methodologies more highly, a representative from the American College of Physicians wrote, 'A haemoglobin A_{1c} level less than 7% based on individualized assessment is a reasonable goal for many but not all patients'.[53]

In general, guidelines advocate initiating therapy with metformin in overweight individuals, with the addition of subsequent agents as indicated by blood glucose levels. With respect to individual drugs, achievement of blood glucose lowering, rather than using specific therapies, guides most recommendations.

Future research questions relate largely to the ability of newer blood glucose-lowering therapies to reduce the risk of cardiovascular complications and to defining the target level of glycaemia at which the benefits of therapy exceed the side-effects and financial costs. Long-term trials of blood glucose lowering which also cause weight loss are essential. Since drugs may have effects beyond blood glucose lowering for which they receive authorization, trials must test specific drugs in addition to blood glucose lowering *per se*.

References

1 Stratton IM, Adler AI, Neil HAW, Matthews DR, Manley SE, Cull CA, Hadden D, Turner RC, Holman RR, on behalf of the UKPDSG. Association of glycaemia with macrovascular and microvascular complications of type 2 diabetes (UKPDS 35): prospective observational study. *BMJ* 2000;**321**:405–411.

2 Selvin E, Marinopoulos S, Berkenblit G, Rami T, Brancati FL, Powe NR, Golden SH. Meta-analysis: glycosylated hemoglobin and cardiovascular disease in diabetes mellitus. *Ann Intern Med* 2004;**141**(6):421–431.

3 Brownlee M. The pathobiology of diabetic complications: a unifying mechanism. *Diabetes* 2005;**54**(6):1615–1625.

4 Meinert C, Knatterud G, Prout T, Klimt C. A study of the effects of hypoglycemic agents on vascular complications in patients with adult-onset diabetes. *Diabetes* 1970; **19**:789–830.

5 University Group Diabetes Program. A study of the effects of hypoglycemic agents on vascular complications in patients with adult-onset diabetes. *Diabetes* 1970;**19**:789–830.

6 Feinglos M, Bethel M. Therapy of type 2 diabetes, cardiovascular death and the UGDP. *Am Heart J* 1999;**138**:346–352.

7 Seltzer HS. Avoiding the pitfalls of long-term therapeutic trials: lessons learned from the UGDP study. *J Clin Pharmacol New Drugs* 1972;**12**(10):393–398.

8 Kilo C, Miller J, Williamson J. The Achilles heel of the University Group Diabetes Program. *JAMA* 1980;**243**: 450–457.

9 Schwartz TB Meinert CL. The UGDP controversy: thirty-four years of contentious ambiguity laid to rest. *Perspect Biol Med* 2004;**47**(4):564–574.

10 Abraira C, Colwell J, Nuttall F, Sawin C, Nagel N, Comstock J, Emanuele N, Levin S, Henderson W, Lee H. Veterans Affairs Cooperative Study on glycemic control and complications in type II diabetes (VA CSDM). Results of the

feasibility trial. Veterans Affairs Cooperative Study in Type II Diabetes. *Diabetes Care* 1995;**18**:1113–1123.

11 Kirkman MS McCarren M, Shah J, Duckworth W, Abraira C. The association between metabolic control and prevalent macrovascular disease in Type 2 diabetes: the VA Cooperative Study in diabetes. *J Diabetes Complications* 2006;**20**(2): 75–80.

12 Abraira C, Duckworth W, McCarren M, Emanuele N, Arca D, Reda D, Henderson W. Design of the cooperative study on glycemic control and complications in diabetes mellitus type 2: Veterans Affairs Diabetes Trial. *J Diabetes Complications* 2003;**17**(6):314–322.

13 Shichiri M, Kishikawa H, Ohkubo Y, Wake N. Long-term results of the Kumamoto Study on optimal diabetes control in type 2 diabetic patients. *Diabetes Care* 2000;**23**(Suppl 2): B21–B29.

14 UKPDS Group. Intensive blood-glucose control with sulphonylureas or insulin compared with conventional treatment and risk of complications in patients with type 2 diabetes (UKPDS 33). *Lancet* 1998;**352**:837–853.

15 UKPDS Group. Effect of intensive blood-glucose control with metformin on complications in overweight patients with type 2 diabetes (UKPDS 34). *Lancet* 1998;**352**:854–865.

16 Holman R, Paul S, Bethel M, Matthews D, Neil H. 10-year follow-up of intensive glucose control in type 2 diabetes. *N Engl J Med* 2008;**359**:1577–1589.

17 Gæde P, Vedel P, Larsen N, Jensen G, Parving H, Pedersen O. Multifactorial intervention and cardiovascular disease in patients with type 2 diabetes. *N Engl J Med* 2003;**348**: 383–393.

18 Gæde P, Lund-Andersen H, Parving HH Pedersen O. Effect of a multifactorial intervention on mortality in type 2 diabetes. *N Engl J Med* 2008;**358**:580–591.

19 Charbonnel B, Dormandy J, Erdmann E, Massi-Benedetti M, Skene A. The prospective pioglitazone clinical trial in macrovascular events (PROactive): can pioglitazone reduce cardiovascular events in diabetes? Study design and baseline characteristics of 5238 patients. *Diabetes Care* 2004;**27**: 1647–1653.

20 Dormandy JA, Charbonnel B, Eckland DJ, Erdmann E, Massi-Benedetti M, Moules IK, Skene AM, Tan MH, Lefebvre PJ, Murray GD, Standl E, Wilcox RG, Wilhelmsen L, Betteridge J, Birkeland K, Golay A, Heine RJ, Koranyi L, Laakso M, Mokan M, Norkus A, Pirags V, Podar T, Scheen A, Scherbaum W, Schernthaner G, Schmitz O, Skrha J, Smith U, Taton J. Secondary prevention of macrovascular events in patients with type 2 diabetes in the PROactive Study (PROspective pioglitAzone Clinical Trial In macroVascular Events): a randomised controlled trial. *Lancet* 2005;**366**(9493): 1279–1289.

21 Gerstein HC, Riddle MC, Kendall DM, Cohen RM, Goland R, Feinglos MN, Kirk JK, Hamilton BP, Ismail-Beigi F, Feeney P. Glycemia treatment strategies in the Action to Control Cardiovascular Risk in Diabetes (ACCORD) trial. *Am J Cardiol* 2007;**99**(12A):34i–43i.

22 Gerstein HC, Miller ME, Byington RP, Goff DC Jr, Bigger JT, Buse JB, Cushman WC, Genuth S, Ismail-Beigi F, Grimm RH Jr, Probstfield JL, Simons-Morton DG, Friedewald WT. Effects of intensive glucose lowering in type 2 diabetes. *N Engl J Med* 2008;**358**(24):2545–2559.

23 Chalmers J, Perkovic V, Joshi R, Patel A. ADVANCE: breaking new ground in type 2 diabetes. *J Hypertens Suppl* 2006;**24** (5):S22–S28.

24 Pittas AG, Siegel RD, Lau J. Insulin therapy and in-hospital mortality in critically ill patients: systematic review and meta-analysis of randomized controlled trials. *J Parenter Enteral Nutr* 2006;**30**(2):164–172.

25 Diaz R, Goyal A, Mehta SR, Afzal R, Xavier D, Pais P, Chrolavicius S, Zhu J, Kazmi K, Liu L, Budaj A, Zubaid M, Avezum A, Ruda M, Yusuf S. Glucose–insulin–potassium therapy in patients with ST-segment elevation myocardial infarction. *JAMA* 2007;**298**(20):2399–2405.

26 Gray CS, Hildreth AJ, Sandercock PA, O'Connell JE, Johnston DE, Cartlidge NE, Bamford JM, James OF, Alberti KG. Glucose–potassium–insulin infusions in the management of post-stroke hyperglycaemia: the UK Glucose Insulin in Stroke Trial (GIST-UK). *Lancet Neurol* 2007;**6** (5):397–406.

27 Malmberg K. Prospective randomised study of intensive insulin treatment on long term survival after acute myocardial infarction in patients with diabetes mellitus. DIGAMI (Diabetes Mellitus, Insulin Glucose Infusion in Acute Myocardial Infarction) Study Group. *BMJ* 1997;**314**:1512–1515.

28 Malmberg K, Ryden L, Wedel H, Birkeland K, Bootsma A, Dickstein K, Efendic S, Fisher M, Hamsten A, Herlitz J, Hildebrandt P, MacLeod K, Laakso M, Torp-Pedersen C, Waldenstrom A. Intense metabolic control by means of insulin in patients with diabetes mellitus and acute myocardial infarction (DIGAMI 2): effects on mortality and morbidity. *Eur Heart J* 2005;**26**(7):650–661.

29 Langley J, Adams G. Insulin-based regimens decrease mortality rates in critically ill patients: a systematic review. *Diabetes Metab Res Rev* 2007;**23**(3):184–192.

30 Chalk C, Benstead T, Moore F. Aldose reductase inhibitors for the treatment of diabetic polyneuropathy. *Cochrane Database Syst Rev* 2007; (4): Art. No.: CD004572. DOI: 10.1002/ 14651858. CD004572.pub2.

31 Way KJ, Katai N, King GL. Protein kinase C and the development of diabetic vascular complications. *Diabet Med* 2001;**18**(12):945–959.

32 The, PKC-DRS, Study Group. The effect of ruboxistaurin on visual loss in patients with moderately severe to very severe nonproliferative diabetic retinopathy: initial results of the Protein Kinase C beta Inhibitor Diabetic Retinopathy Study (PKC-DRS) multicenter randomized clinical trial. *Diabetes* 2005;**54**(7):2188–2197.

33 Sjostrom L, Narbro K, Sjostrom CD, Karason K, Larsson B, Wedel H, Lystig T, Sullivan M, Bouchard C, Carlsson B, Bengtsson C, Dahlgren S, Gummesson A, Jacobson P, Karlsson J, Lindroos AK, Lonroth H, Naslund I, Olbers T, Stenlof K, Torgerson J, Agren G, Carlsson LM. Effects of bariatric surgery on mortality in Swedish obese subjects. *N Engl J Med* 2007;**357**(8):741–752.

34 Brooks MM, Frye RL, Genuth S, Detre KM, Nesto R, Sobel BE, Kelsey SF, Orchard TJ. Hypotheses, design and methods for the Bypass Angioplasty Revascularization Investigation 2 Diabetes (BARI 2D) Trial. *Am J Cardiol* 2006;**97**(12A):9G–19G.

35 Milicevic Z, Raz I, Strojek K, Skrha J, Tan MH, Wyatt JW, Beattie SD, Robbins DC. Hyperglycemia and its effect after acute myocardial infarction on cardiovascular outcomes in

patients with Type 2 diabetes mellitus (HEART2D) Study design. *J Diabetes Complications* 2005;**19**(2):80–87.

36 Look, AHEAD, Research Group. Look AHEAD (Action for Health in Diabetes): design and methods for a clinical trial of weight loss for the prevention of cardiovascular disease in type 2 diabetes. *Controll Clin Trials* 2003;**24**:610–628.

37 Look, AHEAD, Research Group. Reduction in weight and cardiovascular disease risk factors in individuals with type 2 diabetes: one-year results of the look AHEAD trial. *Diabetes Care* 2007;**30**:1374–1383.

38 Look, AHEAD, Protocol Review, Committee. Protocol, Action for Health in Diabetes Look AHEAD Clinical Trial. https://wwwlookaheadtrialorg/public/LookAHEADProtocolpdf, 2005.

39 DECODE, Study Group. Glucose tolerance and cardiovascular mortality: comparison of fasting and 2-hour diagnostic criteria. *Arch Intern Med* 2001;**161**:397–405.

40 Barr EL, Zimmet PZ, Welborn TA, Jolley D, Magliano DJ, Dunstan DW, Cameron AJ, Dwyer T, Taylor HR, Tonkin AM, Wong TY, McNeil J, Shaw JE. Risk of cardiovascular and all-cause mortality in individuals with diabetes mellitus, impaired fasting glucose and impaired glucose tolerance: the Australian Diabetes, Obesity and Lifestyle Study (AusDiab). *Circulation* 2007;**116**(2):151–157.

41 ORIGIN, Trial Investigators. Rationale, design and baseline characteristics for a large international trial of cardiovascular disease prevention in people with dysglycemia: The ORIGIN Trial (Outcome Reduction with an Initial Glargine Intervention). *Am Heart J* 2008;**155**(26):26–32.

42 Chiasson JL, Josse RG, Gomis R, Hanefeld M, Karasik A, Laakso M. Acarbose for prevention of type 2 diabetes mellitus: the STOP-NIDDM randomised trial. *Lancet* 2002; **359**(9323):2072–2077.

43 Holman R. A new era in the secondary prevention of CVD in prediabetes – the Acarbose Cardiovascular Evaluation (ACE) trial. *Diabetes Vasc Dis Res* **4**(Suppl 1.): 2007.

44 Home PD, Pocock SJ, Beck-Nielsen H, Gomis R, Hanefeld M, Dargie H, Komajda M, Gubb J, Biswas N, Jones NP. Rosiglitazone Evaluated for Cardiac Outcomes and Regulation of Glycaemia in Diabetes (RECORD): study design and protocol. *Diabetologia* 2005;**48**(9):1726–1735.

45 Nissen SE, Wolski K. Effect of rosiglitazone on the risk of myocardial infarction and death from cardiovascular causes. *N Engl J Med* 2007;**356**(24):2457–2471.

46 Home PD, Pocock SJ, Beck-Nielsen H, Gomis R, Hanefeld M, Jones NP, Komajda M, McMurray JJ. Rosiglitazone evaluated for cardiovascular outcomes – an interim analysis. *N Engl J Med* 2007;**357**(1):28–38.

47 Kahn SE, Haffner SM, Heise MA, Herman WH, Holman RR, Jones NP, Kravitz BG, Lachin JM, O'Neill MC, Zinman B, Viberti G. Glycemic durability of rosiglitazone, metformin or glyburide monotherapy. *N Engl J Med* 2006;**355**(23): 2427–2443.

48 Norris S, Zhang X, Avenell A, Gregg E, Schmid C, Lau J. Pharmacotherapy for weight loss in adults with type 2 diabetes mellitus. *Cochrane Database Syst Rev* (1):2005; Issue 1. Art. No.: CD004096. DOI:10.1002/14651858.CD004096.pub2.

49 Torp-Pedersen C, Caterson I, Coutinho W, Finer N, Van Gaal L, Maggioni A, Sharma A, Brisco W, Deaton R, Shepherd G, James P. Cardiovascular responses to weight management and sibutramine in high-risk subjects: an analysis from the SCOUT trial. *Eur Heart J* 2007;**28**(23):2915–2923.

50 Scheen AJ, Finer N, Hollander P, Jensen MD, Van Gaal LF. Efficacy and tolerability of rimonabant in overweight or obese patients with type 2 diabetes: a randomised controlled study. *Lancet* 2006;**368**(9548):1660–1672.

51 Home P, Mant J, Diaz J, Turner C. Management of type 2 diabetes: summary of updated NICE guidance. *BMJ* 2008;**336** (7656):1306–1308.

52 Scottish Intercollegiate Guidelines Network. Management of Diabetes, Report No. 55, SIGN, Edinburgh, 2001.

53 Qaseem A, Vijan S, Snow V, Cross JT, Weiss KB, Owens DK. Glycemic control and type 2 diabetes mellitus: the optimal hemoglobin A_{1c} targets. A guidance statement from the American College of Physicians. *Ann Intern Med* 2007; **147**(6):417–422.

54 Canadian Diabetes Association Clinical Practice Guidelines Expert Committee. Canadian Diabetes Association 2003 Clinical Practice Guidelines for the Prevention and Management of Diabetes in Canada. *Can J Diabetes* 2003;**27**(Suppl 2): S1–S152.

11 Glycaemic control and other interventions in the treatment of gestational diabetes

David R. McCance

Regional Centre for Endocrinology and Diabetes, Belfast, UK

Introduction

Some 50 years on from the originally published description of gestational diabetes mellitus, debate continues as to the significance of minor degrees of glucose intolerance during pregnancy for maternal/fetal outcome.[1] Confusion has been compounded by different diagnostic practices and a growing number of studies pointing to a continuum of glycaemic risk. A fundamental lack of robust evidence is reflected in the lack of consensus among published guidelines. The picture has further been complicated by the current sophistication of obstetric and neonatal intensive care, the potential for confounding by established risk factors and traditional obstetric practice. Until recently, the therapeutic options have largely rested on a combination of diet and exercise with our without the addition of insulin. Evolution of the therapeutic armamentarium to include insulin analogues and oral hypoglycaemic agents has presented new challenges in terms of both efficacy and safety. We are only just beginning to appreciate the impact of the intrauterine milieu for future generations, and it is vital that clearly defined and meaningful short- and long-term outcomes are considered in intervention trials and economic equations.

This chapter reviews the role of glycaemic control and other interventions in the treatment of gestational diabetes mellitus. The key focus is on data from randomized trials, but, given a limited literature, observational and prospective data are also reviewed. The primary question is whether treatment can be justified by its ability to improve adverse health outcomes. The possibilities for the future are discussed.

Background

Gestational diabetes mellitus (GDM) is defined as carbohydrate intolerance with onset or first recognition during pregnancy.[2] This definition, however, provides little insight into underlying pathophysiology, the spectrum of associated glycaemia and the impact of such a diagnosis for maternal/fetal outcome.

GDM is the commonest medical condition of pregnancy, with estimates varying between 2 and 7%.[3,4] Recognized risk factors for developing GDM include increasing maternal age, a family history of diabetes, a history of GDM in a previous pregnancy and increased body mass index (BMI) preceding pregnancy.[5] The prevalence of GDM is directly proportional to the prevalence of type 2 diabetes in a given population or ethnic group[3] and is more common among African American, Hispanic and American Indian women and less common among Asian women and with the use of different diagnostic criteria. Prevalence rates range from 1.4 to 2.8% among women at low risk,[6,7] while higher rates (3.3–6.1%) among those with defined high risk factors have been reported.[6] Despite this variation, screening and diagnostic approaches generally highlight women with asymptomatic glucose intolerance in the upper end of the population distribution during pregnancy; the presumption being

The Evidence Base for Diabetes Care, Second Edition, Edited by William H. Herman, Ann Louise Kinmonth, Nicholas J. Wareham and Rhys Williams.
© 2010 John Wiley & Sons, Ltd

that only a small minority would have glucose levels diagnostic of diabetes outside pregnancy. There is a consensus that the prevalence of GDM is increasing globally.

Pathophysiology

In normal pregnancy, the fasting levels of glucose range from 3.3 to 5.0 mmol l^{-1} (from 60 to 90 mg dl^{-1}); 1 and 2 h post-prandial levels of glucose are less than 7.8 mmol l^{-1} (140 mg dl^{-1}) and 6.7 mmol l^{-1} (120 mg dl^{-1}), respectively.[8] Pregnant women demonstrate a spectrum of glucose intolerance exemplified by prolonged post-prandial hyperglycaemia and hyperinsulinaemia, but with mild fasting hypoglycaemia.

Pregnancy is normally associated with progressive insulin resistance that begins near mid-pregnancy and progresses to levels approximating that seen in individuals with type 2 diabetes by the end of pregnancy. The insulin resistance seems to result from a combination of increased maternal adiposity and the insulin-antagonizing effects of placental hormones (supported by the rapid abatement of insulin resistance after delivery). Pancreatic beta cells normally increase their insulin secretion to compensate for the insulin resistance of pregnancy, with the result that changes in circulating glucose levels during pregnancy are fairly small compared with the large changes in insulin sensitivity.[9] However, the increase occurs along an insulin sensitivity–secretion curve that is approximately 50% lower (i.e. 50% less insulin for any degree of insulin resistance) than that of normal women (Figure 11.1).

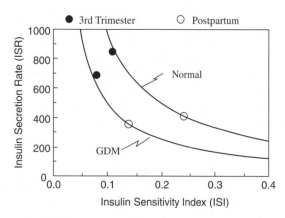

Figure 11.1 Insulin sensitivity–secretion relationships in normal women and women with GDM during the third trimester and postpartum. Pre-hepatic insulin secretion was assessed during steady-state hyperglycaemia using plasma insulin and c-peptide kinetics in individual patients. Insulin sensitivity was calculated as the ratio of glucose disposal rate to plasma insulin during steady-state hyperglycaemia. Reproduced with permission from the Endocrine Society (Ref. 9)

In late pregnancy, when insulin requirements are high and differ only slightly between normal women and women with GDM, reduced responses to nutrients have been consistently reported in women with GDM.[10] Studies conducted before and after pregnancy reveal that both lean and obese women with prior GDM[11,12] are usually more insulin resistant than normal women. Insulin responses in these two groups may be similar or reduced only slightly in women with prior GDM,[11,12] but the latter group show a large defect in beta cell function when each individual response is expressed in relation to individual insulin resistance.[9]

The causes of inadequate beta cell function are incompletely understood but, extrapolating from mechanisms outside pregnancy, might include autoimmune beta cell destruction, monogenic diabetes and beta cell dysfunction which occurs on a background of chronic insulin resistance (the majority of women with GDM). An appreciation of these various aetiologies is needed to direct appropriate treatment strategies both during and after pregnancy. Only a small number of potential mediators of the chronic insulin resistance that frequently accompanies GDM have been examined. Several small studies documenting alterations in cytokines and inflammatory markers would be consistent with obesity-related insulin resistance,[13] and there are analogies which can be drawn between the biochemical abnormalities of pregnancy and the metabolic syndrome.

The exaggerated insulin resistance of pregnancy does not appear to result from defects in binding of insulin to its receptor in skeletal muscle.[13] Although various abnormalities in skeletal muscle or fat cells of women with GDM or previous GDM have been reported, whether these defects are primary or the result of defects in insulin action is unknown.[9]

Relevant outcomes

Relevant short- and long-term outcomes for both mother and infant are listed in Table 11.1. Detection and intervention strategies for GDM are justified by their impact on these outcomes. Most studies, however, have focused on macrosomia as the outcome of interest and possibly the only factor reversible by treatment. The key issue is whether excess fetal growth is associated with an increased risk of adverse neonatal outcomes such as brachial plexus injuries (most of which are temporary) and clavicular fracture.[14] Data on the overall impact of GDM screening and treatment on these outcomes are limited because most babies with macrosomia are born to mothers without GDM,[15–17] and most cases of injuries related

Table 11.1 Relevant maternal and fetal outcomes

Mother	Offspring
Caesarean delivery	Perinatal mortality
Third- and fourth-degree lacerations	Brachial plexus injury or clavicular fracture secondary to fetal macrosomia resulting in shoulder dystocia
Pre-eclampsia	Hypoglycaemia
Later development of type 1 and type 2 diabetes	Hyperbilirubinaemia
	Polycythaemia

to shoulder dystocia occur in pregnancies with infants of normal birth weight. The relationship between GDM and adverse outcomes is further confounded by the fact that maternal obesity is an independent risk factor for many of the same outcomes.[18–20] The association between GDM and fetal macrosomia persists but is decreased after controlling for maternal weight.[21] Much less is known about the association between morbidities such as neonatal hypoglycaemia and hyperbilirubinaemia with maternal glucose levels in GDM. Long-term outcomes (obesity, cardiovascular risk) have been relatively ignored, but are of major public health significance.

Obstetric outcomes may be simple to define but more difficult to standardize and still tend to reflect traditional obstetric practice rather than significant metabolic antecedents.[20] Perinatal mortality is now uncommon, most likely as a direct reflection of improved obstetric/neonatal care, and it may not be possible to reduce existing rates further.[22] It is now generally accepted that gestational diabetes is a risk factor for diabetes after pregnancy.[1,23–26] Relevant risk factors include obesity, advanced maternal age and the use of insulin, but widely differing rates are reported and comparisons are made difficult by variable periods of follow-up and by the use of differing criteria inside and outside pregnancy.[14]

Diagnosis of GDM

Type 1 diabetes preceding pregnancy is usually associated with the highest maternal blood glucose levels. Here the diagnosis is not in doubt and these pregnancies are at increased risk of multiple complications for both mother and fetus, which are improved by current treatment. The relation between hyperglycaemia during pregnancy and adverse outcome would appear to be continuous.[20,27–30] The point on this

continuum of glucose intolerance that defines 'gestational diabetes' is controversial and there is no universally accepted 'gold standard'. Different diagnostic criteria are used in North America and Europe. In the United States, the O'Sullivan and Mahan criteria[24,31] endorsed by the National Diabetes Data Group are currently used. These criteria employ a 100 g 3 h glucose tolerance test, with the requirement that two or more cutpoints are exceeded for diagnosis.[1] These criteria, however, were originally developed for their ability to predict the subsequent development of diabetes in the mother rather than adverse neonatal outcomes.[23,24] More recently, alternative figures have been proposed by Carpenter and Coustan [endorsed by the 4th GDM Workshop and the American Diabetes Association (ADA)],[2,32] correcting not only for the change from venous whole blood to plasma, but also for the use of glucose oxidase or hexokinase methodology, which yields values approximately $0.27 \, \text{mmol} \, \text{l}^{-1}$ ($5 \, \text{mg} \, \text{dl}^{-1}$) lower than the Somogi–Nelson criteria (Table 11.2). In several studies, the revised criteria identified more patients with GDM whose infants had perinatal morbidity.[1] These latter, more inclusive, criteria may increase the number of women diagnosed with GDM by more than 50% but may not reduce the prevalence of fetal macrosomia.[2]

By contrast, in 1985, the World Health Organization (WHO) defined GDM using a 75 g OGTT on the basis of criteria used for non-pregnant adults.[33] These criteria include an additional category of impaired glucose tolerance (G-IGT) (venous plasma glucose fasting $>7.8 \, \text{mmol} \, \text{l}^{-1}$ and at 2 h $7.8–11.1 \, \text{mmol} \, \text{l}^{-1}$) with the onset or first recognition during pregnancy (Table 11.3). From 1998, the fasting glucose cutoff was reduced to $7 \, \text{mmol} \, \text{l}^{-1}$ with any glucose value above this level being indicative of diabetes.[34] In addition, a new category of impaired fasting plasma glucose (IFG) [$6.0–6.9 \, \text{mmol} \, \text{l}^{-1}$ ($108–125 \, \text{mg} \, \text{dl}^{-1}$)] was created. More recently, the lower limit of IFG was reduced further by the ADA to $5.6 \, \text{mmol} \, \text{l}^{-1}$ ($100 \, \text{mg} \, \text{dl}^{-1}$).[35] Both IFG and IGT have been officially termed 'pre-diabetes'; both are risk factors for future diabetes and cardiovascular disease. The WHO criteria identify twice as many women with GDM as do NDDG criteria; ADA criteria give an intermediate prevalence.[2]

By way of compromise, the 4th International Workshop Conference on Gestational Diabetes Mellitus suggested that the same numerical values be used for the fasting, 1 and 2 h time points in both the 75 g OGTT and the Carpenter–Coustan 100 g test (again with two being exceeded for diagnosis); the cutpoints were justified on the basis that they represented the mean ± 1.5 SDs of the OGTT in a study by Sacks *et al*.[27]

Table 11.2 Diagnostic scheme for gestational mellitus as defined by the Fourth Gestational Diabetes Workshop–Conference on Gestational Diabetes Mellitus in 1998[2]

| Venous plasma glucose | 100 g OGTT diagnostic test[a] | | | |
| | Carpenter and Coustan | | 4th GDM Workshop | |
	mmol l^{-1}	mg dl^{-1}	mmol l^{-1}	mg dl^{-1}
Fasting	5.3	95	5.3	95
1 h	10.0	180	10.0	180
2 h	8.6	155	8.6	155
3 h	7.8	140		

[a]The cutoff values for the diagnosis of GDM with a 100 g oral glucose load proposed by the 4th GDM Workshop and ADA are those of Carpenter and Coustan. The 4th GDM Workshop also proposed that the 1 h and 2 h cut-off values be used for diagnosis of GDM after a 75 g oral glucose load (see text). Using a 75 g load, two or more of the venous plasma concentrations must be met or exceeded for a positive diagnosis. These cut-off values are of necessity arbitrary.

but with the 2 h value being raised to 8.6 mmol l^{-1} to provide consistency with the 100 g OGTT.[2]

It was against this background that the Hyperglycaemia in Pregnancy Outcome (HAPO) Study[30,36] was conceived. The HAPO Study was a multicentre, multicultural, observational study, specifically designed to examine whether maternal hyperglycaemia, less severe than that in diabetes mellitus, is associated with increased risks of adverse maternal fetal outcome. The study comprised 25 000 individuals who underwent a 75 g OGTT at 28 weeks gestation with caregivers blinded to the results unless the fasting glucose was >5.8 mmol l^{-1} or the 2 h level was above 11.1 mmol l^{-1}. The primary results of this study have been published[36] and demonstrated a continuum of risk, without clear thresholds, between glucose levels during pregnancy (fasting, 1 and 2 h glucose during the OGTT) and increased birth weight and cord-blood c-peptide levels. Weaker associations were found

between glucose levels and primary Caesarean delivery and neonatal hypoglycaemia (Figure 11.2). The associations persisted after controlling for multiple confounding variables including field centre, maternal BMI, previous macrosomia and previous gestational diabetes mellitus. Positive associations were also found between increasing plasma glucose levels and each of the five secondary outcomes examined: premature delivery, shoulder dystocia or birth injury, intensive neonatal care, hyperbilirubinaemia and pre-eclampsia. Individual glucose measures from the OGTT were not highly correlated and no single measure was clearly superior in predicting the primary outcomes. The large study size, broad inclusion criteria and similarity across centres in the associations between maternal glycaemia and outcomes, support the development of universal outcome-based criteria for classifying glucose metabolism in pregnancy. However, in the absence of clear

Table 11.3 1997/2003 ADA and 1998 WHO criteria for the diagnosis of diabetes mellitus[a]

Normoglycaemia	IFG and IGT//G-IGT	Diabetes mellitus
FPG <6.1 mmol l^{-1}	FPG ≥5.6 mmol l^{-1} (100 mg dl^{-1}) but <7.0 mmol l^{-1} (125 mg dl^{-1}) (IFG)	FPG ≥7.0 mmol l^{-1} (126 mg dl^{-1})
2 h PG <7.8 mmol l^{-1}	2 h PG ≥7.8 mmol l^{-1} (140 mg dl^{-1}) but <11.1 mmol l^{-1} (200 mg dl^{-1}) (IGT)	2 h PG ≥11.1 mmol l^{-1} (200 mg dl^{-1})
		Symptoms of diabetes and casual plasma glucose ≥11.1 mmol l^{-1} (200 mg dl^{-1})

[a]Plasma glucose (PG) values in mmol l^{-1} (mg dl^{-1}); FPG (fasting plasma glucose), 2 h PG (2 h post-load plasma glucose); impaired fasting glucose (IFG), impaired glucose tolerance (IGT). 1997 ADA recommendations included a reduction in FPG cutpoint from 7.8 to 7.0 mmol l^{-1} and creation of a new IFG category; the lower limit of this category was recently reduced from 6.0 to 5.6 mmol l^{-1} (see text). A diagnosis of diabetes must be confirmed on a subsequent day by any one of the three methods included in the chart. Fasting is defined as no caloric intake for at least 8 h. The term gestational diabetes is retained but now encompasses the groups formerly classified as gestational impaired glucose tolerance (G-IGT) and gestational diabetes mellitus.

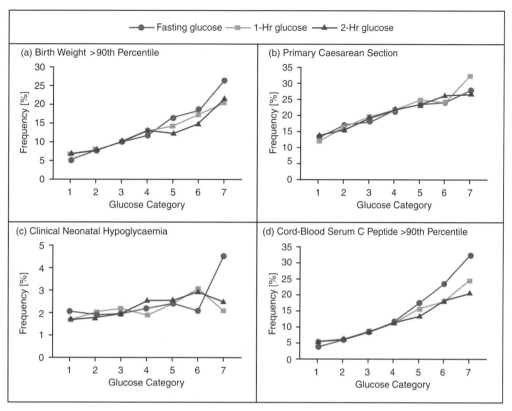

Figure 11.2 Frequency of primary outcomes across the glucose categories. Glucose categories are defined as follows. Fasting plasma glucose level: category 1, 4.2 mmol l^{-1} or less; category 2, 4.2–4.4 mmol l^{-1}; category 3, 4.5–4.7 mmol l^{-1}; category 4, 4.8–4.9 mmol l^{-1}; category 5, 5.0–5.2 mmol l^{-1}; category 6, 5.3–5.5 mmol l^{-1}; category 7, 5.6 mmol l^{-1} or more. 1 h plasma glucose: category 1, 5.8 mmol l^{-1} or less; category 2, 5.9–7.3 mmol l^{-1}; category 3, 7.4–8.6 mmol l^{-1}; category 4, 8.7–9.5 mmol l^{-1}; category 5, 9.6–10.7 mmol l^{-1}; category 6, 10.8–11.7 mmol l^{-1}; category 7, 11.8 mmol l^{-1} or more. 2 h plasma glucose: category 1, 5.0 mmol l^{-1} or less; category 2, 5.1–6.0 mmol l^{-1}; category 3, 6.1–6.9 mmol l^{-1}, category 4, 7.0–7.7 mmol l^{-1}; category 5, 7.8–8.7 mmol l^{-1}; category 6.8.8–9.8 mmol l^{-1}; category 7, 9.9 mmol l^{-1} or more. Reproduced with permission from the *New England Journal of Medicine* (Ref. 30)

thresholds for risk and given the fact that the four primary outcomes are not necessarily of equal importance, direct translation of the HAPO Study results into clinical practice clearly will require an international consensus.

Screening strategies for GDM

In the absence of a 'gold standard' diagnostic test, defining the characteristics of a screening test is problematic. In North America, screening traditionally has been based on a 50 g 1 h non-fasting glucose challenge test, usually performed between the 24 and 28th week of gestation. Two abnormal thresholds were proposed by different groups: a venous plasma glucose of 7.2 mmol l^{-1} (130 mg dl^{-1})[25] (usually positive for 20–25% of all pregnant women and identifying more than 90% of women with a positive 100 g 3 h OGTT) and a higher cutpoint of 7.8 mmol l^{-1} (140 mg dl^{-1})[31] (positive in 14–18% of women and detecting 80% of women with an abnormal OGTT).[2] The latter

figure results in a reduced rate of false positives – a common feature with the GCT. Less than 20% with a positive GCT will have GDM diagnosed on a full OGTT.[37] Methodological limitations, including the poor reproducibility of the OGTT, non-fasting status and the optimal timing for the test, are well recognized.[1] Diagnosis ideally should be made at a time when the greatest number of women can be identified and meaningful intervention implemented.

Other screening approaches include the use of fasting or random glucose measurements,[1,38] a fixed dose of simple sugar (such as jelly beans)[39] or a single-step 75 or 100 g oral glucose challenge test.[4] A single report suggested that it may be possible to avoid the glucose challenge test in parous women with negative GDM screening during a previous pregnancy occurring within 4 years; the risk for recurrent GDM in these circumstances is <1%.[40] A relatively simple and pragmatic universal screening approach has been adopted by Diabetes UK[41] involving the testing of urine at each visit with the addition of a timed random laboratory plasma glucose measurement at booking, 28 weeks

Table 11.4 Screening consensus statement

Organization	Recommendation
Canadian Task Force on the Periodic Health Examination (1992)[44]	Insufficient evidence for or against screening
	Evidence for screening is poor
US Preventive Services Task Force (1996)[45]	Insufficient evidence for or against routine screening
Fourth International Workshop–Conference on Gestational Diabetes Mellitus (1998)[2]	Selective screening based on risk factors
Australian Diabetes in Pregnancy Society (1998)[34]	Selective screening based on risk factors
American Diabetes Association (1999)[31]	Selective screening based on risk factors
American College of Obstetricians and Gynaecologists (2001)[3]	No definite recommendation
	No data to support the benefit of screening
	Selective screening in some settings; universal in others
Diabetes UK[41]	Universal screening
National Institute of Clinical Excellence (UK) (2003)[47]	No evidence to justify routine screening

gestation and whenever $\geq 1+$ glycosuria is detected. A 75 g OGTT is performed if the timed random blood glucose concentrations are (a) >6 mmol l^{-1} fasting or 2 h after food or (b) > 7 mmol l^{-1} within 2 h of food.

Despite the universal consensus that the prevalence if GDM is increasing globally, national bodies and expert groups disagree as to whether or not to recommend screening. (Table 11.4).[2–4,14,15,42–48] A 1994 ACOG Technical Bulletin on Diabetes in Pregnancy failed to endorse a universal screening programme.[15] Both the American Diabetes Association and the 4th International Workshop on Gestational Diabetes Mellitus recommend selective screening (screening all women with risk factors and no glucose testing of women who do not meet specific criteria).[2,43] This was subsequently endorsed in more recent position statements[4] and would exempt only around 10% of a predominantly white population.[3] In the mid-1990s, the US Preventive Services Task Force[45] and earlier the Canadian Task Force on the Periodic Health Examination[44] concluded that the evidence was insufficient to recommend for or against routine screening. Others have concluded that routine screening in pregnancy is not indicated[47] and, except for research purposes, should be abandoned.[48]

Justification for intervention

Discussion of treatment options is predicated on the assumption that GDM is a disease entity which justifies screening and is associated with significant adverse outcomes.

Screening

In the only RCT, Griffin et al.[49] examined the effect of selective screening (based on risk factors at 32 weeks gestation) or universal screening (between 26 and 28 weeks gestation) for gestational diabetes on maternal and neonatal outcomes. The prevalence of GDM was 2.7% in the universal screening group and 1.45% in the selective screening group ($p < 0.03$). Women with GDM in the universal screening group had improved health outcomes (spontaneous vaginal deliveries, Caesarean delivery, prematurity, pre-eclampsia and admissions to neonatal intensive care units) compared with women found to have GDM in the selective group and to a combination of women found not to have diabetes from both screening groups. The study was flawed by differences in the timing and duration of treatment, the lack of an intention-to-screen analysis or statistical comparison between the universal and selective groups, the composition of the control group and the lack of blinding of obstetric management. In summary, this study did not answer the question of whether universal screening offers benefits beyond selective screening or whether either is more effective than no screening at all.

Retrospective studies comparing screened with unscreened populations are also flawed;[50,51] those that found no significant differences in macrosomia or birth trauma do not definitively exclude a benefit of screening because of insufficient size and the fact that that women screened for GDM are more likely to be at high risk.[50] Moreover, generally improved outcomes, irrespective of screening, seen with more recent cohorts, suggest that any previous association between GDM and perinatal mortality may be diminished by current day obstetric practice. Alternatively, better glycaemic control may account for this improved outcome.

A prospective cohort study (The Toronto Tri-Hospital Gestational Diabetes Project)[21] compared (1) non-GDM (blinded caregivers), (2) women with carbohydrate intolerance who did not meet criteria for GDM by NDDG criteria (caregivers blinded), which can essentially be viewed as an unscreened group, and (3) women diagnosed with GDM (caregivers unblinded and GDM treated). The borderline untreated group had higher rates of macrosomia (28.7 vs 13.7%, $p < 0.001$) and Caesarean delivery (29.6 vs 20.2%, $p = 0.03$) compared with the normoglycaemic group. Treatment of GDM normalized the birth weights but the rate of Caesarean delivery (33%) (controlled for multiple risk factors) remained significantly increased compared with normoglycaemic controls, whether macrosomia was present or not. Other maternal outcomes such as lacerations, peripheral nerve injuries or fractures did not differ between the groups.

One ecological study found no evidence that a programme of universal screening compared with a geographic area without such a programme reduced macrosomia, Caesarean delivery or other diabetes-related complications.[52]

Adverse outcomes and untreated or undiagnosed GDM

Determining the existence and magnitude of a causal association between GDM (of various degrees) and adverse health outcomes is complicated by traditional obstetric practice and by interventions to treat GDM. Moreover, if the risk of adverse health outcomes with hyperglycaemia is continuous, as some studies suggest,[2,27,28,30,43] then considering GDM as a dichotomous variable may underestimate or miss the association altogether.

Although some (and particularly older) studies found an association between untreated GDM and increased perinatal mortality,[24,53–55] perinatal rates have declined in both groups and more recent studies have generally failed to confirm this.[20,51,56–58] No still births were reported in three large studies including untreated women with GDM since 1985,[20,56,58] but one occurred among 131 women with a 2 h glucose between 7.8 and 8.9 mmol l^{-1}.[54] The extent to which GDM is associated with perinatal mortality remains unclear – the reduced perinatal mortality in these studies may be attributable to small size, the actual lack of an association or improved obstetric care.

Several large recent studies of untreated women with GDM reported rates of macrosomic infants (greater than 4000 g) between 17 and 29%[20,56,57] and LGA (≥90th centile) from 22 to 42%;[54,58,59] these compare with general population figures of 10%[52] and 1.5%,[6] respectively. Most infants with macrosomia, however, are born to women without GDM.[16] Other risk factors for macrosomia are well recognized;[14]

maternal obesity, for example, is an important potential confounding factor associated both with GDM and (independently) with macrosomia.[21]

Langer et al.[60] reported rates of perinatal morbidity among 555 gravidas (GDM diagnosed after 37 weeks) compared with 1110 patients treated for GDM and 1110 non-diabetic control individuals matched for delivery year, obesity, parity, ethnicity, gestational age at delivery and prenatal visits. Women were treated with both intermediate- and/or short-acting insulin if they failed to achieve established levels of glycaemic control after 2 weeks on diet [fasting >5.3 mmol l^{-1} (95 mg dl^{-1}), 2 h >6.7 mmol l^{-1} (120 mg dl^{-1}) and mean >5.5 mmol l^{-1} (100 mg dl^{-1})]. A composite adverse outcome (stillbirth, neonatal macrosomia/LGA, neonatal hypoglycaemia, erythrocytosis and hyperbilirubinaemia with at least one of the five components present for positive diagnosis) occurred in 59% of untreated, 18% of treated and 11% of non-diabetic patients. A 2–4-fold increase in metabolic complications, macrosomia/LGA and neonatal morbidity (not associated with obesity) was found in the untreated group compared with the other two groups. It was concluded that untreated GDM carried significant risk for perinatal morbidity in all disease severity levels and timely and effective treatment may substantially improve outcome.

The significance of macrosomia is through its linkage to birth trauma. Recent observational studies have shown that the incidence of injury related to shoulder dystocia is 1.6 and 5.7% for neonates greater than 4000 and 4500 g, respectively.[61,62] Clavicular fracture occurs in 0.3–0.7% of all deliveries and is increased approximately 10-fold for macrosomic infants. Three large observational studies of non-diabetic mothers reported rates of birth-related brachial plexus injuries among vaginally born infants with birth weights ≥4000 g ranging from 0.6 to 1.1% compared with 2.1–5% for infants (of similar birth weight) born to diabetic mothers.[61,63,64] The best available data on untreated GDM women reveal no differences in the rates of brachial plexus injury or clavicular fracture between untreated women with GDM and the non-GDM population.[20] One study, however, of only 16 patients[54] found increased rates for both of these outcomes above the general population percentage of less than 1%. Recent data suggest that women with higher levels of hyperglycaemia treated for GDM may have a 2% increase in brachial plexus injury and 6% in clavicular fracture.[54,65] Most often brachial plexus injuries do not lead to permanent disability with 80–90% having resolved by 1 year of life.[14]

GDM may be a risk factor for other complications such as pre-term birth, hypoglycaemia, hyperbilirubinaemia and polycythaemia, but the literature is limited.[56,66–70] The evidence is possibly strongest for neonatal hypoglycaemia, where higher rates among untreated than treated women with GDM have been reported,[56] but the magnitude of clinically significant hypoglycaemia is unclear and increased surveillance of infants of GDM mothers may contribute to increased detection.

Some studies have suggested that GDM may have long-term implications for the offspring, such as impaired glucose tolerance, childhood obesity and neuropsychological disturbances,[71–75] but the results are variable, the studies do not always differentiate women with GDM[71,72] and in two studies the populations had a high genetic predisposition to obesity and diabetes, making the findings difficult to generalize.[71,72] Two studies found no association between GDM and childhood obesity,[73,74] while Vohr et al.,[75] using multivariate analyses, showed that infant BMI and maternal prepregnancy BMI predicted 7-year-old BMI in the GDM group, whereas maternal prepregnancy BMI and weight gain during pregnancy were positive predictors for control individuals. Overall data on obesity in the offspring of mothers with GDM are limited and the mixed results may be explained by methodological flaws, including parental obesity.[73–75] No data are available on offspring from women with GDM subjected to intervention.

Maternal health outcomes

Fetal macrosomia may lead to maternal trauma by increasing the risk of Caesarean delivery[17,18,62] and third- and fourth-degree perineal lacaerations.[76] Limited data on unrecognized or untreated women with GDM over the last 25 years reveal Caesarean delivery rates of 22%[18] to 30%[20] compared with around 17% for non GDM women, but some studies are limited by lack of adjustment for maternal obesity and the impact of the diagnosis of GDM on clinical decision making. Limited evidence is available on the rate of perineal lacerations. The single study that found a substantial percentage of women with GDM who had such lacerations had only 16 individuals;[54] another study found equally low rates among women with and without GDM.[20]

An association between GDM and a higher risk of pre-eclampsia has been reported in some studies but not in others.[14] Jensen et al. found a rate of 20% of maternal hypertension in women treated for GDM compared with 11% in controls.[77] A positive association was reported in two large cohort studies[78,79] controlled for confounding variables. Obesity is also a risk factor for pre-eclampsia and may confound this relationship.[67] Recent data from untreated women with GDM[20] reported a rate of around 9% (similar to

that of treated women and women in the non-GDM group).[80–83] In the HAPO Study, the adjusted odds ratios (95% CI) for the association between maternal glycaemia and pre-eclampsia for a one standard deviation increase in glucose were 1.21 (1.13 to 1.29), 1.28 (1.20 to 1.37) and 1.28 (1.20 to 1.37) for the fasting, 1 h and 2 h OGTT glucose values, respectively.[30]

The diagnosis of GDM is now generally recognized to be associated with a higher risk for the future development of diabetes after pregnancy.[23–26] Observational studies have suggested that of women with GDM, 2% may develop type 2 diabetes within 6 months of delivery, 40% of Hispanic American women will develop diabetes over 6 years and 20–40% of white Europeans will develop it over 20 years. Overall, 17–68% of women with GDM will develop diabetes within 5–16 years after delivery,[1] most likely because pregnancy serves as a provocative test for uncovering women with subclinical degrees of glucose intolerance. As noted above, these studies are confounded by low participation rates, retrospective design, variable follow-up and differing diagnostic criteria within and outside pregnancy.

Intervention trials

A small number of randomized trials have examined the impact of glycaemic control on health outcomes in women with GDM. Unfortunately, the validity of these studies is often limited because of failure to recognized the following three factors. First, there is the degree of hyperglycaemia in study participants – as some adverse outcomes increase with the degree of hyperglycaemia, absolute risk reductions may be larger with higher glycaemic levels. Over 70% of women diagnosed with GDM have a mild degree of hyperglycaemia and are usually treated with diet alone.[51,84] Second, the hypothesis that improved glycaemic control results in improved outcomes can only be tested if there is a reasonable degree of separation of glycaemic control between the treatment and control groups. Third, there is a need to focus on relevant outcomes. Most studies to date have focused on short-term outcomes such as fetal macrosomia or biochemical outcomes such as neonatal hypoglycaemia. The problem with macrosomia is that only a small percentage of these cases lead to maternal or fetal trauma. Alternatively, few studies reporting biochemical endpoints such as glucose or bilirubin document the percentage of abnormalities that required treatment. In most of these studies, there is a lingering suspicion that differences attributed to improved glycaemic control may rather have reflected more intense surveillance of offspring of GDM pregnancies or bias created by knowledge of GDM status.[20,58,85] Few studies have examined the impact of intensive compared with less intensive therapy among GDM women with lower levels of glycaemia.

Medical nutritional therapy

Once the diagnosis has been made, a stepwise approach to management is usually initiated involving, first, advice about diet and exercise, followed by the introduction of pharmacotherapy if unsuccessful. The goal of therapy is to approach normoglycaemia.

A detailed review of the limited evidence for this treatment strategy was published by Dornhorst and Frost in 2002.[86] Few studies have examined the effect of intensive compared with less intensive glycaemic control in women with GDM who have mild hyperglycaemia. In the Cochrane database, a meta analysis of four randomized clinical trials involving 612 women examining the role of dietary therapy for impaired glucose tolerance in pregnancy revealed no significant reduction in offspring weighing more than 4000 g (OR 0.78, 95% CI 0.45 to 1.35) or for Caesarean deliveries (OR 0.97, 95% CI 0.65 to 1.44).[87] In an RCT by Li et al.,[58] participants were randomly assigned into three groups on the basis of the OGTT results: (1) mild GDM ($n = 75$) on the basis of the National Diabetes Data Group criteria, who remained untreated; (2) a group diagnosed by WHO criteria who were treated; and (3) a non-diabetic control group. There was no blinding of either the caregivers or the women to the OGTT results. The untreated GDM women had 29% LGA that was comparable to the rate of non-diabetic controls and treated GDM individuals; this may have reflected the inability of treated individuals to achieve glycaemic targets. Jovanovic et al. reported the effect of treatment of 83 female individuals with a positive glucose challenge test but a negative 100 g OGTT. The 35 individuals who were randomized to dietary counselling and home glucose monitoring had a lower prevalence of macrosomia than did controls; maternal complications did not differ between the groups.[88]

Despite this limited evidence, it should be noted that may studies have shown that maternal diet can influence maternal metabolism and fetal growth. In addition, the effectiveness of dietary and lifestyle measures post-partum were demonstrated among women with previous GDM in the DPP programme.[89] The optimal caloric content of a diet for a woman with GDM is uncertain. Obesity is a frequent accompaniment of GDM and treatment should be individualized and response assessed by regular monitoring of blood glucose. The ADA recommendations are based on ideal body weight (IBW): 36–40 kcal kg^{-1} for IBW <90%; 30 kcal kg^{-1} for IBW 90–120%; 24 kcal kg^{-1} for IBW 121–150%; and 12–18 kcal kg^{-1} for pre-pregnancy IBW >150%.[4,86] The literature suggests that it is the type rather than the absolute amount of carbohydrate and fat that dictates the metabolic response to diet. Dietary management needs to focus on reducing post-prandial glycaemia, thereby reducing fetal exposure to hyperglycaemia. Complex carbohydrate is consistently recommended over simple sugars, but the percentage of carbohydrate within the diet is debated. In one study, restricting carbohydrate content to 35–40% of calories decreased maternal post-prandial glucose levels.[90] In a prospective study of women with GDM, those assigned to a low (<42% carbohydrate) versus high (>42%) diet were likely to require insulin or to have a baby weighing >4 kg.[90] Diets that limit the proportion of carbohydrate over fat seem unwise given the fact that these women are already at increased risk of future diabetes and vascular disease. Use of low glycaemic index carbohydrate diets (recommended by the British guidelines) allows up to 60% of the total dietary energy with no detrimental effect on glucose tolerance.[86] Modest calorie restriction in obese GDM women (20–25 kcal kg^{-1} day^{-1}) resulted in fewer LGA infants compared with obese glucose-tolerant women on no diet,[86] and the published evidence supports limiting weight gain in all GDM pregnancies to the bottom rather than the top of that recommended for non-diabetic pregnancies.[86]

Exercise

Exercise is integral to the general management of diabetes and is considered safe for most women during pregnancy. The literature is limited and not infrequently the studies are combined with diet and insulin. Surrogate endpoints such as avoidance of the need for insulin therapy may be reported rather than clinical endpoints. Bung et al.[91] randomized 41 individuals with GDM requiring insulin to an exercise programme. Seventeen of the 21 individuals completed the programme while maintaining normoglycaemia and obviating insulin therapy. Maternal and neonatal complications did not differ between the study and control groups. Jovanovic-Peterson and Peterson et al.[92] applied arm ergometer training to a population of women with GDM and compared their glycaemia with that of women receiving only dietary instruction. The two groups' glycaemic levels started to diverge by the fourth week of the programme and by the sixth week the women in the exercise group had normalized their HbA$_{1c}$, fasting plasma glucose and their response to a glucose challenge test compared with no change in glucose levels in those women treated with diet alone. In a study of 12 women with GDM, 30 min of low- and moderate-intensity cycling (35 and 55% of estimated maximum oxygen consumption, respectively) reduced blood glucose progressively;[93] after 45 min, blood glucose levels or insulin levels did not differ between the groups.[94] No data are available that indicate that exercise during pregnancy can impact on neonatal birth weight.

Insulin

The usual approach, supported by the ADA and ACOG, is to consider insulin if medical nutritional therapy fails to maintain fasting plasma glucose ≤ 5.8 mmol l^{-1} (105 mg dl^{-1}), and/or 2 h post-prandial values ≤ 6.7–7.2 mmol l^{-1} (120–130 mg dl^{-1}).[4] No ideal insulin dosage or regimen has been identified for the management of GDM and many different approaches have been utilized. The ADA simply recommends that 'self-monitoring of blood glucose should guide doses and timing of the insulin regimen'.

Prospective studies of insulin treatment for GDM have generally shown a reduction in the likelihood of macrosomia.[95,96] There would appear to be an optimum level of glycaemic control. In a prospective study of 334 women with GDM treated with insulin, Langer et al.[95] showed that those with a mean plasma glucose level of 4.8–5.8 mmol l^{-1} (87–104 mg dl^{-1}) had an incidence of large for gestational age (LGA) and small for gestational age (SGA) neonatal birth weights similar to those of non-diabetic control women. A mean glucose level >7.8 mmol l^{-1} (140 mg dl^{-1}) was associated with a greater incidence of LGA infants and a mean level <4.8 mmol l^{-1} (87 mg dl^{-1}) was associated with a doubling of the risk (20%) for SGA birth weight.

Several observational studies without randomized controls have suggested improved intermediate health outcomes with more intensive management of women with GDM,[97–101] but the improvements in health outcomes may be attributable to factors other than glycaemic control.

Randomized controlled trials of insulin therapy in GDM

The validity of a number of early trials[102–104] comparing diet and insulin with diet alone is flawed by small sample size, inadequately described randomization including historical controls, discrepancies involving diagnostic criteria and patient characteristics and variable definitions of the outcomes reviewed.

O'Sullivan et al. in Boston[102] randomized women prospectively during two times periods (1954–1960; 1962–1970) to diet and insulin management ($n = 305$), routine prenatal care ($n = 306$) and compared these with a group of women with normal glucose tolerance ($n = 324$). Insulin treatment (10 units isophane insulin) each morning from 32 weeks gave a macrosomia rate of 4.3% compared with 13.1% (no treatment, $p < 0.01$)

and 3.7% (controls). A small study by Coustan and Lewis[103] randomized 38 women with GDM to diet and insulin (20 units NPH and 10 units regular) ($n = 27$), diet alone ($n = 11$) or neither ($n = 34$). Rates of offspring weighing more than 8.5 lb (3.9 kg) in each of the three categories were 2 (7%), 4 (36.4%) and 17 (50%), respectively (NS). Thompson et al.[104] randomized 108 women with GDM to either diet alone or diet plus insulin (20 units NPH and 10 units regular) with weekly blood glucose evaluated at weekly intervals. Among 68 women treated for a minimum of 6 weeks, the mean birth weight (3170 ± 522 vs 3584 ± 543 g, $p < 0.002$), macrosomia rate (5.9 vs 26.5%, $p < 0.05$) and ponderal index were reduced significantly in the insulin group versus the control group, respectively. There was no difference in neonatal morbidity, nor did glucose values differ between the two groups.

A number of other randomized controlled clinical trials for the management of GDM are shown in Table 11.5. Garner et al.[56] and Bancroft et al.[85] compared intensive with less intensive glycaemic control. Some degree of glycaemic separation was achieved among GDM women with varying degrees of hyperglycaemia but entry fasting glucose and HbA_{1c} levels were generally low. Both studies were limited by small size. In the study of Garner et al.,[56] patients were unblinded and untreated individuals were instructed in capillary self-monitoring. In the study of Bancroft et al.,[85] the unmonitored group had more severely abnormal glucose metabolism at baseline. None of these studies found clear differences in health outcomes, although Garner et al. reported a higher incidence of hypocalcaemia in the treatment group.

Two other studies examined tight and less tight glycaemic control among women with higher glycaemic levels.[80,101] The only difference between the groups reported by Persson et al.[80] was a small absolute reduction in neonatal hypoglycaemia in the treatment group. Langer et al.[101] achieved a larger glycaemic separation between groups [1.3 mmol l^{-1} (23 mg dl^{-1})]; the infants of the more intensively treated women had a lower mean birth weight and lower rates of neonatal hypoglycaemia and polycythaemia (Table 11.5).

Of particular significance is the study by Crowther et al.,[105] in which 1000 women with gestational IGT (recruited over a 10 year period, 1993–2003) were randomized to dietary advice, blood glucose monitoring and insulin therapy compared with no treatment (blinded). The intervention group were asked to perform four times daily monitoring, aiming for target fasting values ≥ 3.5 mmol l^{-1} (63 mg dl^{-1}) and <5.5 mmol l^{-1} (99 mg dl^{-1}), pre-meal values <5.5 mmol l^{-1} and target 2 h post-prandial values

Table 11.5 Randomized controlled clinical trials in the treatment of gestational diabetes mellitus

	Li et al.[58] (1987)	Garner et al.[56] (1997)	Bancroft et al.[85] (2000)	Persson et al.[80] (1985)	Langer et al.[101] (1989)
No. of patients	158	300	68	202	272
Controls	A ($n = 73$) No treatment	A ($n = 150$) Routine care; self glucose monitoring	A ($n = 36$) Diet and no monitoring	A ($n = 105$) Diet; add insulin for high glucose	A ($n = 146$) No treatment
Treatment	B ($n = 85$) Diet, monitoring	B ($n = 149$) Strict glycaemic control and tertiary care	B ($n = 32$) Diet and intensive diabetic monitoring	B ($n = 97$) Diet and insulin	B ($n = 126$) Diet and/or insulin
GDM inclusion criteria	GDM by NDDG criteria and normal or IGT by WHO criteria	Hatem and Dennis (1987) criteria Controls treated	WHO criteria FPG 7.0 mmol l^{-1}; 2 h PG 7.8–11.1 mmol l^{-1}	IGT	NDDG criteria One abnormal value on 3 h OGTT
Treatment details		Controls treated with insulin if FPG >7.8 and/or 1 h post-prandial >11.1 mmol l^{-1} ($n = 16$)	Obstetric care blinded	Insulin started if FPG >7 or 1 h post-prandial >9 mmol l^{-1}	B: goal of glucose 5.3 mmol l^{-1}
Glucose separation	Not recorded	Lower in treated group by 0.3–0.5 mmol l^{-1} 1 h post-prandial	HbA$_{1c}$ 0.2–0.7% 2 h PG 0.3 mmol l^{-1} ($p = 0.03$)	No difference	1.3 mmol l^{-1} difference in mean capillary blood glucose
Still births (%)	Not recorded	A:0 B:0, NS	A:0 B:0, NS	A:0 B:0, NS	Not recorded
Birth weight >4000 g (%)	A: 7 B: 4, NS	A: 18.7 B: 16.1, NS	Not recorded	Not recorded	Not recorded
LGA (%)	A: 22 B: 18, NS	Not recorded	Not recorded	Not recorded	A: 26 B: 6, $p < 0.05$
Brachial plexus injury (%)	A: 0 B: 0, NS	A: 0 B: 0, NS	Not recorded	Not recorded	Not recorded
Clavicular fracture (%)	A: 0 B: 0, NS	A: 0 B: 0, NS	Not recorded	Not recorded	Not recorded
Hypoglycaemia (%)	No difference	A: 8.7 B: 14.1, NS	Not recorded	A: 13 B: 2; $p < 0.02$ Lab. diagnosis	A: 13 B: 2, $p < 0.02$ Lab. diagnosis
Hyperbilirubinaemia (%)	Not recorded	A: 6.6 B: 5.4, NS	Not recorded	A: 14 B: 6, NS Lab. diagnosis	A:14 B: 6, NS Lab. diagnosis
Hypocalcaemia (%)	Not recorded	A: 30 B: 40.9, $p = 0.048$	Not recorded	Not recorded	Not recorded
Caesarean section delivery (%)	A: 26 B: 27, NS	A: 18.6 B: 20.1, NS	A: 31 B: 31, NS	A: 11 B: 10, NS	A: 11 B: 10, NS

<7.0 mmol l^{-1} (126 mg dl^{-1}) with insulin adjusted on the basis of these results. The intervention group had a reduced rate of a composite endpoint (death, shoulder dystocia, bone fracture and nerve palsy) of 4% compared with 1% in the control group ($p = 0.01$). These benefits were associated with an increased use of induction of labour (39 vs 29%, $p < 0.001$) for the mother and an increased rate of admission to the neonatal nursery for the infant (71 vs 61%, $p = 0.01$), both of which may have been related to the knowledge of the diagnosis by the attending physician. It was suggested that the earlier age at birth, as a consequence of induction of labour, may have contributed to the reduction in serious perinatal outcomes. Caesarean delivery was similar in the two groups. Rates of macrosomia (10 vs 21%, $p < 0.001$) and large for gestational age (13 vs 22%, $p < 0.001$) were significantly reduced in the intervention group. Differences in primary outcomes between groups remained significant after adjustment for known confounders (maternal age, race, ethnicity and parity) and for analyses involving multiple endpoints. There was also some evidence that treatment improved health-related quality of life and the incidence of

depression both during the antenatal period and 3 months after birth. The ACHOIS trial demonstrated a significant reduction in a composite endpoint; however, the number of individual adverse outcomes was small, most of these events (64%) involved shoulder dystocia (which some have questioned as a serious complication) and knowledge of the condition was attended by more induction of labour and more admissions to a neonatal nursery.

Frequency and type of glucose monitoring

There are no uniform recommendations regarding the frequency of serum glucose monitoring or an ideal 'target' range for glycaemic control. It would be expected that more frequent monitoring would highlight greater instances of hyperglycaemia. In a study comparing home glucose monitoring and weekly plasma glucose monitoring at office visits, the former identified more frequent hyperglycaemia, leading to a higher insulin usage and a lower incidence of macrosomia but no other difference in outcomes.[106]

Recognition that the primary manifestation of hypoinsulinaemia in GDM is post-prandial hyperglycaemia and the correlation of the latter with birth weight have focused attention on the relative importance of post-prandial versus pre-prandial home blood glucose monitoring in relation to outcome. De Veciana et al.[82] randomized 66 insulin-requiring Latino women at <30 weeks gestation to pre- or post-prandial monitoring and found that the post-prandial group had a lower mean HbA_{1c} pre-delivery (8.1 vs 6.5%), a lower rate of Caesarean section due to cephalopelvic disproportion (12 vs 36%) and had offspring who were less likely to be LGA (12 vs 42%). There was a non-significant trend towards more neonatal hypoglycaemia and shoulder dystocia in the pre-prandial monitoring group. This study reported the largest separation in HbA_{1c} (1.6%) and some of the largest reductions in fetal macrosomia, but the women had severe hyperglycaemia (including some who had frank diabetes) and its relevance for GDM is therefore uncertain. The study is also limited by the small number of individuals, the lack of masking and the use of an unproven strategy for elective Caesarean section deliveries.

In a small study of women with GDM randomized to receive only porcine regular insulin before each meal or a morning dose of neutral protamine Hagedorn (NPH) insulin, those receiving pre-meal short-acting insulin had infants with lower birth weight (3.079 ± 0.722 vs 3.943 ± 0.492 kg) and a lower rate of macrosomia.[107] All individuals performed home glucose monitoring at least 2 days per week with insulin adjustment if two pre-prandial glucose values

exceeded 5.5 mmol l^{-1} (100 mg dl^{-1}) (NPH group) or if one 2 h post-prandial value exceeded 7.9 mmol l^{-1} (142 mg dl^{-1}) (regular insulin group).

A randomized trial by Nachum et al.[81] involved the randomization of insulin-requiring pregnant individuals with type 1 diabetes preceding pregnancy and those with GDM (NDDG criteria) to insulin given four times daily (GDM group, $n = 138$) versus twice daily (GDM group, $n = 136$) prior to 35 weeks gestation. The former regimen was associated with better glycaemic control, lower rates of neonatal hypoglycaemia (0.7 vs 5.9%, $p = 0.02$) and hyperbilirubinaemia (11 vs 21%, $p = 0.02$) but no other differences in individual outcomes were observed. There was a lower overall rate of neonatal morbidity with the four times daily regimen [relative risk (RR) 0.59, 95% CI 0.38 to 0.92], but this was a composite variable including respiratory distress syndrome, hypoglycaemia, hyperbilirubinaemia and birth trauma, and it seemed likely that this statistic was influenced by the biochemical abnormalities.

Randomized trials based on asymmetric fetal growth

Buchanan et al.[108] randomized 59 Latino women with GDM, who at 29–33 weeks of gestation had a fetal ultrasound abdominal circumference of greater than or equal to the 75th percentile for gestational age either to diet therapy ($n = 29$) or to diet plus twice daily insulin ($n = 30$). The diet-only group had a higher mean birth weight (3878 g compared with 3647 g, $p < 0.04$), a higher LGA rate (45 vs 13%, $P < 0.01$) but a lower Caesarean section rate (14–21% using the range for three diet groups compared with 43%, $p < 0.05$). Rates of birth weights greater than 4000 or 4500 g were not provided and there was no significant birth trauma in this study. This study is limited, however, by a lack of power for many of the important health outcomes, a lack of comparability (including obstetric management) between the two groups and a large percentage of refusals for which no information is provided.

Kjos et al.[65] in a pilot study randomized 98 women with fasting plasma glucose concentrations of 5.8–6.7 mmol l^{-1} (105–120 mg dl^{-1}) to either insulin and diet therapy (standard group, $n = 48$) or insulin added to diet therapy only if the abdominal circumference (AC) on ultrasound (measured monthly) was ≥ 70 centile and/or if any venous FPG measurements (measured every 1–2 weeks) were >6.7 mmol l^{-1} (120 mg dl^{-1}) (experimental group, $n = 49$). Thirty of 49 women in the experimental group received insulin therapy (21 at the start of the trial). Mean fasting plasma glucose was lower at 4.7–4.9 mmol l^{-1} (84.9 vs 88.1 mg dl^{-1}, $p < 0.003$) in the standard group but the targets were different for the two groups: ≤ 5.0 mmol l^{-1} (90 mg dl^{-1}) before meals and ≤ 6.7 mmol l^{-1} (120 mg dl^{-1}) 2 h post-prandial level (standard) and ≤ 4.4 mmol l^{-1} (80 mg dl^{-1}) before meals and 2 h post-prandial ≤ 6.1 mmol l^{-1} (110 mg dl^{-1}) 2 h (experimental). There was also a lower incidence of Caesarean section delivery (14.6 vs 33.3%, $p < 0.03$) in the standard group, but there were more individuals in the experimental group who had a prior Caesarean section delivery (nine versus four individuals) and other obstetric differences existed between the two groups seemingly unrelated to maternal diabetes. There were no statistical differences in gestational weeks at delivery, macrosomia, polycythaemia, neonatal hypoglycaemia or hyperbilirubinaemia requiring treatment. The experimental group had more LGA neonates (8.3 vs 6.3%). Problems with the study include its lack of statistical power to determine important health outcomes, the fact that the groups differed in obstetric risk factors and the lack of blinding of the obstetricians.

In a related study, Schaefer-Graf et al.[109] compared management of women with GDM who attained fasting capillary glucose <6.7 mmol l^{-1} (120 mg dl^{-1}) [and 2 h post-prandial capillary glucose <11.1 mmol l^{-1} (200 mg dl^{-1})] after 1 week of diet with management based on either maternal glycaemia alone (standard) or glycaemia plus ultrasound. Insulin was initiated if the fasting capillary glucose was >5.0 mmol l^{-1} (90 mg dl^{-1}) or 2 h capillary glucose >6.7 mmol l^{-1} (120 mg dl^{-1}) (standard group) or if the fasting and 2 h values were >6.7 mmol l^{-1} (120 mg dl^{-1}) and 11.1 mmol l^{-1} (200 mg dl^{-1}), respectively (or fetal abdominal circumference $>$75th centile in the USS group). Maternal and neonatal outcomes were similar between the groups, leading to the suggestion that inclusion of fetal growth might provide the opportunity to reduce glucose testing in low-risk pregnancies.

A major criticism of these trials is that they have too few participants to be able to detect differences among treatment groups in such uncommon health outcomes as perinatal mortality or brachial plexus injury; in addition, they have even less power to determine if the health benefit is different for GDM women with high levels of hyperglycaemia compared with lower levels. By contrast, the results of the ACHOIS trial are of major significance, but adverse outcomes in this study were few in number and the significance of the composite nature of the endpoint seemed largely related to a reduction in the rate of shoulder dystocia. Moreover, the results were obtained among GDM women, the majority of whom (over 80%) were treated with diet alone, findings which are generally not supported by previous literature.

Although some studies have shown that insulin therapy reduces the incidence of fetal macrosomia, this was generally only seen in individuals with more severe hyperglycaemia or those targeted because of asymmetric fetal growth; moreover, the magnitude of any benefit is not clear. The current evidence is insufficient to determine the magnitude of benefit among GDM patients with milder degrees of hyperglycaemia.

Ante-partum surveillance

If non-stress testing (NST) or biophysical profile (BPP) were to provide justification for GDM screening, data would need to show clearly that use of these tests reduced stillbirths among women with GDM who had no other indication for these tests. As most women with GDM have a low risk for stillbirth, this would require a large RCT. Observational studies have found that use of these tests in GDM is associated with either absent or very low rates of stillbirth,[110–113] but without control groups it is uncertain whether these results can be attributed to the additional procedures.[112] Non-stress tests or BPPs have high false-positive rates[110,113] and may lead to unnecessary interventions.[112]

Those RCTS which have utilized ultrasound assessment of abdominal circumference to target insulin therapy found no significant difference in health outcomes (and lacked power to do so); in addition, the obstetricians were not blinded to the intervention group.[65,108,109]

Benefits and risks of screening and treatment

This area is not well researched, but the potential for adverse psychological effects from screening seems real; more than 80% of all positive glucose challenge tests are false positives[114] and some evidence suggests that labelling may negatively influence a woman's perception of her health during pregnancy[114,115] and possibly in the longer term.[115,116] It is clear that the diagnosis of GDM may lower the threshold for Caesarean section and may also unnecessarily increase the use of NSTs or BPPS, again prompting operative delivery triggered by the false-positive results – all resulting in increased additional costs. Concerns have also been raised regarding the possibility that excessively low glycaemic thresholds may result in increased rates of infants with starvation ketosis[117] or small for gestational age, but limited evidence makes the magnitude of this risk difficult to quantify.[95] By making various assumptions, the number needed to screen to prevent one case of brachial plexus injury varied from 3300 to 8900.[14]

Trials in progress

An ongoing randomized trial by Landon et al.[118] is designed to determine whether a benefit exists for the treatment of mild carbohydrate intolerance during pregnancy. The study is comparing individuals randomized to diet and insulin therapy as required between 24 and 29 weeks of gestation with those randomized to no specific treatment. Mild GDM is defined as a 1 h 50 g glucose loading test result between 7.5 and 11.1 mmol l^{-1} (135 and 200 mg dl^{-1}) followed by a 3 h OGTT with normal fasting glucose level <5.4 mmol l^{-1} (95 g dl^{-1}) and two of three timed glucose determinations exceeding thresholds established by the 4th GDM Workshop. The primary outcome is a composite of neonatal morbidity in the treatment and control groups (perinatal mortality and morbidities including still birth, neonatal hypoglycaemia, neonatal hyperinsulinaemia, neonatal hyperbilirubinaemia and birth trauma). Secondary outcomes include large for gestational age and/or macrosomia (birth weight >4000 g), admission to neonatal intensive care and maternal complications including Caesarean section and pre-eclampsia. Macrosomia rates will also be compared with the incidence in a normal non-diabetic population. It has been estimated that a total of 950 individuals will allow the detection of a reduction of 30% in the composite outcome.

Insulin analogues

The advent of both short- and more recently long-acting insulin analogues has provided the possibility to reproduce more closely the normal physiological mode of insulin secretion. In particular, these agents have the potential to address fasting hyperglycaemia and the post-prandial hyperglycaemic spike (without the tendency for hypoglycaemia before the next meal). The rapid onset and short duration of action of both lispro and aspart theoretically compensate for the decline in beta cell function. In addition, given the evidence from a number of studies in both type 1 and GDM showing that fetal growth is more closely related to post-prandial than pre-prandial glycaemia,[82,119–121] it is conceivable that short-acting analogues might contribute to more favourable pregnancy outcomes.

Three short-acting human insulin analogues are currently commercially available. Insulin lispro [(Lys (B28)(Pro (B29)] and insulin aspart [Asp (B29)] include modifications at amino acid sites on the B chain which are not critical in binding to the insulin receptor. Glulisine has lysine at the B3 position and glutamine at the B29 position. These structural

modifications inhibit self-association into dimers and hexamers, leading to more rapid absorption after subcutaneous injection.

In addition, two long-acting insulin analogues are also commercially available. Glargine is where human insulin has been modified by extending the C-terminal end of the B chain with two arginine residues and substituting glycine for arginine at amino acid position 21 on the A chain. These modifications shift the isoelectric point from pH 5.4 to 6.7, making insulin glargine less soluble at physiological pH. Insulin glargine precipitates in the subcutaneous tissue following injection, delaying absorption and prolonging its duration of action. Detemir, another long-acting insulin analogue, has the threonine at the B30 position removed and myristoyl fatty acid is acylated to lysine at B29. Its prolonged action is believed to be due to a combination of hexamer formation and reversible albumin binding. When evaluated by HbA$_{1c}$ and mean blood glucose levels, these analogues are at least as effective as regular and NPH insulin in individuals with type 1[122] and type 2 diabetes.[123] Their main advantage when used in intensive therapy is the lower incidence of severe and nocturnal hypoglycaemia.[122]

Randomized trials

Clinical experience with these newer insulins in pregnancy (and particularly the long-acting analogues) is very limited and mostly retrospective. Few randomized trials have been published of insulin lispro in pregnancy. Among women with GDM[124,125] or type 1 diabetes treated from week 15,[126] both in addition to basal NPH insulin, those receiving insulin lispro had fewer hypoglycaemic episodes[124] and lower 1 h post-prandial glucose levels[125,126] but no difference in overall blood glucose levels or HbA$_{1c}$.[124,126] Birth weight, macrosomia, Caesarean delivery, neonatal hypoglycaemia and anti-insulin antibody levels[124] were similar between the two groups.[124,126] Carr et al.[127] performed a randomized controlled trial of insulin lispro given before or after meals in pregnant women with nine women with type 1 diabetes and found no difference in glucose excursion or fetal compromise between the two groups.

Retrospective data

Cypryk et al.[128] reported pregnancy outcome among 25 women with type 1 diabetes treated with lispro compared with 46 controls (who had maintained the same treatment there were on pre-pregnancy); outcomes in the two groups were similar.

Two studies have been reported using insulin aspart.[129,130] In the first, insulin aspart was compared with regular insulin or diet in terms of its capacity to lower post-prandial glycaemia. Regular insulin was given 30 min and lispro 5 min prior to the meal. The AUC for glucose did not differ significantly between the regular insulin and diet groups, whereas with aspart it was significantly smaller.[128] In the second, the efficacy and perinatal outcome were examined during a randomized trial comparing insulin aspart with human insulin (each with NPH as basal insulin) in 322 individuals with type 1 diabetes. Treatment with aspart was associated with a lower rate of major hypoglycaemia (although not significant) and similar overall glycaemic control; perinatal outcomes were similar in the two groups and it was concluded that aspart was at least as safe as human insulin regarding perinatal outcome.[130]

Safety issues

Short-acting analogues

In a pooled analysis of data from clinical trials, Glazer et al.[131] demonstrated the clinical safety of insulin lispro among non-pregnant patients. *In vitro* studies also support the safety of short-acting insulin analogues. The mitogenic potential of insulin analogues correlates with their relative affinity for the insulin-like growth factor(IGF-1) receptor and with occupancy time at the insulin receptor.[132,133] Because the mitogenic response to insulin requires stimulation by insulin for over 14.5 h,[133] short-acting insulins such as lispro and aspart would not be expected to exert a mitogenic influence. Both analogues, with insulin receptor affinity less than that of human insulin, also have mitogenic potencies less than that of human insulin[132] (Table 11.6).

Three retrospective studies did not find any unfavourable pregnancy outcomes. Bhattacharyya et al.[134] reviewed 138 pregnancies treated with regular insulin and 75 treated with lispro. HbA$_{1c}$ in the lispro group was significantly lower (5.8 vs 6.1%) at the end of pregnancy and patients were more satisfied with the treatment. The second study in 33 pregnant patients treated with lispro and 27 treated with regular insulin did not show any higher risk of malformations or unusual pregnancy outcomes in patients treated with lispro.[135] The third summarized outcomes of 78 pregnancies treated with lispro.[136] The frequencies of abortion, congenital malformations, perinatal mortality, glycaemic control and retinopathy progression were similar to those in other large studies in pregnant women with diabetes.

Some concern has been raised regarding the potential relationship between insulin lispro and the development of proliferative retinopathy. In one retrospective report of pregnant women treated with insulin lispro either before or early in pregnancy, three of 10 progressed from no retinopathy to proliferative retinopathy;[137] however, this was not confirmed in two larger studies[138,139] and other pregnancy factors may have been relevant. The three women who developed proliferative retinopathy received insulin lispro for 20–23 weeks, which would not be the custom in GDM and overall no significant risk for retinopathy with lispro seems likely.

Long-acting analogues

Around 98% of detemir in plasma is bound to albumin and only the free fraction can activate the insulin receptor. Detemir has a lower receptor affinity than human insulin and even lower IGF-1 affinity and mitogenic potential.[133] The long-acting insulin glargine has an IGF-1 receptor affinity and mitogenic potency approximately seven times greater than human regular insulin (Table 11.7); the clinical implications of these findings remains to be determined.[132]

Clinical data on the use of long-acting insulin analogues are negligible, but of note are the results or a retrospective multicentre study which found no difference in outcomes among individuals receiving isophane insulin and glargine.[140] In *in vitro* studies, five fetuses from two litters of rabbits exposed to insulin glargine developed cerebral ventriculmegaly. These teratogenicity issues do not arise in GDM, where insulin does not cross the placenta and treatment is instituted during the latter half of pregnancy.

Table 11.6 Pharmacokinetic properties of regular human insulin and rapid-acting analogues

Type of insulin	Onset of action	Peak plasma values (h)	Duration of action (h)
Regular human insulin	30–60 min	1–3	5–7
NPH insulin	60–90 min	8–12	18–24
Insulin lispro	15–60 min	0.5–1	2–4
Insulin aspart	10–20 min	1–3	3–5
Glargine	4–5 h	No peak	>24
Detemir	4–6 h	No peak	20

Table 11.7 Receptor binding and metabolic potencies of insulin analogues relative to insulin[a]

Analogue	Insulin receptor affinity (%)	Insulin receptor off-rate (%)	Metabolic potency (lipogenesis) (%)	IGF-1 receptor affinity (%)	Mitogenic potency (%)
Human insulin	100	100	100	100	100
Aspart	92 ± 6	81 ± 8	101 ± 2	81 ± 9	58 ± 22
Lispro	84 ± 6	100 ± 11	82 ± 3	156 ± 16	66 ± 10
Glargine	86 ± 3	152 ± 13	60 ± 3	641 ± 51	783 ± 132
Detemir	18 ± 2	204 ± 9	~27	16 ± 1	~11

[a]Data are means ± SE, except for metabolic potency data which are means ± 95% confidence limits. Binding assays for insulin detemir were performed in albumin-free buffer systems. Estimated potencies of free (not albumin-bound) insulin detemir are reported.
Source: adapted from Ref. 132.

The literature to date suggests that short-acting analogues are at least as safe as regular insulin in pregnancy with their major impact being on post-prandial hyperglycaemia and nocturnal hypoglycaemia. More information is needed on the role and safety of longer acting analogues in pregnancy, but this may be a less critical consideration given the fact that in GDM patients these analogues are prescribed after the period of organogenesis.

Oral hypoglycaemic agents

Traditionally, insulin has been considered the treatment of choice in the management of GDM when dietary therapy has proved insufficient. A particular attraction is its ability to achieve tight blood glucose control and the fact that it does not cross the placenta except as an insulin–antibody complex in women who have developed insulin antibodies. For some women, however, insulin therapy during pregnancy is inconvenient and stressful, adding further complexity to capillary glucose monitoring. In other circumstances, insulin treatment is unaffordable; each of these factors may influence compliance. Treatment with oral hypoglycaemic drugs has a strong logistical basis given that both type 2 diabetes and GDM are characterized by insulin resistance and declining beta cell function, usually in the context of mild hyperglycaemia.

Traditionally, these drugs have been avoided in pregnancy because of concern regarding transplacental passage[141] and the possibility of fetal teratogenesis[142] and prolonged neonatal hypoglycaemia.[143,144] With few exceptions, knowledge of their tolerability and efficacy has largely been gleaned from case reports and retrospective data, much of which have been confounded by poor glycaemic control during conception and pregnancy. It should also be noted that both glyburide and metformin have been widely prescribed in Europe and South Africa for many years

without reported adverse effects to the fetus. The need for a definitive answer has become more pertinent given the rising tide of obesity and type 2 diabetes in women of childbearing age and the more widespread prescribing of metformin to women with PCOS, many of whom (up to 46%) may develop GDM during pregnancy. To date, these drugs are not licensed for use in pregnancy.

Drug categories

The first-generation sulfonylureas were discovered in the 1950s followed by the development of other agents in this class. Second-generation sulfonylureas in use today include glyburide and glipizide. Sulfonylureas bind to specific receptors in the plasma membrane of the pancreatic beta cell that trigger the release of insulin. In 1997, a new class of oral insulin secretagogues (meglitinides) was approved for clinical use. Biguanides were recognized as early as 1920; phenformin was withdrawn in the 1950s because of lactic acidosis. Its replacement metformin, although widely used in Europe for many years, has only approved for use in the United States since 1995. Biguanides reduce hepatic glucose output and increase peripheral glucose disposal in muscle and adipose tissue.

Pharmacokinetics and placental passage

First-generation sulfonylureas, such as tolbutamide and chloropropamide, were found to be associated with congenital malformations in the majority of animal studies; chloropropamide is embryotoxic to mouse embryos in culture. To date, no animal studies have been performed to evaluate second- and third-generation sulfonylureas and their association with malformations. Denno and Sadler[145] found that metformin produced no alterations in embryonic growth and no major malformations, but the drug delayed neural tube closure and also reduced yolk sac protein values at two different concentrations.

Placental transfer is inversely correlated with the molecular weight of each of these drugs. Using the recirculating single cotyledon human placenta model,[146,147] however, placental passage of glyburide was found to be minimal. In addition, a recent study by the same group found that metformin, despite its low molecular weight, did not affect human placental glucose transfer, suggesting that the potential of increasing glucose delivery to the fetus is less than expected.[148] Metformin does not promote placental glucose uptake or transport, as demonstrated with an *in vitro* human placental perfusion model.[148]

Congenital malformations

Of particular initial concern is a frequently cited paper by Piacquadio *et al.*,[142] which highlighted a possible teratogenic risk for first trimester chloropropamide in which 10 of 20 women had babies with birth defects compared with 15% in the control group. The majority of these were minor; four of the six had external malformations and had been exposed to chloropropamide. Most of the women in this study, however, had poor control around conception. By contrast, reports from South Africa (where both metformin and sulfonylureas have had considerable clinical use) have not shown an increased risk of congenital malformations.[149–151]

Three studies in the last decade are also reassuring in this regard. Towner *et al.*[152] treated 332 type 2 diabetic patients with oral hypoglycaemic agents or insulin prior to pregnancy. Using stepwise logistic regression analysis, they showed that the mode of therapy did not have an adverse effect, while the level of glycaemia and maternal age were significant contributing factors to the rate of anomalies. A retrospective study of 850 patients by Langer *et al.*[153] reported similar findings. Finally, Konen[154] presented the results of eight studies and concluded that the use of oral agents had no effect on the rate of fetal anomalies due to a very narrow confidence interval (odds ratio 1.0, 95% CI 1.05 to 1.85).

A meta-analysis of 471 women exposed to oral agents (sulfonylureas and/or biguanides) in the first trimester compared with 1344 women not exposed found no significant difference in the rates of major malformations.[155] In the largest retrospective cohort study to date ($n = 342$), congenital anomalies were associated with poor glycaemic control rather than the specific oral hypoglycaemic agent used (glyuride/glibenclamide or metformin).[156]

Clinical outcomes

Some, but not all, early reports on the use of first-generation sulfonylurea agents during pregnancy demonstrated an increased risk for neonatal hypoglycaemia.[143,144] Hypoglycaemia in adults was already recognized as a common adverse effect of these drugs most likely on the basis of their ability to stimulate insulin secretion by the beta cell. In South Africa, Coetzee and Jackson treated more than 150 pregnant women with diabetes with metformin and glyburide between 1974 and 1983.[150,151] They found no cases of serious hypoglycaemia and a very acceptable rate of perinatal morbidity rates in the offspring of women with type 2 diabetes and GDM. In a further review of their management strategy of women with type 2 diabetes, involving rapid recourse to insulin if metformin did not result in good diabetic control, they found that if the objective of strict blood glucose control was achieved, the perinatal mortality rate was similar to that of type 1 diabetes.[150,151] More recently, in a retrospective review by the same group, the use of oral hypoglycaemic drugs throughout pregnancy (glyburide alone or in combination with metformin) was associated with increased perinatal mortality;[156] however, there were no perinatal deaths in infants of women taking metformin exclusively. The perinatal mortality rate was significantly higher in the group that used oral agents throughout compared with those who switched to insulin at the beginning of pregnancy or those who were treated with insulin alone. This could not be explained by differences in glycaemic control, maternal age, BMI, parity, booking gestational age or co-morbidities between the groups.

In Scandinavia, Helmuth *et al.* reported that among 50 obese women with gestational or type 2 diabetes, treatment with metformin, but not a sulfonylurea, was associated with an increased prevalence of pre-eclampsia (32%) and perinatal mortality (8%).[157] These data, however, are retrospective, non-randomized, based on weight and the treatment of GDM may have been obscured by the fact that one-third of the patients had type 2 diabetes. There were, however, no differences in rates of neonatal morbidity, including neonatal hypoglycaemia, between the groups. More recently, an audit by Hughes *et al.*[158] of 214 pregnancies in women with type 2 diabetes between 1998 and 2003 found that outcome measures did not differ between the metformin and control groups.

Experience with metformin has also accrued from treatment of insulin resistance in non-pregnant women with the polycystic ovarian syndrome (PCOS). Among 28 non-diabetic women with PCOS in whom metformin was started before conception and continued throughout pregnancy, there was a greatly reduced incidence of GDM (OR 0.115, 95% CI 0.014 to 0.938) compared with a retrospective cohort of women with PCOS who did not receive the drug during pregnancy.[159] No fetal malformations or neonatal hypoglycaemia was reported. Glueck *et al.* compared 90 women with PCOS who conceived on metformin with healthy control women and found no major birth defects and similar rates of pre-eclampsia even though the PCOS women were older and heavier.[160] The same group found no difference among offspring of mothers who conceived and continued on metformin compared with control offspring over the first 18 months of life in terms of growth and motor-social development.[161] In addition, during a prospective observational study of 42 women with PCOS treated with metformin and diet pre-conception, women reduced their weight by 5.8% and weight continued to fall in the first trimester; fasting serum insulin levels were also reduced by 40%.[162]

Oral hypoglycaemic agents and gestational diabetes mellitus

Here the issue of anomalies is simpler as patients are diagnosed and commence treatment after the first trimester (period of organogenesis). The remaining concerns pertain to neonatal hypoglycaemia and stimulation of macrosomia if the drug crosses the placenta (although this appears to be minimal with glyburide).

Few randomized studies have been reported in the literature. Notolovitz[163] examined the utility of tolbutamide, chlorpropamine, diet and insulin in a small study (50 patients in each group) of limited statistical power. There was no significance difference for perinatal mortality or congenital anomalies. Good glycaemic control [defined as $<8.3 \, \text{mmol} \, \text{l}^{-1}$ $(150 \, \text{mg} \, \text{dl}^{-1})$] was achieved by 80% of the individuals on oral agents or diet and 36% for those on insulin. In another trial, Langer *et al.*[69] randomized 404 GDM women with fasting hyperglycaemia to receive either insulin or glyburide starting at 11 to 33 weeks gestation. The outcomes in the two groups were similar with no differences in achieved blood glucose control [mean blood glucose levels around $5.8 \, \text{mmol} \, \text{l}^{-1}$ $(105 \, \text{mg} \, \text{dl}^{-1})$] daily. In addition, the glyburide and insulin groups had similar rates of large for gestational age infants ($\geq$90th centile) (12 vs 13%), macrosomia ($\geq$4 kg) (7 vs 4%), birth weight, congenital anomalies (both 2%) or hypoglycaemia (9 vs 6%). Satisfactory control was achieved in 88% of the drug group and 84% of the insulin group. Glyburide was not detected in the cord serum of any infant in the glyburide group.[69]

A recently published Australian study, the Metformin versus Insulin for the Treatment of Gestational Diabetes (MIG) Study,[164] randomized 751 women aged 18–45 years with gestational diabetes to treatment with metformin (up to 2500 g daily with supplemental insulin if required) or insulin, from 20 to 33 weeks gestation. The primary outcome was a composite of neonatal hypoglycaemia, respiratory distress, need for phototherapy, birth trauma, 5 min Agpar score less than 7 or prematurity. The rate of the primary composite outcome was 32.0% in the metformin group and 32.2% in the insulin group (RR 0.99, 95% CI 0.80 to 1.23). More women in the metformin group compared with the insulin group indicated that they would choose to receive their assigned treatment again (76.6 vs 27.2%, $p < 0.001$). The frequency of preterm birth was higher in the metformin group (12.1%) than the insulin group (7.6%, $p = 0.04$), but the difference was associated with a greater frequency of spontaneous (rather than iatrogenic) prematurity that could have been due to chance or to an unrecognized effect of metformin on the labour process. The increased rate of preterm birth was not associated with higher rates of other complications, probably because the difference between the two groups in mean gestational age at delivery was clinically insignificant. The rates of other secondary outcomes (neonatal anthropometric measurements, maternal glycaemic control, maternal hypertensive complications, post-partum glucose tolerance) did not differ significantly between the groups. There were no serious adverse events associated with the use of metformin.

In the MIG study, 46.3% of women taking metformin required supplemental insulin. In the study of Langer *et al.*[69] comparing glyburide and insulin among 404 GDM women, 4% required supplemental insulin. Subsequent experience with glyburide has shown that approximately 20% of women change to insulin.

Breast feeding and pharmacokinetics

The first-generation sulfonylureas, tolbutamide and chlorpropamide, cross into breast milk. To date, only one study has looked at the transfer of glyburide and glipizide into breast milk.[165] In this study, eight women with type 2 diabetes received a single oral dose of 5 or 10 mg of glyburide and five women were given 5 mg of glyburide daily from the first day post-partum. Neither drug was detected in the breast milk of any of the women. In the study of Glueck *et al.*, at 6 months of age, the height, weight and motor-social development of infants of mothers taking metformin while breast feeding did not differ from those of formula-fed infants.

In three studies which examined the transfer of metformin into breast milk, all three found that metformin crosses into breast milk, albeit in very small quantities.[166–168] Metformin has negligible plasma protein binding and is eliminated unchanged in urine. Renal clearance exceeds the glomerular filtration rate, suggesting active tubular secretion.[169] In pregnancy, gastrointestinal motility is reduced and the glomerular filtration rate is increased by 40–50%, thus potentially altering the pharmacokinetics of metformin significantly. In a small study of seven women taking metformin in pregnancy, Hughes et al.[170] demonstrated that the clearance of metformin increased as a result of enhanced renal elimination and suggested that dose adjustment of 20% or more might be needed in late pregnancy to maintain the therapeutic effect, but these data require confirmation. As peak plasma concentrations are unchanged across the entire dosing interval, there is no virtue in avoiding breast feeding for a few hours after maternal dose ingestion.

Other drugs

One case series from Mexico reported on the use of acarbose during pregnancy.[171] Six women with GDM and moderately elevated fasting and post-prandial glucose levels were treated with acarbose (25 mg) three times per day before meals. All women achieved adequate glucose control and delivered healthy offspring. However, the women experienced intestinal discomfort which persisted throughout pregnancy. Acarbose was also used in a small trial of GDM women unsuccessfully controlled on diet who were randomized to insulin ($n = 27$), glyburide ($n = 24$) or acarbose ($n = 19$).[172] No differences were observed in the maternal glucose levels achieved, rate of LGA or birth weight among the three groups. Larger RCTs are needed to examine further the benefits of acarbose in pregnancy.

Data on newer agents such as PPAR-gamma agonists are few, but it is likely that more women will conceive while undergoing treatment with these agents. In a study of 31 women between 8 and 12 weeks gestation, two doses of rosiglitazone 4 mg were given prior to surgical termination of pregnancy.[173] Rosiglitazone was detected in fetal tissue, especially after 10 weeks gestation, suggesting that the drug crosses the placenta. No teratogenic effects have been noted in studies of rats and rabbits.[174] Two cases of exposure of rosiglitazone have been reported in the first trimester and a third case in the second trimester with no congenital anomalies or neonatal complications described.[175,176] Rosiglitazone was used in two randomized trials of women with PCOS for ovulation induction ($n = 25$ in each trial); one trial compared rosiglitazone and clomiphene versus metformin plus clomiphene and the other compared rosiglitazone plus placebo versus rosiglitazone plus clomiphene.[177,178] In the first trial, rosiglitazone improved ovulatory rates whereas in the second the addition of clomiphene to rosiglitazone was superior. No congenital anomalies were described in the 14 pregnancies although there were three early fetal losses.

Summary of current position on prescribing of oral hypoglycaemic agents in pregnancy

In summary, randomized trial data suggest that metformin (alone or with supplemental insulin) and glyburide are effective and safe treatment options for women with GDM who meet the usual criteria for starting insulin. Data on these agents in the first trimester are more limited but the results of small, retrospective studies and the increasing use of metformin in PCOS are generally reassuring. Caution is necessary, however, until safety in the first trimester has been evaluated more fully. Follow-up data focusing on both short- and long-term neonatal outcomes are required. Glyburide, glipizide and metformin appear compatible with breast feeding but their use is still not recommended in all practice guidelines.[179] PPAR-gamma agonists cross the placenta and to date there are few data on the safety of these drugs in pregnancy. At present, it would seem advisable that their use be confined to ovulation induction if potential benefits outweigh the potential risk to the fetus.

Diabetes after pregnancy

Long-term follow up studies, reviewed by Kim et al.,[180] reveal that relatively few (around 10%) individuals develop diabetes soon after delivery and the rate of incident cases if thereafter fairly constant over the first 10 years; the few studies where follow-up has extended beyond 10 years reveal a long-term risk of approximately 70% within 5–63 years after the index pregnancy.[1]

Subtyping

Attempts to classify individuals into one of the three major subtypes of GDM has been largely neglected but can facilitate clinical management. Lean patients are less likely to be insulin resistant than overweight or obese patients, so autoimmune and monogenic type of diabetes should be considered in these individuals. This may include the measurement of GAD antibodies, especially in women where type 1 diabetes is relatively common in their ethnic group or whether there is no apparent family history of diabetes. Alternatively, those women with a history of early onset diabetes with a relevant family history (autosomal dominant for MODY, maternal inheritance for mitochondrial mutations) may suggest the diagnosis of monogenic diabetes. Ellard et al.[181] suggested four clinical criteria with relatively high specificity for identification of women with the glucokinase mutations that cause MODY2: (1) persistent fasting hyperglycaemia 5.8–8.0 mmol l^{-1} (105–145 mg dl^{-1}) after pregnancy, (2) a small [less than 4.6 mmol l^{-1} (82 mg dl^{-1})] increment in glucose above the fasting level during the 75 g OGTT, (3) insulin treatment during at least one pregnancy but subsequently controlled on diet and (4) a first-degree relative with type 2 diabetes, GDM or a fasting serum or plasma glucose greater than 5.5 mmol l^{-1} (100 mg dl^{-1}). While this constellation is uncommon in the UK, some 80% of women who met all four criteria had glucokinase mutations. Genotyping for these mutations is now available. The diagnosis is also important for genetic counselling and possibly also treatment.

By contrast, there is no clinical role for genetic testing in the more common form of polygenic diabetes. Here, the key at present is an understanding of the basic pathophysiology. The short-term responses in beta cell function during pregnancy seem to occur on a background of long-term deterioration of beta cell function that over years leads to progressive hyperglycaemia and diabetes. Longitudinal studies of lean and obese women before, at the beginning of the second trimester and in the third trimester show that although the increase in insulin secretion is less that which occurs in normal pregnant women despite somewhat greater insulin resistance in women with GDM, insulin secretion is still responsive to changing sensitivity. Utilization of this knowledge presents a possible approach to long-term prevention strategies.

Recognized risk factors that are known to be associated with type 2 diabetes, including obesity, weight gain and increased age, are well recognized. Higher glucose levels during pregnancy, necessitating the use of insulin, also correlate with increased risk, possibly because they represent a later stage on the pathway to the development of diabetes. Elegant longitudinal studies on the pathophysiology of GDM that develop in one ethnic group of Hispanic women have revealed that chronic and acute insulin resistance associated with declining beta cell function increase the risk of developing diabetes.[182,183] The impact of reduced beta cell function on glucose levels is relatively small until the acute insulin response to glucose in relation to insulin resistance is approximately 10–15% of normal; thereafter, relatively small differences in beta cell function are associated with disproportionately large

increases in glucose levels.[183] The same group have also shown that treatment of insulin resistance at the stage of impaired glucose tolerance results in reciprocal downregulation of insulin secretion,[184] which in turn is associated with a reduction in the risk of diabetes and with preservation of beta cell function.[185] These findings need to be explored in other ethnic groups, but the general principle of prevention of diabetes by lifestyle change in a number of major trials suggests that broadly similar mechanisms are operative and similar benefits might accrue. Two studies have included women with a history of GDM. In the US DPP Trial,[89] intensive lifestyle modification to promote weight loss and increase physical activity resulted in a 58% reduction in the risk of type 2 diabetes in adults with impaired glucose tolerance. Treatment with metformin also reduced the risk of diabetes but to a lesser extent and primarily in the younger and overweight individuals. In the Troglitazone in Prevention of Diabetes (TRIPOD) study,[185] conducted exclusively among Hispanic women with recent GDM, the insulin-sensitizing drug was associated with a 55% reduction in the incidence of diabetes. Similar findings have been reported for beta cell function with pioglitzone in individuals with previous GDM.[186] Protection of diabetes was closely linked to initial reductions in endogenous insulin requirements and ultimately associated with stabilization of pancreatic beta cell function.[185] Stabilization of beta cell function was also observed when the drug was started at the time of initial detection of diabetes by annual glucose tolerance testing.[187] These two trials suggest that the post-partum management of individuals with GDM must include a documentation of glucose tolerance, a careful assessment of risk factors for diabetes and cardiovascular disease, aggressive treatment of insulin resistance and continuing long-term follow up.

Conclusions

It seems clear from the HAPO Study and other observational data that there is a continuum of risk between hyperglycaemia and maternal and neonatal morbidity. Justification for screening and intervention is based on their ability to impact on intermediate health outcomes. The evidence for this at various levels of glycaemic control is not directly available, but is likely to be small among the many GDM women with mild hyperglycaemia. Treatment of women with more severe hyperglycaemia may reduce macrosomia, but whether this translates into reductions in birth trauma is uncertain. The ACHOIS trial demonstrated a significant reduction in a composite endpoint, but most of these women were treated with diet alone and by inference had mild hyperglycaemia, which contrasts with previous data. In general, research in this area is limited by the small number of studies, low patient numbers, lack of masking of obstetric care and the focus on macrosomia as the outcome of interest.

Future needs and directions

Diagnosis

In the light of the continuum of glycaemic risk reported by the HAPO Study, an international consensus on the diagnosis of hyperglycaemia during pregnancy is clearly indicated and is currently in progress. While maternal OGTT glucose levels in the HAPO Study were most strongly associated with cord c-peptide, this endpoint is generally considered more of a physiological occurrence, generally providing support for the Pedersen hypothesis. In contrast, Caesarean section as an endpoint was only moderately increased with maternal glucose levels. Other more robust endpoints such as pre-eclampsia or traumatic delivery must also be considered. Preliminary inspection of the results suggests that fasting glucose is strongly associated with primary outcome variables such as birth weight and it will be necessary to review whether additional sampling at the 1 and 2 h OGTT time points offers significant additional information. Pragmatically, an abridged or even abandoned OGTT test would generally be welcomed.

Nomenclature

There is a need to review the nomenclature of diabetes in pregnancy and this should be facilitated by the HAPO Study. The term GDM (gestational diabetes mellitus) is confusing and made more so by the recent WHO criteria, which now include individuals with a 2 h glucose above $7.8 \, mmol \, l^{-1}$ (no upper limit). A term such as hyperglycaemia in pregnancy would seem preferable to include both gestational IFG and IGT; the term gestational diabetes would then be applied only to individuals where the fasting or 2 h glucose levels are in the frank diabetic range.

Screening

Screening for any condition is based on its significance, a valid diagnostic test and the value of intervention. At present, there is no well-conducted RCT that provides direct evidence for the health benefits of screening in GDM. Screening strategies will have to be evaluated in relation to new HAPO diagnostic criteria. The demonstration by the HAPO Study that even levels of fasting glucose as low as $5.0 \, mmol \, l^{-1}$ result in an increased incidence of macrosomia may well support a universal approach to screening. Pragmatically, a single screening and diagnostic test would be appealing.

Effect of treatment RCTs

Efforts to optimize hyperglycaemia in pregnancy must target clinically relevant short- and long-term health outcomes. The ACHOIS trial has provided RCT evidence that treatment of GDM can significantly reduce adverse outcomes, but adverse endpoints in this study were few and most women were treated with diet alone. The RCT of Landon *et al.* currently in progress, involving the randomization of women with mild GDM to treatment or not, will provide important supplementary information. Future randomized trials should compare various insulin regimens (including the use of insulin analogues) in relation to relevant outcomes and against different glycaemia targets. The utilization of fetal abdominal circumference as a means of facilitating the identification of individuals sensitive to hyperinsulinism needs further exploration.

Oral hypoglycaemic agents

Two large randomized trials have now shown that among women with GDM, treatment with glyburide or metformin results in similar glycaemic control to that of insulin. Of note is the fact that in the MIG trial 46% of individuals in the metformin group required supplemental insulin compared with only 4% of individuals in a trial involving treatment with glyburide. These differences could be the result of varying populations and protocols, but deserve further evaluation. Not surprisingly patients prefer pills to insulin. The main remaining question is whether metformin is better or worse then glyburide, an acceptable alternative pill. Carefully conducted and adequately powered randomized trials involving the use of metformin and glyburide in GDM and PCOS associated with pregnancy and with long-term follow-up of both mother and offspring are needed. On the basis of data now available, these drugs are likely to become more widely used in GDM.

Long-term outcomes

The transgenerational effects of GDM need to be fully elucidated and all interventions must also be evaluated in relation to long-term health outcomes. GDM is analogous to the metabolic syndrome and should be viewed as a condition of cardiovascular risk frequently compounded by obesity. Although polygenic diabetes is the most common, continuing awareness of monogenic diabetes and latent autoimmune diabetes is needed. The detection of diabetes during pregnancy offers the possibility of prevention or at least postponement of future diabetes, as has been demonstrated in studies outside pregnancy. Lifestyle advice to the mother post-partum and careful follow-up are critical in this regard.

References

1 McCance DR. Gestational diabetes mellitus. In: *The Evidence Base for Diabetes Care* (eds R Williams, W Herman, AL Kinmonth, NJ Wareham,), John Wiley & Sons, Ltd, Chichester, 2002, pp. 245–288.

2 Metzger BE, Coustan DM. Summary and recommendations of the Fourth International Workshop–Conference on Gestational Diabetes Mellitus. *Diabetes Care* 1998; **211**(Suppl 2): B161–B167.

3 ACOG Practice Bulletin. Clinical management guidelines for obstetrician-gynecologists. Number 30, September 2001. *Obstet Gynecol* 2001;**98**:525–538.

4 American Diabetes Association. Gestational diabetes mellitus. *Diabetes Care* 2004;**27**(Suppl 1): S88–S90.

5 Solomon CG, Willett WC, Carey VJ, Richards J, Hunter DJ, Colditz GA *et al.* A prospective study of pregravid determinants of gestational diabetes mellitus. *JAMA* 1997;**278**: 1078–1083.

6 Marquette GP, Klein VR, Niebyl JR. Efficacy of screening for gestational diabetes. *Am J Perinatol* 1985;**2**:7–9.

7 Moses RG, Moses J, Davis WS. Gestational diabetes: do lean young Caucasian women need to be tested?. *Diabetes Care* 1998;**21**:1803–1806.

8 Parretti E, Mecacci F, Papini M *et al.* Third-trimester maternal glucose levels from diurnal profiles in nondiabetic pregnancies. *Diabetes Care* 2001;**24**:1319–1323.

9 Buchanan TA. Pancreatic beta-cell defects in gestational diabetes: implications for the pathogenesis and prevention of type 2 diabetes. *J Clin Endocrinol Metab* 2001;**86**:989–993.

10 Xiang AH *et al.* Multiple metabolic defects during late pregnancy in women at high risk for type 2 diabetes mellitus. *Diabetes* 1999;**48**:848–854.

11 Catalano PM Huston L, Amini SB Kalahan SC. Longitudinal changes in glucose metabolism during pregnancy in obese women with normal glucose tolerance and gestational diabetes mellitus. *Am J Obstet Gynecol* 1999;**180**:903–916.

12 Catalano PM *et al.* Carbohydrate metabolism during pregnancy in control subjects and women with gestational diabetes. *Am J Physiol* 1993;**264**:E60–E67.

13 Buchanan TA Xiang AH. Gestational diabetes mellitus. *J Clin Invest* 2005;**115**:485–491.

14 Brody S, Harris R, Whitener BL, Krasnov C, Lux LJ, Sutton SF, Lohr K. *Screening for Gestational Diabetes*: Systematic Evidence Review. Agency for Health Care Research and Quality, Rockville, MD, 2003;www.ahrq.gov.

15 American College of Obstetricians, Gynecologists. *Management of Diabetes Mellitus in Pregnancy*. ACOG Technical Bulletin No. 200. AGOG, Washington, DC, 1994.

16 Gross TL, Sokol RJ, Williams T, Thompson K. Shoulder dystocia? A fetal-physician risk. *Am J Obstet Gynecol* 19897;**156**:1408–1418.

17 Mondalou HD, Dorchester WL, Thorosian A, Freeman RK. Macrosomia – maternal, fetal and neonatal implications. *Obstet Gynecol* 1980;**55**:420–424.

18 Spellacy WN, Miller S, Winegar A, Peterson PQ. Macrosomia – maternal characteristics and infant complications. *Obstet Gynecol* 1985;**66**:158–161.

19 Lucas MJ, Lowe TW, McIntyre DD. Class A1 gestational diabetes: a meaningful diagnosis. *Obstet Gynecol* 1993;**82**:260–265.

20 Naylor CD, Sermer M, Chen E, Sykora K. Caesarean delivery in relation to birth weight and gestational glucose tolerance: pathophysiology or practice style? Toronto Tri-Hospital Gestational Diabetes Investigators. *JAMA* 1996;**275**:1165–1170.

21 Sermer M, Naylor CD, Farine D *et al.* The Toronto Tri-Hospital Gestational Diabetes Project. A preliminary review. *Diabetes Care* 1998;**21**:B33–B42.

22 Blank A, Grave G, Metzget BE. Effects of gestational diabetes on perinatal morbidity reassessed: report of the International Workshop on Adverse Perinatal Outcomes of Gestational Diabetes Mellitus, December 3-4, 1992. *Diabetes Care* 1995;**18**:127–129.

23 O'Sullivan JB, Gelliss SS, Dandrow RV, Tenney BO. The potential diabetic and her treatment in pregnancy. *Obstet Gynecol* 1966;**27**:683–689.

24 O'Sullivan J, The Boston Gestational Diabetes Studies. In: *Carbohydrate Metabolism in Pregnancy and the Newborn* (eds HW Sutherland, JM Stowers, DWM Pearson), Springer, London, 1989, pp. 287–294.

25 MacNeill S, Dodds L, Hamilton DC, Armson BA, Vandenhof M. Rates and risk factors for recurrence of gestational diabetes. *Diabetes Care* 2001;**24**:659–662.

26 Major CA, deVeciana M, Weeks J, Morgan MA. Recurrence of gestational diabetes: who is at risk? *Am J Obstet Gynecol* 1998;**179**:1038–1042.

27 Sacks DA, Greenspoon JS, Abu-Fadil S, Henry HM, Wolde-Tsadik G, Yao JFF. Towards universal criteria for gestational diabetes: the 75-gram glucose tolerance test in pregnancy. *Am J Obstet Gynecol* 1995;**172**:607–614.

28 Sermer M, Naylor CD, Gare DJ, Kenshole AB, Ritchie JW, Farine D *et al.* Impact of increasing carbohydrate intolerance on maternal–fetal outcomes in 3637 women without gestational diabetes: The Toronto Tri-Hospital Gestational Diabetes Project. *Am J Obstet Gynecol* 1995;**173**:146–156.

29 Langer I, Leevy J, Brustman L, Anyaegbunam A, Merkatz R, Divon M. Glycemic control in gestational diabetes mellitus – how tight is tight enough: small for gestational age vs large for gestational age? *Am J Obstet Gynecol* 1989;**161**:646–653.

30 The HAPO Study Cooperative Research Group. Hyperglycemia and pregnancy outcomes. *N Engl J Med* 2008;**358**: 1991–2002.

31 National Diabetes Data Group. Classification and diagnosis of diabetes mellitus and other categories of glucose intolerance. *Diabetes* 1979;**28**:1039–1057.

32 American Diabetes Association. Gestational diabetes: position statement. *Diabetes Care* 1999;**22**(Suppl 1): S74–S76.

33 World Health Organization. Diabetes mellitus: report of a World Health Organization study group. *WHO Tech Rep Ser* 1985;**727**:1–113.

34 Alberti KG, Zimmett PZ. Definition, diagnosis and classification of diabetes mellitus and its complications. Part 1: diagnosis and classification of diabetes mellitus: provisional report of a WHO consultation. *Diabet Med* 1998;**15**:539–553.

35 Expert Committee on the Diagnosis, Classification of Diabetes Mellitus. Report of the Expert Committee on the Diagnosis and Classification of Diabetes Mellitus. *Diabetes Care* 1997;**20**:1183–1197.

36 The HAPO Study Cooperative Research Group. The Hyperglycemia and Adverse Pregnancy Outcome (HAPO) Study. *Int J Obstet Gynaecol Obstet* 2002;**78**(1):69–77.

37 Sermer M, Naylor CD, Gare DJ, Kenshole AB, Ritchie JW, Farine D *et al.* Impact of time since last meal on the gestational glucose challenge test. The Toronto Tri-Hospital Gestational Diabetes Project. *Am J Obstet Gynecol* 1994; **171**:607–616.

38 Perucchini D, Fischer U, Spinas GA *et al.* Using fasting plasma glucose concentrations to screen for gestational diabetes mellitus: prospective population-based study. *BMJ* 1999;**181**:812–815.

39 Lamar ME, Kuehl TJ, Cooney AT *et al.* Jelly beans as an alternative to a fifty-gram glucose beverage for gestational diabetes screening. *Am J Obstet Gynecol* 1999;**181**:1154–1157.

40 Young C, Kuehl TJ, Sulak PJ *et al.* Gestational diabetes screening in subsequent pregnancies of previously healthy patients. *Am J Obstet Gynecol* 2000;**182**:1024–1026.

41 Recommendations for the management of pregnant women with diabetes (including gestational diabetes): *Diabetes UK* (online): www.diabetes.org.uk.

42 Hoffman L, Nolan CC, Wilson JD, Oats J, Simmons D. Gestational diabetes mellitus – management guidelines: the Australasian Diabetes in Pregnancy Society. *Med J Aust* 1998;**16**:93–97.

43 American Diabetes Association. Gestational diabetes mellitus. *Diabetes Care* 2002;**25**(Suppl 1): S94–S96.

44 Canadian Task Force on the Periodic Health Examination. Periodic health examination, 1992; update 1. Screening for gestational diabetes mellitus. *CMAJ* 1992;**147**:435–443.

45 Preventative Services Task Force. Screening for diabetes mellitus. In: *Guide to Clinical Preventive Services*: Report of the US Preventative Services Task Force, 2nd edn; Williams and Wilkins, Baltimore, 1996, pp. 193–208.

46 Scott DA, Loveman E, McIntyre L, Waugh N. Screening for gestational diabetes: a systematic review and economic evaluation. *Health Technol Assess* 2002;**6**:1–161.

47 National Institute for Clinical Excellence. *CG6 Antenatal Care: Routine Care for the Healthy Pregnant Woman – NICE Guideline*, National Institute for Clinical Excellence, London, 2003; http://www.nice.org.uk.

48 Hunter DJS, Kierse MJNC. Gestational diabetes. In: *Effective Care in Pregnancy and Childbirth*, Vol 1 (eds I Chalmers,

M Enkin, MJNC Keirse), Oxford University Press, Oxford, 1989, pp. 565–572.

49 Griffin ME, Coffey M, Johnson H *et al.* Universal vs risk factor based screening for gestational diabetes mellitus: detection rates, gestation at diagnosis and outcome. *Diabet Med* 2000;**17**:26–32.

50 Santini DL, Ales KL. The impact of universal screening for gestational glucose intolerance on outcome of pregnancy. *Surg Gynecol Obstet* 1990;**170**:427–436.

51 Beischer NA, Wein P, Sheedy MT, Steffen B. Identification and treatment of women with hyperglycaemia diagnosed during pregnancy can significantly reduce perinatal mortality rates. *Aust NZ J Obstet Gynecol* 1996;**36**:239–247.

52 Wen SW, Kramoer M, Joseph KS, Levitt C, Marcoux S, Liston R. Impact of prenatal glucose screening on the diagnosis of gestational diabetes and on pregnancy outcomes. *Am J Epidemiol* 2000;**152**:1009–1116.

53 Pettitt DJ, Knowler WC, Baird HR, Bennett PH. Gestational diabetes: infant and maternal complications of pregnancy in relation to third-trimester glucose tolerance in Pima Indians. *Diabetes Care* 1980;**3**:458–464.

54 Adams KM, Li H, Nelson RL *et al.* Sequelae of unrecognised gestational diabetes. *Am J Obstet Gynecol* 1998;**178**: 1321–1323.

55 Schmidt MA, Duncan BB, Reichelt AJ *et al.* Gestational diabetes mellitus diagnosed with a 2-hour oral glucose tolerance test and adverse pregnancy outcome. *Diabetes Care* 2001;**24**:1151–1155.

56 Garner P, Okun N, Keely E, Wells G, Perkins S, Sylvain K *et al.* A randomized controlled trial of strict glycaemic control and tertiary level obstetric care versus routine obstetric obstetric care in the management of gestational diabetes: a pilot study. *Am J Obstet Gynecol* 1997;**177**: 190–195.

57 Lu G, Rouse D, Dubard M, Cliver S. The impact of lower threshold values for the detection of gestational diabetes mellitus. *Obstet Gynecol* 2000;**95**:S44.

58 Li DF, Wong VC, O'Hoy KM, Yeung CY, Ma HK. Is treatment needed for mild impairment of glucose tolerance in pregnancy? A randomised controlled trial. *Br J Obstet Gynaecol* 1987;**107**:959–963.

59 Lu GC, Rouse DJ, Dubard M, Cliver S, Kimberlin D, Hauth JC. The effect of the increasing prevalence of maternal obesity on perinatal morbidity. *Am J Obstet Gynecol* 2001; **185**:845–849.

60 Langer O, Yogev Y, Most O, Xenakis EMJ. Gestational diabetes: the consequences of not treating. *Am J Obstet Gynecol* 2005;**192**:989–997.

61 Kolderup LB, Laros RK Jr, Musci TJ. Incidence of persistent birth injury in macrosomic infants: association with mode of delivery. *Am J Obstet Gynecol* 1997;**177**:37–41.

62 Berard J, Dufour P, Vinatier D *et al.* Fetal macrosomia: risk factors and outcome. A study of the outcome concerning 100 cases >4500 g. *Eur J Obstet Gynecol Reprod Biol* 1998;**77**:51–59.

63 Bryant DR, Leonardi MR, Landwehr JB, Bottoms SF. Limited usefulness of fetal weight in predicting neonatal brachial plexus injury. *Am J Obstet Gynecol* 1998; **179**:686–689.

64 Ecker JL, Greenburg JA, Norwitz ER, Nadel AS, Repke JT. Birth weight as a predictor of brachial plexus injury. *Obstet Gynecol* 1997;**89**:643–647.

65 Kjos SL, Schaefer-Graf U, Sardesi S, Peters RK, Buley A, Xiang AH *et al.* A randomised controlled trial using glycemic plus fetal ultrasound parameters versus glycemic parameters to determine insulin therapy in gestational diabetes with fasting hyperglycemia. *Diabetes Care* 2001; **24**:1904–1910.

66 Magee MS, Walden CE, Benedetti TJ, Knopp RH. Influence of diagnostic criteria on the incidence of gestational diabetes and perinatal morbidity. *JAMA* 1993;**269**:609–615.

67 Xiong X, Saunders LD, Wang FL, Demianczuk NN. Gestational diabetes mellitus: prevalence, risk factors and infant outcomes. *Int J Gynaecol Obstet* 2001;**75**:221–228.

68 Langer O. Management of gestational diabetes. *Clin Obstet Gynecol* 2000;**43**:106–115.

69 Langer O, Conway D, Berkus M, Xenakis E, Gonzales O. A comparison of glyburide and insulin on women with gestational diabetes mellitus. *N Engl J Med* 2000;**343**:1134–1138.

70 Ogata E. Perinatal morbidity in offspring of diabetic mothers. *Diabetes Rev* 1995;**3**:652–657;Silverman B, Metzger B, Cho N, Loeb C. Impaired glucose tolerance in adolescent offspring of diabetic mothers. Relationship to fetal hyperinsulinism. *Diabetes Care* 1995;**18**:611–617.

71 Pettitt DJ, Bennett PH, Knowler WC, Baird HR, Alec KA. Gestational diabetes mellitus and impaired glucose tolerance during pregnancy. Long-term effects ion obesity and glucose tolerance in the offspring. *Diabetes* 1985;**34**:119–122.

72 Silverman BL, Rizzo T, Green OC *et al.* Long-term prospective evaluation of offspring of diabetic mothers. *Diabetes* 1991;**40**:196–199.

73 Whitaker RC, Pepe MS, seidel KD, Wright KA, Knopp RH. Gestational diabetes and the risk of offspring obesity. *Pediatrics* 1998;**101**:E9.

74 Persson B, Gentz J, Moller E. Follow up of children of insulin dependent (type 1), and gestational diabetic mothers. Growth pattern, glucose tolerance, insulin response and HLA types. *Acta Paediatr Scand* 1984;**73**:778–784.

75 Vohr BR, McGarvey ST, Tucker R. Effects of maternal gestational diabetes on offspring adiposity at 4–7 years of age. *Diabetes Care* 1994;**17**:832–834.

76 Lipscomb KR, Gregory K, Shaw K. The outcome of macrosomic infants weighing at least 4500 grams: Los Angeles County and University of Southern California experience. *Obstet Gynecol* 1995;**85**:558–564.

77 Jensen DM, Sorensen B, Feilberg-Jorgensen N, Westergaardt JG, Beck-Neilsen H. Maternal and perinatal outcomes in 143 Danish women with gestational diabetes mellitus and 143 controls with a similar risk profile. *Diabet Med* 2000;**17**:281–286.

78 Casey BM, Lucas MJ, McIntyre DD, Leveno KJ. Pregnancy outcomes in women with gestational diabetes compared with the general obstetric population. *Obstet Gynecol* 1997;**90**:869–873.

79 Roach VJ, Hin LY, Tam WH, Ng KB, Rogers MS. The incidence of pregnancy-induced hypertension among patients with carbohydrate intolerance. *Hypertens Pregnancy* 2000;**19**:183–189.

80 Persson B, Strangenberg M, Hansson U, Norlander E. Gestational diabetes mellitus (GDM) comparative evaluation of two treatment regimens, diet versus insulin and diet. *Diabetes* 1985;**11**:101–105.

81 Nachum Z, Ben-Shlomo I, Weiner E, Shalev E. Twice daily versus four times daily insulin dose regimens for diabetes in pregnancy: randomised controlled trial. *BMJ* 1999;**319**: 1223–1227.

82 De Veciana M, Major CA, Morgan MA *et al.* Postprandial versus pre-prandial glucose monitoring in women with gestational diabetes mellitus requiring insulin therapy. *N Engl J Med* 1995;**333**:1237–1241.

83 Naylor CD, Sermer M, Chen E, Farine D. Selective screening for gestational diabetes mellitus. Tronto Tri-Hospital Gestational Diabetes Project Investigators. *N Engl J Med* 1997; **337**:1591–1596.

84 Langer O. Maternal glycemic criteria for insulin therapy in gestational diabetes mellitus. *Diabetes Care* 1998;**21** (Suppl 2): B91–B98.

85 Bancroft K, Tuffnell DJ, Masson GC, Rogerson LJ, Mansfield M. A randomised controlled pilot study of the management of gestational impaired glucose. *Br J Obstet Gynecol* 2000; **107**:959–963.

86 Dornhorst A, Frost G. The principles of dietary management of gestational diabetes: reflection on current evidence. *J Hum Nutr Dietet* 2002;**15**:145–156.

87 Walkinshaw SA. Dietary regulation for 'gestational diabetes'. *Cochrane Database Syst Rev* 2000;(2):CD000070.

88 Jovanovic L, Durak EP, Peterson CM. Randomised trial of diete versus diet plus cardiovascular conditioning on glucose levels in gestational diabetes. *Am J Obstet Gynecol* 1989;**161**:415–419.

89 Diabetes Prevention Program Research Group. Reduction in the incidence of type 2 diabetes with lifestyle intervention or metformin. *N Engl J Med* 2002;**346**:393–403.

90 Major CA, Henry MJ, de Veciana M *et al.* The effects of carbohydrate restriction in patients with diet-controlled gestational diabetes. *Obstet Gynecol* 1998;**91**:600–604.

91 Bung P, Artal R, Rhodiguian N, Kjos S. Exercise in gestational diabetes. An optional therapeutic approach. *Diabetes* 1991;**40**(Suppl 2): 182–185.

92 Jovanovic-Peterson L, Peterson CM. Is exercise safe or useful for gestational diabetic women?. *Diabetes* 1991;**40** (Suppl 1): 179–181.

93 Avery MD, Walker AJ. Acute effect of exercise on blood glucose and insulin levels in women with gestational diabetes. *J Matern Fetal Neonatal Med* 2001;**10**:52–58.

94 Avery MD. Leon AS, Kopher RA. Effects of a partially home-based exercise program for women with gestational diabetes. *Obstet Gynecol* 1997;**89**:10–15.

95 Langer I, Levy J, Brustman L *et al.* Glycaemic control in gestational diabetes mellitus: how tight is tight enough for gestational age versus large for gestational age? *Am J Obstet Gynecol* 1989;**161**:646–653.

96 Langer O, Berkus M, Brustman L *et al.* Rationale for insulin management in gestational diabetes mellitus. *Diabetes* 1991;**40**(Suppl 2): 186–190.

97 Drexel H, Bichler A, Sailer S, Breier C, Lisch HJ, Braunsteiner H *et al.* Prevention of perinatal morbidity by tight

metabolic control in gestational diabetes mellitus. *Diabetes Care* 1988;**11**:761–768.

98 Shushan A, Ezra Y, Samuelloff A. Early treatment of gestational diabetes reduces the rate of fetal macrosomia. *Am J Perinatol* 1997;**14**:253–256.

99 Kalhoff RK. Therapeutic results of insulin therapy in gestational diabetes mellitus. *Diabetes* 1985;**34**(Suppl 2): 97–100.

100 Coustan DR, Imarah J. Prophylactic insulin treatment of gestatinal diabetes reduces the incidence of macrosomia, operative delivery and birth trauma. *Am J Obstet Gynecol* 1984;**150**:836–842.

101 Langer O, Anyaegbunam A, Brustman L, Divon M. Management of women with one abnormal glucose tolerance test value reduces adverse outcome in pregnancy. *Am J Obstet Gynecol* 1989;**161**:593–599.

102 O'Sullivan JB, Mahan CM, Charles D, Dandrow RV. Medical treatment of the gestational diabetic. *Obstet Gynecol* 1974;**43**:817–821.

103 Coustan DR, Lewis SB. Insulin therapy for gestational diabetes. *Obstet Gynecol* 1978;**51**:306–310.

104 Thompson DJ, Porter KB, Gunnells DJ. Prophylactic insulin in the management of gestational diabetes. *Obstet Gynecol* 1990;**75**:960–964.

105 Crowther CA, Hiller JE, Moss JR *et al.* Effect of treatment of gestational diabetes mellitus on pregnancy outcomes. *N Engl J Med* 2005;**352**:2477–2486.

106 Goldberg JD, Franklin B, Lasser D *et al.* Gestational diabetes: impact of home glucose monitoring on neonatal birth weight. *Am J Obstet Gynecol* 1986;**154**:546–550.

107 Poyhonen-Alho M, Teramo K, Kaaja R. Treatment of gestational diabetes with short- or long-acting insulin and neonatal outcome: a pilot study. *Acta Obstet Gynecol Scand* 2002;**81**:258–259.

108 Buchanan TS, Kjos SL, Montoro MN *et al.* Use of fetal ultrasound to select metabolic therapy for pregnancies complicated by mild gestational diabetes. *Diabetes Care* 1994;**17**:275–283.

109 Schaefer-Graf UM, Kjos SL, Fauzan OH, Buhling KJ, Siebert G, Buhrer C, Ladendorf B, Dudenhausen JW, Vetter K. A randomised trial evaluating a predominantly fetal growth-based strategy to guide management of gestational diabetes in Caucasian women. *Diabetes Care* 2004;**27**:297–302.

110 Landon MB, Gabbe SG. Antepartum fetal surveillance in gestational diabetes mellitus. *Diabetes* 1985;**34**(Suppl 2): 50–52.

111 Girz BA, Divon MY, Merkatz IR. Sudden fetal death in women with well controlled, intensively monitored gestational diabetes. *J Perinatol* 1992;**12**:229–233.

112 Kjos SL, Leung A, Henry OA. Antepartum surveillance in diabetic pregnancies. Predictors of fetal distress in labor. *Am J Obstet Gynecol* 1995;**173**:1532–1539.

113 Johnson JM, Lange IR, Harman CR, Torchia MG, Manning FA. Biophysical profile scoring ni the management of the diabetic pregnancy. *Obstet Gynecol* 1988;**72**:841–846.

114 Kerbel D, Glazier R, Holzapfel S, Yeung M, Lofsky S. Adverse effects of screening for gestational diabetes: a prospective cohort study in Toronto, Canada. *J Med Screen* 1997;**4**:128–132.

115 Syogren B, Robeus B, Hansson U. Gestational diabetes: a case–control study of women's experience of pregnancy, health and the child. *Psychosom Res* 1994;**38**: 815–822.

116 Feig DS, Chen E, Naylor CD. Self-perceived health status of women three to five years after the diagnosis of gestational diabetes: a survey of cases and matched controls. *Am J Obstet Gynecol* 1998;**178**:386–393.

117 Knopp RH, Magee MS, Raisys V, Benedetti T, Bonet B. Hypocaloric diets and ketogenesis in the management of obese gestational diabetic women. *J Am Coll Nutr* 1991;**10**: 649–667.

118 Landon MB, Thom E, Spong CY, Gabbe SG, Leindecker S, Johnson F, Lain K, Miodovnik M, Carpenter M. A planned randomised clinical trial of treatment for mild gestational diabetes mellitus. *J Matern Fetal Neonatal Med* 2002; **11**:226–231.

119 Manderson JG, Patterson CC, Hadden DR, Traub AI, Ennis C, McCance DR. Preprandial versus post-prandial blood glucose monitoring in type 1 diabetic pregnancy. *Am J Obstet Gynecol* **189**:(2):2003;507–512.

120 Combs CA, Gunderson E, Kitzmiller JL *et al.* Relationship of fetal macrosomia to maternal post-prandial glucose control during pregnancy. *Diabetes Care* 1992;**15**:1251–1257.

121 Jovanovic L, Peterson CM, Reed GF *et al.* Maternal post-prandial glucose levels and infant birth weight: the Diabetes in Early Pregnancy Study. *Am J Obstet Gynecol* 1991;**164**:103–111.

122 Brunelle RL, Llewelyn J, Anderson JH *et al.* Meta-analysis of the effect of insulin lispro on severe hypoglycaemia in patients with type 1 diabetes. *Diabetes Care* 1998;**21**: 1726–1731.

123 Yki-Yarvinen H, Dressler A, Ziemen M. Less nocturnal hypoglycaemia and better post-dinner glucose control with bedtime insulin glargine compared with bedtime NPH insulin during insulin combination therapy in type 2 diabetes. HOE 901/3002 Study Group. *Diabetes Care* 2003;**26**:1490–1496.

124 Jovanovic L, Ilic S, Pettitt DJ. Metabolic and immunologic effects of insulin lispro in gestational diabetes. *Diabetes Care* 1999;**22**:1422–1427.

125 Mecacci F, Carignani L, Cioni R, Bartoli E, Parretti E, La Torre P, Scarselli G, Mello G. Maternal metabolic control and perinatal outcome in women with gestational diabetes treated with regular or lispro insulin: comparison with non-diabetic women. *Eur J Obstet Gynecol* Reprod Biol 2003; **111**:19–24.

126 Persson B, Swahn ML, Hjertberg R *et al.* Insulin lispro therapy in pregnancies complicated by type 1 diabetes mellitus. *Diabetes Res Clin Pract* 2002;**58**:115–121.

127 Carr KJE, Idama TO, Masson EA, Ellis K, Lindow SW. A randomized controlled trial of insulin lispro given before or after meals in pregnant women with type 1 diabetes – the effect of glycaemic excursion. *J Obstet Gynaecol* 2004; 24382–386.

128 Cypryk K, Sobczak M, Pertynska-Marczewska M, Zawodniak- Szatapska M, Szymczak W, Wilczynski J, Lewinski A. Pregnancy complications and perinatal outcomes in diabetic women treated with Humalog (insulin

lispro) or regular human insulin during pregnancy. *Med Sci Mont* 2004;**10**:129–132.

129 Pettitt DJ, Ospina P, Kolaczynski JW, Jovanovic L. Comparison of an insulin analog, insulin aspart and regular human insulin with no insulin in gestational diabetes mellitus. *Diabetes Care* 2003;**26**:183–1096.

130 Mathiesen E, Kinsley B, McCance D, Heller S, Raben AMaternal hypoglycaemia and glycaemic control in pregnancy: a randomized trial comparing insulin aspart with human insulin in 322 subjects with type 1 diabetes. Abstract. Presented at the 66th Annual Meeting of the American Diabetes Association, 2006.

131 Glazer NB, Zalani S, Anderson JH *et al.* Safety of insulin lispro: pooled data from clinical trials. *Am J Health Syst Pharm* 1999;**56**:542–547.

132 Kurtzhals P, Schaffer L, Sorensen A *et al.* Correlations of receptor binding and metabolic and mitogenic potencies of insulin analogs designed for clinical use. *Diabetes* 2000;**49**:999–1005.

133 Reid TW, Reid WA. The labile nature of the insulin signal(s) for the stimulation of DNA synthesis in mouse lens epithelial and 3T3 cells. *J Biol Chem* 1987;**262**:229–233.

134 Bhattacharyya A, Brown S, Hughes S *et al.* Insulin lispro and regular insulin in pregnancy. *Q J Med* 2001;**94**:255–260.

135 Scherbaum WA, Lamkisch MR, Pawlowski B. Insulin lispro in pregnancy: retrospective analysis of 33 cases and matched controls. *Exp Clin Endocrinol Diabetes* 2002;**110**:6–9.

136 Masson EA, Patmore JE, Brash PD *et al.* Pregnancy outcome in type 1 diabetes mellitus trreated with insulin lispro. *Diabet Med* 2003;**20**:46–50.

137 Kitzmiller JL, Main E, Ward B *et al.* Insulin lispro and the development of proliferative retinopathy during pregnancy. *Diabetes Care* 1999;**22**:874–876.

138 Buchbinder A, Midovnik M, McElvvy S *et al.* Is insulin lispro associated with the development or progression of proliferative retinopathy during pregnancy? *Am J Obstet Gynecol* 2000;**183**:1162–1165.

139 Loukovaara S, Immonen I, Teramo KA *et al.* Progression of retinopathy during pregnancy in type 1 diabetic women treated with insulin lispro. *Diabetes Care* 2003;**26**:1193–1198.

140 Gallen IW, Jaap A. Insulin glargine use in pregnancy is not associated with adverse maternal or fetal outcomes. Presented at the 66th Annual Meeting of the American Diabetes Association, 2006;1804P.

141 Sivan E, Feldman B, Dolitzki M *et al.* Glyburide crosses the placenta *in vivo* in pregnant rats. *Diabetologia* 1995;**38**:753–756.

142 Piacquadio K, Hollingsworth DR, Murphy H. Effects of *in-utero* exposure to oral hypoglycaemic drugs. *Lancet* 1991;**338**:866–869.

143 Kemball ML, McIvert C, Milner C, Milner RDG *et al.* Neonatal hypoglycaemia in infants of diabetic mothers given sulphyonylurea drugs in pregnancy. *Arch Dis Child* 1970;**45**:696–701.

144 Zucker P, Simon G. Prolonged symptomatic neonatal hypoglycaemia associated with maternal chhloropropamide therapy. *Paediatrics* 1968;**42**:824–825.

145 Denno KM, Sadler TW. Effects of the biguanide class of oral hypoglycemic agents on mouse embryogenesis. *Teratology* 1994;**49**:260–266.

146 Elliott BD, Langer O, Schenker S, Johnson R. Insignificant transfer of glyburide across the human placenta. *Am J Obstet Gynecol* 1991;**165**:807–812.

147 Elliott BD, Schenker S, Langer O, Johnson R, Prihoda T. Comparative placental transport of oral hypoglycaemic agents in humans: a human model of placental drug transfer. *Am J Obstet Gynecol* 1994;**171**:653–660.

148 Elliott BD, Langer O, Schuessling F. Human placental glucose uptake and transport are not altered by the oral antihyperglycaemic agent metformin. *Am J Obstet Gynecol* 1997;**176**:527–530.

149 Coetzee EJ, Jackson WPU. Metformin in management of pregnant insulin-dependent diabetics. *Diabetologia* 1979;**16**: 241–245.

150 Coetzee EJ, Jackson WPU. Oral hypoglycaemic in the first trimester and fetal outcome. *S Afr Med J* 1984;**65**:635–637.

151 Coetzee EJ, Jackson WPU. The management of non insulin-dependent diabetes during pregnancy. *Diabetes Res Clin Pract* 1986;287; **1**:281–287.

152 Towner D, Kjos SL, Montoro MM *et al.* Congenital malformations in pregnancies complicated by NIDDM. *Diabetes Care* **18**:1995;1446–1451.

153 Langer O, Conway D, Berkus M, Xenakis EMJ. There is no association between hypoglycaemic use and fetal anomalies. *Am J Obstet Gynecol* 1999;**180**:S38 (abstract).

154 Konen G. Presented at the NIH/FDA Toxicology in Pregnancy Conference, Toronto, 2000.

155 Gutzin SJ, Kozer E, Magee LA, Feig DS, Koren G. The safety of oral hypoglyemic agends in the first trimester of pregnancy: a meta-analysis. *Can J Clin Pharmacol* 2003;**10**:179–183.

156 Ekpebegh CO, Coetzee EJ, van der Merwe L, Levitt NS. A 10-year retrospective analysis of pregnancy outcome in pregestational type2 diabetes: comparison of insulin and oral glucose-lowering agents. *Diabet Med* 2007;**24**:253–258.

157 Helmuth E, Damm P, Molsted-Pedersen L. Oral hypoglycaemic agents in 118 diabetic pregnancies. *Diabet Med* 2000;**17**:507–511.

158 Hughes RCE, Gardiner SJ, Begg EJ, Zhang M. Effect of pregnancy on the pharmacokinetics of metformin. *Diabet Med* 2006;**23**:324–327.

159 Glueck CJ, Wang P, Kobayashi S, Phillips H, Sieve-Smith L. Metformin therapy throughout pregnancy reduces the development of gestational diabetes in women with polycystic ovarian syndrome. *Fertil Steril* 2002;**77**:520–525.

160 Glueck CJ, Bornovali S, Prannikoff J, Goldenberg N, Dharashivkar S, Wang P. Metformin, pre-eclampsia and pregnancy outcomes in women with polycystic ovary syndrome. *Diabet Med* 2004;**21**:829–836.

161 Glueck CJ, Goldenberg N, Pranikoff J, Loftspring M, Sieve L, Wang P. Height, weight and motor-social development during the first 18 months of life in 126 infants born to 109 mothers with polycystic ovary syndrome who conceived on and continued metformin through pregnancy. *Hum Reprod* 2004;**19**:1323–1330.

162 Glueck CJ, Goldenberg N, Wang P, Loftspring M, Sherman A. Metformin during pregnancy reduces insulin, insulin resistance, insulin secretion, weight, testosterone and development of gestational diabetes: prospective longitudinal

assessment of women with polycystic ovary syndrome from preconception throughout pregnancy. *Hum Reprod* 2004;**19**:510–521.

163 Notelowitz M. Sulphonylurea therapy in the treatment of the pregnant diabetic. *S Afr Med J* 1971;**45**:226–229.

164 Rowan JA, Hague WM, Wanzhen G, Battin MR, Moore MP. Metformin versus insulin for the treatment of gestational diabetes. *N Engl J Med* 2008;**358**:2003–2015.

165 Feig DS, Briggs GG, Kraemer JM *et al*. Transfer of glyburide and glipizide into breast milk. *Diabetes Care* 2005;**28**:1851–1855.

166 Hale TW, Fristensen JH, Hackett LP, Kohan R, Ilett KF. Transfer or metformin into human milk. *Diabetologia* 2002;**45**:1509–1514.

167 Briggs CG, Ambrose PJ, Nageotte MP *et al*. Excretion of metformin into breast milk and the effect on nursing infants. *Obstet Gynecol* 2005;**105**:1437–1441.

168 Gardiner SJ, Kirkpatrick CM, Begg EJ *et al*. Transfer of metformin into human milk. *Clin Pharmacol Ther* 2003;**743**:71–77.

169 Bailey CJ, Turner RC. Metformin. *N Engl J Med* 1996;**334**:574–579.

170 Hughes RCE, Gardiner SJ, Begg EJ, Zang M. Effect of pregnancy on pharmacokinetics of metformin. *Diabet Med* 2006;**23**:324–327.

171 Zarate A, Ochoa R, Hernandez M *et al*. Effectiveness of acarbose in the control of glucose tolerance worsening in pregnancy. *Ginecol Obstet Mex* 2000;**68**:42–45.

172 Bertini AM, Silva JC, Tamborda W *et al*. Perinatal outcomes and the use of oral hypoglycemic agents. *J Perinat Med* 2005;**33**:519–523.

173 Yik-Si Chan L, Hok-Keung J, Kin Lau T *et al*. Placental transfer of rosiglitazone in the first trimester of human pregnancy. *Fertil Steril* 2005;**83**:955–980.

174 Briggs CG, Freeman RK, Yaffe SJ. *Drugs in Pregnancy and Lactation*, 7th edn, Lippincott Williams and Wilkins, Philadelphia, PA, 2005, pp. 1316 and 1438.

175 Brooks Vaughan T, Bell DSH. Stockpiling of ovarian follicles and the response to rosiglitazone. *Diabetes Care* 2005;**28**:2333–2334.

176 Kalyoncu NI, Yaris F, Ulku C *et al*. A case of rosiglitazone exposure in the second trimester of pregnancy. *Reprod Toxicol* 2005;**19**:563–564.

177 Rouzi AA, Ardawi MSM. A randomised controlled trial of the efficacy of rosiglitazone and clomiphene citrate versus metformin and clomiphene citrate in women with clomiphene citrate-resistant polycystic ovary syndrome. *Fertil Steril* 2006;**85**:428–435.

178 Ghazeeri G, Kutteh WH, Bryer-Ash M, Haas D, Ke RW. Effect of rosiglitazone on spontaneous and clomiphene citrate-induced ovulation in women with polycystic ovary syndrome. *Fertil Steril* 2003;**779**:562–566.

179 National Institute of Health and Clinical Excellence. *Guidelines for Management of Diabetes in Pregnancy*, NICE, London, 2008.

180 Kim C, Newton KM, Knopp RH. Gestational diabetes and the incidence of type 2 diabetes. *Diabetes Care* 2002;**25**:1862–1868.

181 Ellard S *et al*. A high prevalence of glucokinase mutations in gestational diabetic subjects selected by clinical criteria. *Diabetologia* 2000;**43**:250–253.

182 Peters RK, Kjos SL, Ziang A, Buchanan TA. Long-term diabetogenic effect of a single pregnancy in women with prior gestational diabetes mellitus. *Lancet* 1996;**347**:227–230.

183 Buchanan TA *et al*. Changes in insulin secretion and sensitivity during the development of type 2 diabetes after gestational diabetes in Hispanic women. *Diabetes* 2003;**52** (Suppl 1): A34.

184 Buchanan TA *et al*. Response of pancreatic beta-cells to improved insulin sensitivity in women at high risk for type 2 diabetes. *Diabetes* 2000;**49**:782–788.

185 Buchanan TA, Xiang AH, Peters RK, Marroquin A *et al*. Preservation of pancreatic beta-cell function and prevention of type 2 diabetes by pharmacological treatment of insulin resistance in high-risk Hispanic women. *Diabetes* 2002;**51**:2796–2803.

186 Buchanan TA, Xiang AH, Kjos SL, Peters RK, Marroquin A, Goici J *et al*. Diabetes rates and beta-cell function in the Pioglitazone Prevention of Diabetes (PIPOD) study. *Diabetes* 2005;**28**:A39.

187 Xiang AH *et al*. Pharmacological treatment of insulin resistance at two different stages in the evolution of type 2 diabetes: impact on glucose tolerance and beta-cell function. *J Clin Endocrinol Metab* 2004;**89**:2846–2851.

12 Antihypertensive therapy to prevent the cardiovascular complications of diabetes mellitus

Tonya L. Corbin, Alan B. Weder

Division of Cardiovascular Medicine, Department of Internal Medicine, University of Michigan, Ann Arbor, MI, USA

Introduction

Hypertension is a common co-morbidity of type 2 diabetes mellitus (hereafter referred to as diabetes), occurring in up to 75% of patients with diabetes.[1] Some 65% of patients with type 2 diabetes eventually die of cardiovascular events.[2] The evidence base supporting the efficacy of antihypertensive therapy for the prevention of macrovascular disease complications in type 2 diabetes is now extensive and consistent: in addition to placebo-controlled trials, we now have many drug–drug comparisons and others comparing more versus less aggressive therapeutic targets for blood pressure. There is complete consensus that antihypertensive drug treatment improves outcomes compared with placebo and strong support for the contention that lower blood pressure treatment targets are desirable.

Mechanisms of atherosclerosis in diabetes and hypertension

Diabetes mellitus is a powerful risk factor for atherosclerotic cardiovascular disease (CVD), conferring a risk equivalent to that of established coronary artery disease.[3] Part of the association of diabetes and CVD is the result of its concordance with other cardiovascular risk factors: as noted above, the development of hypertension is the rule in type 2 diabetes and many patients with diabetes also have dyslipidaemia. Obesity, which plays a major role in diabetes, may further increase cardiovascular risk. The need to address the obesity epidemic has been the subject of a recent 'call to action' issued jointly by the American Heart Association and the American Diabetes Association.[4] However, even when the effects of these other risk factors are accounted for, diabetes itself still contributes independently to CVD.[5]

Our understanding of the mechanisms initiating and accelerating atherosclerosis and its complications has undergone substantial change over the past decade, with a growing appreciation of the importance of endothelial injury as an early initiating mechanism and of inflammation as a key process promoting atherosclerotic plaque formation and growth.[6] Explanations commonly offered to explain how hypertension and diabetes jointly increase atherosclerotic risk have focused on the impact of both high blood pressure and hyperglycaemia on endothelial dysfunction and oxidative stress. In addition, some of the specific mechanisms underlying the diseases, particularly increased activity of the renin–angiotensin–aldosterone system and the hyperinsulinaemia resulting from insulin resistance, increase the production of oxygen free radicals and further impair endothelial function.[7] Key aspects of endothelial dysfunction include increased permeability, which compromises the normal endothelial barrier function, decreased cell–cell adhesion, which promotes macrophage infiltration into the subendothelial space, and enhanced expression and elaboration of growth factors. A damaged endothelium also permits increased rates of retention of low-density lipoprotein (LDL) particles in the subendothelial space, enhanced LDL oxidation and increased expression of the macrophage lectin-like oxidized LDL receptor, all of which contribute to foam

The Evidence Base for Diabetes Care, Second Edition, Edited by William H. Herman, Ann Louise Kinmonth, Nicholas J. Wareham and Rhys Williams.
© 2010 John Wiley & Sons, Ltd

cell formation and elaboration of cytokines and growth factors. These changes promote the development of the fatty streak and its progression to the formation of the fibrofatty lesion and ultimately to the complicated lesion of advanced atherosclerosis with its lipid core and fibrous cap.

The importance of inflammation in promoting the progression of atherosclerosis is now well established. While we regard its role in atherosclerosis as harmful, inflammation evolved to counter infectious, primarily bacterial, threats to an organism.[7] It is an ancient and powerful mechanism with numerous pathways that serve to reinforce each other and provide a multifaceted defence that contributes to the phenotype of the infectious illness. In addition to its role in infectious illness, the inflammatory response is part of many other non-infectious diseases, including arthritidies, vasculitis, allergies and some cancers. In these cases, inflammation usually does more harm than good and the medical perspective is that suppression of the inflammatory response is beneficial.

Inflammation in the atherosclerotic plaque can be thought of as a non-specific response to a perceived infectious trigger. In this case, rather than a bacterial cell, the trigger is oxidized LDL particles. Circulating LDL particles traverse the endothelium and enter the subendothelial space where lipoproteins and lipids undergo the chemical process of oxidation. Oxidized LDL particles are treated by the body as if they were bacteria and are removed from contact with the vessel by macrophages. Macrophages are a key element in the inflammatory response, since they serve not only to remove invaders but also to elaborate cytokines that signal other inflammatory cells to migrate to the area and reinforce the defence response. Small numbers of oxidized LDL particles can be metabolized by macrophages, but as the cells continue to take up more and more particles, macrophages eventually become overloaded and become 'foam cells', a term that reflects the histological appearance of a macrophage stuffed with oxidized LDL particles. Accumulations of foam cells elaborate inflammatory and growth-promoting substances that cause expansion of the early atherosclerotic lesion and production of a cap of fibrous tissue, which serves to wall off the foam cells from the circulation and to stabilize the complex. This complex of cap and core is the mature atherosclerotic plaque and to a great degree the relative size and thickness of the cap and the size and composition of the core determine whether a plaque is relatively stable or unstable and therefore prone to rupture.

Identification of plaque rupture as the precipitating event is another change in our thinking about what causes CVD events. We currently distinguish between the stable occlusive plaque, which is characterized by a thick fibrous cap covering a relatively small core of cholesterol, and the more dynamic unstable plaque characterized by a thin cap with a large core and active inflammation and growth factor production. Occlusive plaques are most commonly associated with stable angina, the effort-induced chest pain the arises from a mismatch of myocardial oxygen need and delivery. These stable lesions can cause coronary occlusion and heart attack, but a more common scenario is the rupture of an unstable non-occlusive plaque, which results in the exudation of the lipid-rich inflammatory core into the lumen of the coronary vessel. This highly thrombogenic material triggers the clotting sequence and the resulting blood clot can block the artery and cut off blood flow. Beyond this obstruction, tissue damage begins and, if the area is not reperfused, heart tissue dies. Both diabetes and hypertension are associated with increased activity of processes promoting plaque instability, including heightened expression of the proinflammatory Cox-2 enzyme in the shoulder of the atherosclerotic plaque and increased activity of metalloproteases, which break down collagen and destabilize the plaque.

Advanced glycation endproducts and increased risk for cardiovascular complications in diabetes

A diabetes-specific mechanism of endothelial injury is the formation of advanced glycation endproducts (AGEs), a process aggravated by hyperglycaemia and increased oxidative stress. AGEs are formed by a process of non-enzymatic glycation known as the Millard reaction, during which a reducing sugar attaches to an amino group to form a Schiff base. This product then undergoes rearrangement, dehydration and condensation steps, which eventually result in the irreversible formation of AGEs. These AGEs have both direct effects and actions medicated by interactions with a specific receptor for AGEs (RAGE).

Non-receptor-mediated actions of AGEs include the cross-linking of a variety of membrane proteins, including collagen. This process accelerates vascular ageing by decreasing vascular compliance, which results in increased systolic blood pressure and pulse pressure, both of which are associated with increased CVD risk. As described above, oxidation of LDL-C particles is an important trigger for atherosclerosis, and in diabetes AGEs accelerate the oxidation of lipids and apolipoprotein B.[8] AGE-mediated oxidative modification of LDL particles results in decreased LDL recognition by cellular LDL receptors and increased expression of the macrophage scavenger receptor with increased accumulation of oxidized LDL. Increased levels of AGE-modified lipids thereby promote the formation of the lipid-laden foam cells characteristic of fatty streaks. The AGEs resulting from non-enzymatic glycation of lipids and proteins also accumulate in diabetic atherosclerotic plaques and result in increased oxidant stress and stimulation of inflammation, including the increased Cox-2 activity and upregulation of matrix metalloprotease expression noted above, in addition to increased elaboration of prostaglandins and leukotrienes. All these effects accelerate atherosclerosis and promote macrovascular diabetic complications.[9]

In addition to the direct actions of AGEs, RAGE is upregulated in the presence of AGEs. RAGE is one of the immunoglobulin superfamily of receptors and is expressed primarily on endothelial cells. When occupied by AGEs, RAGE stimulates the production of tissue necrosis factor and VCAM-1 by macrophages, resulting in increased vascular permeability and increased lipoprotein flux into the subendothelium. The monocyte–macrophage cascade of adhesion mediators such as cytokines and growth factors further facilitates the migration of inflammatory cells into the nascent plaque, promoting plaque instability and increasing the risk of plaque rupture and coronary thrombosis.[10] The interaction of AGE and RAGE markedly stimulates the production of reactive oxygen species and increases oxidative stress, the effects of which are aggravated by reductions of natural antioxidants: levels of reduced glutathione and vitamins C and E are all reduced in diabetic patients. Increased concentrations of reactive oxygen species resulting from increased production and decreased removal result in decreased activity of endothelial nitric oxide, which contributes to endothelial dysfunction.

A number of inhibitors of AGE production, including aminoguanidine, pimagedine and pyradoxamine, have demonstrated anti-atherosclerotic effects in animal models, although no human data are available. Proposed mechanisms of benefit include the inhibition of AGE-mediated fatty acid oxidation by inhibition of lipid advanced glycosylation and by direct reaction with reactive aldehydes that form during fatty acid oxidation.[8]

Clinical trials for the prevention of macrovascular disease in patients with diabetes and hypertension

Placebo-controlled trials and comparisons of more versus less intensive treatment regimens definitely established that active treatment is superior to placebo and that lower achieved blood pressure is beneficial. Fuller has previously comprehensively reported the early experience with antihypertensive therapy in diabetes to 2001 in an earlier edition of this volume,[11] and the reader is referred to that report for a more detailed discussion of these studies. Summary tables from that review are included in the Appendix to this chapter.

Placebo-controlled trials or trials comparing different blood pressure targets

Prior to 1998, only two trials of antihypertensive therapy, the Hypertension Detection and Follow-up Program trial[12,13] and the Systolic Hypertension in the Elderly Program trial,[14,15] included moderately sized diabetic sub-groups and both showed that antihypertensive therapy was associated with significant reductions in CVD rates but not in mortality. In 1998, the results of the first large trial to examine specifically the effects of antihypertensive treatment on CVD outcomes, the United Kingdom Prospective Diabetes Study (UKPDS), were published and demonstrated that a lower achieved blood pressure level results in substantial reductions in cardiovascular and non-cardiovascular event rates.[16,17] The UKPDS trial was primarily a comparison of strategies for glycaemic control in diabetes, but it included 1148 hypertensive patients who were randomized in a comparison of 'tight' versus 'less tight' blood pressure control; the design also incorporated a comparison of captopril- and atenolol-based treatment regimens. Although the targets for 'tight' (<150/85 mmHg) and 'less tight' (<180/105 mmHg) blood pressure control, and also achieved blood pressures (averaging 144/82 and 154/87 mmHg in the 'tight' and 'less tight' groups, respectively), were well above contemporary consensus recommendations, there was a significant reduction in the combined primary endpoint (comprised of sudden death, death from hyper- or hypoglycaemia, fatal or non-fatal myocardial infarction (MI) or stroke, new-onset angina, heart failure, renal failure, amputation, vitreous haemorrhage, need for retinal photocoagulation, unilateral blindness or cataract extraction) in the more aggressively treated group. Individual components of this combined endpoint demonstrated substantial reductions, although only stroke rates were statistically significantly reduced. Overall, the benefits of more intensive blood pressure control substantially outweighed those attributable to tight glucose control [mean haemoglobin A_{1c} (HbA$_{1c}$) of 7.0% versus 7.9%] Of considerable interest was the effect of 'tight' control of blood pressure on microvascular endpoints previously thought to relate mainly to hyperglycaemia; the effect was mostly due to reduction in the need for retinal photocoagulation.

At about the same time as the UKPDS report, results for the diabetic sub-group of the Hypertension Optimal Treatment (HOT) trial were reported.[18] The

HOT trial was designed to address the 'J-point' controversy, that is, the question of whether there was a blood pressure level below which CVD rates begin to increase, presumably as the result of myocardial hypoperfusion due to fixed coronary artery obstruction. In the HOT trial, hypertensive patients were randomized to three groups with blood pressure treatment targets of <80, <85 or <90 mmHg: the trial included a sub-group of 1501 patients with diabetes. Achieved in-study blood pressures averaged 81.1, 83.2 and 85.2 mmHg for the three randomized groups, with considerable overlap between the population distributions of values. For patients with diabetes (although not for those without), the 80 mmHg target group had significantly reduced risk of cardiovascular death and major cardiovascular events and a trend (not statistically significant) for reduced total mortality compared with the 90 mmHg target group. Further analysis of the blood pressures achieved in the total population of trial participants suggested that the nadir for event rates occurs at a diastolic blood pressure of about 83 mmHg. In the HOT trial, systolic blood pressure was reduced by only 4 mmHg in the lowest and highest target groups (144 vs 140 mmHg), but even though that figure suggests that a goal systolic blood pressure somewhat greater than the currently recommended guideline-based target of <130/80 mmHg[19] can be defended, the recommended guideline still seems reasonable.[20]

Two major placebo-controlled trials of calcium channel blocker-based therapy in elderly patients with isolated systolic hypertension (systolic 160–219 mmHg and diastolic <95 mmHg) also demonstrated benefits of active treatment. The SYST-EUR trial compared nitrendipine with placebo and included 492 diabetic patients.[21] The results clearly demonstrated improvements in the rates of several cardiovascular endpoints and also for total mortality. A closely related study, SYST-CHINA, included only 98 diabetic patients (of a total of 2394 hypertensive patients), but showed trends in CVD events and mortality that were strikingly similar to those in SYST-EUR.[22]

Finally, the Heart Outcomes Prevention Evaluation (HOPE) trial was designed as a placebo-controlled study of the efficacy of the ACE inhibitor ramipril for the prevention of CVD in high-risk patients.[23] A specific blood pressure target was not part of the HOPE design, and following randomization a placebo or ramipril (at a fixed 10 mg dose taken at bedtime) was simply added to existing therapy. The primary report of the study showed significant reductions in fatal and non-fatal MI and the investigators contended that the magnitude of the observed benefits could not be fully attributed to an antihypertensive effect of ramipril, as blood pressure was reported to be reduced by only 2.4/1.0 mmHg in the ramipril

compared with the placebo group.[23] That conclusion has, however, been criticized based on the lack of standardization of the methodology for blood pressure determination (which was never described in either the design[24] or the results reports) and because of the results of a sub-study in which 24 h automated blood pressure determinations showed a much greater decline in blood pressure of 10/4 mmHg, which if generalized to the entire study population could explain all of the apparent benefit of ramipril.

Results for the diabetic sub-group of the HOPE trial (3577 patients out of a total of 9297 in the parent trial) were reported separately as the MICRO-HOPE study.[25,26] Patients with diabetes mellitus in MICRO-HOPE had a significant 25% reduction in the risk of the primary composite endpoint of MI, stroke and cardiovascular death and also significant reductions in each of the individual components (MI 22%, stroke 33% and cardiovascular death 37%). All-cause mortality was also significantly decreased by 24%, largely due to the reduction in cardiovascular deaths. Microvascular endpoints also were ameliorated by ramipril treatment. The development of overt nephropathy (24 hour urinary albumin $\geq$200 mg min^{-1} or $\geq$300 mg day^{-1} or a 24 hour urine protein >500 mg day^{-1}) was 22% lower in the ramipril-treated group ($p = 0.045$) and total microvascular complications (overt nephropathy, dialysis and the requirement for laser therapy of retinopathy) were reduced by 15% ($p = 0.050$).

Recent clinical trials: placebo-controlled trials or trials comparing different blood pressure targets

Table 12.1 lists the more recent trials of antihypertensive therapy in diabetes and Tables 12.2 and 12.3 describe selected trial design features and results. The EURopean trial On reduction of cardiac events with Perindopril in stable coronary Artery disease (EUROPA) evaluated the effect of the ACE inhibitor perindopril versus placebo in 13 655 individuals with stable coronary artery disease treated with aspirin, beta-blockers and lipid-lowering drugs.[27] Perindopril lowered overall CV event rates by some 20% (8.0 vs 9.9%, perindopril vs placebo) with statistically significant benefits favouring perindopril for fatal and non-fatal acute MI (5.2 vs 6.8%), CV mortality and acute MI (7.9 vs 9.8%) and heart failure requiring hospitalization (1.0 vs 1.7%). In addition, perindopril showed favourable, although not statistically significant, effects for cardiovascular mortality (3.5 vs 4.1%), cardiac arrest (0.1 vs 0.2%) and total mortality (6.1 vs 6.9%).

The risk reductions in acute MI and CV deaths with ACE inhibitor treatment in EUROPA (20%) were very

Table 12.1 Names and acronyms of recent randomized controlled trials evaluating the effects of antihypertensive therapy on cardiovascular outcomes in diabetes

Acronym	Trial name
DIAMBHYCAR	Non-insulin-dependent diabetes, hypertension, microalbuminuria or proteinuria, cardiovascular events and ramipril
EUROPA	EURopean trial On reduction of cardiac events with Perindopril in stable coronary Artery disease
DREAM	Dream REduction Assessment with ramipril and rosiglitazone Medication
TRANSCEND	The Telmisartan Randomized AssessmeNt Study in aCE iNtolerant subjects with cardiovascular Disease
INDT	Irbesartan Diabetic Nephropathy Trial
INVEST	International Verapamil–Trandolapril Study
LIFE	Losartan Intervention For Endpoint reduction in hypertension study
ALLHAT	Antihypertensive and Lipid-Lowering Treatment to Prevent Heart Attack Trial
ONTARGET	The Ongoing Telmisartan Alone and in Combination with Ramipril Global Endpoint Trial

similar to those observed in the HOPE trial (21%). Thus, the EUROPA and HOPE trials support the efficacy of ACE inhibitors for reducing CVD outcomes in a spectrum of patients at high risk for coronary events, despite differences the study populations (the EUROPA trial included only younger Europeans with CAD, whereas the HOPE trial included participants with atherosclerosis and diabetes with one other risk factor[28]). The similarity of the magnitude of the benefits observed in HOPE and EUROPA suggests that the benefits of ACE inhibition may be a class effect, since ramipril was studied in HOPE and perindopril in EUROPA. Whether the benefits of ACE inhibitors

are dose dependent is unknown. Both HOPE and EUROPA used single doses of ACE inhibitor (ramipril 10 mg in HOPE and perindopril 8 mg in EUROPA), but a lower dose of ramipril (1.25 mg) compared with placebo in the non-insulin-dependent diabetes, hypertension, microalbuminuria or proteinuria, cardiovascular events and ramipril (DIABHYCAR) study did not result in a significant benefit for any of the components of the primary endpoint for cardiovascular risk (combined incidence of cardiovascular death, non-fatal MI, stroke, heart failure leading to hospitalization and end-stage renal disease) despite a slight decrease in blood pressure and urinary albumin in the ramipril group.[29] Results from the recently completed DREAM trial did not detect significant effects of ramipril (up to $15\,\mathrm{mg\,day^{-1}}$) on the incidence of death.[30]

Notwithstanding the inconsistencies, the HOPE, MICRO-HOPE and EUROPA trials have created considerable enthusiasm for the routine administration of ramipril or perindopril in diabetic patients with multiple CV risk factors or extant CVD and were a consideration when ACE inhibitor (ACEI) and angiotensin II receptor blocker (ARB) therapies were endorsed in recent guideline recommendations.

Comparisons of active therapies

With the benefits of antihypertensive therapy compared with placebo in patients with diabetes and hypertension well established, attention turned to the issue of whether drug-specific pharmacodynamic mechanisms are important determinants of outcomes. The question of greatest interest is whether ACEIs and ARBs confer benefits beyond their blood pressure-lowering actions.

Table 12.2 Studies of antihypertensive therapies in diabetes: comparisons of active treatment versus placebo

Study[a]	Year	Total sample (n)	Diabetes sample[b] (n)	Age (years) (mean)	Entry criteria[c]	Intervention (first step)	Duration (years) (median/mean)
DIAMBHYCAR	2001	4912	4912	65.2	DM, MCA	Ramipril vs placebo	4
EUROPA	2003	13 655	1502	60	Hypertension, DM, CAD	Perindopril vs placebo	4.2
DREAM	2006	5269	4527 (IGT) 739 (IFG)	54.7	Hypertension, DM, dyslipidaemia	Ramipril vs placebo with rosiglitazone	3
TRANSCEND	2007	5926	35.4%	66.9	CAD	Telmisartan vs placebo	4

[a]See Table 12.1.
[b]IGT = impaired glucose tolerance; IFG = impaired fasting glucose.
[c]MCA = microalbuminuria; DM = diabetes mellitus; CAD = coronary artery disease.

Table 12.3 Studies of antihypertensive therapies in diabetes: comparisons of active treatment versus placebo

Study[a]	Endpoints[b]	Events		Relative risk (95% CI)
DIABHYCAR		*Ramipril (n = 2443)*	*Placebo (n = 2469)*	
	CVD combined	362	377	0.97 (0.85 to 1.11)
	MI	52	59	0.89 (0.61 to 1.29)
	CVA	89	84	1.07 (0.80 to 1.44)
	CVD	141	133	1.07 (0.85 to 1.35)
EUROPA		*Perinodopril (n = 6110)*	*Placebo (n = 6108)*	
	MI	320	418	0.76 (0.77 to 1.02)
	CVA	98	102	0.96 (0.75 to 1.29)
	CVD	904	1043	0.86 (0.86 to 1.02)
DREAM		*Rosiglitazone (n = 2635)*	*Placebo (n = 2634)*	
	CVD combined	75	55	1.36 (0.81 to 1.61)
	MI	15	9	1.66 (0.55 to 2.85)
	CVA	7	5	1.39 (0.37 to 3.64)
	CVD	32	23	1.39 (0.68 to 1.97)
TRANSCEND	MI	Results pending		—
	CVA	Results pending		—
	CVD	Results pending		—

[a]See Table 12.1.
[b]CVD = cardiovascular disease; CVA = cardiovascular accident; MI = myocardial infarction.

As noted above, the UKPDS trial incorporated a comparison of atenolol- and captopril-based treatments in patients with diabetes and hypertension and the results of that sub-study showed no difference in outcomes between the treatment regimes despite similar blood pressure reductions.[16] This result contrasted somewhat with that of the Captopril Prevention Project (CAPP), which compared captopril with conventional therapies of beta-blockers, diuretics or both in a sub-group of 572 patients.[31] In CAPP, captopril was associated with a 66% reduction in fatal and non-fatal MI.

Other trials compared ACEIs or ARBs with calcium channel blockers and sometimes included additional limbs of other drug classes. The Appropriate Blood Pressure Control in Diabetes (ABCD) trial compared the ACE inhibitor enalapril with the calcium channel blocker nisoldipine.[32] ABCD was actually two studies: one examined hypertensive patients and the other normotensive patients. The hypertensive ABCD study was terminated prematurely when the nisoldipine group was found to have a significantly higher rate of MI compared with the enalapril group. The Fosinopril Amlodipine Cardiovascular Events Trial (FACET) was an open-label randomized comparison of the ACE inhibitor fosinopril and the calcium channel blocker amlodipine in 380 diabetic patients with hypertension.[33] At the end of the 3.5 year follow-up period, although diastolic blood pressures were comparable in the two groups, systolic blood pressure control was somewhat better in the amlodipine arm. However, despite the higher systolic blood pressure, patients assigned to fosinopril had fewer cardiovascular events for the combined endpoint of acute MI, stroke or hospitalization for angina.

The Swedish Trial in Old Patients with Hypertension-2 (STOP-2) extended the comparison to three drug groups: calcium blockers, ACEIs and beta-blockers plus diuretics.[34] Total mortality and total CV events did not differ between the groups, but as in ABCD, the rate of MI was lower in ACEI-treated patients than in those receiving the calcium blocker, although not lower than in those who received conventional beta-blocker plus diuretic treatment. A similar result was observed in the Nordic Diltiazem (NORDIL) study, which compared the calcium channel blocker diltiazem with traditional therapy of diuretics and beta-blockers.[35] In the sub-group of 727 patients with diabetes, there were no differences in combined cardiovascular endpoints or total mortality. Finally, the International Nifedipine GITS Study: Intervention as a Goal in Hypertension Treatment (INSIGHT) trial, which compared a long-acting nifedipine formulation with the diuretic combination coamilozide, included a sub-set of 1302 hypertensive diabetic patients: there were no differences in CVD endpoints or total mortality.[36]

Recent clinical trials: comparisons of active therapies

Tables 12.4 and 12.5 list the studies in which drugs of different classes were compared for similar degrees of blood pressure lowering. The largest comparative trial was the Antihypertensive and Lipid-Lowering treatment to prevent Heart Attack Trial (ALLHAT), which compared treatments based on randomized assignment to initial treatment with the thiazide diuretic chlorthalidone, the ACE inhibitor lisinopril or the calcium channel blocker nifedipine.[37,38] A sub-group analysis of the 12 063 patients with diabetes revealed no significant differences between groups for the primary outcome of non-fatal MI plus CHD death or for total mortality.[39] Similarly, the diabetic sub-group (6400 out of a total of 22 576) in the International Verapamil–Trandolapril Study (INVEST) demonstrated no difference in a primary outcome consisting of death (all-cause), non-fatal MI and

non-fatal stroke for randomized treatments beginning with long-acting calcium channel blocker (verapamil) plus the ACEI trandolapril compared with a regimen initiated with the beta-blocker atenolol plus trando-lapril.[40] Finally, in the Irbesartan type II Diabetic Nephropathy Trial (IDNT), the outcomes of MI, stroke and cardiovascular death did not differ between those randomized to the angiotensin receptor blocker irbe-sartan and those who received the calcium channel blocker amlodipine.[41]

Two large ongoing trials are under way to compare the benefits of ACE inhibitors and ARBs. The On-going Telmisartan Alone and in Combination with Ramipril Global Endpoint Trial (ONTARGET) will compare the ARB telmisartan, the ACEI ramipril and the combination of telmisartan plus ramipril for prevention of cardiovascular outcomes.[42–44] The study population is comprised of individuals at high risk for CVD and is similar to that of the HOPE trial. The companion TRANSCEND trial will enrol pa-tients intolerant of ACEIs and will compare telmi-sartan with placebo. The pending primary endpoints of both ONTARGET and TRANSCEND will include death, acute MI, stroke and hospitalization for con-gestive heart failure.

Table 12.4 Studies of antihypertensive therapies in diabetes: comparisons of active treatments

Study[a]	Year	Total sample (n)	Diabetes sample (n)	Age (years) (mean)	Entry criteria[b]	Intervention (first step)	Duration (years) (median/mean)
IDNT	2001	1715	1650	59.1	SBP > 135 DBP > 85 DM Cr (1.0–3.0 mg dl^{-1} women; 1.2–3.0 mg dl^{-1} men)	Irbesartan vs amlodipine vs placebo	2.6
LIFE	2002	9193	1195	66.9	Hypertension, LVH	Losartan ± HCT vs atenolol ± HCT	4.8
INVEST	2003	22476	6400	66.0	CAD	Verapamil vs atenolol Step treatment trandolapril/ hydrochlorothiazide	2
ALLHAT	2002	33357	5528	66.9	Hypertension	Amlopidine vs lisinopril vs chlorthalidone vs doxazosin (stopped early)	4.9
ONTARGET	2007	25620	–	66.4	Age >55 years, CAD, PAD,CVA, DM	Telmisartan vs ramipril vs temisartan + ramipril	5.5

[a]See Table 12.1.

[b]SBP = systolic blood pressure; DBP = diastolic blood pressure; DM = diabetes mellitus; Cr = serum creatinine; LVH = left ventricular hypertrophy; CAD = coronary artery disease; PAD = peripheral artery disease.

Table 12.5 Studies of antihypertensive therapies in diabetes: comparisons of active treatment versus placebo or alternative active drug

Study[a]	Endpoints[b]	Events			Relative risk (95% CI)
IDNT		*Irbesartan (n = 579)*	*Amlodipine (n = 567)*	*Placebo (n = 569)*	
	CV combined	172	161	—	1.05 (0.85 to 1.22)
		172	—	185	0.88 (0.81 to 1.14)
		—	161	185	0.87 (0.81 to 1.14)
	MI	44	27	—	1.59 (0.77 to 1.95)
		44	—	46	0.94 (0.65 to 1.45)
		—	27	46	0.59 (0.50 to 1.26)
	CVA	28	15	—	1.83 (0.70 to 2.41)
		44	—	28	1.54 (0.76 to 1.91)
		—	15	28	0.54 (0.41 to 1.41)
	CVD	52	37	—	1.37 (0.76 to 1.72)
		52	—	46	1.11 (0.72 to 1.53)
LIFE		*Losartan (n = 4605)*	*Atenolol (n = 4588)*		
	MI	198	188		1.05 (0.84–1.24)
	CVA	232	309		0.75 (0.75–1.04)
	CVD	204	234		0.87 (0.78–1.13)

[a]See Table 12.1.
[b]CVD = cardiovascular disease; CVA = cardiovascular accident; MI = myocardial infarction.

Is there a preferred way to treat hypertension in patients with diabetes?

Antihypertensive therapy has evolved without a clear understanding of why lowering blood pressure improves outcomes. Early epidemiological observations proved that hypertension is a risk factor for heart attack and stroke and, after considerable effort, drugs were developed that lower blood pressure without producing disabling side-effects.[45] The advent of thiazide diuretics ushered in the modern era of antihypertensive therapy and, shortly after their introduction into clinical practice, the randomized, controlled clinical trial was established as the preferred way of testing the efficacy of blood pressure lowering for the prevention of cardiovascular events. Early trials quickly established the benefits of antihypertensive drug treatment in severe hypertension, where event rates were high and risk reductions dramatic. It took longer to perform the larger trials necessary to demonstrate improved outcomes in lower risk milder hypertension. These larger trials included substantial sub-groups of patients with diabetes and hypertension, who were, as reviewed above, quickly shown to benefit from blood pressure lowering regardless of the particular drugs used.

The recent trials have not yet provided definitive proof of the superiority of any agent or class of agents for the prevention of macrovascular complications of diabetes. Nonetheless, guidelines developed by the American Diabetes Association[19] and the American Association of Clinical Endocrinologists[46] recommend beginning antihypertensive therapy with an ACEI or an ARB in all patients with diabetes and hypertension (Table 12.6).

The appeal of ACEI- and ARB-based therapies is predicated on three possible advantages of those agents. First, some 30% of type 2 diabetic patients will eventually develop renal disease and ACEIs and ARBs have proven efficacy for delaying the progression of diabetic kidney disease to end-stage renal disease. Although there is no clinical trial evidence, it is hoped that initiation of treatment with ACEIs or ARBs may primarily prevent or at least delay the development of renal disease.[47] Second, a number of pharmacological treatment trials of patients with hypertension alone have shown decreased rates of new-onset diabetes when these groups were treated with ACEIs or ARBs compared with those receiving diuretics or beta-blockers.[48] Presumably this represents differences in the effect of the drugs on insulin resistance, a precursor of diabetes commonly associated with hypertension.[49] Results of the DREAM trial have called this explanation into question as there was no decrease in the incidence of diabetes in groups with impaired fasting glucose and impaired glucose tolerance treated with ramipril compared with those receiving placebo (there was a benefit of ramipril

Table 12.6 Recommendations for hypertension diagnosis and control in patients with diabetes mellitus[19]

- Blood pressure should be measured at every routine diabetes visit. Patients found to have systolic blood pressure ≥130 mmHg or diastolic blood pressure ≥80 mmHg should have blood pressure confirmed on a separate day
- Patients with diabetes should be treated to a systolic blood pressure <130 mmHg and a diastolic blood pressure <80 mmHg
- Patients with a systolic blood pressure of 130–139 mmHg or a diastolic blood pressure of 80–89 mmHg should initiate lifestyle modification alone (weight control, increased physical activity, alcohol moderation, sodium reduction and emphasis on increased consumption of fresh fruits, vegetables and low-fat dairy products) for a maximum of 3 months. If, after these efforts, targets are not achieved, treatment with pharmacological agents should be initiated
- Patients with hypertension (systolic blood pressure ≥140 mmHg or diastolic blood pressure ≥90 mmHg) should receive drug therapy in addition to lifestyle and behavioural therapy
- All patients with diabetes and hypertension should be treated with a regimen that includes either an ACEI or an ARB. If one class is not tolerated, the other should be substituted. Other drug classes demonstrated to reduce CVD events in patients with diabetes (beta-blockers, thiazide diuretics and calcium channel blockers) should be added as needed to achieve blood pressure targets
- If ACEIs, ARBs or diuretics are used, renal function and serum potassium levels should be monitored within the first 3 months. If levels are stable, follow-up could occur every 6 months thereafter
- Multiple drug therapy generally is required to achieve blood pressure targets
- In elderly hypertensive patients, blood pressure should be lowered gradually to avoid complications
- Orthostatic measurement of blood pressure should be performed in people with diabetes and hypertension when clinically indicated
- Persons who do not achieve target blood pressure despite multiple drug therapy should be referred to a physician specializing in the care of patients with hypertension

---

compared with placebo for the number of patients in whom glucose levels were restored to normal).[50] Finally, the HOPE trial raised the possibility that treatment with ACEIs might decrease the rate of adverse CVD outcomes beyond what could be attributed to blood pressure lowering alone.[25] Although HOPE has flaws in its outcome ascertainment (see above), the report captured the attention of physicians and is now widely regarded as compelling evidence supporting a salutary effect of ACEIs, specifically ramipril, beyond its antihypertensive action.

The issue of whether the clinical incidence of diabetes differs with exposure to different antihypertensive drugs deserves careful consideration. There is remarkable consistency among trials that diuretics and beta-blockers are associated with higher rates of new-onset diabetes compared with ACEIs, ARBs and calcium antagonists,[48] although none of these trials demonstrated any increase in cardiovascular events or mortality associated with new-onset diabetes. As pointed out by Mancia *et al.*, however, it is likely that the failure to find any adverse consequences of drug-related new-onset diabetes is the result of the relative brevity of antihypertensive drug trials compared with the time course of the macrovascular complications of diabetes, which typically requires a decade or more to develop.[48] Thus, although the evidence is not conclusive, the recommendation for preferential initiation of antihypertensive therapy with ACEIs and ARBs in diabetes seems prudent.

It has been assumed that the benefit of ACEI/ARB therapy on incident diabetes reflects improvement in insulin-mediated glucose disposal, that is, a decrease in insulin resistance. Multiple mechanisms have been proposed as mediators of improved insulin action, although there is no agreement as to which is predominant in the clinical setting. The effects are probably modest and, as noted above, in a recent comparison of ramipril and rosiglitazone in incident diabetes and glucose metabolism, ramipril was ineffective in preventing the development of diabetes.[30] In addition, whether any effect of ACEI/ARB therapy on insulin sensitivity is maintained when additional agents are added to achieve optimal blood pressure control is uncertain. Since virtually all patients with diabetes and hypertension will eventually receive diuretic therapy, the arguments about differential impact of monotherapies may be moot.

This last point is relevant to how clinical trial results are applied in clinical practice. In all of the trials we have reviewed, participants were randomized to alternative initial antihypertensive drug treatments, but multiple drugs were eventually required to achieve blood pressure goals in most subjects. Thus, the results of trials of antihypertensive drug treatment in patients with diabetes reflect not only the action of the initial drug assigned but also the net impact of the total regimen used, and when considering multiple drug therapy, clinicians should not be reluctant to use whatever drug classes are necessary to reach target blood pressures.[51] For example, observations of increased rates of new-onset diabetes in groups treated with diuretics or beta-blockers compared with ACEIs, ARBs or calcium blockers does not mean that the use of the older agents is inappropriate, particularly when they are required as add-on agents to achieve good blood pressure control. Similarly, the preference for non-dihydropyridine calcium blockers over dihydropyridines in proteinuric patients with diabetes does not preclude the use of the latter in patients already treated with ACEIs or ARBs. Finally, the recommendations of JNC 7 for the treatment of hypertension with 'compelling' concomitant conditions, for example, beta-blockers for patients with prior MI, are still valid in patients with diabetes.[52] Also, as pointed out by Vijan *et al.*,[53] many experts have advocated 'evidence-based' recommendations rather uncritically. The most important goal of antihypertensive therapy is tight blood pressure control, regardless of the specific agents required to achieve it.[20,54]

The challenge of controlling hypertension in diabetes

Despite clear evidence that patients with diabetes and hypertension are at high risk of developing CVD and that antihypertensive treatment is effective in preventing complications, national surveys reveal that distressingly few patients actually receive effective treatment.[55,56] In part, this represents the generally poor control rates of hypertension in general, in part the more aggressive targets established for diabetes (<130/80 mmHg) and perhaps a variety of other reasons.[57,58] Regardless of the causes, the fact is that we are realizing very little of the achievable benefit of antihypertensive therapy in diabetes.[59,60] In addition, it is abundantly clear that optimal management of the other risk factors, particularly dyslipidaemia, is also necessary to reduce overall cardiovascular risk:[61] the current emphasis on the importance of global cardiovascular risk management is especially pertinent in diabetes, where the risk factor burden is typically greatest. Now that we have the evidence that treatment works and the pharmacological tools at our command, we must set ourselves to the task.

References

1 National Institute of Diabetes and Kidney, Diseases. *National Diabetes Statistics Fact Sheet: General Information and National Estimates on Diabetes in the United States, 2003.* US Department of Health and Human Services, National Institutes of Health, Bethesda, MD, 2004.

2 Gu K, Cowie CC, Harris MI. Mortality in adults with and without diabetes in a national cohort of the US population, 1971–1993. *Diabetes Care* 1998;**21**:1138–1145.

3 Haffner SM, Lehto S, Ronnemaa T, Pyorala K, Laakso M. Mortality from coronary heart disease in subjects with type 2 diabetes and in nondiabetic subjects with and without prior myocardial infarction. *N Engl J Med* 1998;**339**: 229–234.

4 Eckel RH, Kahn R, Robertson RM, Rizza RA. Preventing cardiovascular disease and diabetes: a call to action from the American Diabetes Association and the American Heart Association. *Diabetes Care* 2006;**29**:1697–1699.

5 Calkin AC, Allen TJ. Diabetes mellitus-associated atherosclerosis. Mechanisms involved and potential for pharmacological intervention. *Am J Cardiovasc Drugs* 2006;**6**: 15–40.

6 Esper RJ, Nordaby RA, Vilarino JO, Paragano A, Cacharron JL, Machado RA. Endothelial dysfunction: a comprehensive review. *Cardiovasc Diabetol* 2006;**5**:4.

7 Nesse RM, Weder AB. What evolutionary medicine offers to endothelium researchers. In *Endothelial Biomedicine* (ed. WC Aird), Cambridge University Press, Cambridge, 2007, pp. 122–128.

8 Bucala R, Makita Z, Koschinsky T, Cerami A, Vlassara H, Lipid advanced glycosylation: pathway for lipid oxidation *in vivo. Proc Natl Acad Sci USA* 1993;**90**:6434–6438.

9 Rong LL, Gooch C, Szabolcs M, Herold KC, Lalla E, Hays AP, Fang S, Yan SSD, Schmidt AM. RAGE: a journey from the complications of diabetes to disorders of the nervous system striking a fine balance between injury and repair. *Restor Neurol Neurosci* 2005;**23**:355–365.

10 Aronson D, Rayfield RJ. How hyperglycemia promotes atherosclerosis: molecular mechanisms. *Cardiovasc Diabetol* 2002;**1**:1–10.

11 Fuller J. Prevention of hypertension. in *The Evidence Base of Diabetes Care* (eds R Williams, W Herman, AL Kinmouth, NJ Wareham), John Wiley & Sons, Ltd, Chichester, 2002, pp. 389–411.

12 Hypertension Detection and Follow-up Program Cooperative Group. Five-year findings of the Hypertension Detection and Follow-up Program. 1. Reduction in mortality of persons with high blood pressure, including mild hypertension. *JAMA* 1979;**242**:2562–2571.

13 Hypertension Detection and Follow-up Program Cooperative Research Group. Mortality findings for steped-care and referred-care participants in the hypertension detection and follow-up program, stratified by other risk factors. *Prevent Med* 1985;**14**:312–335.

14 SHEP Cooperative Research Group. Prevention of stroke by antihypertensive drug treatment in older persons with isolated systolic hypertension. Final results of the systolic hypertension in elderly program (SHEP). *JAMA* 1991;**265**: 3255–3264.

15 Curb JD, Pressel SL, Cutler JA, Savage PJ, Applegate WB, Camel G, Davis BR, Frost PH, Gonzales N, Gutnrie G, Oberman A, Rutan GH, Stamler J. Effect of diuretic-based antihypertensive treatment on cardiovascular disease risk in older diabetic patients with isolated systolic hypertension. *JAMA* 1996;**276**:1886–1892.

16 UK Prospective Diabetes Study Group. Tight blood pressure control and risk of macrovascular complications in type 2 diabetes: UKPDS 28. *BMJ* 1998;**317**:703–713.

17 UK Prospective Diabetes Study Group. Efficacy of atenolol and captopril in reducing risk of macrovascular and microvascular complications in type 2 diabetes: UKPDS 39. *BMJ* 1998;**317**:713–720.

18 Hansson L, Zanchetti A, Carruthers SG, Dahlof D, Julius S, Menard J, Rahn KH, Wedel H, Westerling S. Effects of intensive blood-pressure lowering and low-dose aspirin in patients with hypertension: principal results of the Hypertension Optimal Treatment (HOT) randomized trial. *Lancet* 1998;**35**:1755–1762.

19 American Diabetes Association. Standards of medical care in diabetes – 2007. *Diabetes Care* 2007;**30**(Suppl 1): S4–S41.

20 Vijan S, Hayward RA. Treatment of hypertension in type 2 diabetes mellitus: blood pressure goals, choice of agents and setting priorities in diabetes care. *Ann Intern Med* 2003;**138**: 593–602.

21 Tuomilehto J, Rastenyte D, Birkenhager WH, Thijs L, Antikainen R, Bulpitt CJ, Fletcher AE, Forette F, Goldhaber A, Palatini P, Sarti C, Fagard R. for the Systolic Hypertension in Europe Trail Investigators. Effects of calcium-channel blockade in older patients with diabetes and systolic hypertension. *N Engl J Med* 1999;**340**:677–684.

22 Wang JG, Staessen JA, Gong L, Liu L, *et al.* Chinese trial isolated systolic hypertension in the elderly. Systolic Hypertension in China (Syst-China) Collaborative Group. *Arch Intern Med* 2000;**160**:211–220.

23 The Heart Outcomes Prevention Evaluation Study Investigators. Effects of an angiotensin-converting-enzyme inhibitor, ramipril, on cardiovascular events in high-risk patients. *N Engl J Med* 2000;**342**:145–153.

24 The HOPE Study Investigators. The HOPE (Heart Outcomes Prevention Evaluation) study: the design of a large, simple randomized study of an angiotensin-converting enzyme inhibitor (ramipril) and vitamin E in patients at high risk of cardiovascular events. *Can J Cardiol* 1996;**12**:127–137.

25 The Heart Outcomes Prevention Evaluation (HOPE) Study Investigators. Effects of ramipril on cardiovascular and microvascular outcomes in people with diabetes mellitus: results of the HOPE study and MICRO-HOPE substudy. *Lancet* 2000;**355**:253–259.

26 HOPE/HOPE-TOO Study Investigators. Long-term effects of ramipril on cardiovascular events and on diabetes: results of the HOPE study extension. *Circulation* 2005;**112**:1339–1346.

27 The EURopean trial On reduction of cardiac events with Perindopril in stable coronary Artery disease Investigators. Efficacy of perindopril in reduction of cardiovascular events among patients with stable coronary artery disease: randomized, double-blind, placebo-controlled, muticentre trial (the EUROPA study). *Lancet* 2003;**362**:783–788.

28 Liebson PR. Clinical Trial Update: the EUropean trial of reduction of cardiac events with Perindopril in stable coronary Artery disease Investigators. Efficacy of perindopril in reduction of cardiovascular events among patients with stable coronary artery disease: randomized, double-blind, placebo-controlled, multicentre trial (the EUROPA study). *Prev Cardiol* 2004;**7**:42–44.

29 Marre M, Lievre M, Chatellier G, Mann JFE, Passa P, Menard J on behalf of the DIABHYCAR Study Investigators. Effects of low dose ramipril on cardiovascular and renal outcomes in patients with type 2 diabetes and raised excretion of urinary albumin: randomized, double blind, placebo controlled trial (the DIABHYCAR study). *BMJ* 2004;**328**:495–500.

30 The DREAM Trial Investigators. Effect of ramipril on the incidence of diabetes. *N Engl J Med* 2006;**355**:1551–1562.

31 Hansson L, Lindholm LH, Niskanen L, Lanke J, Hedner T, Niklason A, Luomanmaki K, Dahlof B, de Faire U, Morlin C, Karlberg BE, Wester PO, Bjorck J-E for the Captopril Prevention Project (CAPP) Study Group. Effect of angiotensin-converting-enzyme inhibition compared with conventional therapy on cardiovascular morbidity and mortality in hypertension: the Captopril Prevention Project (CAPP) randomized trial. *Lancet* 1999;**353**:611–616.

32 Estacio RO, Jeffers BW, Hiatt WR, Biggerstaff SL, Gifford N, Schrier RW. The effect of nisoldipine as compared with enalapril on cardiovascular outcomes in patients with non-insulin-dependent diabetes and hypertension. *N Engl J Med* 1998;**338**:645–652.

33 Tatti P, Pahor M, Byington RP, Di Mauro P, Guarisco R, Strollo G, Strollo F. Outcome results of the Fosinopril versus Amlodipine Cardiovascular Events Randomized Trial (FACET) in patients with hypertension and NIDDM. *Diabetes Care* 1998;**21**:597–603.

34 Hanson L, Lindholm LH, Ekbom T, Dahlöf B, Lanke J, Scherstén B, Wester P-O, Hedner T, de Faire U for the STOP-Hypertension-2 Study Group. Randomized trial of old and new antihypertensive drugs in elderly patients: cardiovascular mortality and morbidity. The Swedish Trial in Old Patients with Hypertension-2 study. *Lancet* 1999; **354**:1751–1756.

35 Hansson L, Hedner T, Lund-Johansen P, Kjeldsen SE, Lindholm LH, Syvertsen JO, Lanke J, de Faire U, Dahlof B, Karlberg BE. Randomized trial of effects of calcium antagonists compared with diuretics and β-blockers on cardiovascular morbidity and mortality in hypertension: the Nordic Diltiazem (NORDIL) study. *Lancet* 2000;**356**: 359–365.

36 Svensson P, de Faire U, Sleight P, Yusuf S, Ostergrean J. Comparative effects of ramipril on ambulatory and office blood pressures. A HOPE substudy. *Hypertension* 2001;**38**: e28–e32.

37 Davis BR, Cutler JA, Gordon DJ, Furberg CD, Wright JT Jr., Cushman WC, Grimm RH, LaRosa J, Whelton PK, Perry HM, Alderman MH, Ford CE, Oparil S, Francis C, Proschan M, Pressel S, Black HR, Hawkins CM. Rationale and design for the Antihypertensive and Lipid Lowering Treatment of Prevent Heart Attack Trial (ALLHAT). ALLHAT Research Group. *Am J Hypertens* 1996;**9**:342–360.

38 The ALLHAT Officers and Coordinator for the ALLHAT Collaborative Research Group. Major cardiovascular events in hypertensive patients randomized to doxazosin vs. chlorthalidone. The Antihypertensive and Lipid-Lowering Treatment to prevent Heart Attack Trial (ALLHAT). *JAMA* 2000;**283**:1967–1975.

39 Barzilay JI, Jones CL, Davis BR, Basile JN, Goff DC Jr, Ciocon JO, Sweeney ME, Randall OS for the ALLHAT Collaborative Research group Baseline characteristics of the diabetic participants in the Antihypertensive and Lipid-Lowering treatment to prevent Heart Attack Trial (ALLHAT). *Diabetes Care* 2001;**24**:654–658.

40 Pepine CJ, Handberg EM, Cooper-DeHoff R, Marks RG, Kowey P, Messerli FH, Mancia G, Cangiano JL, Garcia-Barreto D, Keltai M, Erdine S, Bristol HA, Kolb HR, Bakris GL, Cohen JD, Parmley WW for the INVEST Investigators. A calcium antagonist vs a non-calcium antagonist hypertension treatment strategy for patients with coronary artery disease. The International Verapamil–Trandolapril Study (INVEST): a randomized controlled trial. *JAMA* 2003;**290**: 2805–2816.

41 Berl T, Hunsicker LG, Lewis JB, Pfeffer MA, Porush JG, Rouleau J-L, Drury PL, Esmatjes E, Hricik D, Pohl M, Raz I, Vanhille P, Wiegmann TB, Wolfe BM, Locatelli F, Goldhaber SZ, Lewis EJ, for the Collaborative Study Group. Impact of achieved blood pressure on cardiovascular outcomes in the Irbesartan Diabetic Nephropathy Trial. *J Am Soc Nephrol* 2005;**16**:2170–2179.

42 Sleight P. The ONTARGET/TRANSCEND Trial Programme: baseline data. *Acta Diabetol* 2005;**42**:s50–s56.

43 Unger T. The Ongoing Telmisartan Alone in the Combination with Ramipril Global Endpoint Trial Program. *Am J Cardiol* 2003;**91**(Suppl): 28G–34G.

44 The ONTARGET/TRANSCEND Investigators. Rationale, design and baseline characteristics of 2 large, simple, randomized trials evaluating telmisartan, ramipril and their combination in high-risk patients: The Ongoing Telmisartan Alone and in Combination with Ramipril Global Endpoint Trial; Telmisartan Randomized Assessment Study in ACE Intolerant Subjects with Cardiovascular Disease (ONTARGET/TRANSCEND) trial. *Am Heart J* 2004;**148**:52–61.

45 Weder AB, Julius S. Pathophysiology of hypertension and treatment. In: *Cardiovascular Pharmacology and Therapeutics* (eds by BN Singh, VJ Dzau, PM Vanhoutte, RL Woosley), Churchill Livingstone, New York, 1994, pp. 861–883.

46 AACE Hypertension Task Force. American Association of Clinical Endocrinologists medical guidelines for clinical practice for the diagnosis and treatment of hypertension. *Endocr Pract* 2006;**12**:193–222.

47 Bakris GL. ACE inhibitors and ARBs: are they better than other agents to slow nephropathy progression? *J Clin Hypertens* 2007;**9**:413–415.

48 Mancia G, Grassi G, Zanchetti A. New-onset diabetes and antihypertensive drugs. *J Hypertens* 2006;**24**:3–10.

49 McFarlane SI, Kumar A, Sowers JR. Mechanisms by which angiotensin-converting enzyme inhibitors prevent diabetes and cardiovascular disease. *Am J Cardiol* 2003;**91**:H30–H37.

50 Fonseca VA. Rosiglitazone reduces incident type 2 diabetes and increases regression to normoglycemia in patients with prediabetes: clinical implications of the Dream trial. www.medscape.com/viewarticle/546709. (accessed 14 May 2007).

51 Buse JB, Ginsberg HN, Bakris GL, Clark NG, Costa F, Eckel R, Fonseca V, Gerstein HC, Grundy S, Nesto RW, Pigone MP, Plutzky J, Porte D, Redberg R, Stitzel KF, Stone NJ. Primary prevention of cardiovascular diseases in people with diabetes mellitus. A scientific statement from the American Heart Association and the American Diabetes Association. *Diabetes Care* 2007;**30**:162–172.

52 Chobanian AV, Bakris GL, Black HR, Cushman WC, Green LA, Izzo JL Jr, Jones DW, Materson BJ, Oparil S, Wright JT Jr, Rochella EJ and National Heart, Lung and Blood Institute Joint National Committee on Prevention, Detection, Evaluation and Treatment of High Blood, National High Blood Pressure Education Program Coordinating Committee. The seventh report of the Joint National Committee on Prevention, Detection, Evaluation and Treatment of High Blood Pressure: the JNC 7 report. *JAMA* 2003;**289**:2560–2572.

53 Vijan S, Kent DM, Hayward RA. Are randomized controlled trials sufficient evidence to guide clinical practice in type II (non-insulin-dependent) diabetes mellitus? *Diabetologia* 2000;**43**:125–130.

54 Snow V, Weiss KB, Mottur-Pilson C for the Clinical Efficacy Assessment Subcommittee of the American College of Physicians. The evidence base for tight blood pressure control in the management of type 2 diabetes mellitus. *Ann Int Med* 2003;**138**:587–592.

55 Boero R, Prodi E, Elia F, Porta L, Martelli S, Ferraro L, Quarello F. How well are hypertension and albuminuria treated in type II diabetic patients? *J Hum Hypertens* 2003;**17**:413–418.

56 Chin MH, Su AW, Jin L, Nerney MP. Variations in the care of elderly persons with diabetes among endocrinologists, general internists and geriatricians. *J Genontol A Biol Sci Med Sci* 2000;**55**:M601–M606.

57 Duggirala MK, Cuddihy RM, Cuddihy M-T, Naessens JM, Cha SS, Mandrekar JN, Leibson CL. Predictors of blood pressure control in patients with diabetes and hypertension seen in primary care clinics. *Am J Hypertens* 2005;**18**:833–838.

58 Greenberg JD, Tiwari A, Rajan M, Miller D, Natarajan S, Pogach L. Determinants of sustained uncontrolled blood pressure in a national cohort of persons with diabetes. *Am J Hypertens* 2006;**19**:161–169.

59 Berlowitz DR, Ash AS, Hickey EC, Glickman M, Friedman R, Kader B. Hypertension management in patients with diabetes: the need for more aggressive therapy. *Diabetes Care* 2003;**26**:355–359.

60 Borzecki AM, Berlowitz DR. Management of hypertension and diabetes: treatment goals, drug choices, current practice and strategies for improving care. *Curr Hypertens Rep* 2005;**7**:439–449.

61 Rodgers PT, Fuke DC. New and emerging strategies for reducing cardiometabolic risk factors. *Pharmacology* 2006;**26**: 13S–31S.

APPENDIX

Table 12.A1 Names and acronyms of completed randomised controlled trials evaluating the effect of antihypertensive therapy on cardiovascular outcomes in type 2 diabetes (to 2001)

Acronym	Trial name
ABCD[A1]	Appropriate Blood Pressure Control in Diabetes
CAPP[A2]	Captopril Prevention Project
FACET[A3]	Fosinopril versus Amlodipine Cardiovascular Events Randomised Trial
HDFP[A4]	Hypertension Detection and Follow-up Program
HOPE[A5]	Heart Outcomes Prevention Evaluation Study
HOT[A6]	Hypertension Optimal Treatment Trial
NORDIL[A7]	Nordic Diltiazem Study
SHEP[A8]	Systolic Hypertension in the Elderly Program
STOP-2[A9]	Swedish Trial in Old Patients with Hypertension
SYST-EUR[A10]	Systolic Hypertension in Europe Trial
SYST-CHINA[A11]	Systolic Hypertension in China
UKPDS[A12,A13]	United Kingdom Prospective Diabetes Study

Table 12.A2 Studies of antihypertensive therapies in type 2 diabetes: comparisons of active treatments with a placebo or less actively treated group

Study	Year	Total sample size	Diabetes sample size	Age range (years)	Entry criteria	Intervention (first step)	Duration (years) (median/mean)
HDFP[A14,A15]	1979	10940	772	30–69	Diast. BP ≥90 mmHg	Stepped care versus referred care	5
SHEP[A8]	1996	4736	583	60+	Syst. BP ≥160 mmHg and Diast BP <90 mmHg	Chlorthalidone versus placebo	4.5
UKPDS[A12]	1998	1148	1148	25–65	BP ≥160/90 mmHg or BP ≥150/85 mmHg on treatment	Tight versus less tight BP control	8.4
HOT[A6]	1998	18790	1501	50–80	Diast. BP 100–115 mmHg	Feladipine + other agents. Target Diast BP ≤90, ≤85, ≤80 mmHg	3.8
SYST-EUR[A10]	1999	4695	492	60+	Syst. BP 160–219 mmHg and Diast. BP <95 mmHg	Nitrendipine versus placebo	2
SYST-CHINA[A11]	2000	2394	98	60+	Syst. BP 160–219 mmHg and Diast. BP <95 mmHg	Nitrendipine versus placebo	3
HOPE[A8]	2000	9297	3577	55+	History of CVD or diabetes plus one other cardiovascular risk factor	Ramipril versus placebo	4.5

Table 12.A3 Studies of antihypertensive therapies in type 2 diabetes: comparisons of active treatments

Study	Year	Total sample size	Diabetes sample size	Age range (years)	Entry criteria	Intervention (first step)	Duration (years) (median/mean)
ABCD[A1]	1998	470	470	47–74	Diast. BP ≥90 mmHg	Enalapril versus Nisoldipine	5
FACET[A3]	1998	380	380	Mean 63	BP >140/90 mmHg	Fosinopril versus amlodipine	3.5
UKPDS[A13]	1998	758	758	25–65	BP ≥160/90 mmHg or BP ≥150/85 mmHg on treatment	Captopril versus atenolol	8.4
CAPP[A2]	1999	10985	572	25–66	Diast. BP ≥100 mmHg	Captopril versus Conv.[a]	6.1
STOP-2[A9]	1999	6614	719	70–84	BP ≥180/105 mmHg	ACEI vs CCB versus Conv.	4
NORDIL[A7]	2000	10916	727	50–74	Diast. BP ≥100 mmHg	Diltiazem versus Conv.	4.5

[a]Conv. = β-blocker/diuretic.

Table 12.A4 Studies of antihypertensive therapies in type 2 diabetes: Comparisons of active treatment with a placebo or less active treatment

Study	Endpoints	Event rates (/10³ person-year)		Absolute risk reduction (/10³ person-year)	Relative risk reduction[a] (95% CI)
		Active treatment	Less active treatment		
HDFP[A14,A15]	Total CVD	35.2	51.2	16.3	0.62 (0.44 to 0.57)
	Total mortality	22.0	25.0	3.0	0.86 (0.56 to 1.34)

(continued)

Table 12.A4 *(Continued)*

Study	Endpoints	Event rates (/10³ person-year)		Absolute risk reduction (/10³ person-year)	Relative risk reduction[a] (95% CI)
		Active treatment	**Less active treatment**		
SHEP[A8]	MI	12.8	22.7	9.9	0.46 (0.24 to 0.88)
	Stroke	17.7	24.0	6.3	0.78 (0.45 to 1.31)
	Total CVD	40.3	55.3	15.0	0.66 (0.46 to 0.94)
	Total mortality	27.6	32.0	4.4	0.84 (0.53 to 1.32)
UKPDS[A12]	MI	18.6	23.5	0.59 ($p = 0.13$)	0.79 (0.59 to 1.07)
	Stroke	6.5	11.6	0.59 ($p = 0.013$)	0.56 (0.35 to 0.89)
	Total mortality	22.4	27.2	4.8 ($p = 0.17$)	0.82 (0.63 to 1.08)
HOT[A6]	MT	NA	NA	NA	0.50 (NS)[b]
	Stroke	NA	NA	NA	0.70 (NS)[b]
	Total CVD	NA	NA	NA	0.50 ($p = 0.04$)[b]
SYST-EUR[A10]	MI	11.7	27.1	15.4 ($p = 0.06$)	0.37 ($p = 0.12$)[c]
	Stroke	8.3	26.6	18.3 ($p = 0.02$)	0.27 ($p = 0.13$)[c]
	Total CVD	22.0	57.6	35.6 ($p = 0.002$)	0.31 ($p = 0.01$)[c]
	Total mortality	26.4	45.1	18.7 ($p = 0.09$)	0.45 ($p = 0.04$)[c]
SYST-CHINA[A11]	Cardiac (MI, heart failure or sudden death)	NA	NA	NA	0.90 ($p = 0.08$)
	Stroke	NA	NA	NA	0.45 ($p = 0.42$)
	Total CVD	32.1	76.4	NA	0.74 ($p = 0.03$)
	Total mortality	NA	NA	NA	0.59 ($p = 0.15$)
HOPE[A5]	MI	NA	NA	NA	0.88 (0.64 to 0.94)
	Stroke	NA	NA	NA	0.67 (0.50 to 0.90)
	Total CVD	NA	NA	NA	0.75 (0.64 to 0.88)
	Total mortality	NA	NA	NA	0.76 (0.63 to 0.92)

[a]Active versus untreated or less actively treated group.
[b]Approximate risk reductions for target group ≤80 mmHg versus ≤90 mmHg.
[c]Adjusted relative hezards. *p*-values are for the interaction between treatment and diabetes.
NA, not available; NS, not significant.

Table 12.A5 Studies of antihypertensive therapies in type 2 diabetes: Comparisons of active treatment with a placebo or less active treatment

Study	Endpoints	Event rates (/10³ person-years)		Absolute risk reduction[a] (/10³ person-years)	Relative risk reduction[a] (95% CI)
		Newer treatment	**Comparison treatment**		
ABCD[A1]	MI	NA	NA	NA	0.18 (0.07 to 0.48)
	Stroke	NA	NA	NA	0.63 (0.24 to 1.67)
	Total CVD	NA	NA	NA	0.50 (0.16 to 1.43)
	Total mortality	NA	NA	NA	0.77 (0.36 to 1.67)
FACET[A3]	MI	NA	NA	NA	0.77 (0.34 to 1.75)
	Stroke	NA	NA	NA	0.39 (0.12 to 1.23)
	Total CVD	NA	NA	NA	0.49 (0.26 to 0.95)
	Total mortality	NA	NA	NA	0.81 (0.22 to 3.02)
UKPDS[A13]	MI	20.2	16.9	−3.3 ($p = 0.35$)	1.20 (0.82 to 1.76)
	Stroke	6.8	6.1	−0.7 ($p = 0.74$)	1.12 (0.59 to 2.12)
	Total mortality	23.8	20.8	−3.0 ($p = 0.44$)	1.14 (0.81 to 1.61)
CAPP[A2]	MI	NA	NA	NA	0.34 (0.17 to 0.67)
	Stroke	NA	NA	NA	1.02 (0.55 to 1.88)
	Fatal CVD	NA	NA	NA	0.48 (0.21 to 1.10)
	Total mortality	NA	NA	NA	0.54 (0.31 to 0.96)

(continued)

Table 12.A5 *(Continued)*

Study	Endpoints	Event rates (/10³ person-years)		Absolute risk reduction[a] (/10³ person-years)	Relative risk reduction[a] (95% CI)
		Newer treatment	Comparison treatment		
STOP-2[A9]	Fatal CVD	NA	NA	NA	(No significant differences)
NORDIL[A7]	MI	11.2	11.1	−0.1 ($p = 0.99$)	0.99 (0.51 to 1.94)
	Stroke	13.3	12.3	−1.0 ($p = 0.92$)	0.97 (0.52 to 1.81)
	Total CVD	29.8	27.7	−2.1 ($p = 0.98$)	1.01 (0.66 to 1.53)
	Total mortality	18.1	15.6	−2.5 ($p = 0.80$)	1.07 (0.63 to 1.84)

[a]ACEI versus comparison treatment except CCB versus comparison treatment in NORDIL.

NA, not available.

References

A1 Estacio RO, Jeffers BW, Hiatt WR, Biggerstaff SL, Gifford N, Schrier RW. The effect of nisoldipine as compared with enalapril on cardiovascular outcomes in patients with non-insulin-dependent diabetes and hypertension. *N Engl J Med* 1998;**338**:645–52.

A2 Hansson L, Lindholm LH, Niskanen L, Lanke J, Hedner T, Niklasan A, Luomunmaki K, Dahlof B, de Faire U, Morlin C, Karlberg BE, Wester PO, Bjorck J-E, for the Captopril Prevention Project (CAPP) Study Group. Effect of angiotensin-converting-enzyme inhibition compared with conventional therapy on cardiovascular morbidity and mortality in hypertension: the Captopril Prevention Project (CAPP) randomised trial. *Lancet* 1999;**353**:611–616.

A3 Tatti P, Pahor M, Byington RP, Di Mauro P, Guarisco R, Strollo F. Outcome results of the Fosinopril versus Amlodipine Cardiovascular Events Randomised Trial (FACET) in patients with hypertension and NIDDM. *Diabetes Care* 1998;**21**:597–603.

A4 Hypertension Detection and Follow-up Program Cooperative Group. Five-year findings of the hypertension detection and follow-up program. 1. Reduction in mortality of persons with high blood pressure, including mild hypertension. *JAMA* 1997;**242**:2562–2571.

A5 Heart Outcomes Prevention Evaluation (HOPE) Study Investigators. Effects of ramipril on cardiovascular and microvascular outcomes in people with diabetes mellitus: results of the HOPE study and MICRO-HOPE substudy. *Lancet* 2000;**355**:253–259.

A6 Hansson L, Zanchetti A, Carruthers SG, Dahlof D, Julius S, Menard J, *et al*. Effects of intensive blood-pressure lowering and low dose aspirin in patients with hypertension: principal results of the Hypertension Optimal Treatment (HOT) randomised trial. *Lancet* 1998;**351**:1755–1762.

A7 Hansson L, Hedner T, Lund-Johansen P, Kjeldsen SE, Lindholm LH, Syvertsen JO, Lanke J, de Faire U, Dahlof B, Karlberg BE. Randomised trial of effects of calcium antagonists compared with diuretics and β-blockers on cardiovascular morbidity and mortality in hypertension: the Nordic Diltiazem (NORDIL) study. *Lancet* 2000;**356**:359–365.

A8 Curb JD, Pressel SL, Cutler JA, Savage PJ, Applegate WB, Camel G, Davis BR, Frost PH, Gonzalez N, Gutnrie G, Oberman A, Rutan GH, Stamler J. Effect of diuretic-based antihypertensive treatment on cardiovascular disease risk in older diabetic patients with isolated systolic hypertension. *JAMA* 1996;**276**:1886–1892.

A9 Hansson L, Lindholm LH, Ekbom T, Dahlöf B, Lanke J, Scherstén B, Wester P-O, Hedner T, de Faire U, for the STOP-Hypertension-2 Study Group. Randomised trial of old and new antihypertensive drugs in elderly patients: cardiovascular mortality and morbidity. The Swedish Trial in Old Patients with Hypertension-2 study. *Lancet* 1999;**354**:1751–1756.

A10 Tuomilehto J, Rastenyte D, Birkenhanger WH, Thijs L, Antikainen R, Bulpitt CJ, Fletcher AE, Forette F, Goldhaber A, Palatini P, Sarti C, Fagard R, for the Systolic Hypertension in Europe Trial Investigators. Effects of calcium-channel blockade in older patients with diabetes and systolic hypertension. *N Engl J Med* 1999;**340**:677–684.

A11 Wang JG, Staessen JA, Gong L, Liu L. Chinese trial on isolated systolic hypertension in the elderly. Systolic Hypertension in China (Syst-China) Collaborative Group. *Arch Intern Med* 2000;**160**:211–220.

A12 UK Prospective Diabetes Study Group. Tight blood pressure control and risk of macrovascular and microvascular complications in type 2 diabetes: UKPDS 38. *BMJ* 1998;**317**:703–713.

A13 UK Prospective Diabetes Study Group. Efficacy of atenolol and captopril in reducing risk of macrovascular and microvascular complications in type 2 diabetes: UKPDS 39. *BMJ* 1998;**317**:713–720.

A14 The Hypertension Detection and Follow-up Program Cooperative Research Group. Mortality findings for stepped-care and referred-care participants in the hypertension detection and follow-up program, stratified by other risk factors. The Hypertension Detection and Follow-up Program Cooperative Research Group. *Prevent Med* 1985;**4**:312–335.

A15 Fuller J, Stevens LK, Chaturvedi N, Holloway JF. Antihypertensive therapy in diabetes mellitus (Cochrane Review). *The Cochrane Library* 1999;1–13.

13 Does treating hyperlipidaemia with medication prevent complications?

Helen M. Colhoun

Department of Genetic Epidemiology, University College Dublin, Belfield, Dublin, Ireland

Introduction

In this chapter, the current evidence base for lipid-lowering therapy for preventing diabetic complications is reviewed, current guidelines are summarized and some controversial issues are discussed. First we will focus on the evidence that cardiovascular disease can be prevented by treating lipids. We will focus only on trials that have actual clinical cardiovascular disease (CVD) endpoints and not those with surrogate endpoints such as carotid intima medial thickness. Then we will briefly consider the impact of such therapy on microvascular complications.

There is now available a strong evidence base to support prescribing to reduce lipid levels in secondary prevention and increasing evidence in relation to primary prevention.

The major secondary prevention trials with cardiovascular endpoints include an influential group reporting before 2002,[1] the Scandinavian Simvastatin Survival Study (4S),[2] the Cholesterol and Recurrent Events Trial (CARE),[3] the Long-Term Intervention with Pravastatin in Ischemic Disease (LIPID)[4] and the Veterans Affairs High-Density Lipoprotein Intervention Trial (VA-HIT),[5] and after 2002 several key trials of lipid lowering using statins and fibrates that have included large numbers of diabetic patients have reported, including the Heart Protection Study (HPS).

For primary prevention for CVD, the evidence that it now rests on was sparse, based on less than 500 patients with type 2 diabetes who had been included in the Helsinki Heart Study (HHS),[6] the St Mary's, Ealing, Northwick Park Diabetes Cardiovascular Disease Prevention Study (SENDCAP)[7] and the Air Force/Texas Coronary Atherosclerosis Prevention Studies (AFCAPS/TEXCAPS)[8] for those with existing vascular disease.

These trials have answered some questions definitively but have also raised some new questions.

Hyperlipidaemia in diabetes and its relationship to CVD risk

The lipid profile of patients with type 2 diabetes differs from the non-diabetic population in that plasma triglycerides are often higher, high-density lipoprotein cholesterol (HDL-C) often lower, small dense low-density lipoprotein (LDL) particle concentration higher and there is greater post-prandial lipaemia.[9,10] LDL cholesterol (LDL-C) concentrations are often similar to those in the non-diabetic population. However, about 40–50% of patients with type 2 diabetes have increased levels of small dense LDL even when LDL-C levels are apparently normal.[10] Secondary causes of dyslipidaemia that are more common in people with than without diabetes include hypothyroidism, chronic renal failure and drug side-effects such as increased triglycerides secondary to diuretic use. In patients with at least moderate glycaemic control, severe hypertriglyceridaemia or hypercholesterolaemia are not usually attributable solely to diabetes and other causes should be sought.

In type 1 diabetes, the lipid profile is different to that in type 2 diabetes. HDL-C is often higher than, triglycerides often lower than and LDL-C similar to the levels in the general population.[11,12] As nephropathy develops or when glycaemic control is poor, HDL-C levels are reduced and triglycerides elevated and there is an increase in the level of atherogenic small dense LDL.[13]

The Evidence Base for Diabetes Care, Second Edition, Edited by William H. Herman, Ann Louise Kinmonth, Nicholas J. Wareham and Rhys Williams.
© 2010 John Wiley & Sons, Ltd

The objective of lipid-altering therapy in diabetes is to reduce CVD risk, not to treat 'hyperlipidaemia'. Despite the typical dyslipidaemia of diabetes, reduction of LDL-C is the first-line objective of treatment. The reason for this is that there is substantially more trial evidence to support the effect of lowering LDL-C on improving cardiovascular outcomes than there is for altering HDL-C or triglycerides. (see below). Furthermore, LDL-C is often a stronger predictor of vascular disease risk than HDL-C, triglycerides or small dense LDL. In the United Kingdom Prospective Diabetes Study, for example, the strongest predictor of coronary heart disease (CHD) was LDL-C followed by HDL-C.[14] Triglycerides did not predict CHD independently of total: HDL-C ratio.[15] However, there is considerable disparity in the literature, with some studies finding triglycerides to be the most important predictor[16] and some finding non-HDL-C more useful than LDL-C.

Therapeutic options for altering lipids in diabetes and the evidence base to support their use

Lifestyle change, medical nutrition therapy and pharmaceutical therapies that improve glycaemic control all have some impact on hyperlipidaemia and are discussed elsewhere in this book. Here we focus on drug treatments. The current options available and their relative potency for altering lipids are summarized in Table 13.1.

Table 13.1 Typical range of effects of lipid altering drugs on cholesterol components and triglycerides

Drug	Change (%)		
	LDL-C	Triglycerides	HDL-C
Statins	↓18–55	↓7–30	↑0–15
Niacin	↓5–25	↓20–50	↑15–35
Fibrates	↓0–20	↓20–50	↑2–35
Omega-3 fatty acids	↑5–45	↓25–45	↑1–3
Colestipol (bile acid resins)	↓15–30	Possible increase	↑3–5
Ezetimibe	↓15–20	↓2–8	↑0–3

Lowering LDL-C

The most potent agents for lowering LDL-C are statins and bile acid sequestrants, with newer cholesterol absorption inhibitors having a substantial but lesser effect. Niacin and, to a lesser extent, fibrates also lower LDL-C modestly. As described below, statins have by far the largest evidence base to support their efficacy for LDL-C lowering and CVD prevention.

Statins

More than 20 000 patients with diabetes have been included in trials with statins that have CVD endpoints. The main trials and their principal results are shown in Table 13.2. The largest secondary prevention trials in terms of numbers of events in patients with diabetes were 4S, CARE, LIPID and the Heart

Table 13.2 Major statin trials in patients with diabetes

Trial[a]	No. of subjects with diabetes	Primary endpoint	Drug	Difference in primary endpoint with treatment (%)	p-Value
Secondary prevention					
4S	202	CHD	Simvastatin 20 mg	↓55	0.002
CARE	586	CHD	Pravastatin 40 mg	↓25	0.005
LIPID	782	CHD	Pravastatin 40 mg	↓19	ns
PROSPER	623	CVD	Pravastatin 40 mg	↑27	ns
HPS	3051	CVD	Simvastatin 20 mg	↓15	<0.01
ASPEN	505	CVD	Atorvastatin 10 mg	↓18	ns
Primary prevention					
HPS	2912	CVD	Simvastatin 20 mg	↓33	0.0003
ASCOT	2527	CHD	Atorvastatin 10 mg	↓16	ns
ALLHAT-LLT[b]	3638	CHD	Pravastatin 40 mg	↓11	ns
CARDS	2838	CVD	Atorvastatin 10 mg	↓37	0.001
ASPEN	1903	CVD	Atorvastatin 10 mg	↓3	ns

[a]Other statin trials with small numbers of patients with diabetes include WOSCOPS (n = 76), Post CABG (n = 116), AFCAPS/TEXCAPS (n = 155), LIPS (n = 202).

[b]ALLHAT-LLT: 14% were secondary prevention.

Protection Study (HPS).[17] In the 4S study, a *post hoc* analysis of the efficacy of simvastatin 20 mg in a subgroup of 202 diabetic patients showed a significant 55% reduction in the secondary endpoint of major coronary heart disease events; the hazard ratio (HR) with treatment was 0.45, 95% CI 0.27 to 0.74 ($p = 0.002$) and a 43% reduction in the primary endpoint of total mortality which did not reach conventional significance (HR 0.57, 95% CI 0.30 to 1.08, $p = 0.09$).[2] LDL-C was reduced by 36%, HDL-C increased by 7% and triglycerides were reduced by 11%. In the CARE trial, treatment with pravastatin 40 mg in 586 patients with diabetes and prior CHD reduced LDL-C by 27%, increased HDL-C by 4% and decreased triglycerides by 13%.[3] The primary endpoint of major CHD was reduced by 25% ($p = 0.05$), an effect that did not differ significantly from the effect in the total 4159 patients with existing CHD. In the LIPID study of 9014 patients with prior CHD, there was no heterogeneity of effect by diabetes ($n = 782$) with a 19% non-significant reduction in major CHD and a significant 21% reduction in risk of any CVD event ($p = 0.003$) associated with pravastatin 40 mg daily.[4] In the PROspective Study of Pravastatin in the Elderly at Risk Trial (PROSPER), 5804 older participants (70–84 years) with prior vascular disease were studied, of whom 623 had diabetes.[18] Overall, the primary endpoint of major CVD was reduced by 15% with treatment and CHD was reduced by 19%. There was no significant heterogeneity of effect by diabetes, but among the diabetic subgroup the primary endpoint of major CVD was non significantly higher in those on pravastatin than placebo (HR 1.27, 95% CI 0.90 to 1.80).

In the Antihypertensive and Lipid Lowering Treatment to Prevent Heart Attack Trial (ALLHAT-LLT), 10 355 older patients were randomized to usual care or placebo 40 mg daily.[19] Most (86%) had no prior CHD. Treatment was associated with a modest 17% reduction in LDL-C, as expected given high rates (30%) of lipid lowering drug use in the usual care arm. Overall, CHD was not significantly reduced (relative risk 0.91, $p = 0.2$). In the sub-group of 3638 patients with diabetes, there was a similar 11% reduction in CHD which was also non-significant.

The HPS was the first definitive primary prevention trial of lipid lowering in type 2 diabetes. It included 5963 people with diabetes, of whom 2912 had no prior vascular disease. Simvastatin 40 mg daily reduced major CVD by about 15% in the secondary prevention group and by 33% ($p = 0.0003$) in the primary prevention arm, with the overall reduction being 22% ($p < 0.0001$). In the Collaborative Atorvastatin Diabetes Study (CARDS), 2838 patients with type 2 diabetes were randomized to receive atorvastatin 10 mg daily or placebo. The primary endpoint was major cardiovascular events.[20] The trial was stopped early as an interim analysis had shown unequivocal evidence of benefit. At the median 3.9 years follow-up, major CVD was reduced by 37% ($p = 0.001$), CHD by 36% and stroke rates by 48%.[20] Substantial lipid differences were observed in the study, with LDL-C reduced by 40% and triglycerides by 19%, but with little change in HDL-C. The Anglo-Scandinavian Cardiac Outcomes Study lipid-lowering arm (ASCOT-LLA), was also terminated early because of treatment benefit.[21] In this study, 10 305 patients were randomized to atorvastatin 10 mg daily or placebo, of whom 2527 had type 2 diabetes. Overall treatment reduced acute CHD by 36% ($p = 0.0005$) and total CVD by 21%. There was no heterogeneity of effect by diabetes, although within the diabetes group the 16% primary endpoint reduction was not statistically significant. Total CVD events were significantly reduced in the diabetic sub-group by 23%.[22] The Atorvastatin for the Prevention of Coronary Heart Disease Endpoints in Non-insulin-dependent diabetes (ASPEN) trial also examined the effect of atorvastatin 10 mg in patients with type 2 diabetes and included both a primary and a secondary prevention arm.[23] The lipid differences achieved were lower than in CARDS, as expected given the high rate of dropout in statin use during the study (27% in the placebo arm compared with 15% in the placebo arm at year 4 on CARDS). LDL-C was reduced by 29% and triglycerides by 6%. There was no significant reduction in major CVD events (10% reduction, $p = 0.3$) overall or in either arm examined separately. The observed LDL-C lowering of about 1 mmol l^{-1} might have been expected to reduce CVD by about 20% and ASPEN had just 60% power to detect such an effect on CVD. Furthermore, softer endpoints of CABG and revascularization and hospitalization for angina comprised a greater proportion of the primary endpoint on ASPEN, and this may have contributed to the lack of a treatment effect.

The Cholesterol Treatment Trialists Collaboration (CTTC) have summarized almost all the available data on statins in diabetes in a recent meta-analysis. Data from 18 686 individuals with diabetes were included (1466 with type 1 and 17 220 with type 2) in the context of a further 71 370 without diabetes in 14 randomized trials of statin therapy with follow-up to 5 years. They reported that, among patients with diabetes, the proportional effects of statin therapy were similar irrespective of whether there was a prior history of vascular disease or not. Effects on outcomes were similar among participants with and without diabetes and amongst those with type 1 or type 2 diabetes. Amongst those with diabetes, there was a 9% proportional reduction in all-cause mortality per 1 mmol l^{-1}

reduction in LDL-C [rate ratio (RR) 0·91, 99% CI 0·82 to 1·01, $p = 0·02$]. This finding reflected a significant reduction in vascular mortality (RR 0·87, 95% CI 0·76 to 1·00, $p = 0·008$) with no effect on non-vascular mortality (RR 0·97, 95% CI 0·82 to 1·16, $p = 0·7$). There was a significant 21% proportional reduction in major vascular events per 1 mmol l^{-1} reduction in LDL-C (RR 0·79, 95% CI 0·72–0·86, $p < 0·0001$), There were also significant reductions in myocardial infarction or coronary death (RR 0·78, 95% CI 0·69 to 0·87, $p < 0·0001$), coronary revascularization (RR 0·75, 95% CI 0·64 to 0·88, $p < 0·0001$) and stroke (RR 0·79, 95% CI 0·67 to 0·93, $p = 0·0002$). There was no evidence that the relative effects of statin therapy differed by diabetes type (type 1 or 2), gender, age, blood pressure, smoking, body mass index, renal function, predicted annual risk of a major vascular event or baseline lipid profile.

The main trial not yet included in these analyses is ASPEN. The inclusion of ASPEN in the meta-analysis would be expected to reduce the estimate for CVD prevention for every 1 mmol l^{-1} by a few percentage points at most. The ASPEN data demonstrate the important point that a very large evidence base with several trials is really needed to evaluate any class of drugs and individual drugs reliably. Overall, there is clear and reliable evidence that statins have substantial effects on reducing CVD in patients with diabetes. The extent to which this is true in patients with diabetes and severe cardiovascular or renal complications is less clear. Of the CVD endpoint trials of the newer statin, rosuvastatin, the Study to evaluate the Use of Rosuvastatin in subjects On Regular Haemodialysis: an Assessment of Survival and Cardiovascular events (AURORA)[24] and the Controlled Rosuvastatin Multinational Study in Heart Failure (CORONA) trials in patients with renal and heart failure,[25] respectively, include some patients with type 2 diabetes. The latter trial has recently reported and rosuvastatin did not reduce the composite cardiovascular outcome or the number of deaths from any cause in older patients with systolic heart failure. In terms of primary prevention, the large ($n = 15\,000$) Justification for the Use of Statins in Primary Prevention: an Intervention Trial Evaluating Rosuvastatin (JUPITER) trials excludes diabetes.[26]

The large numbers of patients studied in statin trials with several years of follow-up has also allowed precise quantification of adverse effects. Statins are generally safe and well-tolerated drugs. The most life-threatening adverse event is rhabdomyolysis, which occurs rarely at three events per 100 000 person-years of use. Fatal rhabdomyolysis occurs at one-tenth this rate.[27] Peripheral neuropathy is estimated to occur at a rate of 12 events per 100 000 person-years of use.

Ezetimibe

Ezetimibe is a cholesterol absorption inhibitor that lowers LDL-C modestly, by about 20% in comparison with about 35% at starting doses of many statins. This is similar to the LDL-C-lowering effect with niacin, but ezetimibe has much less effect than niacin on triglycerides or HDL-C. Its likely main usefulness may be in allowing sparing of statin dose in patients where concern about side-effects from highest statin doses is of particular concern. However, there are as yet no CVD endpoint data from ezetimibe clinical trials. The Improved Reduction of Outcomes: VYTORIN Efficacy International Trial (IMPROVE IT) will compare the effectiveness of ezetimibe/simvastatin combination 10/40 mg with simvastatin 40 mg on major CVD events in 10 000 patients with acute coronary syndrome, a substantial number of whom would be expected to have type 2 diabetes. Similarly, the SHARP trial is testing whether a combination of simvastatin and ezetimibe can prevent heart disease and strokes in patients with kidney disease (http://clinicaltrials.gov/ct/show/NCT00202878?order=1; accessed 26 October 2008).

Bile acid resins

Bile acid sequestrants (anion-exchange resins) are highly effective at reducing LDL-C and can raise HDL-C slightly, but can increase triglycerides. Large-scale evidence for the effectiveness of bile acid resins in preventing CVD in diabetes is lacking. In the Lipid Research Clinics Coronary Primary Prevention Trial (LRC-CPPT), men without CHD were randomized to cholestyramine or placebo. The 13% reduction in LDL-C achieved was associated with a 19% reduction in acute CHD events, but this trial did not include patients with diabetes. Due to the potential for worsening triglyceride levels, bile acid sequestrants are not recommended for use as monotherapy in patients with triglycerides above 2 mmol l^{-1}. Given the potency of statins for lowering LDL-C, bile acid sequestrants have limited use in patients with diabetes, mainly being of use in patients with statin intolerance.

Lowering triglyceride and raising HDL-C

Although the statins and cholesterol absorption inhibitors can reduce triglycerides substantially, niacin, fibrates and omega-3 fatty acids have more potent effects on triglycerides and the evidence base for their use is summarized here. For raising HDL-C, niacin is the most potent currently available agent. In many studies fibrates are also potent agents for raising HDL-C although, as described below, the Fenofibrate Intervention and Event Lowering in Diabetes (FIELD) data call into question whether such effects are seen and maintained with all fibrates.[28]

Omega-3 fatty acids

N-3 (omega) fatty acids, eicosapentaenoic acid (EPA) and docosahexaenoic acid (DHA), consumed either through dietary oily fish intake or through fish oil capsules, lower triglycerides substantially. However, at large doses, marine oil intake can increase LDL-C in patients with hypertriglyceridaemia. The National Cholesterol Education Program Adult Treatment Panel III (NCEP-ATPIII) guidelines state that higher dietary intakes of n-3 omega fatty acids are an option for reducing CHD but refrain from recommending dietary or fish oil capsules in the treatment of high triglyceride.[29] In contrast, the American Heart Association states that 2–4 g of EPA + DHA per day provided as capsules under a physician's care may be useful in the treatment of high triglycerides.[30] However, a Cochrane systematic review of 48 randomized controlled trials (36 913 participants) and 41 cohort analyses concluded that there was no reduction in the risk of total mortality or combined cardiovascular events in those taking additional omega-3 fats (with significant statistical heterogeneity). Restricting analysis to trials increasing fish-based omega-3 fats did not suggest significant effects on mortality or cardiovascular events in either group.[31] Since then, a large Japanese study ($n = 18\,645$) including patients with and without prior CVD reported on the effect of EPA oil given as an additional treatment to patients taking HMG-CoA reductase inhibitors for hypercholesterolaemia. Treatment was associated with a 19% reduction in major coronary events (95% CI 0.69 to 0.95). In this study, 16% had diabetes. However, despite being presented in November 2005 at the American Heart Association Congress, the full report of this trial is not yet published.32 Important trials in patients with type 2 diabetes are under way. The ASCEND Trial (A Study of Cardiovascular Events in Diabetes) will examine the efficacy and safety of 100 mg daily aspirin and/or supplementation with 1 g capsules containing 90% omega-3 fatty acids (0.4 g EPA, 0.3 g DHA) in the primary prevention of CVD in patients with diabetes (http://clinicaltrials.gov/ct/show/NCT00135226?order=26, accessed 5 March 2007).

The study is recruiting at least 10 000 patients with diabetes and no clinical evidence of occlusive arterial disease and is not expected to complete until at least 2012. In the recently reported Atorvastatin in Factorial with Omega-3 fatty acids Risk Reduction in Diabetes (AFORRD) study results, presented at the 2006 IDF Congress, omega-3 EE90 reduced serum triglycerides by 5.6% in type 2 diabetic patients (http://www.dtu.ox.ac.uk/aforrd/AFORRDPressRelease.pdf, accessed 5 March 2007).

The endpoint of the trial was estimated rather than observed CVD risk, and this was unaffected by omega-3 EE90.

Nicotinic acid (niacin)

Niacin lowers triglycerides by 20–50% while increasing HDL-C levels (by 15–35%). It also lowers levels of free fatty acids and lipoprotein. At high doses it lowers LDL-C by up to 25%. It is the most potent agent available at present for raising HDL-C. The common side-effect of flushing has limited its use and hepatotoxicity is a concern at higher doses. Flushing can be decreased by pretreatment with aspirin or nonsteroidal anti-inflammatory drugs and is less with newer extended- and slow-release preparations. Niacin also worsens glycaemic control. For example, in the Assessment of Diabetes Control and Evaluation of the Efficacy of Niaspan Trial (ADVENT) study, the higher 1500 mg dose of niacin-ER was associated with a 0.3% net increase in HbA_{1c} and a greater requirement for glucose-lowering therapy at 16 weeks of use.[33]

Trial evidence for the efficacy of niacin in preventing CVD in patients with diabetes is inadequate at present. The main efficacy data come from the Coronary Drug Project reported in 1975. The Coronary Drug Project included 8341 men with prior coronary disease and initially involved comparisons of two oestrogen regimens and dextrothyroxine (subsequently discontinued) and clofibrate and niacin.

No evidence of efficacy was found for the clofibrate treatment. The trial excluded patients on insulin but about 40% of study entrants had raised fasting plasma glucose. At the initial 6 years follow-up, niacin was associated with a 17% decrease in acute CHD events ($p < 0.005$) and there was no heterogeneity of effect by baseline glucose status.[34] However, whether all of the effect can be attributed to niacin *per se* is unclear since aspirin use is likely to have been higher in those on niacin. Two important trials started in 2006/2007 that will evaluate the benefit of combination statin + niacin against statin therapy alone, but will not report until at least 2012. The Niacin Plus Statin to Prevent Vascular Events (AIM-HIGH) study will compare simvastatin alone with extended-release niacin plus simvastatin in just over 3000 patients with established vascular disease, 40% of whom are expected to have the metabolic syndrome (http://clinicaltrials.gov/ct/show/NCT00120289, accessed 2 March 2007).

The trial will exclude any effect of pre-administration of aspirin by prescribing this in both arms of the study. In the Treatment of HDL to Reduce the Incidence of Vascular Events Study (HPS-2 THRIVE), 20 000 patients with vascular disease, 7000 of whom will also have diabetes, will have statin therapy to achieve the LDL-C goal and will then be randomized to receive a niacin–prostaglandin D2 receptor 1 antagonist combination tablet or placebo (www.ctsu.ox.ac.uk/pressreleases/2006-05-31/hps2-thrive-press-release, accessed 5 March 2007). The prostaglandin D2 receptor 1 antagonist reduces niacin-induced flushing but trials of its efficacy and safety such as in HPS-2 THRIVE are needed.[35]

Fibrates

Fibrates typically lower triglycerides to a similar extent to that found with niacin. They also raise HDL-C substantially in some studies (by up to 35%). However, in the FIELD study detailed below, a disappointing 5% initial rise in HDL-C was observed that fell to 2% by the study end. This demonstrates the importance of having long-term studies for establishing the effects of lipid-lowering agents on lipids.

The main cardiovascular endpoint data on the efficacy and safety of fibrates in type 2 diabetes comes from the VA-HIT and FIELD studies. Other fibrate trials such as the HHS ($n = 135$)[6] have included too few patients with diabetes to be informative or had too few events.[7] In the Bezafibrate Infarct Prevention (BIP) study,[36] 3122 patients with existing vascular disease and low HDL-C ($<1.15 \, \mathrm{mmol}\,l^{-1}$) were randomized to bezafibrate 400 mg versus placebo. HDL-C increased by 18% and triglycerides decreased by 21% and LDL-C decreased about 4%. There was no reduction in the primary endpoint of acute CHD. Only in a *post hoc* analysis in those with triglycerides above $2.25 \, \mathrm{mmol}\,l^{-1}$ was there some evidence for a reduction in CHD, but no formal test of treatment by triglyceride level was reported. Only 299 patients had type 2 diabetes.

In the VA-HIT, patients with established CHD were randomized to receive either gemfibrozil $1.2 \, \mathrm{g}\,\mathrm{day}^{-1}$ or placebo. The trial included 769 patients with diabetes and 1748 without diabetes.[5] The lipid levels at entry in those with diagnosed diabetes were triglycerides $1.85 \, \mathrm{mmol}\,l^{-1}$, HDL $0.8 \, \mathrm{mmol}\,l^{-1}$ and LDL-C $2.8 \, \mathrm{mmol}\,l^{-1}$. There was a significant 22% reduction in the primary endpoint of acute CHD and a significant 24% reduction in major CVD. Although differences in drug effect between those with and without diabetes were non-significant, when examined separately CHD was reduced by 32% in those with diabetes and 18% in those without, consistent with a possible

differential effect. Importantly, HDL-C was raised just 5% and triglycerides were lowered by 20% and there was no treatment effect on LDL-C so that VA-HIT is one of the few trials that gives an indication of the efficacy of altering triglycerides and HDL-C while not changing LDL-C. Also, just under half of those in the study were already at the $2.6 \, \mathrm{mmol}\,l^{-1}$ target for LDL-C at entry.

In FIELD, patients with type 2 diabetes were randomized to receive fenofibrate 200 mg or placebo.[28] The study included 2131 patients with prior CVD and 7664 without. At entry, mean LDL-C was 3.07 mmol l^{-1}, mean HDL-C was $1.1 \, \mathrm{mmol}\,l^{-1}$ and median triglycerides were $1.7 \, \mathrm{mmol}\,l^{-1}$. During follow-up, initially LDL-C was reduced by 12% and triglycerides by 29% and HDL-C was raised by just 5%. By the study close, these treatment differences had narrowed to a 6% reduction in LDL-C, a 22% reduction in triglycerides and just a 1.2% rise in HDL-C. On average, 17% of the placebo group and 8% of the fenofibrate group had add-in lipid-lowering therapy, predominately with statins, during follow-up. After 5 years of follow-up there was a non-significant 11% reduction in the primary endpoint of CHD events and a significant 11% reduction in total CVD events overall. A difficult issue in interpreting the FIELD data was the potential impact of add-in therapy on the results. If patients were censored at the time of starting -n therapy, then there was a slightly higher 14% effect on CHD. The 11% reduction in CHD events comprised a significant 25% reduction in those without previous CVD and a non-significant 8% increase in those with previous CVD. Total CVD events fell by 19% in those without a history of CVD, but there was no effect in those with previous CVD. These differences in treatment effects between CVD groups in FIELD were of borderline significance ($p = 0.05$ for CHD, $p = 0.03$ for CVD), making interpretation of the data very difficult. Importantly, the FIELD investigators noted that rates of additional statin use did not account for the difference in treatment effect by CVD status. Thus, although the data are consistent with a modest treatment effect in those with established CVD, they do not provide convincing evidence that such a benefit exists, in marked contrast to the VA-HIT data using gemfibrozil. Conversely, although the 25% reduction in CHD in the primary prevention group was much greater than the overall 11% reduction, the evidence was not sufficiently clear to suggest that fibrates could be used instead of statins for primary prevention. There were also some safety concerns raised by FIELD including absolute differences in the cumulative incidence rates of pulmonary embolism of 0.3%. There was a significant rise in plasma homocysteine level of $4 \, \mu\mathrm{mol}\,l^{-1}$. The authors noted that observational epidemiological studies suggest a difference of 10–20% in CVD risk with this level of homocysteine level. However, it remains unclear whether such drug-induced differences would really be causal for CVD or not.

Taken together, the data from VA-HIT and FIELD are difficult to interpret since for secondary prevention of CVD with a fibrate they give directly opposing results. Whereas the VA-HIT data suggest that in patients with existing CVD fibrates may be potent at reducing CVD, the FIELD data suggest that there is no such benefit and raise the possibility of important adverse effects. Whether these data reflect important drug-specific differences within the class of fibrates is not known. Put simply, the difficulty in establishing the role of fibrates in patients with diabetes is that there are not enough data. Of note, more than three times more patients with type 2 diabetes have been evaluated in endpoint trials of statins than fibrates and further trials of fibrate therapy would be needed to give more reliable estimates of benefit in different subgroups of patients. However, given the strength of data on LDL-C lowering with statins, placebo-controlled trials of fibrates will no longer be done. The practical clinical question is now whether adding fibrate therapy on top of statin therapy in patients at goal for LDL-C is efficacious in reducing LDL-C. Although it did not address this question directly, the VA-HIT data would favour the use of gemfibrozil rather than fenofibrate in this situation. However, in many countries the combination of gemfibrozil and a statin is specifically contraindicated because of a reportedly higher incidence of muscle-related side-effects.[37] Data on efficacy and safety of using a statin and a fibrate in combination will have to await the Action to Control Cardiovascular Risk in Diabetes (ACCORD) trial, due to report in 2010 (http://www.accordtrial.org/public/protocol_2005-05-11.pdf, accessed 19 February 2007; http://clinicaltrials.gov/ct/show/NCT00000620. accessed 2 March 2007).[13] This trial of 10 000 patients has a 2×2 factorial design. One arm will assess whether, in the context of good glycaemic control, a therapeutic strategy that uses a fibrate to raise HDL-C/lower triglyceride levels and uses a statin for treatment of LDL-C reduces the rate of CVD events compared with a strategy that only uses a statin for treatment of LDL-C.

Current lipid-altering guidelines and lipid targets in diabetes

Current guidelines

There are a number of authoritative guidelines on lipid lowering in diabetes. In the United States, the main guidelines are the NCEP-ATPIII and the American Diabetes Association (ADA) Guideline.[38,39] In Europe, the Joint Societies' Guideline is available,[40] but within some European countries national guidelines are in common use, for example The UK Joint Societies guideline.[37] The main lipid-altering recommendations of these guidelines are summarized in Table 13.3. All the major guidelines agree that the first priority of lipid-lowering therapy in diabetes is to use a potent LDL-C-lowering agent. and they agree that statins have the best evidence base for this. All the guidelines agree that all patients with established CVD warrant lipid-lowering therapy. All the guidelines also agree that at least for patients with type 2 diabetes aged over 40 years, the risk of CVD is sufficient that they should be considered for lipid-lowering therapy. However, the guidelines differ on the target or goal set for LDL-C lowering and whether triglycerides and HDL-C should be targeted. They also differ in the finer detail of which patients warrant primary preventive therapy. Some aspects of the guidelines and their evidence base are discussed below.

Target LDL-C

As shown in Table 13.3, there is some disagreement on what the target LDL-C should be. For secondary prevention, the target or goal LDL-C varies from an optional target of $1.8\,\text{mmol}\,\text{l}^{-1}$ in the ATPIII guideline to a target of $2.5\,\text{mmol}\,\text{l}^{-1}$ in the European Joint Societies guidelines. For primary prevention, there is greater consensus on a target of $2.5/2.6\,\text{mmol}\,\text{l}^{-1}$ but within the UK the Joint Societies recommend a lower target of $2\,\text{mmol}\,\text{l}^{-1}$. Note, however, that the ADA and UK Joint Societies guidelines do allow for lipid lowering beyond these targets if the pretreatment cholesterol level is already low. Trial evidence certainly supports a target as low as $2\,\text{mmol}\,\text{l}^{-1}$ as described below.

Among the 5963 patients with diabetes included in the HPS study,[17] 2426 had an LDL-C below $3\,\text{mmol}\,\text{l}^{-1}$ at baseline. In those with an initial LDL-C below $3\,\text{mmol}\,\text{l}^{-1}$, the on-treatment values for LDL-C were below $2\,\text{mmol}\,\text{l}^{-1}$. These patients experienced as much CVD benefit from lipid lowering (a 27% reduction, $p = 0.0007$) as patients with initial levels of LDL-C above $3\,\text{mmol}\,\text{l}^{-1}$. Among the sub-set of these patients with an LDL-C $<3\,\text{mmol}\,\text{l}^{-1}$ who had no prior vascular disease at baseline there was also a 30% reduction in major CVD of borderline significance ($p = 0.05$). Among the diabetic and non-diabetic participants, 3421 had an LDL-C below $2.6\,\text{mmol}\,\text{l}^{-1}$ at entry and even among these patients there was a highly significant ($p = 0.0006$) reduction in CVD. Their

Table 13.3 Current guidelines on LDL-C goals in diabetes

LDL-C		Goal
Secondary prevention		
European Joint Societies	All patients with diabetes with above goal LDL-C	LDL-C <2.5 mmol l^{-1}
UK Joint Societies	All patients with diabetes	<2 mmol l^{-1} or a reduction of 30%, whichever is lower
ADA	Reduce LDL-C by 30–40% regardless of baseline	LDL-C <2.6 mmol l^{-1}
		But <1.8 mmol l^{-1} an option
NCEP-ATP III R	Treat all patients with diabetes and CVD to goal LDL-C	LDL-C <1.8 mmol l^{-1}
Primary prevention		
European Joint Societies	Treat if above goal and type 2 diabetes or type 1 diabetes with albuminuria	LDL-C <2.5 mmol l^{-1}
	Or estimated 10 year fatal CVD risk is at least 5%	
UK Joint Societies	All patients with diabetes aged over 40 years. Those under 40 years if one other risk factor	<2 mmol l^{-1} or a reduction of 30%, whichever is lower
ADA	Over age 40 years reduce LDL-C by 30–40% regardless of baseline	LDL-C <2.6 mmol l^{-1}
	Under age 40 years treat if other risk factors present if above goal after lifestyle change	
NCEP-ATP III R	Treat if 10 year CHD risk is ≥20% and LDL-C is ≥2.6 mmol l^{-1}	LDL-C <2.6 mmol l^{-1}
	Treat if 10 year CHD risk is 10–20% and LDL-C is ≥3.35 mmol l^{-1}	
	If 10 year CHD risk is ≥20% and LDL-C is <2.6 mmol l^{-1} use clinical judgement	
	If 10 year CHD risk is 10–20% and LDL-C is <3.35 mmol l^{-1} use clinical judgement	

on-treatment LDL-C was on average 1.7 mmol l^{-1}. Hence the HPS data certainly support a lower LDL-C target than 2.6 mmol l^{-1} and demonstrate the safety of reducing LDL-C to much lower levels.

In the CARDS trial,[20] the median LDL-C at entry was 3.02 mmol l^{-1} and 25% of patients already had an LDL-C of 2.5 mmol l^{-1} or lower prior to randomization. In the atorvastatin 10 mg arm, the median achieved LDL-C during follow up was 2.0 mmol l^{-1}, with 75% having an LDL-C of less than 2.5 mmol l^{-1} and 25% having an LDL-C below 1.7 mmol l^{-1}. Thus CARDS is essentially a trial of the benefits and safety of going below the current 2.5 mmol l^{-1} primary prevention target for LDL-C. Among those with an LDL-C at or below 3 mmol l^{-1} at baseline, a similar treatment effect was observed to those with higher LDL-C and the treatment effect was significant ($p = 0.025$). Even among the 743 patients in the bottom quartile for LDL-C at entry (i.e. those with an LDL-C below 2.5 mmol l^{-1}), there was a similar reduction in major CVD (26% reduction). Taken with the HPS data, these data provide strong supportive evidence that a targeting LDL-C down to at least 2 mmol l^{-1} is effective and safe in reducing CVD. The practical therapeutic implication is that even if pretreatment LDL-C

is near 2.5 mmol l^{-1}, further lowering with statin therapy is beneficial.

Of course, both HPS and CARDS showed that modest doses of simvastatin and atorvastatin, respectively, could achieve the current target LDL-C and beyond in a large proportion of patients. They did not directly assess the benefits of higher versus lower doses of statins. In the Treating to New Targets (TNT) trial,[41] 10 001 patients with existing CVD were treated with atorvastatin 10 mg to achieve an LDL-C of no more than 3.4 mmol l^{-1} (the mean achieved was 2.5 mmol l^{-1}) and were then randomized to either continue atorvastatin 10 mg or to start atorvastatin 80 mg. The trial included 1501 patients with type 2 diabetes for whom the data were reported separately. In this group, the median achieved LDL-C in the atorvastatin 80 mg arm was 2 mmol l^{-1} and in the atorvastatin 10 mg arm it was 2.5 mmol l^{-1}. Over a median follow-up of 4.9 years, there was a significant 25% reduction in major CVD ($p = 0.025$) with this greater reduction in LDL-C. In the Incremental Decrease in End Points Through Aggressive Lipid Lowering Study (IDEAL), among patients with existing CVD and at mean LDL-C of 2.5 mmol l^{-1} at randomization,[42] 80 mg of atorvastatin was compared with

40 mg of simvastatin. The mean on-treatment LDL-C levels were 2.1 and 2.7 mmol l^{-1}, respectively. The effect of this difference in LDL-C on CVD was less than in TNT with the primary endpoint of major CHD being reduced by 11% (a non-significant effect, $p = 0.07$) and the secondary endpoint of major CVD being reduced by 13% ($p = 0.02$). Myalgia occurred in 2.2% of the atorvastatin 80 mg group and in 1.1% of the simvastatin 40 mg group. There were more than 1000 patients with diabetes in IDEAL but no diabetes-specific analysis has been reported as yet. These data suggest a net benefit in achieving a lower target LDL-C in patients with established CVD, even when it requires higher doses of statin, and establish that this is safe but that patients should be monitored carefully when higher doses are initiated.

Target triglyceride and HDL-C levels

The evidence base for the use of target triglyceride and HDL-C levels in diabetes is much weaker than for LDL-C. Although LDL-C is most consistently the strongest predictor of CVD in diabetes., the constellation of low HDL-C, raised triglycerides and increased small dense LDL also contributes to CVD risk.[16,43,44] As shown in Table 13.4, there is disagreement between the current guidelines on whether there should

be specific therapeutic targets set for triglycerides and HDL-C. Only the ADA guideline says that patients should be treated to achieve an explicit target for triglycerides and HDL-C and suggests that combination therapy of a statin with niacin or a fibrate might be used. The main evidence that altering triglycerides (or the lipoproteins with which they are correlated) or HDL-C, without affecting LDL-C, is effective in altering CVD risk in diabetes comes from the VA-HIT study as described above. In VA-HIT, allocation to gemfibrozil 1200 mg daily was associated with a 5% increase in HDL-C and a 20% reduction in triglycerides but no change in LDL-C. In the ATP III guideline, rather than targets for triglycerides, a target for non-HDL-C in those with elevated triglycerides is used. This is in part to emphasize that in those at goal for LDL-C, achieving a non-HDL-C goal could indicate either additional statin therapy or therapy aimed at triglyceride lowering, namely niacin or fibrate. As described above for patients with diabetes and established CVD, there is direct evidence from the TNT study to support benefits of additional statin beyond an LDL-C goal of 2.5 mmol l^{-1}, but otherwise there is no good evidence base on which to base a choice between additional statin therapy or combination with niacin, fibrate or ezetimibe. Hence the results of the ACCORD, HPS-2 Thrive and other endpoint

Table 13.4 Current guidelines on HDL-C- and triglyceride-related goals in diabetes

		Goal
Triglycerides		
European Joint Societies	No target set but fasting TG >1.7 mmol l^{-1} is a marker of increased CVD risk	
UK Joint Societies	No target set but fasting TG >1.7 mmol l^{-1} is a marker of increased CVD risk	Non-HDL-C < 3 mmol l^{-1} and TG <1.7 mmol l^{-1} are preferred values but not targets
ADA	Treat all patients with diabetes to goal	Lower TG to <1.7 mmol l^{-1}
NCEP-ATP III R	In patients with triglycerides >200 mg dl^{-1} treatment target should encompass atherogenic remnant lipoproteins – therefore non HDL-C is set as a target since it encompasses VLDL-C, which is correlated with atherogenic remnants	If TG >200 mg dl^{-1} non HDL-C should be no more than LDL-C target + 30 mg dl^{-1}
HDL-C		
European Joint Societies	No target set but HDL-C <1 mmol l^{-1} in men or <1.2 mmol l^{-1} in women is a marker of increased CVD risk	
UK Joint Societies	No target set but HDL-C <1 mmol l^{-1} in men or <1.2 mmol l^{-1} in women is a marker of increased CVD risk	
ADA	Treat all patients with diabetes to goal	Goal is >1mmol l^{-1}, but in women >1.3 mmol l^{-1} can be considered
NCEP-ATP III R	No target set but HDL-C <1 mmol l^{-1} is a marker of increased CVD risk	

studies of combination therapies are badly needed (http://www.ctsu.ox.ac.uk/projects/hps2-thrive, accessed 2 March 2007).

Lipid lowering to prevent CVD in patients with type 1 diabetes

The evidence base to support lipid lowering for preventing CVD in type 1 diabetes comes primarily from the HPS Study. In that study there were 615 patients with type 1 diabetes and the effect of treatment was the same as for the total group of patients with diabetes with a major CHD event rate of 13.7% in those on romvastatin compared with 17.5% in those on placebo ($p = 0.9$ for heterogeneity of effect by type of diabetes). This provides some reassurance that type 1 diabetic patients receive a similar magnitude of benefit from lipid lowering as found in type 2 diabetes. This is confirmed in the recent meta-analysis from the Cholesterol Treatment Trialists Collaboration (CTTC), which collated data from 1466 patients with type 1 diabetic patients included in the HPS and other statin trials.

There is a lack of clarity in the current guidelines on the role of lipid-altering treatments in patients with type 1 diabetes. This reflects not just the lack of clinical trials data but also the lack of precise estimates of CVD in type 1 diabetes, particularly at younger ages and in patients who are normoalbuminuric. The UK Joint Societies guideline specifically recommends lipid lowering in all type 1 diabetic patients above age 40 years and in those aged 18–40 years if there is one additional CVD risk factor. The ADA guideline states that consideration should be given for similar lipid-lowering therapy in type 1 and type 2 diabetes. The European Joint Societies guideline explicitly states that patients with type 1 diabetes who are albuminuric are a priority group for lipid-lowering interventions. However, it also states that the increased risk of CVD in type 1 diabetes is almost entirely confined to patients developing diabetic renal disease. In our view, this latter statement needs qualification. The study that the statement cites in fact showed that the relative mortality from CVD compared with the general population in type 1 diabetes patients without proteinuria is 4.2.[45] This is a substantial increased risk despite being dwarfed by the extraordinarily higher 37-fold relative mortality in patients with proteinuria. Furthermore, we and others have demonstrated increased levels of coronary atherosclerosis at a young age in normoalbuminuric type 1 diabetes patients.[12] The European Joint Societies guideline also encourages the idea of looking beyond a 10 year time horizon for younger patients and projecting their risk

at age 60 years as a means of deciding on whether intervention is warranted. In a recent analysis from a large General Practice research database in the United Kingdom, we reported that typically type 1 diabetic women have a CVD risk similar to that seen in non-diabetic individuals who are at least 15 years older.[46] In type 1 diabetic men, the risk is typical of non-diabetic men who are 10–15 years older. A Canadian study also recently reported that diabetes was associated with about a 15 year ageing effect in terms of CVD rates with the group rate for patients with diabetes becoming high risk, that is, >20% 10 year risk for CVD at age 42 years in men and age 48 years in women.[47] However, it was not possible to establish nephropathy status in either of these cohorts. Hence better data on the absolute risk of CVD at different ages in type 1 diabetic patients who are normoalbuminuric are badly needed to inform clinical decision making for when preventive therapies should be introduced.

Lipid lowering to prevent CVD in patients with chronic kidney disease

In the presence of chronic kidney disease, there are vasculopathic changes that may not be strongly related to cholesterol levels, including vascular calcification. In many observational studies of chronic kidney disease patients, there is no relationship between cholesterol and CVD outcomes. Therefore, consideration has been given to whether or not such patients would derive significant benefits from lipid-lowering therapy. Relatively few of the statin trials have explicitly reported on efficacy by baseline glomerular filtration rate, although this will be part of the forthcoming meta-analysis report from the CTTC. In the HPS, 1019 non-diabetic and 310 diabetic patients had elevated plasma creatinine at baseline, too few to establish treatment effect within the sub-group with precision. However, there was no significant difference in treatment effect by creatinine status.

In the ALERT (Assessment of LEscol in Renal Transplantation) study, 2102 renal transplant recipients were randomized to placebo or fluvastatin 40 mg, increasing to 80 mg with an achieved average LDL-C difference of 1 mmol l^{-1} during the study.[48] Overall, 19% of those randomized had diabetes and 13% of those randomized had diabetic nephropathy as the reason for transplantation. At the study close there was a non-significant 17% reduction in major CVD and a significant 35% reduction in the secondary endpoint of acute CHD, with no effect on stroke. Two years beyond the end of the study, the difference in major CVD and CHD events between the original treatment groups was maintained. No diabetes-specific analyses or test of heterogeneity were carried out, appropriately given the small numbers of patients with diabetes. Overall, 13% of those randomized died during the 5 year follow-up study.

In contrast to these data, in the Deutsche Diabetes-Dialyse-Studie (4D), 1255 patients with type 2 diabetes undergoing haemodialysis were randomized to receive atorvastatin 20 mg or placebo and were followed up for a median of 4 years.[49] A striking difference between the 4D study and ALERT is that in the 4D study 50% of those randomized died during follow-up. The achieved LDL-C difference decreased during follow-up from about 1.3 mmol l^{-1} initially to about 0.9 mmol l^{-1} at 3 years. There was no significant difference in major CVD observed (8% lower in the atorvastatin group, $p = 0.4$), there was an 18% reduction in all cardiac events combined ($p = 0.03$) and no significant effect on total deaths (7% lower in the atorvastatin group, $p = 0.3$). The report highlighted an analysis of the sub-set of fatal stroke events which occurred in 2% of the placebo group and 4% of the atorvastatin group ($p = 0.04$). However, this needs to be interpreted in the context of no overall difference in the incidence of total stroke in the two groups and no difference in total deaths. A sensible interpretation of these data is that although there may be a modest effect on coronary events overall, there is insufficient effect on total morbidity and mortality to consider treatment to be of benefit.

Taking account of these data, the recent guidelines from the National Kidney Foundation – KDOQI in the United States recommended that in type 2 diabetic patients on haemodialysis statin therapy should not be initiated 'unless there is a specific cardiovascular indication'. The interpretation of specific cardiovascular indication is not clear.[50] Although the National Kidney Foundation – KDOQI graded the evidence for this statement as 'strong', in fact much more trial data on statin efficacy in renal disease are needed. This is particularly so given that complex patterns of treatment effect over time are more plausible in trials in patient groups with very large competing mortality risks, as seen in 4D. Hence forthcoming data from the AURORA and SHARP trials are needed. The Study of Heart and Renal Protection (SHARP)[51] will examine the effect of lowering blood cholesterol with a combination of simvastatin (20 mg daily) and the cholesterol absorption inhibitor ezetimibe (10 mg daily) on the risk of major vascular events among patients on dialysis or at pre-dialysis renal failure stage. It is not expected to report until at least 2010. AURORA is a double-blind, randomized, multicentre, Phase IIIb, parallel-group study comparing the effects of rosuvastatin (10 mg once daily) with placebo on survival

and cardiovascular events in ESRD patients on chronic haemodialysis.[24] It was expected to report in 2007/2008.

Microvascular complications

A number of observational studies have examined the relationship between lipids and diabetic microvascular complications. For retinopathy, cohort analyses have shown mixed results. Although in several studies cholesterol and triglyceride levels are associated with retinal outcomes in univariate analyses, in only a few studies have they remained independent predictors of outcomes in multivariate analyses. However, many of the studies were small and underpowered and in the two largest cohorts, the Early Treatment of Diabetic Retinopathy Study (ETDRS) which studied both type 1 and type 2 diabetes ($n > 2600$), cholesterol predicted the development of hard exudates and triglycerides predicted retinopathy.[52] In the EURODIAB Prospective Complications Study (EURODIAB PCS) cohort of type 1 diabetic patients ($n = 764$), triglycerides were an independent predictor of retinopathy.[53] For nephropathy, the situation is complicated by the fact that changes in lipids can occur secondary to renal disease. However, the results are more consistent than for retinopathy with most cohort analyses showing some relationship for both total or LDL-C and triglycerides.[1,54–58] There are fewer data on diabetic neuropathy, but cholesterol and triglycerides predict distal symmetric neuropathy in several large diabetic cohorts including EURODIAB PCS[59] and triglycerides predict cardiac autonomic neuropathy in several cohorts.[55] Hence the epidemiological data are consistent with a role for lipids in the pathogenesis of microvascular disease and data in animal and cell biology studies support this idea.

The evidence on whether lipid-lowering drugs alter microvascular complications is sparse. In a meta-analysis of small trials pre-2001 in patients with existing renal disease, there was evidence that lipid lowering reduced deterioration in GFR (net benefit 1.9 ml min^{-1} per year), although the results between studies were heterogenous.[60] Since then, there have been several further trial reports and systematic reviews of the effect of lipid lowering on microvascular outcomes. In the HPS, treatment with simvastatin 20 mg daily was associated a lesser rise in plasma creatinine (by 2.18 µmol l^{-1} less) during follow-up in those with diabetes ($p < 0.05$). Using the MDRD equation, among those with diabetes eGFR fell by -1.4 ml min^{-1} less in those on simvastatin over a mean 4.8 years of follow-up.[17] No retinal outcome data were reported from HPS. Atorvastatin treatment was associated with an improvement in creatinine clearance in the Greek Atorvastatin and Coronary Heart Disease Evaluation (GREACE) study.[61] In a recent combined analysis across the West of Scotland Coronary Prevention Study (WOSCOPS), CARE and LIPID trials that included 1334 patients with diabetes, pravastatin was associated with a significant but small $0.24\,ml\,min^{-1}$ per $1.73\,m^2$ per year net benefit in eGFR. The effect within the diabetic sub-group was not reported separately.[62] Douglas et al. conducted a recent meta-analysis of statin studies with albuminuria outcomes. The meta-analysis was dominated by a single pravastatin study that showed no benefit on albuminuria and included very few diabetic subjects.[63,64] Sandhu et al. reported a significant benefit for eGFR (1.22 ml min per year slower in statin recipients than placebo) and a reduction in albuminuria in a meta-analysis of statin trials that included 39 704 participants, but the analysis within the diabetic sub-group showed no significant effect.[65] Overall, the evidence that statins have any beneficial impact on the progression of albuminuria is weak and there is some evidence of small effects on GFR of unclear clinical significance. At higher doses, some statins may actually increase proteinuria through inhibition of proximal tubular protein uptake [66,67] However, in their recent systematic review of statin safety, Law and Rudnicka[27] concluded that there was no evidence of any adverse effect on renal status from statins at currently marketed doses. There are much fewer data from large clinical trials on the effect of statins in diabetic retinopathy. Small underpowered studies suggest there may be an effect, but the data are inadequate to be able to draw any firm conclusion.[68] Similarly for diabetic neuropathies, there are no adequate trial data on whether lipid lowering has any beneficial impact. As reviewed by Law and Rudnicka, statin-induced peripheral neuropathy is rare, occurring at about 12 events per 100 000 person-years of use.[27]

With regard to the effects of other lipid-lowering drugs on diabetic microvascular complications, there are surprisingly few data. In the recent FIELD Study[28] there was some evidence of a beneficial effect on albuminuria with fenofibrate with a net difference of 2.6% in the proportion of patients whose albuminuria regressed or did not worsen. However, there was a significant increase in plasma creatinine of $10\,\mu mol\,l^{-1}$ that resolved at study cessation. Interestingly, reports of new photocoagulation in FIELD were reduced by 30% with fenofibrate, but firm conclusions on benefit need to wait for the full analysis of retinal photographs from FIELD.

From a clinical decision-making point of view, whether lipid lowering alters microvascular outcomes is now largely a moot point. Almost all patients with type 2 diabetes will warrant lipid-lowering therapy anyway. However, in younger type 1 diabetic patients it would be of interest to know whether those whose absolute risk of CVD in a given time period is deemed too low to warrant initiation of lipid lowering might benefit from it from a microvascular perspective.

Conclusion

There is now a good evidence base supporting the efficacy and safety of LDL-C lowering for CVD prevention in patients with diabetes, particularly with statin therapy. Almost all patients with type 2 diabetes will warrant such therapy. The extent to which lowering triglycerides and raising HDL-C with currently available drugs reduces CVD risk remains less clear. Trials of fibrates in patients with diabetes and established CVD have given conflicting results. In patients without CVD, lowering LDL-C with a statin seems more efficacious than focusing on triglycerides and HDL-C with a fibrate. The effect of sole therapy with niacin on CVD risk in diabetes is untested. Trials are under way to provide an evidence base for some important outstanding questions, in particular the role of combination therapy (statin plus fibrate, statin plus niacin, statin plus ezetimibe) in patients at goal for LDL-C and the efficacy of lipid lowering in advanced renal disease.

References

1 Orchard T, Fried L. Prevention of hyperlipidaemia. In: *The Evidence Base for Diabetes Care* (eds Williams R, Herman W, Kinmonth AL, Wareham NJ,), John Wiley & Sons, Ltd, Chichester, 2002, pp. 413–448.

2 Pyorala K, Pedersen TR, Kjekshus J, Faergeman O, Olsson AG, Thorgeirsson G. Cholesterol lowering with simvastatin improves prognosis of diabetic patients with coronary heart disease. A sub-group analysis of the Scandinavian Simvastatin Survival Study (4S). *Diabetes Care* 1997; **20**:614–620.

3 Goldberg RB, Mellies MJ, Sacks FM, Moye LA, Howard BV, Howard WJ et al. Cardiovascular events and their reduction with pravastatin in diabetic and glucose-intolerant myocardial infarction survivors with average cholesterol levels: subgroup analyses in the cholesterol and recurrent events (CARE) trial. The Care Investigators. *Circulation* 1998; **98**:2513–2519.

4 Keech A, Colquhoun D, Best J, Kirby A, Simes RJ, Hunt D et al. Secondary prevention of cardiovascular events with long-term pravastatin in patients with diabetes or impaired fasting glucose: results from the LIPID trial. *Diabetes Care* 2003; **26**:2713–2721.

5 Rubins HB, Robins SJ, Collins D, Nelson DB, Elam MB, Schaefer EJ et al. Diabetes, plasma insulin and cardiovascular

disease: sub-group analysis from the Department of Veterans Affairs high-density lipoprotein intervention trial (VA-HIT). *Arch Intern Med* 2002; **162**:2597–2604.

6 Tenkanen L, Manttari M, Kovanen PT, Virkkunen H, Manninen V. Gemfibrozil in the treatment of dyslipidemia: an 18-year mortality follow-up of the Helsinki Heart Study. *Arch Intern Med* 2006; **166**:743–748.

7 Elkeles RS, Diamond JR, Poulter C, Dhanjil S, Nicolaides AN, Mahmood S *et al.* Cardiovascular outcomes in type 2 diabetes. A double-blind placebo-controlled study of bezafi-brate: the St. Mary's, Ealing, Northwick Park Diabetes Cardiovascular Disease Prevention (SENDCAP) Study, *Diabetes Care* 1998; **21**:641–648.

8 Downs JR, Clearfield M, Weis S, Whitney E, Shapiro DR, Beere PA *et al.* Primary prevention of acute coronary events with lovastatin in men and women with average cholesterol levels: results of AFCAPS/TexCAPS. Air Force/Texas Coronary Atherosclerosis Prevention Study. *JAMA* 1998; **279**:1615–1622.

9 Betteridge DJ. Diabetic dyslipidemia. *Am J Med* 1994; **96**:25S–31S.

10 Taskinen MR. Diabetic dyslipidaemia: from basic research to clinical practice. *Diabetologia* 2003; **46**:733–749.

11 Nikkila EA, Hormila P. Serum lipids and lipoproteins in insulin-treated diabetes. Demonstration of increased high density lipoprotein concentrations. *Diabetes* 1978; **27**:1078–1086.

12 Colhoun HM, Rubens MB, Underwood SR, Fuller JH. The effect of type 1 diabetes mellitus on the gender difference in coronary artery calcification. *J Am Coll Cardiol* 2000; **36**:2160–2167.

13 Soedamah-Muthu SS, Colhoun HM, Taskinen MR, Idzior-Walus B, Fuller JH. Differences in HDL-cholesterol: apoA-I + apoA-II ratio and apoE phenotype with albuminuric status in Type I diabetic patients. *Diabetologia* 2000; **43**:1353–1359.

14 Turner RC, Millns H, Neil HA, Stratton IM, Manley SE, Matthews DR *et al.* Risk factors for coronary artery disease in non-insulin dependent diabetes mellitus: United Kingdom Prospective Diabetes Study (UKPDS: 23). *BMJ* 1998; **316**:823–828.

15 Stevens RJ, Kothari V, Adler AI, Stratton IM. The UKPDS risk engine: a model for the risk of coronary heart disease in Type II diabetes (UKPDS 56). *Clin Sci (Lond)* 2001; **101**:671–679.

16 Lehto S, Ronnemaa T, Haffner SM, Pyorala K, Kallio V, Laakso M. Dyslipidemia and hyperglycemia predict coronary heart disease events in middle-aged patients with NIDDM. *Diabetes* 1997; **46**:1354–1359.

17 Collins R, Armitage J, Parish S, Sleigh P, Peto R. MRC/BHF Heart Protection Study of cholesterol-lowering with simvastatin in 5963 people with diabetes: a randomised placebo-controlled trial. *Lancet* 2003; **361**:2005–2016.

18 Shepherd J, Blauw GJ, Murphy MB, Bollen EL, Buckley BM, Cobbe SM *et al.* Pravastatin in elderly individuals at risk of vascular disease (PROSPER): a randomised controlled trial. *Lancet* 2002; **360**:1623–1630.

19 Furberg CJT, Davis B, Cutler J. Major outcomes in moderately hypercholesterolemic, hypertensive patients randomized to pravastatin vs usual care: The Antihypertensive and Lipid-Lowering Treatment to Prevent Heart Attack Trial (ALLHAT-LLT). *JAMA* 2002; **288**:2998–3007.

20 Colhoun HM, Betteridge DJ, Durrington PN, Hitman GA, Neil HA, Livingstone SJ *et al.* Primary prevention of cardiovascular disease with atorvastatin in type 2 diabetes in the Collaborative Atorvastatin Diabetes Study (CARDS): multicentre randomised placebo-controlled trial. *Lancet* 2004; **364**:685–696.

21 Sever PS, Dahlof B, Poulter NR, Wedel H, Beevers G, Caulfield M *et al.* Prevention of coronary and stroke events with atorvastatin in hypertensive patients who have average or lower-than-average cholesterol concentrations, in the Anglo-Scandinavian Cardiac Outcomes Trial – Lipid Lowering Arm (ASCOT-LLA): a multicentre randomised controlled trial. *Lancet* 2003; **361**:1149–1158.

22 Sever PS, Poulter NR, Dahlof B, Wedel H, Collins R, Beevers G *et al.* Reduction in cardiovascular events with atorvastatin in 2,532 patients with type 2 diabetes: Anglo-Scandinavian Cardiac Outcomes Trial – Lipid-Lowering Arm (ASCOT-LLA). *Diabetes Care* 2005; **28**:1151–1157.

23 Knopp RH, d'Emden M, Smilde JG, Pocock SJ. Efficacy and safety of atorvastatin in the prevention of cardiovascular end points in subjects with type 2 diabetes: the Atorvastatin Study for Prevention of Coronary Heart Disease Endpoints in non-insulin-dependent diabetes mellitus (ASPEN). *Diabetes Care* 2006; **29**:1478–1485.

24 Fellstrom B, Holdaas H, Jardine A, Rose H, Schmieder R, Zannad F on behalf of the AURORA Study Group. Effect of rosuvastatin on outcomes in chronic haemodialysis patients – Baseline data from the AURORA study. *Kidney Blood Press Re.* 2007; **30**:314–322.

25 Kjekshus J, Apetrei E, Barrios V, Bohm M, Cleland JGF *et al.* for the CORONA Group. Rosuvastatin in older patients with systolic heart failure. *N Engl J Med* 2007; **22**:2248–2261.

26 Mora S, Ridker PM. Justification for the Use of Statins in Primary Prevention: an Intervention Trial Evaluating Rosuvastatin (JUPITER) – can C-reactive protein be used to target statin therapy in primary prevention? *Am J Cardiol* 2006; **97**:33A–41A.

27 Law M, Rudnicka AR. Statin safety: a systematic review. *Am J Cardiol* 2006; **97**:52C–60C.

28 Keech A. Fenofibrate Intervention and Event Lowering in Diabetes (FIELD) study, a randomized, placebo-controlled trial: baseline characteristics and short-term effects of fenofibrate. *Cardiovasc Diabetol* 2005; **4**:13.

29 National Institutes of Health. Third Report of the National Cholesterol Education Program (NCEP) Expert Panel on Detection, Evaluation and Treatment of High Blood Cholesterol in Adults (Adult Treatment Panel III) final report. *Circulation* 2002; **106**:3421.

30 Kris-Etherton PM, Harris WS, Appel LJ. Omega-3 fatty acids and cardiovascular disease: new recommendations from the American Heart Association. *Arterioscler Thromb Vasc Biol* 2003; **23**:151–152.

31 Hooper L, Thompson RL, Harrison RA, Summerbell CD, Ness AR, Moore HJ *et al.* Risks and benefits of omega 3 fats for mortality, cardiovascular disease and cancer: systematic review. *BMJ* 2006; **332**:752–760.

32 Yokoyama M. Effects of eicosapentaenoic acid (EPA) on major cardiovascular events in hypercholesterolemic patients: the Japan EPA Lipid Intervention Study (JELIS). Presented at the American Heart Association Scientific

Sessions 2005, 13–16 November 2005, Dallas, TX; Late Breaking Clinical Trials II, 2005.

33 Grundy SM, Vega GL, McGovern ME, Tulloch BR, Kendall DM, Fitz-Patrick D et al. Efficacy, safety and tolerability of once-daily niacin for the treatment of dyslipidemia associated with type 2 diabetes: results of the assessment of diabetes control and evaluation of the efficacy of niaspan trial. Arch Intern Med 2002; **162**:1568–1576.

34 Canner PL, Furberg CD, Terrin ML, McGovern ME. Benefits of niacin by glycemic status in patients with healed myocardial infarction (from the Coronary Drug Project). Am J Cardio. 2005; **95**:254–257.

35 Cheng K, Wu TJ, Wu KK, Sturino C, Metters K, Gottesdiener K et al. Antagonism of the prostaglandin D2 receptor 1 suppresses nicotinic acid-induced vasodilation in mice and humans. Proc Natl Acad Sci USA 2006; **103**:6682–6687.

36 BIP Study Group. Secondary prevention by raising HDL cholesterol and reducing triglycerides in patients with coronary artery disease: the Bezafibrate Infarction Prevention (BIP) study. Circulation 2000; **102**:21–27.

37 Joint British Societies. JBS 2: Joint British Societies' guidelines on prevention of cardiovascular disease in clinical practice. Heart 2005; **91**(Suppl 5): v1–v52.

38 Grundy SM, Cleeman JI, Bairey NM, Brewer HB, Clark LT, Hunninghake DB et al. Implications of recent clinical trials for the National Cholesterol Education Program Adult Treatment Panel III Guidelines. Circulation 2004; **110**:227–239.

39 American Diabetes Association. Standards of medical care in diabetes. Diabetes Care 2005;**28**:S4–S36.

40 De Backer G, Ambrosioni E, Borch-Johnsen K, Brotons C, Cifkova R, Dallongeville J et al. European guidelines on cardiovascular disease prevention in clinical practice. Third Joint Task Force of European and Other Societies on Cardiovascular Disease Prevention in Clinical Practice. Eur Heart J 2003; **24**:1601–1610.

41 Shepherd J, Barter P, Carmena R, Deedwania P, Fruchart JC, Haffner S et al. Effect of lowering LDL cholesterol substantially below currently recommended levels in patients with coronary heart disease and diabetes: the Treating to New Targets (TNT) study. Diabetes Care 2006; **29**:1220–1226.

42 Pedersen TR, Faergeman O, Kastelein JJ, Olsson AG, Tikkanen MJ, Holme I et al. High-dose atorvastatin vs usual-dose simvastatin for secondary prevention after myocardial infarction: the IDEAL study: a randomized controlled trial. JAMA 2005; **294**:2437–2445.

43 Laakso M, Lehto S, Penttila I, Pyorala K. Lipids and lipoproteins predicting coronary heart disease mortality and morbidity in patients with non-insulin-dependent diabetes. Circulation 1993; **88**:1421–1430.

44 Fontbonne A, Eschwege E, Cambien F, Richard JL, Ducimetiere P, Thibult N et al. Hypertriglyceridaemia as a risk factor of coronary heart disease mortality in subjects with impaired glucose tolerance or diabetes. Results from the 11-year follow-up of the Paris Prospective Study. Diabetologia 1989; **32**:300–304.

45 Borch-Johnsen K, Kreiner S. Proteinuria: value as predictor of cardiovascular mortality in insulin dependent diabetes mellitus. Br Med J (Clin Res Ed) 1987; **294**:1651–1654.

46 Soedamah-Muthu SS, Fuller JH, Mulnier HE, Raleigh VS, Lawrenson RA, Colhoun HM. High risk of cardiovascular disease in patients with type 1 diabetes in the U.K.: a cohort study using the general practice research database. Diabetes Care 2006; **29**:798–804.

47 Booth GL, Kapral MK, Fung K, Tu JV. Relation between age and cardiovascular disease in men and women with diabetes compared with non-diabetic people: a population-based retrospective cohort study. Lancet 2006; **368**:29–36.

48 Holdaas H, Fellstrom B, Jardine AG, Holme I, Nyberg G, Fauchald P et al. Effect of fluvastatin on cardiac outcomes in renal transplant recipients: a multicentre, randomised, placebo-controlled trial. Lancet 2003; **361**:2024–2031.

49 Wanner C, Krane V, Marz W, Olschewski M, Mann JF, Ruf G et al. Atorvastatin in patients with type 2 diabetes mellitus undergoing hemodialysis. N Engl J Med 2005; **353**:238–248.

50 KDOQI. KDOQI clinical practice guidelines and clinical practice recommendations for diabetes and chronic kidney disease. Am J Kidney Dis 2007; **49**:S12–S154.

51 Baigent C, Landry M. Study of Heart and Renal Protection (SHARP). Kidney Int Suppl 2003; S207–S210.

52 Chew EY, Klein ML, Ferris FL III, Remaley NA, Murphy RP, Chantry K et al. Association of elevated serum lipid levels with retinal hard exudate in diabetic retinopathy. Early Treatment Diabetic Retinopathy Study (ETDRS) Report 22. Arch Ophthalmol 1996; **114**:1079–1084.

53 Chaturvedi N, Sjoelie AK, Porta M, Aldington SJ, Fuller JH, Songini M et al. Markers of insulin resistance are strong risk factors for retinopathy incidence in type 1 diabetes. Diabetes Care 2001; **24**:284–289.

54 Retnakaran R, Cull CA, Thorne KI, Adler AI, Holman RR. Risk factors for renal dysfunction in type 2 diabetes: U.K. Prospective diabetes study 74. Diabetes 2006; **55**:1832–1839.

55 Colhoun HM, Lee ET, Bennett PH, Lu M, Keen H, Wang SL et al. Risk factors for renal failure: the WHO Multinational Study of Vascular Disease in Diabetes. Diabetologia 2001; **44** (Suppl 2): S46–S53.

56 Yishak AA, Costacou T, Virella G, Zgibor J, Fried L, Walsh M et al. Novel predictors of overt nephropathy in subjects with type 1 diabetes. A nested case control study from the Pittsburgh Epidemiology of Diabetes Complications cohort. Nephrol Dial Transplant 2006; **21**:93–100.

57 Fagot-Campagna A, Nelson RG, Knowler WC, Pettitt DJ, Robbins DC, Go O et al. Plasma lipoproteins and the incidence of abnormal excretion of albumin in diabetic American Indians: the Strong Heart Study. Diabetologia 1998; **41**:1002–1009.

58 Goldfarb-Rumyantzev AS, Pappas L. Prediction of renal insufficiency in Pima Indians with nephropathy of type 2 diabetes mellitus. Am J Kidney Dis 2002; **40**:252–264.

59 Tesfaye S, Chaturvedi N, Eaton SE, Ward JD, Manes C, Ionescu-Tirgoviste C et al. Vascular risk factors and diabetic neuropathy. N Engl J Med 2005; **352**:341–350.

60 Fried LF, Orchard TJ, Kasiske BL. Effect of lipid reduction on the progression of renal disease: a meta-analysis. Kidney Int 2001; **59**:260–269.

61 Athyros VG, Mikhailidis DP, Papageorgiou AA, Symeonidis AN, Pehlivanidis AN, Bouloukos VI et al. The effect of statins versus untreated dyslipidaemia on renal

function in patients with coronary heart disease. A sub-group analysis of the Greek atorvastatin and coronary heart disease evaluation (GREACE) study. *J Clin Pathol* 2004; **57**:728–734.

62 Tonelli M, Isles C, Craven T, Tonkin A, Pfeffer MA, Shepherd J *et al*. Effect of pravastatin on rate of kidney function loss in people with or at risk for coronary disease. *Circulation* 2005; **112**:171–178.

63 Douglas K, O'Malley PG, Jackson JL. Meta-analysis: the effect of statins on albuminuria. *Ann Intern Med* 2006; **145**:117–124.

64 Asselbergs FW, Diercks GF, Hillege HL, van Boven AJ, Janssen WM, Voors AA *et al*. Effects of fosinopril and pravastatin on cardiovascular events in subjects with micro-albuminuria. *Circulation* 2004; **110**:2809–2816.

65 Sandhu S, Wiebe N, Fried LF, Tonelli M. Statins for improving renal outcomes: a meta-analysis. *J Am Soc. Nephrol* 2006; **17**:2006–2016.

66 Wolfe SM. Dangers of rosuvastatin identified before and after FDA approval. *Lancet* 2004; **363**:2189–2190.

67 Agarwal R. Effects of statins on renal function. *Am J Cardiol* 2006; **97**:748–755.

68 Leiter LA. The prevention of diabetic microvascular complications of diabetes: is there a role for lipid lowering? *Diabetes Res Clin Pract* 2005; **68**(Suppl 2): S3–S14.

14 Other cardiovascular risk factors

Stephen Thomas, GianCarlo Viberti

Diabetes Centre St Thomas' Hospital, London, UK
Department of Diabetes and Endocrinology, KCL Guy's Hospital, London, UK

Introduction

The development of diabetes significantly increases an individual's cardiovascular risk. In some population studies, diabetes carries an equivalent or even higher cardiovascular risk than prior evidence of coronary heart disease (CHD) in non-diabetic individuals.[1-3] Traditional risk factors such as increased concentrations of low-density lipoprotein cholesterol, decreased concentrations of high-density lipoprotein cholesterol, raised blood pressure, hyperglycaemia and smoking are important in diabetes.[4] The challenge is to identify other risk factors which may explain the mechanisms by which diabetes increases cardiovascular risk and which may be amenable to therapeutic intervention (Figure 14.1).

Microalbuminuria

The development of diabetic kidney disease is associated with increased cardiovascular risk and the greater the degree of kidney damage, the greater is the risk. Thus, the mortality rises as the glomerular filtration rate falls, particularly at glomerular filtration rates $<60\,\mathrm{ml\,min^{-1}}$ (Stage 3 and 4 chronic kidney disease).[5,6] Estimation of kidney function by measurement of cystatin C may add additional benefits in predicting cardiovascular risk but is not part of routine clinical practice.

Microalbuminuria, first described in the 1960s, was identified as a cardiovascular risk factor in type 2 diabetes in 1980, when a re-analysis of a cohort of 44 patients with type 2 diabetes studied in 1966–67 revealed that 15 had died of cardiovascular disease

(CVD) and that risk of mortality was related to the baseline albumin excretion rate.[7] Currently, microalbuminuria is defined by convention as a urinary albumin excretion of $20–200\,\mathrm{mg\,min^{-1}}$ or $30–300\,\mathrm{mg}$ $\mathrm{day^{-1}}$. There is significant day-to-day variability in urinary albumin levels, hence two positive levels out of three are required before an individual is deemed to have microalbuminuria. Interpretation is further complicated by the variety of different assessments possible from 24 h collections to random or early morning spot urine albumin:creatinine ratio estimation. Most centres use a spot urine albumin:creatinine ratio in everyday clinical practice. Currently, yearly estimation is recommended as a screening procedure in the UK.

Microalbuminuria and cardiovascular disease in type 2 diabetes

Several prospective studies have described microalbuminuria as a predictor of mortality in type 2 diabetes.[7-13] In 1988, in a 10 year follow-up study of ~500 patients with type 2 diabetes, microalbuminuria was associated with cardiovascular mortality.[9] Microalbuminuria was the best predictor of long-term mortality in type 2 diabetes in an 8–9 year follow-up of 228 patients with type 2 diabetes.[10]

Similarly, in a 9 year follow-up Finnish study of 134 patients with type 2 diabetes, the baseline predictors of death were higher HbA$_{1c}$, higher low-density lipoprotein, lower high-density lipoprotein cholesterol, higher non-esterified fatty acid concentrations and higher urinary albumin. About 45% of the patients who died had microalbuminuria compared with 6% of the survivors.[12] An 8 year prospective follow-up

The Evidence Base for Diabetes Care, Second Edition, Edited by William H. Herman, Ann Louise Kinmonth, Nicholas J. Wareham and Rhys Williams.

Microalbuminuria

Timed Albumin Excretion Rate	≥ 20 mg min^{-1} (30 mg day^{-1})
Albumin:Creatinine Ratio (Usually on spot urine sample)	≤ 2.5 (men) ≤ 3.5 (women)

C-Reactive Protein

Low risk	<1 mg l^{-1}
Average risk	1–3 mg l^{-1}
High risk	>3 mg l^{-1}

Figure 14.1 Cutoffs for risk markers

UK study comparing 153 patients with type 2 diabetes and an abnormal urinary albumin excretion with 153 patients with type 2 diabetes with a urinary albumin excretion in the 'normal' range suggested that the increased cardiovascular risk operates at levels of urinary albumin below those conventionally termed 'microalbuminuria'. In this study, higher vascular mortality (odds ratio 1.7) was detectable at albumin excretion rates >10 μg min^{-1}.[11]

Even in high-risk patients with known vascular disease and other risk factors, the presence of microalbuminuria is associated with increased risk.

In patients with hypertension, urinary albumin excretion is an independent predictor of both total and cardiovascular mortality. In 439 men with treated hypertension, the increased risk became evident only at higher levels of urinary albumin (over 300 mg day^{-1}) in those without diabetes, whereas in those with diabetes there was increased risk at the stage of microalbuminuria.[14]

Similarly, the presence of microalbuminuria is associated with higher risk in those with established reduced kidney function. In an analysis of 2966 participants in the Framingham offspring cohort, those with reduced eGFR and with microalbuminuria were at increased risk for combined CVD and all-cause mortality compared with those with neither condition (hazard ratio 1.7), The coexistence of reduced eGFR and microalbuminuria was associated with increased risk for CVD and all-cause mortality, in part because of a heavy burden of CVD risk factors.[15]

A sub-analysis of 804 patients with type 2 diabetes and known vascular disease from the Second Manifestation of Arterial Disease (SMART) study followed up for 4 years demonstrated that, even in patients with established cardiovascular disease, coronary artery, cerebrovascular and peripheral vascular disease, microalbuminuria was still an independent predictor of new cardiovascular events (hazard ratio 1.4).[16]

In a systematic review of microalbuminuria and cardiovascular disease in type 2 diabetes; 11 cohort studies were included with a total of 2138 patients followed up for around 6 years. The overall prevalence of microalbuminuria was around 30% with an odds ratio for death of 2.4 [95% confidence interval (CI) 1.8 to 3.1] and for cardiovascular morbidity or mortality of 2 (95% CI 1.4 to 2.7) in those with microalbuminuria.[17]

Association in different ethnicities

The relationship between microalbuminuria and CVD is generally consistent between populations. In those of South Asian descent, microalbuminuria may be more prevalent than in European populations[18] but is also associated with a higher cardiovascular risk.[19–21] In Japanese populations, the relationship with CVD appears weaker but the development of microalbuminuria is still associated with an excess mortality.[22] There is some evidence that the risks of microalbuminuria differ between different ethnicities, at least from studies in populations predominantly without diabetes. A combined analyses of two population-based cohorts suggested that albumin excretion rates were significantly higher in those of African–Caribbean descent as compared with South Asian and European individuals. In men of South Asian descent, microalbuminuria was associated with CHD mortality. The same was true in European women but not in those of African–Caribbean descent. This may relate, of course, to the background ethnic risk of CHD, which tends to be lower in those of African–Caribbean descent.[23]

Microalbuminuria and cardiovascular disease in type 1 diabetes

In type 1 diabetes, microalbuminuria is predictive of the development of excess of coronary, cerebrovascular and peripheral arterial disease. In a 23 year follow-up study of UK patients with type 1 diabetes, those with microalbuminuria had significantly higher cardiovascular mortality (relative risk 2.94).[24] Similarly, in a 10 year observational follow-up of 939 Scandinavian patients with type 1 diabetes, microalbuminuria, smoking and heavier proteinuria were all significant predictors of cardiovascular mortality.[25] The increased cardiovascular mortality is seen even in populations who develop microalbuminuria after a long duration of diabetes although there is less risk of renal progression.[26,27]

Other cardiovascular associations of microalbuminuria

Diabetes is associated not only with myocardial infarction and stroke, but also with other increasingly important cardiac causes of morbidity and premature mortality, congestive heart failure and autonomic neuropathy.

The DIABHYCAR (type 2 DIABetes, Hypertension, CArdiovascular Events and Ramipril) study reported an association between diabetes and the development of congestive heart failure.[28] There is also an association with cardiac autonomic neuropathy in type 2 diabetes with lower heart rate variability and altered baroreflex sensitivity, cardiac [^{123}I]-m-iodobenzyl-guanidine (MIBG) scintigraphy.[29]

Microalbuminuria is also associated with an increase in left ventricular mass index in both type 1 and type 2 diabetes. This is related, at least in part, to greater blood pressure load with increased nocturnal systolic blood pressure.[30]

Even in populations predominantly without diabetes, the development of microalbuminuria is associated with extra risk. In a population of around 8000 patients of average age 66 years with hypertension, microalbuminuria was present in 23%. Urinary albumin was positively related to voltage markers of left ventricular hypertrophy independent of age, blood pressure, diabetes, race, serum creatinine or smoking.[31]

Microalbuminuria and other cardiovascular risk factors

Higher urinary albumin excretion rates are associated with conventional cardiovascular risk factors (Figure 14.2). Microalbuminuria is related to increasing age, higher systolic blood pressure and markers of systemic inflammation.[32] Furthermore, microalbuminuria and cardiovascular disease may have common antecedents. In prospective studies, the excess risk of cardiovascular death with microalbuminuria is at least in part dependent on glycaemic control and cholesterol levels.[33]

There may be a shared familial predisposition to both the development of kidney disease and CVD in diabetes.[34] Those with a positive family history of hypertension or CVD are more likely to develop microalbuminuria than those without. Similarly, children with one hypertensive parent have on average a higher AER than children of a normotensive parent whereas normotensive adults with at least one hypertensive parent have elevated AER compared with normotensive adults with a negative family history for arterial hypertension.[35]

Blood pressure

In both type 1 and type 2 diabetes, high blood pressure is associated with microalbuminuria. In particular, in the Hypertension in Diabetes Study within UKPDS, intensive treatment of blood pressure (mean 144/82 mmHg) resulted in a significant 29% reduction in the risk of microalbuminuria after 6 years, compared with less tight control (mean 154/87 mmHg).[36]

During the phase of microalbuminuria in both type 1 and type 2 diabetes, systolic and diastolic blood pressure, whether office or 24 hour measurements, rise with the albumin excretion rate. In type 1 diabetes,

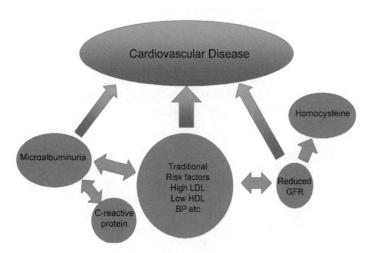

Figure 14.2 Markers of kidney disease are related to traditional and non-traditional risk factors

the sitting blood pressure rises in the phase of micro-albuminuria by an average of 3–4 mmHg per year, compared with 1 mmHg per year in long-term nor-moalbuminuric and healthy controls.

Smoking

Smoking is an independent risk factor for the devel-opment of microalbuminuria in both type 1 and type 2 diabetes, albeit a relatively weak one unlikely to explain much of the excess cardiovascular risk.[37,38]

Lipid abnormalities

The concentrations of total cholesterol, VLDL choles-terol, LDL cholesterol, triglycerides and fibrinogen rise with increasing AER in patients with type 1 diabetes, being 11–14% higher in microalbuminuria and 26–87% higher in macroalbuminuria.[39] In addi-tion, there is an increase in LDL mass and atherogenic small dense LDL particles and HDL levels are lower with a disadvantageous alteration in their composi-tion.[40] An altered composition of HDL particles with a low ratio of HDL particles containing apolipoprotein (apo) A-I but not apo A-II [lipoprotein (Lp) A-I] to those containing both apo A-I and A-II (Lp A-I:A-II) is associated with a fourfold increased risk of new-onset CVD (odds ratio 4.2, 95% CI 1.4 to 13.4), a risk that is additive to that of kidney disease.[41]

Insulin resistance

Microalbuminuria is associated with insulin resis-tance in those with and without diabetes.[29,42,43] Hence microalbuminuria may form part of a metabolic syn-drome predisposing to accelerated vascular disease.

Endothelial dysfunction and haemostatic abnormalities

Levels of Von Willebrand factor (vWF), PAI1, Factor VII and fibrinogen are higher in patients with micro-albuminuria, suggesting endothelial activation and a hypercoagulable state,[44,45] It is also suggested that an increase in vWF, marking endothelial dysfunction, may precede the onset of microalbuminuria.[46]

In addition, there is a generalized increase in vascular permeability in both the non-diabetic and diabetic population with microalbuminuria[47,48] and evidence of greater impairment of endothelium-dependent and endothelium-independent vasodilation than the abnormality already present in type 2 diabetes.[49]

Treatment of microalbuminuria: Cardiovascular benefits

Reduction of urinary albumin excretion and particu-larly the normalization of urinary albumin excretion are associated not only with a significant reduction in the risk of loss of eGFR but also with cardiovascular events.[50] Other studies have similarly described that the rate of change of urinary albumin excretion is associated with cardiovascular risk in those with microalbuminuria independent of other cardiovascu-lar risk factors.[51]

Further evidence comes from the beneficial effects of treatment of microalbuminuria with inhibitors of the renin–angiotensin system, which lower urinary albumin excretion rates to a greater degree than other anti-hypertensive treatments.

The Microalbuminuria, Cardiovascular and Renal Outcomes sub-study of the Heart Outcomes Preven-tion Evaluation (MICRO-HOPE) study randomized 3577 patients with type 2 diabetes and microalbumi-nuria who were aged 55 years or older and had at least one other cardiovascular risk factor (lipid abnormal-ities, hypertension, microalbuminuria or current smoking). Treatment with an angiotensin-converting enzyme inhibitor lowered the risk of the primary combined endpoint of myocardial infarction, stroke or CVD death by 25% and total mortality by 24% (Figure 14.3).[52]

The Steno-2 Study randomized 160 patients with type 2 diabetes and microalbuminuria to a targeted, intensified, multifactorial intervention or conven-tional treatment. Treatment goals in the intensively treated group were blood pressure less than 130/80, $HbA_{1c} < 6.5$, total cholesterol < 4.5 mmol l^{-1}, triglycer-ide < 1.7 mmol l^{-1}, treatment with angiotensin-converting enzyme inhibitor irrespective of blood pressure and treatment with aspirin for those with a previous cardiovascular event. Urinary albumin excretion fell by one-third and this was associated with a significantly lower risk of cardiovascular dis-ease (hazard ratio 0.47, 95% CI 0.24 to 0.73), and also reduced progression of microvascular complications (Figure 14.4).[53]

Conclusion

The evidence clearly suggests that patients with type 1 or type 2 diabetes who develop microalbuminuria are at increased cardiovascular risk and should benefit from aggressive treatment, including

- blood pressure treatment aiming at systolic blood pressures at least less than 130;
- therapy with either an angiotensin-converting enzyme inhibitor, angiotensin II antagonist or both;
- cholesterol-lowering therapy usually with a high-dose statin aiming for total cholesterol levels < 4 mmol l^{-1} and LDL levels < 2 mmol /l^{-1};
- low-dose aspirin therapy where tolerated;
- individualized 'tight' glycaemic control.

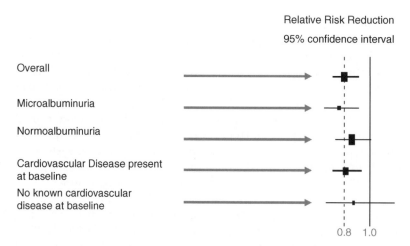

Figure 14.3 ACE inhibitor-based therapy reduces cardiovascular risk in those with type 2 diabetes and microalbuminuria. The use of an ACE inhibitor has most cardioprotective effect in those with microalbuminuria or baseline cardiovascular disease presumably as they had the highest risk. Modified from Ref. 52

Inflammatory markers

There has been much focus on the relationship of low-grade inflammation, in particular activation of the innate immune system, to cardiovascular risk in diabetes. Alteration of markers of chronic inflammation such as C-reactive protein, sialic acid, tumour necrosis factor-α and other cytokines are all associated with increased cardiovascular risk and greater cardiovascular mortality in the general population.

Serum sialic acid

Sialic acid is the terminal sugar of the oligosaccharide chain of acute-phase proteins. It is a molecule attached to many acute-phase proteins and is bound to fibrinogen. It is therefore closely associated with rises in many inflammatory markers. In prospective studies,

higher levels were associated with a 1.5–2-fold increased risk of cardiovascular mortality.[54]

In early studies, serum total and lipid-associated sialic concentrations were elevated in patients with type 2 diabetes.[55,56] Subsequently, serum sialic acid concentrations were found to be significantly higher in patients with type 1 diabetes and microalbuminuria compared with those with normal urinary albumin excretion.[57] The relationship with heavier proteinuria is uncertain.[58]

Elevated plasma sialic acid concentrations are associated with risk factors for vascular disease, namely diabetes duration, HbA$_{1c}$, plasma triglyceride and cholesterol concentrations, waist-to-hip ratio, hypertension smoking and low physical exercise. It is also independently related to microvascular complications such as proliferative retinopathy and urinary albumin excretion.[59] Serum sialic acid levels are

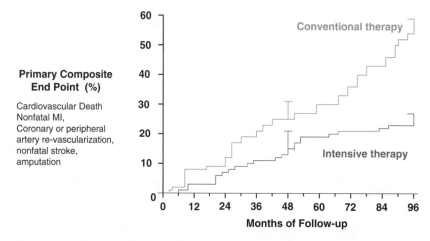

Figure 14.4 Aggressive treatment of risk factors lowers cardiovascular risk in those with microalbuminuria. Modified from Ref. 53

associated with blood coagulability and with fibrinogen levels.[60]

Elevated serum sialic acid concentrations are associated with CHD and predict cardiovascular and all-cause mortality in type 2 diabetes.[61] In a sub-set of over 2000 participants in the EURODIAB study of type 1 diabetes, serum sialic acid concentrations and serum fibrinogen were strong predictors of CHD and were, at least in univariate analysis, associated with microvascular complications of diabetes.[58]

There appears to be a gender difference in the predictive value of sialic acid which usually appears in type 2 diabetes to be a stronger cardiovascular risk factor in men.[58,62] To date, there is little evidence that sialic acid levels are modifiable with a beneficial effect on cardiovascular events in diabetes.

C-reactive protein

C-reactive protein is an acute-phase plasma protein produced by the liver and by adipocytes. It plays a role in innate immunity – the non-specific mechanisms that defend from infection. Elevations of C-reactive protein are associated with cardiovascular risk in the general population. As C-reactive protein is an acute-phase reactant, there should be at least two measurements in order to define an individual as having a high level. A C-reactive protein level $<1 \, mg \, l^{-1}$ is defined as low risk, $1–3 \, mg \, l^{-1}$ as average risk and $>3 \, mg \, l^{-1}$ as high risk. A rise in C-reactive protein from 1 to $3 \, mg \, l^{-1}$ is associated in type 2 diabetes with a significant increased risk of carotid intima-media thickening independently of features of the metabolic syndrome and other markers of endothelial dysfunction.[63]

Serum C-reactive protein is associated with microalbuminuria (Table 14.1[64]), particularly if the blood pressure is elevated.[65] In cross-sectional studies in the general population, a one unit increase in C-reactive protein concentration was associated with a 2% increased odds of microalbuminuria.[66] There is a suggestion in the non-diabetic population that C-reactive protein may predict different types of vascular disease, possibly having greater predictive value for peripheral vascular disease.[67]

There are few prospective data to address whether C-reactive protein predicts cardiovascular events in patients with diabetes. In the Health Professionals Follow-Up Study, a cohort of 746 men aged 46–81 years free of CVD at baseline were followed for an average of 5 years. Higher C-reactive protein levels were associated with an increased risk of cardiovascular events (myocardial infarction, coronary revascularization and strokes) independently of conventional risk factors including lipids and glycaemic control.[68]

Similarly, in an add-on to a previous study, 878 patients with type 2 diabetes free from known coronary artery disease were followed for 7 years. Those with a C-reactive protein level $>3 \, mg \, l^{-1}$ had a higher risk for CHD death than those with a C-reactive protein $3 \, mg \, l^{-1}$ (adjusted relative risk 1.84).[69]

Conversely, in a series of case–cohort studies, within the prospective Atherosclerosis Risk in Communities (ARIC) Study, C-reactive protein or other markers of inflammation or endothelial dysfunction did not add significantly to the cardiovascular risk prediction derived from the traditional risk markers: age, race, sex, total and high-density lipoprotein cholesterol levels, systolic blood pressure, antihypertensive medication use, smoking status and diabetes.[70]

To date there are no effective treatments to lower C-reactive protein. Trials with low-dose aspirin did not affect C-reactive protein levels.[71]

Overall, there is insufficient evidence to recommend the routine use of C-reactive protein as a marker of cardiovascular risk. Nor does it appear to be modifiable given current therapies.

Homocysteine

Homocysteine is related to the amino acid cysteine and the plasma levels are under the influence of genetic and environmental factors, including diet, plasma folic acid levels, age, systolic blood pressure and vitamin B_{12}.[72] Plasma homocysteine levels were first reported to be elevated in diabetes in association with kidney disease[73] at the stage of proteinuria and reduced kidney function. Individuals with diabetes

Table 14.1 Microalbuminuria and other non-traditional cardiovascular risk factors are associated

	Without microalbuminuria	With microalbuminuria	*p*-Value
Albumin:creatinine ratio (mg mmol^{-1})	8.38 ± 0.2	41.6 ± 2.9	
C-reactive protein (mg l^{-1})	3.8 ± 0.15	5.37 ± 0.47	0.0018
Fibrinogen (mg dl^{-1})	278.2 ± 1.6	295.7 ± 4	0.0001

Source: modified from Ref. 64.

may have lower folic acid levels which contribute to the higher homocysteine levels.[74] Plasma homocysteine may be associated with vascular damage and generation of endogenous reactive oxygen species.

There is controversy as to whether the association between plasma homocysteine and cardiovascular mortality is independent. Plasma homocysteine levels are higher in those with microalbuminuria and reduced kidney function.[75] In patients with type 2 diabetes, the association between higher plasma homocysteine levels and CHD[75] may be mediated by glycaemic control and reduced kidney function.[76] In a prospective study in 211 white patients with type 2 diabetes followed for around 6 years, homocysteine was a predictor of cardiovascular mortality in univariate analysis but this association was not independent of other risk factors, particularly pre-existing CHD, AER and age.[77] However, in a Finnish study of around 800 patients, plasma homocysteine 15 mmol l^{-1} at baseline compared with <15 mmol l^{-1} was associated with a higher risk for CHD death, independent of other factors, including reduced creatinine clearance.[78] In a *post hoc* analysis of 1575 individuals enrolled in the Irbesartan Diabetic Nephropathy Trial (IDNT), a significant univariate association was found between total plasma homocysteine levels and congestive heart failure, but this was attenuated after adjustment for kidney function as assessed by plasma creatinine level.[79]

Folic acid supplementation has been hypothesized to lower homocysteine levels. In one short-term study in 26 patients with type 2 diabetes, 5 mg day^{-1} of oral folic acid supplementation enhanced endothelium-dependent vasodilatation measured as forearm arterial blood flow during local intra-arterial administration of acetylcholine. In multiple regression analysis, changes in folic acid concentrations were independently associated with changes in maximum endothelium-dependent vasodilatation. However, this was not associated with lowering of homocysteine.[80]

Thus the current evidence suggests that although homocysteine levels are related to cardiovascular disease, it may be mostly mediated by the coexistence of other risk factors, particularly kidney disease.

Other risk factors

There is some evidence that the use of multiple biomarkers including C-reactive protein, troponin I, N-terminal pro-brain natriuretic peptide and cystatin C, most of them markers of myocardial or kidney damage, increases the predictive value,[81] although this is yet to be tested in diabetes. Other factors may also be related to cardiovascular mortality in diabetes.

In the Atherosclerosis Risk in Communities (ARIC) Study of 1676 people with diabetes but no known heart disease, albumin, fibrinogen and Von Willebrand factor, factor VIII activity and leukocyte count were all independently associated with the risk of new CHD over an 8 year follow-up.[82]

Adiponectin

Adiponectin is a plasma protein produced by adipocytes with anti-atherogenic properties. To date, despite much plausibility that low adiponectin levels are related to atherosclerosis, there is little prospective evidence suggesting that it is useful in diabetes in predicting cardiovascular risk.

Conclusion

Premature cardiovascular disease accounts for most of the increased mortality seen in diabetes. Traditional cardiovascular risk factors predict risk in people with diabetes, in whom there is enhanced additive risk. Of the non-traditional risk factors, increased urinary albumin excretion comes the closest to fulfilling the requirements of a risk worth screening for in diabetes. This is particularly true for those with a progressively increasing urinary albumin excretion as there is evidence of a clear biological gradient with those with the highest urinary albumin levels being at greater risk. In addition, there are effective treatment strategies. The development of consensus about the measurement of increased urinary albumin excretion and simplification of the definitions and terms may facilitate its use as a cardiovascular screening tool.

Detection of and aggressive targeting of cardiovascular risk factors including reduction or normalization of urinary albumin excretion in those with microalbuminuria should be undertaken. Future directions may include the use of more complex prediction models, perhaps incorporating some of the other risk factors discussed here.

References

1 Juutilainen A, Lehto S, Ronnemaa T, Pyorala K, Laakso M. Type 2 diabetes as a 'coronary heart disease equivalent': an 18-year prospective population-based study in Finnish subjects. *Diabetes Care* 2005;**28**(12):2901–2907.

2 Whiteley L, Padmanabhan S, Hole D, Isles C. Should diabetes be considered a coronary heart disease risk equivalent?: results from 25 years of follow-up in the Renfrew and Paisley survey. *Diabetes Care* 2005;**28**(7):1588–1593.

3 Ninomiya JK, L'Italien G, Criqui MH, Whyte JL, Gamst A, Chen RS. Association of the metabolic syndrome with history

of myocardial infarction and stroke in the Third National Health and Nutrition Examination Survey. *Circulation* 2004;**109**(1):42–46.

4 Turner RC, Millns H, Neil HA, Stratton IM, Manley SE, Matthews DR *et al.* Risk factors for coronary artery disease in non-insulin dependent diabetes mellitus: United Kingdom Prospective Diabetes Study (UKPDS: 23). *BMJ* 1998;**316**(7134):823–828.

5 Astor BC, Coresh J, Heiss G, Pettitt D, Sarnak MJ. Kidney function and anemia as risk factors for coronary heart disease and mortality: the Atherosclerosis Risk in Communities (ARIC) Study. *Am Heart J* 2006;**151**(2):492–500.

6 Astor BC, Hallan SI, Miller ER III, Yeung E, Coresh J. Glomerular filtration rate, albuminuria and risk of cardiovascular and all-cause mortality in the US population. *Am J Epidemiol* 2008;**167**(10):1226–1234.

7 Jarrett RJ, Viberti GC, Argyropoulos A, Hill RD, Mahmud U, Murrells TJ. Microalbuminuria predicts mortality in non-insulin-dependent diabetics. *Diabet Med* 1984;**1**(1):17–19.

8 Mogensen CE. Microalbuminuria predicts clinical proteinuria and early mortality in maturity-onset diabetes. *N Engl J Med* 1984;**310**(6):356–360.

9 Schmitz A, Vaeth M. Microalbuminuria: a major risk factor in non-insulin-dependent diabetes. A 10-year follow-up study of 503 patients. *Diabet Med* 1988;**5**(2):126–134.

10 Damsgaard EM, Froland A, Jorgensen OD, Mogensen CE. Microalbuminuria as predictor of increased mortality in elderly people. *BMJ* 1990;**300**(6720):297–300.

11 MacLeod JM, Lutale J, Marshall SM. Albumin excretion and vascular deaths in NIDDM. *Diabetologia* 1995;**38**(5):610–616.

12 Forsblom CM, Sane T, Groop PH, Totterman KJ, Kallio M, Saloranta C *et al.* Risk factors for mortality in Type II (non-insulin-dependent) diabetes: evidence of a role for neuropathy and a protective effect of HLA-DR4. *Diabetologia* 1998;**41**(11):1253–1262.

13 Gerstein HC, Mann JF, Yi Q, Zinman B, Dinneen SF, Hoogwerf B *et al.* Albuminuria and risk of cardiovascular events, death and heart failure in diabetic and nondiabetic individuals. *JAMA* 2001;**286**(4):421–426.

14 Agewall S, Wikstrand J, Ljungman S, Fagerberg B. Usefulness of microalbuminuria in predicting cardiovascular mortality in treated hypertensive men with and without diabetes mellitus. Risk Factor Intervention Study Group. *Am J Cardiol* 1997;**80**(2):164–179.

15 Foster MC, Hwang SJ, Larson MG, Parikh NI, Meigs JB, Vasan RS *et al.* Cross-classification of microalbuminuria and reduced glomerular filtration rate: associations between cardiovascular disease risk factors and clinical outcomes. *Arch Intern Med* 2007;**167**(13):1386–1392.

16 Soedamah-Muthu SS, Visseren FL, Algra A, van der Graaf Y. The impact of Type 2 diabetes and microalbuminuria on future cardiovascular events in patients with clinically manifest vascular disease from the Second Manifestations of ARTerial disease (SMART) study. *Diabet Med* 2008;**25**(1):51–57.

17 Dinneen SF, Gerstein HC. The association of microalbuminuria and mortality in non-insulin-dependent diabetes mellitus. A systematic overview of the literature. *Arch Intern Med* 1997;**157**(13):1413–1418.

18 Mather HM, Chaturvedi N, Kehely AM. Comparison of prevalence and risk factors for microalbuminuria in South

Asians and Europeans with type 2 diabetes mellitus. *Diabet Med* 1998;**15**(8):672–677.

19 Mather HM, Chaturvedi N, Fuller JH. Mortality and morbidity from diabetes in South Asians and Europeans: 11-year follow-up of the Southall Diabetes Survey, London. UK. *Diabet Med* 1998;**15**(1):53–59.

20 Tindall H, Tin P, Nagi D, Pinnock S, Stickland M, Davies JA. Higher levels of microproteinuria in Asian compared with European patients with diabetes mellitus and their relationship to dietary protein intake and diabetic complications. *Diabet Med* 1994;**11**(1):37–41.

21 Wu AY, Kong NC, de Leon FA, Pan CY, Tai TY, Yeung VT et al. An alarmingly high prevalence of diabetic nephropathy in Asian type 2 diabetic patients: the MicroAlbuminuria Prevalence (MAP) Study. *Diabetologia* 2005;**48**(1):17–26.

22 Araki S, Haneda M, Togawa M, Sugimoto T, Shikano T, Nakagawa T *et al.* Microalbuminuria is not associated with cardiovascular death in Japanese NIDDM. *Diabetes Res Clin Pract* 1997;**35**(1):35–40.

23 Tillin T, Forouhi N, McKeigue P, Chaturvedi N. Microalbuminuria and coronary heart disease risk in an ethnically diverse UK population: a prospective cohort study. *J Am Soc Nephrol* 2005;**16**(12):3702–3710.

24 Messent JW, Elliott TG, Hill RD, Jarrett RJ, Keen H, Viberti GC. Prognostic significance of microalbuminuria in insulin-dependent diabetes mellitus: a twenty-three year follow-up study. *Kidney Int* 1992;**41**(4):836–839.

25 Rossing P, Hougaard P, Borch-Johnsen K, Parving HH. Predictors of mortality in insulin dependent diabetes: 10 year observational follow up study. *BMJ* 1996;**313**(7060):779–784.

26 Allen KV, Walker JD. Microalbuminuria and mortality in long-duration type 1 diabetes. *Diabetes Care* 2003;**26**(8): 2389–2391.

27 Arun CS, Stoddart J, Mackin P, MacLeod JM, New JP, Marshall SM. Significance of microalbuminuria in long-duration type 1 diabetes. *Diabetes Care* 2003;**26**(7):2144–2149.

28 Vaur L, Gueret P, Lievre M, Chabaud S, Passa P. Development of congestive heart failure in type 2 diabetic patients with microalbuminuria or proteinuria: observations from the DIABHYCAR (type 2 DIABetes, Hypertension CArdiovascular Events and Ramipril) study. *Diabetes Care* 2003; **26**(3):855–860.

29 Takahashi N, Anan F, Nakagawa M, Yufu K, Ooie T, Nawata T et al. Microalbuminuria, cardiovascular autonomic dysfunction and insulin resistance in patients with type 2 diabetes mellitus. *Metab Clin Exp* 2004;**53**(10): 1359–1364.

30 Rutter MK, McComb JM, Forster J, Brady S, Marshall SM. Increased left ventricular mass index and nocturnal systolic blood pressure in patients with Type 2 diabetes mellitus and microalbuminuria. *Diabet Med* 2000;**17**(4):321–325.

31 Wachtell K, Olsen MH, Dahlof B, Devereux RB, Kjeldsen SE, Nieminen MS *et al.* Microalbuminuria in hypertensive patients with electrocardiographic left ventricular hypertrophy: the LIFE study. *J Hypertens* 2002;**20**(3):405–412.

32 Barzilay JI, Peterson D, Cushman M, Heckbert SR, Cao JJ, Blaum C et al. The relationship of cardiovascular risk factors to microalbuminuria in older adults with or without diabetes mellitus or hypertension: the cardiovascular health study. *Am J Kidney Dis* 2004;**44**(1):25–34.

33 Uusitupa MI, Niskanen LK, Siitonen O, Voutilainen E, Pyorala K. Ten-year cardiovascular mortality in relation to risk factors and abnormalities in lipoprotein composition in type 2 (non-insulin-dependent) diabetic and non-diabetic subjects. *Diabetologia* 1993;**36**(11):1175–1184.

34 Earle K, Walker J, Hill C, Viberti G. Familial clustering of cardiovascular disease in patients with insulin-dependent diabetes and nephropathy. *N Engl J Med* 1992;**326**(10): 673–677.

35 Earle K, Viberti GC. Familial, hemodynamic and metabolic factors in the predisposition to diabetic kidney disease. *Kidney Int* 1994;**45**(2):434–437.

36 UK Prospective Diabetes Study Group. Tight blood pressure control and risk of macrovascular and microvascular complications in type 2 diabetes: UKPDS 38. UK Prospective Diabetes Study Group. *BMJ* 1998;**317**(7160):703–713.

37 Mattock MB, Barnes DJ, Viberti G, Keen H, Burt D, Hughes JM *et al.* Microalbuminuria and coronary heart disease in NIDDM: an incidence study. *Diabetes* 1998;**47**(11):1786–1792.

38 Predictors of the development of microalbuminuria in patients with Type 1 diabetes mellitus: a seven-year prospective study. The Microalbuminuria Collaborative Study Group. *Diabet Med* 1999;**16**(11):918–925.

39 Jensen T, Stender S, Deckert T. Abnormalities in plasmas concentrations of lipoproteins and fibrinogen in type 1 (insulin-dependent) diabetic patients with increased urinary albumin excretion. *Diabetologia* 1988;**31**(3):142–145.

40 Jones SL, Close CF, Mattock MB, Jarrett RJ, Keen H, Viberti GC. Plasma lipid and coagulation factor concentrations in insulin dependent diabetics with microalbuminuria. *BMJ* 1989;**298**(6672):487–490.

41 Groop PH, Thomas MC, Rosengard-Barlund M, Mills V, Ronnback M, Thomas S *et al.* HDL composition predicts new-onset cardiovascular disease in patients with type 1 diabetes. *Diabetes Care* 2007;**30**(10):2706–2707.

42 Yip J, Mattock MB, Morocutti A, Sethi M, Trevisan R, Viberti G. Insulin resistance in insulin-dependent diabetic patients with microalbuminuria. *Lancet* 1993;**342**(8876):883–887.

43 Bianchi S, Bigazzi R, Quinones Galvan A, Muscelli E, Baldari G, Pecori N *et al.* Insulin resistance in microalbuminuric hypertension. Sites and mechanisms. *Hypertension* 1995; **26**(5):789–795.

44 Gruden G, Cavallo-Perin P, Bazzan M, Stella S, Vuolo A, Pagano G. PAI-1 and factor VII activity are higher in IDDM patients with microalbuminuria. *Diabetes* 1994;**43**(3):426–429.

45 Wakabayashi I, Masuda H. Association of D-dimer with microalbuminuria in patients with type 2 diabetes mellitus. *J Thromb Thrombol* 2007.

46 Stehouwer CD, Nauta JJ, Zeldenrust GC, Hackeng WH, Donker AJ, den Ottolander GJ. Urinary albumin excretion, cardiovascular disease and endothelial dysfunction in non-insulin-dependent diabetes mellitus. *Lancet* 1992;**340**(8815): 319–323.

47 Feldt-Rasmussen B. Increased transcapillary escape rate of albumin in type 1 (insulin-dependent) diabetic patients with microalbuminuria. *Diabetologia* 1986;**29**(5):282–286.

48 Jensen JS, Borch-Johnsen K, Jensen G, Feldt-Rasmussen B. Microalbuminuria reflects a generalized transvascular albumin leakiness in clinically healthy subjects. *Clin Sci (Lond)* 1995;**88**(6):629–633.

49 Papaioannou GI, Seip RL, Grey NJ, Katten D, Taylor A, Inzucchi SE *et al.* Brachial artery reactivity in asymptomatic patients with type 2 diabetes mellitus and microalbuminuria (from the Detection of Ischemia in Asymptomatic Diabetics – brachial artery reactivity study). *Am J Cardiol* 2004;**94**(3): 294–299.

50 Araki S, Haneda M, Koya D, Hidaka H, Sugimoto T, Isono M *et al.* Reduction in microalbuminuria as an integrated indicator for renal and cardiovascular risk reduction in patients with type 2 diabetes. *Diabetes* 2007;**56**(6):1727–1730.

51 Yilmaz G, Yilmaz FM, Aral Y, Yucel D. Levels of serum sialic acid and thiobarbituric acid reactive substances in subjects with impaired glucose tolerance and type 2 diabetes mellitus. *J Clin Lab Anal* 2007;**21**(5):260–264.

52 Heart Outcomes Prevention Evaluation Study Investigators. Effects of ramipril on cardiovascular and microvascular outcomes in people with diabetes mellitus: results of the HOPE study and MICRO-HOPE substudy. Heart Outcomes Prevention Evaluation Study Investigators. *Lancet* 2000;**355** (9200):253–259.

53 Gaede P, Vedel P, Larsen N, Jensen GV, Parving HH, Pedersen O. Multifactorial intervention and cardiovascular disease in patients with type 2 diabetes. *N Engl J Med* 2003; **348**(5):383–393.

54 Lindberg G, Rastam L, Gullberg B, Eklund GA. Serum sialic acid concentration predicts both coronary heart disease and stroke mortality: multivariate analysis including 54,385 men and women during 20. 5 years follow-up. *Int J Epidemiol* 1992;**21**(2):253–257.

55 Crook MA, Tutt P, Simpson H, Pickup JC. Serum sialic acid and acute phase proteins in type 1 and type 2 diabetes mellitus. *Clin Chim Acta* 1993;**219**(1–2):131–138.

56 Crook MA, Tutt P, Pickup JC. Elevated serum sialic acid concentration in NIDDM and its relationship to blood pressure and retinopathy. *Diabetes Care* 1993;**16**(1):57–60.

57 Crook MA, Earle K, Morocutti A, Yip J, Viberti G, Pickup JC. Serum sialic acid, a risk factor for cardiovascular disease, is increased in IDDM patients with microalbuminuria and clinical proteinuria. *Diabetes Care* 1994;**17**(4):305–310.

58 Soedamah-Muthu SS, Chaturvedi N, Pickup JC, Fuller JH. Relationship between plasma sialic acid and fibrinogen concentration and incident micro- and macrovascular complications in type 1 diabetes. The EURODIAB Prospective Complications Study (PCS). *Diabetologia* 2008;**51**(3):493–501.

59 Crook MA, Pickup JC, Lumb PJ, Giorgino F, Webb DJ, Fuller JH. Relationship between plasma sialic acid concentration and microvascular and macrovascular complications in type 1 diabetes: the EURODIAB Complications Study. *Diabetes Care* 2001;**24**(2):316–322.

60 Wakabayashi I, Masuda H. Relation of serum sialic acid to blood coagulation activity in type 2 diabetes. *Blood Coagul Fibrinol* 2002;**13**(8):691–696.

61 Pickup JC, Mattock MB. Activation of the innate immune system as a predictor of cardiovascular mortality in Type 2 diabetes mellitus. *Diabet Med* 2003;**20**(9):723–726.

62 Pickup JC, Mattock MB, Crook MA, Chusney GD, Burt D, Fitzgerald AP. Serum sialic acid concentration and coronary heart disease in NIDDM. *Diabetes Care* 1995;**18**(8):1100–1103.

63 Alizadeh Dehnavi R, Beishuizen ED, van de Ree MA, Le Cessie S, Huisman MV, Kluft C *et al.* The impact of

metabolic syndrome and CRP on vascular phenotype in type 2 diabetes mellitus. *Eur J Intern Med* 2008;**19**(2):115–121.

64 Festa A, D'Agostino R, Howard G, Mykkanen L, Tracy RP, Haffner SM. Inflammation and microalbuminuria in non-diabetic and type 2 diabetic subjects: The Insulin Resistance Atherosclerosis Study. *Kidney Int* 2000;**58**(4):1703–1710.

65 Stuveling EM, Bakker SJ, Hillege HL, Burgerhof JG, de Jong PE, Gans RO *et al.* C-reactive protein modifies the relationship between blood pressure and microalbuminuria. *Hypertension* 2004;**43**(4):791–796.

66 Kshirsagar AV, Bomback AS, Bang H, Gerber LM, Vupputuri S, Shoham DA *et al.* Association of C-reactive protein and microalbuminuria (from the National Health and Nutrition Examination Surveys, 1999 to 2004). *Am J Cardiol* 2008;**101**(3): 401–406.

67 Stuveling EM, Hillege HL, Bakker SJ, Asselbergs FW, de Jong PE, Gans RO *et al.* C-reactive protein and microalbuminuria differ in their associations with various domains of vascular disease. *Atherosclerosis* 2004;**172**(1):107–114.

68 Schulze MB, Rimm EB, Li T, Rifai N, Stampfer MJ, Hu FB. C-reactive protein and incident cardiovascular events among men with diabetes. *Diabetes Care* 2004;**27**(4):889–894.

69 Soinio M, Marniemi J, Laakso M, Lehto S, Ronnemaa T. High-sensitivity C-reactive protein and coronary heart disease mortality in patients with type 2 diabetes: a 7-year follow-up study. *Diabetes Care* 2006;**29**(2):329–333.

70 Folsom AR, Chambless LE, Ballantyne CM, Coresh J, Heiss G, Wu KK *et al.* An assessment of incremental coronary risk prediction using C-reactive protein and other novel risk markers: the atherosclerosis risk in communities study. *Arch Intern Med* 2006;**166**(13):1368–1373.

71 Hovens MM, Snoep JD, Groeneveld Y, Frolich M, Tamsma JT, Huisman MV. Effects of aspirin on serum C-reactive protein and interleukin-6 levels in patients with type 2 diabetes without cardiovascular disease: a randomized placebo-controlled crossover trial. *Diabetes Obes Metab* 2007.

72 Russo GT, Di Benedetto A, Giorda C, Alessi E, Crisafulli G, Ientile R *et al.* Correlates of total homocysteine plasma concentration in type 2 diabetes. *Eur J Clin Invest* 2004; **34**(3):197–204.

73 Agardh CD, Agardh E, Andersson A, Hultberg B. Lack of association between plasma homocysteine levels and microangiopathy in type 1 diabetes mellitus. *Scand J Clin Lab Invest* 1994;**54**(8):637–641.

74 Rudy A, Kowalska I, Straczkowski M, Kinalska I. Homocysteine concentrations and vascular complications in patients with type 2 diabetes. *Diabetes Metab* 2005;**31**(2):112–117.

75 Abdel Aziz MT, Fouad HH, Mohsen GA, Mansour M, Abdel Ghaffar S. TNF-alpha and homocysteine levels in type 1 diabetes mellitus. *East Mediterr Health J* 2001;**7**(4–5): 679–688.

76 Abdella NA, Mojiminiyi OA, Akanji AO, Moussa MA. Associations of plasma homocysteine concentration in subjects with type 2 diabetes mellitus. *Acta Diabetol* 2002;**39**(4): 183–190.

77 Stehouwer CD, Gall MA, Hougaard P, Jakobs C, Parving HH. Plasma homocysteine concentration predicts mortality in non-insulin-dependent diabetic patients with and without albuminuria. *Kidney Int* 1999;**55**(1):308–314.

78 Soinio M, Marniemi J, Laakso M, Lehto S, Ronnemaa T. Elevated plasma homocysteine level is an independent predictor of coronary heart disease events in patients with type 2 diabetes mellitus. *Ann Intern Med* 2004;**140**(2):94–100.

79 Friedman AN, Hunsicker LG, Selhub J, Bostom AG. Total plasma homocysteine and arteriosclerotic outcomes in type 2 diabetes with nephropathy. *J Am Soc Nephrol* 2005;**16**(11): 3397–2402.

80 Mangoni AA, Sherwood RA, Asonganyi B, Swift CG, Thomas S, Jackson SH. Short-term oral folic acid supplementation enhances endothelial function in patients with type 2 diabetes. *Am J Hypertens* 2005;**18**(2 Pt 1): 220–226.

81 Zethelius B, Berglund L, Sundstrom J, Ingelsson E, Basu S, Larsson A *et al.* Use of multiple biomarkers to improve the prediction of death from cardiovascular causes. *N Engl J Med* 2008;**358**(20):2107–2116.

82 Saito I, Folsom AR, Brancati FL, Duncan BB, Chambless LE, McGovern PG. Nontraditional risk factors for coronary heart disease incidence among persons with diabetes: the Atherosclerosis Risk in Communities (ARIC) Study. *Ann Intern Med* 2000;**133**(2):81–91.

15 Prevention of the consequences of diabetes – a commentary

Hertzel C. Gerstein

Department of Medicine and the Population Health Research Institute, McMaster University and Hamilton Health Sciences, Hamilton, ON, Canada

Introduction

Diabetes mellitus is a serious, life-shortening disease that is rapidly increasing in prevalence and that currently affects approximately 5% of adults globally and up to 10% of adults in western populations.[1–3] If neglected, people with both type 1 and type 2 diabetes have a reduced quality of life, which is attributable in part to the symptoms of labile blood sugar levels, burden of managing the disease, lost work and the symptoms of various co-morbidities. They also have serious health-related consequences including blindness, renal failure, amputations, chronic neuropathic pain, ulceration and infections, heart attacks, strokes, peripheral vascular disease, cirrhosis, cognitive decline, fractures and early mortality.[4–8] Indeed, the 6 year incidence of death in people with diabetes is similar to the 6 year incidence of death in people with a recent myocardial infarction and no diabetes.[9] The reasons why diabetes increases the incidence of all of these problems remains unclear and has fuelled a tremendous amount of literature.[10] Gluco-metabolic, lipid, haemodynamic, inflammatory, autonomic, hormonal and other explanations have all been implicated to various degrees although no clear single underlying cause has emerged. This is perhaps not surprising in the light of the fact that diabetes is so common and, to a large extent, may itself reflect a consequence of some of the processes that culminate in cardiovascular and other chronic consequences of diabetes. In this light, diabetes is perhaps best viewed as both a disease with its own specific morbidities and as an independent risk factor for many other clinical and preclinical abnormalities, some of which may be responsive targets for intervention.

Earlier chapters are concerned with these serious chronic consequences and carefully review the relevant literature related to the clinical effects of lifestyle interventions, smoking cessation, glucose, blood pressure and lipid therapies and targeting emerging cardiovascular risk factors such as microalbuminuria. A review of the effects of glycaemic management in women with gestational diabetes – which is essentially a prodrome of type 2 diabetes – is also included. Key features of these chapters are highlighted within this chapter.

Lifestyle interventions

There is universal agreement that both excess weight and inactivity are strong risk factors for the development of type 2 diabetes and the magnitude of this risk is fairly large. Indeed, men and women whose body mass index is $\geq 30\,kg\,m^{-2}$ are more than 10 times as likely to develop diabetes than people whose body mass index is $<25\,kg\,m^{-2}$,[11,12] and inactivity increases the risk of diabetes by approximately 30%.[13] Moreover, several randomized controlled trials conducted in people from different regions of the world have consistently shown that modest degrees of weight reduction and increases in physical activity can profoundly reduce the risk of developing type 2 diabetes.[14–16] Thus, not only are excess weight and inactivity risk factors for diabetes, they are modifiable risk factors, suggesting that they are closely related to the underlying cause. Many studies have also shown that once

The Evidence Base for Diabetes Care, Second Edition, Edited by William H. Herman, Ann Louise Kinmonth, Nicholas J. Wareham and Rhys Williams.
© 2010 John Wiley & Sons, Ltd

people develop diabetes, regardless of its cause, metabolic control can be easily influenced by both dietary and activity, changes. These data are summarized very nicely in Chapter 7, which highlights the fact that lifestyle approaches can effect significant weight loss, especially when combined with physical activity. The chapter also points out that physical activity alone is usually ineffective at accomplishing weight loss but can certainly improve metabolic control.

To date, most of the research on weight loss, diet and physical activity has comprised lifestyle interventions. There has recently been a focus on surgical approaches, which have produced remarkable results and which are discussed in this chapter. Undoubtedly, surgery will have its place in selected individuals with significant obesity and poorly controlled type 2 diabetes. However, despite some notable results from recent trials, the paucity of information regarding the long-term risks of surgery for diabetes suggests that much more research is needed before such a therapeutic strategy can be recommended in any but the most specific cases.

As in other areas of research, the literature describing the effectiveness of lifestyle intervention comprises studies in which there was a fairly high degree of adherence to these interventions by the participants. However, the reality of clinical medicine is such that it is difficult for patients to change their lifestyle and it is even more difficult for clinicians to facilitate adherence to these interventions with the limited resources that are typically available in most clinical environments. Recent literature has suggested that simple behavioural approaches can clearly increase the acceptance and the adherence to lifestyle changes.[17,18] Although the literature describing how to implement behavioural modification has not typically captured the attention of the medical community, this is an area which clearly needs to change if clinicians are going to be able to start translating into clinical practice all of the growing data on the efficacy and the benefits of lifestyle interventions. Indeed, the application of several behavioural approaches has the potential to not only facilitate lifestyle changes but also many other behaviours that have been shown to reduce the long-term consequences of diabetes, including medication adherence, regular foot examinations, regular eye examinations and home glucose monitoring where appropriate.

Smoking cessation

Cigarette smoking has clearly been established as a risk factor for many serious health outcomes. As discussed in Chapter 8, it is also associated with lower socioeconomic class, other unhealthy behaviours and less access to medical care – themselves risk factors for poor health consequences. Smoking also negatively affects other risk factors for diabetes-related consequences, including glycated haemoglobin, abnormal fat distribution, lipid abnormalities and blood pressure, both in people with diabetes and in those without diabetes. The data summarized in Chapter 8 clearly show that the risk for cardiovascular disease and mortality in smokers with diabetes is similar to the risk in smokers without diabetes. However, as the absolute incidence of these consequences in people with diabetes is 2–3 times higher than it is in people without diabetes,[19] the doubling of incidence related to smoking would lead to a much higher absolute incidence in smokers who also have diabetes. This observation and the fact that smoking is itself a risk factor for incident diabetes[13] highlight its major importance with respect to serious health consequences. In this context, the lack of a clear association between smoking and retinopathy, documented in this review, is puzzling, especially since retinopathy itself is a strong risk factor for cardiovascular disease. This clearly requires more research.

In this light, it is surprising that 10–20% of people with diabetes continue to smoke, although it is encouraging that the numbers are falling with time in response to public health measures. It is to be hoped that this trend will continue and, if it does, it may reduce both the incidence of diabetes and also some of the consequences of diabetes, particularly early mortality and cardiovascular disease.

Glucose lowering

Much epidemiological evidence shows that dysglycaemia is a risk factor for morbidity and mortality in the general population.[20] The relationship between progressively higher glucose levels and adverse outcomes has been observed both in people with diabetes and in those without diabetes, and has been noted for various measures of glycaemia, including fasting glucose, postload glucose and HbA_{1c}.[21–26] Several epidemiological studies have also suggest that the risk factor–response relationship differs depending on the outcome being assessed.[4] Thus, for retinopathy, the relationship may be most marked within the diabetes range of dysglycaemia, whereas for cardiovascular disease it may be more pronounced in the non-diabetic range. These observations provide the basis for the hypothesis that amelioration of the abnormal glucose levels or the underlying cause for the abnormal glucose levels may reduce these outcomes. This hypothesis is addressed in several completed and ongoing studies of (a) more versus less intensive glucose lowering using a variety of medications, (b) fasting versus post-prandial glucose lowering, (c) one versus another therapeutic strategy targeting similar glucose levels and (d) gluco-metabolic interventions within the larger context of reduction of multiple risk factors at the same time.

As noted in the chapter, results from intervention studies in type 2 diabetes have raised more questions than answers. The UKPDS study, which is the only trial done in people with newly diagnosed diabetes (and, as pointed out in the chapter, which included some individuals who would today be classified as having impaired fasting glucose and not diabetes), strongly suggests that a policy of lower versus higher glucose goals for at least 10 years after diabetes is diagnosed reduces the 20 year incidence of several diabetes-related consequences, including myocardial infarction and death.[27] Other trials done in patients with established diabetes and a high cardiovascular risk have supported a benefit on major kidney disease[28] but have not clearly shown a cardiovascular effect,[12,29] and one trial suggested a mortality risk in people with well-established type 2 diabetes and high cardiovascular risk.[12] The most dramatic finding came from a small but long-term follow-up trial of the effects of multiple risk factor reduction and evidence-based therapy within a comprehensive clinic compared with family practice care: it clearly showed a profound long-term benefit on almost all diabetes-related outcomes.[30] The small sample size and multiplicity of interventions preclude dissection of the results and the open nature of the trial and the different settings (specialty clinic versus family practice) within which the interventions were delivered make it impossible to discern if it was the environment, one or more of the interventions, the changes in risk factors or some combination that was responsible for the findings. Nevertheless, a similar trial done in another environment with similar results[31] supports such an approach.

The last 10 years have seen the introduction of a large variety of gluco-metabolic interventions for the management of diabetes. Some of these have been included in the trials to date but many more are being studied in ongoing trials and in other trials currently being planned. The world of glucose lowering is, therefore, akin to the world of blood pressure lowering in the 1970s and it is likely to take another 10 years of research and intervention studies to increase certainty around the best way of managing gluco-metabolic abnormalities, both in people with diabetes and in those without diabetes.

can reduce cardiovascular and other outcomes overall and in people with diabetes. This evidence has been nicely reviewed in Chapter 12, which summarizes the data showing that antihypertensive drugs reduce the risk of cardiovascular outcomes by 15–25%. Guidelines based on this evidence have recommended target blood pressure levels less than 130/80 in people with diabetes. However, the evidence from clinical trials completed to date supports systolic blood pressure lowering to <135 mmHg systolic.[32] Nevertheless, ACE inhibitors, ARBs, beta-blockers, thiazides and calcium channel blockers all have robust clinical trial evidence showing that their use to lower blood pressure can reduce cardiovascular outcomes in people with diabetes and various co-morbidities.

It has been recognized for many years that both hypertension and diabetes coexist in 70% or more of individuals. Such concordance is almost certainly related to the fact that both are confounded with cardiovascular disease and the high blood pressure likely represents vascular functional and anatomic abnormalities. Indeed, blood pressure-lowering agents may reduce outcomes by ameliorating some of these abnormalities. However, the debate regarding whether it is the agent or the blood pressure lowering that is responsible for benefit remains unresolved. For example, in a recent large trial the combination of telmisartan and ramipril lowered blood pressure more than ramipril but did not further reduce cardiovascular events (with no difference in the diabetes versus the non-diabetes group).[33] This suggests that the means by which blood pressure lowering is achieved may be as relevant as or more relevant than the actual blood pressure achieved – a conclusion that certainly applies to modification of other risk factors such as lipids, glucose, weight or albuminuria. This supports the importance of measuring cardiovascular outcomes in trials of putative therapies and not relying on the change in the risk factor as a surrogate measure of clinical benefit.

Finally, this chapter highlights the fact that many people with diabetes continue to have poorly controlled blood pressure. This, and the fact that those with the highest blood pressure will have the largest absolute reduction in events in response to blood pressure lowering, identify an important need for therapy in people with diabetes. The fact that most of the blood pressure drugs are very well tolerated and many are inexpensive identifies a simple opportunity to practice preventive medicine in people with diabetes.

Blood pressure lowering

It has been clearly established that blood pressure lowering using a variety of therapeutic approaches

Lipid lowering

That statin therapies (particularly simvastatin, atorvastatin and pravastatin) reduce cardiovascular outcomes in the general population and in people with diabetes, have a greater benefit at higher doses and are well tolerated is clearly reviewed in Chapter 13. Chapter 13 also provides a comprehensive review of many ongoing trials of a variety of therapies (including omega-3 fatty acids[34]) that are addressing these additional questions. The paucity of evidence for non-statin lipid-modifying therapies, including bile acid sequestrants, cholesterol absorption inhibitors, fibrates, niacin and omega-3 fatty acids, in people with diabetes precludes drawing definitive conclusions regarding whether these agents consistently reduce cardiovascular outcomes in people with diabetes.

All of the statin trials were masked comparisons of one statin versus a control therapy. Thus, the most conservative conclusion is that they reflect the benefits of statins *per se*. That is, the inference that they reflect the benefits of achieving lower versus higher LDL levels therapy is indirect and comes from trials which compared a higher with a lower statin dose. Whether lower LDL target and higher statin doses are interchangeable constructs cannot be answered by these trials. If ongoing trials of different ways of lowering LDL cholesterol show results that are similar to the statin trials for similar degrees of lowering, this would provide strong evidence in support of the concept of more aggressive LDL lowering. However, if they do not, then it is possible that all the results to date may simply reflect a dose–response effect of statins. Until more is known, LDL cholesterol levels are certainly a reliable and convenient measure of adherence to statin therapy.

Finally, Chapter 13 reminds us that individuals with diabetes have similar LDL cholesterol concentrations to individuals without diabetes, but they have higher numbers of LDL particles in addition to higher triglyceride and lower HDL levels. Whether changes in these metabolic abnormalities by statins are related to the proven cardiovascular benefits of statin therapy and/or whether they can predict the cardiovascular effect of other lipid-modifying drugs is not answered by the clinical trials.

Targeting emerging cardiovascular risk factors

It is well known that dysglycaemia is accompanied by a wide range of physiological abnormalities including, but not limited to, (a) insufficient insulin action due either to a relative or absolute lack of insulin; (b) abnormal fat metabolism; (c) abnormalities in secretion or action of other hormones secreted from the pancreas, gut, fat cells and elsewhere; (d) abnormal cytokine secretion; and (e) renal disease.[10] Dysglycaemia is also associated with microalbuminuria, endothelial dysfunction, somatic and autonomic nervous system dysfunction, haemodynamic abnormalities and a host of other problems. Whether many of these abnormalities develop before or after the gluco-metabolic abnormalities is not clear. In this light, the safest inference is that diabetes is associated with a large cluster of abnormalities which may themselves mediate, magnify or be confounded with the consequences of diabetes. For example, a growing number of epidemiological studies report that many of the abnormalities associated with diabetes also predict cardiovascular outcomes independently of diabetes, and also of each other. Indeed, a recent review identified close to 100 independent risk factors of cardiac disease in the general population. of which diabetes was only one.[35] These data make it difficult, if not impossible, to identify an underlying cause of cardiovascular outcomes in people with diabetes. Moreover, the large variety of risk factors (and therapeutic targets) and the growing number of interventions that can modify these risk factors present a growing number of interventions that need to be individually tested to determine if they can safely reduce cardiovascular risk.

Chapter 14 catalogues some of these other risk factors and highlights microalbuminuria as a possible modifiable risk factor in people with diabetes. This is supported by trials showing that some interventions, such as ACE inhibitors and blood pressure lowering, also reduce both albuminuria and cardiovascular risk. As noted earlier with respect to blood pressure lowering, changes in a risk factor such as albuminuria in response to an intervention may simply be a marker of the effect of the intervention and may not be the mediator of any benefit. It is therefore appropriate to be very cautious before embracing any one or another risk factor as being an ideal target for therapy.

In this light, the simplest and most effective therapeutic approach seems to be a comprehensive implementation of all proven therapies within an appropriate practice environment as discussed earlier.[30] Such an approach may yield the greatest benefit when high-risk individuals such as those with microalbuminuria are selected. However, whether such an approach works as a result of reducing the risk factor or as a result of increased attention and early detection of pathology or a combination may never be known. Indeed, short of completely eliminating diabetes and dysglycaemia completely, there is unlikely to be a magic bullet that will eliminate the associated excess cardiovascular risk.

Glucose control in gestational Diabetes

The type 2 diabetes epidemic is matched by a similar epidemic of gestational diabetes. Up to 7% of pregnancies are complicated by gestational diabetes – making it the most common medical complication of pregnancy. Risk factors for gestational diabetes are essentially the same as those for type 2 diabetes and, as noted in Chapter 11, the pathophysiology of gestational diabetes to a large extent mirrors the pathophysiology of type 2 diabetes. That is, women with gestational diabetes have pancreatic beta cells that are unable to meet the progressively increasing insulin needs associated with pregnancy; the resulting relative insufficiency of insulin is reflected in a rising glucose level, along with other associated metabolic abnormalities. Pregnancy can, therefore, be thought of as a 'stress test' of gluco-metabolic physiology in a woman. This is reflected in the well-known relationship between a history of gestational diabetes and future type 2 diabetes, occurring at a rate of 4–10% per year with no preventive intervention. However, the facts that the gluco-metabolic abnormalities resolve in most women post-partum and that some studies have suggested that interventions can reduce the risk of type 2 diabetes following gestational diabetes suggest that this natural history can be modified. Perhaps more importantly, resolution of diabetes after pregnancy in response to changes in some of its pathophysiological determinants in post-partum women may provide important clues to research directed at ways to resolve type 2 diabetes in older populations.

Chapter 11 also clearly points out that in addition to identifying women at long-term risk for type 2 diabetes, gestational diabetes has clinically important consequences for pregnant women, post-partum women and newborns. The risk of most of these consequences has been reduced with modern obstetric and ante-partum care; however, both maternal and perinatal morbidity persist even today. Although much observational research has been done on this population, there has been a paucity of clinical trial work, probably because of heightened concerns regarding safety in the light of the emotionally charged pregnant state. Fortunately, this experimental research deficit is being addressed[36] by studies which are providing further insights into the diagnosis and treatment of this increasingly prevalent condition.

Conclusion

The early 21st century has seen a global pandemic of diabetes. The rapid increase in prevalence throughout both the developed and the developing world and the alarming number of people affected by this serious disease is highlighted by the 20 December 2006 United Nations resolution that formally recognized diabetes as a 'chronic, debilitating and costly disease', which 'poses severe risks for families, countries and the entire world', and that encouraged countries 'to develop national policies for the prevention, treatment and care of diabetes'.[37] The impact of diabetes is huge and cannot be disputed. For example, the estimated direct and indirect costs of diabetes in the United States approached $200 billion in 2007[38] – costs that were to a large part due to the consequences described in these chapters. These considerations highlight the importance of reducing the incidence of diabetes globally. Indeed in the first decade of the 21st century, well-done research studies have shown that it is clearly possible to reduce dramatically the incidence of diabetes with a variety of non-pharmacological and, in some cases, pharmacological therapies.

The evidence documented in these chapters has shown that the consequences of diabetes can be dramatically reduced by simple and generally inexpensive therapies. Not discussed in these chapters is the importance of societal changes to reduce the high prevalence and the consequences of the disease. As the environment clearly has a strong influence on the incidence of diabetes, a major part of the solution to the problem lies in innovative food policies, transportation policies, new approaches to urban planning and development and changes in the way that healthcare is delivered, so as to be more responsive to chronic disease management versus reacting to acute complaints.

The most important message is that medical science today has a tremendous amount of knowledge regarding how to reduce both the incidence and the consequences of the disease. The task at hand is to implement things that we already know can work in an efficient and sustainable way.

References

1 International Diabetes Federation. Prevalence estimates of diabetes 2007. In: *Diabetes Atlas*, 3rd edn, International Diabetes Federation, Brussels, 2006.

2 Lipscombe LL, Hux JE. Trends in diabetes prevalence, incidence and mortality in Ontario, Canada, 1995–2005: a population-based study. *Lancet* 2007;**369**:750–756.

3 Centers for Disease Control and Prevention. *Prevalence of Diagnosed Diabetes by Age, United States, 1980–2005*, www.cdc.gov/diabetes/statistics/prev/; accessed 13 June 2008.

4 Stratton IM, Adler AI, Neil HA *et al.* Association of glycaemia with macrovascular and microvascular complications of type 2 diabetes (UKPDS 35): prospective observational study. *BMJ* 2000;**321**:405–412.

5 Cukierman T, Gerstein HC, Williamson JD. Cognitive decline and dementia in diabetes-systematic overview of prospective observational studies. *Diabetologia* 2005;**48**:2460–2469.

6 Tolman KG, Fonseca V, Tan MH, Dalpiaz A. Narrative review: hepatobiliary disease in type 2 diabetes mellitus. *Ann Intern Med* 2004;**141**:946–956.

7 Ivers RQ, Cumming RG, Mitchell P, Peduto AJ. Diabetes and risk of fracture: The Blue Mountains Eye Study. *Diabetes Care* 2001;**24**:1198–1203.

8 Nicodemus KK, Folsom AR. Type 1 and type 2 diabetes and incident hip fractures in postmenopausal women. *Diabetes Care* 2001;**24**:1192–1197.

9 Booth GL, Kapral MK, Fung K, Tu JV. Relation between age and cardiovascular disease in men and women with diabetes compared with non-diabetic people: a population-based retrospective cohort study. *Lancet* 2006;**368**:29–36.

10 Punthakee Z, Werstuck GH, Gerstein HC. Diabetes and cardiovascular disease: explaining the relationship. *Rev Cardiovasc Med* 2007;**8**:145–153.

11 van Dam RM, Rimm EB, Willett WC, Stampfer MJ, Hu FB. Dietary patterns and risk for type 2 diabetes mellitus in U.S. men. *Ann Intern Med* 2002;**136**:201–209.

12 Action to Control Cardiovascular Risk in Diabetes Study Group., Gerstein HC, Miller ME *et al.* Effects of intensive glucose lowering in type 2 diabetes. *N Engl J Med* 2008;**358**:2545–2559.

13 Hu FB, Manson JE, Stampfer MJ *et al.* Diet, lifestyle and the risk of type 2 diabetes mellitus in women. *N Engl J Med* 2001;**345**:790–797.

14 Knowler WC, Barrett-Connor E, Fowler SE *et al.* Reduction in the incidence of type 2 diabetes with lifestyle intervention or metformin. *N Engl J Med* 2002;**346**:393–403.

15 Tuomilehto J, Lindstrom J, Eriksson JG *et al.* Prevention of type 2 diabetes mellitus by changes in lifestyle among sub-jects with impaired glucose tolerance. *N Engl J Med* 2001;**344**:1343–1350.

16 Ramachandran A, Snehalatha C, Mary S, Mukesh B, Bhas-kar AD, Vijay V. The Indian Diabetes Prevention Pro-gramme shows that lifestyle modification and metformin prevent type 2 diabetes in Asian Indian subjects with impaired glucose tolerance (IDPP-1). *Diabetologia* 2006;**49**: 289–297.

17 Jones H, Edwards L, Vallis TM *et al.* Changes in diabetes self-care behaviors make a difference in glycemic control: the Diabetes Stages of Change (DiSC) study. *Diabetes Care* 2003;**26**:732–737.

18 Wing RR, Hamman RF, Bray GA *et al.* Achieving weight and activity goals among diabetes prevention program lifestyle participants. *Obes Res* 2004;**12**:1426–1434.

19 Huxley R, Barzi F, Woodward M, Excess risk of fatal cor-onary heart disease associated with diabetes in men and women: meta-analysis of 37 prospective cohort studies. *BMJ* 2006;**332**:73–78.

20 Gerstein HC, Yusuf S. Dysglycaemia and risk of cardiovas-cular disease. *Lancet* 1996;**347**:949–950.

21 Held C, Gerstein HC, Yusuf S *et al.* Glucose levels predict hospitalization for congestive heart failure in patients at high cardiovascular risk. *Circulation* 2007;**115**:1371–1375.

22 Gerstein HC, Pogue J, Mann JF *et al.* The relationship between dysglycaemia and cardiovascular and renal risk in diabetic and non-diabetic participants in the HOPE study: a prospective epidemiological analysis. *Diabetologia* 2005;**48**:1749–1755.

23 Gerstein HC, Swedberg K, Carlsson J *et al.* The hemoglobin A1c level as a progressive risk factor for cardiovascular death, hospitalization for heart failure or death in patients with chronic heart failure: an analysis of the Candesartan in Heart failure: Assessment of Reduction in Mortality and Morbidity (CHARM) program. *Arch Intern Med* 2008;**168**: 1699–1704.

24 Lawes CM, Parag V, Bennett DA *et al.* Blood glucose and risk of cardiovascular disease in the Asia Pacific region. *Diabetes Care* 2004;**27**:2836–2842.

25 Brunner EJ, Shipley MJ, Witte DR, Fuller JH, Marmot MG. Relation between blood glucose and coronary mortality over 33 years in the Whitehall Study. *Diabetes Care* 2006;**29**:26–31.

26 Khaw KT, Wareham N, Bingham S, Luben R, Welch A, Day N. Association of hemoglobin A1c with cardiovascular disease and mortality in adults: the European prospective investigation into cancer in Norfolk. *Ann Intern Med* 2004;**141**: 413–420.

27 Holman RR, Paul SK, Bethel MA, Matthews DR, Neil HA. 10-year follow-up of intensive glucose control in type 2 diabetes. *N Engl J Med* 2008;**359**:1577–1589.

28 Patel A, MacMahon S, Chalmers J *et al.* Intensive blood glucose control and vascular outcomes in patients with type 2 diabetes. *N Engl J Med* 2008;**358**:2560–2572.

29 Duckworth W, Abraira C, Moritz T *et al.* Glucose control and vascular complications in veterans with type 2 diabetes. *N Engl J Med* 2009;**360**:129–139.

30 Gaede P, Lund-Andersen H, Parving HH, Pedersen O. Effect of a multifactorial intervention on mortality in type 2 dia-betes. *N Engl J Med* 2008;**358**:580–591.

31 Rachmani R, Slavachevski I, Berla M, Frommer-Shapira R, Ravid M. Teaching and motivating patients to control their risk factors retards progression of cardiovascular as well as microvascular sequelae of Type 2 diabetes mellitus – a randomized prospective 8 years follow-up study. *Diabet Med* 2005;**22**:410–414.

32 Patel A, MacMahon S, Chalmers J *et al.* Effects of a fixed combination of perindopril and indapamide on macro-vascular and microvascular outcomes in patients with type 2 diabetes mellitus (the ADVANCE trial): a randomised controlled trial. *Lancet* 2007;**370**: 829–840.

33 Yusuf S, Teo KK, Pogue J *et al.* Telmisartan, ramipril or both in patients at high risk for vascular events. *N Engl J Med* 2008;**358**:1547–1559.

34 Origin Trial Investigators. Rationale, design and baseline characteristics for a large international trial of cardiovascular disease prevention in people with dysglycemia: the ORIGIN Trial (Outcome Reduction with an Initial Glargine Interven-tion). *Am Heart J* 2008;**155**:26–32.

35 Brotman DJ, Walker E, Lauer MS, O'Brien RG. In search of fewer independent risk factors. *Arch Intern Med* 2005;**165**: 138–145.

36 Crowther CA, Hiller JE, Moss JR, McPhee AJ, Jeffries WS, Robinson JS. Effect of treatment of gestational diabetes mellitus on pregnancy outcomes. *N Engl J Med* 2005;**352**: 2477–2486.

37 International Diabetes Federation. *Unite for Diabetes. 2009*, http://www.worlddiabetesday.org/the-campaign/unite-for-diabetes; accessed 1 September 2008.

38 Economic costs of diabetes in the U.S. in 2007. *Diabetes Care* 2008;**31**:596–615.

Part 4: Treatment of established complications

16 Treatment of diabetic retinopathy

Ayad Al-Bemani[1], Roy Taylor[2]

[1]*Department of Opthamology, Royal Victoria Infirmary, Newcastle upon Tyne, UK*
[2]*School of Clinical Medical Sciences, Medical School, Newcastle University, Newcastle upon Tyne, UK*

Diabetic retinopathy is a potentially blinding disease which has been studied extensively. This chapter reviews the epidemiology of the condition, its progression and the effect of various treatment modalities using information from randomized controlled trials, case series and other forms of evidence.

Risk factors for diabetic retinopathy

The development and progression of diabetic retinopathy are each influenced by several factors. Some of these factors are modifiable but others are not. Genetic factors and duration of diabetes are important non-modifiable factors. There is a clear genetic component of susceptibility to retinopathy. A meta-analysis of 88 studies has suggested at least eight candidate genes which could underlie the familial tendency to develop diabetic retinopathy.[1] The duration of diabetes is the strongest single influence on the prevalence of retinopathy.[2] Patients who have had type 1 diabetes mellitus for less than 5 years rarely show evidence of sight-threatening diabetic retinopathy, although background diabetic retinopathy may already be present.[3,4] However, after 20 years, the prevalence of background diabetic retinopathy rises to 95% and 30–50% of these patients have proliferative diabetic retinopathy.[5] Around 37% of patients with type 2 diabetes have retinopathy at the time of diagnosis.[6] After 10 years, 67% of type 2 patients have some retinopathy and 10% have proliferative diabetic retinopathy. These data come from cohort studies which recruited participants many years ago and the current prevalence and incidence of diabetic retinopathy may be different because of improvements in the control of blood pressure and blood glucose. However, the general pattern of rising prevalence of diabetic retinopathy with time since diagnosis of disease is unlikely to have changed.

The factors which may be modified by patient and physician are described below.

Good glycaemic control

Strict glycaemic control reduces both the incidence and the progression of early retinopathy.[7,8] In the United Kingdom Prospective Diabetes Study (UKPDS) of type 2 diabetes, a 1% reduction in glycated haemoglobin resulted in a 25% reduction in microvascular endpoints, a 37% decrease in laser treatment and a 10% reduction in cataract extraction.[9] Furthermore, the EDIC study showed that the effect of good blood glucose control conferred a prolonged beneficial effect even during a subsequent period of less good control. Specifically, the risk of deterioration of retinopathy and of progression to proliferative or severe non-proliferative retinopathy was decreased by 74 and 78%, respectively, despite the change in glycaemic control.[10]

Several large randomized studies have shown that rapid tightening of blood glucose control brings about an initial worsening of diabetic retinopathy.[7,11] This phenomenon is likely to be secondary to a fall in retinal blood flow as near-normoglycaemic blood glucose levels are attained. This may result in hypoperfusion in areas of marginal perfusion. Although the worsening of retinopathy is potentially reversible, proliferation can be induced in cases of pre-existing severe non-proliferative retinopathy. A study of 294 poorly controlled type 2 diabetes patients[12] commenced on insulin showed that over the first 3 years

The Evidence Base for Diabetes Care, Second Edition, Edited by William H. Herman, Ann Louise Kinmonth, Nicholas J. Wareham and Rhys Williams.

of insulin therapy, significant progression occurred in 5/193 (2.6%) without any retinopathy at baseline, 22/77 (28.5%) with minimal NPDR and 6/11 with moderate NPDR (54.5%) ($\chi^2 = 56.1$, $p < 0.001$). In a control group of 70 patients who remained on oral hypoglycaemic agents, only nine had significant worsening of retinopathy over 3 years.

Good blood pressure control

In the UKPDS, over half of the patients had high blood pressure or were receiving antihypertensive treatment. A total of 758 patients were allocated to a tight blood pressure (BP) control policy with angiotensin-converting enzyme inhibitor or beta-blockers as the main therapy; 390 were allocated to a less tight BP control policy. Tight control of the blood pressure, aiming at below 150/90, had a significant beneficial effect, reducing the incidence of retinopathy and progression to photocoagulation. For every 10 mm reduction in the systolic blood pressure, there was an 11% reduction in the need for laser treatment. The cumulative incidence of the endpoint of blindness in one eye was 18/758 (2.37%) for the tight BP control group compared with 12/390 (3.08%) for the less tight BP control group ($p < 0.05$). The effect was similar whether beta-blocker or angiotensin-converting enzyme inhibitor was used.[13] Overall, the effect of tight BP control was greater than tight glycaemic control.

The importance of the effect of good BP control upon progression of retinopathy is hard to overstate. This is particularly so as tight blood glucose control is genuinely difficult to achieve using the current imperfect tools, whereas tight BP control merely requires appropriate use of existing agents in combination.

Renal disease

Renal disease, as evidenced by proteinuria, elevated blood urea nitrogen and elevated blood creatinine, is a reliable predictor of the presence of retinopathy.[2] Even patients who have microalbuminuria, the earliest detectable stage of diabetic nephropathy, are at high risk of developing retinopathy.[14] This is explicable in terms of shared susceptibility to two microvascular complications of diabetes, but also as those developing nephropathy tend to be more hypertensive than the rest of the diabetic population.

Pregnancy

Three cohort studies on a total of 409 pregnant women have observed that pregnancy is associated with progression of diabetic retinopathy.[15–17] In each study, the risk of progression of retinopathy was approximately doubled by pregnancy.

A cohort study of 155 pregnant women with type 1 diabetes found that those with more severe retinopathy prior to conception were more likely to progress during pregnancy, 10.3% in those with no retinopathy compared with 54.8% of those with moderate background retinopathy. Furthermore, those with non-proliferative diabetic retinopathy at the onset of pregnancy and those who have or who develop systemic hypertension were more likely to progress. About 4% of pregnant women who have non-proliferative diabetic retinopathy progress to proliferative diabetic retinopathy.[18]

Classification of diabetic retinopathy

Sight-threatening changes in diabetic retinopathy arise either from the growth of new vessels with all the complications that it can cause, such as vitreous haemorrhage, retinal detachment and rubeotic glaucoma, or from localized damage to the fovea from vascular incompetence with loss of central visual acuity.

There are two approaches to the classification of diabetic retinopathy, the first of which is aimed at ophthalmologists and covers the full range of retinopathy. This classification is derived from the Early Treatment Diabetic Retinopathy Study (ETDRS) and defines three stages of low-risk non-proliferative retinopathy, a fourth stage of severe non-proliferative retinopathy and a fifth grade of proliferative retinopathy. Macular oedema is classified as present or absent and further sub-classified based on the involvement of the centre of the macula (Table 16.1).[19,20] The second approach is for population screening, which is simple and clinically effective in practice.[21] It is aimed at detecting a level of retinopathy sufficient to merit referral to an ophthalmologist and can readily be used by retinal screeners or other non-ophthalmologists. It identifies four parameters: retinopathy (R), maculopathy (M), photocoagulation (P) and unclassifiable (U). Retinopathy is sub-classified into R1 or background diabetic retinopathy, R2 or preproliferative diabetic retinopathy and R3 or proliferative diabetic retinopathy[22] (Table 16.2). The M and P parameters are expressed as present or absent (e.g. M0 or M1). Hence any retinal image can be classified by a few letters and numbers (e.g. R1 M0 P0).

Screening for diabetic retinopathy

Optimal treatment of sight-threatening changes in patients with diabetic retinopathy requires the treatment to be carried out before loss of vision from either maculopathy or vitreous haemorrhage. Therefore,

Table 16.1 Full diabetic retinopathy grading based on the ETDRS

Stage	Retinal findings[a]
Mild non-proliferative diabetic retinopathy	MAs only
Moderate non-proliferative diabetic retinopathy	Extensive MAs with or without CWS, IRMA and venous beading
Severe non-proliferative diabetic retinopathy	Extensive MAs, haemorrhages, CWS, venous beading, or IRMA
Early proliferative diabetic retinopathy	Mild NVD or NVE, without vitreous haemorrhage
High-risk proliferative diabetic retinopathy	Moderate NVD or NVE, with vitreous haemorrhage
Non-clinically significant macular oedema	Retinal thickening/hard exudates within 1 DD of the centre of macula
Clinically significant macular oedema	Retinal thickening/hard exudates less than 500 μm from the centre of fovea or an area greater than 1 DD within 1 DD of the centre of fovea

[a]MAs, microaneurysms; CWS, cotton-wool spots; IRMA, intra-retinal microvascular abnormalities; NVD, neovascularization around the disc; NVE, neovascularization elsewhere; DD, disc diameter.

there is a need for regular retinal examination for all people with diabetes. The current consensus is that screening should be carried out annually as this is simple to organize, even though individuals with no retinopathy at diagnosis of type 2 diabetes could theoretically be left for 3 years with minimal risk.[23] Screening programmes carried out for patients with diabetes (Table 16.3) need to be simple to operate and to provide complete population coverage in order to achieve their targets successfully.

It is clear that the use of the ophthalmoscope is inadequate in most circumstances, probably because of the need to spend adequate time dilating the pupil and examining each retina in a darkened room in the context of a busy clinic.[24] Retinal photography using digital imaging is now established as the method of choice for regular screening.[25] Even the use of retinal photography without mydriasis is superior to ophtha-moscopy.[26] Polaroid retinal photography has a sensitivity of 83% and a specificity of 98% for detection of referable retinopathy.[27] However, digital retinal ima-ging has brought further benefits as the intensity of the flash is less than for Polaroid photography and films from previous years can readily be retrieved from storage for clinical decision making and quality assurance. Using two digital images per eye, a quality assurance system built into the routine screening system has shown sensitivity and specificity to be 94 and 98%, respectively.[28a] An important feature of this screening system is that the retinal screeners acquire the images, grade the images and give immediate results to patients, thus maximizing the incentive to return for screening the following year. Population coverage is the most important single factor in determining the success of any retinal screening system to reduce blindness in any population. A successful screening system relies heavily on properly trained retinal screeners and a training manual for the new profession of retinal screeners has been published.[28b]

Screening should be performed annually for most people with diabetes and certainly all with

Table 16.2 UK national guidelines on screening for diabetic retinopathy – grading protocol

Level	Grade	Description
Retinopathy (R)		
R0	None	
R1	Background	MA(s), retinal haemorrhage(s) with or without any exudates
R2	Preproliferative	Venous beading, looping or reduplication, IRMA, multiple deep, round or blot haemorrhages and CWS
R3	Proliferative	NVD, NVE, pre-retinal or vitreous haemorrhage, pre-retinal fibrosis with or without tractional retinal detachment
Maculopathy (M)		Exudate within 1DD of the centre of the fovea, group of exudates within the macula, retinal thickening within 1 DD of the centre of the fovea, any MA or haemorrhage within 1 DD the centre of the fovea only with visual acuity of 6/12 or better
Photocoagulation (P)		Macular focal/Grid or peripheral scatter
Unclassifiable (U)		

MAs, microaneurysms; CWS, cotton-wool spots; IRMA, intra-retinal microvascular abnormalities; NVD, neovascularization around the disc; NVE, neovascularization elsewhere; DD: disc diameter.

Table 16.3 Management of cases after completion of grading in the UK national guidelines on screening for diabetic retinopathy

Grade	Management
Retinopathy (R)	
R0	Annual screening.
R1	Annual screening.
R2	Refer to hospital eye service.
R3	Fast track referral to hospital eye service
Maculopathy (M)	
M	Refer to hospital eye service
Photocoagulation (P)	
P	New screenee – refer to hospital eye service
	Quiescent post-treatment – annual screening
Other lesions (OL)	Refer to hospital eye service or inform physician
Ungradable/unobtainable (U)	Poor view but gradable on biomicroscopy – refer to hospital eye service
	Unscreenable – discharge, inform GP (option to recall for photographs if purely a technical failure)

background retinopathy. Less frequent screening may be appropriate for patients with no retinopathy. Similarly, more frequent targeted screening may be appropriate for patients with intermediate levels of retinopathy and maculopathy.[3] The current recommendation is that all patients aged over 12 years should be screened because significant diabetic retinopathy does not occur in persons under the age of 11 years, but puberty is a time of increasing risk of retinopathy. Screening should be increased in frequency during pregnancy.[17,29]

The effectiveness of regular retinal screening has been demonstrated in a cohort study of the entire population of people with diabetes in a single health district where a decrease of more than one-third in the incidence of diabetes-related blindness in patients was observed after 15 years of annual screening and appropriate laser therapy.[21]

No discussion of screening would be complete without mention of the need for mydriasis for adequate screening by any method.[30] Tropamide is adequate for this purpose, although its use is occasionally limited by the persistent and erroneous belief that this agent may precipitate glaucoma in susceptible individuals. A systematic review has established that this is extremely unlikely to occur.[31] There is no excess risk of angle closure in people with chronic, open-angle glaucoma. People with treated acute glaucoma are not at risk. Tropicamide may be used for all in a population screening programme.

Investigations in diabetic retinopathy

Visual acuity

Visual acuity is the simplest and most important measurement of visual function. It assesses the optics of the eye, the retina and the central nervous functions of the foveal region. Testing the visual acuity of patients with diabetes at presentation and further testing at each follow-up visit provides a screen for disease progression. The test should be carried out with patients wearing their most up-to-date spectacles.

Snellen charts are the most commonly used test for visual acuity and are very suitable for screening populations. The test types should be clearly printed, legible and uniformly illuminated. The patient should be sat at 6 m or at 3 m using a reverse test type placed above the patient's head observed as a reflection in a mirror hung on the opposite wall. The Bailey–Lovie chart,[32] which forms the basis for the (ETDRS) visual acuity chart, is more suitable for the differentiation between degrees of loss of visual acuity. This design has several advantages. The letters used are of approximately equal detectability whereas earlier charts had some letters that were more legible than others. Each line has an equal number of letters and the spacing between letters is proportional to the letter size, unlike older acuity charts which had unequal spacing between letters. Finally, the change in visual acuity from one line to another is in equal logarithmic steps. Older eye charts had very small changes for different lines at the small-letter end of the chart and rather large changes for the big-letter end of the chart.

Fluorescein angiography of the fundus

Sodium fluorescein is a yellow–red dye used as a 10 or 25% solution injected intravenously. When subjected to blue light it emits green–yellow light. A specially designed fundus camera with light filters is used to capture this fluorescence phenomenon. The pupil has to be dilated in order to obtain optimal images and the cooperation of the patient is critical.

This test is valuable in identifying diabetic retinopathy, particularly in demonstrating leaking microaneurysms which can be targeted in laser treatment. It can also demonstrate the status of the retinal vasculature that may affect the decision to carry out macula laser and pan-retinal photocoagulation.[33,34]

Optical coherence tomography

Optical coherence tomography (OCT) is a new technique for high-resolution cross-sectional imaging of retinal architecture. It is based on the principle of low-coherence interferometry. In this technique, the distances and sizes of different structures in the eye are determined by measuring the 'echo' time it takes for light to be backscattered from different structures at various axial distances. Using a modified standard slit-lamp or a specially designed fundus camera, imaging can be carried out without direct contact with the eye.

OCT can provide quantitative estimates of retinal thickness caused by the accumulation of intraretinal fluid to within 10 μm. Although clinically significant macular oedema continues to be a clinical diagnosis, OCT images can quantify the retinal thickening which correlates with visual acuity. This measure can be used to follow the clinical response to focal laser treatment for clinically significant macular oedema.[35–37]

Treatment of diabetic retinopathy

Treatment of patients with diabetic retinopathy may be grouped into three stages:

1 Reduction of risk factors in order to modify the progression of diabetic retinopathy.
2 Treatment of established complications of diabetic retinopathy by laser photocoagulation and vitrectomy.
3 Treatment of the consequences of visual impairment: patients who fail to respond and progress to severe visual impairment require support to enable them to lead as normal a life as possible. Low visual aids for use at home and at work, including various magnifiers and closed-circuit television, can maximize personal and social effectiveness.

Pan-retinal photocoagulation

Light amplification by stimulated emission of radiation (laser) involves light of a single wavelength, travelling in one direction with the light waves being coherent, each component wave reaching its peaks simultaneously with all other waves. The clinical use of laser is based on light–tissue interactions. Photocoagulation involves light absorption by tissues with pigmented cells (e.g. erythrocytes, retinal pigment epithelial cells) and conversion to heat coagulates the cells and surrounding tissues.

Treatment of diabetic retinopathy using photocoagulation is delivered by instruments which have evolved over the years into a small, portable instrument which uses argon gas. More advanced lasers include the double-frequency Nd:YAG laser, which has comparable efficacy.[38] The power, time exposure and spot size can be changed to suit different requirements.

Pan-retinal photocoagulation (PRP) is carried out by placing 1500–2000 laser burns, each 200–500 μm in diameter depending upon the type of lens used. The burns need to be intense enough to cause whitening of the retina and this is achieved by modifying the power and duration of laser delivery. Burns are scattered throughout the peripheral part of the retina, which is less vital for general visual function. More burns may be required for non-responsive eyes until regression is reached. Laser light is delivered through contact or non-contact fundal lenses into eyes with pupils dilated by topical mydriatics. Topical, periocular or even general anaesthesia may be required. Treatment is carried out in one or more sessions. Extensive PRP delivered in one session may increase the possibility of causing choroidal effusion or macular oedema.

PRP has significant complications. It often causes temporary decreased visual acuity by increasing macular oedema[39–41] or by causing macular pucker. The oedema frequently regresses spontaneously over 6 months. The visual field is usually moderately decreased but is sufficiently well preserved to permit driving in most cases.[42] Colour vision and dark adaptation, which are often already impaired, are worsened by the technique.[43]

Retinal circulation is improved by PRP and there is better regulatory response to hypoxia and decreased blood flow.[44,45] The exact mechanism by which PRP works remains unknown. It may decrease the production of vasoproliferative factors by (1) eliminating some of the hypoxic retina or (2) stimulating the release of antiangiogenic factors from the retinal pigment epithelium.[46] PRP may bring about an increase in vasoinhibitors, either by stimulating the retinal pigment epithelium to produce inhibitors of vasoproliferation[47–50] or by causing a breakdown in the blood–retina barrier so that the serum vasoinhibitors can diffuse into the vitreous.[51]

The Early Treatment Diabetic Retinopathy Study (ETDRS) found that PRP significantly reduces the progression to severe visual loss in high-risk eyes. Approximately two-thirds of eyes that received PRP have regression of their high-risk characteristics by 3 months. Eyes with high-risk characteristics have (1) NVD greater than half the disc area; (2) any NVD and vitreous haemorrhage; or (3) NVE greater than half the disc area and vitreous or pre-retinal haemorrhage. The main findings of the Diabetic Retinopathy Study are summarized in Table 16.4. The study found that

Table 16.4 Results of the Diabetic Retinopathy Study at 3 years

High-risk characteristics	Patients with final visual acuity < 5/200 = 6/240 (%)	
	With PRP	**Without PRP**
NVD less than $^1/_2$ DD with vitreous haemorrhage	4.3	25.6
NVD more than $^1/_2$ DD without vitreous haemorrhage	8.5	26.2
NVD more than $^1/_2$ DD with vitreous haemorrhage	20.1	36.9
NVE more than $^1/_2$ DD with vitreous haemorrhage	7.2	29.7

NVD, neovascularization of the disc; NVE, neovascularization elsewhere; DD, disc diameter; PRP, panretinal photocoagulation.

PRP retards the development of high-risk characteristics in eyes with severe non-proliferative diabetic retinopathy and macular oedema.[52] After 7 years of follow-up, 25% of eyes that received PRP developed high-risk characteristics compared with 75% of eyes in which PRP was deferred until high-risk characteristics developed. Nevertheless, the ETDRS concluded that treatment of non proliferative diabetic retinopathy and proliferative diabetic retinopathy in the absence of high-risk characteristics was not indicated, based on the following findings:

1 After 7 years of follow-up, 25% of eyes assigned to deferral of PRP never developed high- risk characteristics.
2 When patients are closely monitored and PRP is given as soon as high-risk characteristics develop, severe visual loss is prevented. After 7 years of follow-up, 4% of eyes that did not receive PRP until high-risk characteristics developed had a visual acuity of 5/200 (6/240) or less, compared with 2.5% of eyes assigned to immediate PRP. The difference was neither clinically nor statistically significant. Therefore, many eyes with severe non-proliferative diabetic retinopathy that received PRP would be unnecessarily treated.
3 The complications described above.

PRP is considered in patients in the non-high-risk category of proliferative diabetic retinopathy when there are concerns about patient compliance with follow-up or when the treatment is aimed at the second eye in patients who have already had a poor outcome in the other eye. Rubeosis iridis and rubeotic glaucoma, manifestations of severe retinal ischaemia, should be treated with PRP in the presence of clear eye optical media as regression can be induced.[53] However, rubeosis is often associated with advanced proliferative diabetic retinopathy, making it impossible to use further laser treatment due to vitreous haemorrhage. In these circumstances, prompt vitreous surgery is required to enable peroperative photocoagulation to be carried out.

Before PRP was available, the prognosis for patients with proliferative diabetic retinopathy was poor, with blindness developing within 5 years in more than 50% of patients. Rates of blindness in ETDRS patients following the development of proliferative retinopathy are remarkably lower. The risk of progression to legal blindness is reduced to less than 5% in 5 years for patients with proliferative retinopathy. Severe vision loss is reduced to 1%. Furthermore, if visual acuity is stable 3 months after PRP, then visual function is likely to be preserved at 10 years.[54]

Treatment of macular oedema

The ETDRS recommends treating all leaking microaneurysms which are further than 500 μm from the centre of the macula, placing a grid of 100–200 μm burns in areas of either diffuse capillary leakage or capillary non-perfusion. Burns here are gentle, compared with PRP. After 3 years of follow-up, 15% of eyes with clinically significant macular oedema had doubling of the visual angle, as opposed to 32% of non-treated control eyes. Recent sub-group analysis showed that treatment can be deferred in eyes in which the centre of the fovea is not thickened provided that hard exudates are not threatening the centre. Such eyes must be closely observed.[55]

In people with diabetic maculopathy, ETDRS found a significant improvement in visual acuity in eyes treated with grid photocoagulation versus untreated eyes at 12 and 24 months. Photocoagulation versus no photocoagulation reduced the risk of moderate visual loss by 50–70%.[56]

Severe diffuse macular oedema which is non-responsive to grid laser photocoagulation or repeated grid laser photocoagulation may benefit from vitrectomy with removal of the attached posterior vitreous face. Evidence for the value of vitrectomy in tractional diabetic macular oedema comes mostly from interventional case series in cases of severe clinically significant macular oedema refractory to laser therapy.[57–59]

Intra-ocular injections of crystalline steroid preparations (Triamcinolone)

Triamcinolone has been used for treatment of refractory clinically significant macular oedema which has not responded to laser therapy.[60–62] The evidence to date is that retinal thickening, evaluated clinically and by OCT, can be reduced and there is some improvement in vision in some cases. Diff...

Table 16.5 DRVS, diabetic retinopathy vitrectomy study – results of vitrectomy for non clearing vitreous haemorrhage

Visual acuity	Patients (%)
20/20–20/40	25
20/50–20/100	29
20/120–20/300	5
20/400–CF	7
HM–LP	10
NLP	25

CF, counting fingers; HM–LP, hand movements–light perception; NLP, no light perception.

If a patient has a vitreous haemorrhage severe enough to cause a visual acuity of 5/200 (6/240) or less, the chances of visual recovery within 1 year are only about 17%.[68] The DRVS randomized patients who had a visual acuity of 5/200 (6/240) or less for more than 6 months into two groups: those who received an immediate vitrectomy and those whose vitrectomy was deferred for 6 months.[69] Of those who had a deferred vitrectomy, 15% had a final visual acuity of 20/40 (6/12) or better, as opposed to 25% of those who had an immediate vitrectomy. In patients with type I diabetes, 12% of those who had a deferred vitrectomy had a final visual acuity of 20/40 (6/12) or better, as opposed to 36% of those who had an immediate vitrectomy. The reason for this discrepancy was believed to be excessive growth of fibrovascular proliferation during the waiting period. For this reason, the DRVS concluded that strong consideration should be given to immediate vitrectomy, especially in patients with type 1 diabetes. In patients with type 2 diabetes, the final visual results were similar.

If surgery is deferred, then B scan ultrasonography should be performed at regular intervals to make sure that traction retinal detachment is not developing behind the haemorrhage. The goals of surgery are to release all anteroposterior vitreous traction and to perform a complete panretinal photocoagulation to reduce the incidence of recurrent haemorrhage. The results of vitrectomy for non-clearing vitreous haemorrhage are excellent (Table 16.5).

References

mann K, Kovacs P, Boettcher Y, Hammes HP, Paschke R. Genetics of diabetic retinopathy. *Exp Clin Endocrinol Diabetes* 2006;**114**(6):275–294.

2 Klein R, Klein BEK. Epidemiology of proliferative diabetic retinopathy. *Diabetes Care* 1992;**15**:1875–1891.

...y do not benefit from early vitrectomy but they should be observed closely so that vitrectomy, when indicated, can be undertaken promptly.

3 Younis N, Broadbent DM, Harding SP, Vora JP. Incidence of sight-threatening retinopathy in Type 1 diabetes in a systematic screening programme. *Diabet Med* 2003;**20**(9): 758–765.

4 Malone JI, Morrison AD, Pavan PR, Cuthbertson DD; Diabetic Control and Complications Trial. Prevalence and significance of retinopathy in subjects with type 1 diabetes of less than 5 years duration screened for the diabetes control and complications trial. *Diabetes Care* 2001;**24**(3):522–526.

5 Klein R, Klein BE, Moss SE, Cruickshanks KJ. The Wisconsin epidemiologic study of diabetic retinopathy. XIV. Ten-year incidence and progression of diabetic retinopathy. *Arch Ophthalmol* 1994;**112**:1217–1228.

6 Stratton IM, Kohner EM, Adlington S, Mathews DR, Turner RC. Prevalence of diabetic retinopathy at diagnosis of NIDDM in 2964 white Caucasian subjects and association with hypertension, hyperglycaemia and impaired B cell function. *Diabetes* 1995;**44**:117a.

7 Diabetes Control and Complications Trial Research Group. The effect of intensive treatment of diabetes on the development and progression of long term complications in insulin dependent diabetes mellitus. *N Engl J Med* 1993;**32**:977–986.

8 United Kingdom Prospective Diabetes Study Group. Intensive blood glucose control with sulphonylureas or insulin compared with conventional treatment and risk of complications in patients with type 2 diabetes (UKPDS 33). *Lancet* 1998;**352**:837–853.

9 Stratton IM, Adler AI, Neil HA, Matthews DR, Manley SE, Cull CA *et al.* Associaion of glycaemia with macrovascular and microvascular complications of type 2 diabetes (UKPDS 35). *BMJ* 2000;**321**:405–412.

10 White NH, Cleary PA, Dahms W, Goldstein D, Malone J, Tamborlane WV and Diabetes Control and Complications Trial (DCCT)/Epidemiology of Diabetes Interventions and complications (EDIC) Research Group. Beneficial effects of intensive therapy of diabetes during adolescence: outcomes after the conclusion of the Diabetes Control and Complications Trial (DCCT). *J Pediatr* 2001;**139**(6): 804–812.

11 Dahl-Jorgensen K, Brinchmann-Hansen O, Hanssen KF, Sandvik L, Aagenaes O. Rapid tightening of blood glucose control leads to transient deterioration of retinopathy in insulin dependent diabetes mellitus: the Oslo study. *Br Med J (Clin Res Ed)* 1985;**290**(6471):811–815.

12 Arun CS, Pandit R, Taylor R. Long term progression of retinopathy after initiation of insulin therapy in type 2 diabetes. *Diabetologia* 2004;**47**:1380–1384.

13 Matthews DR, Stratton IM, Aldington SJ, Holman RR, Kohner EM. Risks of progression of retinopathy and vision loss related to tight blood pressure control in type 2 diabetes mellitus: UKPDS 69. *Arch Ophthalmol* 2004;**122** (11):1631–1640.

14 Klein R, Klein BEK, Moss SE, Davis MD, DeMets DL. The Wisconsin epidemiologic study of diabetic retinopathy. II. Prevalence and risk of diabetic retinopathy when age is less than 30 years. *Arch Ophthalmol* 1984;**102**:520–526.

15 DCCT Research Group. Effect of pregnancy on microvascular complications in the DCCT research group. *Diabetes Care* 2000;**23**:1084–1091.

16 Maayah J, Shammas A, Haddadin A. Effect of pregnancy on diabetic retinopathy. *Bahrain Med Bull* 2001;**23**:163–165.

17 Klein BE, Moss SE, Klein R. Effect of pregnancy on progression of diabetic reinopathy. *Diabetes Care* 1990;**13**:34–40.

18 Rosenn B, Miodovnik M, Kranias G *et al.* Progression of diabetic retinopathy in pregnancy: association with hypertension in pregnancy. *Am J Obstet Gynecol* 1992;**166**: 1214–1218.

19 Early Treatment Diabetic Retinopathy Study Research Group. Grading diabetic retinopathy from stereoscopic color fundus photographs – an extension of the Airlie House classification. ETDRS report No. 10. *Ophthalmology* 1991;**98**: 786.

20 Wilkinson CP, Ferris FL III, Klein RE, Lee PP, Agardh CD, Davis M, Dills D, Kampik A, Pararajasegaram R, Verdaguer JT and the Global Diabetic Retinopathy Group. Proposed international clinical diabetic retinopathy and diabetic macular edema disease severity scales. *Ophthalmology* 2003;**110**: 1677.

21 Arun CS, Ngugi N, Taylor R. Effectiveness of screening in preventing blindness due to diabetic retinopathy. *Diabet Med* 2003;**20**:186–190.

22 Harding S, Greenwood R, Aldington S, Gibson J, Owens D, Taylor R, Kohner E, Scanlon P, Leese G. Grading and disease management in national screening for diabetic retinopathy in England and Wales. *Diabet Med* 2003;**20**:965.

23 Stratton IM, Kohner EM, Aldington SJ, Turner RC, Holman RR, Manley SE, Matthews DR. UKPDS 50: risk factors for incidence and progression of retinopathy in Type II diabetes over 6 years from diagnosis. *Diabetologia* 2001;**44**(2): 156–163.

24 Harding SP, Broadbent DM, Neoh C, White MC, Vora J. Sensitivity and specificity of photography and direct ophthalmoscopy in screening for sight threatening eye disease: the Liverpool Diabetic Eye Study. *BMJ* 1995;**311**(7013):1131–1135.

25 Scanlon PH, Malhotra R, Greenwood RH, Aldington SJ, Foy C, Flatman M, Downes S. Comparison of two reference standards in validating two field mydriatic digital photography as a method of screening for diabetic retinopathy. *Br J Ophthalmol* 2003;**87**(10):1258–1263.

26 Taylor R, Lovelock L, Tunbridge WM, Alberti KG, Brackenridge RG, Stephenson P, Young E. Comparison of non-mydriatic retinal photography with ophthalmoscopy in 2159 patients: mobile retinal camera study. *BMJ* 1990;**301** (6763):1243–1247.

27 Pandit RJ, Taylor R. Quality assurance in screening for sight-threatening diabetic retinopathy. *Diabet Med* 2002;**19** (4):285–291.

28 (a) Arun CS, Young D, Batey D, Shotton M, Mitchie D, Stannard K, Taylor R. Establishing an ongoing quality assurance in retinal screening programme. *Diabet Med* 2005;**23**:629–634; (b) Taylor R. *Handbook of Retinal Screening,* John Wiley & Sons Ltd, Chichester, 2006.

29 Maloney JBM, Drury MI. The effect of pregnancy on the natural course of diabetic retinopathy. *Am. J. Ophthalmol* 1982;**93**:745.

30 Scanlon PH, Foy C, Malhotra R, Aldington SJ. The influence of age, duration of diabetes, cataract and pupil size on image quality in digital photographic retinal screening. *Diabetes Care* 2005;**28**(10):2448–2453.

31 Pandit R, Taylor R. Mydriasis and glaucoma: exploding the myth. *Diabet Med* 2000;**17**:693–699.

32 Bailey IL, Lovie JE. New design principles for visual acuity letter charts. *Am J Optom Physiol Opt* 1976;**53**: 740–745.

33 JDM. *Stereoscopic Atlas of Macular Diseases: Diagnosis and Treatment*, 4th edn, Mosby Year Book, St. Louis, MO, 1997.

34 Rabb MF, Burton TC, Schatz H, Yannuzzi LA. Fluorescein angiography of the fundus: a schematic approach to interpretation. *Surv Ophthalmol* 1978;**22**:387–403.

35 Huang D, Swanson EA, Lin CP *et al.* Optical coherence tomography. *Science* 1992;**254**:1178.

36 Swanson EA, Izatt JA, Hee MR *et al. In vivo* retinal imaging by optical coherence tomography. *Opt Lett* 1993;**18**: 1864.

37 Hee MR, Izatt JA, Swanson EA *et al.* Optical coherence tomography of the human retina. *Arch Ophthalmol* 1995;**113**: 325.

38 Bandello F, Brancato R, Lattanzio R, Trabucchi G, Azzolini C, Malegori A. Double-frequency Nd:YAG laser vs. argon-green laser in the treatment of proliferative diabetic retinopathy: randomized study with long-term follow-up. *Laser Surg Med* 1996;**19**(2):173–176.

39 Meyers SM. Macular edema after scatter laser photocoagulation for proliferative diabetic retinopathy. *Am J Ophthalmol* 1980;**90**:210.

40 Ferris FL, Podgor MJ, Davis MD. The Diabetic Retinopathy Research Group: macular edema in diabetic retinopathy study patients. *Ophthalmology* 1987;**94**:754.

41 Kleiner RC, Elman MJ, Murphy RP *et al.* Transient severe visual loss after panretinal photocoagulation. *Am J Ophthalmol* 1988;**106**:298.

42 Cambie E., Functional results following argon laser photocoagulation in eyes with diabetic retinopathy. In: *Diabetic Renal— Retinal Syndrome* (eds EA Friedman, FA L'Esperance,), Grune and Stratton, New York, 1980, pp. 295–307.

43 Henson DB, North RV. Dark adaptation in diabetes mellitus. *Br J Ophthalmol* 1979;**63**:539.

44 Patel V, Rassam S, Newsom R *et al.* Retinal blood flow in diabetic retinopathy. *BMJ* 1992;**305**:678.

45 Grunwald JE, Brucker AJ, Petrig BL *et al.* Retinal blood flow regulation and the clinical response to panretinal photocoagulation in proliferative diabetic retinopathy. *Ophthalmology* 1989;**96**:1518.

46 Glaser BM, Campochiaro PA, Davis DL Jr, Sato M. Retinal pigment epithelial cells release an inhibitor of neovascularization. *Arch Ophthalmol* 1985;**103**:1870.

47 Stefansson E, Landers MB III, Wolbarsht ME. Oxygenation and vasodilation in relation to diabetic and other proliferative retinopathies. *Ophthalmic Surg* 1983;**17**:209.

48 Wolbarsht ML, Landers MB III, Stefansson E. Vasodilation and the etiology of diabetic retinopathy: a new model. *Ophthalmic Surg* 1981;**12**(2):104–107.

49 Wolbarsht ML, Landers MB. The rationale of photocoagulation therapy for proliferative diabetic retinopathy: a review and a model. *Ophthalmic Surg* 1980;**11**:235.

50 Stefansson E, Machemer R, de Juan E Jr *et al.* Retinal oxygenation and laser treatment in patients with diabetic retinopathy. *Am J Ophthalmol* 1992;**113**:36.

51 Schiodte N. Ocular effects of panretinal photocoagulation. *Acta Ophthalmol* 1988;**66**(Suppl): 9.

52 Early Treatment Diabetic Retinopathy Study Research Group. Early photocoagulation for diabetic retinopathy: ETDRS report number 9. *Ophthalmology* 1991;**98**:766.

53 Murphy RP, Egbert PR. Regression of iris neovascularization following panretinal photocoagulation. *Arch Ophthalmol* 1979;**97**(4):700–702.

54 Kohner EM, Porta M. Diabetic retinopathy: preventing blindness in the 1990's. *Diabetologia* 1991;**34**(11):844–845.

55 Early Treatment Diabetic Retinopathy Study Research Group. Focal photocoagulation treatment of diabetic macular edema: relationship of treatment effect to fluorescein angiographic and other retinal characteristics at baseline: ETDRS report No. 19. *Arch Ophthalmol* 1995;**113**(9): 1144–1155.

56 Olk RJ. Modified grid argon (blue–green) laser photocoagulation for diffuse diabetic macular edema. *Ophthalmology* 1986;**93**:938.

57 Massin P, Duguid G, Erginay A, Haouchine B, Gaudric A. Optical coherence tomography for evaluating diabetic macular edema before and after vitrectomy. *Am J Ophthalmol* 2003;**135**:169.

58 Yamamoto T, Hitani K, Tsukahara I, Yamamoto R, Kawasaki R, Yamashita H, Takeuchi S. Early postoperative retinal thickness changes and complications after vitrectomy for diabetic macular edema. *Am J Ophthalmol* 2003;**135**: 14.

59 Lewis H, Abrams GW, Blumenkranz S, Campochiaro PV. Resolution of diabetic macular oedema associated with a thickened and taut posterior hyaloid after vitrectomy (abstract). *Ophthalmology* 1991;**98**(Suppl): 146.

60 Jonas JB, Kreissig I, Sofker A, Degenring RF. Intravitreal injection of triamcinolone for diffuse diabetic macular edema. *Arch Ophthalmol* 2003;**121**:57.

61 Jonas JB, Sofker A. Intraocular injection of crystalline cortisone as adjunctive treatment of diabetic macular edema. *Am J Ophthalmol* 2001;**132**:425.

62 Beer PM, Bakri SJ, Singh RJ, Liu W, Peters GB III, Miller M. Intraocular concentration and pharmacokinetics of triamcinolone acetonide after a single intravitreal injection. *Ophthalmology* 2003;**110**:681.

63 Cunningham ET Jr, Adamis AP, Altaweel M, Aeillo LP *et al.* Macugen diabetic retinopathy study group. A phase II randomized double-masked trial of pegaptanib, an anti-vascular endothelial growth factor aptamer, for diabetic macular edema. *Ophthalmology* 2005;**112**(10): 1747–1757.

64 Lewis H, Abrams GW, Blumenkranz MS, Campo RV. Vitrectomy for diabetic macular traction and edema associated with posterior hyaloidal traction. *Ophthalmology* 1992;**99**:753.

65 Harbour JW, Smiddy WE, Flynn HW, Rubsamen PE. Vitrectomy for diabetic macular edema associated with a thickened and taut posterior hyaloid membrane. *Am J Ophthalmol* 1996;**121**:405.

66 Ramsay RC, Knobloch WH, Cantrill HL. Timing of vitrectomy for active proliferative diabetic retinopathy. *Ophthalmology* 1986;**93**:283.

67 Diabetic Retinopathy Vitrectomy Study Research Group. Early vitrectomy for severe proliferative diabetic retinopathy in eyes with useful vision: results of a randomized trial – Diabetic Retinopathy Vitrectomy Study report 3. *Ophthalmology* 1988;**95**:1307.

68 Diabetic Retinopathy Vitrectomy Study Research Group. Two year course of visual acuity in severe proliferative diabetic retinopathy with conventional management. *Ophthalmology* 1985;**92**:492.

69 Diabetic Retinopathy Vitrectomy Study Research Group. Early vitrectomy for severe vitreous hemorrhage in diabetic retinopathy: two year results of a randomized trial – Diabetic Retinopathy Vitrectomy Study report 2. *Arch Ophthalmol* 1985;**103**:1644.

17 Prevention and treatment of diabetic nephropathy: the role of blood pressure lowering

Carl Erik Mogensen

Department of Internal Medicine M (Diabetes and Endocrinology), Aarhus University Hospital, Aarhus, Denmark

Introduction

Several factors are important in determining the rate of progression of diabetic renal disease from microalbuminuria,[1,2] with elevated blood pressure being a major factor, in both type 1 and type 2 diabetes.[3] Although the prognosis for diabetic nephropathy has improved in the last two decades, proteinuric patients still have a very poor prognosis. Patients with type 2 diabetes and proteinuria often die from cardiovascular disease before progression to end-stage renal disease (ESRD), even more than patients with type 1 diabetes and albuminuria.[3] For both types of diabetes, elevated blood pressure, glycaemic control and albuminuria are major factors in progression of nephropathy[3] Individual case histories of patients with unilateral renal arterial stenosis demonstrate the role of local blood pressure (BP) level in generating structural damage, which was not seen in post-stenotic kidney.[4,5]

Hence there can be no doubt that high BP is a major factor in progression of diabetic nephropathy in the two types of diabetes. Agents that block the renin–angiotensin system (RAS), angiotensin-converting enzyme inhibitors (ACE-i) or angiotensin II receptor blockers (ARBs), now dominate antihypertensive treatment in these patients.[3,6] In the management of patients, not only renal prognosis, including the rate of decline in glomerular filtration rate (GFR), should be considered, but also cardiovascular endpoints. Obviously, cost–benefit considerations must also be taken into account. It should also be considered whether the so-called dual blockade with both

ACE-i and ARB may further improve risk factors and prognosis as compared with single blockade of RAS.[6] Another important question remains to be answered: is traditional antihypertensive treatment inferior to agents that block the RAS system in inhibiting progression of diabetic nephropathy? It can be concluded that there is not a substantial difference between risk factors and progression promoters in the two types of diabetes and the same strategy for treatment seems warranted, but early treatment is essential.[1,2] As the result of more intensified treatment, the incidence of ESRD seems now to have declined, at least for type 1 diabetes. However, the epidemic rise in the prevalence of type 2 diabetes is likely to be followed by an epidemic in renal and other complications.[3,7,8]

New meta-analysis of BP lowering

Recently, two major meta-analyses of the effect of BP lowering on renal outcomes and major cardiovascular events have been published.[9,10] The principal message from these two important studies based on randomized trials is that the main effect of BP lowering is in fact the BP lowering itself and not the specific method or type of BP-lowering medication. This is clearly the case for major cardiovascular events.[9] The studies indicate that the benefits from ACE inhibition or ARBs on renal outcomes in placebo-controlled trials probably result from the effective BP-lowering effect of these agents. The renal meta-analysis concludes[10] that

The Evidence Base for Diabetes Care, Second Edition, Edited by William H. Herman, Ann Louise Kinmonth, Nicholas J. Wareham and Rhys Williams.
© 2010 John Wiley & Sons, Ltd

in patients with diabetes, additional renal protection action of these agents beyond BP lowering remains unproved. It is important to point out, however, that lowering of urinary albumin concentration is seen with RAS inhibition. This is considered as a positive effect in patients with diabetes as in people without diabetes.

The positive effect of blocking the RAS is clearly related to BP. If the BP is reduced by a mean of 6.8 mmHg, there is a major benefit in using agents that block the RAS. With only a minor reduction in BP, the effect is almost neutral, suggesting that it is the BP lowering *per se* associated with RAS inhibition that is important.[10]

This clearly points to the old observation[11] that increased BP is a major risk factor for progression of diabetic renal disease and that treatment of BP reduces the later decline in GFR and also ESRD. The use of ACE-i and ARBs is thus beneficial by lowering BP. Casas *et al.* argue that their study shows that there is an absence of evidence to support renoprotective effects of renin–angiotensin inhibitors independently of BP lowering.[12] Further studies are needed, but may be difficult to conduct.

Blocking the RAS seems to have a beneficial effect by reducing the risk of type 2 diabetes in some studies, but not in all.[13,14] Beyond the prevention of nephropathy, the use of ACE-i is beneficial in diabetic patients with heart disease, which is commonly seen in conjunction with nephropathy.[15,16] The mechanisms remain to be explained.

Meta-analysis and the effect of ACE-i and ARBs on renal outcomes and mortality

It would be of interest to compare ACE-i with ARBs, because we know that ACE-i are effective in type 1 and type 2 diabetes (Table 17.1).[16] The question put forward in a recent meta-analysis was whether there was a difference between ACE-i and ARBs in the risk of adverse renal outcomes and all-cause mortality in patients with diabetic nephropathy. The data extracted from the meta-analysed studies including a total of about 7500 patients focused on renal outcomes and mortality, which were:

1 prevention of progression of micro- and macroalbuminuria and regression to normoalbuminuria;
2 doubling of serum creatinine concentration;
3 ESRD and the final outcome in all studies: mortality.

Both agents had similar effect on renal outcomes when confounding factors were taken into consideration. Comparing ACE-i directly with ARBs was at that time difficult, but results from a new study [the Diabetics Exposed to Telmisartan And enalapriL (DETAIL) trial] are now available.[17] ACE-i had a significant effect on overall mortality, mainly driven by the MICRO-HOPE study.[18,19] The test for the overall effect on mortality had a *p*-value of 0.04. A similar result was seen in a large Chinese study.[20] In contrast, the ARBs had no significant effect on mortality, with a *p*-value of 0.95.[16] This is important because patients with renal disease may not die from ESRD (they undergo dialysis) and the cause of death, especially in type 2 diabetes, is primarily cardiac mortality. A similar result was seen in a large Chinese study.[21]

This issue has been further addressed by the DETAIL trial.[17] DETAIL was a much-needed, long-term study comparing an ACE-i with an ARB head-to-head in a diabetic population. The 5 year, prospective, multicentre, double-blind study directly compared the ACE-i enalapril with the ARB telmisartan in patients with type 2 diabetes, hypertension and evidence of early nephropathy and in many cases microalbuminuria. DETAIL was also the first study of its kind to monitor the progression of kidney disease by directly measuring the GFR, now recognized as the best indicator of overall kidney function and ESRD.

The fall in GFR at 5 years – the main endpoint – was the same in patients treated with either drug, with

Table 17.1 Inhibition of the renin–angiotensin system in diabetes[a]

	Prevention of microalbuminuria	Treating microalbuminuria	Treating macroalbuminuria	Left ventricular hypertrophy	Heart failure
ACE-i	+++ BENEDICT[28]	T1 +++[2] T2 +++ (DETAIL)[17]	T1 +++[2] T2 +[13]		+++[15]
ARBs	Roadmap study[45] (in progress) (DIRECTrenal, *Ann Int Med* 2009; in press)	T1 –T2 +++ (DETAIL)[17]	T1 – T2 +++ (RENAAL) IDNT[38–40]	T2 +++ (LIFE)[22]	+[15]

[a] +, ++, +++, increasing levels of strength of evidence.

changes in GFR from baseline of around $-17\,\mathrm{ml\,min^{-1}}$ per $1.73\,\mathrm{m^2}$ in the telmisartan group and $-15\,\mathrm{ml\,min^{-1}}$ per $1.73\,\mathrm{m^2}$ in the enalapril group. Analysis of the secondary endpoint of the yearly change in GFR revealed an initial steep decline in GFR in both groups, of around $-8\,\mathrm{ml\,min^{-1}}$ per $1.73\,\mathrm{m^2}$, which then stabilized to around $-2\,\mathrm{ml\,min^{-1}}$ per $1.73\,\mathrm{m^2}$ beyond 3 years.

BP was lowered to a comparable extent in each treatment group and cardiovascular (CV) mortality was much lower than would be expected at 5 years, with three and five CV-related deaths in the telmisartan and enalapril groups, respectively. Other adverse event rates were similar between the two groups, since ACE-i-intolerant patients were excluded from the study. There were no cases of ESRD in either group.

Other shorter studies have indicated that the ACE-i and ARBs produce similar effects as far as albuminuria and BP are concerned.[31–36] Furthermore, dual blockade using a drug of each class is a possible approach in patients who do not respond well to single blockade, especially in microalbuminuric patients.[34,36]

Thus, with the latest results from DETAIL in mind, the clinician may choose either an ACE inhibitor or an ARB or even the two in combination. However, questions remain regarding the longer term benefits in advanced nephropathy. The strong endpoint studies, namely the RENAAL study and the IDNT study, in patients with type 2 diabetes and overt nephropathy are important.[37,39] The results of these studies would favour the use of ARBs and as yet there are no similar studies comparing ACE-i with ARBs to provide further information in this patient group. Indeed, compared with advanced disease intervention in microalbuminuric patients may prove much more effective.[2]

Another impressive finding of the meta-analysis is that there was a very significant effect on regression from microalbuminuria to normoalbuminuria by ACE-i – an effect that has been observed earlier for type 1 diabetes.[22]

Strippoli et al.[16] finally pointed out the need for more comparative trials. For instance, the ARB losartan was compared positively with a β-blocker in hypertensive diabetic (and non-diabetic) patients with left ventricular hypertrophy in the LIFE study.[22] In addition, it was concluded that combination therapy, including the use of diuretics, is important.

Preventing microalbuminuria in diabetes

Prevention of microalbuminuria is the initial step in preventing diabetic kidney disease.[25] Ravid et al. examined type 2 diabetic patients with normoalbuminuria treated with an ACE-i.[26] The ACE-i

prevented the development of microalbuminuria.[26,27] Kvetny et al. showed the same for type 1 diabetes using perindopril.[27] The Bergamo Nephrologic Diabetes Complications Trial (BENEDICT) was recently published.[28] It is important to distinguish between normo- and microalbuminuria and renal insufficiency, as confirmed in the study by Adler et al. of UKPDS.[29] Clearly, patients with normoalbuminuria have the best prognosis and there is evidence to show that preventing progression is associated with a much better prognosis, which was also documented in the recent paper by Gæde et al. of the Steno Diabetes Centre. They showed that regression to normoalbuminuria is associated with much better preservation of renal function in terms of GFR fall, which is stabilized.[30,31]

The BENEDICT study is the largest study conducted so far. It also compared an ACE-i with a calcium channel blocker, verapamil. This large study in Northern Italy included 1204 patients randomly designated to 3 years of treatment with trandolapril alone, trandolapril + verapamil, verapamil alone and placebo.[28] Interestingly, hypertension was defined as a BP above $130/85\,\mathrm{mmHg}$ or ongoing antihypertensive treatment. The primary endpoint was development of persistent microalbuminuria with an overnight albumin excretion rate higher than $20\,\mathrm{mg\,min^{-1}}$ on two consecutive occasions.

The primary outcome was seen in 6% of the patients treated with the ACE-i alone and in 10% of the patients receiving placebo ($p = 0.01$) Treatment with verapamil alone was not different from placebo. The authors also estimated the so-called acceleration factors, which were clearly in favour of the use of the ACE-i. There were only minor differences in BP between the treatment arms, but this may still have played a role for the positive results with the ACE-i. There were few serious events in the two treatment groups. The conclusion was clear: in patients with type 2 diabetes and hypertension (above $130/85\,\mathrm{mmHg}$) but with normoalbuminuria, treatment with an ACE-i was clearly beneficial in preventing the development of microalbuminuria, which is the first sign of renal damage in these patients. Microalbuminuria is a major risk factor for vascular events and for advanced renal disease and death.[2,29]

In conclusion, there is now fairly good evidence from clinical trials that treatment with an ACE-i should be started early in patients with type 2 diabetes and normoalbuminuria. Treatment should be initiated when the systolic BP is more than $130\,\mathrm{mmHg}$. Systolic BP elevation is very common in patients with type 2 diabetes and metabolic syndrome. This means that most type 2 diabetic patients would qualify for this type of treatment. These patients also often show sodium retention and therefore a combination of an

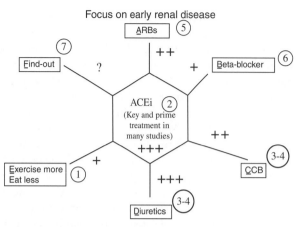

+ indicate the level of evidence
The numbers indicate sequence of treatment (1-7) (vary from patient to patient)
Remember sufficient doses, clinical, and laboratory control

Figure 17.1 The BP-lowering hexagon (ABCDEF) in diabetes

ACE-i and diuretics seems to be most effective in reducing microalbuminuria and BP. There now seems to be a very good foundation for substantial improvements in the prognosis for patients with type 2 diabetes.[2,3] Early treatment of hypertension leads to better prognosis, as does, but maybe to a lesser extent, improved glycaemic control.[29] Treatment with statins is also important, as documented in many studies, including the Steno 2 study.[30,31] Now we have apparently completed the paradigm shift: it is essential to normalize glycaemia BP, and dyslipidaemia in all patients with type 2 diabetes. The BP-lowering hexagon (Figure 17.1) summarizes antihypertensive treatment in diabetes.

Regression of albuminuria: a new paradigm shift

It is well known to diabetologists that patients with 'proteinuria' or 'albuminuria' have a poor prognosis. The same is true, to a lesser extent, for microalbuminuria. Indeed, the higher the level of albuminuria, the greater is the risk of renal progression and the risk of all complications including early mortality.[3] These results come from studies of the natural history of diabetic nephropathy, in both type 1 and type 2 diabetes. The next question is, of course, whether regression or remission of albuminuria is of clinical relevance. Is it really associated with better prognosis? Blocking the RAS as well as dual blockade should be considered along with several other BP-lowering strategies.

This question was recently discussed by Hovind et al., who analysed whether remission of nephrotic-range albuminuria is associated with a better prognosis.[41] This, indeed, seems to be the case. It is now clear also from other studies that remission of albuminuria[41–43] signifies a good prognosis, also in microalbuminuric patients. The results from the LIFE study,[22] including diabetic patients, and the RENAAL study clearly document that reduction of albuminuria and microalbuminuria really indicates a prognosis.[37,39]

Hence it is important to screen for microalbuminuria, but also to follow up the assessment of albuminuria. Physicians should look for reduction by means of better BP control, especially ACE inhibition or other blockade of the RAS.

This is indeed a second paradigm shift. The first paradigm shift[1,2] was to screen for microalbuminuria and the next is now to follow up on the level of albuminuria.[41–43]

It is not difficult to screen for microalbuminuria. In our unit, for example, we use the first morning or a random urine sample. This is used for screening using the albumin to creatinine ratio, which is a good measure of the albumin excretion rate, both in the short term and over 24 h. There are good and reliable reference values.[2] It could be argued that the classification into the categories of normo-, macro- and microalbuminuria is somewhat artificial because albuminuria, like many other parameters including glycaemic control, BP and cholesterol, is a continuously distributed variable. However, it is practical in the screening process to classify people into these categories. Microalbuminuria is associated not only with progression to renal disease, but also with early mortality.

Part of the explanation for the improved outcome associated with reduction in albuminuria or microalbuminuria relates to reduction of BP and treatment with agents that block the RAS, but this may not be the whole story. Reduction in albuminuria means that the pressure over the glomerular membrane is specifically reduced and there is good evidence to indicate that pressure-induced damage is an important factor for the deterioration in renal function observed in diabetic patients with proteinuria. Patients with microalbuminuria usually have well-preserved renal function and thus, by reducing microalbuminuria by better treatment, both glycaemic and antihypertensive treatment translate into better preservation of GFR[30,31] and, in this situation, preservation of renal function before the decline in GFR. With proteinuria there is normally a decline in GFR, which is related to a traditional risk factors, namely elevated BP, microalbuminuria and HbA$_{1c}$ – risk markers that are clearly modifiable.

It is clear that early antihypertensive treatment has improved the prognosis for diabetic patients dramatically and the prognosis may further improve with early screening for microalbuminuria and follow-up to monitor whether microalbuminuria is reduced. On the other hand, it may seem a paradox that we still have an increase in the number of patients developing end-stage renal failure due to diabetes. However, this is explained by the fact that many more patients develop type 2 diabetes and that these patients have a longer period of survival, because of better cardiovascular management, but further studies are needed.

References

1 Mogensen CE. Prediction of clinical diabetic nephropathy in type 1 diabetic patients: alternatives to microalbuminuria? Messages related to the microalbuminuria concept: 1990–2006. *Diabetes Care* 2006;**29**:113–115.

2 Mogensen CE. Microalbuminuria and hypertension with focus on type 1 and type 2 diabetes. *J Intern Med* 2003;**254**:45–66.

3 Thomas AC, Atkins RC. Blood pressure lowering for the prevention and treatment of diabetic kidney disease. Submitted.

4 Berkman J, Rifkin H. Unilateral nodular diabetic glomerulosclerosis (Kimmelstiel–Wilston): report of a case. *Metabolism* 1973;**22**:715–722.

5 Beronoiade VC, Lefebvre R, Falardeau P. Unilateral nodular diabetic glomerulosclerosis: Recurrence of and experiment of nature. *Am J Nephrol* 1987;**7**:55–59.

6 Wolf G, Ritz E. Combination therapy with ACE inhibitors and angiotensin II receptor blockers to halt progression of chronic renal disease: Pathophysiology and indications. *Kidney Int* 2005;**67**:799–812.

7 Astrup AA, Tarnow L, Rossing P et al. Improved prognosis in type 1 diabetic patients with nephropathy: a prospective follow-up study. *Kidney Int* 2005;**68**:1250–1257.

8 Finne P, Reunanen A, Stenman S et al. Incidence of end-stage renal disease in patients with type 1 diabetes. *JAMA* 2005;**294**:1782–1787.

9 Blood Pressure Lowering Treatment Trialists' Collaboration. Effects of different blood pressure-lowering regimens on major cardiovascular events in individuals with and without diabetes mellitus. *Arch Intern Med* 2005;**165**:1410–1419.

10 Casas JP, Chua W, Loukogeorgakis S et al. Effect of inhibitors of the renin–angiotensin system and other antihypertensive drugs on renal outcomes: systematic review and meta-analysis. *Lancet* 2005;**36**:2026–2033.

11 Mogensen CE. Diabetic renal disease: the quest for normotension – and beyond. *Diabet Med* 1995;**12**:756–769.

12 Casas JP, Vallance P, Smeeth L et al. Authors' reply. *Lancet* 2006;**367**:900–901.

13 Scheen AJ. Renin–angiotensin system inhibition prevents type 2 diabetes mellitus. Part 2. Overview of physiological and biochemical mechanisms. *Diabetes Metab* 2004;**39**: 498–505.

14 Mancia G, Grassi G, Zanchetti A. New-onset diabetes and antihypertensive drugs. *J Hypertens* 2006;**24**:3–10.

15 Mogensen CE, Andersen NH. Diabetic renal and related heart diesease. ACE-inhibitors and/or angiotensin receptor blockers: does it matter? In: Contemporary Diabetes: the Diabetic Kidney (eds P Cortes, CE Mogensen), Humana Press, Totowa, NJ, 2006, pp. 435–351.

16 Strippoli GF, Craig M, Deeks JJ et al. Effect of angiotensin converting enzyme inhibitors and angiotensin II receptor antagonists on mortality and renal outcomes in diabetic nephropathy: systematic review. *BMJ* 2004;**329**:828–831.

17 Barnett AH, Bain SC et al. Angiotensin-receptor blockade versus converting-enzyme inhibition in type 2 diabetes and nephropathy. *N Engl J Med* 2004;**351**:1952–1961.

18 Heart Outcomes Prevention Evaluation Study Investigators. Effects of ramipril on cardiovascular and microvascular outcomes in people with diabetes mellitus: results of the HOPE study and MICRO-HOPE substudy. *Lancet* 2000;**355**: 253–259.

19 HOPE/HOPE-TOO Study Investigators. Long-term effects of ramipril on cardiovascular events and on diabetes. *Results of the HOPE study extension. Circulation* 2005;**112**: 1339–1346.

20 So WY, Ozaki R, Chan NN et al. Effect of angiotensin-converting enzyme inhibition on survival in 3773 Chinese type 2 diabetic patients. *Hypertension* 2004;**44**:294–299.

21 ACE-Inhibitors in Diabetic Nephropathy Trialist Group. Should all patients with type 1 diabetes mellitus and microalbuminuria receive angiotensin-converting-enzyme inhibitors? A meta-analysis of individual patient data. *Ann Intern Med* 2001;**134**:370–379.

22 Ibsen H, Olsen MH, Wachtell K et al. Does albuminuria predict cardiovascular outcomes on treatment with losartan versus atenolol in patients with diabetes, hypertension and left ventricular hypertrophy? The LIFE Study. *Diabetes Care* 2006;**29**:595–600.

23 The DREAM Trial Investigators. Rationale, design and recruitment characteristics of a large, simple international trial of diabetes prevention; The DREAM Trial. *Diabetologia* 2004;**47**:1519–1527.

24 Unger T. The ongoing telmisartan alone and in combination with Ramipril Global Endpoint Trial program. *Am J Cardiol* 2003;**91**(Suppl): 28G–34G.

25 Strippoli GFM, Craig M, Schena FP, Craig JC. Antihypertensive agents for primary prevention of diabetic nephropathy. *J Am Soc Nephrol* 2005;**16**:3081–3091.

26 Ravid M, Brosh D, Levi Z *et al.* Use of enalapril to attenuate decline in renal function in normotensive patients with type 2 diabetes mellitus. *Ann Intern Med* 2009;**128**:982–988.

27 Kvetny J, Gregersen G, Pedersen RS. Randomized pacebo-controlled trial of perindopril in normotensive, normoalbuminuric patients with type 1 diabetes mellitus. *Q J Med* 2001;**94**:89–94.

28 Ruggenenti P, Fassi A *et al.* Preventing microalbuminuria in type 2 diabetes. *N Engl J Med* 2004;**351**:1941–1951.

29 Adler AI, Stevens RJ *et al.* Development and progression of nephropathy in type 2 diabetes: the United Kingdom Prospective Diabetes Study. *Kidney Int* 2003;**63**:225–232.

30 Gæde P, Lund-Andersen H, Parving H-H, Pedersen O. Effect Multifactorial intervention on mortality in type 2 diabetes. *N Engl J Med*. 2008;**358**:580–591.

31 Gæde P, Tarnow L, Vedel P, Parving H-H, Pedersen O. Remission to normoalbuminuria during multifactorial treatment preserves kidney function in patients with type 2 diabetes and microalbuminuria. *Nephrol Dial Transplant* 2004;**19**: 2784–2788.

32 Lacourcière Y, Bélanger A, Godin C *et al.* Long-term comparison of losartan and enalapril on kidney function in hypertensive Type 2 diabetics with early nephropathy. *Kidney Int* 2000;**58**:762–769.

33 Derosa G, Cicero AFG, Ciccareeli L, Fogari R, A randomized, double-blind, controlled parallel-group comparison of perindopril and candesartan in hypertensive patients with type 2 diabetes mellitus. *Clin Ther* 2003;**25**:2006–2021.

34 Muirhead N, Feagan BF, Mahon J *et al.* The effects of valsartan and captopril on reducing microalbuminuria in patients with Type 2 diabetes mellitus: a placebo-controlled trial. *Curr Ther Res* 1999;**60**:650–660.

35 Mogensen CE, Neldam S, Tikkanen I *et al.* Randomised controlled trial of dual blockade of renin-angiotensin system in patients with hypertension, microalbuminuria and non-insulin dependent diabetes: the candesartan and lisinopril microalbuminuria (CALM) study. *BMJ* 2000;**321**: 1440–1444.

36 Izzo JL, Weinberg MS *et al.* Antihypertensive efficacy of candesartan–lisinoprilincombination vs. up-titration of lisinopril:theAMAZEtrials. *J Clin Hypertens* 2004;**6**:485–493.

37 Fujisawa T, Ikegami H, Ono M *et al.* Combination of half doses of angiotensin type 1 receptor antagonist and angiotensin-converting enzyme inhibitor in diabetic nephropathy. *Am J Hypertens* 2005;**18**:13–17.

38 Brenner BM, Cooper ME *et al.* Effects of losartan on renal and cardiovascular outcomes in patients with type 2 diabetes and nephropathy. *N Engl J Med* 2001;**345**:861–869.

39 Lewis EJ, Hunsicker LG *et al.* Renoprotective effect of the angiotensin-receptor antagonist irbesartan in patients with nephropathy due to type 2 diabetes. *N Engl J Med* 2001;**345**: 851–860.

40 Parving H-H, Lehnert H, Brochner-Mortensen JK *et al.* The effect of irbesartan on the development of diabetic nephropathy in patients with type 2 diabetes. *N Engl J Med* 2001;**345**:870–878.

41 Hovind P, Tarnow L *et al.* Improved survival in patients obtaining remission of nephrotic range albuminuria in diabetic nephropathy'. *Kidney Int* 2004;**66**:1180–1186.

42 Yuyun MF, Dinnesen SF *et al.* Absolute level and rate of change of albuminuria over 1 year independently predict mortality and cardiovascular events in patients with diabetic nephropathy. *Diabet Med* 2003;**20**:277–282.

43 Spoelstra-de Man AM, Brouwer CB *et al.* Rapid progression of albumin excretion is an independent predictor of cardiovascular mortality in patients with type 2 diabetes and microalbuminuria. *Diabetes Care* 2001;**24**:2097–2101.

44 American Diabetes Association. Clinical Practice Recommendations 2005. *Diabetes Care* 2005;**28**(Suppl 1): S1–S79.

45 Haller H, Viberti CG, Mimran A *et al.* Preventing microalbuminuria in patients with diabetes – rationale and design of the Randomised Olmesartan and Diabetes Microalbuminuria Prevention study. *J Hypertens* 2006;**24**:403–408.

18 Treatment of established complications: periodontal disease

George W. Taylor, Wenche S. Borgnakke

Department of Cariology, Restorative Sciences and Endodontics, University of Michigan School of Dentistry, Ann Arbor, MI, USA

Introduction

Clinicians have long assumed diabetes and periodontal diseases are biologically linked. The cumulative evidence from cross-sectional and longitudinal studies supports a causal relationship. The increased susceptibility of people with diabetes to many types of infections has carried over to the presumed link between diabetes mellitus and periodontitis.[1] Although this concept has been questioned,[2,3] population-based studies support diabetes as a risk factor for developing, in addition to dying from, infectious diseases.[4] Some reports have suggested that diabetes adversely affects host resistance to certain infections which influence the endocrinological–metabolic status of the patient with diabetes. Gram-negative anaerobes, several of which have been recognized as periodontal pathogens, have been implicated in this latter set of infections.[5–8] Although studies have not established different periodontal pathogenic flora in people with diabetes,[9–11] results have suggested that diabetes and persistent hyperglycaemia lead to an exaggerated immuno-inflammatory response to the periodontal pathogenic bacterial challenge,[12,13] resulting in more rapid and severe periodontal tissue destruction.

Gingivitis and periodontitis are the most common periodontal diseases. Gingivitis is an inflammatory condition of the gingiva in which the junctional epithelium is altered by the disease but remains attached to the tooth at its original level.[14] In otherwise healthy individuals, gingivitis is most often caused by supragingival bacterial plaque and is reversible. However, if untreated, gingivitis may progress to more destructive periodontitis.[15] Periodontitis is a chronic, potentially progressive bacterial infection that results in inflammation and destruction of tooth-supporting tissues. The most common form of destructive periodontal disease is chronic periodontitis, a bacterially induced, chronic inflammatory disease in which Gram-negative anaerobes, including *Porphyromonas gingivalis* and *Prevotella intermedia* (classified in the genus Bacteroides until 1988 and 1990, respectively[16,17]), *Tannerella forsythia*, spirochetes and occasionally the microaerophilic organism *Actinobacillus actinomycetemcomitans*, are prominent microorganisms in subgingival bacterial plaque. These organisms are considered putative periodontopathogens.[18–27] Chronic periodontitis is characterized by destruction of periodontal tissues (gingiva, periodontal ligament, alveolar bone and cementum) and loss of connective tissue attachment.[14]

Typically, chronic periodontitis begins in adolescence[28] and, in its most common presentation, has a cyclic pattern of progression followed by periods of remission.[29,30] If untreated, chronic periodontitis progresses over time, typically from the initial lesions confined to interdental areas of the posterior teeth to a general pattern involving the entire dentition.[31] Chronic periodontitis may occur without noticeable symptoms. Severe periodontitis can lead to oral pain, suppuration and tooth loss and may affect proper dietary intake and overall quality of life.

Gingivitis is common. Approximately 50% of the United States population in all age groups exhibit reversible gingival inflammation.[32] Moderate or severe periodontitis with destruction of periodontal attachment tissues is much less common, affecting approximately 5–15% of any population.[33,34]

The Evidence Base for Diabetes Care, Second Edition, Edited by William H. Herman, Ann Louise Kinmonth, Nicholas J. Wareham and Rhys Williams.
© 2010 John Wiley & Sons, Ltd

Our review of the evidence supporting the link between diabetes mellitus and periodontal diseases comes from the English language literature published since 1960. Identification of reports to include involved PubMed/Medline electronic searches and reviewing the reference lists of papers obtained from the searches to find primary research reports on the relationships between diabetes/diabetes control and periodontal diseases/periodontal treatment. Although the literature review is extensive, no formal assessment of the quality of the reports is presented. All reports are displayed in table form and the description is organized according to (1) the effects of having diabetes on periodontal diseases in studies that include control groups without diabetes (Table 18.1); (2) the effect of glycaemic control, usually measured by level of glycosylated or glycated haemoglobin, on periodontal status (Table 18.2); and (3) the effects of periodontal disease and periodontal treatment on glycaemic control (Table 18.3).

Diabetes and periodontal disease

Table 18.1 is restricted to studies which compared periodontal health in subjects with and without diabetes. The studies were conducted on all continents with almost half (28) of the 63 studies reported from the United States. The subject has attracted increasing attention; six studies were reported in the 1960s, eight in the 1970s, 12 in the 1980s and 20 in the 1990s. To date, 17 studies have been published in the decade starting in 2000.

In Table 18.1, studies are broadly classified by level of evidence, type of diabetes and age of subjects. Using this classification scheme makes it obvious that most studies (56) are cross-sectional and thus of evidence level III. Only seven were prospective or case–control designs and of evidence level II.

There were 10 reports focusing principally on children and adolescents with type 1 diabetes[35,42–45,47,49–52] and all except one[45] reported greater prevalence, extent or severity of at least one measure of periodontal disease in subjects with diabetes. Six studies were of subjects between the ages of 15 and 35 years with type 1 diabetes and all reported greater prevalence, extent or severity of at least one measure or index of periodontal disease.[36,46,48,53–55] Five studies included adults between 20 and 70 years of age[37,56–59] with type 1 diabetes. All five studies reported greater prevalence, extent or severity of at least one measure or index of periodontal disease in the diabetic group.

We identified 17 reports examining the relationship between type 2 diabetes and periodontitis. One report comprised 15 to 45 + year olds[61] and 11 included only adults.[41,63–72] The remaining five reports are from an epidemiological study in the Pima Indians of the Gila River Indian Community, Arizona, USA and include subjects aged 5 years and older[60] or 15 years and older.[38–40,62]. Fourteen of these 17 studies reported significantly poorer periodontal health in subjects with type 2 diabetes. No significant difference in periodontal disease was discerned in a study of mostly older Taiwanese dialysis patients with and without 'insulin-dependent (type II) diabetes'[69] or well-controlled (mean $HbA_{1c} = 7.3\%$) subjects with diabetes and subjects without diabetes in a study of US university clinic patients 60 + years of age with good medical and dental care.[71] In a study of Mexicans 60 + years of age, there was a marginally significantly ($p = 0.09$) greater prevalence of periodontitis in the group with diabetes (61.5%) than in the group without diabetes (49.5%).[72] A small sub-set of these reports provided additional epidemiologic parameter estimates of association and risk. Emrich's group reported that the odds were approximately three times greater for people with diabetes to have destructive periodontal disease after controlling for other important factors;[62] Nelson's group found a 2.6-fold greater risk of advanced periodontal disease incidence[39] and Taylor's group reported that subjects with type 2 diabetes had a four-fold greater risk for more severe alveolar bone loss progression.[40]

Several reports did not distinguish between type 1 and type 2 diabetes. All these studies were cross-sectional. One study included children only.[74] The other studies included adult subjects, although three also included children or adolescents.[73,75,76] Ten of these 13 studies reported greater prevalence, extent or severity of periodontal disease for at least one measure or index of periodontal disease in people with diabetes.[74–78,80–84] Three reports did not find significant differences in periodontal disease between subjects with and without diabetes.[73,79,85]

Two studies examined NHANES III data from over 4000 women with histories of gestational diabetes mellitus (GDM). One report included women 15–44 years of age[86] and the other women 20–59 years of age.[87] Both concluded that there is a strong relationship between diabetes and periodontal disease. Xiong et al. found periodontitis in 45% of pregnant women with GDM versus 14% in the group without diabetes, with an adjusted odds ratio of 9.11.[86] In non-pregnant women, 40% of those with type 1 or 2 diabetes, 25% of those with a history of GDM and 14% of those without diabetes had periodontal disease. The odds ratio for those with type 1 and 2 diabetes was 2.76. Novak et al. found the prevalence of periodontal disease to be higher in women with a history of GDM[87] and concluded that women with a history of GDM may be

Table 18.1 Effects of diabetes on periodontal diseases in studies including a non-diabetes control group, ordered by level of evidence, diabetes type and subject age[†]

Study	Country	Study design	Diabetes type[a]	No. of subjects a. Diabetes b. Control	Ages (years)[b] a. Diabetes b. Control	Periodontal measure: diabetes effect[c]	Other diabetes-related variables considered	Evidence level[d]
Firatli, 1997[35]	Turkey	Prospective	1	a. 44 b. 20	a. 12.2 (mean) b. 12.3 (mean)	Ging: 0s Ppd: 0s Lpa: 1s	Glycaemic control Duration of diabetes	II-2
Cohen et al., 1970[36]	USA	Prospective	1*	a. 21 b. 18	a. 18–35 b. 18–35	Ging: 1s Lpa: 1r, 1s	None	II-2
Tervonen and Karjalainen, 1997[37]	Finland	Prospective	1	a. 36 b. 10	a. 24–36 b. 24–36	Ging: 0e Ppd: 1r Lpa: 1e	Glycaemic control Duration of diabetes Diabetes complications	II-2
Taylor et al., 1998[38]	USA	Prospective	2	a. 21 b. 338	a. 15–49 b. 15–49	XRBL: 1i, 1r	Glycaemic control	II-2
Nelson et al., 1990[39]	USA	Prospective	2	a. 720 b. 1553	a. 15–55+ b. 15–55+	XRBL: 1i, 1p	None	II-2
Taylor et al., 1998[40]	USA	Prospective	2	a. 24 b. 338	a. 15–57 b. 15–57	XRBL: 1i, 1r	None	II-2
Novaes et al., 1996[41]	Brazil	Prospective	2	a. 30 b. 30	a. 30–77 b. 30–67	Ppd: 1s, 1r Lpa, 1s, 1r	Glycaemic control	II-2
Harrison and Bowen, 1987[42]	USA	Cross-sectional	1	a. 30 b. 30	a. 4–19 b. 4–19	Ging: 1s Lpa: 1p	Glycaemic control	III
Faulconbridge et al., 1981[43]	England	Cross-sectional	1	a. 94 b. 94	a. 5–17 b. 5–17	Ging: 1s	Duration of diabetes	III
Novaes AB et al., 1991[44]	Brazil	Cross-sectional	1	a. 30 b. 30	a. 5–18 b. 5–18	Ging: 1s Ppd: 0s XRBL: 1s	None	III
Goteiner et al., 1986[45]	USA	Cross-sectional	1	a. 169 b. 80	a. School ages b. 5–18	Ging: 0s Lpa: 0p, 0s PDI: 0s	None	III
Galea et al., 1986[46]	Malta	Cross-sectional	1*	a. 82 b. Unknown	a. 5–29 b. 5–29	Ppd: 1p	Glycaemic control Duration of diabetes Diabetes complications	III
Pinson et al., 1995[47]	USA	Cross-sectional	1	a. 26 b. 24	a. 7–18 b. 7–18	Ging: 1s Ppd: 0s Lpa: 0s	Glycaemic control Duration of diabetes	III

(continued)

Table 18.1 (Continued)

Study	Country	Study design	Diabetes type[a]	No. of subjects a. Diabetes b. Control	Ages (years)[b] a. Diabetes b. Control	Periodontal measure: diabetes effect[c]	Other diabetes-related variables considered	Evidence level[d]
Sznajder et al., 1978[48]	Argentina	Cross-sectional	1*	a. 20 / b. 26	a. 9–29 / b. 9–29	Ging: 1s; Lpa: 0s	None	III
Cianciola et al., 1982[49]	USA	Cross-sectional	1	a. 263 / b. 208	a. <10–19+ / b. <10–19+	Ging: 1p; Lpa: 1p; XRBL: 1p, 1s; JPS: 1p,1s	Duration of diabetes	III
Ringleberg et al., 1977[50]	USA	Cross-sectional	1	a. 56 / b. 41	a. 10–16 / b. 10–12	Ging: 1s; MGI: 1s	None	III
de Pommereau et al., 1992[51]	France	Cross-sectional	1	a. 85 / b. 38	a. 12–18 / b. 12–18	Ging: 1e; Lpa: 0e, 0p, 0s; XRBL: 0e, 0p, 0s	Glycaemic control; Duration of diabetes	III
Firatii et al., 1996[52]	Turkey	Cross-sectional	1	a. 77 / b. 77	a. 12.5 (mean) / b. 12.6 (mean)	Ging: 0s; Ppd: 1s; Lpa: 1s	Duration of diabetes	III
Kjellman et al., 1970[53]	Sweden	Cross-sectional	1*	a. 105 / b. 52	a. 15–24 / b. 15–24	Ging: 1e; Ppd: 0s; XRBL: 0s	Glycaemic control; Diabetes complications	III
Guven et al., 1996[54]	Turkey	Cross-sectional	1	a. 10 / b. 52	a. 18–27 / b. 19–22	Ging: 1e	None	III
Rylander et al., 1987[55]	Sweden	Cross-sectional	1	a. 46 / b. 41	a. 18–26 / b. 19–25	Ging: 1e, 1p; Ppd: 0e; Lpa: 1e, 1p; XRBL: 0p	Diabetes complications	III
Glavind et al., 1968[56]	Denmark	Cross-sectional	1*	a. 51 / b. 51	a. 20–40 / b. 20–40	Ging: 0s; Ppd: 0s; Lpa: 1s; XRBL: 1s	Duration of diabetes; Diabetes complications	III
Hugoson et al., 1989[57]	Sweden	Cross-sectional	1	a. 154 / b. 77	a. 20–70 / b. 20–70	Ging: 1e; Ppd: 1e, 1p, 1s; XRBL: 1s	Duration of diabetes	III
Tervonen et al., 2000[58]	Finland	Cross-sectional	1	a. 35 / b. 10	a. 29.7 (mean) / b. 29.0 (mean)	XRBL: 1e	Glycaemic control; Duration of diabetes; Diabetes severity based on presence of complications	III

Study	Country	Design	Diabetes type	n	Age	Periodontal measures	Diabetes variables	Evidence
Thorstennsson and Hugoson 1993[59]	Sweden	Cross-sectional	1	a. 117 / b. 99	a. 40–70 / b. 40–70	Ging: 0e / Ppd: 1e, 1s / XRBL: 1s	Duration of diabetes / Onset age	III
Shlossman et al., 1990[60]	USA	Cross-sectional	2	a. 736 / b. 2483	a. 5–45+ / b. 5–45+	Lpa: 1p / XRBL: 1p	None	III
Endean et al., 2004[61]	Australia	Cross-sectional	2	a. 58 / b. 231	All: 15–45+ / a. Unknown / b. Unknown	Ppd: 1p, 1s	None	III
Emrich et al., 1990[62]	USA	Cross-sectional	2	a. 254 / b. 1088	a. 15–55+ / b. 15–55+	Lpa: 1p, 1s / XRBL: 1p, 1s	None	III
Morton et al., 1995[63]	Mauritius	Cross-sectional	2	a. 24 / b. 24	a. 26–76 / b. 25–73	Ging: 1p / Ppd: 1s / Lpa: 1s	None	III
Mattout et al., 2006[64]	France	Cross-sectional	2	a. 71 / b. 2073	All: 35 – 75 / a. 54.5 (mean) / b. 49.0 (mean)	Ging: 1p, 1s / Ppd: 0p, 0s / Lpa: 1p, 1s	Fasting blood glucose	III
Campus et al., 2005[65]	Italy	Cross-sectional	2	a. 71 / b. 141	a. 36–75 / b. 35–75	Ging: 1e / Ppd: 1e, 1s	Glycaemic control	III
Orbak et al., 2002[66]	Turkey	Cross-sectional	2	a. 40 / b. 20	a1. 46 (mean) / a2. 43 (mean) / b. 41 (mean)	Ging: 1e, 1p, 1s	Glycaemic control / Diabetes complications	III
Tsai et al., 2002[67]	USA	Cross-sectional	2	a. 502 / b. 3841	a1. 45+ / a2. 45+ / b. 45+	Lpa and Ppd: 1p	Glycaemic control	III
Lu and Yang, 2004[68]	Taiwan	Cross-sectional	2	a. 72 / b. 92	a. 54.3 (mean) / b. 54.9 (mean)	Ging: 1p, 1e, 1s / Lpa: 1p, 1e, 1s	Glycaemic control / Duration of diabetes	III
Chuang et al., 2005[69]	Taiwan	Cross-sectional	2	a. 43 / b. 85	All: 28–85 / a. 60.2 (mean) / b. 56.1 (mean)	Ppd: 0s	Glycaemic control	III
Sandberg et. al., 2000[70]	Sweden	Cross-sectional	2	a. 102 / b. 102	a. 64.8 (mean) / b. 64.9 (mean)	Ging: 1e / Ppd: 1e / XRBL: 1p	Glycaemic control / Duration of diabetes	III
Zielinski et al., 2002[71]	USA	Cross-sectional	2	a. 32 / b. 40	All: 60+ / a. 71 (mean) / b. 74 (mean)	Ppd: 0e, 0p, 0s	Glycaemic control / Duration of diabetes	III
Borges-Yáñez et al., 2006[72]	Mexico	Cross-sectional	2	a. 247 / b. 78	All: 60+ / a. 73.4 (mean) / b. Unknown	Lpa: 0p	Fasting blood glucose	III
Benveniste et al., 1967[73]	USA	Cross-sectional	1, 2*	a. 53 / b. 71	a. 5–72 / b. 5–72	Ging: 0s / Ppd: 0p, 0s	None	III

(continued)

Table 18.1 (*Continued*)

Study	Country	Study design	Diabetes type[a]	No. of subjects a. Diabetes b. Control	Ages (years)[b] a. Diabetes b. Control	Periodontal measure: diabetes effect[c]	Other diabetes-related variables considered	Evidence level[d]
Lalla et al., 2007[74]	USA	Cross-sectional	1, 2	a. 350 b. 350	a. 6–18 b. 6–18	Ging: 1e, 1p, 1s Ppd: 1e, 1p, 1s Lpa: 1e, 1p, 1s	Duration of diabetes Glycaemic control	III
Arrieta-Blanco et al., 2003[75]	Spain	Cross-sectional	1, 2	a. 70 b. 74	a. 11–81 b. 11–75	Ging: 1e Ppd: 0s, 0e Lpa: 1e, 1s XRBL:0 s, 0 e	Glycaemic control Duration of diabetes Diabetes complications	III
Wolf, 1977[76]	Finland	Cross-sectional	1, 2	a. 186 b. 156	a. 16–60 b. 16–60	Ging: 1s Lpa: 1s XRBL: 1s	Glycaemic control Duration of diabetes Diabetes complications	III
Bacic et al., 1988[77]	Yugoslavia	Cross-sectional	1, 2	a. 222 b. 189	a. <20–60 + b. <20–60 +	Ppd: 1e, 1p, 1s	Glycaemic control Duration of diabetes Diabetes complications	III
Yavuzyilmaz et al., 1996[78]	Turkey	Cross-sectional	1, 2	a. 17 b. 17	a. 25–74 b. 19–29	Ppd: 1s	None	III
Hove and Stallard, 1970[79]	USA	Cross-sectional	1, 2*	a. 28 b. 16	a. 20–40 + b. 20–40 +	Ging: 0s Ppd: 0s XRBL: 0s	Duration of diabetes Diabetes severity	III
Oliver and Tervonen, 1993[80]	USA	Cross-sectional	1, 2	a. 114 b. 15 132	a. 20–64 b. 20–64	Ppd: 1e, 1p Lpa: 1e, 0p, 0s	None	III
Sandler and Stahl, 1960[81]	USA	Cross-sectional	1, 2*	a. 100 b. 3894	a. 20–69 b. 20–69	PDR: 1e	None	III
Finestone and Booruiy, 1967[82]	USA	Cross-sectional	1, 2*	a. 189 b. 64	a. 20–79 b. 20–79	Pl: 1s	Glycaemic control Duration of diabetes Diabetes complications	III
Belting et al., 1964[83]	USA	Cross-sectional	1, 2*	a. 78 b. 79	a. 20–79 b. 20–79	Pl: 1s	Diabetes severity	III
Bridges et al., 1996[84]	USA	Cross-sectional	1, 2	a. 118 b. 115	a. 24–78 b. 24–78	Ging: 0s Ppd: 0s Lpa: 1s	Glycaemic control Duration of diabetes	III
Ogunbodede et al., 2005[85]	Nigeria	Cross-sectional	1, 2	a. 65 b. 54	a. 25–82 b. 25–82	Ppd: 0p	Duration of diabetes	III
Xiong et al., 2006[86]	USA	Cross-sectional	1, 2, GDM	a. 81 b. 4339	All: 15–44 a. Unknown b. Unknown	Ppd or Lpa: 1p	None	III

Reference	Country	Study type	Diabetes type[a]	N	Ages[b]	Measure[c]	Glycaemic control / Duration of diabetes	Quality[d]
Novak et al., 2006[87]	USA	Cross-sectional	2, GDM	a. 113 / b. 4131	All: 20–59	Ging and Ppd and Lpa: 1p, 1s	Glycaemic control / Duration of diabetes	III
Mittas et al., 2006[88]	Greece	Cross-sectional	GDM	a. 64 / b. 88	a. Unknown / b. Unknown	Ging: 1s	None	III
Szpunar et al. (NHANES I) 1989[89]	USA	Cross-sectional	9	a. 474 / b. 15 174	a. 31.1 (mean) / b. 26.5 (mean)	PI: 1s	None	III
Szpunar et al. (HHANES), 1989[89]	USA	Cross-sectional	9	a. 322 / b. 8040	a. 6–65+ / b. 6–65+	PI: 1s	None	III
Albrecht et al., 1988[90]	Hungary	Cross-sectional	9	a. 1360 / b. 625	a. 15–65+ / b. 12–65+	Ging: 1s / PI: 0s	None	III
Campbell, 1972[91]	Australia	Cross-sectional	9	a. 70 / b. 102	a. 15–65+ / b. 15–65+	PI: 1p, 1s	None	III
Grossi et al., 1994[92]	USA	Cross-sectional	9	a. 1426 / b. 69	a. 17–39 / b. 17–39	Lpa: 1s, 1p	None	III
Tervonen and Knuuttila, 1986[93]	Finland	Cross-sectional	9	a. 50 / b. 53	All: 25–74 / a. Unknown / b. Unknown	Ppd: 0e, 0p / XRBL: 0s	Glycaemic control	III
Sznajder et al., 1978[48]	Argentina	Cross-sectional	9	a. 63 / b. 39	a. <30–40+ / b. <30–40+	Ging: 1s	None	III
Mackenzie and Millard, 1963[94]	USA	Cross-sectional	9	a. 124 / b. 92	a. 30–49 / b. 30–50; a. 32–78 / b. 32–78	Lpa: 1s / XRBL: 0s	None	III
Dolan et al., 1997[95]	USA	Cross-sectional	9	Weighted a. 107 / b. 554	a. 45–75+ / b. 45–75+	Lpa: 1e, 1p, 1s	None	III

[a]Diabetes type: 1 = type 1 diabetes mellitus; 2 = type 2 diabetes mellitus; 1, 2 = both subjects with type 1 and type 2 diabetes mellitus included; GDM = gestational diabetes mellitus; 9 = diabetes type not specified and not clearly ascertainable from other information in the report; * = diabetes type not specified but ascertained by reviewers from other information in the report or from other sources, such as direct communication with the authors.

[b]Ages: subjects' ages presented as minimum–maximum reported for those with (a) diabetes and (b). controls unless specified otherwise.

[c]Measure of periodontal disease status. Measures used include Ging = gingivitis or gingival bleeding, Ppd = probing pocket depth, Lpa = loss of periodontal attachment, XRBL = radiographic bone loss, JPS = juvenile periodontal score, MGI = modified gingival index, PI = Russell's Periodontal Index, PDR = periodontal disease rate (proportion of teeth affected by periodontal disease). The number following the measure corresponds to greater disease in those with diabetes (1) or no difference between those with diabetes and controls (0). The letters following the number correspond to the parameter(s) assessed in the study: e = extent, i = incidence, p = prevalence, s = severity, r = progression.

[d]Hierarchy of evidence based on classification scheme used by US Preventive Services Task Force,[96] where: I = evidence obtained from at least one properly randomized controlled trial; II-1 = evidence obtained from well-designed controlled trial without randomization; II-2 = evidence obtained from well-designed cohort or case–control analytical studies, preferably from more than one centre or research group; II-3 = evidence obtained from multiple time series with or without the intervention; dramatic results in uncontrolled experiments (such as the results of the introduction of penicillin treatment in the 1940s) could also be regarded as this type of evidence; III = opinions of respected authorities, based on clinical experience, descriptive studies and case reports or reports of expert committees.

†Please note acknowledgment for this table on p. 309.

Table 18.2 Effect of degree of glycaemic control on periodontal status, ordered by level of evidence, diabetes type and subject age†

Study	Country	Study design	Diabetes type[a]	Age group	Effect[b]	Non-DM comparison group[c]	Evidence level[d]
Karjalainen and Knuuttila, 1996[97]	Finland	Prospective	1	Children	1	No	II-2
Firatli, 1997[35]	Turkey	Prospective	1	Children	1	Yes	II-2
Seppala et al., 1993[98]	Finland	Prospective	1	Adults	1	No	II-2
Tervonen and Karjalainen, 1997[37]	Finland	Prospective	1	Adults	1	Yes	II-2
Taylor et al., 1998[38]	USA	Prospective	2	Mixed ages	1	Yes	II-2
Novaes et al., 1996[41]	Brazil	Prospective	2	Adults	1	Yes	II-2
Wolf, 1977[76]	Finland	Prospective	1, 2	Mixed ages	0	Yes	II-2
Seppala and Ainamo, 1994[99]	Finland	Prospective	1, 2	Adults	1	No	II-2
Karikoski and Murtomaa, 2003[100]	Finland	Prospective	1, 2, other	Adults	0	No	II-2
Gusberti et al., 1983[101]	USA	Cross-sectional	1	Children	1	No	III
Barnett et al., 1984[102]	USA	Cross-sectional	1	Children	0	No	III
Harrison and Bowen, 1987[42]	USA	Cross-sectional	1	Children	1	Yes	III
Sandholm et al., 1989[103]	Finland	Cross-sectional	1	Children	0	Yes	III
de Pommereau et al., 1992[51]	France	Cross-sectional	1	Children	0	Yes	III
Pinson et al., 1995[47]	USA	Cross-sectional	1	Children	0	Yes	III
Kjellman et al., 1970[53]	Sweden	Cross-sectional	1	Children, young adults	1	Yes	III
Galea et al., 1986[46]	Malta	Cross-sectional	1	Children, young adults	1	Yes	III
Rylander et al., 1987[55]	Sweden	Cross-sectional	1	Mixed ages	0	Yes	III
Safkan-Seppala and Ainamo, 1992[104]	Finland	Cross-sectional	1	Mixed ages	1	No	III
Sastrowijoto et al., 1989[105]	Netherlands	Cross-sectional	1	Adults	0	No	III
Moore et al., 1999[106]	USA	Cross-sectional	1	Adults	0	No	III
Tervonen et al., 2000[58]	Finland	Cross-sectional	1	Adults	1	Yes	III
Ainamo et al., 1990[107]	Finland	Prospective (case report)	2	Adults (N = 2)	1	No	III

Study	Country	Study design	Diabetes type[a,c]	Age group	Effect[b]	[†]	Hierarchy[d]
Unal et al., 1993[108]	Turkey	Cross-sectional	2	Adults	1	Yes	III
Sandberg et al., 2000[70]	Sweden	Cross-sectional	2	Adults	0	Yes	III
Tsai et al., 2002[67]	USA	Cross-sectional	2	Adults	1	Yes	III
Lu and Yang, 2004[68]	Taiwan	Cross-sectional	2	Adults	1	Yes	III
Campus et al., 2005[65]	Italy	Cross-sectional	2	Adults	1	Yes	III
Chuang et al., 2005[69]	Taiwan	Cross-sectional	2	Adults	0	No	III
Peck et al., 2006[109]	South Africa	Cross-sectional	2	Adults	1	No	III
Jansson et al., 2006[110]	Sweden	Cross-sectional	2	Adults	1	No	III
Finestone and Boorujy, 1967[82]	USA	Cross-sectional	1, 2	Adults	1	Yes	III
Bacic et al., 1988[77]	Yugoslavia	Cross-sectional	1, 2	Adults	0	Yes	III
Oliver and Tervonen, 1993[80]	USA	Cross-sectional	1, 2	Adults	1	No	III
Tervonen and Oliver, 1993[111]	USA	Cross-sectional	1, 2	Adults	1	No	III
Bridges et al., 1996[84]	USA	Cross-sectional	1, 2	Adults	0	Yes	III
Arietta-Blanco et al., 2003[75]	Spain	Cross-sectional	1, 2	Mixed ages	0	Yes	III
Guzman et al., 2003[112]	USA	Cross-sectional	1, 2*	Adults	1	No	III
Negishi et al., 2004[113]	Japan	Cross-sectional	1, 2*[e]	Adults	1	No	III
Hove and Stallard, 1970[79]	USA	Cross-sectional	9	Adults	0	Yes	III
Nichols et al., 1978[114]	USA	Cross-sectional	9	Adults	0	No	III
Tervonen and Knuuttila, 1986[93]	Finland	Cross-sectional	9	Adults	1	Yes	III
Albrecht et al., 1988[90]	Hungary	Cross-sectional	9	Mixed ages	0	Yes	III
Hayden and Buckley, 1989[115]	Ireland	Cross-sectional	9	Mixed ages	0	No	III

[a]Diabetes type: 1 = type 1 diabetes mellitus; 2 = type 2 diabetes mellitus; 1, 2 = both subjects with type 1 and type 2 diabetes mellitus; 9 = diabetes type not specified and not clearly ascertainable from other information in the report; * = diabetes type not specified but ascertained by reviewers from other information in the report or from other sources, such as direct communication with the authors.

[b]Effect: 1 = subjects with poorer glycaemic control had poorer health than the comparison group(s); 0 = no difference in the periodontal health status between subjects with poorer glycaemic control and comparison group(s).

[c]Diabetes types are 1 and 2 for all but one subject who had drug-induced diabetes mellitus.

[d]Hierarchy of evidence based on classification scheme used by US Preventive Services Task Force[96], where: I = evidence obtained from at least one properly randomized controlled trial; II-1 = evidence obtained from well-designed controlled trial without randomization; II-2 = evidence obtained from well-designed cohort or case–control analytical studies, preferably from more than one centre or research group; II-3 = evidence obtained from multiple time series with or without the intervention; dramatic results in uncontrolled experiments (such as the results of the introduction of penicillin treatment in the 1940s) could also be regarded as this type of evidence; III = opinions of respected authorities, based on clinical experience, descriptive studies and case reports or reports of expert committees.

[e]Drug-induced diabetes mellitus.

[†]Please note acknowledgment for this table on p. 309.

at greater risk for developing more severe periodontal disease. A smaller Greek study of pregnant women at 34–36 weeks concluded that gingival inflammation was more prevalent in the women with GDM.[88]

Finally, we identified a set of cross-sectional studies in which the type of diabetes was not specified and was not easily determined from the information provided. Five of the nine reports included only adults.[48,92–95] The other four included subjects with ages ranging from childhood to older adulthood.[89–91] Seven of the eight studies based on clinical assessment found subjects with diabetes to have increased prevalence, extent or severity of periodontal disease. The one study relying on radiographic measurements only[94] did not find any difference in severity of periodontal disease. This was also the case in the one report that included both clinical and radiographic assessment.[93] In two of the population-based surveys, Grossi's and Dolan's groups provided epidemiological estimates of the association between diabetes and attachment loss severity.[92,95] Individuals with diabetes were approximately twice as likely to have more severe attachment loss than those without diabetes after controlling for other variables.

Glycaemic control and periodontal disease

Poorer glycaemic control appears to contribute to poorer periodontal health. Primary research reports investigating the relationships between glycaemic control and periodontal disease have included subjects with type 1 diabetes exclusively (17 studies), a combination of individuals with either type 1 or type 2 diabetes (11 studies) or with unspecified type of diabetes (five studies) (Table 18.2).

Only 11 of the 44 reports studied patients with type 2 diabetes exclusively.[38,41,65,67–70,107–110] Nine of the latter found poorer glycaemic control to be a significant factor for poorer periodontal health. The association was of borderline significance in one study of dialysis patients[699] and no difference was found in the remaining study.[70] Most of the reports on glycaemic control and periodontal disease have been cross-sectional, with 26 of 44 publications reporting more prevalent or more severe periodontal disease in those with poorer glycaemic control[35,37,38,41,42,46,53,58,65,67,68,80,82,93,97–99,101,104,107–113] and 18 reporting no differences.[47,51,55,69,70,75–77,79,84,90,100,102,103,105,106,114,115] Of the published follow-up studies (evidence level II-2), eight of 10 reported poorer periodontal health in subjects with poorer glycaemic control.[35,37,38,41,95,97,99,107] Among reports published before 1990, six of 16 reported more frequent or severe periodontal disease in subjects with poorer glycaemic control.[42,46,53,82,93,101] Twelve of 16 papers published in the 1990s reported that poorer glycaemic control was associated with or contributed to more severe or frequent periodontal disease.[35,37,38,41,80,97–99,104,107,108,111] Eight of 12 studies published since 2000 also found such an association.[58,65,67,68,109,110,112,113]

Although most of the studies included in this review are cross-sectional and involve convenience samples of patients, principally from hospitals and clinics, the smaller sub-set of longitudinal and population-based studies support the association between diabetes and periodontal disease. Studies were conducted in different settings and different countries, with different ethnic populations and age mixes and with a variety of measures of periodontal disease status (i.e. gingival inflammation, pathological probing pocket depth, loss of periodontal attachment or radiographic evidence of alveolar bone loss). They used different parameters to assess periodontal disease occurrence (prevalence, incidence, extent, severity or progression). Hence this inevitable variation in methodology and study populations limits the possibility that the same biases or confounding factors apply in all the studies and provides support for concluding that diabetes is a risk factor for periodontal disease incidence, progression and severity. In addition, there is substantial evidence to support a 'dose–response' relationship, that is, as glycaemic control worsens, the adverse effects of diabetes on periodontal health become greater. Finally, there are no studies with superior design features to refute this conclusion.

The findings and conclusions from the preceding narrative review are consistent with two published meta-analyses that have provided quantitative summaries of the adverse effects of diabetes on periodontal health.[116,117]

Cellular and molecular dynamics

This section reviews biological mechanisms considered to explain the increased risk for destructive periodontal disease in people with diabetes.

As with other complications of diabetes, biological mechanisms important in diabetes-associated periodontitis are probably multi-factorial, arising from cellular and molecular interactions resulting from the metabolic abnormalities that characterize diabetes. Microangiopathy, alterations in the composition of gingival crevicular fluid found in the space

Table 18.3 Effects of periodontal disease and its treatment on glycaemic control: clinical and epidemiological evidence, ordered by level of evidence and diabetes type[†]

Study	Study design	Diabetes type[a]	No. of subjects a. Treatment (age, years) b. Control (age, years)	Follow-up time	Periodontal treatment a. Treatment group b. Control group	Metabolic control outcome measure	Effects on metabolic control	Evidence level[b]
Aldridge et al.: Study 1, 1995[196]	RCT	1	a. 16 (16–40) b. 15 (16–40)	2 months	a. Oral hygiene instruction, scaling, adjustment of restoration margins and reinforcement after 1 month. b. No treatment	Glycated haemoglobin Fructosamine	Periodontal treatment had no effect on change in glycated haemoglobin	I
Aldridge et al.: Study 2, 1995[196]	RCT	1	a. 12 (20–60) b. 10 (20–60)	2 months	a. Oral hygiene instruction, scaling and root planing, extractions, root canal therapy b. No treatment	Glycated haemoglobin	Periodontal treatment had no effect on change in glycated haemoglobin	I
Skaleric et al., 2004[197]	RCT	1	All: 26–58 (41.8 = mean) a. 10 (42.0 = mean) b. 10 (41.6 = mean)	24 weeks	a. Scaling and root planing + minocycline microspheres (Arestin) in pockets ≥5 mm at baseline and at 12 weeks b. Scaling and root planing	Glycated haemoglobin	Decreased glycated haemoglobin in test and control groups Adjunct local Arestin treatment is significantly more effective than scaling and root planing only	I
Grossi et al., 1997[198]	RCT	2	a. 89 (25–65) b. 24 (25–65)	12 months	a. Either systemic doxycycline or placebo and ultrasonic bactericidal curettage with irrigation using either H$_2$O, chlorhexidine or povidone–iodine b. Ultrasonic bacterial curettage with H$_2$O irrigation and placebo	Glycated haemoglobin	The three groups receiving doxycycline and ultrasonic bacterial curettage showed significant reductions ($p \leq 0.04$) in mean glycated haemoglobin at 3 months	I
Kiran et al., 2005[199]	RCT	2	a. 22 (31–79) (56 = mean) b. 22 (31–79) (53 = mean)	3 months	a. Scaling and root planing Oral hygiene instruction b. No treatment	Glycated haemoglobin Fasting plasma glucose 2 h post-prandial glucose	Decreased glycated haemoglobin and 2 h post-prandial glucose levels in treatment group only	I

Table 18.3 (*Continued*)

Study	Study design	Diabetes type[a]	No. of subjects a. Treatment (age, years) b. Control (age, years)	Follow-up time	Periodontal treatment a. Treatment group b. Control group	Metabolic control outcome measure	Effects on metabolic control	Evidence level[b]
Rodrigues et al., 2003[200]	RCT	2	a. 15 (unknown) b. 15 (unknown)	3 months	a. Initial full-mouth scaling and root planing Systemic amoxicillin/clavulanic acid 875 mg Oral hygiene instruction at baseline. Control/re-instruction and prophylaxis every 2 weeks b. Same as (a), except no medication	Glycated haemoglobin Fasting plasma glucose	Periodontal therapy was associated with improved glycaemic control expressed as glycated haemoglobin and fasting plasma glucose [but only significant improvement in glycated haemoglobin in (b)]	I
Jones et al., 2007[201]	RCT	2[*,c]	a. 82 (59 = mean) b. 83 (60 = mean)	4 months	a. Early treatment: scaling/root planing; 100 mg doxycycline daily for 14 days; two daily 30 cm³ chlorhexidine rinses for 4 months. b. Usual care: usual dental and medical care	Glycated haemoglobin Insulin use	'The results . . . suggest that the addition of periodontal therapy to current medical therapy may have promise in regard to improvement of glycaemic control' No significant differences between early treatment and usual care groups	I
Talbert et al., 2006[202]	Treatment study, non-RCT	2	a. 25 (16–64) b. 0	3 months	a. Scaling and root planing b. No control group	Glycated haemoglobin Fasting insulin Fasting glucose	Periodontal treatment did not decrease HbA₁c levels	II–2
Smith et al., 1996[203]	Treatment study, non-RCT	1	a. 18 (26–57) b. 0	2 months	a. Scaling and root planing with ultrasonic and curettes; oral hygiene instruction b. No control group	Glycated haemoglobin	Found no statistically or clinically significant change in glycated haemoglobin	II–1
Westfelt et al., 1996[204]	Treatment study, non-RCT	1, 2	a. 20 (45–65) b. 20 (45–65)[e]	5 years	a. Baseline oral hygiene instruction, scaling and root planing followed by periodic prophylaxes, OHI, localized subgingival plaque removal and surgery at sites with bleeding on probing and PPD >5 mm	Glycated haemoglobin	'The mean value of HbA₁c between BL–24 months was not significantly different from that between 24–60 months'	II–1

Reference	Study design	Group	Sample	Duration	Intervention	Outcome measure	Results	Level
					b. Same as group (a)			(Continued)
Christgau et al., 1998[205]	Treatment study, non-RCT	1, 2	a. 20 (30–66) b. 20 (30–66)[e]	2 months	a. Scaling/root planing; subgingival irrigation with chlorhexidine; OHI; and extractions b. Same as group (a)	Glycated haemoglobin	No effect on glycated haemoglobin	II-1
Taylor et al., 1996[206]	Historical prospective cohort	2	a, b. No treatment or control subjects 49 (severe periodis.) 56 (less severe periodis.)	2–4 years	Not applicable	Glycated haemoglobin	Those with severe periodontitis were ~6 times more likely to have poor glycaemic control at follow-up	II-2
Collin et al., 1998[207]	Retrospective cohort	2	a, b. No subjects received treatment 25 with diabetes (aged 58–76) 40 without diabetes (aged 59–77)	2–3 years	Not applicable	Glycated haemoglobin	Among subjects with type 2 diabetes the HbA_{1c} level significantly increased in those with advanced periodontitis, but not in those without advanced periodontitis	II-2
Schara et al., 2006[208]	Treatment study, non-RCT	1	a. 10 (26–55) (38.6 = mean) b. 0	12 months	a. At baseline: full-mouth disinfection. At 6 months: ultrasonic debridement; scaling and root planing; crown polishing; chlorhexidine gel, rinse and irrigation followed by 14 days of chlorhexidine rinsing b. No control group	Glycated haemoglobin	Reduction in HbA_{1c} 3 months after each treatment, but not at 6 months post-treatment. [Baseline mean $HbA_{1c} = 10.5\%$ (range 8.4–16.4%)]	III
Seppala et al., 1993, 1994[98,99]	Treatment study, non-RCT	1	a. 38-1 y; 22-2 y[d] 26 PIDD-1 y (48 ± 6)[d] 12 CIDD-1 y (43 ± 5) 16 PIDD-2 y 6 CIDD-2 y b. 0	1–2 years	a. Scaling and root planing, periodontal surgery and extractions b. No control group	Glycated haemoglobin Blood glucose	Reported an improvement of the HBA_1 levels of the PIDD and CIDD subjects ($p < 0.068$, t-test).	III
Miller et al., 1992[209]	Treatment study, non-RCT	1	a. 10 (unknown) b. 0	8 weeks	a. Scaling and root planing, systemic doxycycline b. No control group	Glycated haemoglobin Glycated albumin	Found decrease in glycated haemoglobin and glycated albumin in patients with improvement in gingival inflammation ($p < 0.01$)	III

(continued)

Table 18.3 (*Continued*)

Study	Study design	Diabetes type[a]	No. of subjects a. Treatment (age, years) b. Control (age, years)	Follow-up time	Periodontal treatment a. Treatment group b. Control group	Metabolic control outcome measure	Effects on metabolic control	Evidence level[b]
							Patients with no improvement in gingival inflammation had either no change or increase in glycated haemoglobin post treatment	
Wolf, 1977[76]	Treatment study, non-RCT	1, 2	a. 117 (16–60) b. 0	8–12 months	a. Scaling and home care instruction; periodontal surgery; extractions; endodontic treatment; restorations; denture replacement or repair b. No control group	Blood glucose, 24 h urinary glucose Insulin dose	Compared 23 subjects with improved oral infect with 23 who had no improvement after treatment for oral infection and inflammation. The subjects with improved oral inflammation and infection tended to demonstrate diabetes control improvement ($p < 0.1$). However, author states in discussion, 'treatment of periodontal inflammation and periapical lesions … does little to improve the control of diabetes'	III
Iwamoto, 2001[210]	Treatment study, non-RCT	2	a. 13 (19–65) b. 0	1 month	a. Local minocycline in every periodontal pocket and mechanical debridement once per week for 1 month b. No control group	Glycated haemoglobin	Anti-infectious treatment is effective in improving metabolic control	III
Faria-Almeida et al., 2006[211]	Treatment study, non-RCT	2	All: 35–70 a. 10 (unknown) b. 10 (unknown)[e]	6 months	a. Scaling and root planing b. Same as group (a)	Glycated haemoglobin	Significant reductions in HbA$_{1c}$ values from baseline to 3 and 6 months follow-up, respectively	III

Study	Study type	Diabetes type	Number (age range)	Duration	Intervention	Outcomes	Results	Evidence
Stewart et al., 2001[212]	Treatment study, non-RCT	2	a. 36 (DM+) (62 = mean) b. 36 (DM+) (67 = mean)	18 months	a. Scaling, sub-gingival curettage and root planing Oral hygiene instruction b. No intervention	Glycated haemoglobin Changes in medications/dosages	Periodontal therapy was associated with improved glycaemic control	III
Promsudthi et al., 2005[213]	Treatment study, non-RCT	2	a. 27 (55–80) b. 25 (55–73)	3 months	a. Mechanical perio treatment and systemic doxycycline 100 mg daily for 15 days b. No intervention	Glycated haemoglobin Fasting plasma glucose	Test group: the reductions in the levels of fasting plasma glucose and HbA$_{1c}$ did not reach significance; 'no association between periodontal treatment with adjunctive antimicrobial treatment and changes in HbA$_{1c}$ levels'	III
Williams and Mahan, 1960[214]	Descriptive clinical study	9	a. 9 (20–32) b. 0	3–7 months	a. Extractions, scaling and curettage, gingivectomy, systemic antibiotics b. No control group	Insulin requirement Diabetes control (not operationally defined)	7/9 subjects had 'significant' reduction in insulin requirements	III

[a]Diabetes type: 1 = type 1 diabetes mellitus; 2 = type 2 diabetes mellitus; 1, 2 = both subjects with type 1 and type 2 diabetes mellitus included; 9 = diabetes type not specified and not clearly ascertainable from other information in the report; * = diabetes type not specified but ascertained by reviewers from other information in the report or from other sources, such as direct communication with the authors.

[b]Hierarchy of evidence based on classification scheme used by US Preventive Services Task Force[96], where: I = evidence obtained from at least one properly randomized controlled trial; II-1 = evidence obtained from well-designed controlled trial without randomization; II-2 = evidence obtained from well-designed cohort or case–control analytic studies, preferably from more than one centre or research group; II-3 = evidence obtained from multiple time series with or without the intervention; dramatic results in uncontrolled experiments (such as the results of the introduction of penicillin treatment in the 1940s) could also be regarded as this type of evidence; III = opinions of respected authorities, based on clinical experience; descriptive studies and case reports; or reports of expert committees.

[c]Five subjects at most might have diabetes type 1, but the majority have type 2.

[d]38 subjects were followed for 1 year (y) and 22 for 2 years. PIDD = poorly controlled insulin-dependent diabetes; CIDD = controlled insulin-dependent diabetes.

[e]Control group consists of healthy subjects without diabetes mellitus, not of subjects with diabetes.

[†]Please note acknowledgment for this table on p. 309.

between the tooth and the free gingiva, alterations in collagen metabolism and impaired wound healing, altered host immuno-inflammatory response, altered subgingival microflora and hereditary predisposition have been proposed to contribute to increased periodontal inflammation and alveolar bone loss in diabetes.[118–124] Hence a biological explanation for more frequent and more severe periodontal infection in diabetes involves synthesis of observations from several perspectives.

In the stable periodontal environment where there is effective oral hygiene and a systemically healthy host, protective cellular and molecular interactions occur in response to the bacterial challenge associated with dental plaque biofilm. In this 'normal' situation, neutrophils, which are the principal host defence cell, accumulate at the surface of the dental plaque biofilm and limit its lateral and apical extension.[125] Normal host defences, accompanied by effective daily oral hygiene practices, prevent extension of bacterial proliferation into the gingival sulcus and the subsequent initiation of chronic inflammation and periodontal pocket formation.[125] In the uncompromised state, the immuno-inflammatory response is tightly regulated to act in concert with normal tissue turnover, regeneration and repair. The colonizing bacteria in the dental plaque biofilm and their metabolic processes subject the gingiva to repetitive pathological injury and repair. This continual healing process is necessary to maintain structural integrity. When tissue healing cannot keep pace with tissue injury, progressive gingivitis develops and may lead to destructive periodontitis.

In the susceptible individual in whom the bacterial plaque biofilm is not effectively removed, bacteria colonize the teeth, forming an adherent plaque that progressively becomes more Gram-negative, anaerobic and virulent in composition as it matures. Substances released from the surface of the dental plaque, such as bacterial lipopolysaccharides (LPS), activate a destructive inflammatory response that includes periodontal epithelial cell proliferation, increased inflammatory cell infiltration and heightened secretion of inflammatory mediators and matrix metalloproteinases. This net catabolic response results in degradation of collagen and the components of the connective tissue extracellular matrix and destruction of the collagen fibres attached to the root surface, followed by lateral and apical extension of the sulcular epithelium.[125] This process results in deepening of the periodontal pockets, gingival recession, clinical attachment loss, increased tooth mobility and, ultimately, tooth loss.

Impaired neutrophil function has been observed in diabetes. The impaired chemotaxis,[126–130] adher-

ence,[131,132] phagocytosis and bacteriocidal activity[133–135] could result in an increased propensity for colonization and proliferation of periodontal pathogens in the dental plaque biofilm. Recent evidence also suggests that chronic hyperglycaemia in diabetes contributes to defects in neutrophil function that mediate diabetes-related tissue damage to the periodontium by stimulating exaggerated production of inflammatory mediators and superoxide release by neutrophils, enhanced leukocyte rolling and attachment to the vascular endothelium in periodontal vessels and impaired transendothelial migration.[136,137]

Several studies have provided additional insight into potential metabolic and genetic factors that could contribute to the increased risk and severity of periodontal tissue destruction in diabetes. Persistent hyperglycaemia causes non-enzymatic glycation and oxidation of proteins and lipids and subsequent formation of advanced glycation end-products (AGEs), which accumulate in the plasma and tissues.[138–140] Hyperglycaemia and resultant AGE formation are considered to be a major causal factor in the pathogenesis of diabetic complications.[138,141] In subjects with diabetes who also have periodontitis, AGEs and increased oxidant stress have been demonstrated in gingiva.[142] Cell surface binding sites or receptors for AGE (RAGE) have been identified on the cell surfaces of several cell types exhibiting a heightened inflammatory response and involved with the pathogenesis of complications of diabetes including mononuclear phagocytes, endothelial cells, fibroblasts, smooth muscle cells, lymphocytes, podocytes and neurons.[140,143] The receptor for AGEs, RAGE, is the principal signal transducer for the AGE ligand.[144]

Enhanced oxidant stress in the gingival tissues could contribute to more frequent and more severe periodontal tissue destruction in individuals with diabetes. For example, it has been hypothesized that the AGE–RAGE interaction induces an oxidant stress that may contribute to chronic monocytic upregulation, activation of NF-κB and subsequent expression of mRNA and secretion of proinflammatory cytokines such as TNFα, IL-1β and IL-6 by monocytic phagocytes.[139,145–151] These mediators are recognized as effectors in periodontal tissue inflammation and destruction.[152] Blockade of RAGE has been shown to diminish *Porphyromonas gingivalis*-triggered alveolar bone loss in the periodontium and to limit the enhanced inflammatory response in peripheral wounds, accelerating wound closure and facilitating angiogenesis[153,154] Additionally, AGE interaction with endothelial cell RAGE has been shown to enhance endothelial cell vascular hyperpermeability and expression of vascular cell adhesion molecule-1, an adherence molecule capable of attracting mononuclear cells to the vascular wall.[155–157] Hence AGE–RAGE interaction has been proposed to result in pertubation of cellular properties, exaggerated and sustained inflammatory response, impaired wound healing and more severe diabetes-associated periodontal disease.[158]

The ways in which diabetes-enhanced inflammation and apoptosis may specifically impact on periodontal tissues was recently reviewed.[159] Graves and colleagues reported that diabetes adversely affects bone repair by decreasing expression of genes that induce osteoblast differentiation and diminishing growth factor and extracellular matrix production[160–162] One proposed mechanism is through the contribution of AGEs to decreased extracellular matrix production and inhibition of osteoblast differentiation[163–165] AGEs may also delay wound healing by inducing apoptosis of extracellular matrix-producing cells, thus reducing the number of osteoblastic and fibroblastic cells available for the repair of resorbed alveolar bone.[159] In addition to promoting apoptosis, AGEs could affect oral tissue healing by reducing expression of collagen and promoting inflammation. The mechanisms contributing to AGE-enhanced apoptosis include the direct activation of caspase activity and indirect pathways that increase oxidative stress or the expression of pro-apoptotic genes that regulate apoptosis.[159]

In an extensive review, Iacopino[124] provided an additional perspective on metabolic dysregulation in diabetes and the effects of hyperlipidaemia on monocyte/macrophage function in wound signalling. The monocyte/macrophage is considered the major mediator of the inflammatory phase in wound healing, having primary roles in wound signal transduction and in the initiation of the transition of healing from the inflammatory to the granulation phase.[124,166–172] One hypothesized effect of hyperlipidaemia occurs through fatty acid interaction with the monocyte cell membrane causing impaired function of membrane bound receptors and enzyme systems.[124,173,174] This leads to impaired amplification and transduction of the wound signal. Another postulated pathway leading to impaired monocyte function in diabetes and wound signalling is via the non-enzymatic glycosylation of lipids and triglycerides[124,175–177] in addition to proteins. These AGEs are thought to affect normal differentiation and maturation of specific monocyte phenotypes throughout the different stages of wound healing.[124] The net result of both of these pathways is exacerbated host-mediated inflammatory responses and tissue destruction. In impairing monocyte function, diabetes-associated lipid dysregulation leading to high levels of low-density lipoproteins (LDL) and triglycerides (TRG) may be a major factor in the incidence and severity of periodontal disease.[124,178,179]

A substantial sub-set of individuals with type 1 diabetes have a monocytic hyper-responsive phenotype that predisposes them to an exaggerated response to Gram-negative bacterial infections.[180–184] This hyper-responsive monocytic phenotype is genetically determined, possibly regulated by genes in the HLA-DR3/4 and HLA-DQ regions.[118,152,182,184–188] Several important putative periodontal pathogens are Gram-negative anaerobes. Salvi and colleagues[180,181] have reported enhanced peripheral blood monocytic response to LPS challenge, as evidenced by elevated gingival crevicular fluid levels of PGE2, IL-1β and TNFα in individuals with type 1 diabetes and periodontal disease when compared with controls without diabetes. The reported enhanced inflammatory mediator response is functionally consistent with the type and levels of mediators required to induce alveolar bone resorption and other periodontal connective tissue destruction. In addition to the increased monocytic secretory response in the patients with type 1 diabetes, they found significantly greater levels of these inflammatory mediators in the subjects with type 1 diabetes and severe periodontitis. This evidence suggests that the enhanced PGE2, IL-1β and TNFα secretory responsiveness of peripheral blood monocytes in individuals with type 1 diabetes mellitus may contribute to the increased risk for severe periodontal disease.

Periodontal disease and glycaemic control

In addition to the substantial evidence demonstrating that diabetes is a risk factor for poor periodontal health, there is a growing body of evidence suggesting that periodontal infection adversely affects glycaemic control in diabetes and contributes to the risk of diabetic complications. Due to the high vascularity of the inflamed periodontium, this tissue may serve as an endocrine-like source for TNFα and other inflammatory mediators.[123,189] Because of the predominance of Gram-negative anaerobic bacteria in periodontal infection, the ulcerated pocket epithelium may constitute a chronic source of systemic challenge from bacteria, bacterial products and locally produced inflammatory mediators. TNFα, IL-6 and IL-1, all mediators important in periodontal inflammation, have been shown to have important effects on glucose and lipid metabolism, particularly following an acute infectious challenge or trauma.[123,190,191] TNFα interferes with lipid metabolism and is an insulin antagonist.[192,193] IL-6 and IL-1 have also been reported to antagonize insulin action.[190,194,195]

More direct, empirical evidence regarding the adverse effects of periodontal infection on glycaemic control comes from both treatment studies using non-surgical periodontal therapy and observational studies (Table 18.3).

The treatment studies include randomized clinical trials (RCTs) and non-RCTs. The RCTs used control groups that were either non-treated controls,[196,199] positive controls[197,198,200] or controls advised to continue with their usual source of dental care.[201] Of the seven RCTs, four reported a beneficial effect of periodontal therapy on glycaemic control.[197–200]

An important source of variation in the RCTs is the use of adjunctive antibiotics with the non-surgical periodontal therapy. Among the RCTs, four included adjunctive antibiotics administered systemically[198,200,201] or locally.[197] Three of these four RCTs using antibiotics showed beneficial effects on glycaemic control.[197,198,200] The improvement in one study was in the positive control group that did not receive the systemic antibiotic[200] and one of the four RCTs that reported a beneficial effect did not use antibiotics.[199] Hence to date there is no clear-cut evidence that antibiotics are necessary in combination with non-surgical periodontal treatment to improve glycaemic control.

Among the 13 periodontal treatment studies that were not RCTs, eight reported a beneficial effect on glycaemic control[76,98,99,208–211,214] and five did not.[202–205,213] Only two of these studies had control or comparison groups.[212,213] As in the RCTs, there was marked variation in the use of adjunctive antibiotics. Three of the five studies that used systemic antibiotics reported a beneficial effect on glycaemic control.[209,210,214]

As shown in Table 18.3, there is marked heterogeneity in the studies' designs, conduct, length of follow-up, types of participants and periodontal treatment protocols. The details of the variation in this body of literature have been extensively described in several reviews.[123,215,216]

Additional evidence to support the deleterious effect of severe periodontitis on glycaemic control comes from two longitudinal observational studies. A longitudinal epidemiological study of the Pima Indians in Arizona, USA,[206] found that subjects with type 2 diabetes in good to moderate control and with severe periodontitis at baseline were approximately six times more likely to have poor glycaemic control at approximately 2 years follow-up than those without severe periodontitis at baseline. In another observational study of 25 adults with type 2 diabetes, aged 58–77 years, Collin et al. reported an association between advanced periodontal disease and impaired metabolic control.[207]

Poor glycaemic control is a major risk factor for the development and progression of the chronic complications of diabetes. Results from the Diabetes Control and Complications Trial (type 1 diabetes) and the UK Prospective Diabetes Study (UKPDS) (type 2 diabetes) demonstrated that attaining and maintaining good glycaemic control could reduce the risk for and slow the progression of microvascular complications in patients with type 1 and type 2 diabetes[217–219] Additionally, the UKPDS observed a 16% reduction ($p = 0.052$) in the risk of combined fatal or non-fatal myocardial infarction and sudden death. Further epidemiological analysis from the UKPDS showed a continuous association between the risk of cardiovascular complications and glycaemia; each percentage point decrease in HbA_{1c} (e.g. from 9 to 8%) was associated with a 25% reduction in diabetes-related deaths, a 7% reduction in all-cause mortality and an 18% reduction in combined fatal and non-fatal myocardial infarction.[220]

There is emerging evidence from observational studies regarding the association between periodontal disease and the risk for diabetic complications. Thorstensson et al. studied 39 case–control pairs with type 1 and type 2 diabetes for 6 years median follow-up time in Jönköping, Sweden.[221] In each pair, the cases had severe alveolar bone loss and controls had gingivitis or minor alveolar bone loss. They found that cases were significantly more likely to have prevalent proteinuria and cardiovascular complications including stroke, transient ischaemic attacks, angina, myocardial infarction and intermittent claudication than controls at their follow-up assessments.

Two recent reports from the on-going longitudinal study of diabetes and its complications in the Gila River Indian Community in Arizona, USA, conducted by the National Institute of Diabetes and Digestive and Kidney Diseases, address nephropathy and cardiovascular disease. Saremi et al. studied a cohort of 628 individuals for a median follow-up time of 11 years.[222] Individuals with severe periodontal disease had 3.2 times greater risk for cardio-renal mortality (i.e. ischaemic heart disease and diabetic nephropathy combined) than those with no, mild or moderate periodontal disease. This estimate of significantly greater risk persisted after controlling for several major risk factors of cardio-renal mortality, including age, gender, diabetes duration, HbA_{1c}, body mass index (BMI), hypertension, blood glucose, cholesterol, electrocardiographic abnormalities, macroalbuminuria and smoking.

In the second report, Shultis et al. investigated the effect of periodontitis on risk of overt nephropathy (macroalbuminuria) and end-stage renal disease (ESRD) in a group of 529 Gila River Indian Community adults with type 2 diabetes.[223] After adjusting for age, gender, diabetes duration, BMI and smoking, periodontitis and edentulism were significantly associated with overt nephropathy and ESRD. The incidence of macroalbuminura was 2.0, 2.1 and 2.6 times greater in individuals with moderate or severe periodontitis or in those who were edentulous, respectively, than those with none/mild periodontitis. The incidence of ESRD was also 2.3, 3.5 and 4.9 times greater for individuals with moderate or severe periodontitis or for those who were edentulous than for those with none/mild periodontitis.

The clinical and epidemiological evidence reviewed provides support for the concept that periodontal infection contributes to poorer glycaemic control and the risk for diabetic complications in people with diabetes mellitus. Rigorous, controlled trials in diverse populations are warranted to establish firmly that treating periodontal infections increases glycaemic control and reduces the burden of complications of diabetes.

Conclusion

Diabetes is associated with increased occurrence and progression of periodontitis. Periodontal infection is associated with poorer glycaemic control in people with diabetes. Periodontal disease may be associated with increased risk for diabetic complications. Although treating periodontal infection in people with diabetes is clearly an important component of oral health, it may also be important for establishing and maintaining glycaemic control and in delaying the onset or progression of diabetic complications. Additional rigorous, systematic studies in diverse populations are needed to confirm that treating periodontal infections improves glycaemic control and reduces the burden of complications of diabetes mellitus.

Acknowledgements

Portions of this text and the tables have been adapted, with permission, from the Surgeon General's Report on Oral Health (US Department of Health and Human Services, 2000) and papers published in the *Journal of Public Health Dentistry* (Taylor *et al.*, 2000) and *Ann Periodontol* (Taylor, 2001).

References

1 Mealey BL, Ocampo GL. Diabetes mellitus and periodontal disease. *Periodontology 2000* 2007;**44**:127–153.

2 Kaslow RA. Infections in diabetics. In: *Diabetes in America* (ed. MI Harris), US Government Printing Office, Washington, DC, 1985.

3 Wilson RM. Infection and diabetes mellitus. In: *Textbook of Diabetes* (eds JC Pickup, W Williams), Blackwell Scientific, London, 1991.

4 Shah BR, Hux JE. Quantifying the risk of infectious diseases for people with diabetes. *Diabetes Care* 2003;**26**:510–513.

5 Rayfield EJ, Ault MJ, Keusch GT, Brothers MJ, Nechemias C, Smith H. Infection and diabetes: the case for glucose control. *Am J Med* 1982;**72**:439–450.

6 Wheat LJ. Infection and diabetes mellitus. *Diabetes Care* 1980;**3**:187–197.

7 Lewis RP, Sutter VL, Finegold SM. Bone infections involving anaerobic bacteria. *Medicine* 1978;**57**:279–305.

8 Joshi N, Caputo GM, Weitekamp MR, Karchmer AW. Infections in patients with diabetes mellitus. *N Engl J Med* 1999;**341**:1906–1912.

9 Tervonen T, Oliver RC, Wolff LF, Bereuter J, Anderson L, Aeppli DM. Prevalence of periodontal pathogens with varying metabolic control of diabetes mellitus. *J Clin Periodontol* 1994;**21**:375–379.

10 Yuan K, Chang CJ, Hsu PC, Sun HS, Tseng CC, Wang JR. Detection of putative periodontal pathogens in non-insulin-dependent diabetes mellitus and non-diabetes mellitus by polymerase chain reaction. *J Periodontal Res* 2001;**36**:18–24.

11 Lalla E, Kaplan S, Chang S-M J, Roth GA, Celenti R, Hinckley K, Greenberg E, Papapanou PN Periodontal infection profiles in type 1 diabetes. *J Clin Periodontol* 2006;**33**:855–862.

12 Southerland JH, Taylor GW, Moss K, Beck JD, Offenbacher S. Commonality in chronic inflammatory diseases: periodontitis, diabetes and coronary artery disease. *Periodontology 2000* 2006;**40**:130–143.

13 Nishimura F, Iwamoto Y, Soga Y. The periodontal host response with diabetes. *Periodontology 2000* 2007;**43**:245–253.

14 Genco RJ. Classification and clinical and radiographic features of periodontal disease. In: *Contemporary Periodontics* (eds RJ Genco, HM Goldman, DW Cohen), Mosby, St Louis, MO, 1990.

15 Page RC. Gingivitis. *J Clin Periodontol* 1986;**13**:345–359.

16 Shah HN, Collins MD. Proposal for reclassification of *Bacteroides asaccharolyticus*, *Bacteroides gingivalis* and *Bacteroides endodontalis* in a new genus, Porphyromonas. *Int J Syst Bacteriol* 1988;**38**:128.

17 Shah HN, Collins DM. Prevotella, a new genus to include *Bacteroides melaninogenicus* and related species formerly classified in the genus Bacteroides. *Int J Syst Bacteriol* 1990;**40**:205–208.

18 Dzink JL, Socransky SS, Haffajee AD. The predominant cultivable microbiota of active and inactive lesions of destructive periodontal diseases. *J Clin Periodontol* 1988;**15**:316–323.

19 Loesche WJ, Syed SA, Schmidt E, Morrison EC. Bacterial profiles of subgingival plaques in periodontitis. *J Periodontol* 1985;**56**:447–456.

20 Slots J, Genco RJ. Black-pigmented *Bacteroides* species, *Capnocytophaga* species and *Actinobacillus actinomycetemcomitans* in human periodontal disease: virulence factors in

colonization, survival and tissue destruction. *J Dent Res* 1984;**63**:412–421.

21 Moore WE. Microbiology of periodontal disease. *J Periodontal Res* 1987;**22**:335–341.

22 Zambon JJ. *Actinobacillus actinomycetemcomitans* in human periodontal disease. *J Clin Periodontol* 1985;**12**:1–20.

23 Kornman KS, Robertson PB. Clinical and microbiological evaluation of therapy for juvenile periodontitis. *J Periodontol* 1985;**56**:443–446.

24 Slots J, Hafstrom C, Rosling B, Dahlen G. Detection of *Actinobacillus actinomycetemcomitans* and *Bacteroides gingivalis* in subgingival smears by the indirect fluorescent-antibody technique. *J Periodontal Res* 1985;**20**:613–620.

25 Genco RJ, Zambon JJ, Christersson LA. The origin of periodontal infections. *Adv Dent Res* 1988;**2**:245–259.

26 Socransky SS, Haffajee AD, Cugini MA, Smith C, Kent RL, JR. Microbial complexes in subgingival plaque. *J Clin Periodontol* 1998;**25**:134–144.

27 Tanner AC. R, Izard J. *Tannerella forsythia*, a periodontal pathogen entering the genomic era. *Periodontology 2000* 2006;**42**:88–113.

28 Loe H, Morrison E. Periodontal health and disease in young people: screening for priority care. *Int Dent J* 1986;**36**: 162–167.

29 Socransky SS, Haffajee AD, Goodson JM, Lindhe J. New concepts of destructive periodontal disease. *J Clin Periodontol* 1984;**11**:21–32.

30 Gilthorpe MS, Zamzuri AT, Griffiths GS, Maddick IH, Eaton KA, Johnson NW. Unification of the 'burst' and 'linear' theories of periodontal disease progression: a multilevel manifestation of the same phenomenon. *J Dent Res* 2003;**82**:200–205.

31 Loe H, Anerud A, Boysen H, Morrison E. Natural history of periodontal disease in man. Rapid, moderate and no loss of attachment in Sri Lankan laborers 14 to 46 years of age. *J Clin Periodontol* 1986;**13**:431–445.

32 Albandar JM, Kingman A. Gingival recession, gingival bleeding and dental calculus in adults 30 years of age and older in the United States, 1988–1994. *J Periodontol* 1999;**70**:30–43.

33 Albandar JM, Brunelle JA, Kingman A. Destructive periodontal disease in adults 30 years of age and older in the United States, 1988–1994. *J Periodontol* 1999;**70**:13–29.

34 Burt B, and Research, Science and Therapy Committee of the American Academy of Periodontology. Position paper: epidemiology of periodontal diseases. *J Periodontol* 2005;**76**: 1406–1419.

35 Firatli E. The relationship between clinical periodontal status and insulin-dependent diabetes mellitus. Results after 5 years. *J Periodontol* 1997;**68**:136–140.

36 Cohen DW, Friedman LA, Shapiro J, Kyle GC, Franklin S. Diabetes mellitus and periodontal disease: two-year longitudinal observations. I. *J Periodontol* 1970;**41**:709–712.

37 Tervonen T, Karjalainen K. Periodontal disease related to diabetic status. A pilot study of the response to periodontal therapy in type 1 diabetes. *J Clin Periodontol* 1997;**24**: 505–510.

38 Taylor GW, Burt BA, Becker MP, Genco RJ, Shlossman M. Glycaemic control and alveolar bone loss progression in type 2 diabetes. *Ann Periodontol* 1998;**3**:30–39.

39 Nelson RG, Shlossman M, Budding LM, Pettitt DJ, Saad MF, Genco RJ, Knowler WC. Periodontal disease and NIDDM in Pima Indians. *Diabetes Care* 1990;**13**:836–840.

40 Taylor GW, Burt BA, Becker MP, Genco RJ, Shlossman M, Knowler WC, Pettitt DJ. Non-insulin dependent diabetes mellitus and alveolar bone loss progression over 2 years. *J Periodontol* 1998;**69**:76–83.

41 Novaes AB Jr, Gutierrez FG, Novaes AB. Periodontal disease progression in type II non-insulin-dependent diabetes mellitus patients (NIDDM). Part I – Probing pocket depth and clinical attachment. *Braz Dent J* 1996;**7**:65–73.

42 Harrison R, Bowen WH. Periodontal health, dental caries and metabolic control in insulin-dependent diabetic children and adolescents. *Pediatr Dent* 1987;**9**:283–286.

43 Faulconbridge AR, Bradshaw WC, Jenkins PA, Baum JD. The dental status of a group of diabetic children. *Br Dent J* 1981;**151**:253–255.

44 Novaes AB Jr, Pereira AL, De Moraes N, Novaes AB. Manifestations of insulin-dependent diabetes mellitus in the periodontium of young Brazilian patients. *J Periodontol* 1991;**62**:116–122.

45 Goteiner D, Vogel R, Deasy M, Goteiner C. Periodontal and caries experience in children with insulin-dependent diabetes mellitus. *J Am Dent Assoc* 1986;**113**:277–279.

46 Galea H, Aganovic I, Aganovic M. The dental caries and periodontal disease experience of patients with early onset insulin dependent diabetes. *Int Dent J* 1986;**36**:219–224.

47 Pinson M, Hoffman WH, Garnick JJ, Litaker MS. Periodontal disease and type I diabetes mellitus in children and adolescents. *J Clin Periodontol* 1995;**22**:118–123.

48 Sznajder N, Carraro JJ, Rugna S, Sereday M. Periodontal findings in diabetic and nondiabetic patients. *J Periodontol* 1978;**49**:445–448.

49 Cianciola LJ, Park BH, Bruck E, Mosovich L, Genco RJ. Prevalence of periodontal disease in insulin-dependent diabetes mellitus (juvenile diabetes). *J Am Dent Assoc* 1982;**104**:653–660.

50 Ringelberg ML, Dixon DO, Francis AO, Plummer RW. Comparison of gingival health and gingival crevicular fluid flow in children with and without diabetes. *J Dent Res* 1977;**56**:108–111.

51 de Pommereau V, Dargent-Pare C, Robert JJ, Brion M. Periodontal status in insulin-dependent diabetic adolescents. *J Clin Periodontol* 1992;**19**:628–632.

52 Firatli E, Yilmaz O, Onan U. The relationship between clinical attachment loss and the duration of insulin-dependent diabetes mellitus (IDDM) in children and adolescents. *J Clin Periodontol* 1996;**23**:362–366.

53 Kjellman O, Henriksson CO, Berghagen N, Andersson B. Oral conditions in 105 subjects with insulin-treated diabetes mellitus. *Svensk Tandlakaretidskrift* 1970;**63**:99–110.

54 Guven Y, Satman I, Dinccag N, Alptekin S. Salivary peroxidase activity in whole saliva of patients with insulin-dependent (type-1) diabetes mellitus. *J Clin Periodontol* 1996;**23**:879–881.

55 Rylander H, Ramberg P, Blohme G, Lindhe J. Prevalence of periodontal disease in young diabetics. *J Clin Periodontol* 1987;**14**:38–43.

56 Glavind L, Lund B, Loe H. The relationship between periodontal state and diabetes duration, insulin dosage and retinal changes. *J Periodontol* 1968;**39**:341–347.

57 Hugoson A, Thorstensson H, Falk H, Kuylenstierna J. Periodontal conditions in insulin-dependent diabetics. *J Clin Periodontol* 1989;**16**:215–223.

58 Tervonen T, Karjalainen K, Knuuttila M, Huumonen S. Alveolar bone loss in type 1 diabetic subjects. *J Clin Periodontol* 2000;**27**:567–571.

59 Thorstensson H, Hugoson A. Periodontal disease experience in adult long-duration insulin-dependent diabetics. *J Clin Periodontol* 1993;**20**:352–358.

60 Shlossman M, Knowler WC, Pettitt DJ. Genco RJ. Type 2 diabetes mellitus and periodontal disease. *J Am Dent Assoc* 1990;**121**:532–536.

61 Endean et al. 2004.

62 Emrich LJ, Shlossman M, Genco RJ. Periodontal disease in non-insulin-dependent diabetes mellitus. *J Periodontol* 1991;**62**:123–131.

63 Morton AA, Williams RW, Watts TL. Initial study of periodontal status in non-insulin-dependent diabetics in Mauritius. *J Dent* 1995;**23**:343–345.

64 Mattout C, Bourgeois D, Bouchard P. Type 2 diabetes and periodontal indicators: epidemiology in France, 2002–2003. *J Periodontal Res* 2006;**41**:253–258.

65 Campus G, Salem A, Uzzau S, Baldoni E, Tonolo G. Diabetes and periodontal disease: a case-control study. *J Periodontol* 2005;**76**:418–425.

66 Orbak R, Tezel A, Canakci V, Demir T. The influence of smoking and non-insulin-dependent diabetes mellitus on periodontal disease. *J Int Med Res* 2002;**30**:116–125.

67 Tsai C, Hayes C, Taylor GW. Glycaemic control of type 2 diabetes and severe periodontal disease in the US adult population. *Commun Dent Oral Epidemiol* 2002;**30**:182–192.

68 Lu HK, Yang PC. Cross-sectional analysis of different variables of patients with non-insulin dependent diabetes and their periodontal status. *Int J Periodont Restor Dent* 2004;**24**:71–79.

69 Chuang SF, Sung JM, Kuo SC, Huang JJ, Lee SY. Oral and dental manifestations in diabetic and nondiabetic uremic patients receiving hemodialysis. *Oral Surg Oral Med Oral Pathol Oral Radiol Endod* 2005;**99**:689–695.

70 Sandberg GE, Sundberg HE, Fjellstrom CA, Wikblad KF. Type 2 diabetes and oral health: a comparison between diabetic and non-diabetic subjects. *Diabetes Res Clin Pract* 2000;**50**:27–34.

71 Zielinski MB, Fedele D, Forman LJ, Pomerantz SC. Oral health in the elderly with non-insulin-dependent diabetes mellitus. *Special Care Dent* 2002;**22**:94–98.

72 Borges-Yanez SA, Irigoyen-Camacho ME, Maupome G. Risk factors and prevalence of periodontitis in community-dwelling elders in Mexico. *J Clin Periodontol* 2006;**33**:184–194.

73 Benveniste R, Bixler D, Conneally PM. Periodontal disease in diabetics. *J Periodontol* 1967;**38**:271–279.

74 Lalla E, Cheng B, Lal S, Kaplan S, Softness B, Greenberg E, Goland RS, Lamster IB. Diabetes mellitus promotes periodontal destruction in children. *J Clin Periodontol* 2007;**34**:294–298.

75 Arrieta-Blanco JJ, Bartolome-Villar B, Jimenez-Martinez E, Saavedra-Vallejo P, Arrieta-Blanco FJ. Dental problems in patients with diabetes mellitus (II): gingival index and periodontal disease. *Med Oral* 2003;**8**:233–247.

76 Wolf J. Dental and periodontal conditions in diabetes mellitus. A clinical and radiographic study. *Proc Finn Dent Soc* 1977;**73**:1–56.

77 Bacic M, Plancak D, Granic M. CPITN assessment of periodontal disease in diabetic patients. *J Periodontol* 1988;**59**:816–822.

78 Yavuzyilmaz E, Yumak O, Akdoganli T, Yamalik N, Ozer N, Ersoy F, Yeniay I. The alterations of whole saliva constituents in patients with diabetes mellitus. *Aust Dent J* 1996;**41**:193–197.

79 Hove KA, Stallard RE. Diabetes and the periodontal patient. *J Periodontol* 1970;**41**:713–718.

80 Oliver RC, Tervonen T. Periodontitis and tooth loss: comparing diabetics with the general population. *J Am Dent Assoc* 1993;**124**:71–76.

81 Sandler HC, Stahl SS. Prevalence of periodontal disease in a hospitalized population. *J Dent Res* 1960;**39**:439–449.

82 Finestone AJ, Boorujy SR. Diabetes mellitus and periodontal disease. *Diabetes* 1967;**16**:336–340.

83 Belting CM, Hiniker JJ, Dummett CO. Influence of diabetes mellitus on the severity of periodontal disease. *J Periodontol* 1964;**35**:476–480.

84 Bridges RB, Anderson JW, Saxe SR, Gregory K, Bridges SR. Periodontal status of diabetic and non-diabetic men: effects of smoking, glycaemic control and socioeconomic factors. *J Periodontol* 1996;**67**:1185–1192.

85 Ogunbodede EO, Fatusi OA, Akintomide A, Kolawole K, Ajayi A. Oral health status in a population of Nigerian diabetics. *J Contemp Dent Pract [Electronic Resource]* 2005;**6**:75–84.

86 Xiong X, Buekens P, Vastardis S, Pridjian G. Periodontal disease and gestational diabetes mellitus. *Am J Obstet Gynecol* 2006;**195**:1086–1089.

87 Novak KF, Taylor GW, Dawson DR, Ferguson JE II, Novak MJ, Periodontitis and gestational diabetes mellitus: exploring the link in NHANES III. *J Public Health Dent* 2006;**66**:163–168.

88 Mittas E, Erevnidou K, Koumantakis E, Papavasileiou S, Helidonis E. Gingival condition of women with gestational diabetes on a Greek island. *Spec Care Dentist* 2006;**26**:214–219.

89 Szpunar S, Ismail A, Eklund S. Diabetes and periodontal disease: analyses of NHANES I and HHANES. *J Dent Res* 1989;**68**:383 (Abstr 1605).

90 Albrecht M, Banoczy J, Tamas G Jr. Dental and oral symptoms of diabetes mellitus. *Commun Dent Oral Epidemiol* 1988;**16**:378–380.

91 Campbell MJ. Epidemiology of periodontal disease in the diabetic and the non-diabetic. *Aust Dent J* 1972;**17**:274–278.

92 Grossi SG, Zambon JJ, Ho AW, Koch G, Dunford RG, Machtei EE, Norderyd OM, Genco RJ. Assessment of risk for periodontal disease. I. Risk indicators for attachment loss. *J Periodontol* 1994;**65**:260–267.

93 Tervonen T, Knuuttila M. Relation of diabetes control to periodontal pocketing and alveolar bone level. *Oral Surg Oral Med Oral Pathol* 1986;**61**:346–349.

94 Mackenzie RS, Millard HD. Interrelated effects of diabetes, arteriosclerosis and calculus on alveolar bone loss. *J Am Dent Assoc* 1963;**66**:191–198.

95 Dolan TA, Gilbert GH, Ringelberg ML, Legler DW, Antonson DE, Foerster U, Heft MW. Behavioral risk indicators of attachment loss in adult Floridians. *J Clin Periodontol* 1997;**24**:223–232.

96 US Preventive Services Task Force. *Guide to Clinical Preventive Services*, 2nd edn, US Government Printing Office, Washington, DC, 1996.

97 Karjalainen KM, Knuuttila ML. The onset of diabetes and poor metabolic control increases gingival bleeding in children and adolescents with insulin-dependent diabetes mellitus. *J Clin Periodontol* 1996;**23**:1060–1067.

98 Seppala B, Seppala M, Ainamo J. A longitudinal study on insulin-dependent diabetes mellitus and periodontal disease. *J Clin Periodontol* 1993;**20**:161–165.

99 Seppala B, Ainamo J. A site-by-site follow-up study on the effect of controlled versus poorly controlled insulin-dependent diabetes mellitus. *J Clin Periodontol* 1994;**21**: 161–165.

100 Karikoski A, Murtomaa H. Periodontal treatment needs in a follow-up study among adults with diabetes in Finland. *Acta Odontol Scand* 2003;**61**:6–10.

101 Gusberti FA, Syed SA, Bacon G, Grossman N, Loesche WJ. Puberty gingivitis in insulin-dependent diabetic children. I. Cross-sectional observations. *J Periodontol* 1983;**54**:714–720.

102 Barnett ML, Baker RL, Yancey JM, MacMillan DR, Kotoyan M. Absence of periodontitis in a population of insulin-dependent diabetes mellitus (IDDM) patients. *J Periodontol* 1984;**55**:402–405.

103 Sandholm L, Swanljung O, Rytomaa I, Kaprio EA, Maenpaa J. Periodontal status of Finnish adolescents with insulin-dependent diabetes mellitus. *J Clin Periodontol* 1989;**16**: 617–620.

104 Safkan-Seppala B, Ainamo J. Periodontal conditions in insulin-dependent diabetes mellitus. *J Clin Periodontol* 1992;**19**:24–29.

105 Sastrowijoto SH, Hillemans P, van Steenbergen TJ, Abraham-Inpijn L, de Graaff J. Periodontal condition and microbiology of healthy and diseased periodontal pockets in type 1 diabetes mellitus patients. *J Clin Periodontol* 1989;**16**:316–322.

106 Moore PA, Weyant RJ, Mongelluzzo MB, Myers DE, Rossie K, Guggenheimer J, Block HM, Huber H, Orchard T. Type 1 diabetes mellitus and oral health: assessment of periodontal disease. *J Periodontol* 1999;**70**:409–417.

107 Ainamo J, Lahtinen A, Uitto VJ. Rapid periodontal destruction in adult humans with poorly controlled diabetes. A report of 2 cases. *J Clin Periodontol* 1990;**17**:22–28.

108 Unal T, Firatli E, Sivas A, Meric H, Oz H. Fructosamine as a possible monitoring parameter in non-insulin dependent diabetes mellitus patients with periodontal disease. *J Periodontol* 1993;**64**:191–194.

109 Peck T, Price C, English P, Gill G. Oral health in rural South African type 2 diabetic patients. *Trop Doct* 2006;**36**:111–112.

110 Jansson H, Lindholm E, Lindh C, Groop L, Bratthall G. Type 2 diabetes and risk for periodontal disease: a role for dental health awareness. *J Clin Periodontol* 2006;**33**:408–414.

111 Tervonen T, Oliver RC. Long-term control of diabetes mellitus and periodontitis. *J Clin Periodontol* 1993;**20**:431–435.

112 Guzman S, Karima M, Wang H-Y, Van Dyke TE. Association between interleukin-1 genotype and periodontal disease in a diabetic population. *J Periodontol* 2003;**74**: 1183–1190.

113 Negishi J, Kawanami M, Terada Y, Matsuhashi C, Ogami E, Iwasaka K, Hongo T. Effect of lifestyle on periodontal disease status in diabetic patients. *J Int Acad Periodontol* 2004;**6**:120–124.

114 Nichols C, Laster LL, Bodak-Gyovai LZ. Diabetes mellitus and periodontal disease. *J Periodontol* 1978;**49**:85–88.

115 Hayden P, Buckley LA. Diabetes mellitus and periodontal disease in an Irish population. *J Periodontal Res* 1989;**24**: 298–302.

116 Papapanou PN. Periodontal diseases: epidemiology. *Ann Periodontol* 1996;**1**:1–36.

117 Khader YS, Dauod AS, El-Qaderi SS, Alkafajei A, Batayha WQ. Periodontal status of diabetics compared with non-diabetics: a meta-analysis [see comment in *Evid Based Dent* 2006; 7(2): 45; PMID: 16858380]. *J Diabetes Complications* 2006;**20**:59–68.

118 Salvi GE, Lawrence HP, Offenbacher S, Beck JD. Influence of risk factors on the pathogenesis of periodontitis. *Periodontology* 1997;**14**:173–201.

119 Wilton JM, Griffiths GS, Curtis MA, Maiden MF, Gillett IR, Wilson DT, Sterne JA, Johnson NW. Detection of high-risk groups and individuals for periodontal diseases. Systemic predisposition and markers of general health. *J Clin Periodontol* 1988;**15**:339–346.

120 Murrah VA. Diabetes mellitus and associated oral manifestations: a review. *J Oral Pathol* 1985;**14**:271–281.

121 Manouchehr-Pour M, Bissada NF. Periodontal disease in juvenile and adult diabetic patients: a review of the literature. *J Am Dent Assoc* 1983;**107**:766–770.

122 Oliver RC, Tervonen T. Diabetes – a risk factor for periodontitis in adults? *J Periodontol* 1994;**65**:530–538.

123 Grossi SG, Genco RJ. Periodontal disease and diabetes mellitus: a two-way relationship. *Ann Periodontol* 1998;**3**: 51–61.

124 Iacopino AM. Diabetic periodontitis: possible lipid-induced defect in tissue repair through alteration of macrophage phenotype and function. *Oral Dis* 1995;**1**:214–229.

125 Page RC. The pathobiology of periodontal diseases may affect systemic diseases: inversion of a paradigm. *Ann Periodontol* 1998;**3**:108–120.

126 Brayton RG, Stokes PE, Schwartz MS, Louria DB. Effect of alcohol and various diseases on leukocyte mobilization, phagocytosis and intracellular bacterial killing. *N Engl J Med* 1970;**282**:123–128.

127 Hill HR, Sauls HS, Dettloff JL, Quie PG. Impaired leukotactic responsiveness in patients with juvenile diabetes mellitus. *Clin Immunol Immunopathol* 1974;**2**:395–403.

128 Mowat A, Baum J. Chemotaxis of polymorphonuclear leukocytes from patients with diabetes mellitus. *N Engl J Med* 1971;**284**:621–627.

129 Miller ME, Baker L. Leukocyte functions in juvenile diabetes mellitus: humoral and cellular aspects. *J Pediatr* 1972;**81**:979–982.

130 Molenaar DM, Palumbo PJ, Wilson WR, Ritts RE Jr. Leukocyte chemotaxis in diabetic patients and their non-diabetic first-degree relatives. *Diabetes* 1976;**25**:880–883.

131 Bagdade JD, Stewart M, Walters E. Impaired granulocyte adherence. A reversible defect in host defense in patients with poorly controlled diabetes. *Diabetes* 1978;**27**:677–681.

132 Bagdade JD, Walters E. Impaired granulocyte adherence in mildly diabetic patients: effects of tolazamide treatment. *Diabetes* **29**:309–311.

133 Bagdade JD, Nielson KL, Bulger RJ. Reversible abnormalities in phagocytic function in poorly controlled diabetic patients. *Am J Med Sci* 1972;**263**:451–456.

134 Bagdade JD, Root RK, Bulger RJ. Impaired leukocyte function in patients with poorly controlled diabetes. *Diabetes* 1974;**23**:9–15.

135 Walters MI, Lessler MA, Stevenson TD. Oxidative metabolism of leukocytes from nondiabetic and diabetic patients. *J Lab Clin Med* 1971;**78**:158–166.

136 Collison KS, Parhar RS, Saleh SS, Meyer BF, Kwaasi AA, Hammami MM, Schmidt AM, Stern DM, Al-Mohanna FA. RAGE-mediated neutrophil dysfunction is evoked by advanced glycation end products (AGEs). *J Leukoc Biol* 2002;**71**:433–444.

137 Gyurko R, Siqueira CC, Caldon N, Gao L, Kantarci A, Van Dyke TE. Chronic hyperglycemia predisposes to exaggerated inflammatory response and leukocyte dysfunction in Akita mice. *J Immunol* 2006;**177**:7250–7256.

138 Brownlee M, Lilly Lecture 1993. Glycation and diabetic complications. *Diabetes* 1994;**43**:836–841.

139 Schmidt AM, Hori O, Cao R, Yan SD, Brett J, Wautier JL, Ogawa S, Kuwabara K, Matsumoto M, Stern D. RAGE: a novel cellular receptor for advanced glycation end products. *Diabetes* 1996;**45**:S77–S80.

140 Ramasamy R, Vannucci SJ, Yan SS. D, Herold K, Yan SF, Schmidt AM. Advanced glycation end products and RAGE: a common thread in aging, diabetes, neurodegeneration and inflammation. *Glycobiology* 2005;**15**:16R–28R.

141 Vlassara H. Recent progress on the biologic and clinical significance of advanced glycosylation end products. *J Lab Clin Med* 1994;**124**:19–30.

142 Schmidt AM, Weidman E, Lalla E, Yan SD, Hori O, Cao R, Brett JG, Lamster IB. Advanced glycation end-products (AGEs) induce oxidant stress in the gingiva: a potential mechanism underlying accelerated periodontal disease associated with diabetes. *J Periodontal Res* 1996;**31**:508–515.

143 Brett J, Schmidt AM, Yan SD, Zou YS, Weidman E, Pinsky D, Nowygrod R, Neeper M, Przysiecki C, Shaw, A *et al.* Survey of the distribution of a newly characterized receptor for advanced glycation end products in tissues. *Am J Pathol* 1993;**143**:1699–1712.

144 Schmidt AM, Yan SD, Yan SF, Stern DM. The biology of the receptor for advanced glycation end products and its ligands. *Biochim Biophys Acta* 2000;**1498**:99–111.

145 Yan SD, Schmidt AM, Anderson GM, Zhang J, Brett J, Zou YS, Pinsky D, Stern D. Enhanced cellular oxidant stress by the interaction of advanced glycation end products with their receptors/binding proteins. *J Biol Chem* 1994;**269**: 9889–9897.

146 Schmidt AM, Hasu M, Popov D, Zhang JH, Chen J, Yan SD, Brett J, Cao R, Kuwabara K, Costache, G *et al.* Receptor for advanced glycation end products (AGEs) has a central role in vessel wall interactions and gene activation in response to circulating AGE proteins. *Proc Natl Acad Sci USA* 1994;**91**:8807–8811.

147 Moughal NA, Adonogianaki E, Thornhill MH, Kinane DF. Endothelial cell leukocyte adhesion molecule-1 (ELAM-1) and intercellular adhesion molecule-1 (ICAM-1) expression in gingival tissue during health and experimentally-induced gingivitis. *J Periodontal Res* 1992;**27**:623–630.

148 Baeuerle PA. The inducible transcription activator NF-kappa B: regulation by distinct protein subunits. *Biochim Biophys Acta* 1991;**1072**:63–80.

149 Schreck R, Rieber P, Baeuerle PA. Reactive oxygen intermediates as apparently widely used messengers in the activation of the NF-kappa B transcription factor and HIV-1. *EMBO J* 1991;**10**:2247–2258.

150 Collins T. Endothelial nuclear factor-kappa B and the initiation of the atherosclerotic lesion. *Lab Invest* 1993;**68**: 499–508.

151 Takahashi K, Takashiba S, Nagai A, Takigawa M, Myoukai F, Kurihara H, Murayama Y. Assessment of interleukin-6 in the pathogenesis of periodontal disease. *J Periodontol* 1994;**65**:147–153.

152 Salvi GE, Beck JD, Offenbacher S. PGE2, IL-1 beta and TNF-alpha responses in diabetics as modifiers of periodontal disease expression. *Ann Periodontol* 1998;**3**:40–50.

153 Goova MT, Li J, Kislinger T, Qu W, Lu Y, Bucciarelli LG, Nowygrod S, Wolf BM, Caliste X, Yan SF, Stern DM, Schmidt AM. Blockade of receptor for advanced glycation end-products restores effective wound healing in diabetic mice. *Am J Pathol* 2001;**159**:513–525.

154 Lalla E, Lamster IB, Feit M, Huang L, Spessot A, Qu W, Kislinger T, Lu Y, Stern DM, Schmidt AM. Blockade of RAGE suppresses periodontitis-associated bone loss in diabetic mice. *J Clin Invest* 2000;**105**:1117–1124.

155 Lalla E, Lamster IB, Schmidt AM. Enhanced interaction of advanced glycation end products with their cellular receptor RAGE: implications for the pathogenesis of accelerated periodontal disease in diabetes. *Ann Periodontol* 1998;**3**:13–19.

156 Wautier JL, Zoukourian C, Chappey O, Wautier MP, Guillausseau PJ, Cao R, Hori O, Stern D, Schmidt AM. Receptor-mediated endothelial cell dysfunction in diabetic vasculopathy. Soluble receptor for advanced glycation end products blocks hyperpermeability in diabetic rats. *J Clin Invest* 1996;**97**:238–243.

157 Schmidt AM, Hori O, Chen JX, Li JF, Crandall J, Zhang J, Cao R, Yan SD, Brett J, Stern D. Advanced glycation endproducts interacting with their endothelial receptor induce expression of vascular cell adhesion molecule-1 (VCAM-1) in cultured human endothelial cells and in mice. A potential mechanism for the accelerated vasculopathy of diabetes. *J Clin Invest* 1995;**96**:1395–1403.

158 Lalla E, Lamster IB, Feit M, Huang L, Schmidt AM. A murine model of accelerated periodontal disease in diabetes. *J Periodontal Res* 1998;**33**:387–399.

159 Graves DT, Liu R, Alikhani M, Al-Mashat H, Trackman PC. Diabetes-enhanced inflammation and apoptosis – impact on periodontal pathology. *J Dent Res* 2006;**85**:15–21.

160 Bouillon R. Diabetic bone disease. *Calcified Tissue Int* 1991;**49**:155–160.

161 Kawaguchi H, Kurokawa T, Hanada K, Hiyama Y, Tamura M, Ogata E, Matsumoto T. Stimulation of fracture repair by recombinant human basic fibroblast growth factor in normal and streptozotocin-diabetic rats. *Endocrinology* 1994;**135**:774–781.

162 Lu H, Kraut D, Gerstenfeld LC, Graves DT. Diabetes interferes with the bone formation by affecting the expression of transcription factors that regulate osteoblast differentiation. *Endocrinology* 2003;**144**:346–352.

163 McCarthy AD, Etcheverry SB, Cortizo AM. Effect of advanced glycation endproducts on the secretion of insulin-like growth factor-I and its binding proteins: role in osteoblast development. *Acta Diabetol* 2001;**38**:113–122.

164 Cortizo AM, Lettieri MG, Barrio DA, Mercer N, Etcheverry SB, McCarthy AD. Advanced glycation end-products (AGEs) induce concerted changes in the osteoblastic expression of their receptor RAGE and in the activation of extracellular signal-regulated kinases (ERK). *Mol Cell Biochem* 2003;**250**:1–10.

165 Santana RB, Xu L, Chase HB, Amar S, Graves DT, Trackman PC. A role for advanced glycation end products in diminished bone healing in type 1 diabetes. *Diabetes* 2003;**52**: 1502–1510.

166 Clark RAF, Henson PM. *The Molecular and Cellular Biology of Wound Repair*, Plenum Press, New York, 1998.

167 Andreesen R, Kreutz M, Lohr GW. Surface phenotype analysis of human monocyte to macrophage maturation. *J Leuk Biol* 1990;**47**:490–497.

168 Messadi DV, Bertolami CN. General principles of healing pertinent to the periodontal problem. *Dent Clin North Am* 1991;**35**:443–447.

169 Kreutz M, Krause SW, Rehm, A *et al.* Macrophage heterogeneity and differentiation. *Res Immunol* 1992;**143**:107–115.

170 Martin P, Hopkinson-Woolley J, McCluskey J. Growth factors and cutaneous wound repair. *Prog Growth Factor Res* 1992;**4**:25–44.

171 Wikesjo UME, Nilveus RE, Selvig KA. Significance of early healing events on periodontal repair: a review. *J Periodontol* 1992;**63**:158–165.

172 Kiritsy CP, Lynch SE. Role of growth factors in cutaneous wound healing: a review. *Crit Rev Oral Biol Med* 1993;**4**:729–760.

173 Sullivan DR, Conney G, Caterson, I *et al.* The effects of dietary fatty acid in animal models of type 1 and type 2 diabetes. *Diabetes Res Clin Pract* 1990;**9**:225–230.

174 Clarke SD, Jump DB. Regulation of gene transcription by polyunsaturated fatty acids. *Prog Lipid Res* 1993;**32**:139–149.

175 Hicks M, Delbridge L, Yue, D *et al.* Catalysis of lipid peroxidation by glucose and glycosylated proteins. *Biochem Biophys Res Commun* 1988;**151**:649–655.

176 Hunt J, Smith C, Wolff S. Autooxidative glycosylation and possible involvement of peroxides and free radicals in LDL modification by glucose. *Diabetes* 1990;**30**: 1420–1424.

177 Bucala R, Makita Z, Koschinsky, T *et al.* Lipid advanced glycosylation: pathway for lipid oxidation *in vivo*. *Proc Natl Acad Sci USA* 1993;**90**:6434–6438.

178 Salbach PB, Specht E, Von Hodenberg E, Kossmann J, Janssen-Timmen U, Schneider WJ, Hugger P, King WC, Glomset JA, Habenicht AJ. Differential low density lipoprotein receptor-dependent formation of eicosanoids in human blood-derived monocytes. *Proc Natl Acad Sci USA* 1992;**89**:2439–2443.

179 Jambou D, Dejour N, Bayer P, Poiree JC, Fredenrich A, Issa-Sayegh M, Adjovi-Desouza M, Lapalus P, Harter M. Effect of human native low-density and high-density lipoproteins on prostaglandin production by mouse macrophage cell line P388D1: possible implications in pathogenesis of atherosclerosis. *Biochim Biophys Acta* 1993;**1168**: 115–121.

180 Salvi GE, Collins JG, Yalda B, Arnold RR, Lang NP, Offenbacher S. Monocytic TNFα secretion patterns in IDDM patients with periodontal diseases. *J Clin Periodontol* 1997;**24**:8–16.

181 Salvi GE, Yalda B, Collins JG, Jones BH, Smith FW, Arnold RR, Offenbacher S. Inflammatory mediator response as a potential risk marker for periodontal diseases in insulin-dependent diabetes mellitus patients. *J Periodontol* 1997;**68**:127–135.

182 Santamaria P, Gehrz RC, Bryan MK, Barbosa JJ. Involvement of class II MHC molecules in the LPS-induction of IL-1/TNF secretions by human monocytes. Quantitative differences at the polymorphic level. *J Immunol* 1989;**143**: 913–922.

183 Pociot F, Molvig J, Wogensen L, Worsaae H, Dalboge H, Baek L, Nerup J. A tumour necrosis factor beta gene polymorphism in relation to monokine secretion and insulin-dependent diabetes mellitus. *Scand J Immunol* 1991;**33**: 37–49.

184 Pociot F, Wilson AG, Nerup J, Duff GW. No independent association between a tumor necrosis factor-alpha promotor region polymorphism and insulin-dependent diabetes mellitus. *Eur J Immunol* 1993;**23**:3050–3053.

185 Leslie RDG, Lazarus NR, Vergani D. Etiology of insulin dependent diabetes mellitus. *Br Med Bull* 1989;**45**:58–72.

186 Reinhardt RA, Maze CS, Seagren-Alley CD, Dubois LM. HLA-D types associated with type 1 diabetes and periodontitis. *J Dent Res* 1991;**70**:414 (Abstr. 1190).

187 Todd JA. Genetic control of autoimmunity in type 1 diabetes. *Immunol Today* 1990;**11**:122–129.

188 Tsiavou A, Hatziagelaki E, Chaidaroglou A, Manginas A, Koniavitou K, Degiannis D, Raptis SA. TNF-alpha, TGF-beta1, IL-10, IL-6, gene polymorphisms in latent autoimmune diabetes of adults (LADA) and type 2 diabetes mellitus. *J Clin Immunol* 2004;**24**:591–599.

189 Offenbacher S, Katz V, Fertik G, Collins J, Boyd D, Maynor G, McKaig R, Beck J. Periodontal infection as a possible risk factor for preterm low birth weight. *J Periodontol* 1996;**67**:1103–1113.

190 Ling PR, Istfan NW, Colon E, Bistrian BR. Differential effects of interleukin-1 receptor antagonist in cytokine- and endotoxin-treated rats. *Am J Physiol* 1995;**268**: E255–E261.

191 Feingold KR, Soued M, Serio MK, Moser AH, Dinarello CA, Grunfeld C. Multiple cytokines stimulate hepatic lipid synthesis *in vivo*. *Endocrinology* 1989;**125**:267–274.

192 Feingold KR, Grunfeld C. Role of cytokines in inducing hyperlipidemia. *Diabetes* 1992;**41**:97–101.

193 Grunfeld C, Soued M, Adi S, Moser AH, Dinarello CA, Feingold KR. Evidence for two classes of cytokines that stimulate hepatic lipogenesis: relationships among tumor necrosis factor, interleukin-1 and interferon-alpha. *Endocrinology* 1990;**127**:46–54.

194 Pickup JC, Mattock MB, Chusney GD, Burt D. NIDDM as a disease of the innate immune system: association of acute-phase reactants and interleukin-6 with metabolic syndrome X. *Diabetologia* 1997;**40**:1286–1292.

195 Michie HR. Metabolism of sepsis and multiple organ failure. *World J Surg* 1996;**20**:460–464.

196 Aldridge JP, Lester V, Watts TL, Collins A, Viberti G, Wilson RF. Single-blind studies of the effects of improved periodontal health on metabolic control in type 1 diabetes mellitus. *J Clin Periodontol* 1995;**22**:271–275.

197 Skaleric U, Schara R, Medvescek M, Hanlon A, Doherty F, Lessem J. Periodontal treatment by Arestin and its effects on glycaemic control in type 1 diabetes patients. *J Int Acad Periodontol* 2004;**6**:160–165.

198 Grossi SG, Skrepcinski FB, Decaro T, Robertson DC, Ho AW, Dunford RG, Genco RJ. Treatment of periodontal disease in diabetics reduces glycated hemoglobin. *J Periodontol* 1997;**68**:713–719.

199 Kiran M, Arpak N, Unsal E, Erdoan MF. The effect of improved periodontal health on metabolic control in type 2 diabetes mellitus. *J Clin Periodontol* 2005;**32**:266–272.

200 Rodrigues DC, Taba MJ, Novaes AB Jr, Souza SLS, Grisi MFM. Effect of non-surgical periodontal therapy on glycaemic control in patients with type 2 diabetes mellitus [published erratum appears in *J Periodontol* 2004; **75**: 780]. *J Periodontol* 2003;**74**:1361–1367.

201 Jones JA, Miller DR, Wehler CJ, Rich SE, Krall-Kaye EA, McCoy LC, Christiansen CL, Rothendler JA, Garcia RI. Does periodontal care improve glycaemic control? The Department of Veterans Affairs Dental Diabetes Study. *J Clin Periodontol* 2007;**34**:46–52.

202 Talbert J, Elter J, Jared HL, Offenbacher S, Southerland J, Wilder RS. The effect of periodontal therapy on TNF-alpha, IL-6 and metabolic control in type 2 diabetics. *J Dent Hyg* 2006;**80**:7.

203 Smith GT, Greenbaum CJ, Johnson BD, Persson GR. Short-term responses to periodontal therapy in insulin-dependent diabetic patients [published erratum appears in *J Periodontol* 1996; **67**: 1368]. *J Periodontol* 1996;**67**: 794–802.

204 Westfelt E, Rylander H, Blohme G, Jonasson P, Lindhe J. The effect of periodontal therapy in diabetics. Results after 5 years. *J Clin Periodontol* 1996;**23**:92–100.

205 Christgau M, Palitzsch KD, Schmalz G, Kreiner U, Frenzel S. Healing response to non-surgical periodontal therapy in patients with diabetes mellitus: clinical, microbiological and immunologic results. *J Clin Periodontol* 1998;**25**: 112–124.

206 Taylor GW, Burt BA, Becker MP, Genco RJ, Shlossman M, Knowler WC, Pettitt DJ. Severe periodontitis and risk for poor glycaemic control in patients with non-insulin-dependent diabetes mellitus. *J Periodontol* 1996;**67**: 1085–1093.

207 Collin HL, Uusitupa M, Niskanen L, Kontturi-Narhi V, Markkanen H, Koivisto AM, Meurman JH. Periodontal findings in elderly patients with non-insulin dependent diabetes mellitus. *J Periodontol* 1998;**69**:962–926.

208 Schara R, Medvescek M, Skaleric U. Periodontal disease and diabetes metabolic control: a full-mouth disinfection approach. *J Int Acad Periodontol* 2006;**8**:61–66.

209 Miller LS, Manwell MA, Newbold D, Reding ME, Rasheed A, Blodgett J, Kornman KS. The relationship between reduction in periodontal inflammation and diabetes control: a report of 9 cases. *J Periodontol* 1992;**63**:843–848.

210 Iwamoto Y, Nishimura F, Nakagawa M, Sugimoto H, Shikata K, Makino H, Fukuda T, Tsuji T, Iwamoto M, Murayama Y. The effect of antimicrobial periodontal treatment on circulating tumor necrosis factor-alpha and glycated hemoglobin level in patients with type 2 diabetes. *J Periodontol* 2001;**72**:774–778.

211 Faria-Almeida R, Navarro A, Bascones A. Clinical and metabolic changes after conventional treatment of type 2 diabetic patients with chronic periodontitis. *J Periodontol* 2006;**77**:591–598.

212 Stewart JE, Wager KA, Friedlander AH, Zadeh HH. The effect of periodontal treatment on glycaemic control in patients with type 2 diabetes mellitus. *J Clin Periodontol* 2001;**28**:306–310.

213 Promsudthi A, Pimapansri S, Deerochanawong C, Kanchanavasita W. The effect of periodontal therapy on uncontrolled type 2 diabetes mellitus in older subjects. *Oral Dis* 2005;**11**:293–298.

214 Williams RC Jr, Mahan CJ. Periodontal disease and diabetes in young adults. *JAMA* 1960;**172**:776–778.

215 Janket SJ, Wightman A, Baird AE, Van Dyke TE, Jones JA. Does periodontal treatment improve glycaemic control in diabetic patients? A meta-analysis of intervention studies. *J Dent Res* 2005;**84**:1154–1159.

216 Taylor GW. Periodontal treatment and its effects on glycaemic control: a review of the evidence. *Oral Surg Oral Med Oral Pathol Oral Radiol Endod* 1999;**87**:311–316.

217 Diabetes Control and Complications Trial Research Group. The effect of intensive treatment of diabetes on the development and progression of long-term complications in insulin-dependent diabetes mellitus. The Diabetes Control and Complications Trial Research Group. *N Engl J Med* 1993;**329**:977–986.

218 UK Prospective Diabetes Study (UKPDS) Group. Intensive blood-glucose control with sulphonylureas or insulin compared with conventional treatment and risk of complications in patients with type 2 diabetes (UKPDS 33). UK Prospective Diabetes Study (UKPDS) Group [published

erratum appears in *Lancet* 1999; **354**: 602]. *Lancet* 1998;**352**: 837–853.

219 UK Prospective Diabetes Study (UKPDS) Group. Effect of intensive blood-glucose control with metformin on complications in overweight patients with type 2 diabetes (UKPDS 34). UK Prospective Diabetes Study (UKPDS) Group [published erratum appears in *Lancet* 1998; **352**: 1558]. *Lancet* 1998;**352**:854–865.

220 Genuth S, Eastman R, Kahn R, Klein R, Lachin J, Lebovitz H, Nathan D, Vinicor F and the American Diabetes Association. Implications of the United Kingdom Prospective Diabetes Study. *Diabetes Care* 2003;**26**(Suppl 1): S28–S32.

221 Thorstensson H, Kuylenstierna J, Hugoson A. Medical status and complications in relation to periodontal disease experience in insulin-dependent diabetics. *J Clin Periodontol* 1996;**23**:194–202.

222 Saremi A, Nelson RG, Tulloch-Reid M, Hanson RL, Sievers ML, Taylor GW, Shlossman M, Bennett PH, Genco R, Knowler WC. Periodontal disease and mortality in type 2 diabetes. *Diabetes Care* 2005;**28**:27–32.

223 Shultis WA, Weil EJ, Looker HC, Curtis JM, Shlossman M, Genco RJ, Knowler WC, Nelson RG. Effect of periodontitis on overt nephropathy and end-stage renal disease in type 2 diabetes. *Diabetes Care* 2007;**30**:306–311.

19 Treatment of diabetic neuropathy

Rodica Pop-Busui[1], Zachary Simmons[2], Eva L. Feldman[3]

[1]*Department of Internal Medicine, Division of Metabolism, Endocrinology and Diabetes, University of Michigan Medical Center, Ann Arbor, MI, USA*
[2]*Pennsylvania State University College of Medicine, Hershey, PA, USA*
[3]*University of Michigan, Ann Arbor, MI, USA*

Definition

At the San Antonio Consensus Conference in 1988, it was agreed that diabetic neuropathy (DN) 'is a descriptive term meaning a demonstrable disorder, either clinically evident or subclinical, that occurs in the setting of diabetes mellitus without other causes for peripheral neuropathy'.[1] A later international consensus meeting on the outpatient diagnosis and management of DN defined DN as 'the presence of symptoms and/or signs of peripheral nerve dysfunction in people with diabetes after the exclusion of other causes'.[2] This same definition was adopted by the American Diabetes Association in 2005.[3]

Prevalence of diabetic neuropathy

DN is the most common complication of diabetes. In the United States, DN is the leading cause of diabetes-related hospital admissions and non-traumatic amputations and is associated with a poor quality of life.[4,5] The American Diabetes Association estimates that DN costs $22 billion per year (www.diabetes.org).

It is estimated that approximately 50% of patients have DN, although estimates vary from 10 to 100% depending on the diagnostic criteria used.[6] Probably the most frequently cited prospective observational study of DN was completed in an outpatient clinic by Pirart.[7] He examined 4400 patients 10% of whom had neuropathy at the time of diagnosis. After 25 years of diabetes, half (50%) of the patients had neuropathy.[7] A similar prevalence was reported in the Rochester Diabetic Neuropathy Study, in which 59% of type 2 and 66% of type 1 diabetic patients had DN.[8] Another large cross-sectional study of 6487 type 1 and type 2 diabetic patients in the United Kingdom found the prevalence of DN to be 29%.[9] Among type 1 diabetic patients older than 30 years of age followed in the Pittsburgh Epidemiology of Diabetes Study, 58% had DN.[10,11] Prior to entering the Diabetes Control and Complication Trial (DCCT), 39% of 278 otherwise healthy type 1 diabetic patients met the clinical criteria for DN. The EURODIAB IDDM Complications Study found that the prevalence of DN, across 3250 randomly selected type 1 diabetic patients from 16 European countries, was 28% with no significant geographical differences.[12] DN appears to be less common in children, with a prevalence of 2% or less.[6]

The reported differences in prevalence of DN arise partially from differences in age, but primarily from the differences in the criteria used for the diagnosis of DN. In most of these large, prospective studies, the prevalence of DN increased with duration of disease (Table 19.1).

Pathogenesis

The mechanisms underlying the development of DN are under active investigation. The contribution of hyperglycaemia to the pathogenesis of microvascular complications, including DN, in both type 1[15] and type 2 diabetes[16,17] is firmly established. The DCCT provided strong evidence for the importance of

The Evidence Base for Diabetes Care, Second Edition, Edited by William H. Herman, Ann Louise Kinmonth, Nicholas J. Wareham and Rhys Williams.

Table 19.1 Change in the prevalence of diabetic neuropathy over time

Study	Initial prevalence (%)	Time of initial prevalence	Later prevalence (%)	Time of later prevalence
Pirart, 1978[7]	7.5	At diagnosis	50	25 years after diagnosis
Palumbo et al., 1978[13]	4	Within 5 years of diagnosis	15	20 years after diagnosis
Young et al., 1993[9]	20.8	Less than 5 years duration	36.8	Greater than 10 years duration
Partanen et al., 1995[14]	8.3	At diagnosis	41.9	10 years after diagnosis
DCCT, 1995[15]	3.5 primary prevention	At baseline	9.6	6.5 years
	9.4 secondary intervention	At baseline	16.9	6.5 years

hyperglycaemia, insulin deficiency or both in the pathogenesis of DN.[15] Intensive insulin therapy to reduce blood glucose levels to as close to the normal range as possible in subjects with type 1 diabetes and no neuropathy reduced the incidence of clinical DN, confirmed by abnormal nerve conduction studies or autonomic function tests, by 60% after 5 years. A close association between the severity and/or duration of hyperglycaemia and the development and progression of diabetic complications, including DN, is also supported by the results of the Epidemiology of Diabetes Interventions and Complications (EDIC) study, an observational follow-up of the DCCT cohort.[18] Patients in the DCCT intensive therapy arm were protected from the development of DN, despite the fact that their glycaemic control had risen to the same level as those subjects in the conventional arm for at least 8 years following completion of the DCCT.[18]

Prospective studies of patients with type 2 diabetes have established the role of hyperglycaemia in the pathogenesis of DN, but also suggest that other metabolic and vascular factors contribute to the disease. In the United Kingdom Prospective Diabetes Study (UKPDS), intensive treatment lowered HbA_{1c} by 1% and produced a 25% risk reduction in all microvascular endpoints. However, individual surrogate endpoints for DN showed only trends toward improvement in the intensive treatment group in the first 10 years. Only after 15 years was there a significant difference between the two groups in the degree of sensory impairment in the lower extremities (31.2% in the intensive group vs 51.7% in the conventional group, $P = 0.0052$).[19] The authors suggest that hypertension, obesity and smoking contribute to the development of DN in type 2 diabetes. Recent findings from EURODIAB support this idea and suggest that metabolic and vascular factors also promote DN in type 1 diabetic patients. In the EURODIAB cohort of type 1 patients, both hypertension and hyperlipidaemia accelerated the effects of hyperglycaemia on nerve dysfunction and even slight improvements in lipids

were associated with a significantly lower risk of DN.[20]

Data from animal and cell culture models of DN support the concept that both metabolic and vascular factors are involved in the pathogenesis of DN. Animal and *in vitro* experiments implicate enzymatic and non-enzymatic pathways of glucose metabolism in the initiation and progression of DN. These include: increased oxidative and nitrosative stress, redox imbalance secondary to enhanced aldose reductase (AR) activity, non-enzymatic glycation of structural nerve proteins, impaired protein kinase C (PKC) activity, impaired nitric oxide synthesis and endothelial dysfunction, alterations in cyclooxygenase (COX) activity with subsequent perturbations in prostaglandin (PG) metabolism, direct hypoxia and ischaemia of nerve trunks and ganglia, deficiencies in the neurotrophic support of neurons and deficiencies in C-peptide.[21–23] In nerve, this pattern of metabolic and vascular disturbance impairs mitochondrial function and neurotrophic support and mediates injury of neurons and Schwann cells, culminating in progressive damage and loss of peripheral nerve fibres and impaired sensory function.[24]

Classification of DN

DN is associated with a broad spectrum of clinical symptoms and comprises a variety of syndromes.[3,26] Multiple classifications have been proposed. A generally accepted one is shown in Table 19.2. Each classification provides a framework for differential diagnosis. For example, at the time of an initial neuropathy evaluation, it is useful to know whether the neuropathy is compatible with a diabetic aetiology. The less a particular pattern is associated with diabetes, the more vigorously an alternative explanation should be sought. Another value of classification is that it may offer a prognosis to the individual patient. Indolently progressive, distal symmetric

Table 19.2 Classification of diabetic neuropathies

- Distal symmetric sensorimotor polyneuropathy (DN)
- Autonomic neuropathy
- Focal and multifocal neuropathies
  - Cranial neuropathy
  - Limb mononeuropathy
    - Median
    - Ulnar
    - Radial
    - Femoral
    - Peroneal
    - Lateral femoral cutaneous
  - Truncal mononeuropathy
  - Mononeuropathy multiplex
  - Asymmetric lower limb motor neuropathy (amyotrophy)
- Mixed forms

sensorimotor polyneuropathy rarely remits. The subacute, asymmetric proximal neuropathies, on the other hand, usually reach a plateau of maximal deficit and then improve spontaneously.

Distal symmetric sensorimotor polyneuropathy

Distal symmetric sensorimotor polyneuropathy is by far the most common form of DN and in this review DN refers to this form of neuropathy.[3,27] DN usually begins insidiously and may be the presenting feature in type 2 diabetes.[19,28] Indeed, DN may occur in patients with impaired glucose tolerance.[29]

Clinical presentation

In DN, the most distal portions of the longest nerves are affected first. The earliest symptoms typically involve the tip of the toes and fingers and proceed proximally resulting in a 'stocking-glove' pattern of symptoms and sensory loss. If severe DN, the midline chest and abdomen may also be involved.

Symptoms vary according to the class of sensory fibres involved. The most common symptoms are tingling and pain which are induced by the involvement of small fibres. The pain is particularly troubling to most patients and is often the reason why patients with DN seek medical care. The pain may be described as sharp, stabbing, burning or aching. It is often worse at night and may disturb sleep. Involvement of larger fibres produces a tight, band-like feeling around the extremity or an electrical tingling sensation. These symptoms are often similar to those described by patients with lesions in the posterior columns of the spinal cord.

Loss of feeling may also occur in the feet with or without pain or dysaesthesias. If nociceptive fibres are involved, loss of sensation may set the stage for painless injuries. An object may become lodged in the shoe and erode through the skin with normal walking and weight-bearing. Painless ulcers may develop over pressure points, most commonly over the metatarsal heads. In patients with involvement of large sensory fibres, gait ataxia may develop, especially at night or when the patient walks with the eyes closed. Weakness is less common, usually minor and occurs later.

A number of simple screening questionnaires are available to record the presence of symptoms and their severity. The Michigan Neuropathy Screening Instrument (MNSI)[30] and similar symptom scoring systems, used in the European prevalence studies, are useful in clinical practice.[9,31] Both symptoms and deficits may have an adverse effect on quality of life (QoL) in DN.[32] The NeuroQol, a recently developed and validated QoL instrument, includes a symptom checklist and may be used as an outcome measure in clinical studies.[32]

Diagnostic studies

After a careful history, *clinical examination* is the next step to establish the presence of DN. Examination demonstrates a symmetrical distal sensory loss, with reduced or absent ankle reflexes. Among patients who complain only of distal burning, the loss of distal sensation may be very subtle. In patients with severe DN, motor involvement may become clinically apparent with weakness of toe dorsiflexion and of intrinsic hand muscles. This weakness may gradually progress to involve the leg muscles, but it is very rare for weakness to occur proximal to the knee or elbow. Any pronounced motor signs should raise the possibility of a non-diabetic aetiology of the neuropathy, especially if asymmetric.[3] Longitudinal studies have shown that a simple clinical examination using a 10 g monofilament perception and vibration perception is a good predictor of future foot ulcer risk.[34]

Sensory loss is defined in terms of extent, distribution and modality including assessment of pinprick sensation, light touch, vibration and joint position. Evaluation of threshold is probably more reproducible than subjective assessment by the patient of the strength of stimulus.[3]

A variety of scales and composite scores have been used to assess semi-quantitatively sensation, strength and reflexes in clinical trials. Their use was pioneered by Dyck and colleagues,[35,36] who first described the Neuropathy Disability Score and later the Neuropathy Impairment Score. Similarly, the Michigan Diabetes Neuropathy Scale (MDNS), the examination portion of the MNSI and the Toronto Clinical Scoring System are designed to be applicable across a broad range of neuropathy types and severity and balance contribution of sensory and motor findings to the exam score.[30,37]

Electrodiagnostic studies

Electrophysiological studies are usually not required to make a diagnosis of DN. Nerve conduction studies and electromyography (needle electrode examination of muscle) may aid in the clinical evaluation of diabetic patients in several ways: confirmation of the clinical diagnosis of neuropathy, identification of a pattern of electrophysiological changes characteristic of diabetes, monitoring of progression or remission of disease and detection of asymptomatic disease.

Electrophysiological abnormalities are frequently present in completely asymptomatic patients with diabetes. On nerve conduction studies, the lower extremity nerves are affected first and most severely. The earliest and most sensitive findings are changes in sensory nerve conduction, which demonstrate a reduction in conduction velocity and a decrease in amplitude. Motor nerve studies may demonstrate some slowing even when patients have no symptoms or signs of neuropathy, with a greater slowing in symptomatic patients. A decrease in motor amplitudes may be seen in more advanced DN. Needle electromyography may be normal in mild or neurologically asymptomatic subjects, but demonstrates denervation in more severe DN, most prominent distally. With more severe neuropathy, the sensory responses may disappear and findings of axonal degeneration predominate: decreased amplitude of compound muscle action potentials (CMAPs) and sensory nerve action potentials (SNAPs), relative preservation of proximal conduction velocities and evidence of fibrillation potentials and motor unit remodelling on needle examination. Multiple nerves examination usually shows a multifocal pattern of involvement, rather than a completely diffuse symmetric pattern.[38]

Quantitative sensory testing (QST) is an additional measure to assess the loss of protective sensation. QST may be performed with a variety of instruments that deliver specific stimuli at designated intensities, providing a non-invasive parametric gauge of sensory function (i.e. perceptions of light touch or pressure, vibration, heat and cold and pain) and axonal pathology.[39] QST that focuses on the vibration perception threshold (VPT) assessed by using a 128 Hz tuning fork potentially offers a quick, inexpensive and accurate screening instrument to evaluate high-risk patients in the clinic.[40]

Pathology

Histological studies from autopsy and sural nerve biopsy material from patients with DN have identified deficits involving peripheral nerve axons, including progressive damage to and loss of unmyelinated nerve fibres and small and large myelinated fibres. Demyelination is also seen on teased fibre studies. The proximal-to-distal increase in morphological abnormalities suggest a primary axonopathy preferentially involving longer myelinated axons.[41] However, defects in Schwann cells, perineurial cells and endoneurial vascular elements such as basement membrane thickening and reduplication, endothelial cell swelling and proliferation and platelet aggregation resulting in vessel occlusion have been also described.[6]

Acute painful neuropathy is a variant of DN with a distinct mode of onset, signs and prognosis. The natural history of this condition is very different from that of the much more common chronic form of ND. Its onset is acute or subacute and in general the severe symptoms resolve in less than 1 year.[42] Pain is the outstanding complaint in all patients, experienced as a deep aching pain with occasional sudden, sharp, stabbing or 'electric shock'-like sensations in the lower limbs with nocturnal exacerbations. Most patients also experience severe weight loss, depression and, in males, erectile dysfunction. In spite of the dramatic clinical presentation, the clinical examination is usually relatively normal, with allodynia (an exaggerated response to otherwise nonnoxious stimuli) on sensory testing, a normal motor examination and occasionally reduced ankle reflexes.[27]

Treatment

Control of hyperglycaemia

Treatment of DN has traditionally focused on control of hyperglycaemia as a means of delaying the appearance or slowing the progression of neuropathy. Pancreatic transplantation appears to halt the progression of DN, but does not clearly reverse existing neuropathy.[43,44] The DCCT demonstrated that intensive therapy of type 1 diabetes reduced the incidence of neuropathy by 60% over a 5 year period in patients who did not have neuropathy at baseline.[15] An unequivocal benefit of the near-normoglycaemic state on DN was also described in type 1 diabetic patients treated with continuous subcutaneous insulin infusion pumps. Data are less convincing for type 2 diabetic patients.[3]

Experimental therapies

An improved understanding of the pathogenesis of DN affords multiple opportunities for intervention. Therapies being tested in phase two or three clinical trials include aldose reductase inhibitors, the potent antioxidant lipoic acid and a growth factor analogue.

Aldose reductase inhibitors (ARIs)

ARIs have been studied as a means to prevent or improve DN. They act by reducing the flux of glucose through the polyol pathway. There have been many human clinical trials of ARIs since 1981, with mixed results.[45] A recent meta-analysis of 13 randomized controlled clinical trials of ARIs found that the effects on motor nerve conduction velocity were inconsistent on different nerves within trials and between trials, leading the authors to conclude that no clear conclusion can be drawn regarding the benefits of ARIs in the treatment of DN.[46] An analysis of 32 trials of ARIs on patients with DN found that ARIs showed promise for possibly slowing the progression of DN, but that many of these trials were flawed, being of insufficient duration and size.[45] A double-blind, placebo-controlled trial of the ARI zenarestat demonstrated that doses producing >80% suppression of nerve sorbitol content were required to demonstrate efficacy, so that even low residual levels of aldose reductase activity might be neurotoxic.[47]

The benefits associated with the newer ARIs are currently being explored. Recent studies with the potent ARI fidarestat (Sanwa Kagaku KenKyusho, Nagoya, Japan) have shown benefit in animals[48] and in diabetic patients.[49,50] Ranirestat (AS-3201), a novel ARI developed by Dainippon Pharmaceutical (Osaka, Japan), demonstrated that 12 weeks of potent inhibition of the polyol pathway was associated with improved sensory nerve function which was maintained at 60 weeks and improved motor nerve function at 60 weeks.[51] Whether ARIs are effective in the treatment of DN has not yet been established.

α-Lipoic acid (LA)

LA (1,2-dithiolane-3-pentanoic acid), also known as thioctic acid, a derivative of octanoic acid, is present in food and is synthesized by the liver. It is a natural cofactor in the pyruvate dehydrogenase complex, where it binds acyl groups and transfers them from one part of the complex to another. LA plays a role in the antioxidant network as a thiol-replenishing and redox-modulating agent. In its reduced form, LA can regenerate glutathione (GSH).[52] Furthermore, LA can induce the synthesis of GSH by reducing its precursor molecule cysteine to cystine, which is important for the antioxidant network function.[53] LA is probably the most extensively used antioxidant compound. It can be absorbed from the diet and can cross the blood–brain barrier. In rats, LA prevents the development of nerve conduction deficits after 6 weeks of streptozotocin-induced diabetes.[54] Larger multi-centre randomized double-blind placebo trials in Europe and North America have demonstrated limited effects on neuropathic symptoms and electrophysiological testing, suggesting that longer term assessment of neuropathic deficits is merited.[55,56] A recent Phase III clinical trial, the SYDNEY trial, demonstrated that

intravenous administration of LA rapidly and significantly improves several neuropathic symptoms and nerve function in patients with DN.[57] A recent large-scale placebo-controlled multicentre North American trial of oral LA in DN awaits final analysis.

Nerve growth factor (NGF)

Recombinant human NGF (rhNGF) was found to be well tolerated in an open-label Phase I clinical trial.[58] Two randomized, double-blind, placebo-controlled Phase II studies of NGF in the treatment of DN reported improvement in the sensory component of the neurological exam, in quantitative sensory testing and in a symptom score in treated patients when compared with the placebo group.[59] However, a large-scale, 48 week, Phase III clinical trial of 1019 patients randomized to receive either rhNGF or placebo failed to confirm its efficacy. Among the explanations offered for the discrepancy between the two sets of trials was a robust placebo effect, inadequate dosage, different study populations and changes in the formulation of rhNGF for the Phase III trial. As a result of the Phase III outcome, Genentech has decided not to proceed with further development of rhNGF.[60]

Acetyl-L-Carnitine (ALC)

ALC is deficient in diabetes.[61–63] In pre-clinical studies, ALC treatment was shown to correct perturbations of neural Na^+/K^+-ATPase, myoinositol, nitric oxide, prostaglandins and lipid peroxidation.[62–65] Long-term prevention and intervention studies in the diabetic rat revealed therapeutic effects on peripheral nerve function and structural abnormalities.[62–65] In humans, clinical studies have shown modest effects of ALC on painful DN.[66–68] A large multicentre placebo-controlled phase III trial of ALC in patients with mild DN found no efficacy when axonal counts from sural nerve biopsies were used as the primary endpoint (Hoffman-LaRoche, personal communication).

Small-fibre polyneuropathy

Some patients have a selective small-fibre polyneuropathy or small-fibre sensory neuropathy (SFSN).[69–74] The patient with SFSN typically presents with pain as a chief complaint, most commonly in the distal limb, which he or she describes in a variety of terms, including tingling, prickling, burning, coldness, deep aching, jabbing or shooting. Autonomic dysfunction is frequently present. The examination demonstrates distal sensory loss affecting pain and temperature, with relative preservation of large fibre-mediated modalities (vibration and proprioception). Reflexes are generally preserved (although ankle jerks may be decreased or absent) and strength is normal. Nerve

Table 19.3 Summary of treatments for painful diabetic polyneuropathy

Treatment	Double-blind, controlled	Open-label	Other (see text)
Non-steroidal anti-inflammatory agents			×
Tricyclic antidepressants			
Amitriptyline	×		
Imipramine	×		
Desipramine	×		
Nortriptyline			×
Serotonin re-uptake inhibitors			
Paroxetine	×		
Sertraline		×	
Fluoxetine	×		
Dual serotonin–norepinephrine re-uptake inhibitors			
Duloxetine	×	×	
Anticonvulsants			
Gabapentin	×		
Carbamazepine	×	×	
Pregabalin	×	×	
Opioids			
Dextromethorphan	×		
Oxycodone	×		
Tramadol	×		
Other oral agents			
Mexiletine	×		
Levodopa	×		
Clonidine			×
γ-Linolenic acid	×		
Phenothiazines			×
Narcotics			×
α-Lipoic acid	×		
Non-systemic treatment			
Capsaicin cream	×		
Non-pharmacological treatments			
TENS unit		×	×
Acupuncture		×	
Psychological treatment			×

conduction studies are normal or minimally abnormal, since such tests assess primarily the largest, fastest-conducting fibres. Quantitative sensory testing (QST) is abnormal in 60% of patients tested. Autonomic testing may be abnormal. Biopsies of sural nerves show predominantly small fibre loss, but may rarely be normal. Skin biopsies demonstrate abnormalities of intra-epidermal nerves. Treatment is directed towards control of pain, using the agents discussed below. Several studies now point to impaired glucose tolerance or pre-diabetes as a common underlying aetiology for SFSN.[75]

Control of pain

A major goal in the management of DN is control of pain. A large number of agents have been studied in both uncontrolled and controlled clinical trials. Table 19.3 lists the drugs used clinically for the treatment of painful DN.

Non-steroidal anti-inflammatory drugs (NSAIDs)

NSAIDs are often prescribed as a first-line therapy for pain control. A placebo-controlled, single-blind, crossover study demonstrated both ibuprofen 600 mg qid and sulindac 200 mg bid to be more effective than placebo in relieving the pain of DN. The response to sulindac was significantly better than the response to ibuprofen.[76] Caution must be exercised when using NSAIDs in patients with diabetes, due to the risk of nephrotoxicity, hypertension and cardiovascular events.

Antidepressants

Tricyclic antidepressants (TCAs)

TCAs have been studied extensively and for many years have been a first-line treatment for neuropathic pain. They act by blocking neuronal re-uptake of norepinephrine and serotonin, thereby potentiating the inhibitory effect of these neurotransmitters in nociceptive pathways.[77] Amitriptyline, imipramine and desipramine were all found to relieve pain in patients with DN better than placebo in double-blind, placebo-controlled trials. These compounds were effective in both depressed and non-depressed patients and the efficacy appeared to be independent of any antidepressant effect.[78–82] Additional support for the efficacy of TCAs was provided by a meta-analysis of 21 clinical trials.[83] Although nortriptyline as monotherapy might be expected to be effective in treatment of painful DN and is often used in this manner, there is no trial to support its use. When used in combination with fluphenazine, nortriptyline has been shown to be more effective than placebo and as effective as carbamazepine in double-blind, crossover studies.[84,85] The use of neuroleptics may produce extrapyramidal symptoms and are not recommended in the routine treatment of DN pain.

Adverse effects are common with TCAs and may lead to treatment withdrawal. In clinical trials of TCAs, approximately 20% of participants withdrew because of intolerable adverse effects. All of the TCAs may produce sedation, confusion and anticholinergic side-effects such as dry mouth, blurred vision, constipation, urinary hesitancy and orthostatic dizziness. Severe adverse effects include arrhythmias and heart block. These agents are contraindicated in patients with a variety of heart diseases and must be used with great caution in patients with angle-closure glaucoma or orthostatic hypotension. The most commonly used TCAs may be ranked in order from most to least anticholinergic effects. They are amitriptyline, imipramine, nortriptyline and desipramine.[86] Thus, for a patient who does not tolerate amitriptyline, despiramine may be a useful alternative. The usual dosage schedule is 10–25 mg at bedtime initially, increasing as tolerated up to 100 or 150 mg as a single bedtime dose.

Selective serotonin reuptake inhibitors (SSRIs)

SSRIs are another category of antidepressants which may have some efficacy for DN, but the evidence is less convincing than for TCAs. In a randomized, double-blind, crossover study, paroxetine 40 mg day^{-1} reduced symptoms significantly more than placebo, although it was somewhat less effective than imipramine.[87] Fluoxetine at a mean dose of 40 mg day^{-1} was no more effective than placebo except in patients who were depressed.[81] Open-label sertraline up to 150 mg day^{-1} was shown to lead to a reduction in pain from DN in a small study of eight patients, but a placebo-controlled study has not yet been conducted.[88] Trazodone is often used empirically.

Duloxetine hydrochloride

Duloxetine, a selective dual serotonin (5-HT) and norepinephrine (NE) re-uptake inhibitor that is relatively balanced in its affinity for both 5-HT and NE re-uptake inhibition, was the first US Food and Drug Administration (FDA)-approved prescription medication for the management of pain associated with DN. Initial pre-clinical and clinical studies of duloxetine showed that duloxetine was safe and effective in the management of painful DN.[89–91] A recent double-blind study reported that treatment with either duloxetine 60 mg qd or 60 mg bid was associated with significant improvement in the mean score of 24 h average pain severity after 12 weeks in patients with painful DN and no co-morbid depression.[92] Treatment showed a rapid onset of action with separation from placebo beginning at week one.[92] Duloxetine is taken with a meal and begun at a dose of either 20 or 30 mgday^{-1}. The drug can be slowly titrated to 60 mg day^{-1}, taken in one dose. Patients frequently experience nausea with initiation of therapy. A slow titration of the drug can usually avoid this common side-effect. The most common side-effects of duloxetine, besides nausea, are sedation and generalized sleepiness.[93] Duloxetine should not be taken with other serotonin or norepinephrine uptake inhibitors.

Anticonvulsants

Anticonvulsant drugs have been used in the management of pain since the 1960s. The clinical impression is that they are useful for chronic neuropathic pain, especially when the pain is lancinating or burning. Anticonvulsant drugs used for neuropathic pain include pregabalin, gabapentin, carbamazepine, clonazepam, lamotrigine, oxcarbazepine, phenytoin and valproate. Of the listed agents, only pregabalin has been approved by the FDA for use in DN. Phenytoin is not a useful anticonvulsant in the treatment of painful DN. Using identical methods, three simultaneous, placebo-controlled studies of topiramate for painful DN did not show significant benefit.[94] Side-effects of topiramate included diarrhoea, loss of appetite and somnolence. Topiramate significantly reduced body weight versus placebo, suggesting that the beneficial effect of topiramate on weight might be accompanied by other metabolic effects.[95]

Although they are frequently used, the precise mechanisms of action of anticonvulsant medications remain uncertain. The two standard explanations are enhanced γ-aminobutyric acid inhibition or a stabilizing effect on neuronal cell membranes. A third possibility is action via N-methyl-D-aspartate (NMDA) receptor sites.[96]

Pregabalin

Pregabalin is an analogue of gabapentin with multiple modes of action. Pregabalin binds to and modulates voltage-gated calcium channels; pregabalin is a more potent regulator of calcium channels than gabapentin and it is this mode of action that may modulate neuropathic pain. The anticonvulsant action of pregabalin is probably due to its ability to reduce neurotransmitter release from activated epileptogenic neurons, without demonstrated effects on GABAergic receptors or mechanisms.

Several randomized clinical trials explored the effects of pregabalin in painful DN. In a 6 week randomized, double-blind, multicentre study of 246 men and women with painful DN, pregabalin 600 mg day^{-1} significantly decreased mean pain score to 4.3 (vs 5.6 for placebo, $p = 0.0002$) and increased the proportion of patients who had a greater than or equal to 50% decrease from baseline pain (39 vs 15% for placebo, $p = 0.002$). Pregabalin also significantly reduced sleep interference. In this trial, dizziness was the most common side-effect.[97] Another placebo-controlled, multicentre study evaluated the effectiveness of pregabalin in a fixed dose with an open-label extension in alleviating pain associated with DN in 146 diabetic patients. Pregabalin produced significant improvements in pain scores within 1 week of treatment ($p < 0.01$), which persisted for the 8 week duration of the study ($p < 0.01$). About 40% of patients receiving pregabalin reported a 50% or greater reduction in pain compared with 14.5% of the placebo group ($p = 0.001$).[98] Pregabalin also improved mood, sleep disturbance and quality of life and was safe and well tolerated despite a greater incidence of dizziness and somnolence than placebo).[98] Similar effects were described in a 12 week randomized, double-blind, placebo-controlled, parallel-group study evaluating the efficacy and safety of pregabalin in patients with chronic postherpetic neuralgia or painful DN.[99]

Pregabalin is begun at 50–100 mg day^{-1} and can be increased up to 150 mg twice per day. Its side-effects are similar to those of duloxetine, although patients do not frequently experience nausea. Pregabalin is a Schedule Five drug and, unlike its predecessor gabapentin, there is a possibility it could be habit forming. It is consequently recommended that the drug be slowly discontinued if a decision is made to stop therapy. There are no clinical trials comparing the efficacy of pregabalin with duloxetine or other established therapies. It is difficult to make a direct comparison based on the published literature, because study designs vary considerably among the different trials with respect to the primary endpoints and patient selection. Different pain scales were employed in the respective Phase III double-blind, placebo-controlled trials for duloxetine and pregabalin; however, the published data generally suggest that the two therapies are equally efficacious in reducing pain.[91,99]

Unlike duloxetine, pregabalin can be given with serotonin or norepinephrine uptake inhibitors or even with duloxetine, as a dual uptake inhibitor.

Gabapentin

Gabapentin is frequently used in clinical practice for the treatment of painful DN. In the literature, several placebo-controlled studies report various degrees of pain improvement with gabapentin in patients with DN. Backonja[100] reported a 60% improvement on a global scale for patients on gabapentin (up to 3.6 g day^{-1}) after 4 weeks of treatment in a study of 165 participants. The number-needed-to-treat (NNT) for effectiveness compared to placebo was 3.8 (95% CI 2.4 to 8.7). It should be noted that this study used doses significantly higher than the maximum licensed dose of 2.4 g day^{-1}. Another parallel group trial, using doses of up to 1200 mg of gabapentin, reported effectiveness as greater than 50% reduction in pain at 1 month.[101] Two other randomized studies showed that 64% of participants improved on gabapentin compared with 28% on placebo and combined NNT for effectiveness in DN compared with placebo was 2.9 (95% CI 2.2 to 4.3).[102] However the lower end of this dosage range may be relatively ineffective since another placebo-controlled study did not demonstrate efficacy at a dose of 900 mg day^{-1}.[103]

Two small studies with 25 participants each compared gabapentin with amitriptyline. A double blind study reported no significant difference between gabapentin (dose 900 to 1800 mg day^{-1}) and amitriptyline (dose 25 to 75 mg day^{-1}),[104] whereas a second study, which was not blinded, reported a greater reduction in pain with gabapentin (dose 1200–2400 mg day^{-1}) than amitriptyline (30–90 mg day^{-1}), although the difference was not statistically significant.[105]

In practice, gabapentin is begun at 300 mg three times daily and the dose is doubled at weekly intervals until it reaches 900–1200 mg three times daily. Side-effects that may require discontinuation of gabapentin include unsteadiness, somnolence or confusion (especially in the elderly), headache, nausea and diarrhoea. Over the long term, gabapentin is also known to produce weight gain, which may complicate diabetes management.[106]

Carbamazepine

A recent search of the Cochrane Library revealed modest evidence for the effectiveness of carbamazepine in painful DN. One placebo-controlled study of 30 participants with DN[107] found that with 2 weeks of treatment, between 30 and 50% more patients improved on carbamazepine than on placebo. Another active controlled study compared carbamazepine 200 mg versus a nortriptyline 10 mg–fluphenazine 0.5 mg combination.[85] Although both treatments improved paraesthesias and pain, no significant difference was found between carbamazepine and the nortriptyline–fluphenazine combination. Therapy is begun at 100 mg twice daily, increased by 100 mg each week until the patient is taking 200 mg three times daily. The risk of carbamazepine-associated leukopenia and pancytopenia mandates that patients have total blood counts measured after the first month of therapy and monthly for 3 months.

Opioids

Opioids have recently been rediscovered as a treatment for neuropathic pain.[108–110] Opioids suppress pain by activating mu-receptors which are present on the pre- and post-synaptic membranes of primary afferent nerve fibres, second-order neurons in the dorsal horn of the spinal cord and neurons in pain relevant supraspinal centres. Activation of mu-receptors on the presynaptic membrane reduces neurotransmitter release. At the postsynaptic membrane, it causes hyperpolarization due to an increase in potassium conductance.

The efficacy of opioids in controlling neuropathic pain is dose and duration dependent. Tramadol, a weak opioid that acts via low-affinity binding to micro-opioid receptors and weak inhibition of norepinephrine and serotonin reuptake,[111] was found to be effective in treatment of pain in DN in a double-blind, placebo-controlled, randomized trial.[112] It is often good treatment for breakthrough or refractory pain and can be given as 50–100 mg every 4–6 h, up to 400 mg day^{-1}. Dextromethorphan was superior to placebo in a randomized, double-blind, crossover trial of pain control in DN. The initial dose of 30 mg four times per day was increased gradually to 240 mg four times per day. Side-effects were sedation, dizziness, lightheadedness, ataxia and confusion.[113] Another randomized placebo-controlled trial of patients with painful DN reported that CR oxycodone (10 mg every 12 h) resulted in significantly lower mean daily pain ($p = 0.0001$), steady pain and total pain and disability ($p = 0.004$) over 4 weeks compared with placebo.[110]

Pooled data suggest that the maximum tolerated doses of these drugs, administered as single agents, reduce pain by only 26–38%, owing to incomplete efficacy, dose-limiting adverse effects or both.[110,114,115] As with the tricyclic antidepressant and antiepileptic drugs, the side-effects of opioids, especially physical dependence and tolerance, have limited their use.

It has been proposed that a strategy combining mechanistically distinct analgesic agents may result in additivity or synergism and may improve efficacy at lower doses, with fewer side-effects than with the use of one agent alone. Therefore, in a recent randomized, double-blind, active placebo-controlled, four-period crossover trial, patients received daily active placebo (lorazepam), sustained-release morphine, gabapentin and a combination of gabapentin and morphine, each given orally for 5 weeks. Gabapentin and morphine in combination achieved better analgesia at lower doses of each drug and resulted in a lower frequency of adverse effects than either as a single agent.[116]

Other agents

Several other oral agents have been used, as described in the following.

Mexiletine Randomized, double-blind, placebo-controlled trials of the anti-arrhythmic agent mexiletine have demonstrated efficacy in the treatment of painful DN,[117–119] although one small, double-blind study did not demonstrate efficacy.[120] The side-effects most commonly reported are gastrointestinal distress (nausea, vomiting and heartburn), dizziness/lightheadedness, tremor, nervousness and uncoordination. Treatment is initiated with a dose of 150 mg day^{-1}, increasing gradually until there is relief of pain, up to a maximum dose of 600–800 mg day^{-1} in three to four divided doses. An ECG should be obtained to ensure that there are no cardiac contraindications to mexiletine therapy and a cardiologist should be consulted if there are concerns. The response to oral mexiletine can be predicted by an infusion of intravenous lidocaine.[121]

Levodopa Levodopa at a dosage of 100 mg three times per day was used in conjunction with a dopa decarboxylase inhibitor in a 4 week placebo-controlled trial and was found to be more effective than placebo from weeks two to four.[122]

Clonidine The proof of efficacy of clonidine is questionable. Two double-blind, placebo-controlled trials have not shown a significant benefit.[76,123] However, one trial in which the positive responders to clonidine were entered into a second double-blind, placebo-controlled phase demonstrated some benefit, suggesting that perhaps clonidine is effective in a subset of patients.[124]

γ-Linolenic acid   Based on the impaired conversion of linoleic acid to γ-linolenic acid in patients with diabetes, γ-linolenic acid 360 mg day^{-1} was found to be superior to placebo for control of pain in a small, 6 month, randomized, placebo-controlled double-blind trial.[125]

Non-systemic treatments

Capsaicin

Not all agents for pain control must be administered systemically. Topical capsaicin cream stimulates the release and subsequent depletion of substance P from sensory nerve fibres. A placebo-controlled study demonstrated the superiority of capsaicin cream 0.075% over placebo in control of pain and improvement in daily activities.[126,127] Another double-blind study found topical capsaicin to be as effective as amitriptyline.[128] In contrast, a double-blind, placebo-controlled study of capsaicin cream in patients with chronic distal painful neuropathy of various causes demonstrated no benefit over placebo.[129] A meta-analysis of four randomized, double-blind, placebo-controlled trials of capsaicin in DN found capsaicin to be more effective than placebo.[130] Poor compliance is common, due to the need for frequent applications, an initial exacerbation of symptoms and frequent burning and redness at the application site.

Transcutaneous electrical nerve stimulation (TENS) and acupuncture

In a controlled study, TENS was more effective than sham treatment in reducing pain in patients with DN.[131] Uncontrolled studies of TENS and of acupuncture have been reported to decreased pain in over 75% of patients with DN.[132,133] However, the powerful effect of placebo treatment in DN, documented in multiple studies, raises questions about the reliability of such uncontrolled trials.

Psychological treatments

Evidence that the quality of pain is influenced by affective and cognitive processes and the acceptance of the Melzack Gate Control model of pain[134] have led to an increased role for psychological intervention in chronic pain management.[135] Psychological treatments, such as biofeedback, cognitive-behavioural therapy, hypnosis and operant behavioural interventions, may be considered in addition to medications, although clinical trials of psychological intervention in patients with DN are lacking.

A summary of treatments used for painful DN is provided in Table 19.3.

Autonomic neuropathy

Autonomic neuropathy is a consequence of the involvement of the small, lightly myelinated and unmyelinated autonomic nerve fibres. Diabetes mellitus is the most common cause of autonomic neuropathy in developed countries.[136] Visceral autonomic neuropathy was present in 7% of patients with type 1 diabetes and 5% of those with type 2 diabetes in one series.[8] The clinical features of diabetic autonomic neuropathy, which involve the cardiovascular, gastrointestinal, urogenital, sudomotor and pupillomotor systems, may occur in diverse combinations[6,136] and are presented in Table 19.4.

Cardiovascular autonomic neuropathy (CAN) may present as an increased resting heart rate when the cardiac vagus nerve is affected. When sympathetic and parasympathetic fibres are involved, the heart rate is fixed and there is inadequate capacity to increase the heart rate in response to physiological demands.[136] Sympathetic and/or parasympathetic CAN is associated with mortality in patients with diabetes.[137,138] Longitudinal studies of people with CAN have observed 5 year mortality rates between 16 and 50% due to an altered electrical stability with a reduced threshold for malignant arrhythmias and/or impaired regulation of myocardial blood flow.[139]

Table 19.4 Clinical features of diabetic autonomic neuropathy (the majority of these are discussed in the text)

- Pupillary dysfunction
- Cardiovascular autonomic neuropathy
  - Abnormalities of heart rate
  - Orthostatic hypotension
- Gastrointestinal disturbances
  - Oesophageal, gastric, duodenal and colonic atony
  - Gastroparesis
  - Constipation
  - Diarrhoea
  - Gallbladder atony
  - Anal sphincter weakness
- Genitourinary disturbances
  - Bladder dysfunction
  - Retrograde ejaculation
  - Impotence
  - Female sexual dysfunction
- Unawareness of hypoglycaemia
- Abnormalities of sweating

Orthostatic hypotension occurs in diabetes largely as a consequence of efferent sympathetic vasomotor denervation, causing reduced vasoconstriction of the splanchnic and other peripheral vascular beds.[140]

Diabetic gastroparesis is associated with delayed gastric emptying of solids or liquids in the absence of mechanical obstruction. It is present in up to 50% of individuals with diabetes.[141] Dysfunction of the vagus nerve and intrinsic enteric autonomic nerves are involved in this disorder. Patients can present with nausea, post-prandial vomiting, bloating, loss of appetite and early satiety. However, many patients have no symptoms despite impaired gastric motility.[142]

Constipation, which might reflect impaired extrinsic and intrinsic autonomic innervation of the gastrointestinal tract, is the most frequently reported gastrointestinal autonomic symptom and is found in up to 60% of patients with diabetes.[143] Profuse and watery diarrhoea, typically occurring at night and extremely difficult to treat, has been also described especially in patients with type 1 diabetes and may alternate with constipation in these patients.

Symptoms of bladder dysfunction, such as incomplete bladder emptying, increased post-void residual, lower peak urinary flow rate, bladder overdistension and ultimately urinary retention and overflow incontinence, are present in up to 50% of patients with diabetes.[144,145]

Erectile dysfunction is present in 30–75% of diabetic men and can be the earliest symptom of diabetic autonomic neuropathy.[146,147] The aetiology of erectile dysfunction is multifactorial but diabetic autonomic neuropathy and endothelial dysfunction were shown to play a central role.[148] Vascular and psychogenic mechanisms may also contribute to this symptom. It has been also shown that diabetic autonomic neuropathy is associated with aspects of sexual dysfunction in women, although the effect of diabetes on women's sexual function is complex and not yet well understood.[148] Whereas erectile dysfunction is readily quantifiable and directly influences men's subjective arousal, women's genital congestion is more difficult to measure and correlates poorly with their subjective arousal.[148]

Autonomic neuropathy may also cause or contribute to *hypoglycaemia unawareness*, although many argue that unawareness of hypoglycaemia and inadequate counter-regulation occur independently of autonomic neuropathy.[149,150] The spectrum of reduced counter-regulatory hormonal responses (in particular epinephrine) and decreased symptom perception of hypoglycaemia due to decreased autonomic nervous system activation after recent antecedent hypoglycaemia has been termed 'hypoglycaemia-induced autonomic failure'.[151]

Treatment

Treatment of orthostatic hypotension

The treatment of orthostatic hypotension can be challenging and involves the use of both non-pharmacological and pharmacological measures.

Non-pharmacological treatments

Many of the non-pharmacological treatments for orthostatic hypotension are based on commonly-accepted clinical practices, rather than controlled clinical trials.[3,6,152–156] Such measures include (1) avoidance of sudden changes in body posture to the head-up position, particularly in warm weather and after taking a warm bath, both of which produce cutaneous vasodilation; (2) avoiding medications that aggravate hypotension, such as tricyclic antidepressants and phenothiazines; (3) eating small, frequent meals to avoid the post-prandial hypotension which may occur after a large carbohydrate-containing meal; and (4) avoiding activities that involve straining, since increased intra-abdominal and intra-thoracic pressure decrease venous return. Patients with orthostatic hypotension should move from a supine to a standing position in gradual stages, particularly in the morning, when orthostatic tolerance is lowest.[157] In addition, several physical counter-manoeuvres, such as leg crossing, squatting and muscle pumping, can help maintain blood pressure during daily activities by inducing increased cardiac filling pressures and stroke volume with a consequent increase in blood pressure and cerebral perfusion.[158]

The efficacy of some non-pharmacological treatments has been demonstrated in case reports or small uncontrolled studies. Elevation of the head of the bed 18 in (45 cm) at night improved symptoms in a small series of patients with orthostatic hypotension from various causes.[159] The efficacy of a compressive garment over the legs and abdomen has been demonstrated in multiple case reports.[160–163] An inflatable abdominal band was shown to be effective in a small study of six patients with orthostatic hypotension[164] and a low portable chair used by patients as needed for symptoms was found to be effective in one study.[165]

Pharmacological treatments

Some pharmacological treatments for orthostatic hypotension are commonly used in clinical practice, but without studies to document efficacy.[3] Plasma expansion by increased fluid and salt intake is commonly recommended. An increase in dietary sodium to at least 10 g (185 mmol) should be accompanied by an increase in fluid intake of 2–2.5 l (in adults) per day.

Fludrocortisone acetate

Fludrocortisone acetate is a synthetic mineralocorticoid with a long duration of action which induces plasma expansion and may also enhance the sensitivity of blood vessels to circulating catecholamines.[166,167] The earliest report described a single patient.[168] Other case reports followed.[169] A small, open-label study of 14 patients demonstrated both symptomatic and objective improvement.[170] The effects are not immediate, but occur over a 1–2 week period. Supine hypertension, hypokalaemia and hypomagnesaemia may occur. Caution must be used, particularly in patients with congestive heart failure, to avoid fluid overload.[171,172] Treatment with fludrocortisone should begin with 0.05 mg at bedtime and may be titrated upward gradually to a maximum of 0.2 mg daily. The dose can ultimately be titrated up to 0.3–0.4 mg, but at these higher doses there is more of a tendency to develop hypokalaemia and excessive fluid retention with resulting hypertension and congestive heart failure.

Sympathomimetic agents

Mixed α-adrenoreceptor agonists, which act directly on the α-adrenoreceptor and release norepinephrine from the postganglionic sympathetic neuron, include ephedrine, pseudoephedrine and phenylpropanolamine.[136] Typical doses of these indirect agonists are ephedrine 25–50 mg three times per day, pseudoephedrine 30–60 mg three times per day and phenylpropanolamine 12.5–25 mg three times per day. Severe hypertension is an important adverse effect of all sympathomimetic agents. Other side-effects which may limit their use are tremulousness, irritability, insomnia, tachycardia, reduction in appetite and, in males, urinary retention.[154]

The peripheral-selective direct α_1-adrenoreceptor agonist midodrine is the only agent approved by the FDA in the United States for the treatment of orthostatic hypotension. By activating α_1-receptors on arterioles and veins, midodrine increases total peripheral resistance.[173,174] Because it does not cross the blood–brain barrier, it has fewer central side-effects than ephedrine. Several double-blind, placebo-controlled studies have documented its efficacy in the treatment of orthostatic hypotension.[175–177] The main adverse effects are piloerection, pruritis, paraesthesias, urinary retention and supine hypertension. The usual dose of midodrine is 2.5–10 mg three times per day.

There are few head-to-head comparisons of the α-adrenoreceptor agonists. In a small clinical trial, midodrine (mean dose 8.4 mg three times per day) improved standing blood pressure and orthostatic tolerance more than ephedrine (22.3 mg three times per day).[178] In another trial, phenylpropanolamine (12.5 mg) and yohimbine (5.4 mg) produced equivalent increases in standing systolic blood pressure whereas methylphenidate failed to increase standing systolic blood pressure significantly.[179]

All sympathomimetic drugs must be used with caution in patients with ischaemic heart disease, cardiac arrhythmias and peripheral vascular disease.

Erythropoietin

Although erythropoietin may improve standing blood pressure in patients with orthostatic hypotension, the mechanism of action for the pressor effect of this agent is still unresolved. Possibilities include the increase in red cell mass and central blood volume, correction of the normochromic normocytic anaemia that frequently accompanies diabetic autonomic neuropathy[180] and alterations in blood viscosity. There are data to suggest that erythropoietin may also have direct or indirect neurohumoral effects on the vascular wall and vascular tone regulation which are mediated by the interaction between haemoglobin and the vasodilator nitric oxide.[181,182] In general, erythropoietin is administered subcutaneously or intravenously at doses between 25 and 75 U kg^{-1} three times per week until the haematocrit level approaches normal followed by a lower maintenance doses ($\sim$25 U kg^{-1} three times per week).[157]

Dihydroergotamine

Dihydroergotamine in combination with caffeine, indomethacin and the α_2-adrenergic antagonist yohimbine has been used in refractory patients.[139,155] In an experimental animal model of orthostatic hypotension, yohimbine has been found to delay the fall in blood pressure elicited by head-up tilting, but not to modify its magnitude.[183]

Beta-Blockers

Non-selective β-blockers, particularly those with intrinsic sympathomimetic activity such as pindolol and xamoterol, may have a limited role in the treatment of orthostatic hypotension.[184] The suggested mechanism of action of these agents is the blockade of vasodilating β_2-receptors allowing unopposed α-adrenoreceptor-mediated vasoconstrictor. Beta-blockers have shown efficacy in some case reports and open-label studies of patients with orthostatic hypotension due to varying aetiologies.[185–187] A double-blind, placebo-controlled crossover study of eight patients with diabetic autonomic neuropathy and orthostatic hypotension failed to demonstrate efficacy.[117] Congestive heart failure may be a serious side-effect of this medication.

Clonidine

Clonidine is an α_2-antagonist that usually produces a central sympatholytic effect and a consequent decrease in blood pressure. Patients with severe autonomic failure have little central sympathetic efferent activity and clonidine may affect venous postsynaptic α_2-adrenoreceptors. The use of clonidine (0.1–0.6 mg day^{-1}) could therefore result in an increase in venous return without a significant increase in peripheral vascular resistance. However, the use of this agent is limited by the inconsistent hypertensive effect and also serious side-effects.

Caffeine

Caffeine is a methylxanthine with a well-established pressor effect, primarily due to blockade of vasodilating adenosine receptors. Caffeine may improve orthostatic hypotension and attenuate post-prandial hypotension in patients with autonomic failure. Typical caffeine doses are 100–250 mg three times per day, either as tablets or as caffeinated beverages (one cup of coffee contains ~85 mg of caffeine and one cup of tea contains ~50 mg of caffeine). Tachyphylaxis occurs with continuing use of this agent.[157]

Somatostatin and somatostatin analogues

Octreotide and the long-acting synthetic octapeptide may attenuate the post-prandial blood pressure fall and reduce orthostatic hypotension in patients with autonomic failure. Mechanisms of action include a local effect on splanchnic vasculature by inhibiting the release of vasoactive gastrointestinal peptides, enhanced cardiac output and an increase in forearm and splanchnic vascular resistance. Subcutaneous doses of octreotide range from 25 to 200 µg day^{-1}.

Treatment of diabetic gastroparesis

Some treatments for diabetic gastroparesis are based on commonly-accepted clinical practices. These include the use of multiple small feedings and changes in diet such as a decrease in dietary fat and fibre.[139,155,188] The principal pharmacological means of treatment has been the use of a prokinetic agent such as metoclopramide, cisapride or domperidone.

Metoclopramide

Metoclopramide has anti-emetic properties, stimulates acetylcholine release in the myenteric plexus and is a dopamine antagonist.[188] There have been one open trial, two single-blind trials and five double-blind trials. The single- and double-blind trials

demonstrated improvement in gastric emptying, whereas the open trial demonstrated no improvement.[189] Extrapyramidal symptoms such as acute dystonic reactions, drug-induced parkinsonism, akathisia and tardive dyskinesia may be side-effects. Galactorrhoea, amenorrhoea, gynecomastia and hyperprolactinaemia are also potential side-effects. The usual dose is 10 mg given 30 min before meals and at bedtime.

Cisapride

Cisapride increases gut motility by increasing the release of acetylcholine from postganglionic myenteric neurons.[188] There have been 10 open trials and seven double-blind trials which demonstrated improvement in gastric emptying with 10–20 mg of cisapride given 15–30 min before meals and at bedtime.[189] Cisapride appears to maintain efficacy in long-term use[190] and does not have the dopaminergic activity of metoclopramide or the extrapyramidal and other side-effects noted above. However, cisapride has been withdrawn from the United States market as a result of over 200 reported cases of cardiac toxicity attributed to its use.

Domperidone

Domperidone, a peripheral dopamine receptor antagonist, has also been shown to stimulate gastric motility and to possess anti-emetic properties. It acts as a prokinetic agent, increasing the number and/or the intensity of gastric contractions, and improves symptoms in patients suffering from diabetic gastroparesis. It stimulates both liquid- and solid-phase gastric emptying.[191] Its major benefit results from its anti-emetic properties and, to a lesser extent, its motor stimulatory actions.[192] There have been two open trials involving 18 patients and two double-blind trials involving 28 patients, all of which demonstrated improvement in gastric emptying.[189] A double-blind, randomized trial has demonstrated that domperidone and metoclopramide are equally effective.[192] A recent systematic review of all studies using oral domperidone for the treatment of diabetic gastroparesis clearly demonstrates the efficacy of domperidone in treating gastroparesis when compared with placebo and other treatment options available.[193] Its use, however, has recently become controversial owing to safety concerns and it has never been approved for marketing by the US FDA.

Erythromycin

Erythromycin is effective in accelerating gastric emptying. It is believed to act by stimulating motilin receptors in the gut.[194] It may be used orally or intravenously.[195,196] There have been five open trials involving 71 patients, with a mean improvement in gastric emptying of over 40%.[189] One single-blind trial also demonstrated an improvement in gastric emptying of 50%.[189]

An analysis of 36 studies of prokinetic agents found all four of these agents appear to have efficacy in improving gastric emptying times and symptoms.[189] When compared with one another, improvement in gastric emptying time was greatest with erythromycin, followed by domperidone, cisapride and then metoclopramide. Improvement in symptoms was greatest with erythromycin, then domperidone, then metoclopramide, then cisapride. However, with chronic administration of these prokinetic agents, the short-term benefits are frequently lost. The choice of an agent will ultimately be determined by availability, cost and side-effects.

Other treatments

Botulinum toxin injection

The hypothesis that pylorospasm is a contributing factor in the development of diabetic gastroparesis prompted the hypothesis that transient paralysis of the pylorus should accelerate gastric emptying and improve symptoms of nausea and vomiting. Several case reports of patients with severe diabetic gastroparesis, whose symptoms persisted despite dietary changes and the use of high-dose prokinetic agents, describe significant symptomatic improvement after intrapyloric botulinum toxin injection.[197,198] In a recent open-label trial, eight type 1 diabetic subjects who had failed standard therapy were treated with 200 units of botulinum toxin injected into the pylorus during upper gastrointestinal tract endoscopy and followed for 12 weeks. Most of the patients had a significant improvement in mean symptom scores, gastric emptying time and weight following the procedure.[199] However, further investigation with a large, double-blind, placebo-controlled trial is needed.

Ghrelin

Ghrelin is an endogenous ligand of the growth hormone secretagogue receptor and is released from the stomach. Human ghrelin exhibits 36% identity with motilin, while their respective receptors exhibit 50% homology.[200] Animal studies suggest that ghrelin increases gastric emptying and stimulates gastrointestinal motor activity.[200,201] Several recent studies reported that ghrelin significantly decreased a cumulative meal-related symptom score, significantly enhanced liquid emptying and tended to enhance solid emptying.[202,203]

Gastric pacing and gastric stimulation

Gastric pacing (electrical stimulation of gastric smooth muscles) has been investigated for a number of years. Short-term studies in humans and dogs have demonstrated that it is possible to entrain gastric slow waves and normalize myoelectrical activity with pacing.[204,205] All trials were small and unblinded. In one series of nine patients with gastroparesis, five of whom had diabetes, gastric pacing accelerated gastric emptying and improved symptoms.[205]

Gastric stimulation is a potential therapy for patients with refractory gastroparesis. Rather than using a low-frequency, high-amplitude signal to induce muscular contraction, gastric stimulation uses high-frequency, low-amplitude signals that do not alter gastric myoelectrical or muscular activity. Twenty-five patients with gastroparesis, 19 of whom had diabetic gastroparesis, underwent gastric stimulation between 1998 and 2000. Twelve months of follow-up were obtained from 24 of 25 patients in this unblinded, uncontrolled series. Gastric emptying was not significantly improved, but significant reductions in self-report measures for frequency and severity of nausea and vomiting were reported.[206]

Gastrostomy/jejunostomy

Persistent vomiting may require a surgical approach. Placement of a feeding jejunostomy to bypass an atonic stomach has been advocated, based on clinical practice.[188] Radical surgery, consisting of resection of a large portion of the stomach, with performance of a Roux-en-Y loop, has been reported to be successful in a small series of patients.[207]

Treatment of diabetic diarrhoea

Antibiotics

Diarrhoea in diabetic patients is often due to bacterial overgrowth, which can be diagnosed with a hydrogen breath test. An early double-blind study involving a single patient demonstrated that the diarrhoea subsided when the patient was treated with an oral antibiotic preparation (a combination of tetracycline, amphotericin B and potassium metaphosphate), then recurred when placebo was substituted.[208] Broad-spectrum antibiotics are commonly used to treat diabetic diarrhoea, either when the breath test is positive or as an empiric trial. Several different regimens have been advocated: (1) ampicillin or tetracycline 250 mg every 8 h for 14 days;[155,156] (2) amoxicillin 875 mg and clavulanate potassium twice daily for 14 days;[188] (3) metronidazole 500 mg every 6 h or 750 mg every 8 h for 3 weeks.[155,156] Caution must be used since long-term use of metronidazole can lead to neuropathy.

Other treatments have been based largely on accepted clinical practice patterns.[155,156] Cholestyramine can be used in an attempt to chelate bile salts if the hydrogen breath test is normal or if patients fail an empiric trial of broad-spectrum antibiotics. Diphenoxylate with atropine or loperamide can also be used.

Octreotide (a somatostatin analogue) 50–75 µg subcutaneously twice per day was effective in a case report of a single patient with diabetic diarrhoea.[209] A recent study demonstrated that octreotide was effective in accelerating gastric emptying, inhibiting small bowel transit, reducing ileocolonic bolus transfers, inhibiting post-prandial colonic tonic response and increasing colonic phasic pressure activity in healthy volunteers, and thus should be of value in the treatment of diarrhoeal states.[210]

Treatment of the neurogenic bladder

Dysfunction of the lower urinary tract occurs in 26–87% of patients with diabetes.[211] These patients experience a decrease in the ability to sense a distended bladder due to loss of afferent autonomic innervation. As a result, they urinate less frequently and develop a hypocontractile bladder and urinary retention.[211–213] This leads to recurrent urinary tract infections, overflow incontinence, dribbling and poor stream. Recommendations from a number of sources are similar and based largely on commonly-accepted clinical practices.[3,153,155,156] The patient with a neurogenic bladder should be scheduled for an evaluation by a urologist with a cystometrogram. If abnormal, scheduled voiding is recommended, often coupled with Crede's manoeuvre: manual squeezing of the bladder to initiate urination. Bethanechol, a parasympathomimetic agent, 10–30 mg three times per day, may be helpful. Some patients may require intermittent catheterization. Transurethral surgery of the bladder neck may be needed in selected cases and occasional patients may require an indwelling catheter. Based on an animal model, some patients may benefit from surgery to reduce bladder size.[214]

Treatment of impotence

The prevalence of erectile dysfunction in men with diabetes is high, varying from 35 to 75%.[147] The treatment of erectile dysfunction in men is considered in more detail elsewhere.[147] Several case reports have described the use of vacuum devices, rigid penile implants and inflatable prostheses for the treatment of erectile dysfunction.[215,216] Direct injections into the corpus cavernosum of either papaverine or alprostadil represent another option. The success rate of intra-cavernosal injections is high, with nearly 90% of patients achieving erection.[216,217] Yohimbine, an α_2-adrenergic antagonist, is occasionally used. A meta-analysis of seven randomized clinical trials found it to be more effective than placebo.[218]

The current therapy of choice for erectile dysfunction is one of the phosphodiesterase type 5 (PDE-5) inhibitors. However, considering its complex aetiology, phosphodiesterase inhibition produces only moderate benefit in diabetic men.[148] Sildenafil was shown to be significantly more effective than placebo in a randomized, double-blind, placebo-controlled study of 268 men with diabetes and erectile dysfunction.[219] The main side-effects were headache, dyspepsia and respiratory tract disorder. The dose is 25–100 mg taken 1 h before sexual activity. Another multicentre study assessed the efficacy and safety of tadalafil in men with erectile dysfunction and multiple co-morbid conditions including diabetes mellitus. Tadalafil 20 mg significantly increased erectile function and was well tolerated.[220]

A recent review using computerized searches of MEDLINE, EMBASE and the Cochrane Library assessed the effect of PDE-5 inhibitors on the management of erectile dysfunction in diabetic men. In eight randomized, placebo-controlled trials evaluating more than 1600 men, of whom 80% suffered from type 2 diabetes mellitus, PDE-5 treatment was associated with a significant improvement in the frequency of penetration, maintaining erection to completion of intercourse and percentage of successful attempts as compared with placebo.[221] Adverse cardiovascular effects were reported in one study. Headache was the most frequent adverse event reported, flushing was the second most common event, with upper respiratory tract complaints and flu-like syndromes, dyspepsia, myalgias, abnormal vision and back pain also reported in descending order of frequency. Given their known effects on the nitric oxide/cGMP pathway, PDE-5 inhibitors potentiate the hypotensive effects of organic nitrates and nitrites and are therefore contraindicated in patients who are currently on these treatments. In summary, sufficient evidence exists to support the use of PDE-5 inhibitors to improve erectile dysfunction in diabetic men.

Evidence regarding treatment of diabetes-associated sexual dysfunction in women is very scarce. Experience shows that vibrostimulation can help orgasmic dysfunction associated with lost genital sexual sensitivity. A small randomised controlled trial has shown benefit from the investigational use of PDE-5 in genital arousal disorder associated with compromised vulvar congestion.[222]

Cranial neuropathies

Cranial neuropathies affecting extraocular movements occur more frequently in diabetic than non-diabetic patients. Patients are usually over 50 years of age. The onset is typically abrupt and may be painless or associated with a headache. A lesion of the oculomotor nerve (CN III) is the most common single cranial neuropathy in diabetes, often sparing the pupil. Dysfunction of the trochlear nerve (CN IV) is less common. The abducens nerve (CN VI) is rarely involved alone, but may be involved with other cranial nerves. Although facial palsy (CN VII) and other cranial neuropathies occur in patients with diabetes, their relationship to the diabetes is uncertain.[6,223] There is no specific treatment, although gradual recovery typically occurs.

Limb mononeuropathies

Compression and entrapment neuropathies are common in patients both without and with diabetes, and it is uncertain if these are causally related to diabetes. The most commonly involved nerve is the median nerve at the wrist (carpal tunnel syndrome). Symptomatic carpal tunnel syndrome occurs in 11% of patients with type 1 diabetes and 6% of patients with type 2 diabetes. Asymptomatic carpal tunnel syndrome is much more common.[8] Ulnar neuropathy at the elbow also commonly occurs. Typically, such neuropathies are slowly developing lesions characterized by variable amounts of pain and weakness. Treatment has been empirical and may be conservative or surgical. The presence of a superimposed generalized polyneuropathy does not preclude surgical intervention in such patients, but the degree of polyneuropathy which is contributing to the patient's symptoms must be taken into account when making decisions regarding surgery.[224]

Dysfunction of some nerves may be abrupt and painful, likely secondary to nerve infarctions. Common examples include the radial nerve (wrist drop), peroneal nerve (foot drop), femoral nerve (quadriceps weakness) and lateral femoral cutaneous nerve ('meralgia paresthetica'). Electrodiagnostic tests reveal axon loss. Recovery typically occurs over months or years and depends on the extent of axon loss and the site (proximal vs distal) of the lesion. Distal muscle strength is often recovered incompletely. If multiple nerves are affected in this way, a mononeuropathy multiplex will result. There is no specific treatment for these abrupt limb neuropathies, although some have advocated immunomodulating therapy when there is multi-nerve involvement,

similar to that used by some for treatment of diabetic amyotrophy (see below).

Diabetic truncal mononeuropathy

Diabetic truncal mononeuropathy is typically characterized by pain around the abdomen or lower chest. Cutaneous hyperaesthesia may occur, as may abdominal wall weakness. Some cases appear to be a restricted form of diabetic radiculopathy and demonstrate paraspinal muscle denervation on EMG.[38] Once structural abnormalities have been ruled out, treatment consists of pain management. Gradual improvement generally occurs.

Asymmetric lower limb motor neuropathy (diabetic amyotrophy)

There are many names for this syndrome, including proximal diabetic neuropathy, diabetic polyradiculopathy, diabetic femoral neuropathy, diabetic lumbar plexopathy and diabetic lumbosacral plexus neuropathy. Affected individuals have type 2 diabetes mellitus and are usually males over 50 years of age. The initial symptom is pain in most patients, usually in the territory of the lower thoracic and upper lumbar nerve roots. The pain typically is worst at onset and gradually subsides. Paraesthesia and hyperaesthesia are common. Weakness, generally in the upper legs, commonly follows the pain. Weight loss is common. On examination, weakness is most common in the L2–L4 distribution. Thus, the weakness primarily affects the iliopsoas, quadriceps and adductor muscles, usually sparing hip extensors and hamstrings. The weakness may be unilateral or bilateral and when bilateral it is frequently asymmetric. Sensory loss is mild and mainly distal in most patients, consistent with a coexisting distal sensory or sensorimotor polyneuropathy. Knee and/or ankle jerks are lost in most patients.[225]

Progression of symptoms and signs occurs over a very variable period of time, as short as 1–2 weeks and as long as 1 year or more. Most patients experience improvement or resolution of pain or dysaesthesia. Recovery of motor function is often incomplete and usually slower, proceeding for up to 18 months. Nerve conduction studies often reveal evidence of a sensory or sensorimotor polyneuropathy. The needle examination typically reveals fibrillations and positive sharp waves in lower extremity muscles and in thoracic and/or lumbar paraspinal muscles. Most commonly affected are the L2–L4 levels, although low thoracic and L5–S1 levels are abnormal in some patients. The aetiology appears to be microscopic vasculitis producing nerve ischaemia, with multifocal involvement of lumbosacral roots, plexus and peripheral nerves. This has led to the recent use of the term 'diabetic lumbosacral radiculoplexus neuropathy' to characterize this type of neuropathy.[226]

Typically, no treatment is given other than controlling the diabetes. However, the inflammatory changes on biopsy have raised the issue of whether immunomodulating agents might be useful for treatment of this type of diabetic neuropathy. In patients with particularly severe cases, prednisone, intravenous immunoglobulin (IVIg) and plasmapheresis have shown some promise in open-label, uncontrolled studies. Patients appeared to stop worsening and to begin to improve after beginning these treatments. However, since untreated patients also gradually improve, the efficacy of these treatments is so far unproven.[227–230]

Conclusion

DN is the most common complication of both type 1 and type 2 diabetes. In the United States, DN is the leading cause of diabetes-related hospital admissions and non-traumatic amputations and is associated with a poor quality of life. A generally accepted overall prevalence rate is 50%. The mechanisms underlying the development of DN are a source of continued active investigations. Conclusive clinical evidence from randomized prospective trials supports a central role for hyperglycaemia in the pathogenesis of DN, suggesting also that other metabolic and vascular factors contribute to the disease state. The clinical presentation of DN comprises a broad constellation of symptoms and deficits involving all sensory-motor and autonomic nerve fibres. Pain is the outstanding complaint in most patients. DN treatment has traditionally focused on control of hyperglycaemia as a means of slowing progression or delaying its onset and on targeting potential pathogenetic mechanisms. Unfortunately, results from most randomized clinical trials assessing the efficacy of agents such as aldose reductase inhibitors, antioxidants, growth factor analogues or proteinkinase C inhibitors have been disappointing. A large number of agents have been studied for controlling DN associated pain. Duloxetine, a selective dual serotonin/norepinephrine reuptake inhibitor, and pregabalin, a voltage-gated calcium channel modulator, are the only FDA-approved prescription drugs for treating DN pain. Treatment of various forms of autonomic neuropathy continues to be challenging.

Acknowledgements

This work was supported by NIH NS36778, NIH NS38849 and grants from the Juvenile Diabetes Foundation and American Diabetes Association (ELF).

References

1 American Diabetes Association, American Academy of Neurology. Consensus statement: Report and recommendations of the San Antonio Conference on Diabetic Neuropathy. American Diabetes Association and American Academy of Neurology. *Diabetes Care* 1988;**11**(7):592–597.

2 Boulton AJ, Gries FA, Jervell JA. Guidelines for the diagnosis and outpatient management of diabetic peripheral neuropathy. *Diabet Med* 1998;**15**(6):508–514.

3 Boulton AJ, Vinik AI, Arezzo JC *et al*. Diabetic neuropathies: a statement by the American Diabetes Association. *Diabetes Care* 2005;**28**(4):956–962.

4 Vileikyte L, Rubin RR, Leventhal H. Psychological aspects of diabetic neuropathic foot complications: an overview. *Diabetes Metab Res Rev* 2004;**20**(Suppl 1): S13–S18.

5 Vileikyte L, Leventhal H, Gonzalez JS *et al*. Diabetic peripheral neuropathy and depressive symptoms: the association revisited. *Diabetes Care* 2005;**28**(10):2378–2383.

6 Thomas PK, Tomlinson DR. Diabetic and hypoglycemic neuropathy. In: *Peripheral Neuropathy*, 3rd edn (eds PJ Dyck, PK Thomas, JW Griffin, PA Low, JF Poduslo), Saunders, Philadelphia, PA, 1993, pp. 1219–1250.

7 Pirart J. Diabetes mellitus and its degenerative complications: a prospective study of 4,400 patients observed between 1947 and 1973. *Diabetes Care* 1978;**1**:168–188.

8 Dyck PJ, Kratz KM, Karnes JL *et al*. The prevalence by staged severity of various types of diabetic neuropathy, retinopathy and nephropathy in a population-based cohort: the Rochester Diabetic Neuropathy Study [published erratum appears in *Neurology* 1993; **43** (11): 2345]. *Neurology* 1993;**43**(4):817–824.

9 Young MJ, Boulton AJM, Macleod AF *et al*. A multicentre study of the prevalence of diabetic peripheral neuropathy in the United Kingdom hospital clinic populations. *Diabetologia* 1993;**36**:150–154.

10 Maser RE, Steenkiste AR, Dorman JS *et al*. Epidemiological correlates of diabetic neuropathy. Report from Pittsburgh Epidemiology of Diabetes Complications Study. *Diabetes* 1989;**38**:1456–1461.

11 Maser RE, Becker DJ, Drash AL *et al*. Pittsburgh Epidemiology of Diabetes Complications Study. Measuring diabetic neuropathy follow-up study results. *Diabetes Care* 1992;**15**: 525–527.

12 Tesfaye S, Stevens LK, Stephenson JM *et al*. Prevalence of diabetic peripheral neuropathy and its relation to glycaemic control and potential risk factors: the EURODIAB IDDM Complications Study. *Diabetologia* 1996;**39**(11): 1377–1384.

13 Palumbo PJ, Elveback LR, Whisnant JP. Neurologic complications of diabetes mellitus: transient ischemic attack, stroke, and peripheral neuropathy. *Adv Neurol* 1978;**19**:593–601.

14 Partanen J, Niskanen L, Lehtinen J, Mervaala E, Siitonen O, Uusitupa M. Natural history of peripheral neuropathy in patients with non-insulin-dependent diabetes mellitus. *NEJM* 1995;**333**:89–94.

15 Diabetes Control and Complications Trial Research Group. The effect of intensive treatment of diabetes on the development and progression of long-term complications in insulin-dependent diabetes mellitus. The Diabetes Control and Complications Trial Research Group. *N Engl J Med* 1993;**329**:977–986.

16 UK Prospective Diabetes Study (UKPDS) Group. Effect of intensive blood-glucose control with metformin on complications in overweight patients with type 2 diabetes (UKPDS 34). UK Prospective Diabetes Study (UKPDS) Group [published erratum appears in *Lancet* 1998; **352** (9139): 1557]. *Lancet* 1998;**352**:854–865.

17 Shichiri M, Kishikawa H, Ohkubo Y, Wake N. Long-term results of the Kumamoto Study on optimal diabetes control in type 2 diabetic patients. *Diabetes Care* 2000;**23**(Suppl 2): B21–B29.

18 Martin CL, Albers J, Herman WH *et al.* Neuropathy among the diabetes control and complications trial cohort 8 years after trial completion. *Diabetes Care* 2006;**29**(2): 340–344.

19 UK Prospective Diabetes Study (UKPDS) Group Intensive blood-glucose control with sulphonylureas or insulin compared with conventional treatment and risk of complications in patients with type 2 diabetes (UKPDS 33). UK Prospective Diabetes Study (UKPDS) Group. *Lancet* 1998;**352**(9131):837–853.

20 Tesfaye S, Chaturvedi N, Eaton SE *et al.* Vascular risk factors and diabetic neuropathy. *N Engl J Med* 2005;**352**(4):341–350.

21 Stevens MJ, Pop-Busui R, Greene DA *et al.* Pathogenesis of diabetic neuropathy. In: *Ellenberg and Rifkin's Diabetes Mellitus*, 6th edn (eds D Porte, RS Sherwin, A Baron), Appleton and Lange, Stamford, CT, 2002, pp. 747–770.

22 Vincent AM, Russell JW, Low P, Feldman EL. Oxidative stress in the pathogenesis of diabetic neuropathy. *Endocrinol Rev* 2004;**25**(4):612–628.

23 Pop-Busui R, Sima AA, Stevens M. *Diabetes/Metab Res Rev* 2005;**22**(4):257–273.

24 Sullivan KA, Feldman EL. New developments in diabetic neuropathy. *Curr Opin Neurol* 2005;**18**(5):586–590.

25 Low PA, Dotson RM. Symptomatic treatment of painful neuropathy. *JAMA* 1998;**280**(21):1863–1864.

26 Feldman E, Stevens M, Russell J, Peltier A. Somatosensory neuropathy. In: *The Diabetes Mellitus Manual* (eds S Inzucchi, D PorteJr, R Sherwin, A Baron), McGraw-Hill, New York, 2005, pp. 366–384.

27 Boulton AJ, Malik RA, Arezzo JC, Sosenko JM. Diabetic somatic neuropathies. *Diabetes Care* 2004;**27**(6):1458–1486.

28 Oyibo SO, Prasad YD, Jackson NJ *et al.* The relationship between blood glucose excursions and painful diabetic peripheral neuropathy: a pilot study. *Diabet Med* 2002; **19**(10):870–873.

29 Singleton JR, Smith AG, Russell J, Feldman EL. Polyneuropathy with impaired glucose tolerance: implications for diagnosis and therapy. *Curr Treat Options Neurol* 2005; **7**(1):33–42.

30 Feldman EL, Stevens MJ, Thomas PK *et al.* A practical two-step quantitative clinical and electrophysiological assessment for the diagnosis and staging of diabetic neuropathy. *Diabetes Care* 1994;**17**:1281–1289.

31 Cabezas-Cerrato J. The prevalence of clinical diabetic polyneuropathy in Spain: a study in primary care and hospital clinic groups. Spanish Neuropathy Study Group of the Spanish Diabetes Society (SDS) *Diabetologia* 1998;**41** (11): 1263–1269.

32 Vileikyte L. Psychological aspects of diabetic peripheral neuropathy. *Diabetes Rev* 1999;**7**:387–394.

33 Vileikyte L, Peyrot M, Bundy C *et al.* The development and validation of a neuropathy- and foot ulcer-specific quality of life instrument. *Diabetes Care* 2003;**26**(9):2549–2555.

34 Abbott CA, Carrington AL, Ashe H *et al.* The North-West Diabetes Foot Care Study: incidence of and risk factors for, new diabetic foot ulceration in a community-based patient cohort. *Diabet Med* 2002;**19**(5):377–384.

35 Thomas PK. Classification, differential diagnosis and staging of diabetic peripheral neuropathy. *Diabetes* 1997; **46** (Suppl2): S54–S57.

36 Dyck PJ.In: *Textbook of Diabetic Neuropathy* (eds FA Gries, NE Cameron, PA Low, D Ziegler), Georg Thieme, Stuttgart, 2003, pp. 170–175.

37 Bril V, Perkins BA. Validation of the Toronto Clinical Scoring System for diabetic polyneuropathy. *Diabetes Care* 2002;**25**(11):2048–2052.

38 Singleton J, Russell J, Feldman E. Electrodiagnosis of neuromuscular disease. In: *Adult Neurology* (ed. J. Corey-Bloom), Blackwell, Oxford, 2005, pp. 34–49.

39 Siao P, Cros DP. Quantitative sensory testing. *Phys Med Rehabil Clin N Am* 2003;**14**(2):261–286.

40 Armstrong DG, Lavery LA, Vela SA *et al.* Choosing a practical screening instrument to identify patients at risk for diabetic foot ulceration. *Arch Intern Med* 1998;**158** (3): 289–292.

41 Pop-Busui R, London Z, Kellogg A. Diabetes and endocrine disorders. In: *Neurobiology of Disease* (ed. S. Gilman), Elsevier Academic Press, San Diego, CA, 2007, pp. 669–680.

42 Eaton S, Tesfaye S. Clinical manifestations and measurement of somatic neuropathy. *Diabetes Rev* 1997;**7**: 312–325.

43 Kennedy WR, Navarro X, Goetz FC *et al.* Effects of pancreatic transplantation on diabetic neuropathy. *N Engl J Med* 1990;**322**:1031–1037.

44 Navarro X, Sutherland DE, Kennedy WR. Long-term effects of pancreatic transplantation on diabetic neuropathy. *Ann Neurol* 1997;**42**(5):727–736.

45 Pfeifer MA, Schumer MP, Gelber DA. Aldose reductase inhibitors: the end of an era or the need for different trial designs? *Diabetes* 1997;**46**(Suppl 2): S82–S89.

46 Nicolucci A, Carinci F, Cavaliere D *et al.* A meta-analysis of trials on aldose reductase inhibitors in diabetic peripheral neuropathy. The Italian Study Group. The St. Vincent Declaration. *Diabet Med* 1996;**13**(12):1017–1026.

47 Greene DA, Arezzo JC, Brown MB. Effect of aldose reductase inhibition on nerve conduction and morphometry in diabetic neuropathy. Zenarestat Study Group *Neurology* 1999;**53**(3):580–591.

48 Obrosova IG, Minchenko AG, Vasupuram R *et al.* Aldose reductase inhibitor fidarestat prevents retinal oxidative stress and vascular endothelial growth factor overexpression in streptozotocin-diabetic rats. *Diabetes* 2003;**52**(3): 864–871.

49 Hotta N, Toyota T, Matsuoka K *et al.* Clinical efficacy of fidarestat, a novel aldose reductase inhibitor, for diabetic peripheral neuropathy: a 52-week multicenter placebo-controlled double-blind parallel group study. *Diabetes Care* 2001;**24**(10):1776–1782.

50 Asano T, Saito Y, Kawakami M, Yamada N. Fidarestat (SNK-860), a potent aldose reductase inhibitor, normalizes the elevated sorbitol accumulation in erythrocytes of diabetic patients. *J Diabetes Complications* 2002;**16** (2): 133–138.

51 Bril V, Buchanan RA. Long-term effects of ranirestat (AS-3201) on peripheral nerve function in patients with diabetic sensorimotor polyneuropathy. *Diabetes Care* 2006; **29** (1): 68–72.

52 Low PA, Walsh JC, Huang CY, McLeod JG. The sympathetic nervous system in alcoholic neuropathy. A clinical and pathological study. *Brain* 1975;**98**:357–364.

53 Faerman I, Glocer L, Celener D *et al.* Autonomic nervous system and diabetes. Histological and histochemical study of the autonomic nerve fibers of the urinary bladder in diabetic patients. *Diabetes* 1973;**22**:225–237.

54 Cameron NE, Cotter MA, Horrobin DH, Tritschler HJ. Effects of alpha-lipoic acid on neurovascular function in diabetic rats: interaction with essential fatty acids. *Diabetologia* 1998;**41**:390–399.

55 Ziegler D, Hanefeld M, Ruhnau KJ *et al.* Treatment of symptomatic diabetic polyneuropathy with the antioxidant alpha-lipoic acid: a 7-month multicenter randomized controlled trial (ALADIN III Study). ALADIN III Study Group. Alpha-Lipoic Acid in Diabetic Neuropathy *Diabetes Care* 1999;**22**(8):1296–1301.

56 Ziegler D, Reljanovic M, Mehnert H, Gries FA. Alpha-lipoic acid in the treatment of diabetic polyneuropathy in Germany: current evidence from clinical trials. *Exp Clin Endocrinol Diabetes* 1999;**107**(7):421–430.

57 Ametov AS, Barinov A, Dyck PJ *et al.* The sensory symptoms of diabetic polyneuropathy are improved with alpha-lipoic acid: the SYDNEY trial. *Diabetes Care* 2003;**26**(3): 770–776.

58 Petty BG, Cornblath DR, Adornato BT *et al.* The effect of systemically administered recombinant human nerve growth factor in healthy human subjects. *Ann Neurol* 1994;**36**(2):244–246.

59 Apfel SC, Kessler JA, Adornato BT *et al.* Recombinant human nerve growth factor in the treatment of diabetic polyneuropathy. NGF Study Group [In Process Citation]. *Neurology* 1998;**51**:695–702.

60 Apfel SC. Nerve growth factor for the treatment of diabetic neuropathy: what went wrong, what went right and what does the future hold? *Int Rev Neurobiol* 2002;**50**:393–413.

61 Scarpini E, Doneda P, Pizzul S *et al.* L-Carnitine and acetyl-L-carnitine in human nerves from normal and diabetic subjects. *J Peripher Nerv Syst* 1996;**1**(2):157–163.

62 Sima AAF, Ristic H, Merry A *et al.* The primary preventive and secondary interventionary effects of acetyl-L-carnitine on diabetic neuropathy in the BB/W-rat. *J Clin Invest* 1996;**97**:1900–1907.

63 Stevens MJ, Lattimer SA, Feldman EL *et al.* Acetyl-L-carnitine deficiency as a cause of altered nerve myo-inositol content, Na,K-ATPase activity and motor conduction velocity in the streptozotocin-diabetic rat. *Metabolism* 1996;**45**:865–872.

64 Lowitt S, Malone JE, Solem A, Listhals A. Acetylcarnitine improves neuronal function in streptozotocin (STZ) diabetic rats. *Diabetes* 1990;**39**:155A.

65 Pop-Busui R, Marinescu V, Van Huysen C *et al.* Dissection of metabolic, vascular and nerve conduction interrelationships in experimental diabetic neuropathy by cyclooxygenase inhibition and acetyl-L-carnitine administration. *023.*

66 Onofrj M, Fulgente T, Melchionda D *et al.* L-Acetylcarnitine as a new therapeutic approach for peripheral neuropathies with pain. *Int J Clin Pharmacol Res* 1995;**15**(1):9–15.

67 Quatraro A, Roca P, Donzella C *et al.* Acetyl-L-carnitine for symptomatic diabetic neuropathy. *Diabetologia* 1995; **38**(1): 123.

68 Scarpini E, Sacilotto G, Baron P *et al.* Effect of acetyl-L-carnitine in the treatment of painful peripheral neuropathies in HIV+ patients. *J Peripher Nerv Syst* 1997;**2**(3): 250–252.

69 Brown MJ, Martin JR, Asbury AK. Painful diabetic neuropathy. A morphometric study. *Arch Neurol* 1976;**33** (3):164–171.

70 Said G, Slama G, Selva J. Progressive centripetal degeneration of axons in small fibre diabetic polyneuropathy. *Brain* 1983;**106**(Pt 4): 791–807.

71 Kennedy WR, Wendelschafer-Crabb G. Utility of skin biopsy in diabetic neuropathy. *Semin Neurol* 1996;**16**(2): 163–171.

72 Kennedy WR, Wendelschafer-Crabb G, Johnson T. Quantitation of epidermal nerves in diabetic neuropathy. *Neurology* 1996;**47**(4):1042–1048.

73 Holland NR, Crawford TO, Hauer P *et al.* Small-fiber sensory neuropathies: clinical course and neuropathology of idiopathic cases. *Ann Neurol* 1998;**44**(1):47–59.

74 Herrmann DN, Griffin JW, Hauer P *et al.* Epidermal nerve fiber density and sural nerve morphometry in peripheral neuropathies. *Neurology* 1999;**53**(8):1634–1640.

75 Smith AG, Russell J, Feldman EL *et al.* Lifestyle intervention for pre-diabetic neuropathy. *Diabetes Care* 2006;**29**(6): 1294–1299.

76 Cohen K L, Harris S Efficacy and safety of nonsteroidal anti-inflammatory drugs in the therapy of diabetic neuropathy. *Arch Intern Med* 1987;**147**(8):1442–1444.

77 Joss JD. Tricyclic antidepressant use in diabetic neuropathy. *Ann Pharmacother* 1999;**33**(9):996–1000.

78 Kvinesdal B, Molin J, Froland A, Gram LF. Imipramine treatment of painful diabetic neuropathy. *JAMA* 1984; **251**(13):1727–1730.

79 Max MB, Culnane M, Schafer SC *et al.* Amitriptyline relieves diabetic neuropathy pain in patients with normal or depressed mood. *Neurology* 1987;**37**(4):589–596.

80 Max MB, Kishore-Kumar R, Schafer SC *et al.* Efficacy of desipramine in painful diabetic neuropathy: a placebo-controlled trial. *Pain* 1991;**45**(1):3–9; discussion 1–2.

81 Max MB, Lynch SA, Muir J et al. Effects of desipramine, amitriptyline and fluoxetine on pain in diabetic neuropathy. N Engl J Med 1992;326(19):1250–1256.

82 Sindrup SH, Ejlertsen B, Froland A et al. Imipramine treatment in diabetic neuropathy: relief of subjective symptoms without changes in peripheral and autonomic nerve function. Eur J Clin Pharmacol 1989;37(2):151–153.

83 McQuay HJ, Tramer M, Nye BA et al. A systematic review of antidepressants in neuropathic pain. Pain 1996;68(2–3): 217–227.

84 Gomez-Perez FJ, Rull JA, Dies H et al. Nortriptyline and fluphenazine in the symptomatic treatment of diabetic neuropathy. A double-blind cross-over study. Pain 1985;23(4): 395–400.

85 Gomez-Perez FJ, Choza R, Rios JM et al. Nortriptyline––fluphenazine vs carbamazepine in the symptomatic treatment of diabetic neuropathy. Arch Med Res 1996;27(4): 525–529.

86 Richelson E. Pharmacology of antidepressants – characteristics of the ideal drug. Mayo Clin Proc 1994;69(11): 1069–1081.

87 Sindrup SH, Gram LF, Brosen K et al. The selective serotonin reuptake inhibitor paroxetine is effective in the treatment of diabetic neuropathy symptoms. Pain 1990; 42(2):135–144.

88 Goodnick PJ, Jimenez I, Kumar A. Sertraline in diabetic neuropathy: preliminary results. Ann Clin Psychiatry 1997; 9(4):255–257.

89 Iyengar S, Bymaster FP, Wong DT et al. Efficacy of the selective serotonin and norepinephrine reuptake inhibitor, duloxetine, in the formalin model of persistent pain. Eur Neuropsychopharmacol 2002;12(Suppl 3): 215.

90 Goldstein DJ, Lu Y, Detke MJ et al. Effects of duloxetine on painful physical symptoms associated with depression. Psychosomatics 2004;45(1):17–28.

91 Goldstein DJ, Lu Y, Detke MJ et al. Duloxetine vs placebo in patients with painful diabetic neuropathy. Pain 2005; 116(1–2):109–118.

92 Wernicke JF, Pritchett YL, D'Souza DN et al. A randomized controlled trial of duloxetine in diabetic peripheral neuropathic pain. Neurology 2006;67(8):1411–1420.

93 Raskin J, Wang F, Pritchett YL, Goldstein DJ. Duloxetine for patients with diabetic peripheral neuropathic pain: a 6-month open-label safety study. Pain Med 2006;7(5):373–385.

94 Thienel U, Neto W, Schwabe SK, Vijapurkar U. Topiramate in painful diabetic polyneuropathy: findings from three double-blind placebo-controlled trials. Acta Neurol Scand 2004;110(4):221–231.

95 Raskin P, Donofrio PD, Rosenthal NR et al. Topiramate vs placebo in painful diabetic neuropathy: analgesic and metabolic effects. Neurology 2004;63(5):865–873.

96 Wiffen P, Collins S, McQuay H, Carroll D, Jadad A, Moore A. Anticonvulsant drugs for acute and chronic pain (Review). The Cochrane Library 2006, Issue 2, John Wiley & Sons, Ltd.

97 Richter RW, Portenoy R, Sharma U et al. Relief of painful diabetic peripheral neuropathy with pregabalin: a randomized, placebo-controlled trial. J Pain 2005;6(4):253–260.

98 Rosenstock J, Tuchman M, LaMoreaux L, Sharma U. Pregabalin for the treatment of painful diabetic peripheral

neuropathy: a double-blind, placebo-controlled trial. Pain 2004;110(3):628–638.

99 Freynhagen R, Strojek K, Griesing T et al. Efficacy of pregabalin in neuropathic pain evaluated in a 12-week, randomised, double-blind, multicentre, placebo-controlled trial of flexible- and fixed-dose regimens. Pain 2005;115(3): 254–263.

100 Backonja MM. Gabapentin monotherapy for the symptomatic treatment of painful neuropathy: a multicenter, double-blind, placebo-controlled trial in patients with diabetes mellitus. Epilepsia 1999;40(Suppl 6): S57–S59l; discussion S73–S74.

101 Perez HE, Sanchez GF. Gabapentin therapy for diabetic neuropathic pain. Am J Med 2000;108(8):689.

102 Simpson D. Gabapentin and venlafaxine for the treatment of painful diabetic neuropathy. J Clin Neuromusc Dis 2001; 3(2):53–62.

103 Gorson KC, Schott C, Herman R et al. Gabapentin in the treatment of painful diabetic neuropathy: a placebo controlled, double blind, crossover trial. J Neurol Neurosurg Psychiatry 1999;66(2):251–252.

104 Morello CM, Leckband SG, Stoner CP et al. Randomized double-blind study comparing the efficacy of gabapentin with amitriptyline on diabetic peripheral neuropathy pain. Arch Intern Med 1999;159(16):1931–1937.

105 Dallocchio C, Buffa C, Mazzarello P, Chiroli S. Gabapentin vs amitriptyline in painful diabetic neuropathy: an open-label pilot study. J Pain Symptom Manage 2000;20(4): 280–285.

106 Gould HJ. Gabapentin induced polyneuropathy. Pain 1998;74(2–3):341–343.

107 Rull JA, Quibrera R, Gonzalez-Millan H, Lozano Castaneda O. Symptomatic treatment of peripheral diabetic neuropathy with carbamazepine (Tegretol): double blind crossover trial. Diabetologia 1969;5(4):215–218.

108 Dellemijn PL, Vanneste JA. Randomised double-blind active-placebo-controlled crossover trial of intravenous fentanyl in neuropathic pain. Lancet 1997;349(9054):753–758.

109 Rowbotham MC, Twilling L, Davies PS et al. Oral opioid therapy for chronic peripheral and central neuropathic pain. N Engl J Med 2003;348(13):1223–1232.

110 Watson CP, Moulin D, Watt-Watson J et al. Controlled-release oxycodone relieves neuropathic pain: a randomized controlled trial in painful diabetic neuropathy. Pain 2003; 105(1–2):71–78.

111 Raffa RB, Friderichs E, Reimann W, Shank RP, Codd EE and Vaught JL. Opioid and nonopioid components independently contribute to the mechanism of action of tramadol, an 'atypical' opioid analgesic. J Pharmaco Exp Ther 1992;260(1):275–285.

112 Harati Y, Gooch C, Swenson M et al. Double-blind randomized trial of tramadol for the treatment of the pain of diabetic neuropathy. Neurology 1998;50(6):1842–1846.

113 Nelson KA, Park KM, Robinovitz E, Tsigos C, Max MB. High-dose oral dextromethorphan versus placebo in painful diabetic neuropathy and postherpetic neuralgia. Neurology 1997;48:1212–1218.

114 Raja SN, Haythornthwaite JA, Pappagallo M et al. Opioids versus antidepressants in postherpetic neuralgia: a rando-

mized, placebo-controlled trial. *Neurology* 2002;**59**(7): 1015–1021.

115 Dworkin RH, Backonja M, Rowbotham MC *et al.* Advances in neuropathic pain: diagnosis, mechanisms and treatment recommendations. *Arch Neurol* 2003;**60**(11):1524–1534.

116 Gilron I, Bailey JM, Tu D *et al.* Morphine, gabapentin or their combination for 090.

117 Dejgard A, Hilsted J. No effect ofp on postural hypotension in type 1 (insulin-dependent) diabetic patients with autonomic neuropathy. A randomised double-blind controlled study. *Diabetologia* 1988;**31**(5):281–284.

118 Stracke H, Meyer UE, Schumacher H E, Federlin K. Mexiletine in the treatment of diabetic neuropathy. *Diabetes Care* 1992;**15**(11):1550–1555.

119 Oskarsson P, Ljunggren J-G, Lins P-E, Group tMS. Efficacy and safety of mexiletine in the treatment of painful diabetic neuropathy. *Diabetes Care* 1997;**20**:1594–1597.

120 Wright JM, Oki JC, Graves L III. Mexiletine in the symptomatic treatment of diabetic peripheral neuropathy. *Ann Pharmacother* 1997;**31**(1):29–34.

121 Galer BS, Harle J, Rowbotham MC. Response to intravenous lidocaine infusion predicts subsequent response to oral mexiletine: a prospective study. *J Pain Symptom Manage* 1996;**12**(3):161–167.

122 Ertas M, Sagduyu A, Arac N *et al.* Use of levodopa to relieve pain from painful symmetrical diabetic polyneuropathy. *Pain* 1998;**75**(2–3):257–259.

123 Zeigler D, Lynch SA, Muir J *et al.* Transdermal clonidine versus placebo in painful diabetic neuropathy. *Pain* 1992;**48**(3): 403–408.

124 Byas-Smith MG, Max MB, Muir J, Kingman A. Transdermal clonidine compared to placebo in painful diabetic neuropathy using a two-stage 'enriched enrollment' design. *Pain* 1995;**60**(3):267–274.

125 Jamal GA, Carmichael H. The effect of gamma-linolenic acid on human diabetic peripheral neuropathy: a doubleblind placebo-controlled trial. *Diabet Med* 1990;**7**(4): 319–323.

126 Capsaicin Study Group. Treatment of painful diabetic neuropathy with topical capsaicin. A multicenter, doubleblind, vehicle-controlled study. The Capsaicin Study Group. *Arch Intern Med* 1991;**151**(11):2225–2229.

127 Capsaicin Study Group. Effect of treatment with capsaicin on daily activities of patients with painful diabetic neuropathy. The Capsaicin Study Group. *Diabetes Care* 1992;**15** (2):159–165.

128 Biesbroeck R, Bril V, Hollander P *et al.* A double-blind comparison of topical capsaicin and oral amitriptyline in painful diabetic neuropathy. *Adv Ther* 1995;**12**(2):111–120.

129 Low PA, Opfer-Gehrking TL, Dyck PJ *et al.* Double-blind, placebo-controlled study of the application of capsaicin cream in chronic distal painful polyneuropathy. *Pain* 1995;**62**(2):163–168.

130 Zhang WY, Li Wan Po A. The effectiveness of topically applied capsaicin. A meta-analysis. *Eur J Clin Pharmacol* 1994;**46**(6):517–522.

131 Kumar D, Marshall HJ. Diabetic peripheral neuropathy: amelioration of pain with transcutaneous electrostimulation. *Diabetes Care* 1997;**20**(11):1702–1705.

132 Abuaisha BB, Costanzi J. B, Boulton AJ. Acupuncture for the treatment of chronic painful peripheral diabetic neuropathy: a long-term study. *Diabetes Res Clin Pract* 1998;**39**(2): 115–121.

133 Julka IS, Alvaro M, Kumar D. Beneficial effects of electrical stimulation on neuropathic symptoms in diabetes patients. *J Foot Ankle Surg* 1998;**37**(3):191–194.

134 Melzack R, Wall PD. Pain mechanisms: a new theory. *Science* 1965;**150**(699):971–979.

135 Haythornthwaite JA, Benrud-Larson LM. Psychological aspects of neuropathic pain. *Clin J Pain* 2000;**16**(2 Suppl): S101–S105.

136 Freeman R. Autonomic peripheral neuropathy. *Lancet* 2005;**365**(9466):1259–1270.

137 O'Brien OA, McFadden JP, Corrall RJM. The influence of autonomic neuropathy on mortality in insulin-dependent diabetes. *Q J Med* 1991;**290**:495–502.

138 Rathman W, Ziegler D, Jahnke M *et al.* Mortality in diabetic patients with cardiovascular autonomic neuropathy. *Diabet Med* 1993;**10**:820–824.

139 Vinik A, Erbas T, Pfeifer M *et al.* Diabetic autonomic neuropathy. In: *The Diabetes Mellitus Manual* (eds S Inzucchi, D PorteJr, R Sherwin, A Baron), McGraw-Hill, New York, 2005, pp. 347–365.

140 Low PA, Walsh JC, Huang CY, McLeod JG. The sympathetic nervous system in diabetic neuropathy. A clinical and pathological study. *Brain* 1975;**98**(3):341–356.

141 Jones KL, Russo A, Stevens JE *et al.* Predictors of delayed gastric emptying in diabetes. *Diabetes Care* 2001;**24**(7): 1264–1269.

142 Kong MF, Horowitz M, Jones KL *et al.* Natural history of diabetic gastroparesis. *Diabetes Care* 1999;**22**(3):503–507.

143 Maleki D, Locke GR III, Camilleri M *et al.* Gastrointestinal tract symptoms among persons with diabetes mellitus in the community. *Arch Intern Med* 2000;**160**(18): 2808–2816.

144 Frimodt-Moller C, Mortensen S. Treatment of diabetic cystopathy. *Ann Intern Med* 1980;**92**(2 Pt 2): 327–328.

145 Kaplan SA, Te AE, Blaivas JG. Urodynamic findings in patients with diabetic cystopathy. *J Urol* 1995;**153**(2): 342–344.

146 Bacon CG, Hu FB, Giovannucci E *et al.* Association of type and duration of diabetes with erectile dysfunction in a large cohort of men. *Diabetes Care* 2002;**25**(8): 1458–1463.

147 Fedele D. Therapy insight: sexual and bladder dysfunction associated with diabetes mellitus. *Nat Clin Pract Urol* 2005;**2** (6):282–90; quiz 309.

148 Bhasin S, Enzlin P, Coviello A *et al.* Sexual dysfunction in men and women with endocrine disorders. *Lancet* 2007;**369** (9561):597–611.

149 Hepburn DA, Patrick AW, Eadington DW *et al.* Unawareness of hypoglycaemia in insulin-treated diabetic patients: prevalence and relationship to autonomic neuropathy. *Diabet Med* 1990;**7**(8):711–717.

150 Ryder RE, Owens DR, Hayes TM *et al.* Unawareness of hypoglycaemia and inadequate hypoglycaemic counterregulation: no causal relation with diabetic autonomic neuropathy. *BMJ* 1990;**301**(6755):783–787.

151 Cryer PE. Hypoglycemia-associated autonomic failure in diabetes. *Am J Physiol Endocrinol Metab* 2001;**281**(6): E1115–E1121.

152 Onrot J, Goldberg MR, Hollister AS *et al.* Management of chronic orthostatic hypotension. *Am J Med* 1986;**80**(3): 454–464.

153 Hilsted J, Low P. Diabetic autonomic neuropathy. In: *Clinical Autonomic Disorders: Evaluation and Management* (ed. P Low,), Lippincott-Raven, Philadelphia, PA, 1997, pp. 487–507.

154 Mathias CJ, Kimber JR. Treatment of postural hypotension. *J Neurol Neurosurg Psychiatry* 1998;**65**(3):285–289.

155 Vinik AI. Diabetic neuropathy: pathogenesis and therapy. *Am J Med* 1999;**107**(2B):17S–26S.

156 Vinik AI. Diagnosis and management of diabetic neuropathy. *Clin Geriatr Med* 1999;**15**(2):293–320.

157 Freeman R. Treatment of orthostatic hypotension. *Semin Neurol* 2003;**23**(4):435–442.

158 van Lieshout JJ, ten Harkel AD, Wieling W. Physical manoeuvres for combating orthostatic dizziness in autonomic failure. *Lancet* 1992;**339**(8798):897–898.

159 MacLean A, Allen B. Orthostatic hypotension and orthostatic tachycardia. Treatment with head-up bed. *JAMA* 1940;**115**:2162–2167.

160 Schatz IJ, Podolsky S, Frame B. Idiopathic orthostatic hypotension. Diagnosis and treatment. *JAMA* 1963;**186**:537–540.

161 Levin JM, Ravenna P, Weiss M. Idiopathic orthostatic hypotension. Treatment with a commercially available counterpressure suit. *Arch Intern Med* 1964;**114**:145–148.

162 Lewis HD Jr, Dunn M. Orthostatic hypotension syndrome. A case report. *Am Heart J* 1967;**74**(3):396–401.

163 Sheps SG. Use of an elastic garment in the treatment of orthostatic hypotension. *Cardiology* 1976;**61**(Suppl 1): 271–279.

164 Tanaka H, Yamaguchi H, Tamai H. Treatment of orthostatic intolerance with inflatable abdominal band. *Lancet* 1997; **349**(9046):175.

165 Smit AA, Hardjowijono MA, Wieling W. Are portable folding chairs useful to combat orthostatic hypotension? *Ann Neurol* 1997;**42**(6):975–978.

166 Schatz IJ, Miller MJ, Frame B. Corticosteroids in the management of orthostatic hypotension. *Cardiology* 1976;**61** (Suppl 1): 280–289.

167 van Lieshout JJ, ten Harkel AD, Wieling W. Fludrocortisone and sleeping in the head-up position limit the postural decrease in cardiac output in autonomic failure. *Clin Auton Res* 2000;**10**(1):35–42.

168 Hickler RB, Thompson GR, Fox LM, Hamlin JT III. Successful treatment of orthostatic hypotension with 9-alpha-fluorohydrocortisone. *N Engl J Med* 1959;**261**:788–791.

169 Bannister R, Ardill L, Fentem P. An assessment of various methods of treatment of idiopathic orthostatic hypotension. *Q J Med* 1969;**38**(152):377–395.

170 Campbell IW, Ewing DJ, Clarke BF. Therapeutic experience with fludrocortisone in diabetic postural hypotension. *Br Med J* 1976;i (6014):872–874.

171 Chobanian AV, Volicer L, Tifft CP *et al.* Mineralocorticoid-induced hypertension in patients with orthostatic hypotension. *N Engl J Med* 1979;**301**(2):68–73.

172 Robertson D, Davis TL. Recent advances in the treatment of orthostatic hypotension. *Neurology* 1995;**45**(4 Suppl 5): S26–S32.

173 Zachariah PK, Bloedow DC, Moyer TP *et al.* Pharmacodynamics of midodrine, an antihypotensive agent. *Clin Pharmacol Ther* 1986;**39**(5):586–591.

174 McTavish D, Goa KL. Midodrine. A review of its pharmacological properties and therapeutic use in orthostatic hypotension and secondary hypotensive disorders. *Drugs* 1989;**38**(5):757–777.

175 Kaufmann H, Brannan T, Krakoff L *et al.* Treatment of orthostatic hypotension due to autonomic failure with a peripheral alpha-adrenergic agonist (midodrine). *Neurology* 1988;**38**(6):951–956.

176 Low PA, Gilden JL, Freeman R *et al.* Efficacy of midodrine vs placebo in neurogenic orthostatic hypotension. A randomized, double-blind multicenter study. Midodrine Study Group. *JAMA* 1997;**277**(13):1046–1051.

177 Wright RA, Kaufmann HC, Perera R *et al.* A double-blind, dose-response study of midodrine in neurogenic orthostatic hypotension. *Neurology* 1998;**51**(1):120–124.

178 Fouad-Tarazi FM, Okabe M, Goren H. Alpha sympathomimetic treatment of autonomic insufficiency with orthostatic hypotension. *Am J Med* 1995;**99**(6):604–610.

179 Jordan J, Shannon JR, Biaggioni I *et al.* Contrasting actions of pressor agents in severe autonomic failure. *Am J Med* 1998;**105**(2):116–124.

180 Winkler AS, Landau S, Watkins P, Chaudhuri KR. Observations on hematological and cardiovascular effects of erythropoietin treatment in multiple system atrophy with sympathetic failure. *Clin Auton Res* 2002;**12**(3):203–206.

181 Hoeldtke RD, Streeten DH. Treatment of orthostatic hypotension with erythropoietin. *N Engl J Med* 1993;**329**(9):611–615.

182 Perera R, Isola L, Kaufmann H. Effect of recombinant erythropoietin on anemia and orthostatic hypotension in primary autonomic failure. *Clin Auton Res* 1995;**5**(4):211–213.

183 Verwaerde P, Tran MA, Montastruc JL *et al.* Effects of yohimbine, an alpha 2-adrenoceptor antagonist, on experimental neurogenic orthostatic hypotension. *Fundam Clin Pharmacol* 1997;**11**(6):567–575.

184 Cleophas TJ, Grabowsky I, Niemeyer MG *et al.* Paradoxical pressor effects of beta-blockers in standing elderly patients with mild hypertension: a beneficial side-effect. *Circulation* 2002;**105**(14):1669–1671.

185 Chobanian AV, Volicer L, Liang CS *et al.* Use of propranolol in the treatment of idiopathic orthostatic hypotension. *Trans Assoc Am Physicians* 1977;**90**:324–334.

186 Brevetti G, Chiariello M, Giudice P *et al.* Effective treatment of orthostatic hypotension by propranolol in the Shy-Drager syndrome. *Am Heart J* 1981;**102**(5):938–941.

187 Man in 't Veld AJ, Schalekamp MA, Pindolol acts as beta-adrenoceptor agonist in orthostatic hypotension: therapeutic implications. *Br Med J (Clin Res Ed)* 1981;**282**(6268): 929–931.

188 Verne GN, Sninsky CA. Diabetes and the gastrointestinal tract. *Gastroenterol Clin North Am* 1998;**27**(4):861–874, vi–vii.

189 Sturm A, Holtmann G, Goebell H, Gerken G. Prokinetics in patients with gastroparesis: a systematic analysis. *Digestion* 1999;**60**(5):422–427.

190 Kendall BJ, Kendall ET, Soykan I, McCallum RW. Cisapride in the long-term treatment of chronic gastroparesis: a 2-year open-label study. *J Intern Med Res* 1997;**25**(4): 182–189.

191 Horowitz M, Harding PE, Chatterton BE *et al.* Acute and chronic effects of domperidone on gastric emptying in diabetic autonomic neuropathy. *Dig Dis Sci* 1985;**30**(1): 1–9.

192 Patterson D, Abell T, Rothstein R *et al.* A double-blind multicenter comparison of domperidone and metoclopramide in the treatment of diabetic patients with symptoms of gastroparesis. *Am J Gastroenterol* 1999;**94**(5):1230–1234.

193 Ahmad N, Keith-Ferris J, Gooden E, Abell T. Making a case for domperidone in the treatment of gastrointestinal motility disorders. *Curr Opin Pharmacol* 2006;**6**(6):571–576.

194 Peeters T, Matthijs G, Depoortere I *et al.* Erythromycin is a motilin receptor agonist. *Am J Physiol* 1989;**257**(3 Pt 1): G470–G474.

195 Richards RD, Davenport K, McCallum RW. The treatment of idiopathic and diabetic gastroparesis with acute intravenous and chronic oral erythromycin. *Am J Gastroenterol* 1993;**88**(2):203–207.

196 DiBaise JK, Quigley EM. Efficacy of prolonged administration of intravenous erythromycin in an ambulatory setting as treatment of severe gastroparesis: one center's experience. *J Clin Gastroenterol* 1999;**28**(2):131–134.

197 Ezzeddine D, Jit R, Katz N *et al.* Pyloric injection of botulinum toxin for treatment of diabetic gastroparesis. *Gastrointest Endosc* 2002;**55**(7):920–923.

198 Lacy BE, Zayat EN, Crowell MD, Schuster MM. Botulinum toxin for the treatment of gastroparesis: a preliminary report. *Am J Gastroenterol* 2002;**97**(6):1548–1552.

199 Lacy BE, Crowell MD, Schettler-Duncan A *et al.* The treatment of diabetic gastroparesis with botulinum toxin injection of the pylorus. *Diabetes Care* 2004;**27**(10): 2341–2347.

200 Asakawa A, Inui A, Kaga T *et al.* Ghrelin is an appetite-stimulatory signal from stomach with structural resemblance to motilin. *Gastroenterology* 2001;**120**(2): 337–345.

201 Fujino K, Inui A, Asakawa A *et al.* Ghrelin induces fasted motor activity of the gastrointestinal tract in conscious fed rats. *J Physiol* 2003;**550**(Pt 1): 227–240.

202 Murray CD, Martin NM, Patterson M *et al.* Ghrelin enhances gastric emptying in diabetic gastroparesis: a double blind, placebo controlled, crossover study. *Gut* 2005;**54**(12): 1693–1698.

203 Tack J, Depoortere I, Bisschops R *et al.* Influence of ghrelin on gastric emptying and meal-related symptoms in idiopathic gastroparesis. *Aliment Pharmacol Ther* 2005;**22**(9):847–853.

204 Bellahsene BE, Lind CD, Schirmer BD *et al.* Acceleration of gastric emptying with electrical stimulation in a canine model of gastroparesis. *Am J Physiol* 1992;**262**(5 Pt 1): G826–G834.

205 McCallum RW, Chen JD, Lin Z *et al.* Gastric pacing improves emptying and symptoms in patients with gastroparesis. *Gastroenterology* 1998;**114**(3):456–461.

206 Forster J, Sarosiek I, Delcore R *et al.* Gastric pacing is a new surgical treatment for gastroparesis. *Am J Surg* 2001;**182**(6):676–681.

207 Ejskjaer NT, Bradley JL, Buxton-Thomas MS *et al.* Novel surgical treatment and gastric pathology in diabetic gastroparesis. *Diabet Med* 1999;**16**(6):488–495.

208 Green PA, Berge KG, Sprague RG. Control of diabetic diarrhea with antibiotic therapy. *Diabetes* 1968;**17**(6): 385–387.

209 Tsai ST, Vinik AI, Brunner JF. Diabetic diarrhea and somatostatin. *Ann Intern Med* 1986;**104**(6):894.

210 von der Ohe MR, Camilleri M, Thomforde GM, Klee GG. Differential regional effects of octreotide on human gastrointestinal motor function. *Gut* 1995;**36**(5): 743–748.

211 Frimodt-Moller C. Diabetic cystopathy: epidemiology and related disorders. *Ann Intern Med* 1980;**92**(2 Pt 2): 318–321.

212 Buck AC, Reed PI, Siddiq YK *et al.* Bladder dysfunction and neuropathy in diabetes. *Diabetologia* 1976;**12**(3):251–258.

213 Menendez V, Cofan F, Talbot-Wright R *et al.* Urodynamic evaluation in simultaneous insulin-dependent diabetes mellitus and end stage renal disease. *J Urol* 1996;**155**(6): 2001–2004.

214 Watanabe T, Miyagawa I. The effect of partial cystectomy on the residual urine of a large bladder demonstrated in diabetic rats. *J Urol* 1999;**161**(3):1010–1014.

215 Saulie BA, Campbell RK. Treating erectile dysfunction in diabetes patients. *Diabetes Educ* 1997;**23**(1):29–33, 35–36, 38.

216 Spollett GR. Assessment and management of erectile dysfunction in men with diabetes. *Diabetes Educ* 1999; **25**(1):65–73; quiz 75.

217 Virag R, Frydman D, Legman M, Virag H. Intracavernous injection of papaverine as a diagnostic and therapeutic method in erectile failure. *Angiology* 1984;**35**(2):79–87.

218 Ernst E, Pittler MH. Yohimbine for erectile dysfunction: a systematic review and meta-analysis of randomized clinical trials. *J Urol* 1998;**159**(2):433–436.

219 Rendell MS, Rajfer J, Wicker PA, Smith MD. Sildenafil for treatment of erectile dysfunction in men with diabetes: a randomized controlled trial. Sildenafil Diabetes Study Group. *JAMA* 1999;**281**(5):421–426.

220 Goldstein I, Kim E, Steers WD *et al.* Efficacy and safety of tadalafil in men with erectile dysfunction with a high prevalence of co-morbid conditions: results from MOMENTUS: Multiple Observations in Men with Erectile Dysfunction in National Tadalafil Study in the US. *J Sex Med* 2007;**4**(1):166–175.

221 Vardi M, Nini A. Phosphodiesterase inhibitors for erectile dysfunction in patients with diabetes mellitus. *Cochrane Database Syst Rev* 2007;**24**(1):CD002187.

222 Caruso S, Rugolo S, Agnello C *et al.* Sildenafil improves sexual functioning in premenopausal women with type 1 diabetes who are affected by sexual arousal disorder: a double-blind, crossover, placebo-controlled pilot study. *Fertil Steril* 2006;**85**:1496–1501.

223 Low PA, Tuck RR, Takeuchi M. Nerve microenvironment in diabetic neuropathy. In: *Diabetic Neuropathy* (eds PJ Dyck,

PK Thomas, AK Asbury, AI Winegrad, D PorteJr), Saunders, Philadelphia, PA, 1987, pp. 266–278.

224 al-Qattan MM, Manktelow RT, Bowen CV. Outcome of carpal tunnel release in diabetic patients. *J Hand Surg [Br]* 1994;**19**(5):626–629.

225 Dyck PJ, Windebank AJ. Diabetic and nondiabetic lumbosacral radiculoplexus neuropathies: new insights into pathophysiology and treatment. *Muscle Nerve* 2002;**25**(4): 477–491.

226 Dyck PJ, Norell JE. Microvasculitis and ischemia in diabetic lumbosacral radiculoplexus neuropathy. *Neurology* 1999; **53**(9):2113–2121.

227 Krendel DA, Costigan DA, Hopkins LC. Successful treatment of neuropathies in patients with diabetes mellitus. *Arch Neurol* 1995;**52**(11):1053–1061.

228 Krendel DA, Zacharias A, Younger DS. Autoimmune diabetic neuropathy. *Neurol Clin* 1997;**15**(4):959–971.

229 Pascoe MK, Low PA, Windebank AJ, Litchy WJ. Subacute diabetic proximal neuropathy. *Mayo Clin Proc* 1997;**72**(12): 1123–1132.

230 Jaradeh SS, Prieto TE, Lobeck LJ. Progressive polyradiculoneuropathy in diabetes: correlation of variables and clinical outcome after immunotherapy. *J Neurol Neurosurg Psychiatry* 1999;**67**(5):607–612.

20 Treatment of erectile dysfunction

David E. Price[1], Geoffrey Hackett[2]

[1]*ABM University Trust, Morriston Hospital, Swansea, UK*
[2]*Good Hope Hospital, Sutton Coldfield, West Midlands, UK*

Introduction

It is particularly encouraging that we are in a position to review the management of erectile dysfunction (ED) for the evidence base for diabetes care. Historically, the discussion of this subject has been governed more by prejudice and taboo than experimental evidence. Until the 1980s, medical textbooks offered the opinion that, even in diabetic men, impotence usually had a psychogenic cause and as recently as 1990 the guidelines on diabetes care published by the British Diabetic Association (now Diabetes UK) made no mention of the problem.[1] The advent of effective treatments for impotence has changed attitudes considerably. The output of research papers on the subject of ED increased dramatically after effective oral treatments became available, not least because of increased funding for research from the pharmaceutical industry.

Treating ED is easy and rewarding and should be a routine part of managing a diabetes care service. More recently, it has been recognized that the functioning of the erectile tissue is a marker of endothelial function and hence cardiovascular risk. Therefore, an understanding of the pathophysiology and management of ED is important for all diabetes care professionals.

Prevalence of erectile dysfunction in diabetes

ED is a common problem in both diabetic and non-diabetic populations. The Massachusetts Male Aging Study, which is one of the best population-based studies of male sexual function, reported the prevalence of complete erectile failure in the community to be 9.6% in men aged 40–70 years, 5% in men aged less than 40 years and 15% in those aged over 70 years.[2] Studies to date in men with diabetes have reported a wide range for the prevalence of ED but all have shown that it is a very common problem indeed. The prevalence will depend on the population studied and the definition of ED used. A population-based study in Spain reported that diabetes was by far the major risk factor for ED. The overall prevalence of ED was 12.1%. As an independent risk factor the age-adjusted odds ratio for diabetes was 4. In contrast, it was 1.58 for hypertension, 1.63 for elevated serum cholesterol, 2.63 for peripheral vascular disease, 2.93 for prostate disease, 1.79 for heart disease, 2.5 for tobacco use and 1.53 for alcohol consumption[3] (Figure 20.1). A similar population-based study in Iran reported an overall prevalence of ED of 18.8%. Of the risk factors examined, diabetes was associated with the highest risk of ED (odds ratio 3.72).[4] In a diabetic clinic population, McCulloch *et al.* reported an overall prevalence of 35%.[5] In that study, the factors most significantly associated with impotence were age, treatment with either insulin or oral hypoglycaemic agents, retinopathy, symptomatic peripheral neuropathy and symptomatic autonomic neuropathy. In a survey of 428 diabetic men from 10 practices, Hackett reported a prevalence rate of 55%, of whom 39% suffered from the problem all of the time.[6] All studies have shown that the prevalence of ED increases with age so that after the age of 50 years the majority of diabetic men suffer with the problem.

Conversely, ED is a significant risk factor for diabetes. Sun *et al.* reported that men with ED are twice as like to have diabetes.[7] ED may also be the presenting symptom of diabetes.[8] The same group found that the

The Evidence Base for Diabetes Care, Second Edition, Edited by William H. Herman, Ann Louise Kinmonth, Nicholas J. Wareham and Rhys Williams.
© 2010 John Wiley & Sons, Ltd

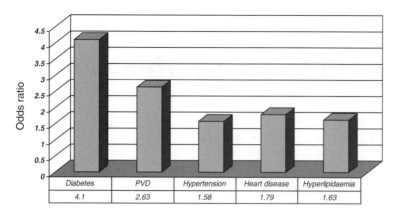

Figure 20.1 Odds ratios for ED in chronic conditions[3]

longer the duration of ED, the lower the subsequent response to therapy.

Pathophysiology of erectile dysfunction in diabetes

Physiology of normal penile erection

An understanding of the anatomy of the penis is necessary before any discussion of the pathophysiology of penile erection. A schematic representation of the processes involved in normal erection is shown in Figure 20.2.[9] Penile erection is predominantly a vascular event under the control of the autonomic nervous system in which relaxation of penile smooth muscle is the key event. The main erectile tissue, the corpus cavernosum, consists of a trabecular meshwork formed by smooth muscle fibre bundles, endothelial cells and connective tissue. In effect, it is a vascular sponge lined by endothelial cells and surrounded in turn by smooth muscle cells. The corpus cavernosum is surrounded by a thick, fibrous sheath,

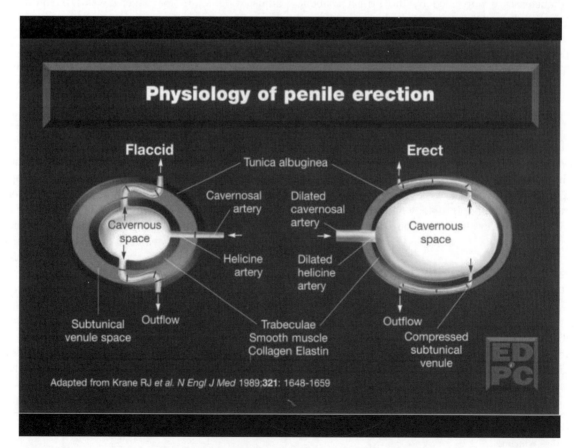

Figure 20.2 Schematic representation of processes involved in normal erection. Adapted from Krane et al.[9]

the tunica albuginea. Under conditions of sexual stimulation there is relaxation of the vascular smooth muscle of the erectile tissue and the inflow arterioles. The resultant expansion of the erectile tissue causes compression of the outflow venules against the firm tunica albuginea. Thus the single phenomenon of smooth muscle relaxation leads to increased arterial inflow and reduced venous outflow and hence tumescence.[10]

Neurophysiology and pharmacology of erection

The process of erection is under the control of the autonomic nervous system. In animal models, parasympathetic stimulation leads to tumescence whereas sympathetic (adrenergic) stimulation induces flaccidity.[11] The search for the neurotransmitter responsible for erection has been a long one; for decades the parasympathethic fibres responsible were known as 'non-adrenergic, non-cholinergic'. It is now clear that nitric oxide (NO), derived from both parasympathetic fibres and the vascular endothelium, plays a central role in the whole process. A model of our current understanding is shown in Figure 20.3. There is some evidence that neuronally derived NO is important in initiation, whereas NO from the endothelium is responsible for maintenance of erection.[12]

Several other neurotransmitters and peptides, such as vaso-active intestinal polypeptide (VIP), acetylcholine and the prostaglandins, may have a role in the physiology of erection, but it is now clear that NO is the central agent leading to the relaxation of smooth muscle in the erectile tissue. Evidence to support this comes from the fact that inhibitors of phosphodiesterase type 5 (PDE 5) are such effective treatments for ED (see below).

The intracellular processes following NO activation are shown in Figure 20.3. NO acts via cyclic guanidine monophosphate (cGMP) as a second messenger; this in turn is broken down by the enzyme PDE 5. This enzyme is discussed further later in the chapter. cGMP acts by opening calcium channels in vascular smooth muscle leading to relaxation.[12]

The pathophysiology of erectile dysfunction in diabetes

The process of tumescence requires intact vasculature, in particular adequate endothelial function, and an intact autonomic nervous supply. For many years there was uncertainty about the relative importance of these two factors. The crucial study which addressed this question was reported by Saenz de Tejada et al. in 1989.[13] In this study, samples of corpus cavernosal tissue, taken from men undergoing implant operations, were studied in vitro. The results suggested that tumescence is produced as a result of direct NO release from nerve terminals and from NO released from endothelial cells mediated by acetylcholine. In those with diabetes, both pathways were impaired compared with those without. In other words, impotence in diabetes is secondary to a failure of NO-mediated smooth muscle relaxation due to both autonomic neuropathy and endothelial dysfunction. Many men with diabetes report that in the early

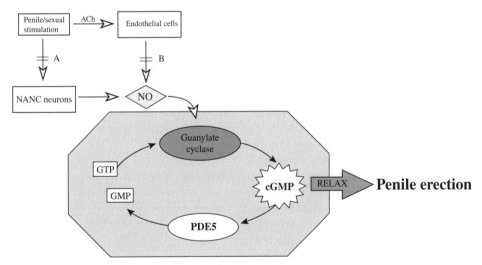

Figure 20.3 Intracellular processes leading to tumescence and the pathophysiology of erectile dysfunction in diabetes. Diagrammatic representation of pathways leading to and within a corpus cavernosal smooth muscle cell. In diabetes there are defects in nitric oxide smooth muscle relaxation due to neuropathy of the NANC fibres (A) and endothelial dysfunction (B). NO = nitric oxide; NANC = non-adrenergic–non-cholinergic neurons; PDE 5 = phosphodiesterase 5; ACh = acetylcholine

stages they do not have a problem initially achieving an erection but that they cannot maintain it. This suggests that in these individuals failure of endothelium-derived NO occurs before significant autonomic neuropathy.

Recently, other potential abnormalities have been described which may contribute to the development of ED in diabetes. Endothelium-derived hyperpolarizing factor (EDHF) plays a role in endothelium-dependent relaxation of human penile arteries[14] and EDHF-mediated endothelium-dependent relaxation is significantly impaired in penile resistance arteries in diabetic men.[15] Impaired EDHF responses might therefore contribute to the endothelial dysfunction of diabetic erectile tissue.

A further body of evidence suggests that increased oxygen free radical levels in diabetes may reduce the vasodilator effect of NO. In particular, non-enzymatic glycosylation produces advanced glycosylation end-products (AGEs) and generates reactive oxygen species, which impairs NO bioactivity.[16] In animal models, inhibition of AGE formation improves endothelium-dependent relaxation and restores erectile function in rats with diabetes.[17,18] Non-enzymatic glycation of proteins has also been reported to impair endothelium-dependent relaxation of the aorta[19] and corpus cavernosum[18] in rats.

Other factors, not limited to diabetes, may also contribute to the development of ED in diabetic men. Structural changes associated with large vessel disease are commonly associated with ED in diabetes. However, this is usually associated with functional changes of widespread endothelial dysfunction in diabetes and it is difficult to separate the relative importance of the two factors.

Hypertension is common in diabetes and is strongly associated with endothelial dysfunction and ED.[20] Many antihypertensive agents cause impotence, especially thiazides and beta-blockers.[21] ACE inhibitors and calcium channel blockers probably have little effect on erectile function and there is some evidence that angiotensin II antagonists may enhance sexual function.[21] It is now recognized that statins, which are widely prescribed to patients with diabetes, may be associated with ED; one uncontrolled study reported that almost one-third of men commencing statin treatment for the first time reported worsening of erectile function.[22] This might suggest a direct effect of erectile function rather than an association between statin use and ED secondary to pre-existing vascular disease, but this awaits confirmation. Conversely, one small study suggested that early lipid-lowering intervention when dyslipidaemia was the only risk factor could improve ED, possibly by effects on endothelial function.[23]

There is also preliminary evidence that dyslipidaemia (particularly raised LDL) may cause ED by impairing the endothelium-dependent relaxation of cavernous smooth muscle.[247] In human subjects, a correlation has been reported between ED and cholesterol and LDL levels.[25]

In summary, the pathophysiology of ED in diabetes is complex but diminished NO production secondary to endothelial dysfunction plays a key role and other factors, including autonomic neuropathy and the presence of oxidative free radicals and advanced glycosylation end-products, contribute.

Testosterone, metabolic syndrome, insulin resistance and type 2 diabetes

Recent research has shown a potential relationship between late-onset hypogonadism and insulin resistance and hence type 2 diabetes and cardiovascular disease.[26] The importance of the moderate reduction in androgen levels seen in late-onset hypogonadism is controversial but it should be considered as a treatable factor in all men with diabetes and sexual dysfunction. This work also raises the possibility that hypogonadism is a treatable causative factor in the development of diabetes and cardiovascular disease. Both hyperinsulinaemia and low testosterone have been shown to predict the development of type 2 diabetes[27] and the metabolic syndrome.[28,29] The results of the Massachusetts Male Aging Study suggested that low serum testosterone and sex hormone binding globulin predict the development of the metabolic syndrome and type 2 diabetes.[30]

Hypogonadism appears to be a common feature of type 2 diabetes in addition to several other chronic conditions associated with the metabolic syndrome[31,32] (Table 20.1). It remains uncertain if there is a causal relationship between hypogonadism and diabetes or the metabolic syndrome, but hypogonadism is a factor that should be considered when managing a man with diabetes and ED.

Table 20.1 Odds ratios for hypogonadism in conditions associated with the metabolic syndrome[31]

Condition	Prevalence (%)	Range (%)	Odds ratio
Obesity	52.4	47.9–56.9	2.38
Diabetes	50	45.5–54.5	2.09
Hypertension	42.4	39.6–45.2	1.84
Hyperlipidaemia	40.4	37.6–43.3	1.47

Impact of erectile dysfunction on the patient

That ED can have a profound affect on quality of life is not in dispute, and it is unfortunate that good research to back up this view is limited. A survey of its members undertaken by the Impotence Association (now the Sexual Function Association) in the United Kingdom reported that psychological symptoms, such as lowered self-esteem and depression, were extremely common in impotent men.[33] These problems were reported by 62% of men in the survey; furthermore, 40% of men expressed concern with either new or established relationships and 21% blamed it for the break-up of a relationship. This type of study undertaken by a patient organization among distressed volunteers has obvious limitations of selection and recall bias. Further analysis of this problem in Hackett's series showed that 45% of men with diabetes stated that they thought about their ED all or most of the time compared with 23% of those without diabetes; 23% felt that it severely affected their quality of life and 10% that it severely affected their relationship with their partner;[6] 80% would like to seek advice and treatment from their doctor if an effective and acceptable treatment was available. There appeared to be a consistent finding that men with diabetes and their partners were more affected by the loss of erectile function that controls.

Cummings *et al.* showed that 38% of men with diabetes and ED felt that their relationship had suffered moderately and 19% severely; 91% would like to seek medical advice if effective treatment was available.[34] However, in 1997, 46% of these men were unaware that treatment was available and in only 17% had a health care professional spontaneously discussed the problem. Of those who were aware, the information that they had obtained had largely been from sources other than primary care or hospital health care professionals and mainly from newspapers, magazines, television and the British Diabetic Association (now Diabetes UK) magazine. In this particular group of patients, those who had discussed the problem were more likely to have done so with their GP (65%) than with the hospital clinic (35%). Successful treatment of ED can have a major impact on distress. A small qualitative study reported great improvement in well-being in men who responded to treatment.[35]

Clinical features

Descriptions of the clinical features of ED in diabetes are limited. ED in men with diabetes is usually gradual in onset and progressive in nature, but the features are variable. The initial problem is usually the inability to sustain an erection long enough for satisfactory intercourse. This can be intermittent initially. The preservation of spontaneous and early morning erections is common and does not necessarily indicate a psychogenic cause.[36] Spontaneous recovery of erectile function in diabetes is rare.[37]

Loss of libido is consistent with hypogonadism but is not a reliable symptom. Many impotent men will understate their sex drive for a variety of reasons, including shame. Others suppress their libidos as a defence mechanism to prevent the disappointment of failure. A history obtained from the partner without the patient present often reveals interesting and useful insight into the problem.

Assessment and investigation of erectile dysfunction in diabetes

The evidence suggests that the likelihood of detecting a significant reversible cause of ED in a man with diabetes, such as pituitary or testicular dysfunction, is low. In one study of over 1000 men with ED of mixed aetiology, routine serum testosterone estimation detected two non-functioning pituitary tumours and one prolactinoma.[38] The detection rate of reversible causes of ED in a population of men with diabetes might be expected to be even lower; however, there are good reasons to undertake certain routine investigations in the management of a man with diabetes and ED. First, ED is a manifestation of endothelial dysfunction and therefore cardiovascular risk (see below). Therefore, an assessment of cardiovascular risk should be considered in all men presenting with ED (with and without diabetes). This should include measurement of blood pressure, lipid profile and urinalysis for microalbuminuria. Second, as discussed above, borderline low serum testosterone levels are a common finding in middle-aged and elderly men and there is some evidence that correction of low serum testosterone can improve the response rate to ED treatments. This will be discussed in more detail below. The suggested investigations to be undertaken in a man with diabetes presenting with ED are shown in Table 20.2.

The management of erectile dysfunction in diabetes

General advice

The management of ED, even in diabetes, used to be the preserve of psychosexual counsellors. The

Table 20.2 Suggested investigation required in the management of ED

- Serum lipids
- Plasma glucose and HbA$_{1c}$
- Serum testosterone, taken in the morning (8–11 am)
- Serum prolactin, FSH and LH if testosterone is borderline or low
- ECG
- Prostate-specific antigen if indicated

---

evidence base for the benefit of counselling in ED management is limited, but there is no doubt that the advice given to impotent men and their partners is extremely important. The available evidence suggests that, in most cases, specialist psychosexual counselling is not required for the management of ED in diabetes. Diabetologists and general practitioners can provide the common sense advice required.[39–43]

The majority of men with diabetes and their partners seeking treatment for impotence are middle aged and have been married for many years and, like all patients, should be treated with respect and dignity. The couple should be told that their problem is largely due to diabetes and they should not blame themselves or each other. It is particularly unhelpful to suggest that sexual intercourse is not essential for a good relationship.

It is important to establish that the couple have maintained a good relationship. Restoring a man's potency in an attempt to save a failing relationship is rarely successful and is more likely to make things worse as it introduces a new tension into the relationship. The assistance of a suitably qualified psychosexual counsellor should be considered in this situation. Referral to a counsellor should also be considered if there is any suggestion of depression, severe anxiety, loss of attraction between partners, fear of intimacy or marked performance anxiety.

Treatment of erectile dysfunction

ED in diabetes is usually irreversible and most impotent men will require a pharmacological or physical treatment in order to restore potency. A reversible cause of ED, although unlikely, should be considered. Endothelial changes are a potentially reversible component of ED and one study has suggested lifestyle modification can improve erectile function by improving endothelial function.[44] Clearly, lifestyle and cardiovascular risk should be addressed in all subjects with ED, but specific treatments should not be withheld pending improvements in lifestyle.

Although concomitant antihypertensive medication could be contributing to the ED, anecdotal experience has shown that changing medication is seldom helpful unless there is a clear temporal relationship between starting the medication and the onset of the ED.

A wide range of effective treatments is available and they are listed in Table 20.3. Information about the available treatments should be given to the patient, who should be allowed to choose his preferred option. However, almost all men will prefer a phosphodiesterase type 5 (PDE 5) inhibitor and the other treatments should be used if these are ineffective or contraindicated.

Phosphodiesterase type 5 inhibitors

The management of ED was transformed when PDE 5 inhibitors became available. The mechanism of action of PDE 5 inhibitors is shown in Figure 20.3. They act via the nitric oxide (NO) pathway. Under conditions of sexual stimulation, there is an increase in the intracellular concentrations of NO which acts via the second messenger cyclic GMP to produce smooth muscle relaxation. Inhibition of PDE 5, which breaks down cGMP, enhances erections under conditions of sexual stimulation. Thus, in theory, these agents only enhance the process of erection if the man is sexually aroused. Conversely, they might not be expected to be as effective in the presence of inadequate nitric oxide tone as would occur in the presence severe endothelial or autonomic dysfunction.

Evidence to support this mode of action of sildenafil comes from work done on human corpus cavernosal tissue *in vitro*.[45] Sildenafil produced a dose-dependent increase in smooth muscle relaxation under conditions of electric field stimulation; in contrast, field stimulation alone produced only modest relaxation.

Table 20.3 Currently available treatments for the management of ED

- Phosphodiesterase 5 inhibitors
  o Sildenafil
  o Tadalafil
  o Vardenafil
- Sublingual apomorphine
- Intracavernosal injection therapy
  o Alprostadil
  o Phenoxybenzamine and VIP (Invicorp)
  o Papaverine (unlicensed)
- Transurethral alprostadil (MUSE)
- Vacuum erection devices

Clinical trial data

Currently, three PDE 5 inhibitors are available, sildenafil (Viagra), vardenafil (Levitra) and tadalafil (Cialis). Sildenafil was the first to be licensed for use and has the largest evidence base. The first study of sildenafil in men with diabetes showed that it was effective in restoring erections in just over 50% of men.[46] It was evident at the time that it represented a revolutionary new treatment for ED and it stimulated an extraordinary degree of interest from the media. There is now considerable evidence that all three PDE 5 inhibitors are effective and safe treatments for ED in both diabetic and non-diabetic men. The most important trials are listed in Table 20.4. Overall, the clinical trial data suggest that response rates to PDE 5 inhibitors are slightly lower in men with diabetes than in other patient groups.

Tadalafil differs from the other two PDE 5 inhibitors as it has a substantially longer half-life (18 versus 4 h). This means that it is a slightly different treatment than the other two drugs. Thus a single tablet of tadalafil has the potential to normalize erectile function for 2 days.

Safety of PDE 5 inhibitors and cardiovascular disease

The launch of sildenafil, the first PDE 5 inhibitor, was soon followed by case reports of cardiovascular events and deaths associated with its use. This caused considerable media interest and concern amongst patients. However, there is now good evidence that PDE 5 inhibitors are not associated with increased cardiovascular risk.[53,54] A questionnaire survey of over 5000 sildenafil users reported that adverse cardiovascular events were no more frequent than expected for a comparable population.[55] A retrospective analysis of 36 clinical trials of tadalafil involving over 14000 men reported no increase in cardiovascular adverse events.[56] Indeed, there is accumulating evidence that PDE 5 inhibitors reduce blood pressure slightly and improve endothelial function.[54,57]

Restoring sexual function however, is not completely without risk. Sexual activity, like any form of physical activity, can precipitate cardiovascular events in those at risk. The amount of exercise during sexual intercourse is often reported to be comparable to that of mowing the lawn, so it should not be surprising that it carries a slight risk of a cardiovascular event. A large case–control study reported that the risk of a cardiovascular event in the 2 h after intercourse was increased by 2.5 in healthy subjects and by 3 if there was a history of previous myocardial infarction.[58] Although the absolute risk remains very small, the issue of cardiovascular safety must be addressed in all men before treating ED. Jackson *et al.* suggested a classification scheme for assessing cardiovascular risk in men undergoing treatment for ED; those with the highest risk should be referred for specialist cardiac evaluation while

Table 20.4 Randomized studies of PDE 5 inhibitors including diabetic men

Trial	PDE 5 inhibitor	n	Population	Response
Price *et al.*, 1998[46]	Sildenafil 25 or 50 mg	21	Men with diabetes	52% reported improved erections sufficient for intercourse
Rendell *et al.*, 1999[47]	Sildenafil titrated up to 100 mg	268	Men with diabetes	56% reported improved erections vs 10% on placebo
	Sildenafil titrated up to 100 mg	329	86% organic or mixed cause for ED; 8% with diabetes	69% of all attempts at intercourse successful vs 22% on placebo
Safarinejad *et al.*, 2004[48]	Sildenafil 100 mg	282	Men with diabetes	51% intercourse successful vs 11% on placebo
Stuckley *et al.*, 2003[49]	Sildenafil 25–100 mg	188	Men with type 1 diabetes	63% intercourse successful vs 33% on placebo
Boulton *et al.*, 2001[50]	Sildenafil 25–100 mg	219	Men with type 2 diabetes	Global Efficacy Score 64.6% vs 10.5% on placebo
Fonseca *et al.*, 2004[51]	Tadalafil 10–20 mg	637	Men with diabetes	53% of intercourse attempts successful vs 22% on placebo
Goldstein *et al.*, 2003[52]	Vardenafil 10–20 mg	452	Men with diabetes	57, 72 and 13% improved erections on 10 mg, 20 mg and placebo, respectively

the lowest risk group could be managed in primary care.[53]

Drug interactions with PDE 5 inhibitors

PDE 5 inhibitors can be used safely in patients taking a wide range of other drugs, but there are several potential important interactions.

Nitrates PDE 5 inhibitors are contraindicated in the presence of any nitrate therapy. Both drugs act via the NO–cGMP pathway and the combination can cause profound hypotension. A patient taking nitrates seeking treatment for ED can be offered alternatives to PDE 5 inhibitors or the nitrates can be stopped or changed to an alternative therapy. Nitrates are a symptomatic treatment with no prognostic implications, so this is possible in most cases but should be done in consultation with a cardiologist in all but the most straightforward cases.

Nitrate therapy should not be given within 24 h of taking sidenafil or vardenafil and at least 48 h of taking tadalafil. If angina develops during or after sexual activity following the use of a PDE 5 inhibitor, the patient should be advised to discontinue any sexual activity and stand up as this reduces the work of the heart by reducing venous return.

Nicorandil PDE 5 inhibitors are contraindicated in the presence of nicorandil, which also acts via the NO–cGMP pathway.[54]

Alpha blockers PDE 5 inhibitors should be used with caution in patients who take alpha-blockers because the combination may lead to symptomatic hypotension in some patients. Patients should be stable on alpha-blocker therapy before initiating sildenafil, which should be initiated at the lowest dose.[54]

Adverse effects of PDE 5 inhibitors

Many of the adverse effects of the PDE 5 inhibitors can be explained by their actions as vasodilators; these include headache and flushing. Dyspepsia or heartburn is also common and may be due to relaxation of the cardiac sphincter of the stomach. The adverse effects of the three currently available PDE 5 inhibitors are listed in Table 20.5. Abnormal vision occurs in about 6% of men taking sildenafil and may be due to the fact it has some activity against PDE 6, which is a retinal isoenzyme. Muscle cramps and back pain appear to be a particular side-effect of tadalafil.

Non-Arteritic anterior ischaemic optic neuropathy Non-arteritic anterior ischaemic optic neuropathy (NAION) is a rare syndrome characterized by sudden, sometimes unilateral, often reversible, visual loss. Since 2002 there have been case reports of this condition occurring in association with the use of PDE 5 inhibitors, particularly sildenafil.[63,64] NAION is rare but potentially serious as it can, exceptionally, lead to blindness. It would appear that it is more common in men with increased cardiovascular risk.[65] The manufacturers of sildenafil estimated the incidence of NAION in 13 000 men receiving sildenafil from pooled safety data from clinical trials and observational studies to be 2.8 cases per 100 000 patient-years of sildenafil exposure.[66] The authors reported this to be similar to estimates reported in general United States population samples (2.52 and 11.8 cases per 100 000 men aged over 50 years). It is therefore unknown if PDE 5 inhibitor use increases the risk of NAION, but is a very rare condition and should not discourage the appropriate use of these agents.

Comparison of PDE 5 inhibitors

The three currently available PDE 5 inhibitors, sildenafil, vardenafil and tadalafil, are all similar in efficacy and safety. Their side-effect profiles differ slightly, as

Table 20.5 Adverse effects of PDE 5 inhibitors (%). The prevalence quoted for each adverse effect is for the top dose used in each study.

Symptom	Sildenafil[59,71]	Tadalafil[60,61,71]	Vardenafil[52,62]
Headache	8.1–9.3	8.0–21	5–11
Flushing	7.4–8.1	3.0–9.0	5.4–10
Back pain	2.5	4.6–9.0	0
Dyspepsia	2.7–3.0	4.1–17	2.3
Nasal congestion	2.7–4.1	2.0–5	10
Dizziness	2.5	1.6	
Diarrhoea	2.5	0.8	
Abnormal vision	1.4	0	
Muscle cramps	4.1	3–7	

described above, but the most notable difference is the longer half-life of tadalafil. This means that it can be used in a different way to the shorter acting agents. A single dose of tadalafil offers the potential to restore erectile function to normal for 2 days. Therefore, a single dose might 'set a man up for the weekend' and thereby remove the need for medication to be taken each time prior to sexual activity. The choice between this form of treatment and on-demand dosing is largely a matter of patient preference. Patient preference studies of agents with differing dosing instructions are difficult to do in a blinded fashion. Several have been reported and have generally shown a preference for tadalafil over sildenafil, but they were less than convincing as there was no assessment of the impact on sexual function.[67–70] More recently, a well-constructed study which included measures of sexual function reported significantly greater patient preference for tadalafil over sildenafil.[71]

Management of PDE 5 non-responsiveness

As listed in Table 20.3, a large proportion of men with diabetes and impotence will not respond to PDE 5 inhibitors and there are many potential reasons for this. PDE 5 inhibitors require a degree of NO tone to be effective, hence severe endothelial dysfunction of autonomic neuropathy might be expected to reduce their efficacy. One study, however, reported that neither autonomic neuropathy nor endothelial dysfunction predicted sildenafil responsiveness. The only significant factor which predicted the response to treatment was the initial degree of ED.[72] In practical terms, no single factor should preclude a trial of PDE 5 inhibitor therapy in a man without a contraindication.

Much has been written on the best approach for dealing with men who do not respond to a PDE 5 inhibitor but, unfortunately, mostly based on limited evidence. It has been suggested that if appropriate advice is given and sufficient attempts at intercourse made, many men previously labelled as non-responders can be treated successfully with PDE 5 inhibitors. One study reported that intercourse success rates reached a plateau after eight attempts, so men with ED should try at least eight times with a PDE 5 inhibitor at the maximum recommended dose before being considered a non-responder.[73]

Hypogonadism should always be considered when dealing with men with ED who do not respond. Hypogonadism due to confirmed pituitary or testicular disease usually responds well to treatment. The management of the borderline hypogonadism of the ageing male is more controversial, but there is some evidence that testosterone replacement in this situation can improve ED as a sole treatment[74] and enhance the response to PDE 5 inhibitors.[75–77]

Other treatments

Vacuum therapy

Vacuum devices became available in the 1970s and, along with self-injection therapy, were the only effective treatment for ED for several years. The early trials of vacuum devices were often done by enthusiastic investigators on selected patients at a time when other effective treatments for impotence were not readily available. It is therefore perhaps not surprising that the reported results were excellent and rather better than more recent experience would suggest.[78] Several subsequent series of vacuum therapy in men with impotence of mixed aetiology have reported success rates between 50 and 90%.[79–82] None of these trials were controlled but the results left little doubt that vacuum devices were an effective treatment for impotence due to various aetiologies.

Trials of vacuum devices in diabetic men have shown results similar to non-diabetic men even in the presence of severe autonomic neuropathy or peripheral vascular disease.[40,41,43]

Complications and contraindications of vacuum therapy
Vacuum therapy would appear to be a remarkably safe treatment for ED; very few serious adverse events have been reported. There has been one reported case of skin necrosis following the use of a vacuum device and one case of penile gangrene.[83,84] Subcutaneous bruising is relatively common but is usually self-limiting. For this reason, most manufacturers advise that bleeding diatheses or anticoagulation therapy are contraindications to the use of vacuum therapy.

Most other side-effects are minor. Discomfort or pain due to the constriction band or during pumping is relatively common and can be the reason for discontinuing treatment. Failure to ejaculate can occur in up to one-third of men but anorgasmia is rare.[43,78,79] Female partners often report that the penis feels cold.

Intracavernosal injection therapy

Intracavernosal injection therapy was first described in 1982 using papaverine, a non-selective phosphodiesterase inhibitor which is a smooth muscle relaxant.[85] It is an unlicensed product and has largely been superseded by alprostadil (prostaglandin E), which was licensed for the treatment of ED in 1996. The principle of self-injection therapy is straightforward. Before intercourse the drug is injected into the corpus cavernosum, the penis is massaged and within a few minutes tumescence should occur. Initial studies of intracavernosal papaverine injection therapy were small and uncontrolled but it was rapidly adopted across the world. Subsequently, intracavernosal alprostadil has been shown to be a highly effective treatment for ED of various aetiologies in large controlled trial.[86] In a smaller uncontrolled study, Alexander reported that a physician can offer self injection therapy as an effective treatment for ED within a diabetic clinic.[39]

Complications of self injection therapy The most important complication of self injection therapy with papaverine is priapism (a sustained unwanted erection).[87,88] Should priapism occur, treatment must be prompt. If the erection persists for more than 2 h then there are several manoeuvres that can be undertaken that may terminate the erection. It has been reported that vigorous leg exercises such as pedalling an exercise bicycle or running up and down stairs can end an erection.[89] Any man using self-injection treatment must be warned to seek urgent medical advice should these manoeuvres fail and the erection persists for more than 6 h. This is made considerably easier if he already has written instructions to take to the nearest hospital emergency department.

Local adverse reactions, such as penile pain, are relatively common with self injection therapy. Prolonged papaverine use may lead to fibrosis in the penis, but this has only rarely been reported with alprostadil.[90]

Other injectable agents

Vaso-active intestinal polypeptide Vaso-active intestinal polypeptide (VIP) is a vasodilator which has a role in the development of erection. When injected into the corpus cavernosum as a single agent, it has only modest effects, producing a limp erection; however, when given in combination with phentolamine, it appears to be a potentially useful treatment for ED.[91] In a study of men with ED of mixed aetiology, the combination produced an erection sufficient for intercourse in all 52 men treated and at 6 months follow-up over 80% of the men were still using the treatment.[92] In a more recent study, the combination of VIP and phentolamine given by injection worked in 67% of men who had failed on other vasoactive agents.[93] At the time of writing, there have been no studies published on this treatment in men with diabetes and it is not yet licensed for the treatment of ED.

Transurethral alprostadil As an alternative to injection therapy, alprostadil can be delivered *per urethram*. A slender applicator is inserted into the urethra to deposit a pellet containing alprostadil in polyethylene glycol (PEG). This gradually dissolves, allowing the prostaglandin to diffuse into the corpus cavernosum.

This preparation has been marketed with the acronym MUSE (Medicated Urethral System for Erection). The applicator is neat and simple to use and most men find it preferable to a needle. In a placebo-controlled study of 1511 men with ED of mixed aetiology, it was reported that 65% were able to have intercourse using MUSE.[94] The results in the 240 diabetic men in the study (presented at a meeting but not yet published) were similar.[95] The most common side-effect was penile pain, which occurred in 10.8% of applications. Hypotension was reported by 3.3% of men receiving alprostadil. Priapism and penile fibrosis were not reported.

Trans-urethral alprostadil is best administered after emptying the bladder to improve lubrication. After administration, the penis should be massaged to improve adsorption of the drug. There is then a delay of approximately 30 min, during which time the man is advised to remain standing. When given the choice, most men prefer trans-urethral alprostadil over self-injection treatment. No comparative studies have been done, but it is the anecdotal experience of most clinicians involved in treating ED that trans-urethral alprostadil does produce the same degree of penile rigidity as self-injection treatment and the long-term usage has been disappointing.[96]

Other oral agents

Several agents have been tried as oral treatments for ED. These include yohimbine, phentolamine, apomorphine and trazodone. The data on all of them is limited and none has stood the test of time.

Surgery

The surgical treatment of ED, in diabetic and non-diabetic men, is usually reserved for those patients in whom more conservative methods have failed or are unacceptable. The most important surgical option remains the insertion of penile prostheses, which is effective in appropriately selected patients. A more detailed discussion of the surgical management of ED is best left to more specialist texts.[97]

References

1 British Diabetic Association. What diabetic care to expect. British Diabetic Association guidelines. *Diabet Med* 2006; 7:554.

2 Feldman HA, Goldstein I, Hatzichristou DG, Krane RJ, McKinlay JB. Impotence and its medical and psychosocial correlates: results of the Massachusetts Male Aging Study. *J Urol* 1994;**151**:54–61.

3 Martin-Morales A, Sanchez-Cruz JJ, Saenz de Tejada I, Rodriguez-Vela L, Jimenez-Cruz JF, Burgos-Rodriguez R.

Prevalence and independent risk factors for erectile dysfunction in Spain: results of the Epidemiologia de la Disfuncion Erectil Masculina Study. *J Urol* 2001;**166**(2):569–574.

4 Safarinejad MR. Prevalence and risk factors for erectile dysfunction in a population-based study in Iran. *Int J Impot Res* 2003;**15**(4):246–252.

5 McCulloch DK, Campbell IW, Wu FC, Prescott RJ, Clarke BF. The prevalence of diabetic impotence. *Diabetologia* 1980;**18**(4):279–283.

6 Hackett GI. Impotence – the most neglected complication of diabetes. *Diabetes Research* 1995;**28**:75–83.

7 Sun P, Cameron A, Seftel A, Shabsigh R, Niederberger C, Guay A. Erectile dysfunction – an observable marker of diabetes mellitus? A large national epidemiological study. *J Urol* 2006;**176**(3):1081–1085.

8 Sairam K, Kulinskaya E, Boustead GB, Hanbury DC, McNicholas TA. Prevalence of undiagnosed diabetes mellitus in male erectile dysfunction. *BJU Int* 2001;**88**(1):68–71.

9 Krane RJ, Goldstein I, Saenz de Tejada I. Impotence. *N Engl J Med* 1989;**321**(24):1648–1659.

10 Aboseif SR, Lue TF. Hemodynamics of penile erection. *Urol Clin North Am* 1988;**15**(1):1–7.

11 Miller M. The pathphysiology of impotence in diabetes. In: *Impotence in Diabetes* (eds DE Price, WD Alexander), Martin Dunitz, London, 2002, pp. 9–53.

12 Saenz de Tejada I, Angulo J, Cellek S, Gonzalez-Cadavid N, Heaton J, Pickard R, *et al.* Physiology of erectile function. *J Sex Med* 2004;**1**(3):254–265.

13 Saenz de Tejada I, Goldstein I, Azadzoi K, Krane RJ, Cohen RA. Impaired neurogenic and endothelium-mediated relaxation of penile smooth muscle from diabetic men with impotence. *N Engl J Med* 1989;**320**:1025–1030.

14 Angulo J, Cuevas P, Fernandez A, Gabancho S, Videla S, Saenz de Tejada I. Calcium dobesilate potentiates endothelium-derived hyperpolarizing factor-mediated relaxation of human penile resistance arteries. *Br J Pharmacol* 2003;**139**(4):854–862.

15 Angulo J, Cuevas P, Fernandez A, Gabancho S, Allona A, Martin-Morales A, *et al.* Diabetes impairs endothelium-dependent relaxation of *human penile vascular tissues mediated by NO and EDHF. Biochem Biophys Res Commun* 2003;**312**(4):1202–1208.

16 Mullarkey CJ, Edelstein D, Brownlee M. Free radical generation by early glycation products: a mechanism for accelerated atherogenesis in diabetes. *Biochem Biophys Res Commun* 1990;**173**(3):932–939.

17 Seftel AD, Vaziri ND, Ni Z, Razmjouei K, Fogarty J, Hampel N, *et al.* Advanced glycation end products in human penis: elevation in diabetic tissue, site of deposition and possible effect through iNOS or eNOS. *Urology* 1997;**50**(6):1016–1026.

18 Cartledge JJ, Eardley I, Morrison JF. Advanced glycation end-products are responsible for the impairment of corpus cavernosal smooth muscle relaxation seen in diabetes. *BJU Int* 2001;**87**(4):402–407.

19 Angulo J, Sanchez-Ferrer CF, Peiro C, Marin J, Rodriguez-Manas L. Impairment of endothelium-dependent relaxation by increasing percentages of glycosylated human hemoglobin. Possible mechanisms involved. *Hypertension* 1996;**28**(4): 583–592.

20 Sharma V, McNeill JH. The etiology of hypertension in the metabolic syndrome part three: the regulation and dysregulation of blood pressure. *Curr Vasc Pharmacol* 2006;**4**(4):321–348.

21 Grimm RH Jr, Flack JM, Grandits GA, Elmer PJ, Neaton JD, Cutler JA, *et al.* Long-term effects on plasma lipids of diet and drugs to treat hypertension. Treatment of Mild Hypertension Study (TOMHS Research Group). *JAMA* 1996;**275**(20): 1549–1556.

22 Solomon H, Samarasinghe YP, Feher MD, Man J, Rivas-Toro H, Lumb PJ, *et al.* Erectile dysfunction and statin treatment in high cardiovascular risk patients. *Int J Clin Pract* 2006;**60**(2):141–145.

23 Saltzman EA, Guay AT, Jacobson J. Improvement in erectile function in men with organic erectile dysfunction by correction of elevated cholesterol levels: a clinical observation. *J Urol* 2004;**172**(1):255–258.

24 Kim SC, Seo KK, Kim HW, Lee MY. The effects of isolated lipoproteins and triglyceride, combined oxidized low density lipoprotein (LDL) plus triglyceride and combined oxidized LDL plus high density lipoprotein on the contractile and relaxation response of rabbit cavernous smooth muscle. *Int J Androl* 2000;**23**(Suppl 2): 26–29.

25 Nikoobakht M, Nasseh H, Pourkasmaee M. The relationship between lipid profile and erectile dysfunction. *Int J Impot Res* 2005;**17**(6):523–526.

26 Kapoor D, Malkin CJ, Channer KS, Jones TH. Androgens, insulin resistance and vascular disease in men. *Clin Endocrinol (Oxf)* 2005;**63**(3):239–250.

27 Oh JY, Barrett-Connor E, Wedick NM, Wingard DL. Endogenous sex hormones and the development of type 2 diabetes in older men and women: the Rancho Bernardo study. *Diabetes Care* 2002;**25**(1):55–60.

28 Kaplan SA, Meehan AG, Shah A. The age related decrease in testosterone is significantly exacerbated in obese men with the metabolic syndrome. What are the implications for the relatively high incidence of erectile dysfunction observed in these men?. *J Urol* 2006;**176**(4 Pt 1): 1524–1527.

29 Kupelian V, Page ST, Araujo AB, Travison TG, Bremner WJ, McKinlay JB. Low sex hormone-binding globulin, total testosterone and symptomatic androgen deficiency are associated with development of the metabolic syndrome in nonobese men. *J Clin Endocrinol Metab* 2006;**91**(3): 843–850.

30 Laaksonen DE, Niskanen L, Punnonen K, Nyyssonen K, Tuomainen TP, Valkonen VP, *et al.* Testosterone and sex hormone-binding globulin predict the metabolic syndrome and diabetes in middle-aged men. *Diabetes Care* 2004;**27**(5):1036–1041.

31 Mulligan T, Frick MF, Zuraw QC, Stemhagen A, McWhirter C. Prevalence of hypogonadism in males aged at least 45 years: the HIM study. *Int J Clin Pract* 2006;**60**(7):762–769.

32 Dhindsa S, Prabhakar S, Sethi M, Bandyopadhyay A, Chaudhuri A, Dandona P. Frequent occurrence of hypogonadotropic hypogonadism in type 2 diabetes. *J Clin Endocrinol Metab* 2004;**89**(11):5462–5468.

33 Impotence Association. Impotence Association Survey. Impotence Association, London, 2007.

34 Cummings MH, Meeking D, Warburton F, Alexander W. *The diabetic male's perception of erectile dysfunction. Practical Diabetes* 1997;**14**:100–102.

35 Tomlinson J, Wright D. Impact of erectile dysfunction and its subsequent treatment with sildenafil: qualitative study. *BMJ* 2004;**328**(7447):1037.

36 Fairburn CG, Wu FC, McCulloch DK, Borsey DQ, Ewing DJ, Clarke BF, *et al.* The clinical features of diabetic impotence: a preliminary study. *Br J Psychiatry* 1982;**140**:447–452.

37 McCulloch DK, Young RJ, Prescott RJ, Campbell IW, Clarke BF. The natural history of impotence in diabetic men. *Diabetologia* 1984;**26**(6):437–440.

38 Buvat J, Lemaire A. Endocrine screening in 1,022 men with erectile dysfunction: clinical significance and cost-effective strategy. *J Urol* 1997;**158**(5):1764–1767.

39 Alexander WD. The diabetes physician and an assessment and treatment programme for male erectile impotence. *Diabet Med* 1990;**7**:540–543.

40 Price DE, Cooksey G, Jehu D, Bentley S, Hearnshaw JR, Osborn DE. The management of impotence in diabetic men by vacuum tumescence therapy. *Diabet Med* 1991;**8**:964–967.

41 Bodansky HJ. Treatment of male erectile dysfunction using the active vacuum assist device. *Diabet Med* 1994;**11**(4):410–412.

42 Ryder RE, Close CF, Moriarty KT, Moore KT, Hardisty CA, Impotence in diabetes: aetiology, implications for treatment and preferred vacuum device. 1992.

43 Wiles PG. Successful non-invasive management of erectile impotence in diabetic men. *Br Med J (Clin Res Ed)* 1988;**296**(6616):161–162.

44 Esposito K, Giugliano F, Di PC, Giugliano G, Marfella R, D'Andrea F, *et al.* Effect of lifestyle changes on erectile dysfunction in obese men: a randomized controlled trial. *JAMA* 2004;**291**(24):2978–2984.

45 Ballard SA, Gingell CJ, Tang K, Turner LA, Price ME, Naylor AM. Effects of sildenafil on the relaxation of human corpus cavernosum tissue *in vitro* and on the activities of cyclic nucleotide phosphodiesterase isozymes. *J Urol* 1998;**159**(6):2164–2171.

46 Price DE, Gingell JC, Gepi-Attee S, Wareham K, Yates P, Boolell M. Sildenafil: study of a novel oral treatment for erectile dysfunction in diabetic men [In Process Citation]. *Diabet Med* 1998;**15**(10):821–825.

47 Rendell MS, Rajfer J, Wicker PA, Smith MD. Sildenafil for treatment of erectile dysfunction in men with diabetes: a randomized controlled trial. Sildenafil Diabetes Study Group. *JAMA* 1999;**281**(5):421–426.

48 Safarinejad MR. Oral sildenafil in the treatment of erectile dysfunction in diabetic men: a randomized double-blind and placebo-controlled study. *J Diabetes Complications* 2004;**18**(4):205–210.

49 Stuckey BG, Jadzinsky MN, Murphy LJ, Montorsi F, Kadioglu A, Fraige F, *et al.* Sildenafil citrate for treatment of erectile dysfunction in men with type 1 diabetes: results of a randomized controlled trial. *Diabetes Care* 2003;**26**(2):279–284.

50 Boulton AJ, Selam JL, Sweeney M, Ziegler D. Sildenafil citrate for the treatment of erectile dysfunction in men with Type II diabetes mellitus. *Diabetologia* 2001;**44**(10):1296–1301.

51 Fonseca V, Seftel A, Denne J, Fredlund P. Impact of diabetes mellitus on the severity of erectile dysfunction and response to treatment: analysis of data from tadalafil clinical trials. *Diabetologia* 2004;**47**(11):1914–1923.

52 Goldstein I, Young JM, Fischer J, Bangerter K, Segerson T, Taylor T. Vardenafil, a new phosphodiesterase type 5 inhibitor, in the treatment of erectile dysfunction in men with diabetes: a multicenter double-blind placebo-controlled fixed-dose study. *Diabetes Care* 2003;**26**(3):777–783.

53 Jackson G, Betteridge J, Dean J, Eardley I, Hall R, Holdright D, *et al.* A systematic approach to erectile dysfunction in the cardiovascular patient: a Consensus Statement – update 2002. *Int J Clin Pract* 2002;**56**(9):663–671.

54 Jackson G, Montorsi P, Cheitlin MD. Cardiovascular safety of sildenafil citrate (Viagra): an updated perspective. *Urology* 2006;**68**(3 Suppl): 47–60.

55 Shakir SA, Wilton LV, Boshier A, Layton D, Heeley E. Cardiovascular events in users of sildenafil: results from first phase of prescription event monitoring in England. *BMJ* 2001;**322**(7287):651–652.

56 Kloner RA, Jackson G, Hutter AM, Mittleman MA, Chan M, Warner MR, *et al.* Cardiovascular safety update of tadalafil: retrospective analysis of data from placebo-controlled and open-label clinical trials of tadalafil with as needed, three times-per-week or once-a-day dosing. *Am J Cardiol* 2006;**97**(12):1778–1784.

57 Rosano GM, Aversa A, Vitale C, Fabbri A, Fini M, Spera G. Chronic treatment with tadalafil improves endothelial function in men with increased cardiovascular risk. *Eur Urol* 2005;**47**(2):214–220.

58 Muller JE, Mittleman A, Maclure M, Sherwood JB, Tofler GH. Triggering myocardial infarction by sexual activity. Low absolute risk and prevention by regular physical exertion. Determinants of Myocardial Infarction Onset Study Investigators. *JAMA* 1996;**275**(18):1405–1409.

59 DeBusk RF, Pepine CJ, Glasser DB, Shpilsky A, DeRiesthal H, Sweeney M. Efficacy and safety of sildenafil citrate in men with erectile dysfunction and stable coronary artery disease. *Am J Cardiol* 2004;**93**(2):147–153.

60 Carson CC, Rajfer J, Eardley I, Carrier S, Denne JS, Walker DJ, *et al.* The efficacy and safety of tadalafil: an update. *BJU Int* 2004;**93**(9):1276–1281.

61 Brock GB, McMahon CG, Chen KK, Costigan T, Shen W, Watkins V, *et al.* Efficacy and safety of tadalafil for the treatment of erectile dysfunction: results of integrated analyses. *J Urol* 2002;**168**(4 Pt 1): 1332–1336.

62 Valiquette L, Young JM, Moncada I, Porst H, Vezina JG, Stancil BN, *et al.* Sustained efficacy and safety of vardenafil for treatment of erectile dysfunction: a randomized, double-blind, placebo-controlled study. *Mayo Clin Proc* 2005;**80**(10):1291–1297.

63 Pomeranz HD, Bhavsar AR. Nonarteritic ischemic optic neuropathy developing soon after use of sildenafil (viagra): a report of seven new cases. *J Neuroophthalmol* 2005;**25**(1):9–13.

64 Pomeranz HD, Smith KH, Hart WM Jr, Egan RA. Sildenafil-associated nonarteritic anterior ischemic optic neuropathy. *Ophthalmology* 2002;**109**(3):584–587.

65 McGwin G Jr, Vaphiades MS, Hall TA, Owsley C. Non-arteritic anterior ischaemic optic neuropathy and the treatment of erectile dysfunction. *Br J Ophthalmol* 2006;**90**(2):154–157.

66 Gorkin L, Hvidsten K, Sobel RE, Siegel R. Sildenafil citrate use and the incidence of nonarteritic anterior ischemic optic neuropathy. *Int J Clin Pract* 2006;**60**(4):500–503.

67 Dean J, Hackett GI, Gentile V, Pirozzi-Farina F, Rosen RC, Zhao Y, et al. Psychosocial outcomes and drug attributes affecting treatment choice in men receiving sildenafil citrate and tadalafil for the treatment of erectile dysfunction: results of a multicenter, randomized, open-label, crossover study. *J Sex Med* 2006;**3**(4):650–661.

68 Govier F, Potempa AJ, Kaufman J, Denne J, Kovalenko P, Ahuja S. A multicenter, randomized, double-blind, crossover study of patient preference for tadalafil 20 mg or sildenafil citrate 50 mg during initiation of treatment for erectile dysfunction. *Clin Ther* 2003;**25**(11):2709–2723.

69 Stroberg P, Murphy A, Costigan T. Switching patients with erectile dysfunction from sildenafil citrate to tadalafil: results of a European multicenter, open-label study of patient preference. *Clin Ther* 2003;**25**(11):2724–2737.

70 von Keitz A, Rajfer J, Segal S, Murphy A, Denne J, Costigan T, et al. A multicenter, randomized, double-blind, crossover study to evaluate patient preference between tadalafil and sildenafil. *Eur Urol* 2004;**45**(4):499–507.

71 Eardley I, Mirone V, Montorsi F, Ralph D, Kell P, Warner MR, et al. An open-label, multicentre, randomized, crossover study comparing sildenafil citrate and tadalafil for treating erectile dysfunction in men naive to phosphodiesterase 5 inhibitor therapy. *BJU Int* 2005;**96**(9):1323–1332.

72 Pegge NC, Twomey AM, Vaughton K, Gravenor MB, Ramsey MW, Price DE. The role of endothelial dysfunction in the pathophysiology of erectile dysfunction in diabetes and in determining response to treatment. *Diabet Med* 2006;**23**(8):873–878.

73 McCullough AR, Barada JH, Fawzy A, Guay AT, Hatzichristou D. Achieving treatment optimization with sildenafil citrate (Viagra in patients with erectile dysfunction. *Urology* 2002;**60**(2 Suppl 2): 28–38.

74 Kalinchenko SY, Kozlov GI, Gontcharov NP, Katsiya GV. Oral testosterone undecanoate reverses erectile dysfunction associated with diabetes mellitus in patients failing on sildenafil citrate therapy alone. *Aging Male* 2003;**6**(2): 94–99.

75 Mulhall JP. Treatment of erectile dysfunction in a hypogonadal male. *Rev Urol* 2004;**6**(Suppl 6): S38–S40.

76 Greco EA, Spera G, Aversa A. Combining testosterone and PDE 5 inhibitors in erectile dysfunction: basic rationale and clinical evidences. *Eur Urol* 2006;**50**(5):940–947.

77 Shamloul R, Ghanem H, Fahmy I, El-Meleigy A, Ashoor S, Elnashaar A, et al. Testosterone therapy can enhance erectile function response to sildenafil in patients with PADAM: a pilot study. *J Sex Med* 2005;**2**(4):559–564.

78 Nadig PW, Ware JC, Blumoff R. Noninvasive device to produce and maintain an erection-like state. *Urology* 1986;**27**(2):126–131.

79 Baltaci S, Aydos K, Kosar A, Anafarta K. Treating erectile dysfunction with a vacuum tumescence device: a retrospective analysis of acceptance and satisfaction. *Br J Urol* 1995;**76**(6):757–760.

80 Korenman SG, Viosca SP. Use of a vacuum tumescence device in the management of impotence in men with a history of penile implant or severe pelvic disease. *J Am Geriatr Soc* 1992;**40**(1):61–64.

81 Sidi AA, Becher EF, Zhang G, Lewis JH. Patient acceptance of and satisfaction with an external negative pressure device for impotence. *J Urol* 1990;**144**(5):1154–1156.

82 Vrijhof HJ, Delaere KP. Vacuum constriction devices in erectile dysfunction: acceptance and effectiveness in patients with impotence of organic or mixed aetiology. *Br J Urol* 1994;**74**(1):102–105.

83 Kaye T, Guay AT. Re: Skin necrosis caused by use of negative pressure device for erectile impotence. *J Urol* 1991;**146**(6):1618–1619.

84 Rivas DA, Chancellor MB. Complications associated with the use of vacuum constriction devices for erectile dysfunction in the spinal cord injured population. *J Am Paraplegia Soc* 1994;**17**(3):136–139.

85 Virag R, Frydman D, Legman M, Virag H. Intracavernous injection of papaverine as a diagnostic and therapeutic method in erectile failure. *Angiology* 1984;**35**(2):79–87.

86 Linet OI, Ogring FG. Efficacy and safety of intracavernosal alprostadil in men with erectile dysfunction. *N Engl J Med* 1996;**334**:873–877.

87 Lomas GM, Jarow JP. Risk factors for papaverine-induced priapism. *J Urol* 1992;**147**(5):1280–1281.

88 Padma-Nathan H, Goldstein I, Krane RJ. Treatment of prolonged or priapistic erections following intracavernosal papaverine therapy. *Semin Urol* 1986;**4**(4):236–238.

89 Alexander W. Detumescence by exercise bicycle. *Lancet* 1989;**I**;(8640):735.

90 Montague DK, Barada JH, Belker AM, Levine LA, Nadig PW, Roehrborn CG, et al. Clinical guidelines panel on erectile dysfunction: summary report on the treatment of organic erectile dysfunction. American Urological Association. *J Urol* 1996;**156**(6):2007–2011.

91 Kiely EA, Bloom SR, Williams G. Penile response to intracavernosal vasoactive intestinal polypeptide alone and in combination with other vasoactive agents. *Br J Urol* 1989;**64**(2):191–194.

92 Gerstenberg TC, Metz P, Ottesen B, Fahrenkrug J. Intracavernous self-injection with vasoactive intestinal polypeptide and phentolamine in the management of erectile failure. *J Urol* 1992;**147**(5):1277–1279.

93 Dinsmore WW, Alderdice DK. Vasoactive intestinal polypeptide and phentolamine mesylate administered by auto-injector in the treatment of patients with erectile dysfunction resistant to other intracavernosal agents. *Br J Urol* 1998;**81**(3):437–440.

94 Padma-Nathan H, Hellstrom WJ, Kaiser FE, Labasky RF, Lue TF, Nolten, et al. Treatment of men with erectile dysfunction with transurethral alprostadil. Medicated Urethral System

for Erection (MUSE) Study Group. *N Engl J Med* 1997;**336**(1):1–7.

95 Nolten WE, Billington CJ, Chiu KC. Treatment of erectile dysfunction (impotence with a novel transurethral drug delivery system: results from a multicenter placeb-controlled trial. [Abstract]. 10th International Congress of Endocrinology, 1996.

96 Fulgham PF, Cochran JS, Denman JL, Feagins BA, Gross MB, Kadesky KT, *et al.* Disappointing initial results with transurethral alprostadil for erectile dysfunction in a urology practice setting. *J Urol* 1998;**160**(6 Pt 1): 2041–2046.

97 Gingell C. The surgical treatment of erectile dysfunction in the diabetic patient. In: *Impotence in Diabetes* (eds DE Price, WD Alexander), Martin Dunitz, London, 2002, pp. 109–119.

21 Cardiac complications and management

Anthony S. Wierzbicki[1], Simon R. Redwood[2]

[1]*Department of Chemical Pathology, Guy's and St Thomas' Hospitals, London, UK*
[2]*Department of Cardiology, Guy's and St Thomas' Hospitals, London, UK*

Introduction

Diabetes is a major risk factor for worldwide coronary heart disease (CHD), with about 10% of population-attributable risk being due to this condition.[1] It is notable that risk factors for diabetes – increased apolipoprotein B_{100}:A1 ratio, central obesity and hypertension – account for about 60% of the remainder (Table 21.1). Patients with type 1 and type 2 diabetes have an increased risk of all cardiovascular disease (CVD),[2–4] not just CHD (Figure 21.1), including stroke, peripheral arterial disease (PAD) and arrhythmias.[5] Patients are also at increased risk of cardiomyopathy and congestive cardiac failure (CCF). Cardiovascular disease accounts for 50% of mortality in diabetes and is a massive cause of morbidity as 75–80% of events and admissions in patients with diabetes are due to CVD, especially acute coronary syndromes (ACS) – unstable angina (UAS) and non-Q wave myocardial infarction (NQMI) and ST elevation myocardial infarction (STEMI).[6,7] Mortality is increased 2-fold in men and 4–5-fold in women.[5,8] Similarly, sudden cardiac death is increased by 50% in men and 3-fold in women. In general terms, diabetes is a cardiovascular risk equivalent as patients with type 2 diabetes without established CHD have a similar CHD risk to patients with established CHD. This is dependent on about 10–15 years of disease;[3,9] otherwise the risk is somewhat lower (Figure 21.2)[10] and global atherosclerotic burdens are similar in angiography trials.

Patients with diabetes show increased carotid plaque inflammation (25 vs 2% plaque macrophage infiltration), increased cytokine levels and reduced collagen and actin.[11,12] Plaques also show internal haemorrhage and a greater prevalence of vasa vasorum with increased leakage and secondary destabilization.[13,14] On non-invasive imaging, patients with diabetes have very high levels of coronary calcium deposition on multi-slice computer tomographic imaging although some of this is adventitial rather than intimal.[15–17] Patients with diabetes have a high prevalence of CHD on angiography, with 55% having significant stenoses as compared with 2–4% in the general population of similar age and sex.[18] The distribution of disease also differs as multi-vessel disease is more common, as are diffuse patterns of arterial involvement.[19–21] Arterial remodelling is altered in diabetes and intimal hyperplasia increases.[22]

The health care burden posed by cardiovascular disease in diabetes is enormous and increasing with the population attributable risk rising in the Framingham cohort from 5.4% in 1952–74 to 8.7% in 1975–98[4] (Figure 21.3). It is about 9.9% in the cross-sectional Inter-HEART study.[1] About 25% of patients presenting with myocardial infarction have type 2 diabetes.[4] This is driven by a number of factors. The largest driver of CVD risk is the rising incidence of the metabolic syndrome paralleling the vast increase in rates of obesity worldwide. Increasing the number of metabolic syndrome risk factors from 1 to 4–5 increases the risk of developing diabetes in men by 23.5-fold compared with a 3.85-fold increase in risk of CHD (Figure 21.4).[23] In addition, as world diet and exercise patterns change, the susceptibility of various high-risk populations including Africans, Latin and South Americans, Micronesians, Turks and Asians (especially South Asians)[24] to diabetes increases even at levels of waist circumference or body

The Evidence Base for Diabetes Care, Second Edition, Edited by William H. Herman, Ann Louise Kinmonth, Nicholas J. Wareham and Rhys Williams.
© 2010 John Wiley & Sons, Ltd

Table 21.1 Risk factors associated with acute myocardial infarction in 50 countries in the InterHEART study[1]

Risk factor	Prevalence Controls (%)	Prevalence Cases (%)	Odds ratio (99% CI) (age, sex, smoking adjusted)	Odds ratio (99% CI) (all risk factors adjusted)	Population attributable risk (99% CI) (age, sex, smoking adjusted)	Population attributable risk (99% CI) (all risk factors adjusted)
ApoB:A1 ratio (quintile 5 vs quintile 1)	20.0	33.5	3.87 (3.39 to 4.42)	3.25 (2.81 to 3.76)	54.1 (49.6 to 58.6)	49.2 (43.8 to 54.5)
Smoking	26.8	45.2	2.95 (2.72 to 3.20)	2.87 (2.58 to 3.19)	36.4 (33.9 to 39.0)	35.7 (32.5 to 39.1)
Diabetes	7.5	18.4	3.08 (2.77 to 3.42)	2.37 (2.07 to 2.71)	12.3 (11.2 to 13.5)	9.9 (8.5 to 11.5)
Hypertension	21.9	39.0	2.48 (2.30 to 2.68)	1.91 (1.74 to 2.10)	23.4 (21.7 to 25.1)	17.9 (15.7 to 20.4)
Abdominal obesity (tertile 3 vs tertile 1)	33.3	46.3	2.22 (2.03 to 2.42)	1.62 (1.45 to 1.80)	33.7 (30.2 to 37.4)	20.1 (15.3 to 26.0)
Psychosocial	—	—	2.51 (2.15 to 2.93)	2.67 (2.21 to 3.22)	28.8 (22.6 to 35.8)	32.5 (25.1 to 40.8)
High fruit and vegetable intake	42.4	35.8	0.70 (0.64 to 0.77)	0.70 (0.62 to 0.79)	12.9 (10.0 to 16.6)	13.7 (9.9 to 18.6)
Exercise	19.3	14.3	0.72 (0.65 to 0.79)	0.86 (0.76 to 0.97)	25.5 (20.1 to 31.8)	12.2 (5.5 to 25.1)
Alcohol intake	24.5	24.0	0.79 (0.73 to 0.86)	0.91 (0.82 to 1.02)	13.9 (9.3 to 20.2)	6.7 (2.0 to 20.2)
All			129 (90 to 185)	129 (90 to 185)		
All combined (extremes)			334 (230 to 484)	333 (230 to 484)	90.4 (88.1 to 92.4)	90.4 (88.1 to 92.4)

Reproduced from Yusuf et al.[1] with permission from Elsevier.

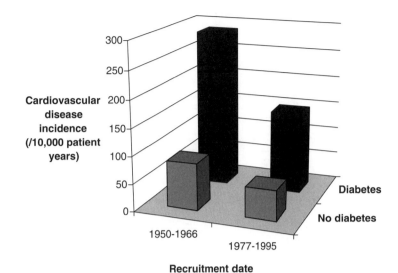

mass index that are low compared with Caucasians[1,25] (Table 21.2). The curvilinear relationship of glycaemic exposure expressed as haemoglobin A_{1c} (HbA$_{1c}$) with CVD risk is increasingly recognized.[26] Successive re-definitions of diabetes have reduced the glucose threshold for diagnosis of diabetes and impaired glucose tolerance/impaired fasting glucose. It could be

argued that glucose or HbA$_{1c}$ should be used in risk calculation rather than imposing arbitrary cut-offs for the diagnosis of diabetes. As world populations age, further increases in age-driven diabetes occur. Lastly, as medical treatment improves and converts diabetes from an acute to a chronic disease and subsequently reduces the rate of massive cardiovascular events while allowing smaller events still to occur, CHD in diabetes is increasingly changing from acute myocardial events to chronic cardiac failure and other long-term myocardial complications of ischaemia.

Factors favouring cardiovascular disease in diabetes

Associated cardiovascular risk factors

Patients with diabetes are subject to the same cardiovascular risk factor influences as the general

(a)

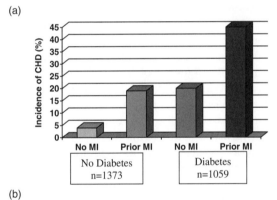

(b)

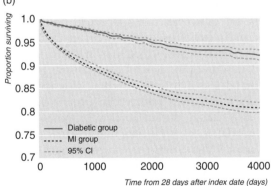

Figure 21.2 Survival curve for time to death from cardiovascular disease for patients with newly diagnosed type 2 diabetes and for those with a recent myocardial infarction. Reproduced from (a) Haffner *et al.*[9] with permission of Massachusetts Medical Society and (b) Evans *et al.*[10] with permission of BMJ Group

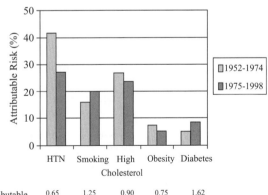

Attributable Risk Ratio (95%CI)	0.65 (0.47-0.84)	1.25 (0.86-2.04)	0.90 (0.42-2.08)	0.75 (0.00-1.68)	1.62 (1.05-2.48)

Figure 21.3 Changes in population attributable risk (PAR) with various cardiovascular risk factors from two cohorts recruited to the Framingham Study.[4] Reproduced with permission from Lippincott

(a)

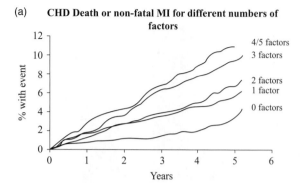

CHD Death or non-fatal MI for different numbers of factors

(b)

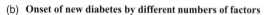

Onset of new diabetes by different numbers of factors

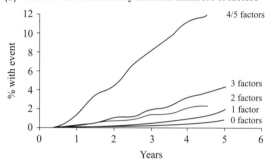

Figure 21.4 Incidence of cardiovascular events and new diabetes assigned by the number of metabolic syndrome risk factors in men in the West of Scotland Coronary Outcomes Prevention Study (WOSCOPS).[23] Reproduced with permission from Lippincott

population but show an increased degree of interaction with other cardiovascular disease risk factors (Figure 21.5). Cigarette smoking is an independent risk factor for cardiovascular disease. In patients with diabetes, smoking is an independent predictor of mortality, especially in women, since it increases

Table 21.2 Definition of the metabolic syndrome by the International Diabetes Federation.[27] This is diagnosed on the presence of abdominal obesity and 2 out of 4 other risk factors

Risk factor	Defining level		
Waist circumference (cm)	USA	Europe	Asia
Men	>102	>94	>90
Women	>88	>80	>80
Triglycerides	>1.70 mmol l^{-1} (150 mg dl^{-1}) or specific treatment for TGs		
HDL-C			
Men	<0.90 mmol l^{-1} (40 mg/dl)		
Women	<1.1 mmol l^{-1} (50 mg dl^{-1}) Or specific treatment for HDL-C		
Blood pressure	>130/>85 mmHg or treatment of hypertension		
Fasting glucose	5.6 mmol l^{-1} (100 mg dl^{-1}) or hypoglycaemic treatment or diabetes		

Reproduced from Alberti *et al.* (Ref. 27) with permission from Elsevier.

their cardiac mortality more than 2-fold.[28] For patients, who continue to smoke despite having diabetes, the benefits of modification of other major cardiovascular risk factors may be reduced.[28]

Hypertension is often associated with diabetes and interacts with nephropathy and albuminuria to increase risks of CVD.[30] It is present in >50% of patients aged >45 years and especially women.[31,32] Through its haemodynamic actions, hypertension promotes the endothelial dysfunction of diabetes, plaque rupture and thus atherothrombotic events. Hypertension also is commonly classified as a part of the metabolic syndrome that predisposes to type 2 diabetes and also to progression of diabetes-related complications. Control of hypertension is a well-recognized intervention for diabetes with targets (130/80 mmHg; 120/80 post-MI) being set lower than for patients without diabetes. Hypertension is also associated with a 2-fold increased risk of progression of nephropathy and renal impairment, both of which are associated with excess cardiovascular risk.[33,34]

Diabetes is associated with abnormalities in lipid metabolism, although these differ between type 1 and type 2 diabetes. Type 2 diabetes is associated with an atherogenic lipid profile of low HDL-cholesterol (HDL-C), raised triglycerides, increased levels of triglyceride-rich remnants, increased apolipoprotein B$_{100}$ and small, dense LDL and HDL particles.[35-37] All of these lipoprotein abnormalities have been associated with increased risks of CVD and some form part of the core definition of the metabolic syndrome.[38] Even at low levels of LDL-C, diabetes is associated with an excess risk of cardiovascular events, probably due to increased small, dense lipoprotein particles that can be measured through apoB levels.[39,40]

In type 1 diabetes, the lipid profile is different, changing from a profile rich in triglyceride-rich remnants in patients with poor glycaemic control to superficially 'normal' levels in well-controlled patients.[41-44] However, this lipoprotein profile shows abnormal metabolism as glycation, carbamylation (in diabetic renal disease), oxidation and advanced glycosylation end-products all cause disintegration of apoB and a switch in its handling to scavenger receptors rather than primary lipoprotein receptors, and also change the metabolism to apolipoprotein A-1 in HDL to favour the cubulin and megalin pathways rather than SR-B1 recycling scavenger receptor.

Hyperinsulinaemia is a feature of insulin resistance in type 2 diabetes and in some studies is associated with increased rates of atherosclerosis independent of other cardiovascular risk factors.[38] There are many studies suggesting that this is not the case. It is another feature of the metabolic syndrome and is associated with central obesity, an atherogenic lipid profile,

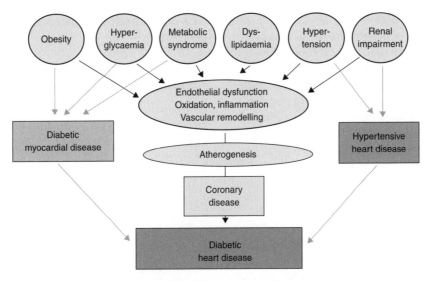

Figure 21.5 Mechanisms and risk factors contributing to heart disease in diabetes.[29] Reproduced with permission from BMJ Group

hyperuricaemia and a prothrombotic state.[45] Hyperinsulinaemia directly interacts with cholesterol synthesis through the sterol receptor element binding protein (SREBP) pathways and has direct effects on atheroma progression through the multiple signalling pathways attached to the insulin receptor.

Microalbuminuria is the first clinical sign of diabetic nephropathy and is associated with increased risk of CVD. The risk of developing coronary artery disease is increased 8-fold in patients with microalbuminuria.[30,46–48] Similarly, the risk of cardiovascular mortality is increased 4-fold in type 2 diabetic patients[47] and 37-fold in type 1 diabetic patients[49] as compared with the general population. Most type 1 diabetic patients over the age of 45 years have over 50% stenosis of one or more of their epicardial coronary arteries.[50] Thus, microalbuminuria or persistent proteinuria is not only a marker of diabetic nephropathy, but also a potent indicator of coronary artery disease.

Clotting-related abnormalities in diabetes

Patients with diabetes have elevated blood viscosity due to increased levels of plasma proteins, increased platelet aggregation and decreased red cell deformity, particularly during periods of metabolic derangement such as diabetic ketoacidosis.[51–53] Haematorheological abnormalities in diabetes are associated with changes in concentrations and functional activities of tissue plasminogen activator (tPA) levels, factors VII, VIII and IX. These changes in clotting-associated proteins are associated with atherosclerosis with an increment of 24–30% per standard deviation[54] and correlate with the degree of insulin sensitivity,[55] the metabolic syndrome and HDL-C levels.[56,57] Hyperviscosity can be due to the dehydra-

tion of osmotic diuresis, increased acute-phase reactant proteins due to increased intercurrent infections and dysfunction of the modified proteins and is associated with an increased risk of thrombosis.[58]

Platelet aggregation is increased in patients with diabetes and correlates with an increase in cardiovascular events.[59,60] Platelet reactivity is consistently elevated throughout the day, without the temporal morning peak seen in the general population.[61] Thromboxane A2 synthesis is increased in the platelets of diabetic patients, particularly in those with poor glycaemic control or vascular complications.[60,62] Platelet function mediated through the protease activated receptor (PAR) pathways is altered in diabetes via PAR-1 and PAR-4 receptor expression through their interaction with inflammation[63] (Figure 21.6).

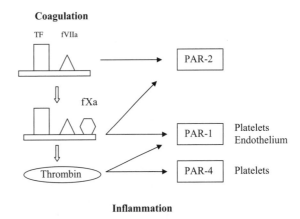

Figure 21.6 Interaction between the coagulation and inflammation pathways demonstrating the role of coagulation proteases and platelet activated receptors (PARs). Abbreviations: TF = tissue factor; fVIIa = activated factor VIIa; fXa = activated factor Xa.[58] Reproduced with permission from the European Society of Cardiology

Platelet consumption is higher in diabetic patients and expression of platelet factor IV is increased, as is release of plasminogen activator inhibitor-1 and von Willebrand factor. The latter tends to help form platelet strings more readily in patients with diabetes. The interaction and mutual activation of platelets and leukocytes (especially neutrophils) in microthrombi is promoted by the intercurrent infections and triglyceride-rich remnants common in diabetes.[64–66]

Fibrinogen levels are elevated in patients with diabetes, possibly as part of a chronic state of activation of the acute-phase reaction.[67–69] Fibrinogen levels are independently associated with myocardial infarction and sudden death in diabetic men and predict vascular complications, especially peripheral arterial disease. Associations between clotting factors and several components of insulin resistance syndrome were seen in the Atherosclerosis Risk In Communities (ARIC) Study.[70]

Endothelial dysfunction or damage precedes both macrovascular and microvascular complications in diabetic patients.[71,72] Endogenous fibrinolysis has also been shown to be deficient in these patients as levels of plasminogen activator inhibitor-1 (PAI-1) are elevated. PAI-1 is the principal physiological inhibitor of endogenous tissue plasminogen activator and PAI-1 levels show parallel elevation to triglycerides. PAI-1 seems to promote progression of diabetes independent of other risk factors.[73,74]

Diabetes and heart muscle metabolism

Abnormalities of metabolism have been described across the spectrum of glycaemic disorders.[75] Patients with impaired glucose tolerance/impaired fasting glucose often show left atrial enlargement – a marker of abnormal filling. Similarly, obese insulin-resistant patients show systolic dysfunction such as strain, diastolic dysfunction and increased reflectivity (backscatter).[76,77]

The disordered glucose and lipid metabolism of diabetes with increased free fatty acids, hyperglycaemia and reduced GLUT-4 transporter expression combine to uncouple oxidative phosphorylation and myocardial oxygen demand.[78] Protein glycation activates protein kinase C inducing nuclear factor kappa-B and inflammatory cytokine release with consequent inflammation, growth factor release and fibrosis.[79–81] Myocyte apoptosis has been shown to be promoted by glucose and angiotensin II and antagonized by insulin-like growth factors.[80] Basement membrane glycation increases vascular permeability and angiogenesis is also increased. All these factors reduce myocardial efficiency.

Specific cardiac diseases in diabetic patients

Coronary artery disease and acute coronary syndromes

Both type 1 and type 2 diabetes are independent risk factors for CHD. Asymptomatic myocardial ischaemia occurs more frequently in patients with diabetes, possibly due to a blunted pain response and small fibre neuropathy.[82] Silent myocardial infarction is commoner in diabetic patients, occurring in 39% of individuals as opposed to 22% in those without diabetes.[83,84] Post mortem data show myocardial scars in the absence of a previous history of myocardial infarction three times more often in autopsies of patients with diabetes.[85] Furthermore, the incidence of painless ST segment depression during exercise stress tests is almost double that seen in patients without diabetes (69 vs 35%).[86] Patients with diabetes experiencing angina often become aware of their symptoms later in the course of ischaemia than do patients without diabetes.[86–88] The delay in time from onset of ST segment depression to angina pain may be doubled in diabetic patients and correlates with the extent of autonomic nervous dysfunction and hence glycaemic control.[86,88] As a result of these changes, clinical diagnosis of infarction based on historical grounds may be difficult, but the presence of a high number of risk factors should always raise suspicions of cardiovascular disease as the primary pathology with any vague symptoms in this group. Atypical symptoms such as confusion, dyspnoea, fatigue or nausea and vomiting (mimicking those from hypo- or hyperglycaemia) may be a presenting complaint in 32–42% of patients with diabetes with myocardial infarction, as opposed to 6–15% of patients without diabetes.[89,90]

These atypical presentations may lower the clinical suspicion of infarction, leading to under-treatment of patients with diabetes and myocardial infarction.[91–95] Atypical symptoms may alter patients' perception of the nature of their illness and interfere with their decision to seek medical advice. Up to 30% of patients with diabetes without chest pain during their infarction wait 24 h or longer to seek medical care. Painless myocardial infarction has been shown to be associated with increased morbidity and mortality. It is likely that the delay in seeking and receiving appropriate medical care may contribute to the observed increase in morbidity and mortality.

Mortality is increased in patients with diabetes presenting with unstable angina or with acute myocardial infarction with a mortality rate of 8.6 versus 2.5% [relative risk (RR) = 3.4)] at 3 months and 16.7 versus 8.6% (RR = 1.94) at 1 year compared with non-diabetic reference groups.[96] One-year mortality rates of 25% after acute myocardial infarction have been reported.[97] Women with diabetes and acute myocardial infarctions have a poorer prognosis than men and double the in-hospital mortality.[5,98–100]

Several factors contribute to this increased in-hospital and long-term mortality. The size of infarct tends to be greater and anterior infarcts are more common in patients with diabetes than in non-diabetic patients.[98,100] Congestive cardiac failure and cardiogenic shock are more common and more severe than can be predicted from the size of infarct in patients with diabetes, with a reduction in both global and regional ejection fractions. Re-infarction, recurrent or persistent ischaemia, myocardial rupture and atrioventricular and intraventricular conduction abnormalities are more common in diabetic than non-diabetic patients.

Diabetic cardiomyopathy

Patients with diabetes are unusually prone to enhanced myocardial dysfunction leading to accelerated heart failure (Figure 21.5).[98,101] In epidemiological studies, the frequency of congestive heart failure was increased 2-fold in men and 5-fold in women.[102,103] Several factors underlie the development of diabetic cardiomyopathy: severe diffuse coronary artery disease, chronic hyperglycaemia, hypertension, microvascular disease, glycosylation of myocardial proteins and autonomic neuropathy. Pathological findings in diabetic cardiomyopathy include myocardial enlargement, hypertrophy and fibrosis. These pathological abnormalities are reflected in a wide spectrum of abnormalities of left ventricular function ranging from asymptomatic diastolic dysfunction to overt decreased systolic function.[104,105] Although diastolic abnormalities are commoner in hypertensive diabetic patients, they are frequently demonstrated in 'normotensive' patients with diabetes (Figure 21.5).[29,78,100] Left ventricular hypertrophy, particularly in women, has been shown to occur in diabetic patients even in the absence of hypertension.[104] Further, decreased contractile reserve, as reflected by lower augmentation of left ventricular ejection fraction with exercise, occurs in diabetes.[87,88,106] Frank systolic dysfunction occurs late in long-standing diabetes with microvascular and macrovascular complications.

Autonomic neuropathy in diabetic patients

Autonomic neuropathy evolves early in the course of diabetes.[107–109] Cardiac parasympathetic nerve fibres are affected before sympathetic fibres, leading to a relative excess of sympathetic tone that initially manifests as tachycardia, reduced heart rate variability at rest and attenuation of heart rate and blood pressure response to exercise.[82,107] Absent parasympathetic tone, allied to endothelial dysfunction, may be responsible for the exaggerated or inappropriate coronary vasoconstriction, which may produce or worsen ischaemia. Sympathetic nervous system dysfunction is evident in 5 years from the onset of parasympathetic abnormalities and manifests as orthostatic hypotension.[82,107,109] Autonomic dysfunction is responsible for the lack of pain perception during ischaemia or exercise testing and for the higher incidence of silent ischaemia, as discussed above. In addition, autonomic neuropathy may be responsible for sudden death in diabetic patients.[110–112] A relationship has been noted between diabetic cardiac autonomic neuropathy and prolonged QT interval on electrocardiogram (ECG), which may predispose to life-threatening ventricular arrhythmia and sudden death.[109,112,113]

Cardiac neuropathy can be identified by reduced heart rate and blood pressure responses to breathing, Valsalva and posture changes and changes in recovery rates after exercise.[114] These effects can be unequivocally demonstrated by the use of single photon emission computed tomography (SPECT) and positron emission tomography (PET).[29,114,107]

Diabetic heart failure

Within the population with heart failure, the prevalence of diabetes is doubled compared with matched controls, particularly those with 'normal' systolic function. Also, diabetes is a risk factor for heart failure as rates of CCF were increased by 2.4-fold in the Framingham study in men and 5.4-fold in women.[102,103,116] These effects occur beyond those of blood pressure as systolic dysfunction and echocardiographic 'backscatter' are increased independent of classical risk factors. Prognosis is also worse, especially in patients with ischaemic cardiomyopathy, and progression to CCF is faster in patients with diabetes suffering an AMI. Hence the supposedly preserved systolic function seen in these patients may be a myth (Figure 21.7) and disturbances of long axis function have been described though these are partially compensated by radial changes.[117–119] Diastolic dysfunction is common in diabetes and impaired relaxation occurs in 26% of young 'fit' patients with diabetes on routine echocardiography.[120] With the use of techniques for assessing pseudo-normal filling (Valsalva response) and tissue Doppler studies, the prevalence rises to 75%.[121] Structural abnormalities may be present, including extracellular fibrosis and myocyte

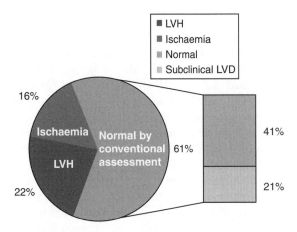

Figure 21.7 Spectrum of cardiac disorders in 101 asymptomatic patients with diabetes. Abbreviations: EF = ejection fraction; LVD = left ventricular dysfunction; LVH = left ventricular hypertrophy.[29] Reproduced with permission from BMJ Group

atrophy and loss, but these are best described in animal models rather than humans.[82,106]

Assessment of coronary risk factors in diabetic patients

Cardiovascular risk assessment in diabetes is similar to that for any patient at risk of coronary artery disease.[122,123] It should begin with assessing the presence of major risk factors, such as

1 hypertension
2 cigarette smoking
3 hyperlipidaemia (cholesterol, triglycerides and HDL-C)
4 family history of pre-mature coronary artery disease
5 glycaemic control
6 renal function.

In addition, factors that contribute to the risk [excess body weight, abdominal obesity (waist circumference), lack of physical activity] should also be sought.

The value of a detailed history, physical examination and appropriate laboratory tests for the identification of these risk factors cannot be overemphasized. Specialized testing such as 24 h monitoring of ambulatory blood pressure through automated techniques may help to detect hypertension.

Laboratory investigation should assess cardiovascular risk factors in addition to glycaemic control. The effectiveness of glycaemic control should be determined by measurement of HbA_{1c} levels. Creatinine should be measured as an index of renal function allied with screening for the presence of micro- or macroalbuminuria. Renal function should be assessed by calculation of estimated glomerular filtration rate by the Modified Diet in Renal Disease (MDRD) formula (Cockcroft–Gault may overestimate renal function in obese patients) and a simultaneous assessment of micro- or macroalbuminuria by albumin:creatinine or protein:creatinine ratios, as these risk factors are associated with greater risk of developing coronary artery disease. Liver function tests have a role beyond assessment of drug safety in diabetes as γ-glutamyl transferase levels and also transaminases correlate with hepatic steatosis and mixed hyperlipidaemia. Hyperuricaemia is part of the metabolic syndrome and a cardiovascular risk factor. Hyperhomocysteinaemia is associated with renal dysfunction and hypertriglyceridaemia, although its role as a cardiovascular risk factor is controversial.

Lipid measurement including a full subfraction profile (total cholesterol, triglycerides, HDL, LDL) should form a routine part of assessment of a patient with diabetes. Although the calculated LDL-C derived from the Freidewald equation is often stated to be accurate in patients with diabetes, doubts remain. The initial study was small and many patients with diabetes are assessed in a non-fasting state in contradiction to the assumptions for the calculation. Thus LDL-C levels may be underestimated by this method. Direct LDL-C methods exist but are more expensive and poorly standardized. There is debate as to whether, given the excess atherogenic risk associated with the increased levels of triglyceride-rich apolipoprotein B-100 containing lipoproteins, it would be preferable to use non-HDL-C (i.e. total – HDL-C) or apolipoprotein B levels as an index of total atherogenic low-density particle burden. There is a strong case for measurement of non-HDL-C or apolipoprotein (apo) B levels, as these can be used to guide LDL-lowering therapy, but the role of lipoprotein particle size measurement is controversial as it seems to add little to apoB levels.

Other cardiovascular biomarkers and risk discrimination tools are being investigated in diabetes, but few add anything significant to current methods.[124]

Detection of clinical and subclinical coronary artery disease

Early diagnosis of coronary artery disease is imperative in patients with diabetes for effective treatment and to decrease the high morbidity and mortality associated with diabetes. A careful history should include the presence of angina, dyspnoea, cerebrovascular events or claudication. The lack of typical symptoms in many patients makes early diagnosis of coronary artery disease difficult and requires a high index of suspicion on the part of physicians for detection of coronary atherosclerotic disease.

Physical examination should include measurement of blood pressure and assessment of carotid and peripheral arteries for bruits that indicate stenosis of these vessels, a marker for coronary artery disease. In patients with extensive risk factors, other markers such as ankle:brachial blood pressure indices[125] and ultrasonic angiology measurements are useful, as many significant stenoses present in patients with diabetes are asymptomatic.[126,127]

An ECG may detect the presence of ischaemia or infarction in some patients and can also reveal gross left ventricular hypertrophy, which has been shown to be associated with increased morbidity and mortality in diabetic patients. A non-invasive test such as an echocardiogram may reveal systolic or diastolic left ventricular dysfunction or regional wall motion abnormality indicative of coronary atherosclerosis and identify left ventricular hypertrophy,[128] but a simple measurement of brain natriuretic peptide (BNP) levels can be used to exclude significant dysfunction and thus preclude the need for imaging. BNP levels can also be used to monitor the success of therapy for ventricular dysfunction. However, the results of studies of BNP in diabetes are controversial and conflicting.[106]

There should be a low threshold for cardiac investigations in patients with diabetes, given the high incidence of silent ischaemia in diabetes. Exercise ECG testing has also been used to assess asymptomatic diabetic patients for coronary artery disease. Prospective screening of 203 patients with diabetes but no chest pain who had normal resting ECGs with exercise ECG tests found that 16% had an abnormal stress test, whereas 9% had silent coronary artery disease as defined by angiography.[129] Most patients (84%) with silent angiographic disease had diabetes. Exercise ECG may be less sensitive in patients with diabetes, but using standard ECG criteria, 38% of 190 patients with diabetes and chest pain had an abnormal exercise test, whereas 69% had coronary artery disease as defined by angiography. The sensitivity of the exercise test among diabetic patients was 47% and the specificity was 81%, which were similar to those in 1092 patients without diabetes (sensitivity 52%, specificity 80%). Among the 638 subjects (87%) with a normal exercise ECG test, the incidence of cardiac events (death, myocardial infarction or angina) was 0.97/100 person-years (95% CI 0.66 to 1.38) compared with 3.85/100 person-years (95% CI 1.84 to 7.07) in those with abnormal stress testing ($p \approx 0.0001$). Although these data are limited by verification bias, they suggest that asymptomatic patients with uncomplicated diabetes mellitus who have a negative exercise ECG test have a lower cardiac event rate and relatively favourable prognosis.[129] In other studies of patients with diabetes and risk factors, resting ECG was a poor discriminator of abnormal coronary angiography results. Coronary disease burden paralleled risk factors, but lesions likely to require intervention were found in 42.5% of patients with diabetes with <1 risk factor and 39.6% of those with >2.[130] A pilot study[131] reported that aggressive screening may reduce events by 30% at 4.3 years ($p = 0.01$). Patients with diabetes have reduced exercise capacities, as evidenced by lower submaximal and peak oxygen consumption rates. In patients with diabetes with positive thallium scans, only 28% have a positive stress exercise ECG compared with 68% of non-diabetic individuals.[90] The Detection of Ischaemia in Asymptomatic Diabetes (DIAD) study showed that screening only patients with diabetes and two other cardiovascular risk factors would miss 40% of patients with significant coronary artery disease. In those patients in whom coronary artery disease was found, 40% had significant ischaemia (40%), of which half affected the anterior wall, and 28% had significant left ventricular dysfunction.[132]

Management of cardiovascular disease in patients with diabetes

Medical management

Early and comprehensive medical intervention in patients with existing coronary artery disease has been shown to decrease the incidence of myocardial infarction, increase survival, improve quality of life and decrease the need for invasive therapies such as coronary angioplasty or bypass surgery. The higher mortality and morbidity in diabetic patients mandates an aggressive approach to secondary prevention in those with known coronary artery disease. The general comprehensive guidelines proposed by specialist societies for the management of patients with known coronary artery disease for risk reduction should be applied to diabetic patients (Table 21.3).[123,133–135]

Antiplatelet agents

The role of aspirin as a secondary prevention therapy following a myocardial infarction (MI) is well established.[136–138] Secondary infarcts in patients on chronic aspirin therapy are likely to be smaller and switch to a non-Q-wave pattern consistent with reduced myocardial damage. Increased platelet reactivity that not only promotes progression of atherosclerosis and the development of occlusive thrombus at the site of

Table 21.3 Ways of improving outcome in diabetic patients with known coronary artery disease

1. Stopping smoking
2. Control of hypertension
3. Lipid-lowering agents in patients to target LDL <100 mg dl^{-1} (<2.5 mmol l^{-1})
4. Aspirin 75–150 mg day^{-1} or clopidogrel 75 mg day^{-1} if genuinely aspirin intolerant
5. Angiotensin-converting enzyme (ACE) inhibitors especially in patients with congestive heart failure and/or left ventricular ejection fraction <35%, but also to prevent and/or slow the progression of nephropathy
6. Oral anticoagulation for increased risk of embolization from left ventricle or left atrium (those with severe LV dysfunction after MI, persistent atrial fibrillation and/or demonstrated mural or left atrial thrombus). Target INR 2–3
7. Beta-blockers (preferably beta 1-selective agents; avoid beta-blockers with intrinsic sympathomimetic activity)
8. Better glycaemic control
9. Diet counselling
10. Physical activity and weight management

plaque rupture has been demonstrated in diabetic patients.[139] However, it should be noted that in the Anti-Platelet Trialists' meta-analysis, aspirin therapy was associated with a 7% non-significant reduction in events in patients with diabetes.[138] As most of the patients received 75–81 mg, it may be that the lower dose is insufficient to counter the prothrombotic state present in diabetes, but this remains to be resolved in clinical trials.[115,136–138]

The thienopyridine ADP-(P2Y$_{12}$)receptor antagonist clopidogrel was compared with aspirin in the CAPRIE (Clopidogrel versus Aspirin in Patients at Risk of Ischemic Events) trial in 19 185 patients and reduced combined cardiovascular events from 5.8 to 5.3%, an 8.7% reduction in relative risk ($p = 0.043$).[140] In sub-group analysis, the greatest differential effect was seen in patients with peripheral arterial disease (RR = 0.77; $p = 0.003$) and a slightly greater benefit (RR = 0.88; $p = 0.04$) was seen in patients with diabetes in a *post hoc* analysis.[141] Rates of gastrointestinal bleeding are reduced with clopidogrel compared with aspirin but better results are obtained with a combination of aspirin with a proton pump inhibitor.[142] Clopidogrel therapy (75 mg) is recommended for those patients with an allergy or genuine intolerance to aspirin. Larger loading doses (300 mg) given for 48 h in addition to aspirin are beneficial in the early treatment of acute coronary syndromes and acute MI and post-PCI.[143,144] The exact length of time to continue clopidogrel therapy post-PCI is controversial and there are no specific data for patients with diabetes, but 1 year is generally accepted. There is no role for chronic aspirin–clopidogrel combination therapy

as it does not result in significant cardiovascular benefits (6.8 vs 7.3%; RR = 0.91; $p = 0.22$) in the Clopidogrel for High Atherothrombotic Risk and Ischemic Stabilization, Management and Avoidance (CHARISMA) trial, which recruited a high-risk population including 42% with diabetes. The combination does slightly increase risks of bruising and haemorrhage (1.7 vs 1.3%; $p = 0.09$). Anti-thrombotic therapies are routinely used in patients with diabetes undergoing intervention, but the evidence base is equivocal. In the Clopidogrel in Unstable angina to prevent Recurrent Events (PCI-CURE) study, major coronary events were not reduced (12.9 vs 16.4%; RR 0.77; $p = 0.12$), in contrast to results in non-diabetic individuals (RR = 0.66; $p = 0.02$).[145] Patients with diabetes more commonly show both aspirin and clopidogrel resistance. Meta-analysis of the abciximab trials showed a survival benefit in diabetes (4.5 vs 2.5%; $p = 0.03$) and better results in the non-Q-wave MI group undergoing PCI.[146] More recently, the TRITON-TIMI 38 study compared the more efficacious ADP-receptor antagonist prasugrel (60 mg loading dose/10 mg maintenance dose) with clopidogrel (300/75) with optimal background therapies in 13 608 patients with acute coronary syndromes. Prasugrel therapy reduced cardiovascular events from 12.1 to 9.8% (19%; $p < 0.001$) with a similar rate of bleeding. In 3146 patients with diabetes, the effects seemed to be greater as events were reduced from 17.0 to 12.2% (30%; $p < 0.001$).[147]

Oral anticoagulants are indicated for patients at risk of embolization from left ventricular or left atrial clot (those with severe left ventricular dysfunction, persistent atrial fibrillation and/or demonstrated mural or left atrial thrombus). The recommended target international normalized ratio (INR) for such patients is 2–3.

Beta-blockers

Beta-blocker therapy has been shown to reduce re-infarction and sudden death in diabetic patients to a greater extent than in non-diabetic patients. Meta-analysis of acute beta-blocker studies in MI showed a 37 versus 13% benefit in mortality in patients with diabetes compared with matched non-diabetic patients.[148] Long-term studies show mortality reductions of 33% in all patients treated with beta-blockers and 48% in patients with diabetes.[148,149] Re-infarction rates are reduced by 55% in diabetic patients compared with 21% in non-diabetics.[149] Beta-blockers may have adverse effects on lipid and glucose profiles and impair glycogenolysis, increase hypoglycaemia, attenuate reflex tachycardia and mask warning symptoms due to hypoglycaemia, worsen claudication, increase fatigue and depression and decrease libido.[150] However, these effects are much less noticeable in patients treated with beta 1-selective agents than in those treated with non-selective agents.[150] However given their benefits these largely theoretical risks should not preclude the use of beta-blockers (preferably beta 1-selective lipid-soluble agents) in patients with diabetes.

Renin–angiotensin system inhibitors

Angiotensin-converting enzyme (ACE) inhibitors (ACEI) have been shown to be beneficial in secondary prevention after acute MI in patients with or without systolic left ventricular dysfunction.[151–153] They decrease symptoms due to heart failure, reduce recurrent ischaemia and infarction, prevent hospitalization and improve survival rates. Furthermore, by reducing blood pressure, they may reduce the risk of stroke. They have also been shown to prevent the development and delay the progression of diabetic nephropathy. Thus, ACEI are currently recommended for all diabetic patients with hypertension, left ventricular dysfunction or congestive heart failure and after large anterior wall MI. In patients who are intolerant or allergic to ACEI, angiotensin-receptor blockers should be used as alternative agents.

Control of high blood pressure

As noted above, hypertension worsens the effects of diabetes on cardiovascular morbidity and mortality and increases the risk of diabetic nephropathy.[123,154] Therefore, every effort should be made to decrease high blood pressure in diabetic patients, with a goal of <130/80 mmHg, although this is difficult to achieve in practice, often being limited by lack of drug efficacy and problems with tolerability and with hypotension. However, it could be argued that the reason why multiple drug treatment is required for hypertension is that, as for glycaemia, the original therapy was not aggressive enough and that drug therapy followed measured blood pressure rather than attempting to prevent it.[155] Although achievement of ideal body weight, exercise and salt restriction should be the first steps towards achieving this goal, usually multiple antihypertensive agents are required. ACEI should be considered the first agents of choice in diabetic patients because of their potential beneficial effect on diabetic nephropathy. It is often necessary to use 3–4 drugs to achieve blood pressure control.

Lipid-lowering therapy

An aggressive attempt at lowering LDL-C with statins to <80–100 mg dl^{-1} (<2.0–2.5 mmol l^{-1}) should be the primary objective, with the secondary aim of achieving at least a 40 mg dl^{-1} (1 mmol l^{-1}) reduction in LDL-C.[122,123,134,156] In intolerant patients, there may be a role of fibrates, but the results of the FIELD trial of fenofibrate therapy in early type 2 diabetes are controversial.[157,158] If triglycerides are persistently elevated to >200 mg dl^{-1} (>2.3 mmol l^{-1}) or HDL-C is reduced to <40 mg/dl (1 mmol l^{-1}), combination statin–fibrate therapy should be considered with appropriate monitoring given the excess risk of rhabdomyolysis, especially with gemfibrozil. It should be noted that the statin–fibrate sub-group in FIELD showed no additional benefit from fibrate therapy.[159] Niacin (nicotinic acid) raises HDL-C and improves general lipid profiles but may exacerbate hyperglycaemia in some patients with overt type 2 diabetes, but this can usually be managed by adjusting the therapy for hyperglycaemia.[160]

Control of hyperglycaemia

Glycaemic control may play a role in the cardiovascular risk of diabetes as there is a continuous relationship between glucose levels and cardiovascular risk. Tight glycaemic control improves microvascular complications such as retinopathy and nephropathy, but there is a lack of conclusive evidence of its beneficial effects in reducing macrovascular complications, especially cardiovascular events.[161,162] In the epidemiological analysis of the United Kingdom Prospective Diabetes Study (UKPDS), a 1% change in HbA$_{1c}$ was associated with a 1.18-fold increased risk of CHD, approximately the same as a 10 mmHg blood pressure increase,[161,162] but these factors also interact to raise risk further.[163] Similar results were seen in ARIC (RR = 1.14).[164]

The Epidemiology of Diabetes Interventions and Complications/Diabetes Control and Complications Trial (EDIC/DCCT) showed that after 17 years of follow-up intensive glycaemic control was associated with a 42% reduction (p = 0.02) in any macrovascular event and a 57% reduction (p = 0.02) in fatal and non-fatal strokes and myocardial infarctions.[165] The UKPDS in type 2 diabetic patients showed a similar improvement in microvascular events, but not in macro-vascular complications with intensive glycaemic control.[166] The DIabetes mellitus Glucose insulin infusion in Acute Myocardial Infarction (DIGAMI) Study showed a significant reduction in 1 year mortality compared with the usual care group (8.6 vs 18%, p = 0.02) in the group allocated to glucose–insulin infusion followed by tight insulin-based glycaemic control.[167] However, in DIGAMI22 there was no survival benefit as mortality between groups 1 (insulin—glucose + later insulin) (23.4%) and 2 (insulin–glucose then oral hypoglycaemic) (22.6%; primary endpoint) did not differ significantly [hazard ratio (HR) 1.03 (95% CI 0.79 to 1.34); $p = 0.83$], nor did mortality between groups 2 (22.6%) and 3 (oral hypoglycaemics/usual care) (19.3%; secondary endpoint) [HR 1.23 (95% CI 0.89 to 1.69); $p = 0.12$]. There were no significant differences in morbidity expressed as non-fatal reinfarctions and strokes among the three groups.[168]

Metformin has been found to be almost as effective as sulfonylurea in controlling hyperglycaemia. The UKPDS study showed that the obese metformin-treated group experienced a 36% reduction in all-cause mortality in comparison with the obese groups receiving sulfonylurea or insulin therapy.[169]

Several concerns have been raised about the use of sulfonylureas and its cardiovascular effects, namely increased propensity for dysrhythmias, induction of vasoconstriction, increased insulin levels and weight, decreases in ischaemic preconditioning and worsening of vascular reactivity. Despite this, trials have failed to demonstrate any increase in cardiac events with these agents.[166]

Thiazolidinediones (glitazones) show numerous beneficial effects on glucose, lipid and myocyte metabolism *in vitro* and in animal studies. However, in the PROspective pioglitAzone Clinical Trial In macro-Vascular Events (PROACTIVE) study of secondary prevention patients with diabetes, the global cardiovascular primary endpoint was negative [RR 0.90 (95% CI 0.80–1.02); $p = 0.09$] but a secondary endpoint excluding revascularization was positive (RR = 0.84; $p = 0.02$).[170] However, the results are controversial as fluid retention, weight gain, peripheral oedema and increased rates of heart failure were observed in the trial.[171]

Hence the role of improved glycaemic control in diabetes above that necessary to prevent microvascular disease remains controversial.

Control of obesity

Obesity is a predisposing cause of type 2 diabetes and exacerbates many of the complications, including hypertension, nephropathy and CVD risk. Most trials of weight-loss strategies have occurred in patients with impaired fasting glucose/impaired glucose tolerance and have included intensive lifestyle modification, metformin, rosiglitazone and orlistat therapy. All these reduce progression to type 2 diabetes by 35–60%.[172] Weight loss therapies are less successful in patients with diabetes than in non-diabetic individuals. For instance, in the Rimonabant in Obesity (RIO) trial series, which all recruited patients of 95–100 kg, the benefit of rimonabant therapy in dia-

betes was 4% compared with 4.8–6.5% in non-diabetic trial populations.[172,173] However, trials of the cardiovascular benefits of weight reduction in diabetes are lacking. Three trials are investigating this area. The Look AHEAD trial has enrolled 5145 obese patients with type 2 diabetes and randomized them to lifestyle intervention or diabetes support and education, with a planned 11.5 year follow-up for cardiovascular events. In contrast, the sibutramine and cardiovascular outcomes trial (SCOUT) in 10 742 patients and the CRESCENDO study with rimonabant in 17 000 patients are under way using pharmacological weight loss strategies.[172]

Reperfusion therapy in patients with acute myocardial infarction

Following an acute MI, diabetic patients continue to have mortality rates that are 1.5–2 times higher than those for non-diabetic individuals, even in the thrombolytic era.[174,175] However, diabetic patients with acute MI treated with thrombolytic therapy have similar reductions in mortality to non-diabetic patients. Meta-analysis of the thrombolytic trials showed a non-significant 21.7% versus 14.3% reduction in 35-day mortality in diabetic compared with non-diabetic patients.[176] Retinal haemorrhage in diabetic patients treated with thrombolytic therapy seems to be rare.[177]

In the Primary Angioplasty in Myocardial Infarction (PAMI) study, in-hospital mortality in diabetic patients randomized to receive tissue plasminogen activator therapy was 20.8% versus 0% in those randomized to have primary percutaneous transluminal coronary angioplasty (PTCA) ($p = 0.01$).[178] Similarly, the rate of death or re-infarction was higher in diabetes treated with thrombolysis than with primary angioplasty (25 vs 4%; $p = 0.03$). Primary stenting in diabetic patients with acute MI improves outcomes, but not as much as bypass grafting.[175] Hence, on the basis of the available data, diabetic patients with acute MIs should receive prompt aggressive reperfusion therapy.

Coronary revascularization

Diabetic patients have similar successes to non-diabetic patients with PTCA.[179] However, as restenosis rates are higher in diabetic patients (reported as between 47 and 71%) than non-diabetic patients (30–45%), thus requiring additional revascularization procedures and increasing late mortality, surgery remains the preferred option[180] (Table 21.4). In the Bypass Angioplasty Revascularization Investigation (BARI), the 7 year survival rate among diabetic

Table 21.4 Trials comparing management of patients with diabetes by stenting and coronary bypass grafts

Trial	Numbers	Follow-up	Primary endpoint	Primary endpoint in diabetes mellitus
ARTS	1205 19% DM	12 months	PCI 74% CABG 88% $p < 0.001$	PCI 63% CABG 84% P < 0.001
SOS	988 14% DM	24 months	PCI 21% CABG 6%	—
ERAC-II	450 17% DM	30 days–5 years	PCI 35% CABG 24% $p = 0.01$	No difference DM vs. non-DM
AWESOME	454 32% DM	37% year survival	PCI 80% CABG 79% $p = NS$	Similar DM vs. non-DM

Abbreviations: CABG = coronary artery bypass graft; DM = diabetes mellitus; PCI = percutaneous coronary intervention; NS = not significant.

patients was significantly better after CABG than angioplasty (76.4 vs 55.7%, $p = 0.001$) and was confined to those receiving internal mammary artery (IMA) grafts to the left anterior descending artery (LAD) as opposed to saphenous vein grafts.[181] At 5 years, the rate of excess death with balloon PTCA was 15% in patients with diabetes and >20% at 7 years, with poor prognosis being associated with insulin therapy, cardiac and renal failure and age.[182] Repeat revascularization rates were similar in all CABG patients in BARI (11.1 vs 13.5%; $p = 0.45$), but PTCA rates were higher in PTCA-treated patients with diabetes (69.9 vs 57.8%; $p = 0.008$). The benefits were due to a reduction in Q-wave MI (RR = 0.09; $p < 0.001$) and was 7-fold in patients with diabetes with a previous Q-wave MI as opposed to those with other MIs.[183] This explained 50% of the variance, with the rest probably being due to a reduction in chronic ischaemia. Both BARI and the Coronary Angioplasty versus Bypass Revascularization Investigation (CABRI) both showed benefits, but some registries do not, possibly due to patient selection bias.[175,184]

Stent studies show similar results. In the Arterial Revascularization Therapy Study, event-free survival was less owing to increased rates of repeat intervention (63.4 vs 84.4%; $p < 0.001$) in patients with diabetes and showed a differential in effectiveness compared with non-diabetic patients.[185] The 5 year mortality was increased in diabetic patients with PTCA compared with non-diabetic patients (13.4 vs 8.3%; RR 1.61; $p < 0.001$). Studies with drug eluting stents (Table 21.5) are confounded by diabetes being a

Table 21.5 Trials comparing drug eluting versus bare metal stents in patients with diabetes

Trial	Numbers and intervention	Follow-up (years)	Primary endpoint	Primary endpoint in diabetes mellitus
SIRIUS	1058; sirolimus 26% DM	0.75	DES 8.6% BMS 21.0% $p < 0.001$	DES 12% BMS 27% $p = 0.003$
TAXUS-IV	1314; pacxilate 24% DM	0.75	DES 4.7% BMS 12.0% $p < 0.001$	DES 11.3% BMS 24.0% $p = 0.004$
DIABETES	160; sirolimus 100% DM	0.75	—	DES 6% BMS 47% $p < 0.001$
SIRTAX	1012; sirolimus DM 20%	0.75	DES 6.2% BMS 10.8% $p = 0.009$	No difference DM vs non-DM
ISAR-DIABETES	250; sirolimus vs pacxilatel	0.50	—	Sirolimus possibly superior to pacxilatel

Abbreviations: BMS = bare metal stent; DM = diabetes mellitus; DES = drug eluting stent.

predictor of revascularization in the SIRolImUS-coated Bx velocity stent (SIRIUS) study[186] and also in TAXUS-IV.[187] The small-scale Diabetes and Sirolimus-eluting stent (DIABETES) study showed benefits for drug-eluting stent (DES) placement in patients with diabetes.[188] Similarly, the IN-Stent Angiographic Restenosis-diabetes (ISAR)[189] and Synergy between percutaneous coronary InteRvention with TAXus and cardiac surgery (SIRTAX)[190] studies showed less in- and para-stent stenosis with DES and less restenosis with Cypher compared with Taxus stents. Larger scale studies are under way to determine the role of DES as opposed to CABG in diabetes. Yet even with DES therapy, rates of restenosis are increased 1.92-fold in patients with diabetes compared with non-diabetic individuals.[191] Compared with non-diabetic patients, rates of morbidity and mortality are increased post-CABG and despite good patency, non-cardiac complications (e.g. stroke) may increase.[175,191] The burden of vein graft disease is increasing and these patients require PTCA as a second intervention given the high risk associated with CABG. However, rates of complication post-PTCA are higher in patients with diabetes and include risks of renal dysfunction and in-stent thrombosis (RR = 3.71) and stenosis (RR = 1.22) caused by intimal fibrosis and increased matrix deposition.[175] Recent meta-analysis shows that DES are associated with lower rates of lumen loss in diabetes [0.18 (95% CI –0.09 to 0.45) vs 0.93 (95% CI 0.51 to 1.35) mm year^{-1}] and thus lower rates of in-stent restenosis [RR = 0.14 (95% CI 0.10 to 0.22); $p < 0.001$] and target lesion revascularization

[RR = 0.34 (95% CI 0.26 to 0.45); $p < 0.001$] compared with bare metal stents.[192]

Conclusion

Diabetes is distinguished by more aggressive CHD. This translates into a poorer prognosis for any atherosclerotic complication of diabetes, including cardiac death, MI and heart failure. In addition, disease is more difficult to detect and more generalized and diffusely located than in patients without diabetes. The cure for cardiac complications in diabetes is principally the prevention of diabetes, as many of the cardiovascular risk factors associated with CHD form part of the metabolic syndrome. Metabolic syndrome shows a stronger predisposition to future diabetes than coronary artery disease. However, the high frequency of low levels of individual risk factors and their synergistic interaction mean that even in the absence of diabetes many patients will unfortunately develop CVD. Once diabetes is established, then all cardiovascular risk factors have to be managed aggressively.[193] Indices of suspicion for CVD have to be low and aggressive intervention has to be pursued, including the use of bypass grafting. Aggressive measures have reduced the prevalence of CVD events in diabetes by 40–50%,[4,194] but rates still remain higher than in non-diabetic patients (Figure 21.7), but the long-term effects of diabetes still tend to attenuate any early benefits they gain from more effective treatments (Figure 21.8).[194]

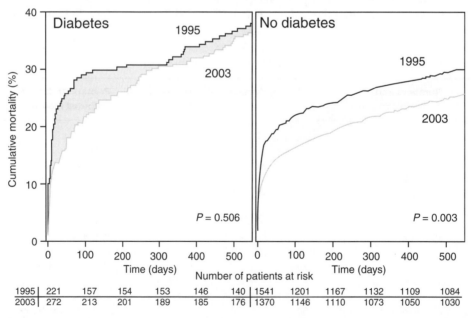

Figure 21.8 Survival trends in diabetes 1995–2003 for cohorts of patients with and without diabetes. Reproduced from Cubbon *et al.*[194] with permission from the European Society of Cardiology

References

1 Yusuf S, Hawken S, Ounpuu S, Dans T, Avezum A, Lanas F, McQueen M, Budaj A, Pais P, Varigos J, Lisheng L. Effect of potentially modifiable risk factors associated with myocardial infarction in 52 countries (the INTERHEART study): case–control study. *Lancet* 2004;**364**(9438):937–952.

2 Fox CS, Coady S, Sorlie PD, Levy D, Meigs JB, D'Agostino RB Sr, Wilson PW, Savage PJ. Trends in cardiovascular complications of diabetes. *JAMA* 2004;**292**(20):2495–2499.

3 Fox CS, Sullivan L, D'Agostino RB Sr, Wilson PW. The significant effect of diabetes duration on coronary heart disease mortality: the Framingham Heart Study. *Diabetes Care* 2004;**27**(3):704–708.

4 Fox CS, Coady S, Sorlie PD, D'Agostino RB Sr, Pencina MJ, Vasan RS, Meigs JB, Levy D, Savage PJ. Increasing cardiovascular disease burden due to diabetes mellitus: the Framingham Heart Study. *Circulation* 2007;**115**(12):1544–1550.

5 Kannel WB, McGee DL. Diabetes and cardiovascular disease. The Framingham study. *JAMA* 1979;**241**(19):2035–2038.

6 Barrett-Connor E. Diabetes and heart disease. *Diabetes Care* 2003;**26**(10):2947–2958.

7 Barrett-Connor E, Orchard TJ. Insulin-dependent diabetes mellitus and ischemic heart disease. *Diabetes Care* 1985;**8** (Suppl 1): 65–70.

8 Kannel WB, McGee DL. Diabetes and cardiovascular risk factors: the Framingham study. *Circulation* 1979;**59**(1):8–13.

9 Haffner SM, Lehto S, Ronnemaa T, Pyorala K, Laakso M. Mortality from coronary heart disease in subjects with type 2 diabetes and in non-diabetic subjects with and without prior myocardial infarction. *N Engl J Med* 1998;**339**(4): 229–234.

10 Evans JM, Wang J, Morris AD. Comparison of cardiovascular risk between patients with type 2 diabetes and those who had had a myocardial infarction: cross sectional and cohort studies. *BMJ* 2002;**324**(7343):939–942.

11 Kockx MM, De Meyer GR, Muhring J, Jacob W, Bult H, Herman AG. Apoptosis and related proteins in different stages of human atherosclerotic plaques. *Circulation* 1998; **97**(23):2307–2315.

12 Marfella R, Di FC, Baldi A, Siniscalchi M, Sasso FC, Crescenzi B, Cirillo F, Nicoletti GF, D'Andrea F, Chiorazzo G, Musacchio E, Rossi F, Verza M, Coppola L, D'Amico M. The vascular smooth muscle cells apoptosis in asymptomatic diabetic carotid plaques: role of glycemic control. *J Am Coll Cardiol* 2006;**47**(10):2118–2120.

13 Barger AC, Beeuwkes R III, Lainey LL, Silverman KJ. Hypothesis: vasa vasorum and neovascularization of human coronary arteries. A possible role in the pathophysiology of atherosclerosis. *N Engl J Med* 1984;**310**(3):175–177.

14 Kolodgie FD, Gold HK, Burke AP, Fowler DR, Kruth HS, Weber DK, Farb A, Guerrero LJ, Hayase M, Kutys R, Narula J, Finn AV, Virmani R. Intraplaque hemorrhage and progression of coronary atheroma. *N Engl J Med* 2003;**349** (24):2316–2325.

15 Hoff JA, Daviglus ML, Chomka EV, Krainik AJ, Sevrukov A, Kondos GT. Conventional coronary artery disease risk factors and coronary artery calcium detected by electron beam tomography in 30,908 healthy individuals. *Ann Epidemiol* 2003;**13**(3):163–169.

16 Hoff JA, Quinn L, Sevrukov A, Lipton RB, Daviglus M, Garside DB, Ajmere NK, Gandhi S, Kondos GT. The prevalence of coronary artery calcium among diabetic individuals without known coronary artery disease. *J Am Coll Cardiol* 2003;**41**(6):1008–1012.

17 Proudfoot D, Davies JD, Skepper JN, Weissberg PL, Shanahan CM. Acetylated low-density lipoprotein stimulates human vascular smooth muscle cell calcification by promoting osteoblastic differentiation and inhibiting phagocytosis. *Circulation* 2002;**106**(24):3044–3050.

18 Fein F, Scheuer J. Heart disease in diabetes mellitus: theory and practice. In: *Diabetes Mellitus: Theory and Practice* (eds H Rifkin, JD Porte), Elsevier, New York, 1990, pp. 812–823.

19 Goraya TY, Leibson CL, Palumbo PJ, Weston SA, Killian JM, Pfeifer EA, Jacobsen SJ, Frye RL, Roger VL. Coronary atherosclerosis in diabetes mellitus: a population-based autopsy study. *J Am Coll Cardiol* 2002;**40**(5):946–953.

20 Mak KH, Moliterno DJ, Granger CB, Miller DP, White HD, Wilcox RG, Califf RM, Topol EJ. Influence of diabetes mellitus on clinical outcome in the thrombolytic era of acute myocardial infarction. GUSTO-I Investigators. Global Utilization of Streptokinase and Tissue Plasminogen Activator for Occluded Coronary Arteries. *J Am Coll Cardiol* 1997;**30** (1):171–179.

21 Natali A, Vichi S, Landi P, Severi S, L'Abbate A, Ferrannini E. Coronary atherosclerosis in Type II diabetes: angiographic findings and clinical outcome. *Diabetologia* 2000;**43**(5):632–641.

22 Kornowski R, Mintz GS, Lansky AJ, Hong MK, Kent KM, Pichard AD, Satler LF, Popma JJ, Bucher TA, Leon MB. Paradoxic decreases in atherosclerotic plaque mass in insulin-treated diabetic patients. *Am J Cardiol* 1998;**81** (11):1298–1304.

23 Sattar N, Gaw A, Scherbakova O, Ford I, O'Reilly DS, Haffner SM, Isles C, Macfarlane PW, Packard CJ, Cobbe SM, Shepherd J. Metabolic syndrome with and without C-reactive protein as a predictor of coronary heart disease and diabetes in the West of Scotland Coronary Prevention Study. *Circulation* 2003;**108**(4):414–419.

24 Forouhi NG, Sattar N, Tillin T, McKeigue PM, Chaturvedi N. Do known risk factors explain the higher coronary heart disease mortality in South Asian compared with European men? Prospective follow-up of the Southall and Brent studies, UK. *Diabetologia* 2006;**49**(11):2580–2588.

25 Cappuccio FP, Cook DG, Atkinson RW, Strazzullo P. Prevalence, detection and management of cardiovascular risk factors in different ethnic groups in south London. *Heart* 1997;**78**(6):555–563.

26 Khaw KT, Wareham N, Luben R, Bingham S, Oakes S, Welch A, Day N. Glycated haemoglobin, diabetes and mortality in men in Norfolk cohort of european prospective investigation of cancer and nutrition (EPIC-Norfolk). *BMJ* 2001;**322**(7277):15–18.

27 Alberti KG, Zimmet P, Shaw J. The metabolic syndrome – a new worldwide definition. *Lancet* 2005;**366**(9491):1059–1062.

28 Moy CS, LaPorte RE, Dorman JS, Songer TJ, Orchard TJ, Kuller LH, Becker DJ, Drash AL. Insulin-dependent

diabetes mellitus mortality. The risk of cigarette smoking. *Circulation* 1990;**82**(1):37–43.

29 Marwick TH. Diabetic heart disease. *Heart* 2006;**92**(3):296–300.

30 Gall MA, Rossing P, Skott P, Damsbo P, Vaag A, Bech K, Dejgaard A, Lauritzen M, Lauritzen E, Hougaard P. Prevalence of micro- and macroalbuminuria, arterial hypertension, retinopathy and large vessel disease in European type 2 (non-insulin-dependent) diabetic patients. *Diabetologia* 1991;**34**(9):655–661.

31 Assmann G, Schulte H. The Prospective Cardiovascular Munster (PROCAM) study: prevalence of hyperlipidemia in persons with hypertension and/or diabetes mellitus and the relationship to coronary heart disease. *Am Heart J* 1988;**116**(6 Pt 2): 1713–1724.

32 Assmann G, Schulte H. Diabetes mellitus and hypertension in the elderly: concomitant hyperlipidemia and coronary heart disease risk. *Am J Cardiol* 1989;**63**(16):33H–37H.

33 Jensen T, Borch-Johnsen K, Kofoed-Enevoldsen A, Deckert T. Coronary heart disease in young type 1 (insulin-dependent) diabetic patients with and without diabetic nephropathy: incidence and risk factors. *Diabetologia* 1987;**30**(3):144–148.

34 Reaven GM, Lithell H, Landsberg L. Hypertension and associated metabolic abnormalities – the role of insulin resistance and the sympathoadrenal system. *N Engl J Med* 1996;**334**(6):374–381.

35 Austin MA, Breslow JL, Hennekens CH, Buring JE, Willett WC, Krauss RM. Low-density lipoprotein subclass patterns and risk of myocardial infarction. *JAMA* 1988;**260**(13):1917–1921.

36 Austin MA, Mykkanen L, Kuusisto J, Edwards KL, Nelson C, Haffner SM, Pyorala K, Laakso M. Prospective study of small LDLs as a risk factor for non-insulin dependent diabetes mellitus in elderly men and women. *Circulation* 1995;**92**(7):1770–1778.

37 Austin MA. Triglyceride, small, dense low-density lipoprotein and the atherogenic lipoprotein phenotype. *Curr Atheroscler Rep* 2000;**2**(3):200–207.

38 Reaven GM. Banting Lecture 1988. Role of insulin resistance in human disease. *Diabetes* 1988;**37**(12):1595–1607.

39 Lamarche B, Tchernof A, Moorjani S, Cantin B, Dagenais GR, Lupien PJ, Despres JP. Small, dense low-density lipoprotein particles as a predictor of the risk of ischemic heart disease in men. Prospective results from the Quebec Cardiovascular Study. *Circulation* 1997;**95**(1):69–75.

40 St-Pierre AC, Cantin B, Dagenais GR, Mauriege P, Bernard PM, Despres JP, Lamarche B. Low-density lipoprotein subfractions and the long-term risk of ischemic heart disease in men: 13-year follow-up data from the Quebec Cardiovascular Study. *Arterioscler Thromb Vasc Biol* 2005;**25**(3):553–559.

41 Christ ER, Carroll PV, Albany E, Umpleby AM, Lumb PJ, Wierzbicki AS, Simpson HL, Sonksen PH, Russell-Ones DL. Normal VLDL metabolism despite altered lipoprotein composition in type 1 diabetes mellitus. *Clin Endocrinol (Oxf)* 2001;**55**(6):777–787.

42 Jenkins AJ, Lyons TJ, Zheng D, Otvos JD, Lackland DT, McGee D, Garvey WT, Klein RL. Lipoproteins in the

DCCT/EDIC cohort: associations with diabetic nephropathy. *Kidney Int* 2003;**64**(3):817–828.

43 Jenkins AJ, Lyons TJ, Zheng D, Otvos JD, Lackland DT, McGee D, Garvey WT, Klein RL. Serum lipoproteins in the diabetes control and complications trial/epidemiology of diabetes intervention and complications cohort: associations with gender and glycemia. *Diabetes Care* 2003;**26**(3):810–818.

44 Karamanos B, Porta M, Songini M, Metelko Z, Kerenyi Z, Tamas G, Rottiers R, Stevens LK, Fuller JH. Different risk factors of microangiopathy in patients with type I diabetes mellitus of short versus long duration. The EURODIAB IDDM Complications Study. *Diabetologia* 2000;**43**(3):348–355.

45 Alberti KG, Zimmet P, Shaw J. The metabolic syndrome – a new worldwide definition. *Lancet* 2005;**366**(9491):1059–1062.

46 Dinneen SF, Gerstein HC. The association of microalbuminuria and mortality in non-insulin-dependent diabetes mellitus. A systematic overview of the literature. *Arch Intern Med* 1997;**157**(13):1413–1418.

47 Mattock MB, Morrish NJ, Viberti G, Keen H, Fitzgerald AP, Jackson G. Prospective study of microalbuminuria as predictor of mortality in NIDDM. *Diabetes* 1992;**41**(6):736–741.

48 Mogensen CE. Microalbuminuria predicts clinical proteinuria and early mortality in maturity-onset diabetes. *N Engl J Med* 1984;**310**(6):356–360.

49 Krolewski AS, Kosinski EJ, Warram JH, Leland OS, Busick EJ, Asmal AC, Rand LI, Christlieb AR, Bradley RF, Kahn CR. Magnitude and determinants of coronary artery disease in juvenile-onset, insulin-dependent diabetes mellitus. *Am J Cardiol* 1987;**59**(8):750–755.

50 Manske CL, Wilson RF, Wang Y, Thomas W. Prevalence of and risk factors for, angiographically determined coronary artery disease in type I-diabetic patients with nephropathy. *Arch Intern Med* 1992;**152**(12):2450–2455.

51 Dunn EJ, Grant PJ. Type 2 diabetes: an atherothrombotic syndrome. *Curr Mol Med* 2005;**5**(3):323–332.

52 MacRury SM, Lowe GD. Blood rheology in diabetes mellitus. *Diabet Med* 1990;**7**(4):285–291.

53 Watala C. Blood platelet reactivity and its pharmacological modulation in (people with) diabetes mellitus. *Curr Pharm Des* 2005;**11**(18):2331–2365.

54 Kannel WB. Overview of hemostatic factors involved in atherosclerotic cardiovascular disease. *Lipids* 2005;**40**(12):1215–1220.

55 Wannamethee SG, Lowe GD, Shaper AG, Rumley A, Lennon L, Whincup PH. Insulin resistance, haemostatic and inflammatory markers and coronary heart disease risk factors in Type 2 diabetic men with and without coronary heart disease. *Diabetologia* 2004;**47**(9):1557–1565.

56 Aloulou I, Varlet-Marie E, Mercier J, Brun JF. Hemorheological disturbances correlate with the lipid profile but not with the NCEP-ATPIII score of the metabolic syndrome. *Clin Hemorheol Microcirc* 2006;**35**:no. 1–2, pp. 207–212.

57 Aloulou I, Varlet-Marie E, Mercier J, Brun JF. The hemorheological aspects of the metabolic syndrome are a combination of separate effects of insulin resistance, hyperinsulinemia and adiposity. *Clin Hemorheol Microcirc* 2006;**35**(1–2):113–119.

58 De Caterina R, Husted S, Wallentin L, Agnelli G, Bachmann F, Baigent C, Jespersen J, Kristensen SD, Montalescot G, Siegbahn A, Verheugt FW, Weitz J. Anticoagulants in heart disease: current status and perspectives. *Eur Heart J* 2007;**28** (7):880–913.

59 Carr ME. Diabetes mellitus: a hypercoagulable state. *J Diabetes Complications* 2001;**15**(1):44–54.

60 Ferroni P, Basili S, Falco A, Davi G. Platelet activation in type 2 diabetes mellitus. *J Thromb Haemost* 2004;**2** (8):1282–1291.

61 Cooke-Ariel H. Circadian variations in cardiovascular function and their relation to the occurrence and timing of cardiac events. *Am J Health Syst Pharm* 1998;**55**(Suppl 3): S5–S11.

62 Davi G, Catalano I, Averna M, Notarbartolo A, Strano A, Ciabattoni G, Patrono C. Thromboxane biosynthesis and platelet function in type II diabetes mellitus. *N Engl J Med* 1990;**322**(25):1769–1774.

63 Serebruany VL, Malinin A, Pokov A, Arora U, Atar D, Angiolillo D. Effects of escalating doses of tirofiban on platelet aggregation and major receptor expression in diabetic patients: hitting the TARGET in the TENACITY trial? *Thromb Haemost* 2007;**119**(2):175–181.

64 Koga H, Sugiyama S, Kugiyama K, Fukushima H, Watanabe K, Sakamoto T, Yoshimura M, Jinnouchi H, Ogawa H. Elevated levels of remnant lipoproteins are associated with plasma platelet microparticles in patients with type–2 diabetes mellitus without obstructive coronary artery disease. *Eur Heart J* 2006;**27**(7):817–823.

65 Tschoepe D, Rauch U, Schwippert B. Platelet–leukocyte-cross-talk in diabetes mellitus. *Horm Metab Res* 1997;**29** (12):631–635.

66 Tuttle HA, Davis-Gorman G, Goldman S, Copeland JG, McDonagh PF. Platelet-neutrophil conjugate formation is increased in diabetic women with cardiovascular disease. *Cardiovasc Diabetol* 2003;**2**:12.

67 Lobo RA. Lipids, clotting factors and diabetes: endogenous risk factors for cardiovascular disease. *Am J Obstet Gynecol* 1988;**158**(6 Pt 2): 1584–1591.

68 Muntner P, He J, Chen J, Fonseca V, Whelton PK. Prevalence of non-traditional cardiovascular disease risk factors among persons with impaired fasting glucose, impaired glucose tolerance, diabetes and the metabolic syndrome: analysis of the Third National Health and Nutrition Examination Survey (NHANES III). *Ann Epidemiol* 2004;**14** (9):686–695.

69 Saito I, Folsom AR, Brancati FL, Duncan BB, Chambless LE, McGovern PG. Nontraditional risk factors for coronary heart disease incidence among persons with diabetes: the Atherosclerosis Risk in Communities (ARIC) Study. *Ann Intern Med* 2000;**133**(2):81–91.

70 Saito I, Folsom AR, Brancati FL, Duncan BB, Chambless LE, McGovern PG. Nontraditional risk factors for coronary heart disease incidence among persons with diabetes: the Atherosclerosis Risk in Communities (ARIC) Study. *Ann Intern Med* 2000;**133**(2):81–91.

71 Guerci B, Bohme P, Kearney-Schwartz A, Zannad F, Drouin P. Endothelial dysfunction and type 2 diabetes. Part 2: altered endothelial function and the effects of treatments

in type 2 diabetes mellitus. *Diabetes Metab* 2001;**27**(4 Pt 1): 436–447.

72 Guerci B, Kearney-Schwartz A, Bohme P, Zannad F, Drouin P. Endothelial dysfunction and type 2 diabetes. Part 1: physiology and methods for exploring the endothelial function. *Diabetes Metab* 2001;**27**(4 Pt 1): 425–434.

73 Juhan-Vague I, Alessi MC. PAI-1, obesity, insulin resistance and risk of cardiovascular events. *Thromb Haemost* 1997;**78** (1):656–660.

74 Mertens I, Verrijken A, Michiels JJ, Van der Planken M, Ruige JB, Van Gaal LF. Among inflammation and coagulation markers, PAI-1 is a true component of the metabolic syndrome. *Int J Obes (Lond)* 2006;**30**(8):1308–1314.

75 Marwick TH. The diabetic myocardium. *Curr Diab Rep* 2006;**6**(1):36–41.

76 Rutter MK, Parise H, Benjamin EJ, Levy D, Larson MG, Meigs JB, Nesto RW, Wilson PW, Vasan RS. Impact of glucose intolerance and insulin resistance on cardiac structure and function: sex-related differences in the Framingham Heart Study. *Circulation* 2003;**107**(3):448–454.

77 Wong CY, O'Moore-Sullivan T, Leano R, Byrne N, Beller E, Marwick TH. Alterations of left ventricular myocardial characteristics associated with obesity. *Circulation* 2004;**110**(19):3081–3087.

78 Watts GF, Marwick TH. Ventricular dysfunction in early diabetic heart disease: detection, mechanisms and significance. *Clin Sci (Lond)* 2003;**105**(5):537–540.

79 Hammes HP. Pathophysiological mechanisms of diabetic angiopathy. *J Diabetes Complications* 2003;**17**(2 Suppl): 16–19.

80 Pfeiffer A, Schatz H. Diabetic microvascular complications and growth factors. *Exp Clin Endocrinol Diabetes* 1995;**103** (1):7–14.

81 Setter SM, Campbell RK, Cahoon CJ. Biochemical pathways for microvascular complications of diabetes mellitus. *Ann Pharmacother* 2003;**37**(12):1858–1866.

82 Fang ZY, Prins JB, Marwick TH. Diabetic cardiomyopathy: evidence, mechanisms and therapeutic implications. *Endocr Rev* 2004;**25**(4):543–567.

83 Niakan E, Harati Y, Comstock JP. Diabetic autonomic neuropathy. *Metabolism* 1986;**35**(3):224–234.

84 Rutter MK, Wahid ST, McComb JM, Marshall SM. Significance of silent ischemia and microalbuminuria in predicting coronary events in asymptomatic patients with type 2 diabetes. *J Am Coll Cardiol* 2002;**40**(1):56–61.

85 Cabin HS, Roberts WC. Quantitative comparison of extent of coronary narrowing and size of healed myocardial infarct in 33 necropsy patients with clinically recognized and in 28 with clinically unrecognized (silent) previous acute myocardial infarction. *Am J Cardiol* 1982;**50** (4):677–681.

86 Regensteiner JG. Type 2 diabetes mellitus and cardiovascular exercise performance. *Rev Endocr Metab Disord* 2004;**5** (3):269–276.

87 Ambepityia G, Kopelman PG, Ingram D, Swash M, Mills PG, Timmis AD. Exertional myocardial ischemia in diabetes: a quantitative analysis of anginal perceptual threshold and the influence of autonomic function. *J Am Coll Cardiol* 1990;**15**(1):72–77.

88 Fang ZY, Sharman J, Prins JB, Marwick TH. Determinants of exercise capacity in patients with type 2 diabetes. *Diabetes Care* 2005;**28**(7):1643–1648.

89 Nesto RW, Phillips RT. Asymptomatic myocardial ischemia in diabetic patients. *Am J Med* 1986;**80**(4C):40–47.

90 Nesto RW, Phillips RT, Kett KG, Hill T, Perper E, Young E, Leland OS Jr. Angina and exertional myocardial ischemia in diabetic and non-diabetic patients: assessment by exercise thallium scintigraphy. *Ann Intern Med* 1988;**108**(2):170–175.

91 Bakhai A, Collinson J, Flather MD, de Arenaza DP, Shibata MC, Wang D, Adgey JA. Diabetic patients with acute coronary syndromes in the UK: high risk and under treated. Results from the prospective registry of acute ischaemic syndromes in the UK (PRAIS-UK). *Int J Cardiol* 2005;**100**(1):79–84.

92 Brown DW, Balluz LS, Giles WH, Beckles GL, Moriarty DG, Ford ES, Mokdad AH. Diabetes mellitus and health-related quality of life among older adults. Findings from the behavioral risk factor surveillance system (BRFSS). *Diabetes Res Clin Pract* 2004;**65**(2):105–115.

93 Maddigan SL, Feeny DH, Johnson JA. Health-related quality of life deficits associated with diabetes and comorbidities in a Canadian National Population Health Survey. *Qual Life Res* 2005;**14**(5):1311–1320.

94 Mehta RH, Ruane TJ, McCargar PA, Eagle KA, Stalhandske EJ. The treatment of elderly diabetic patients with acute myocardial infarction: insight from Michigan's Cooperative Cardiovascular Project. *Arch Intern Med* 2000;**160**(9):1301–1306.

95 Montalescot G, Dabbous OH, Lim MJ, Flather MD, Mehta RH. Relation of timing of cardiac catheterization to outcomes in patients with non-ST-segment elevation myocardial infarction or unstable angina pectoris enrolled in the multinational global registry of acute coronary events. *Am J Cardiol* 2005;**95**(12):1397–1403.

96 Fava S, Azzopardi J, Agius-Muscat H. Outcome of unstable angina in patients with diabetes mellitus. *Diabet Med* 1997;**14**(3):209–213.

97 Savage MP, Krolewski AS, Kenien GG, Lebeis MP, Christlieb AR, Lewis SM. Acute myocardial infarction in diabetes mellitus and significance of congestive heart failure as a prognostic factor. *Am J Cardiol* 1988;**62**(10 Pt 1): 665–669.

98 Bell DS. Heart failure: the frequent, forgotten and often fatal complication of diabetes. *Diabetes Care* 2003;**26**(8):2433–2441.

99 Bibbins-Domingo K, Lin F, Vittinghoff E, Barrett-Connor E, Hulley SB, Grady D, Shlipak MG. Predictors of heart failure among women with coronary disease. *Circulation* 2004;**110**(11):1424–1430.

100 Masoudi FA, Inzucchi SE. Diabetes mellitus and heart failure: epidemiology, mechanisms and pharmacotherapy. *Am J Cardiol* 2007;**99**(4A):113B–132B.

101 Spector KS. Diabetic cardiomyopathy. *Clin Cardiol* 1998;**21**(12):885–887.

102 Kannel WB. Epidemiology and prevention of cardiac failure: Framingham Study insights. *Eur Heart J* 1987;**8**(Suppl F): 23–26.

103 Kannel WB, Hjortland M, Castelli WP. Role of diabetes in congestive heart failure: the Framingham study. *Am J Cardiol* 1974;**34**(1):29–34.

104 Galderisi M, Anderson KM, Wilson PW, Levy D. Echocardiographic evidence for the existence of a distinct diabetic cardiomyopathy (the Framingham Heart Study). *Am J Cardiol* 1991;**68**(1):85–89.

105 Galderisi M. Diastolic dysfunction and diabetic cardiomyopathy: evaluation by Doppler echocardiography. *J Am Coll Cardiol* 2006;**48**(8):1548–1551.

106 Fang ZY, Schull-Meade R, Leano R, Mottram PM, Prins JB, Marwick TH. Screening for heart disease in diabetic subjects. *Am Heart J* 2005;**149**(2):349–354.

107 Nesto RW. Correlation between cardiovascular disease and diabetes mellitus: current concepts. *Am J Med* 2004;**116**(Suppl 5A): 11S–22S.

108 Pfeifer MA, Weinberg CR, Cook DL, Reenan A, Halter JB, Ensinck JW, Porte D Jr. Autonomic neural dysfunction in recently diagnosed diabetic subjects. *Diabetes Care* 1984;**7**(5):447–453.

109 Vinik AI, Ziegler D. Diabetic cardiovascular autonomic neuropathy. *Circulation* 2007;**115**(3):387–397.

110 El-Atat FA, McFarlane SI, Sowers JR, Bigger JT. Sudden cardiac death in patients with diabetes. *Curr Diab Rep* 2004;**4**(3):187–193.

111 Singh N. Diabetes, heart rate and mortality. *J Cardiovasc Pharmacol Ther* 2002;**7**(2):117–129.

112 Veglio M, Chinaglia A, Cavallo-Perin P. QT interval, cardiovascular risk factors and risk of death in diabetes. *J Endocrinol Invest* 2004;**27**(2):175–181.

113 Veglio M, Chinaglia A, Cavallo PP. The clinical utility of QT interval assessment in diabetes. *Diabetes Nutr Metab* 2000;**13**(6):356–365.

114 Vinik AI, Erbas T. Cardiovascular autonomic neuropathy: diagnosis and management. *Curr Diab Rep* 2006;**6**(6):424–430.

115 Tendera M, Wojakowski W. Role of antiplatelet drugs in the prevention of cardiovascular events. *Thromb Res* 2003;**110**(5–6):355–359.

116 Kannel WB. Incidence and epidemiology of heart failure. *Heart Fail Rev* 2000;**5**(2):167–173.

117 Fang ZY, Leano R, Marwick TH. Relationship between longitudinal and radial contractility in subclinical diabetic heart disease. *Clin Sci (Lond)* 2004;**106**(1):53–60.

118 Marwick TH. Tissue Doppler imaging for evaluation of myocardial function in patients with diabetes mellitus. *Curr Opin Cardiol* 2004;**19**(5):442–446.

119 Marwick TH, Wong CY. Role of exercise and metabolism in heart failure with normal ejection fraction. *Prog Cardiovasc Dis* 2007;**49**(4):263–274.

120 Zabalgoitia M, Ismaeil MF, Anderson L, Maklady FA. Prevalence of diastolic dysfunction in normotensive, asymptomatic patients with well-controlled type 2 diabetes mellitus. *Am J Cardiol* 2001;**87**(3):320–323.

121 Boyer JK, Thanigaraj S, Schechtman KB, Perez JE. Prevalence of ventricular diastolic dysfunction in asymptomatic, normotensive patients with diabetes mellitus. *Am J Cardiol* 2004;**93**(7):870–875.

122 Expert Panel on Detection, Evaluation, and Treatment of High Blood Cholesterol in Adults. Executive Summary of

The Third Report of The National Cholesterol Education Program (NCEP) Expert Panel on Detection, Evaluation, and Treatment of High Blood Cholesterol in Adults (Adult Treatment Panel III). *JAMA* 2001;**285**(19):2486–2497.

123 British Cardiac Society, British Hypertension Society, Diabetes UK, HEART UK, Primary Care Cardiovascular Society, The Stroke Association. JBS 2: the Joint British Societies' guidelines for prevention of cardiovascular disease in clinical practice. *Heart* 2005;**91**(Suppl V): v1–v52.

124 St Clair L, Ballantyne CM. Biological surrogates for enhancing cardiovascular risk prediction in type 2 diabetes mellitus. *Am J Cardiol* 2007;**99**(4A):80B–88B.

125 Bagheri R, Schutta M, Cumaranatunge RG, Wolfe ML, Terembula K, Hoffman B, Schwartz S, Kimmel SE, Farouk S, Iqbal N, Reilly MP. Value of electrocardiographic and ankle-brachial index abnormalities for prediction of coronary atherosclerosis in asymptomatic subjects with type 2 diabetes mellitus. *Am J Cardiol* 2007;**99**(7):951–955.

126 Belch JJ, Topol EJ, Agnelli G, Bertrand M, Califf RM, Clement DL, Creager MA, Easton JD, Gavin JR III, Greenland P, Hankey G, Hanrath P, Hirsch AT, Meyer J, Smith SC, Sullivan F, Weber MA. Critical issues in peripheral arterial disease detection and management: a call to action. *Arch Intern Med* 2003;**163**(8):884–892.

127 Lange S, Diehm C, Darius H, Haberl R, Allenberg JR, Pittrow D, Schuster A, von Stritzky B, Tepohl G, Trampisch HJ. High prevalence of peripheral arterial disease and low treatment rates in elderly primary care patients with diabetes. *Exp Clin Endocrinol Diabetes* 2004;**112** (10):566–573.

128 Feinstein SB. Diabetes mellitus and noninvasive imaging of atherosclerosis. *Am J Cardiol* 2007;**99**(4A):89B–95B.

129 Albers AR, Krichavsky MZ, Balady GJ. Stress testing in patients with diabetes mellitus: diagnostic and prognostic value. *Circulation* 2006;**113**(4):583–592.

130 Scognamiglio R, Negut C, Ramondo A, Tiengo A, Avogaro A. Detection of coronary artery disease in asymptomatic patients with type 2 diabetes mellitus. *J Am Coll Cardiol* 2006;**47**(1):65–71.

131 Faglia E, Manuela M, Antonella Q, Michela G, Vincenzo C, Maurizio C, Roberto M, Alberto M. Risk reduction of cardiac events by screening of unknown asymptomatic coronary artery disease in subjects with type 2 diabetes mellitus at high cardiovascular risk: an open-label randomized pilot study. *Am Heart J* 2005;**149**(2):e1–e6.

132 Wackers FJ, Young LH, Inzucchi SE, Chyun DA, Davey JA, Barrett EJ, Taillefer R, Wittlin SD, Heller GV, Filipchuk N, Engel S, Ratner RE, Iskandrian AE. Detection of silent myocardial ischemia in asymptomatic diabetic subjects: the DIAD study. *Diabetes Care* 2004;**27**(8):1954–1961.

133 American Diabetes Association. Standards of medical care in diabetes. *Diabetes Care 2007* 2007;**30**(Suppl 1): S4–S41.

134 Buse JB, Ginsberg HN, Bakris GL, Clark NG, Costa F, Eckel R, Fonseca V, Gerstein HC, Grundy S, Nesto RW, Pignone MP, Plutzky J, Porte D, Redberg R, Stitzel KF, Stone NJ. Primary prevention of cardiovascular diseases in people with diabetes mellitus: a scientific statement from the American Heart Association and the American Diabetes Association. *Circulation* 2007;**115**(1):114–126.

135 Ryden L, Standl E, Bartnik M, Van den BG, Betteridge J, de Boer MJ, Cosentino F, Jonsson B, Laakso M, Malmberg K, Priori S, Ostergren J, Tuomilehto J, Thrainsdottir I, Vanhorebeek I, Stramba-Badiale M, Lindgren P, Qiao Q, Priori SG, Blanc JJ, Budaj A, Camm J, Dean V, Deckers J, Dickstein K, Lekakis J, McGregor K, Metra M, Morais J, Osterspey A, Tamargo J, Zamorano JL, Deckers JW, Bertrand M, Charbonnel B, Erdmann E, Ferrannini E, Flyvbjerg A, Gohlke H, Juanatey JR, Graham I, Monteiro PF, Parhofer K, Pyorala K, Raz I, Schernthaner G, Volpe M, Wood D. Guidelines on diabetes, pre-diabetes and cardiovascular diseases: executive summary. The Task Force on Diabetes and Cardiovascular Diseases of the European Society of Cardiology (ESC) and of the European Association for the Study of Diabetes (EASD). *Eur Heart J* 2007;**28**(1):88–136.

136 Antiplatelet Trialists' Collaboration. Collaborative overview of randomised trials of antiplatelet therapy – I: Prevention of death, myocardial infarction and stroke by prolonged antiplatelet therapy in various categories of patients. *BMJ* 1994;**308**(6921):81–106.

137 Antiplatelet Trialists' Collaboration. Collaborative overview of randomised trials of antiplatelet therapy – II: Maintenance of vascular graft or arterial patency by antiplatelet therapy. *BMJ* 1994;**308**(6922):159–168.

138 Antithrombotic Trialists' Collaboration. Collaborative meta-analysis of randomised trials of antiplatelet therapy for prevention of death, myocardial infarction and stroke in high risk patients. *BMJ* 2002;**324**(7329):71–86.

139 Colwell JA. Antiplatelet agents for the prevention of cardiovascular disease in diabetes mellitus. *Am J Cardiovasc Drugs* 2004;**4**(2):87–106.

140 CAPRIE Steering Committee. A randomised, blinded, trial of clopidogrel versus aspirin in patients at risk of ischaemic events (CAPRIE). *Lancet* 1996;**348**(9038):1329–1339.

141 Bhatt DL, Marso SP, Hirsch AT, Ringleb PA, Hacke W, Topol EJ. Amplified benefit of clopidogrel versus aspirin in patients with diabetes mellitus. *Am J Cardiol* 2002;**90** (6):625–628.

142 Chan FK, Ching JY, Hung LC, Wong VW, Leung VK, Kung NN, Hui AJ, Wu JC, Leung WK, Lee VW, Lee KK, Lee YT, Lau JY, To KF, Chan HL, Chung SC, Sung JJ. Clopidogrel versus aspirin and esomeprazole to prevent recurrent ulcer bleeding. *N Engl J Med* 2005;**352**(3):238–244.

143 Mehta SR, Yusuf S, Peters RJ, Bertrand ME, Lewis BS, Natarajan MK, Malmberg K, Rupprecht H, Zhao F, Chrolavicius S, Copland I, Fox KA. Effects of pretreatment with clopidogrel and aspirin followed by long-term therapy in patients undergoing percutaneous coronary intervention: the PCI-CURE study. *Lancet* 2001;**358**(9281):527–533.

144 Yusuf S, Zhao F, Mehta SR, Chrolavicius S, Tognoni G, Fox KK. Effects of clopidogrel in addition to aspirin in patients with acute coronary syndromes without ST-segment elevation. *N Engl J Med* 2001;**345**(7):494–502.

145 Mehta SR, Yusuf S, Peters RJ, Bertrand ME, Lewis BS, Natarajan MK, Malmberg K, Rupprecht H, Zhao F, Chrolavicius S, Copland I, Fox KA. Effects of pretreatment with clopidogrel and aspirin followed by long-term therapy in patients undergoing percutaneous coronary intervention: the PCI-CURE study. *Lancet* 2001;**358**(9281):527–533.

146 Bhatt DL, Marso SP, Lincoff AM, Wolski KE, Ellis SG, Topol EJ. Abciximab reduces mortality in diabetics following percutaneous coronary intervention. *J Am Coll Cardiol* 2000;**35**(4):922–928.

147 Wiviott SD, Braunwald E, McCabe CH, Montalescot G, Ruzyllo W, Gottlieb S, Neumann FJ, Ardissino D, De Servi S, Murphy SA, Riesmeyer J, Weerakkody G, Gibson CM, Antman EM. Prasugrel versus clopidogrel in patients with acute coronary syndromes. *N Engl J Med* 2007;**357**(20):2001–2015.

148 Smith SC Jr, Allen J, Blair SN, Bonow RO, Brass LM, Fonarow GC, Grundy SM, Hiratzka L, Jones D, Krumholz HM, Mosca L, Pearson T, Pfeffer MA, Taubert KA. AHA/ACC guidelines for secondary prevention for patients with coronary and other atherosclerotic vascular disease: 2006 update endorsed by the National Heart. Lung and Blood Institute. *J Am Coll Cardiol* 2006;**47**(10):2130–2139.

149 McDonald CG, Majumdar SR, Mahon JL, Johnson JA. The effectiveness of beta-blockers after myocardial infarction in patients with type 2 diabetes. *Diabetes Care* 2005;**28**(9):2113–2117.

150 Cruickshank JM. Beta-blockers and diabetes: the bad guys come good. *Cardiovasc Drugs Ther* 2002;**16**(5):457–470.

151 Beckman JA, Creager MA, Libby P. Diabetes and atherosclerosis: epidemiology, pathophysiology and management. *JAMA* 2002;**287**(19):2570–2581.

152 Fonarow GC. The management of the diabetic patient with prior cardiovascular events. *Rev Cardiovasc Med* 2003;**4**(Suppl 6): S38–S49.

153 O'Keefe JH, Lurk JT, Kahatapitiya RC, Haskin JA. The renin–angiotensin–aldosterone system as a target in coronary disease. *Curr Atheroscler Rep* 2003;**5**(2):124–130.

154 European Society of Hypertension, European Society of Cardiology. 2003 European Society of Hypertension–European Society of Cardiology guidelines for the management of arterial hypertension. *J Hypertens.* 2003;**21**(6):1011–1053.

155 Weir MR. Targeting mechanisms of hypertensive vascular disease with dual calcium channel and renin–angiotensin system blockade. *J Hum Hypertens* 2007;**21**(10):770–779.

156 Collins R, Armitage J, Pa*rish S, Sleigh P, Peto R. MRC/BHF Heart Protection Study of cholesterol-lowering with simvastatin in 5963 people with diabetes: a randomised placebo-controlled trial. *Lancet* 2003;**361**(9374):2005–2016.

157 Keech A, Simes RJ, Barter P, Best J, Scott R, Taskinen MR, Forder P, Pillai A, Davis T, Glasziou P, Drury P, Kesaniemi YA, Sullivan D, Hunt D, Colman P, d'Emden M, Whiting M, Ehnholm C, Laakso M. Effects of long-term fenofibrate therapy on cardiovascular events in 9795 people with type 2 diabetes mellitus (the FIELD study): randomised controlled trial. *Lancet* 2005;**366**(9500):1849–1861.

158 Wierzbicki AS. FIELDS of dreams, fields of tears: a perspective on the fibrate trials. *Int J Clin Pract* 2006;**60**(4):442–449.

159 Wierzbicki AS, Mikhailidis DP, Wray R. Drug treatment of combined hyperlipidemia. *Am J Cardiovasc Drugs* 2001;**1**(5):327–336.

160 Chapman MJ, Assmann G, Fruchart JC, Shepherd J, Sirtori C. Raising high-density lipoprotein cholesterol with reduction of cardiovascular risk: the role of nicotinic acid – a position paper developed by the European Consensus Panel on HDL-C. *Curr Med Res Opin* 2004;**20**(8):1253–1268.

161 UK Prospective Diabetes Study Group. Tight blood pressure control and risk of macrovascular and microvascular complications in type 2 diabetes: UKPDS 38. *BMJ* 1998;**317**(7160):703–713.

162 Stratton IM, Adler AI, Neil HA, Matthews DR, Manley SE, Cull CA, Hadden D, Turner RC, Holman RR. Association of glycaemia with macrovascular and microvascular complications of type 2 diabetes (UKPDS 35): prospective observational study. *BMJ* 2000;**321**(7258):405–412.

163 Stratton IM, Cull CA, Adler AI, Matthews DR, Neil HA, Holman RR. Additive effects of glycaemia and blood pressure exposure on risk of complications in type 2 diabetes: a prospective observational study (UKPDS 75). *Diabetologia* 2006;**49**(8):1761–1769.

164 Selvin E, Coresh J, Golden SH, Brancati FL, Folsom AR, Steffes MW. Glycemic control and coronary heart disease risk in persons with and without diabetes: the Atherosclerosis Risk in Communities Study. *Arch Intern Med* 2005;**165**(16):1910–1916.

165 Nathan DM, Cleary PA, Backlund JY, Genuth SM, Lachin JM, Orchard TJ, Raskin P, Zinman B. Intensive diabetes treatment and cardiovascular disease in patients with type 1 diabetes. *N Engl J Med* 2005;**353**(25):2643–2653.

166 UK Prospective Diabetes Study (UKPDS) Group. Intensive blood-glucose control with sulphonylureas or insulin compared with conventional treatment and risk of complications in patients with type 2 diabetes (UKPDS 33). *Lancet* 1998;**352**(9131):837–853.

167 Malmberg K, Ryden L, Hamsten A, Herlitz J, Waldenstrom A, Wedel H. Effects of insulin treatment on cause-specific one-year mortality and morbidity in diabetic patients with acute myocardial infarction. DIGAMI Study Group. Diabetes Insulin–Glucose in Acute Myocardial Infarction. *Eur Heart J* 1996;**17**(9):1337–1344.

168 Malmberg K, Ryden L, Wedel H, Birkeland K, Bootsma A, Dickstein K, Efendic S, Fisher M, Hamsten A, Herlitz J, Hildebrandt P, MacLeod K, Laakso M, Torp-Pedersen C, Waldenstrom A. Intense metabolic control by means of insulin in patients with diabetes mellitus and acute myocardial infarction (DIGAMI 2): effects on mortality and morbidity. *Eur Heart J* 2005;**26**(7):650–661.

169 UK Prospective Diabetes Study (UKPDS) Group. Effect of intensive blood-glucose control with metformin on complications in overweight patients with type 2 diabetes (UKPDS 34). *Lancet* 1998;**352**(9131):854–865.

170 Dormandy JA, Charbonnel B, Eckland DJ, Erdmann E, Massi-Benedetti M, Moules IK, Skene AM, Tan MH, Lefebvre PJ, Murray GD, Standl E, Wilcox RG, Wilhelmsen L, Betteridge J, Birkeland K, Golay A, Heine RJ, Koranyi L, Laakso M, Mokan M, Norkus A, Pirags V, Podar T, Scheen A, Scherbaum W, Schernthaner G, Schmitz O, Skrha J, Smith U, Taton J. Secondary prevention of macrovascular events in patients with type 2 diabetes in the PROactive Study

(PROspective pioglitAzone Clinical Trial In macroVascular Events): a randomised controlled trial. *Lancet* 2005;**366** (9493):1279–1289.

171 Yki-Jarvinen H. The PROactive study: some answers, many questions. *Lancet* 2005;**366**(9493):1241–1242.

172 Wierzbicki AS. Rimonabant: endocannabinoid inhibition for the metabolic syndrome. *Int J Clin Pract* 2006;**60** (12):1697–1706.

173 Scheen AJ, Finer N, Hollander P, Jensen MD, Van Gaal LF. Efficacy and tolerability of rimonabant in overweight or obese patients with type 2 diabetes: a randomised controlled study. *Lancet* 2006;**368**(9548):1660–1672.

174 Berry C, Tardif JC, Bourassa MG. Coronary heart disease in patients with diabetes: part I: recent advances in prevention and noninvasive management. *J Am Coll Cardiol* 2007;**49** (6):631–642.

175 Berry C, Tardif JC, Bourassa MG. Coronary heart disease in patients with diabetes: Part II: recent advances in coronary revascularization. *J Am Coll Cardiol* 2007;**49** (6):643–656.

176 Fibrinolytic Therapy Trialists' (FTT) Collaborative Group. Indications for fibrinolytic therapy in suspected acute myocardial infarction: collaborative overview of early mortality and major morbidity results from all randomised trials of more than 1000 patients. *Lancet* 1994;**343** (8893):311–322.

177 Mahaffey KW, Granger CB, Toth CA, White HD, Stebbins AL, Barbash GI, Vahanian A, Topol EJ, Califf RM. Diabetic retinopathy should not be a contraindication to thrombolytic therapy for acute myocardial infarction: review of ocular hemorrhage incidence and location in the GUSTO-I trial. Global Utilization of Streptokinase and t-PA for Occluded Coronary Arteries. *J Am Coll Cardiol* 1997;**30** (7):1606–1610.

178 Stone GW, Grines CL, Browne KF, Marco J, Rothbaum D, O'Keefe J, Hartzler GO, Overlie P, Donohue B, Chelliah N. Predictors of in-hospital and 6-month outcome after acute myocardial infarction in the reperfusion era: the Primary Angioplasty in Myocardial Infarction (PAMI) trial. *J Am Coll Cardiol* 1995;**25**(2):370–377.

179 Van Belle E, Bauters C, Hubert E, Bodart JC, Abolmaali K, Meurice T, McFadden EP, Lablanche JM, Bertrand ME. Restenosis rates in diabetic patients: a comparison of coronary stenting and balloon angioplasty in native coronary vessels. *Circulation* 1997;**96**(5):1454–1460.

180 Marso SP, Lincoff AM, Ellis SG, Bhatt DL, Tanguay JF, Kleiman NS, Hammoud T, Booth JE, Sapp SK, Topol EJ. Optimizing the percutaneous interventional outcomes for patients with diabetes mellitus: results of the EPISTENT (Evaluation of Platelet IIb/IIIa Inhibitor for Stenting Trial) diabetic substudy. *Circulation* 1999;**100** (25):2477–2484.

181 BARI Investgators. Seven-year outcome in the Bypass Angioplasty Revascularization Investigation (BARI) by treatment and diabetic status. *J Am Coll Cardiol* 2000;**35** (5):1122–1129.

182 Brooks MM, Jones RH, Bach RG, Chaitman BR, Kern MJ, Orszulak TA, Follmann D, Sopko G, Blackstone EH, Califf RM. Predictors of mortality and mortality from cardiac causes in the bypass angioplasty revascularization investigation (BARI) randomized trial and registry. For the BARI Investigators. *Circulation* 2000;**101** (23):2682–2689.

183 Detre KM, Guo P, Holubkov R, Califf RM, Sopko G, Bach R, Brooks MM, Bourassa MG, Shemin RJ, Rosen AD, Krone RJ, Frye RL, Feit F. Coronary revascularization in diabetic patients: a comparison of the randomized and observational components of the Aypass Angioplasty Revascularization Investigation (BARI). *Circulation* 1999;**99**(5):633–640.

184 Kurbaan AS, Bowker TJ, Ilsley CD, Sigwart U, Rickards AF. Difference in the mortality of the CABRI diabetic and non-diabetic populations and its relation to coronary artery disease and the revascularization mode. *Am J Cardiol* 2001;**87**(8):947–950.

185 Abizaid A, Costa MA, Centemero M, Abizaid AS, Legrand VM, Limet RV, Schuler G, Mohr FW, Lindeboom W, Sousa AG, Sousa JE, van HB, Hugenholtz PG, Unger F, Serruys PW. Clinical and economic impact of diabetes mellitus on percutaneous and surgical treatment of multivessel coronary disease patients: insights from the Arterial Revascularization Therapy Study (ARTS) trial. *Circulation* 2001;**104** (5):533–538.

186 Moussa I, Leon MB, Baim DS, O'Neill WW, Popma JJ, Buchbinder M, Midwall J, Simonton CA, Keim E, Wang P, Kuntz RE, Moses JW. Impact of sirolimus-eluting stents on outcome in diabetic patients: a SIRIUS (SIRolImUS-coated Bx Velocity balloon-expandable stent in the treatment of patients with de novo coronary artery lesions) substudy. *Circulation* 2004;**109**(19):2273–2278.

187 Hermiller JB, Raizner A, Cannon L, Gurbel PA, Kutcher MA, Wong SC, Russell ME, Ellis SG, Mehran R, Stone GW. Outcomes with the polymer-based paclitaxel-eluting TAXUS stent in patients with diabetes mellitus: the TAXUS-IV trial. *J Am Coll Cardiol* 2005;**45**(8):1172–1179.

188 Sabate M, Jimenez-Quevedo P, Angiolillo DJ, Gomez-Hospital JA, Alfonso F, Hernandez-Antolin R, Goicolea J, Banuelos C, Escaned J, Moreno R, Fernandez C, Fernandez-Aviles F, Macaya C. Randomized comparison of sirolimus-eluting stent versus standard stent for percutaneous coronary revascularization in diabetic patients: the diabetes and sirolimus-eluting stent (DIABETES) trial. *Circulation* 2005;**112**(14):2175–2183.

189 Dibra A, Kastrati A, Mehilli J, Pache J, Schuhlen H, von BN, Ulm K, Wessely R, Dirschinger J, Schomig A. Paclitaxel-eluting or sirolimus-eluting stents to prevent restenosis in diabetic patients. *N Engl J Med* 2005;**353** (7):663–670.

190 Windecker S, Remondino A, Eberli FR, Juni P, Raber L, Wenaweser P, Togni M, Billinger M, Tuller D, Seiler C, Roffi M, Corti R, Sutsch G, Maier W, Luscher T, Hess OM, Egger M, Meier B. Sirolimus-eluting and paclitaxel-eluting stents for coronary revascularization. *N Engl J Med* 2005;**353** (7):653–662.

191 Stone KE, Chiquette E, Chilton RJ. Diabetic endovascular disease: role of coronary artery revascularization. *Am J Cardiol* 2007;**99**(4A):105B–112B.

192 Boyden TF, Nallamothu BK, Moscucci M, Chan PS, Grossman PM, Tsai TT, Chetcuti SJ, Bates ER, Gurm HS. Meta-analysis of randomized trials of drug-eluting stents versus bare metal stents in patients with diabetes mellitus. *Am J Cardiol* 2007;**99**(10):1399–1402.

193 Gaede P, Vedel P, Larsen N, Jensen GV, Parving HH, Pedersen O. Multifactorial intervention and cardiovascular disease in patients with type 2 diabetes. *N Engl J Med* 2003;**348**(5):383–393.

194 Cubbon RM, Wheatcroft SB, Grant PJ, Gale CP, Barth JH, Sapsford RJ, Ajjan R, Kearney MT, Hall AS. Temporal trends in mortality of patients with diabetes mellitus suffering acute myocardial infarction: a comparison of over 3000 patients between 1995 and 2003. *Eur Heart J* 2007;**28**(5):540–545.

22

The treatment of established complications: cerebrovascular disease

Devin L. Brown[1], Susan L. Hickenbottom[2], Teresa L. Jacobs[3]

[1]*Department of Neurology, University of Michigan, Ann Arbor, MI, USA*
[2]*St Joseph Mercy Hospital, Ann Arbor, MI, USA*
[3]*Departments of Neurosurgery and Neurology, University of Michigan, Ann Arbor, MI, USA*

Stroke is an international problem that creates tremendous personal and economic burdens. Approximately 4.6 million deaths from stroke occur each year, making stroke the second most common cause of death worldwide.[1] Population-based studies in Europe, the United States, Australia and Asia have estimated overall stroke incidence rates to range from 200 to 500 per 100 000.[2–4] Caring for stroke is an expensive undertaking. Stroke accounts for almost 5% of all health service costs in the United Kingdom.[5] In 1997, the estimated direct cost for acute care of stroke was found to be £1.1–1.6 million per 100 000 population per year.[6] In the United States, the total cost for stroke has been estimated at $41 billion per year, which includes both direct costs for hospitalization and indirect costs such as lost productivity at work.[7]

Cerebrovascular disease has been recognized as a complication of diabetes mellitus but, until recently, surprisingly little information regarding the specific epidemiology and pathophysiology of diabetes and stroke has been available. Over the past several years, new information about the nature of stroke in diabetes and potential treatment strategies has become available. Better understanding of the epidemiology, pathophysiology and clinical features of cerebrovascular disease in patients with diabetes can assist physicians in the appropriate management of this condition.

Epidemiology

Ischaemic stroke

Multiple epidemiological studies have demonstrated that diabetes is an independent risk factor for ischaemic stroke, with the vast majority focusing on type 2 diabetes. Table 22.1 outlines prospective studies that have shown an increased relative risk for stroke in people with diabetes.

The Framingham Study initially revealed that the incidence of ischaemic stroke was 2.5–3.5-fold higher in patients with diabetes.[17] Later adjustments for the influence of cofactors such as age, systolic blood pressure, antihypertensive therapy, cigarette smoking, ischaemic cardiovascular disease and atrial fibrillation still found diabetes to be an independent risk factor for stroke.[8] The Honolulu Heart Program demonstrated that men with diabetes were almost 2.5 times more likely to suffer a stroke than men without diabetes.[12] More recent large-scale prospective studies from the United Kingdom and United States have also demonstrated diabetes to be an independent risk factor for stroke with similar relative risks as in the older studies.[15,16] Differences in relative risks between the studies can be explained by differences in definition of diabetes used, type of stroke examined and specific population differences, such as geographic location, race/ethnic mix, age and sex. In retrospective case–control studies, diabetes has also been found to be an independent risk factor for stroke. One study of 1444 ischaemic stroke patients found the odds ratio for stroke in the setting of diabetes to be 1.7 [95% confidence interval (CI) 1.2 to 2.4].[18a] Similar risks for transient ischaemic attack (TIA) were also identified.[18b] Using these data, the investigators estimated the population-attributable risk (PAR) of stroke from diabetes to be 5% (95% CI 2 to 9).[18c] In this model, diabetes appeared to be a less potent risk factor for

The Evidence Base for Diabetes Care, Second Edition, Edited by William H. Herman, Ann Louise Kinmonth, Nicholas J. Wareham and Rhys Williams.

Table 22.1 Relative risk of stroke in diabetic persons according to prospective studies[a]

Location	Study	N	% diabetic	Sex	Stroke type	Relative risk
Framingham, MA, USA	D'Augustino et al., 1994[8]	2372	10.6	Men	All (and TIA)	1.41 (0.97 to 2.04)
		3362	7.9	Women		1.75 (1.25 to 2.45)
Rochester, MN, USA	Davis et al., 1987[9]	686	13.8	Men	ischaemic	2.6 (CI not reported)
		938	combined	Women		n.s.
MRFIT sites, USA	Stamler et al., 1993[10]	347978	1.5	Men	Fatal	2.8 (2.0 to 3.7)
Finland	Tuomilehto et al., 1996[11]	8077	4.6	Men	Fatal	3.35 (1.96 to 5.43)
		8572	18.8	Women		4.89 (2.83 to 8.45)
Honolulu, HI, USA	Abbott et al., 1987[12]	7598	9.1	Men	ischaemic	2.45 (1.73 to 3.47)
Rancho Bernardo, CA, USA	Barrett-Connor et al., 1988[13]	1729	11.2	Men	All	1.7 (1.0 to 2.9)
		2049	6.1	Women		1.3 (0.7 to 2.5)
Finland	Kuuisisto et al., 1994[14]	470	15.7	Men	All	1.36 (0.44 to 4.18)
		828	18.8	Women		2.25 (1.65 to 3.06)
United Kingdom	Wannamethee et al., 1999[15]	7735	5.4	Men	All	2.27 (1.23 to 4.20)
ARIC sites, USA	Folsom et al., 1999[16]	15792	10	Both	ischaemic	3.70 (2.7 to 5.1)

[a]Figures in parentheses indicate 95% confidence intervals; n.s = not statistically significant; MRFIT = Multicenter Risk Factor Intervention Trial; ARIC = Atherosclerosis Risk in Communities; TIA = transient ischaemic attack.
Modified from Lukovits et al. 1999.

ischaemic stroke than cigarette smoking, ischaemic heart disease or hypertension, for which PARs ranged from 12 to 26%. These findings have mirrored results from prospective studies, which have also found diabetes to be a less marked risk factor than those outlined above.[9]

A relatively new development in this arena is the investigation of the relationship between hyperglycaemia, glucose intolerance, hyperinsulinaemia and the incidence of ischaemic stroke in patients without diabetes. Data regarding these possible risk factors for stroke are conflicting. Some studies demonstrate a positive association, although not always statistically significant, between ischaemic stroke and (1) hyperglycaemia,[19] (2) glucose intolerance[12,20,21] and (3) hyperinsulinaemia.[14,16] Other studies have shown no independent association between these factors and stroke: (1) hyperglycaemia,[15] (2) glucose intolerance[22] and (3) hyperinsulinaemia.[15,23,24] Criticisms of the studies that showed a positive association between these factors and stroke have included small number of subjects evaluated, inclusion of subjects with subclinical diabetes and demonstration of increased risk only at the extreme end of the distribution of the population.

Two meta-analyses[25,26] have supported the association between impaired glucose metabolism and

cardiovascular disease, including stroke. Impaired fasting glucose has been shown to be associated with developing a first ischaemic stroke or TIA in the coronary artery disease population without diabetes. The odds ratio of developing a first stroke/TIA was 1.22 for those with fasting glucose of 100–109 mg dl^{-1} and 1.84 for those 110–125 mg dl^{-1}, adjusting for potential confounders.[27]

Few studies have specifically addressed the relationship between type 1 diabetes and stroke. A prospective study of patients who had type 1 diabetes for more than 40 years reported a 10% incidence of stroke and 7% mortality from stroke.[28] Review of death certificates in the United Kingdom found similar rates of death attributable to type 1 diabetes.[29]

Haemorrhagic stroke

Although there is strong evidence that diabetes is an independent risk factor for ischaemic stroke, the few epidemiological studies examining its relationship with haemorrhagic stroke have demonstrated a negative association. In the general population, stroke results from ischaemic infarction approximately 80% of the time and from cerebral haemorrhage approximately 20% of the time. However, in the Rochester

Epidemiologic Project, ischaemic stroke accounted for just over 88% of all strokes among patients with diabetes.[30] Primary intracerebral haemorrhage (ICH) occurred six times less frequently in the Copenhagen Stroke Project.[31] The risk of ICH was not significantly increased in the Honolulu Heart Program.[19] A meta-analysis suggested no association between admission hyperglycaemia and intracerebral haemorrhage mortality in patients with or without diabetes.[32] In a study to examine the association between diabetes and subarachnoid haemorrhage, the University of Iowa-Cooperative Aneurysm Study, a negative correlation was demonstrated.[33]

Pathophysiology

Pathological changes

Autopsy studies have demonstrated a greater frequency of cerebral infarction in individuals with diabetes.[34–37] These studies found a much higher frequency of small vessel ischaemic disease of the penetrating arteries supplying the basal ganglia, thalamus, pons and cerebellum, resulting in 'lacunar' infarction. Smaller autopsy series have not reported an association between diabetes alone and lacunar infarction, but do note the association between diabetes, hypertension and lacunar disease.[38] Other studies have also noted the potentially synergistic effect of hypertension and diabetes on the cerebral vasculature.[39–41] Histopathological changes seen in cerebral small vessels in patients with diabetes include endothelial proliferation and 'hyaline arteriosclerosis', or 'lipohyalinosis'.[34] This condition affects the small penetrating arteries in the brain, in which medial smooth muscle first hypertrophies and is then replaced by extracellular and plasma proteins, eventually leading to vessel occlusion and the production of small, deep lacunar infarcts. There is much less information on large vessel atherosclerotic disease in patients with diabetes. Certainly, systemic atherosclerotic disease occurs earlier and more commonly in patients with diabetes and advances more rapidly, but there has been little pathological documentation of such changes in the cerebral circulation. Some autopsy studies have found large vessel cerebral occlusive disease to be more frequent in people with diabetes, whereas others have not.[34,41] With regard to haemorrhagic stroke, autopsy studies found it to be uncommon in patients with diabetes, mirroring the results of epidemiological studies.[34,35,37,42]

Physiological changes

Numerous investigators have also speculated that other pathogenic factors may be at play in cerebral ischaemia in patients with diabetes. Hyperglycaemia itself is a major determinant of diabetic complications, as has been discussed earlier in this text. In the setting of acute ischaemic stroke, hyperglycaemia may arise as the result of underlying diabetes or serum glucose may increase from physiological stress, or both. However, many authors do argue that hyperglycaemia arises independently of the stress response and thus may be seen to a greater extent in patients with diabetes.[43–45]

Animal models of focal ischaemia indicate that hyperglycaemia increases the extent of ischaemic brain damage in some settings.[46–49] There are several possible explanations for worsening of ischaemic damage in the presence of hyperglycaemia. Under hypoxic conditions, elevated serum glucose levels result in increased anaerobic metabolism, lactic acid production and cellular acidosis, which causes damage to neurons, glial cells and vascular tissue.[50–53] Moreover, hyperglycaemia increases the risk for cerebral oedema formation.[54] The extracellular concentrations of the excitatory neurotransmitters, glutamate and aspartate, are elevated in the presence of hyperglycaemia and hypoxia.[55] These neurotransmitters initiate an extensive cascade of neurotoxic biochemical steps, including increased intracellular calcium levels and free radical production.[56] Finally, animal models have demonstrated that hyperglycaemia promotes the development of haemorrhagic transformation of ischaemic infarcts.[57] Retrospective case–control and case series of human subjects have also reported an association between elevated blood glucose and/or history of diabetes and haemorrhagic transformation of ischaemic infarcts.[58,59]

Pathogenic factors other than hyperglycaemia may also contribute to cerebrovascular disease in patients with diabetes and are outlined in Table 22.2. These mechanisms are not mutually exclusive and many may play a role in worsening ischaemic damage from stroke in patients with diabetes.

Outcome of stroke in diabetes

Patients with diabetes have worse outcome from stroke when it occurs, perhaps because of the pathophysiological derangements described above. Mortality is increased both in patients with previously diagnosed diabetes[11,31,71] and in those with acute hyperglycaemia.[15,45] Recovery is also poorer and proceeds more slowly in those with diabetes or hyperglycaemia.[51,72,73] A meta-analysis of 20 studies concluded that hyperglycaemia is associated with increased 30 day mortality and with worse functional outcome 1 year following stroke.[74] One small study

Table 22.2 Factors that may promote ischaemic cerebrovascular disease in the diabetic patient

Factor	Study
Endothelial dysfunction	Cohen, 1993[60]
	Dandona et al., 1978[61]
	Johnstone et al., 1993[62]
Platelet dysfunction	Colwell et al., 1983[63]
	Davi et al., 1990[64]
Hyperviscosity/	Barnes et al., 1977[65]
hypercoagulability	Biller and Love, 1993[66]
Decreased fibrinolytic activity	McGill et al., 1994[67]
Excessive production of advanced glycation end-products (AGEs)	Lyons, 1993[68]
	Wolffenbuttel and van Haeften, 1995[69]
Upregulation of immediate–early genes	Koistinaho et al., 1999[70]

Table 22.3 Validated stroke risk scoring system for stroke risk in patients with atrial fibrillation off of anticoagulation

Total points[†]	Stroke rate (% per year) (95% CI)	Recommended stroke prevention
0	1.9 (1.2 to 3.0)	Aspirin 81–325 mg
1	2.8 (2.0 to 3.8)	Aspirin or warfarin
2	4.0 (3.1 to 5.1)	Warfarin
3	5.9 (4.6 to 7.3)	Warfarin
4	8.5 (6.3 to 11.1)	Warfarin
5	12.5 (8.2 to 17.5)	Warfarin
6	18.2 (10.5 to 27.4)	Warfarin

[†]1 for recent CHF, hypertension, age ≥75 years, diabetes; 2 for prior stroke/TIA)

demonstrated that an elevated mean capillary glucose and elevated continuous glucose in the acute stroke period were associated with infarct growth between initial MRI and 90 day MRI.[75]

Treatment

Primary stroke prevention

Clearly, the best way to decrease stroke burden is through prevention. Primary stroke prevention in patients with diabetes is achieved through risk factor modification, which has been addressed in previous chapters. It is important to emphasize here, though, that well-established modifiable risk factors for stroke should be sought in the patients with diabetes and treated according to established guidelines. These risk factors include hypertension, ischaemic cardiac disease, atrial fibrillation (AF), hyperlipidaemia and cigarette smoking.[76] An excellent review of guidelines for the prevention of first stroke has been published by the American Stroke Association.[77] Patients should also be questioned for a history of focal neurological symptoms suggestive of TIA or stroke, which would then place them in the category of secondary prevention.

Unlike the other risk factors listed above, non-valvular AF has not traditionally been associated with diabetes. Nevertheless, the United Kingdom Prospective Diabetes Study identified AF as the risk factor most strongly identified with stroke in patients newly diagnosed with diabetes; patients with diabetes and AF were eight times more likely to suffer a stroke than those in sinus rhythm.[78] If AF is detected, patients at high risk for thromboembolism should be started on long-term anticoagulation with warfarin with a goal International Normalized Ratio (INR) of 2.0–3.0, presuming that they have no clear contraindications to anticoagulation. One commonly used scoring system to determine the risk of stroke in AF from anticoagulation is the $CHADS_2$ score.[79] A point is assigned for each of the following: history of hypertension, diabetes, recent heart failure and age >75 years. Two points are assigned for a prior history of stroke or transient ischaemic attack. The points are summed and translated into a yearly stroke risk while not on warfarin using Table 22.3. Warfarin is recommended for 2 or more points and aspirin is recommended for 0 points. Either warfarin or aspirin is acceptable for 1 total point.[77,79]

Finally, it should be noted that although aspirin has been found beneficial in the primary prevention of ischaemic heart disease, its use is more controversial for stroke prevention. Studies have failed to show aspirin's effectiveness for primary stroke prevention in men,[80,81] while the Women's Health Study showed that in women aspirin reduces the risk of first stroke but not the risk of cardiac events.[82] Accordingly, general primary stroke prevention guidelines suggest the use of aspirin for women, but not men, 'whose risk is sufficiently high for the benefits to outweigh the risks associated with treatment'.[77] Some studies raised concern about increased rates of intracranial haemorrhage in patients receiving aspirin.[81,83] However, studies of antiplatelet agent use in diabetes suggest no increased risk for cerebrovascular haemorrhage.[84,85] As such, the American Diabetes Association recommends the use of low-dose enteric coated aspirin (75–162 mg) for primary prevention for patients with type 2 diabetes 'at increased cardiovascular risk, including those who are 40 years of age or who have additional risk factors (family history of CVD, hypertension, smoking, dyslipidaemia or albuminuria)'.[86]

Although there are no data from randomized controlled trials to support tight glucose control specifically for stroke prevention for patients with type 2 diabetes, the Diabetes Control and Complications Trial/Epidemiology of Diabetes Interventions and Complications (DCCT/EDIC) Study showed that a combined cardiovascular and cerebrovascular endpoint was reduced in the intensive treatment group. Although the difference was not significant for any individual component of the main endpoint, the occurrence of each component was lower in the intensive treatment group, including stroke.[87]

Secondary stroke prevention

Once stroke or TIA has occurred, emphasis shifts to preventing recurrent stroke. Patients with diabetes appear to be at higher risk for stroke recurrence. Short-term (30 day) stroke recurrence has been found to be more frequent in patients with than without diabetes (4.88 vs 2.65%, respectively).[88] Other studies have documented increased long-term recurrence rates in diabetes, with a relative risk ratio of approximately 1.7 when compared with people without diabetes.[89–91] Hyperglycaemia at the time of hospitalization for acute ischaemic stroke has also been found to lead to increased risk for stroke recurrence.[92] One relatively large population-based study did not demonstrate an increased risk of stroke recurrence in patients with diabetes, but subjects in this study maintained good glycaemic control following the initial event.[93]

Certainly, risk factor modification as recommended for the primary prevention of stroke should also be pursued in secondary stroke prevention. Detailed descriptions of interventions for glycaemic control, hypertension, hyperlipidaemia, tobacco use and physical inactivity and adiposity are left to other sections of this text. In addition to risk factor modification, specific pharmacological and/or surgical interventions can be implemented to prevent stroke recurrence.

Pharmacological intervention

Antiplatelet agents Until recently, aspirin was the only antiplatelet agent available for secondary stroke prevention. Now, several others – ticlopidine, clopidogrel and dipyridamole – have also been found effective in preventing stroke and other vascular events in patients with cerebrovascular disease. Few of the antiplatelet trials have analysed specific benefit

for patients with diabetes, but data regarding diabetes will be discussed below where available. Otherwise, results from secondary prevention trials in the general stroke population will have to be applied to the management of the diabetic patient.

Aspirin In the Antiplatelet Trialists' (APT) meta-analysis of 145 randomized trials of antiplatelet therapy in non-diabetic and diabetic patients who had already had a major vascular event, the odds reduction for stroke or vascular death attributable to aspirin therapy alone was 25%.[94] This study also analysed differences in response to antiplatelet agents by age, sex and various risk factors. No difference in response was detected based on diabetes status. In a smaller meta-analysis of 10 APT trials that evaluated the benefit of aspirin alone in patients with prior stroke or TIA as entry criteria, aspirin reduced the odds for stroke, myocardial infarction or vascular death by only 16%.[95] Nonetheless, aspirin currently remains the standard initial medical treatment for the secondary prevention of stroke given its low rate of side-effects and low cost.[76] Further trials may help to delineate specific high-risk stroke populations who might benefit more from the selection of alternative antiplatelet agents as an initial step in secondary stroke prevention.

The optimal dose of aspirin for stroke prevention remains somewhat controversial, with doses in randomized clinical trials ranging from 30 mg to 1300 mg daily. Only two trials performed head-to-head comparison of different aspirin doses for general secondary stroke prevention and neither demonstrated difference in efficacy based on aspirin dose.[96,97] Another study performed in the peri-carotid endarterectomy period demonstrated that low-dose aspirin (81 mg and 325 mg groups combined) was superior to high-dose aspirin (650 and 1300 mg groups combined) in preventing stroke, myocardial infarction and death within the first 3 months after endarterectomy.[98] Meta-analysis across all trials of aspirin for secondary stroke prevention has not demonstrated difference in efficacy among high-dose (900–1500 mg day^{-1}), medium-dose (300 mg day^{-1}) and low-dose (50–75 mg day^{-1}) regimens.[99] More favourable side-effect profiles have been seen with low to medium doses, with fewer bleeding events and far fewer gastrointestinal events with lower doses of aspirin.[99] Thus, current guidelines for the use of aspirin in secondary stroke prevention recommend doses between 50 and 325 mg daily.[100,101]

Ticlopidine Ticlopidine is a thienopyridine that inhibits platelet aggregation induced by adenosine phosphate. Two randomized trials have evaluated ticlopidine for secondary stroke prevention. In the Ticlopidine Aspirin Stroke Study (TASS), patients with TIA or minor stroke received ticlopidine 250 mg twice daily or aspirin 650 mg twice daily.[102] The risk for non-fatal stroke or death was 17% in the ticlopidine arm and 19% in the aspirin arm, a small but significant reduction. *Post hoc* analysis of the TASS data examined patient baseline characteristics to determine if treatment effect differed in various subgroups.[103] This analysis indicated that patients with diabetes requiring medical treatment had fewer strokes when treated with ticlopidine (9.4% compared with 17.2% with aspirin). However, caution must be exercised when applying these results clinically since the analysis was not preplanned and included only a small number of patients.

The Canadian American Ticlopidine Study (CATS) compared ticlopidine 250 mg twice daily with placebo in patients with major stroke and demonstrated an absolute risk reduction of 4% for stroke, myocardial infarction and vascular death of in patients treated with ticlopidine (10.8 vs 15.3% with placebo).[104] Taken together, these trials show that ticlopidine significantly reduced the risk for stroke and other vascular outcomes in patients with cerebrovascular disease and TASS demonstrated superiority over aspirin, perhaps with additional benefit seen in patients with diabetes treated with ticlopidine.

In both trials, however, side-effects of diarrhoea and rash were more common in the ticlopidine-treated group and about 4% were unable to tolerate the drug. Severe neutropenia occurred in about 1% of patients receiving ticlopidine, which resulted in recommendations for frequent blood count monitoring during the first 3 months of therapy. More recently, 60 cases of thrombotic thrombocytopenic purpura associated with ticlopidine use have been reported.[105] Ticlopidine's poor side-effect profile and the introduction of newer antiplatelet agents with similar efficacy but minimal adverse effects have led to a substantial reduction in its use for secondary stroke prevention.

Clopidogrel Clopidogrel is a new thienopyridine with a similar mechanism of action as ticlopidine. The Clopidogrel versus Aspirin in Patients at Risk of Ischemic Events (CAPRIE) trial found that the annual combined risk for myocardial infarction, ischaemic stroke or vascular death was 5.32% in clopidogrel-treated patients (75 mg day^{-1}) and 5.83% in patients receiving 325 mg of aspirin daily.[106] The absolute risk reduction of 0.5% for combined vascular endpoints was small but statistically significant. However, for the over 6400 patients entered into CAPRIE with a stroke as the qualifying event, no statistically

significant difference was seen between the treatment groups in the rates of combined endpoint (myocardial infarction, stroke or vascular death). Safety and side-effect profiles were similar for aspirin and clopidogrel. *Post hoc* analysis of the CAPRIE data has been performed to look for additional benefit over aspirin in high-risk patients, but no such analysis specifically examining patients with diabetes has been conducted to date.

The Management of ATherthrombosis with Clopidogrel in High-risk patients (MATCH) study compared the use of clopidogrel alone with the combination of clopidogrel and aspirin.[107] Eligible patients had a recent ischaemic stroke or TIA and one of five factors within the previous 3 years that placed them at high risk of recurrence: previous ischaemic stroke, previous myocardial infarction, angina pectoris, diabetes mellitus or symptomatic peripheral arterial disease. Diabetes was present in 68% of subjects. This study demonstrated no benefit of clopidogrel plus aspirin compared with clopidogrel alone in reducing the primary endpoint of ischaemic stroke, myocardial infarction, vascular death or rehospitalization from a vascular event. The combination did, however, result in a higher risk of life-threatening bleeding complications. Therefore, although there is a role of dual antiplatelet therapy for cardiac prevention, there is no current role in secondary stroke prevention.

Dipyridamole Dipyridamole is a platelet adhesion inhibitor that is postulated to work through interaction with adenosine uptake and inhibition of thromboxane A_2. Until recently, no trials had shown benefit for dipyridamole use in secondary stroke prevention. The Antiplatelet Trialists' meta-analysis found no significant difference in stroke prevention between treatment with dipyridamole and treatment with aspirin, in either patients with or without diabetes, although both agents were superior to placebo.[94] In the European Stroke Prevention Study (ESPS), 216 diabetic patients were treated with dipyridamole and aspirin and had a statistically insignificant reduction in the risk of stroke, all cerebrovascular events and death when compared with placebo.[108] In the VA Cooperative Study, 231 patients with diabetes with recent gangrene and amputation were treated with dipyridamole and aspirin and had a lower incidence of stroke and TIA than the placebo group, but had no reduction in primary vascular endpoints and had a higher mortality rate.[109] More recently, the second European Stroke Prevention Study (ESPS 2) randomized patients with TIA or stroke to one of four treatment arms: placebo, aspirin alone (25 mg twice daily), dipyridamole alone (modified-release formula, 200 mg twice daily) or the combination of aspirin and modified-release dipyridamole.[110] Risk of stroke or death was reduced by 13% with aspirin alone, by 16% with dipyridamole alone and by 24% with the combination therapy, all of which were statistically significant results. However, methodological issues limit the conclusions that can be drawn from this study. No specific subgroup analysis by diabetes status has been performed on the ESPS 2 data. In further support for the combination of aspirin and dipyridamole, the ESPRIT study demonstrated in a non-blinded study that the combination drug was superior to aspirin alone.[111] Interestingly, the study protocol did not specify the exact dose of aspirin or dictate the exclusive use of extended release dipyridamole. One final randomized controlled trial compared the combination of aspirin and dipyridamole with clopidogrel.[112] PRoFESS (Prevention Regimen for Effectively Avoiding Second Strokes) was designed as a non-inferiority study and failed to demonstrate the non-inferiority of aspirin–extended release dipyridamole compared with clopidogrel. The most recent American Heart Association guidelines for secondary stroke prevention state that aspirin alone, aspirin plus extended release dipyridamole and clopidogrel are all 'acceptable options for initial therapy'.[101]

Oral anticoagulant agents As with many of the antiplatelet agents, little is known about the specific role of warfarin in secondary stroke prevention in patients with diabetes. Thus, results from studies of general stroke populations will have to be applied to those with diabetes. The most extensive studies of warfarin for stroke prevention have been done in patients with non-valvular AF and the recommendations for the use of warfarin for primary stroke prevention in the setting of AF, outlined above, should also be applied to secondary prevention. Other indications for warfarin in stroke prevention have been less well studied, such as following myocardial infarction,[113] or with hypercoagulable states.[114] Prospective data are needed before firm treatment recommendations can be made in these clinical settings.

The use of warfarin as compared with aspirin in the general stroke population has been evaluated in a double-blind controlled trial that randomized patients to either low-dose aspirin (30 mg day^{-1}) or relatively high-dose warfarin (INR 3.0–4.5).[115] This trial was terminated prematurely because of a significant excess of major bleeding complications in the warfarin-treated group. The results of this trial clearly indicate that warfarin therapy with an INR between 3.0 and 4.5 is unsafe for secondary prevention in the general stroke population and should not be used in patients with diabetes. Another large, multicentre randomized trial compared the safety and efficacy of moderate-dose warfarin (INR 1.4–2.8) with aspirin 325 mg daily in secondary prevention in the general stroke population (the Warfarin-Aspirin Recurrent Stroke Study).[116] Overall, there was no difference in secondary stroke prevention between the warfarin and aspirin groups. Somewhat surprisingly, there was also no difference in major haemorrhage. The Warfarin and Aspirin for Symptomatic Intracranial Arterial Stenosis (WASID) study, a prospective multicentre, randomized trial, compared warfarin with aspirin in patients with symptomatic intracranial atherosclerotic disease. As would be expected, a sizable minority (over one-third) of patients had diabetes. This study was stopped early due to adverse events in the warfarin group. Although there was no difference by treatment groups in the primary outcome (ischaemic stroke, brain haemorrhage or death from non-stroke vascular cause), death and major haemorrhages were more common in the warfarin group. Therefore, stroke patients with significant symptomatic intracranial atherosclerosis with or without diabetes should not be treated with warfarin for stroke prevention.

Surgical intervention

In addition to risk factor modification and pharmacological therapy, carotid endarterectomy (CEA) may also play a role in secondary stroke prevention in selected patients. Two large, randomized clinical trials, the North American Symptomatic Carotid Endarterectomy Trial (NASCET) and the European Carotid Surgery Trial (ECST), demonstrated marked benefit for CEA in preventing recurrent ipsilateral stroke in symptomatic patients with moderate to severe carotid stenosis.[117–119] The NASCET enrolled patients with 30–99% symptomatic carotid stenosis. In patients with severe (70–99%) stenosis, a dramatic reduction was found in the risk of ipsilateral stroke for patients undergoing CEA and medical treatment as compared with those receiving medical therapy alone (9 vs 26% at 2 years, respectively). The ECST found similar results, although the degree of stenosis for which benefit was documented was somewhat higher (80%). Differences in the outcomes of the two trials are partly explained by the different methods used to calculate degree of stenosis. More recently, the NASCET has also demonstrated a less robust, but statistically significant, benefit for CEA in patients with moderate (50–69%) carotid stenosis: a 15.7% risk of ipsilateral stroke over 5 years among patients treated surgically versus 22.2% in medically managed patients. Patients with less than 50% stenosis did not benefit from CEA.

Although lacunar infarction is thought to be most common in patients with diabetes, extracranial carotid disease may also contribute to cerebrovascular disease among patients with diabetes. A prospective study of patients with diabetes revealed that >50% stenosis was detected in 8.2% of those with diabetes compared with 0.7% of matched controls.[120] Other studies have also documented the association between diabetes and angiographically documented extracranial carotid artery occlusion.[121,122] However, care should be taken in pursuing CEA in some patients with diabetes. *Post hoc* sub group analysis performed on NASCET patients with moderate (50–69%) stenosis revealed that those with diabetes were less likely to benefit from CEA than those without diabetes.[117] Moreover, studies of patients undergoing endarterectomy have shown that diabetics may have increased postoperative mortality, mainly due to higher rates of myocardial infarction.[123]

A possible alternative to CEA is carotid angioplasty and stenting (CAS). Data on stenting compared with CEA are mixed. One study, Stenting and Angioplasty with Protection in Patients at High Risk for Endarterectomy (SAPPHIRE), demonstrated the non-inferiority of stenting compared with CEA for symptomatic patients with >50% stenosis by ultrasound and asymptomatic patients with >80% stenosis by ultrasound who were at high risk for CEA complications.[124] High-risk criteria were based on age >80 years, significant cardiac disease, severe pulmonary disease, contralateral carotid artery occlusion, contralateral larnyngeal nerve palsy, prior neck surgery or radiation and recurrent stenosis after an original CEA. These results support stenting as an alternative to CEA for high-risk symptomatic and asymptomatic patients. Another study, Endarterectomy versus Angioplasty in Patients with Symptomatic Severe Carotid Stenosis (EVA-3S), failed to prove the non-inferiority of stenting in symptomatic patients with carotid stenosis >60%.[125] At 4 years, there were significantly more strokes and death in the stenting group compared with the CEA group.[126] A third study, the Stent-Supported Percutaneous Angioplasty of the Carotid Artery versus Endarterectomy (SPACE), also failed to prove the non-inferiority of stenting for moderate and severe symptomatic patients.[127] Two-year follow-up showed no difference in ipsilateral ischaemic stroke and periprocedural stroke and death.[128] The Carotid Revascularization Endarterectomy Versus Stenting Trial (CREST) is ongoing and should help define the role of stenting in routine use.

Acute stroke treatment

Fundamentals of management
In general, the work-up and treatment of acute stroke in the diabetic patient do not differ greatly from those in the non-diabetic patient. Basic management of the patient with acute stroke begins in the emergency department. The patient should have a rapid evaluation to ensure adequate airway, breathing and circulatory status. Vital signs, including temperature, pulse, blood pressure and oxygen saturation, should be monitored frequently. Endotracheal intubation and mechanical ventilation should be instituted in those patients unable to protect the airway or in those with poor ventilatory drive. Patients with stable respiratory function may receive supplemental oxygen to maintain adequate tissue saturation, since hypoxia may further worsen ischaemia.[129] Rapid determination of blood glucose level should be made in all acute stroke patients to rule out hypo- or hyperglycaemia as a cause for neurological deficit. This is especially important in diabetic patients, who are more predisposed to develop these metabolic abnormalities. Other laboratory work-up includes a complete blood count, chemistry profiles and coagulation studies. A toxicology profile may be ordered in young patients and any others suspected of illicit drug use. An electrocardiogram should be obtained to assess for evidence of arrhythmia or cardiac ischaemia; if clinically indicated, a serum cardiac ischaemia profile may be ordered. A sample emergency department protocol for the initial management of acute ischaemic stroke is provided in Table 22.4.

Treatment of hypertension in acute stroke remains controversial. Mild to moderate elevation of blood pressure is common in the first hours after acute stroke and gradually resolves without intervention.[130,131] Normal cerebral autoregulation is disrupted in acute ischaemia with cerebral perfusion in the ischaemic areas dependent on systemic arterial pressure.[132] Overly aggressive blood pressure reduction to normotensive levels may worsen the ischaemic insult; as such, recent evidence-based guidelines recommend no initial treatment of mild to moderate hypertension in the setting of acute ischaemic stroke.[133] Antihypertensive therapy may be considered, however, in specific clinical settings: prior to and following thrombolytic therapy, in the presence of myocardial ischaemia or aortic dissection or in the setting of hypertensive encephalopathy. For the general ischaemic stroke patient, however, reduction is only necessary for blood pressures >220/120. For potential intravenous thrombolysis candidates, blood pressures should be reduced to just *below* 185/110.

As these general steps are undertaken, specific evaluation for stroke can also begin. History should be obtained to establish time of stroke onset and to elucidate any factors that would preclude treatment with thrombolytics or other agents. Medical history and physical examination, including a careful cardiovascular examination, may suggest stroke

Table 22.4 Emergency department protocol for the initial management of presumed acute ischaemic stroke

1. Obtain vital signs, including temperature, pulse, blood pressure and oxygen saturation; continue to monitor every 15 min
2. Begin continuous cardiac and oxygen saturation monitoring
3. Ensure adequate airway/respiratory status:
   a. Intubate and initiate mechanical ventilation if necessary
   b. Otherwise, begin oxygen at $2\,l\,min^{-1}$ via nasal cannula for O_2 saturation $< 93\%$
4. Intravenous access: 0.9 normal saline at $50-150\,ml\,h^{-1}$ depending on clinical scenario; saline lock in opposite arm
5. STAT laboratory studies:
   a. Serum glucose (may be done at bedside)
   b. Complete blood count with platelet count
   c. Chemistry profile
   d. Coagulation studies (prothrombin time, activated partial thromboplastin time)
   e. Urine pregnancy test for females of childbearing potential
   f. Consider urine toxicology screen
6. Establish patient's weight (measure or estimate)
7. Obtain intravenous pump for possible infusion
8. Order STAT head CT without contrast
9. No aspirin or other antiplatelet agents, heparins or warfarin to be given to potential thrombolytic therapy patients
10. Do not over-treat blood pressure: target $<220/120$ for typical stroke patient and $<185/110$ for thrombolytic candidates.

aetiology. Finally, emergent neuroimaging with computed tomography (CT) should be performed to evaluate for the presence of ICH and for signs of early cerebral oedema.

Acute treatment of hyperglycaemia

Between 25 and 50% of acute stroke patients present with hyperglycaemia,[43,134] and many investigators have questioned whether treatment of hyperglycaemia in this setting might improve outcome. Studies of insulin treatment in animal models of focal ischaemia demonstrate its mitigating effects on infarct volume and neuronal cell loss, both with administration before and after induction of ischaemia.[135] In several models of focal ischaemia, concomitant administration of glucose negated most of the neuroprotective effect of insulin, arguing that almost all the benefit gained from insulin results from reduction of peripheral glucose rather than a primary neuroprotective effect.[136] Moreover, it was shown in a cat model of focal ischaemia that infarct size decreases when normoglycaemia is attained, but increases with hypoglycaemic blood glucose levels.[47] Thus, results from animal stroke models indicate that if insulin is to be used to treat hyperglycaemia in acute stroke, normoglycaemia is the optimal goal.

Hyperglycaemia has also been found to be a marker for mortality in patients with diabetes with acute myocardial infarction, and a randomized trial in patients with diabetes with myocardial infarction demonstrated that glucose–insulin treatment was safe to use in hyperglycaemic patients and also decreased relative mortality rates by 29% (18.6% in the treated group vs 26% in the placebo group).[137,138] Until recently, no similar intervention with insulin–glucose therapy for hyperglycaemia in the setting of acute ischaemic stroke had been attempted. In 1999, the results of the Glucose Insulin in Stroke Trial (GIST) were published.[139] This controlled pilot safety trial randomized 53 acute ischaemic stroke patients who presented within 24 h of symptom onset and had mild to moderate hyperglycaemia (plasma glucose between 7.0 and $17.0\,mmol\,l^{-1}$) to receive either a glucose–potassium–insulin (GKI) infusion or placebo infusion of 0.9% normal saline over 24 h. Patients were excluded if they had cardiac failure, renal failure, severe anaemia, radiographic evidence of pneumonia, coma, previous disabling stroke, haemorrhagic stroke or previously diagnosed insulin-treated diabetes mellitus (type 1 or 2). Treatment consisted of a combined infusion of 500 ml 10% dextrose with 16 U human insulin and 20 mmol potassium chloride, with administration according to a specific protocol based on serum glucose values. Plasma glucose samples were obtained every 8 h and standard bedside glucose strip testing every 2 h, unless serum glucose levels fell below $4\,mmol\,l^{-1}$, in which case monitoring was performed more frequently. Clinical outcomes were assessed using two stroke outcome scales; assessments were not performed in blinded fashion. Fifty patients were included in the final analysis after three were excluded for protocol enrolment violations; 25 patients were in the treatment group and 25 in the placebo group. No significant differences existed between the two groups at baseline.

The main objective of the trial was to assess the feasibility and safety of using a GKI infusion in this acute stroke population. The GKI protocol was not followed accurately in the first two GKI treated patients, but all subsequent patients were treated accurately. The concentration of insulin in the GKI had to be changed at least once in 23 of the 25 GKI patients, with a mean number of changes at 2.5 times (range 1–6). Four of the GKI group required a single dose of 10 ml of 50% glucose for persistent, asymptomatic low test strip glucose values and only one additional patient required similar intervention for symptomatic hypoglycaemia, which resolved promptly with treatment. Plasma glucose levels were non-significantly lowered in the GKI group throughout the infusion period. The 4 week mortality in the GKI group was seven (28%) compared with eight (32%) in the placebo group. There was no statistical difference between the groups in outcome at any time period, although the study was not powered to detect such differences. This study demonstrated that administering a 24 h infusion of GKI was feasible and safe in patients with mild to moderate hyperglycaemia in the setting of acute ischaemic stroke.

The GIST trialists planned a 2400 patient trial to assess the impact of euglycaemia through GKI on all cause mortality at 90 days. Only 933 patients were randomized; trial enrolment ended early due to poor recruitment.[140] Patients had an acute stroke within the prior 24 h and an admission venous plasma glucose concentration between 6.0 and 17.0 mmol l^{-1}. Exclusion criteria included posterior circulation syndrome without physical disability, isolated language dysfunction, insulin-treated diabetes, dementia, symptomatic heart failure, previous disabling stroke, coma, anaemia with a haemoglobin <9 g dl^{-1} and renal failure. The GKI group was treated with a continuous intravenous GKI infusion for a minimum of 24 h to maintain a capillary blood glucose concentration of 4–7 mmol l^{-1}. The control group received 0.9% normal saline at 100 ml h^{-1} for 24 h. If the capillary glucose (assessed every 2 h) exceeded 17 mmol l^{-1}, insulin therapy could be started, at the physician's discretion. Primary intracerebral haemorrhage was present in 11–13%. Mean plasma glucose was significantly lower in the GKI group, with an overall mean difference of 0.57 mmol l^{-1} (95% CI 0.27 to 0.86 mmol l^{-1}). In this underpowered study, there was no difference in deaths at 90 days (30% GKI vs 27% control; $p = 0.37$). The trial did show that the control group had a reduction in glucose with just saline treatment. GKI was shown to reduce glucose but was labour intensive and resulted in hypoglycaemia that required treatment in 16% of patients.

In a recent pilot trial[141] entitled Treatment of Hyperglycaemia In Ischemic Stroke (THIS), 46 patients were randomized to aggressive hyperglycaemic correction (goal blood glucose <130 mg dl^{-1}) versus usual care (goal blood glucose <200 mg dl^{-1}). Those patients treated with aggressive therapy had significantly lower blood glucose results throughout the 72 h trial period but had more hypoglycaemic events. Clinical outcomes were non-significantly better in the aggressive treatment group. A large clinical efficacy trial is currently being planned to test the potential benefits of aggressive hyperglycaemic control in the acute stroke period.

Thrombolytic therapy

Thrombolytic therapy can re-establish cerebral perfusion via recanalization of acutely occluded arteries and may be delivered either intravenously or intra-arterially. To date, only one thrombolytic agent has been approved for use in acute ischaemic stroke. In 1996, the US Food and Drug Administration (FDA) approved recombinant tissue plasminogen activator (rt-PA) for use in specific acute ischaemic stroke patients. The approval was based largely on the results of the National Institute of Neurological Disorders and Stroke (NINDS) rt-PA Stroke Study.[142] Briefly, this was a multicentre, randomized, double-blind, placebo-controlled trial of 624 patients who presented within 3 h of symptom onset. Patients were randomized to receive either intravenous rt-PA (0.9 mg kg^{-1}, maximum dose 90 mg) or placebo. Primary endpoints included 'favourable' outcome (no disability) as measured on four different outcome scales 3 months after stroke. Significantly improved outcome on all four scales was documented for the rt-PA-treated group, with an 11–13% absolute and 30–50% relative increase in favourable outcome and an odds ratio of 1.7 (95% CI 1.2 to 2.8, $p = 0.008$) Treatment with rt-PA was of benefit in all stroke sub-types, including lacunar infarcts. Although there was a statistically significant increase in the rate of symptomatic ICH in the first 36 h in the rt-PA group (6.4 vs 0.6% for the placebo group, $p < 0.001$), there was no difference in mortality between the two groups at 3 months. Following approval of rt-PA in the United States, both the Stroke Council of the American Heart Association and the American Academy of Neurology have issued practice guidelines for the use of rt-PA in acute ischaemic stroke, and these documents outline in detail the inclusion/exclusion criteria for treatment, protocols for delivering the drug and for monitoring and treating hypertension in the setting of thrombolytic therapy.[143,144] In 1997, the NINDS t-PA Stroke Study Group published sub-group analysis from the initial study.[73] Multivariate analysis revealed that diabetes was independently associated with a worse 3 month outcome, but that diabetic patients treated with rt-PA did better than those in the placebo group. This argues that all eligible acute stroke patients in the United States, including diabetic patients, should receive intravenous rt-PA for acute ischaemic stroke. The risk for treatment-associated ICH may be higher in diabetic patients and those patients who present with hyperglycaemia. A recent retrospective study of 138 patients who had received rt-PA for acute ischaemic stroke indicated that elevated baseline serum glucose was an independent predictor of symptomatic ICH, as was a history of diabetes.[145] However, the authors acknowledged that further study of this phenomenon would need to be made before changes in the recommendations for rt-PA use could be made.

The results of European trials of rt-PA for acute ischaemic stroke are conflicting. The initial European Cooperative Acute Stroke Study (ECASS) used a higher dose of rt-PA and a longer 6 h time window for administration; this trial revealed significantly increased ICH rates and no benefit of rt-PA therapy, but the results were compromised by a large percentage of protocol violations.[146] Retrospective analysis of the ECASS intention-to-treat population using the dichotomized NINDS endpoints did reveal a statistically significant improvement in the rt-PA-treated group 3 months after stroke,[147] as did *post hoc* analysis of the ECASS cohort treated within 3 h of symptom onset.[148] The ECASS II study was subsequently undertaken using the lower dose of rt-PA used in the NINDS trial but maintaining the 6 h time window.[149] Like ECASS I, this trial did not demonstrate improved outcome in the rt-PA-treated group at 3 months, although only 158 of the 800 patients were enrolled within 3 h of symptom onset. Symptomatic ICH rates were similar to those seen in the NINDS trial. No subgroup analysis of patients with diabetes was performed for either ECASS trial. As a result of the conflicting results of these trials, no specific recommendations can be made regarding the use of rt-PA in acute stroke patients or in stroke patients with diabetes specifically, outside the United States.

Recently, the ECASS III study results were published.[150] This was the first trial to support the use of intravenous rt-PA for acute ischaemic stroke after 3 h. In ECASS III, patients aged 18–80 years who were last known normal 3–4.5 h prior to treatment were eligible. Exclusion criteria were similar to the European rt-PA treatment criteria, which included an exclusion for patients with a history of both prior stroke and diabetes. Overall, only ~15% of the 821 enrolled subjects had diabetes. Patients enrolled were less severely affected than in the 0–3 h NINDS rt-PA trial. There were more good outcomes at 3 months in the rt-PA group than the placebo group (52.4 vs 45.2%), resulting in a 7% absolute and 16% relative increase in favourable outcome. Use of rt-PA outside the 3 hour window remains off-label and is inconsistent with the most recent AHA guidelines that were published prior to the results of ECASS III.[151] However, a supplement to the guidelines to address the use of rt-PA in the 3–4.5 h window is expected soon.

Several new therapies remain under investigation both in the United States and internationally. Two have completed Phase III trials with promising results: intra-arterial pro-urokinase[152] and an intravenous defibrinogenating agent, ancrod.[153] However, both trials await further scrutiny prior to approval for use in acute ischaemic stroke. Neither trial included pre-planned analysis of a subpopulation with diabetes.

Other acute stroke therapies

A detailed description of other reperfusion, antithrombotic and anticoagulant therapies available for the treatment of acute ischaemic stroke is beyond the scope of this chapter. No sub-group analysis of diabetic patients has been performed in these various trials and further discussion would provide no specific additional information about the acute management of stroke in the diabetic patient. Readers interested in other management therapies available to the general stroke patient are referred to a recent review article on the subject.[154]

References

1 Hankey GJ. Stroke: how large a public health problem and how can the neurologist help? *Arch Neurol* 1999;**56**: 748–754.
2 Broderick J, Brott T, Kothari R, Miller R, Khoury J, Pancioli A, Gebel J, Mills D, Minneci L, Shulka R. The Greater Cincinnati/Northern Kentucky Stroke Study. Preliminary first-ever and total incidence rates of stroke among blacks. *Stroke* 1998;**29**:415–421.
3 Brown RD, Whisnant JP, Sicks JD, O'Fallon WM, Wiebers DO. Stroke incidence, prevalence and survival: secular trends in Rochester, Minnesota, through, 1989. *Stroke* 1996;**27**:373–380.
4 Sudlow CLM, Warlow CP for the International Stroke Incidence Collaboration. Comparable studies of the incidence of stroke and its pathological types. Results from an international collaboration. *Stroke* 1997;**28**:491–499.
5 Isard PA, Forbes JF. The cost of stroke to the National Health Service in Scotland. *Cerebrovasc Dis* 1992;**2**:47–50.
6 Currie CJ, Morgan CL, Gill L, Stott NCH, Peters JR. Epidemiology and costs of acute hospital care for cerebrovascular disease in diabetic and nondiabetic populations. *Stroke* 1997;**28**:1142–1146.
7 American Heart Association. *Heart and Stroke Statistical Update*, American Heart Association, Dallas, TX, 1997.
8 D'Augustino RB, Wolf PA, Belanger AJ, Kannel WB. Stroke risk profile: adjustment for antihypertensive medication. *Stroke* 1994;**25**:40–43.
9 Davis PH, Dambrosia JM, Schoenberg DG, Pritchard BS, Lillienfeld AM, Whisnant JP. Risk factors for ischemic stroke: a prospective study in Rochester. *Minnesota. Ann Neurol* 1987;**22**:40–43.
10 Stamler J, Vaccaro O, Neaton JD, Wentworth D. Diabetes, other risk factors and 12-year cardiovascular mortality for men screened in the Multiple Risk Factor Intervention Trial. *Diabetes Care* 1993;**16**:434–444.
11 Tumilehto J, Rastenyte D, Jousilihti P, Sarti C, Vartiainen E. Diabetes mellitus as a risk factor for death from stroke: prospective study of the middle-aged Finnish population. *Stroke* 1996;**27**:210–215.
12 Abbott RD, Donanue RP, MacMahon SW, Reed DM, Yano K. Diabetes and the risk of stroke: The Honolulu Heart Program. *JAMA* 1987;**257**:949–952.

13 Barrett-Connor E, Khaw KT. Diabetes mellitus: an independent risk factor for stroke? *Am J Epidemiol* 1988;**128**: 116–123.

14 Kuusisto J, Mykkanen L, Pyorala K, Laakso M. Non-insulin dependent diabetes and its metabolic control are important predictors of stroke in elderly subjects. *Stroke* 1994;**25**: 1157–1164.

15 Wannamethee SG, Perry IJ, Shaper AG. Nonfasting serum glucose and insulin concentrations and the risk of stroke. *Stroke* 1999;**30**:1780–1786.

16 Folsom AR, Rasmussen ML, Chambless LE, Howard G, Cooper LS, Schmidt MI, Heiss G. Prospective associations of fasting insulin, body fat distribution and diabetes with risk of ischemic stroke. *Diabetes Care* 1999;**22**: 1077–1083.

17 Kannel WB, McGee DL. Diabetes and cardiovascular disease: The Framingham Study. *JAMA* 1979;**241**:2035–2038.

18 (a) Whisnant JP, Wiebers DO, O'Fallon DM, Sicks JD, Frye RL. A population-based model of risk factors for ischemic stroke: Rochester. Minnesota. *Neurology* 1996;**47**:1420–1428; (b) Whisnant JP, Brown RD, Petty GW, O'Fallon WM, Sicks JD, Wiebers DO. Comparison of population-based models of risk factors for TIA and ischemic stroke. *Nurology* 1999;**53**:532–536; (c) Whisnant JP. Modeling of risk factors for ischemic stroke: The Willis Lecture. *Stroke* 1997;**28**: 1839–1844.

19 Burchfiel CM, Curb JD, Rodriguez BL, Abbott RD, Chiu D, Yano K. Glucose and 22-year stroke incidence: The Honolulu Heart Program. *Stroke* 1994;**25**:951–957.

20 Fuller JH, Shipley MJ, Rose G, Jarrett RJ, Keen H, Mortality from coronary heart disease and stroke in relation to degree of glycaemia: The Whitehall Study. *BMJ* 1983;**287**:861–867.

21 Sandercock PAG, Warlow CP, Jones LN, Starkey IR. Predisposing factors for cerebral infarction: the Oxfordshire Community Stroke Project. *BMJ* 1989;**298**:75–80.

22 Qureshi AI, Giles WH, Croft JB. Impaired glucose tolerance and the likelihood of nonfatal stroke and myocardial infarction. The Third National Health and Nutrition Examination Survey. *Stroke* 1998;**29**:1329–1332.

23 Burchfiel CM, Rodriguea BL, Abbott RD, Sharp DS, Curb JD. Insulin levels and risk of stroke (abstract). *Circulation* 1998;**97**:824.

24 Pyorala M, Miiettinen H, Laakso M, Pyorala K. Hyperinsulinemia and the risk of stroke in healthy middle-aged men: the 22-year follow-up results of the Helsinki Policemen Study. *Stroke* 1998;**29**:1860–1866.

25 Levitan EB, Song Y, Ford ES, Liu S. Is nondiabetic hyperglycemia a risk factor for cardiovascular disease?: a meta-analysis of prospective studies. *Arch Intern Med* 2004;**164**:2147–2155.

26 Coutinho M, Gerstein HC, Wang Y, Yusuf S. The relationship between glucose and incident cardiovascular events. A metaregression analysis of published data from 20 studies of 95,783 individuals followed for 12.4 years. *Diabetes Care* 1999;**22**:233–240.

27 Tanne D, Koren-Morag N, Goldbourt U. fasting plasma glucose and risk of incident ischemic stroke or transient ischemic attacks: a prospective cohort study. *Stroke* 2004;**35**: 2351–2355.

28 Deckert T, Poulsen JE, Larsen M. Prognosis of diabetics with diabetes onset before the age of thirty-one. I. Survival, causes of death and complications. *Diabetologia* 1978;**14**: 363–370.

29 Tunbridge WMG. Factors contributing to deaths of diabetics under fifty years of age. *Lancet* 1981;**ii**(8246): 569–572.

30 Roehmholdt ME, Palumbo PJ, Whisnant JP, Elveback LR. Transient ischemic attack and stoke in a community-based diabetic cohort. *Mayo Clin Proc* 1983;**58**:56–58.

31 Jorgensen HS, Nakayama H, Ranschou HO, Olsen TS. Stroke in patients with diabetes: The Copenhagen Stroke Study. *Stroke* 1994;**25**:1977–1984.

32 Capes SE, Hunt D, Malmberg K, Pathak P, Gerstein HC. Stress hyperglycemia and prognosis of stroke in nondiabetic and diabetic patients: a systematic overview. *Stroke* 2001;**32**:2426–2432.

33 Adams HP, Patman SF, Kassell NF, Torner JC. Prevalence of diabetes mellitus among patients with subarachnoid hemorrhage. *Arch Neurol* 1984;**41**:1033–1035.

34 Alex M, Baron EK, Goldenberg S, Blumenthal HT. An autopsy study of cerebrovascular accident in diabetes mellitus. *Circulation* 1962;**25**:663–673.

35 Aronson SM. Intracranial vascular lesions in patients with diabetes mellitus. *J Neuropathol Exp Neurol* 1973;**32**:183–196.

36 Bell ET. A postmortem study of vascular disease in diabetics. *Arch Pathol* 1952;**53**:444–455.

37 Peress NS, Kane WC, Aronson SM. Central nervous system findings in a tenth decade autopsy population. *Prog Brain Res* 1973;**40**:473–483.

38 Lodder J, Boiten J. Incidence, natural history and risk factors in lacunar infarction. In: *Advances in Neurology, Volume 62: Cerebral Small Artery Disease* (eds P Pullicino, LR Caplan, M Hommel), Raven Press, New York, 1993, pp. 218–219.

39 Arboix A, Marti-Vilalta JL, Garcia JH. Clinical study of 227 patients with lacunar infarcts. *Stroke* 1990;**21**:842–847.

40 Lammie GA, Brannan F, Slattery J, Warlow C. Nonhypertensive cerebral small vessel disease. An autopsy study. *Stroke* 1997;**28**:2222–2229.

41 Lukovits TG, Mazzone T, Gorelick PB. Diabetes mellitus and cerebrovascular disease. *Neuroepidemiology* 1999;**18**: 1–14.

42 Kane WC, Aronson SM. Cerebrovascular disease in an autopsy population. 3. Diminished frequency of cerebral hemorrhage in diabetics. *Trans Am Neur Assoc* 1970;**95**: 266–268.

43 Scott JF, Robinson GM, French JM, O'Connell JE, Alberti KGMM, Gray CS. Prevalence of admission hyperglycemia across clinical subtypes of acute stroke. *Lancet* 1999;**353**: 376–377.

44 van Kooten F, Hoogerbrugge N, Naarding P, Koudstaal PJ. Hyperglycemia in the acute phase of stroke is not caused by stress. *Stroke* 1993;**24**:1129–1132.

45 Weir CJ, Murray GD, Dyker AG, Lees KR. Is hyperglycemia an independent predictor of poor outcome after acute stroke? Results of a long term follow up study. *BMJ* 1997;**314**:1303–1306.

46 Venables G, Miller SA, Gibson G, Hardy J, Strong A. The effects of hyperglycaemia on changes during reperfusion

following focal cerebral ischaemia in cats. *J Neurol Neurosurg Psychiatry* 1985;**48**:663–669.

47 de Courten-Myers GM, Kleinholz M, Wagner KR, Myers RE. Normoglycemia (not hypoglycemia) optimizes outcome from middle cerebral artery occlusion. *J Cereb Blood Flow Metab* 1994;**14**:227–236.

48 Kawai N, Keep RF, Betz AL. Hyperglycemia and the vascular effects of cerebral ischemia. *Stroke* 1997;**28**:149–154.

49 Voll C, Auer R. The effect of postischemic glucose levels on ischemic brain damage in the rat. *Ann Neurol* 1988;**24**:638–644.

50 Collins RC, Dobkin BH, Choi DW. Selective vulnerability of the brain: new insights into the pathophysiology of stroke. *Ann Intern Med* 1989;**110**:992–100.

51 Pulsinelli W, Levy DE, Sigsbee B, Scherer P, Plum F. Increased damage after ischemic stroke in patients with hyperglycemia with or without established diabetes mellitus. *Am J Med* 1983;**74**:540–543.

52 Rehcrona S, Rosen I, Siesjo BK. Brain lactic acidosis and ischemic cell damage: biochemistry and neurophysiology. *J Cereb Blood Flow Metab* 1981;**1**:297–311.

53 Smith ML, VonHanwehr R, Siesjo BK. Changes in extra and intracellular pH in the brain during and following ischemia in hyperglycemic and in moderately hypoglycemic rats. *J Cereb Blood Flow Metab* 1986;**6**:574–583.

54 Berger L, Hakim AM. The association of hyperglycemia with cerebral edema in stroke. *Stroke* 1986;**17**:865–871.

55 Rothman SM, Olaney JW. Glutamate and the pathophysiology of hypoxic–ischemic brain damage. *Ann Neurol* 1986;**19**:105–111.

56 Hickenbottom SL, Grotta JC. Neuroprotective therapy. *Semin Neurol* 1998;**18**:485–492.

57 de Courten-Myers GM, Kleinholz M, Holm P, Schmitt G, Wagner KR, Myers RE. Hemorrhagic infarct conversion in experimental stroke. *Ann Emerg Med* 1992;**21**:120–125.

58 Beghi E, Boglium G, Cavaletti G, Sanguineti I, Tagliabue M, Agostoni F, Macchi I. Hemorrhagic infarction: risk factors, clinical and tomographic features and outcome: a case–control study. *Acta Neurol Scand* 1989;**80**:226–231.

59 Broderick JP, Hagen T, Brott T, Tomsick T. Hyperglycemia and hemorrhagic transformation of cerebral infarcts. *Stroke* 1995;**26**:484–487.

60 Cohen RA. Dysfunction of vascular endothelium in diabetes mellitus. *Circulation* 1993;**87**(Suppl V): V67–V76.

61 Dandona P, James IM, Newburg PA, Wollard ML, Beckett AG. Cerebral blood flow in diabetes mellitus: evidence of abnormal cerebrovascular reactivity. *Br Med J* 1978;ii: 325–326.

62 Johnstone MT, Creager SJ, Scales KM, Cusco JA, Lee BK, Creager MA. Impaired endothelium-dependent vasodilation in patients with insulin-dependent diabetes mellitus. *Circulation* 1993;**88**:2510–2516.

63 Colwell JA, Winocour PD, Halushka PV. Do platelets have anything to do with diabetic microvascular disease? *Diabetes* 1983;**32**(Suppl 2): 14–19.

64 Davi G, Catalano I, Averna M, Notabartolo A, Strano A, Ciabatopi G, Patrono C. Thromboxane biosythesis and platelets in type II diabetes mellitus. *N Engl J Med* 1990;**322**:1769–1744.

65 Barnes AJ, Locke P, Scudder PR, Dormandy TL, Dormandy JA, Slack J. Is hyperviscosity a treatable component of diabetic microcirculatory disease? *Lancet* 1977;**ii**:;789–791.

66 Biller J, Love BB. Diabetes and stroke. *Med Clin North Am* 1993;**77**:95–110.

67 McGill JB, Schneider DJ, Arfken CL, Lucore CL, Sobel BE. Factors responsible for impaired fibrinolysis in obese patients and NIDDM patients. *Diabetes* 1994;**43**:104–109.

68 Lyons TJ. Glycation and oxidation: a role in the pathogenesis of atherosclerosis. *Am J Cardiol* 1993;**71**:26B–31B.

69 Wolffenbuttel BHR, van Haeften TW. Prevention of complications in non-insulin-dependent diabetes mellitus (NIDDM). *Drugs* 1995;**50**:(2):263–288.

70 Koistinaho J, Pasonen S, Yrjanheikki J, Chan PH. Spreading depression-induced gene expression is regulated by plasma glucose. *Stroke* 1999;**30**:114–119.

71 Webster P. The natural history of stroke in diabetic patients. *Acta Med Scand* 1980;**207**:417–424.

72 Bruno A, Biller J, Adams HP, Clarke WWR, Woolson RF, Williams LS, Mansen MD for the Trial of ORG 10172 in Acute Stroke Treatment (TOAST) Investigators. Acute blood glucose level and outcome from ischemic stroke. *Neurology* 1999;**52**:280–284.

73 The NINDS t-PA Stroke Study Group. Generalized efficacy of t-PA for acute stroke: subgroup analysis of the NINDS t-PA Stroke Trial. *Stroke* 1997;**28**:2119–2125.

74 Capes SE. How critical is blood glucose to the outcome of stroke? *Neurol Rev* 1999;**7**:26–30.

75 Baird TA, Parsons MW, Phanh T, Buthcer KS, Desmond PM, Tress BM, Colman PG, Chambers BR, Davis SM. Persistent poststroke hyperglycemia is independently associated with infarct expansion and worse clinical outcome. *Stroke* 2003;**34**:2208–2214.

76 Chaturvedi S, Hickenbottom S, Levine S. Ischemic stroke prevention. *Curr Treat Options Neurol* 1999;**1**:113–125.

77 Goldstein LB, Adams R, Alberts MJ, Appel LJ, Brass LM, Bushnell CD, Culebras A, Degraba TJ, Gorelick PB, Guyton JR, Hart RG, Howard G, Kelly-Hayes M, Nixon JV, Sacco RL. American Heart Association/American Stroke Association Stroke Council, Atherosclerotic Peripheral Vascular Disease Interdisciplinary Working Group, Cardiovascular Nursing Council, Clinical Cardiology Council, Nutrition, Physical Activity and Metabolism Council, Quality of Care and Outcomes Research Interdisciplinary Working Group, American Academy of Neurology. Primary prevention of ischemic stroke: a guideline from the American Heart Association/American Stroke Association Stroke Council: cosponsored by the Atherosclerotic Peripheral Vascular Disease Interdisciplinary Working Group; Cardiovascular Nursing Council; Clinical Cardiology Council; Nutrition, Physical Activity and Metabolism Council; and the Quality of Care and Outcomes Research Interdisciplinary Working Group: the American Academy of Neurology affirms the value of this guideline. *Stroke* 2006;**37**:1583–1633.

78 Davis TME, Millns H, Stratton IM, Holman RR, Turner RC. Risk factors for stroke in type 2 diabetes mellitus: United Kingdom Prospective Diabetes Study (UKPDS) 29. *Arch Int Med* 1999;**159**:1097–1103.

79 Gage BF, Waterman AD, Shannon W, *et al*. Validation of clinical classification schemes for predicting stroke: results from the National Registry of Atrial Fibrillation. *JAMA* 2001;**285**:2864–2870.

80 Peto R, Gray R, Collins R, Wheatley K, Hennekens C, Jamrozik K, Warlow C, Hafner B, Thompson E, Norton S. Randomised trial of prophylactic daily aspirin in British male doctors. *BMJ* 1988;**296**:313–316.

81 Steering Committee of the Physicians' Health Study Research Group. Final report on the aspirin component of the ongoing Physicians' Health Study. *N Engl J Med* 1989;**321**: 129–135.

82 Ridker PM, Cook NR, Lee IM, Gordon D, Gaziano JM, Manson JE, Hennekens CH, Buring JE. A randomized trial of low-dose aspirin in the primary prevention of cardiovascular disease in women. *N Engl J Med* 2005;**352**:1293–1304.

83 He J, Whelton PK, Vu B, Klag MJ, Aspirin and risk for hemorrhagic stroke: a meta-analysis of randomized controlled trials. *JAMA* 1998;**280**:1930–1935.

84 Colwell JA. Aspirin therapy in diabetes. *Diabetes Care* 1997;**20**:1767–1771.

85 Colwell JA. Aspirin and the risk of hemorrhagic stroke. *JAMA* 1999;**282**:731–733.

86 American Diabetes Association. Standards of medical care in diabetes. *Diabetes Care* 2005;**28**:S4–36.

87 The Diabetes Control and Complications Trial/Epidemiology of Diabetes Interventions and Complications (DCCT/EDIC) Study Research Group. Intensive diabetes treatment and cardiovascular disease in patients with type 1 diabetes. *N Engl J Med* 2005;**353**:2643–53.

88 Sacco RL, Foulkes MA, Mohr JP, Worf PA, Hier DB, Price TR. Determinants of early recurrence of cerebral infarction: the Stroke Data Bank. *Stroke* 1989;**20**:983–989.

89 Burn J, Dennis M, Bamford J, Sandercock P, Wade D, Warlow C. Long-term risk of recurrent stroke after a first-ever stroke: the Oxfordshire Community Stroke Project. *Stroke* 1994;**25**:333–337.

90 Hier DB, Foulkes MA, Swiontoniowski M, Sacco RL, Goerlick PB, Mohr JP, Price TR, Wolf PA. Stroke recurrence within 2 years after ischemic infarction. *Stroke* 1991;**22**: 155–161.

91 Petty GW, Brown RD, Whisnant JP, Sicks JD, O'Fallon WM, Wiebers DO. Survival and recurrence after first cerebral infarction: a population-based study in Rochester, Minnesota, 1975–1989. *Neurology* 1998;**50**:208–216.

92 Sacco RL, Shi T, Zamanillo MC, Kargman DE. Predictors of mortality and recurrence after hospitalized cerebral infarction in an urban community: the Northern Manhattan Stroke Study. *Neurology* 1994;**44**:626–634.

93 Lai SM, Alter M, Firday G, Sobel E. A multifactorial analysis of risk factor for recurrence of ischemic stroke. *Stroke* 1994;**25**:958–962.

94 Antiplatelet Trialists' Collaboration. Collaborative overview of randomised trials of antiplatelet therapy. I. Prevention of death, myocardial infarction and stroke by prolonged antiplatelet therapy in various categories of patients. *BMJ* 1994;**308**:81–106.

95 Algre A, van Gijn J. Aspirin at any dose above 30 mg offers only modest protection after cerebral ischaemia. *J Neurol Neurosurg Psychiatry* 1996;**56**:17–25.

96 The Dutch TIA Trial Study Group. A comparison of two doses of aspirin (30 mg vs 283 mg a day) in patients after a transient ischemic attack or minor ischemic stroke. *N Engl J Med* 1991;**325**:1261–1266.

97 UK-TIA Study Group. United Kingdom Transient Ischemic Attack (UK-TIA) aspirin trial: final results. *J Neurol Neurosurg Psychiatry* 1991;**54**:1044–1054.

98 Taylor DW, Barnett HJ, Haynes RB, Ferguson GG, Sackett DL, Thorpe KE, Simard D, Silver FL, Hachinski V, Clagett GP, Barnes R, Spence JD. Low-dose and high-dose acetylsalicylic acid for patients undergoing carotid endarterectomy: a randomised controlled trial. *Lancet* 1999;**353**: 2179–2184.

99 Albers GW, Tijssen JGP. Antiplatelet therapy: new foundations for optimal treatment decisions. *Neurology* 1999;**53**: (Suppl 4): S25–S31.

100 Food and Drug Administration. Internal analgesic, antipyretic and antirheumatic drug products for over-the-counter human use; final rule for professional labeling of aspirin, buffered aspirin and aspirin in combination with antacid drug products. FDA monograph. *Fed Regist* 1998;**63** (205):56802–56819.

101 Sacco RL, Adams R, Albers G, Alberts MJ, Benavente O, Furie K, Goldstein LB, Gorelick P, Halperin J, Harbaugh R, Johnston SC, Katzan I, Kelly-Hayes M, Kenton EJ, Marks M, Schwamm LH, Tomsick T. American Heart Association, American Stroke Association Council on Stroke, Council on Cardiovascular Radiology and Intervention, American Academy of Neurology. Guidelines for prevention of stroke in patients with ischemic stroke or transient ischemic attack: a statement for healthcare professionals from the American Heart Association/American Stroke Association Council on Stroke: co-sponsored by the Council on Cardiovascular Radiology and Intervention: the American Academy of Neurology affirms the value of this guideline. *Stroke* 2006;**37**:577–617.

102 Hass WK, Easton JD, Adams HP, Pryse-Phillips W, Molony BA, Anderson S, Kamm B for the Ticlopidine Aspirin Stroke Study Group. A randomized controlled trial comparing ticlopidine hydrochloride with aspirin for the prevention of stroke in high-risk patients. *N Engl J Med* 1989;**321**: 501–507.

103 Grotta JC, Norris JW, Kamm M and the TASS Baseline and Angiographic Data Subgroup. Prevention of stroke with ticlopidine: who benefits most? *Neurology* 1992;**42**:111–115.

104 Gent M, Blakely JA, Easton JD, Ellis DJ, Hachinski VC, Harbison JW, Panak E, Roberts RS, Sicurella J, Turpie AGG and the CATS Group. The Canadian American Ticlopidine Study (CATS) in thromboembolic stroke. *Lancet* i: 1989;**i**: 1215–1220.

105 Bennett CL, Weinberg PD, Rozenberg-Ben-Dror K, Yarnold PR, Kwaan HC, Green D. Thrombotic thrombocytopenic purpura associated with ticlopidine. A review of 60 cases. *Ann Intern Med* 1998;**128**:541–544.

106 CAPRIE Steering Committee. A randomized, blinded, trial of clopidogrel versus aspirin in patients at risk of ischaemic events (CAPRIE). *Lancet* 1996;**348**:1329–1339.

107 Diener HC, Bogousslavsky J, Brass LM, Cimminiello C, Csiba L, Kaste M, Leys D, Matias-Guiu J, Rupprecht HJ and the MATCH investigators. Aspirin and clopidogrel compared with clopidogrel alone after recent ischaemic stroke or transient ischaemic attack in high-risk patients (MATCH): randomised, double-blind, placebo-controlled trial. *Lancet* 2004;**364**:331–337.

108 Sivenius J, Laakso M, Riekkinen P, Smets P, Lowenthal A. European Stroke Prevention Study: effectiveness of antiplatelet therapy in diabetic patients in secondary prevention of stroke. *Stroke* 1992;**23**:851–854.

109 Colwell JA, Bingham SF, Abraira C, Anderson JW, Comstock JP, Kwaan HC and the Cooperative Study Group. Veterans Administration Cooperative Study on antiplatelet agents in diabetic patients after amputation for gangrene. II. Effects of aspirin and dipyridamole on atherosclerotic vascular disease rates. *Diabetes Care* 1986;**9**:140–148.

110 Diener HC, Cunha L, Forbes C, Sivenius J, Smets P, Lowenthal A. European Stroke Prevention Study 2. Dipyridamole and acetylsalicylic acid in the secondary prevention of stroke. *J Neurol Sci* 1996;**143**:1–13.

111 ESPRIT Study Group. Halkes PH, van Gijn J, Kappelle LJ, Koudstaal PJ, Algra A. Aspirin plus dipyridamole versus aspirin alone after cerebral ischaemia of arterial origin (ESPRIT): randomised controlled trial. *Lancet* 2006;**367**: 1665–1673.

112 Sacco RL, Diener HC, Yusuf S, Cotton D, Ounpuu S, Lawton WA, Palesch Y, Martin RH, Albers GW, Bath P, Bornstein N, Chan BP, Chen ST, Cunha L, Dahlöf B, De Keyser J, Donnan GA, Estol C, Gorelick P, Gu V, Hermansson K, Hilbrich L, Kaste M, Lu C, Machnig T, Pais P, Roberts R, Skvortsova V, Teal P, Toni D, Vandermaelen C, Voigt T, Weber M, Yoon BW and the PRoFESS Study Group. Aspirin and extended-release dipyridamole versus clopidogrel for recurrent stroke. *N Engl J Med* 2008;**359**:1238–1251.

113 Azar AJ, Koudstaal PJ, Wintzen AR, van Bergen PF, Jonker JJ, Deckers JW. Risk of stroke durin long-term anticoagulant therapy in patients after myocardial infarction. *Ann Neurol* 1996;**39**:301–307.

114 Khamashta MA, Cuadrado MJ, Mujic F, *et al.* The management of thrombosis in the antiphospholipid antibody syndrome. *N Engl J Med* 1994;**332**:993–997.

115 The Stroke Prevention in Reversible Ischemia Trials (SPIRIT) Study Group. A randomized trial of anticoagulants versus aspirin after cerebral ischemia of presumed arterial origin. *Ann Neurol* 1997;**42**:857–865.

116 Mohr JP, Thompson JL, Lazar RM, Levin B, Sacco RL, Furie KL, Kistler JP, Albers GW, Pettigrew LC, Adams HP Jr, Jackson CM, Pullicino P and the Warfarin-Aspirin Recurrent Stroke Study Group. A comparison of warfarin and aspirin for the prevention of recurrent ischemic stroke. *N Engl J Med* 2001;**345**:1444–1451.

117 Barnett HJM, Taylor DW, Eliasziw M, Fox AJ, Ferguson GG, Haynes RB, Rankin RN, Clagett GP, Hachinski VC, Sackett DL, Thorpe KE, Meldrum HE for the North American Symptomatic Carotid Endarterectomy Trial Collaborators. Benefit of carotid endarterectomy in patients with symptomatic moderate or severe stenosis. *N Engl J Med* 1998;**339**:1415–1425.

118 European Carotid Surgery Trialists' Collaborative Group. Randomised trial of endarterectomy for recently symptomatic carotid stenosis: final results of the MRC European Carotid Surgery Trial (ECST). *Lancet* 1998;**351**:1379–1387.

119 North American Symptomatic Carotid Endarterectomy Trial Collaborators. Beneficial effect of carotid endarterectomy in symptomatic patients with high-grade carotid stenosis. *N Engl J Med* 1991;**325**:445–453.

120 Kuebler TW, Bendick PJ, Fineberg SE, Markand ON, Norton JA, Vinicor FN, Clark CM. Divetes mellitus and cerebrovascular disease: prevalence and associated risk factors in 482 adult diabetic patients. *Diabetes Care* 1983;**6**:274–278.

121 Bogousslavsky J, Regli F, Van Melle G. Risk factors and concomitants of internal carotid artery occlusion or stenosis. *Arch Neurol* 1985;**42**:864–867.

122 Yasaka M, Yamaguchi T, Shibiri M. Distribution of atherosclerosis and risk factors in atherothrombotic occlusion. *Stroke* 1993;**24**:206–211.

123 Campbell DR, Hoar CS, Wheelock FC. Carotid artery surgery in diabetic patients. *Arch Surg* 1984;**119**:1405–1407.

124 Yadav JS, Wholey MH, Kuntz RE, Fayad P, Katzen BT, Mishkel GJ, Bajwa TK, Whitlow P, Strickman NE, Jaff MR, Popma JJ, Snead DB, Cutlip DE, Firth BG, Ouriel K. Stenting and Angioplasty with Protection in Patients at High Risk for Endarterectomy Investigators. Protected carotid-artery stenting versus endarterectomy in high-risk patients. *N Engl J Med* 2004;**351**:1493–1501.

125 Mas JL, Chatellier G, Beyssen B, Branchereau A, Moulin T, Becquemin JP, Larrue V, Lièvre M, Leys D, Bonneville JF, Watelet J, Pruvo JP, Albucher JF, Viguier A, Piquet P, Garnier P, Viader F, Touzé E, Giroud M, Hosseini H, Pillet JC, Favrole P, Neau JP, Ducrocq X and the EVA-3S Investigators. Endarterectomy versus stenting in patients with symptomatic severe carotid stenosis. *N Engl J Med* 2006;**355**:1660–1671.

126 Mas JL, Trinquart L, Leys D, Albucher JF, Rousseau H, Viguier A, Bossavy JP, Denis B, Piquet P, Garnier P, Viader F, Touzé E, Julia P, Giroud M, Krause D, Hosseini H, Becquemin JP, Hinzelin G, Houdart E, Hénon H, Neau JP, Bracard S, Onnient Y, Padovani R, Chatellier G and the EVA-3S investigators. Endarterectomy Versus Angioplasty in Patients with Symptomatic Severe Carotid Stenosis (EVA-3S) trial: results up to 4 years from a randomised, multicentre trial. *Lancet Neurol* 2008;**7**:885–892.

127 SPACE Collaborative Group, Ringleb PA, Allenberg J, Brückmann H, Eckstein HH, Fraedrich G, Hartmann M, Hennerici M, Jansen O, Klein G, Kunze A, Marx P, Niederkorn K, Schmiedt W, Solymosi L, Stingele R, Zeumer H, Hacke W. 30 day results from the SPACE trial of stent-protected angioplasty versus carotid endarterectomy in symptomatic patients: a randomised non-inferiority trial. *Lancet* 2006;**368**:1239–1247.

128 Eckstein HH, Ringleb P, Allenberg JR, Berger J, Fraedrich G, Hacke W, Hennerici M, Stingele R, Fiehler J, Zeumer H, Jansen O. Results of the Stent-Protected Angioplasty versus Carotid Endarterectomy (SPACE) study to treat symptomatic stenoses at 2 years: a multinational, prospective, randomised trial. *Lancet Neurol* 2008;**7**:893–902.

129 Kwiatkowsi TG, Libman RB. Emergency strategies. In: Primer on *Cerebrovascular Diseases* (eds KMA Welch, LR Caplan, DJ Ries, BK Siesjo, B Weir), Academic Press, San Diego, CA, 1997, p. 672.

130 Broderick J, Brott T, Barsan W, Haley ED, Levy D, Marler J, Sheppard G, Blum C. Blood pressure during the first minutes of focal cerebral ischemia. *Ann Emerg Med* 1993;**22**: 1438–1444.

131 Harper G, Castleden CM, Potter JF. Factors affecting changes in blood pressure after acute stroke. *Stroke* 1994; **25**:1726–1729.

132 Powers W. Acute hypertension after stroke: the scientific basis for treatment decisions. *Neurology* 1993;**43**:461–467.

133 Adams HP, Brott T, Crowell R, Furaln AJ, Gomez CR, Grotta J, Helgason CM, Marler JR, Woolson RF, Zivin JA, Feinberg W, Mayberg M. AHA Medical/Scientific Statement – Guidelines of management of patients with acute ischemic stroke: a statement for healthcare professionals from a special writing committee of the Stroke Council, American Heart Association. *Stroke* 1992;**25**:1901–1914.

134 Scott J, O'Connell J, Gray C. Hyperglycaemia after acute stroke: participants required for trial of treatment with glucose and insulin (letter). *BMJ* 1997;**315**:811.

135 Auer RN. Insulin, blood glucose levels and ischemic brain damage. *Neurology* 1999;**51**(Suppl 3): S39–S43.

136 Hamilton MG, Tranmer BI, Auer RN. Insulin reduction of cerebral infarction due to transient focal ischemia. *J Neurosurg* 1995;**82**:262–268.

137 Malmberg K, Ryden L, Efendic S, Herlitz J, Nicol P, Waldenstrom A, Wedel H, Welin L. Randomized trial of insulin-glucose infusion followed by subcutaneous insulin treatment in diabetic patients with acute myocardial infarction (DIGAMI study). Effects on mortality at 1 year. *J Am Coll Cardiol* 1995;**26**:57–65.

138 Malmberg K, Norhammar A, Wedel H, Ryden L. Glyco-metabolic state at admission: important risk marker of mortality in conventionally treated patients with diabetes mellitus and acute myocardial infarctions. Long-term results from the Diabetes and Insulin–Glucose Infusion in Acute Myocardial Infarction (DIGAMI) study. *Circulation* 1999;**99**:2626–2632.

139 Scott JF, Robinson GM, French JM, O'Connell JE, Alberti KGMM, Gray CS. Glucose potassium insulin infusions in the treatment of acute stroke patients with mild to moderate hyperglycemia. The Glucose Insulin in Stroke Trial (GIST). *Stroke* 1999;**39**:793–799.

140 Gray CS, Hildreth AJ, Sandercock PA, O'Connell JE, Johnston DE, Cartlidge NE, Bamford JM, James OF, Alberti KG and the GIST Trialists Collaboration. Glucose–potassium–insulin infusions in the management of post-stroke hyperglycaemia: the UK Glucose Insulin in Stroke Trial (GIST-UK). *Lancet Neurol* 2007;**6**:397–406.

141 Bruno A, Kent TA, Coull BM, Shankar RR, Saha C, Becker KJ, Kissela BM, Williams LS. Treatment of Hyperglycemia in Ischemic Stroke (THIS). *Stroke* 2007;**39**:384–389.

142 The National Institute of Neurologic Disorders and Stroke (NINDS) rt-PA Stroke Study Group. Tissue plasminogen activator for acute ischemic stroke. *N Engl J Med* 1995;**333**:1581–1587.

143 Adams HP, Brott T, Furlan AJ, Gomez CR, Grotta J, Helgason CM, Kwiatkowski T, Lyden PD, Marler JR, Torner J, Feinberg W, Mayberg M, Thies W. Guidelines for thrombolytic therapy for acute stroke: a supplement for the guidelines for the management of patients with acute ischemic stroke. A statement for healthcare professionals from a special writing group of the Stroke Council of the American Heart Association. *Stroke* 1996;**27**:1711–1718.

144 Quality Standards Subcommittee of the American Academy of Neurology. Report of the Quality Standards Subcommittee of the American Academy of Neurology. Practice advisory: thrombolytic therapy for acute ischemic stroke – summary statement. *Neurology* 1996;**47**:834–839.

145 Demchuk AM, Morgenstern LB, Krieger DW, Chi TL, Hu W, Wein TH, Hardy RJ, Grotta JC, Buchan AM. Serum glucose level and diabetes predict tissue plasminogen activator-related intracerebral hemorrhage in acute ischemic stroke. *Stroke* 1999;**30**:34–39.

146 The European Cooperative Acute Stroke Study (ECASS). Intravenous thrombolysis with recombinant tissue plasminogen activator for acute hemispheric stroke. *JAMA* 1995;**274**:1017–1025.

147 Hacke W, Bluhmki E, Steiner T, Tatlisumark T, Mahagne MH, Sacchetti ML, Meier D. Dichotomized efficacy end points and global end-point analysis applied to the ECASS intention-to-treat data set: *post hoc* analysis of ECASS I. *Stroke* 1998;**29**:2073–2075.

148 Steiner T, Bluhmki E, Kaste M, Toni D, Trouillas P, von Kummer R, Hacke W. The ECASS 3-hour cohort. Secondary analysis of ECASS data by time stratification. ECASS Study Group. European Cooperative Acute Stroke Study. *Cerebrovasc Dis* 1998;**8**:198–203.

149 Hacke W, Kaste M, Fieschi C, von Kummer R, Davalos A, Meier D, Larrue V, Bluhmki E, Davis S, Donnan G, Schneider D, Diez-Tejedor E, Trouillas P. Randomised, double-blind, placebo-controlled trial of thrombolytic therapy with intravenous alteplase in acute ischemic stroke. (ECASS II). Second European–Australian Acute Stroke Study Investigators. *Lancet* 1998;**352**:1245–1251.

150 Hacke W, Kaste M, Bluhmki E, Brozman M, Dávalos A, Guidetti D, Larrue V, Lees KR, Medeghri Z, Machnig T, Schneider D, von Kummer R, Wahlgren N, Toni D, ECASS Investigators. Thrombolysis with alteplase 3 to 4.5 hours after acute ischemic stroke. *N Engl J Med* 2008;**359**:1317–1329.

151 Adams HP, Jr., del Zoppo G, Alberts MJ, Bhatt DL, Brass L, Furlan A, Grubb RL, Higashida RT, Jauch EC, Kidwell C, Lyden PD, Morgenstern LB, Qureshi AI, Rosenwasser RH, Scott PA, Wijdicks EFM. Guidelines for the Early Management of Adults With Ischemic Stroke: A Guideline From the American Heart Association/American Stroke Association Stroke Council, Clinical Cardiology Council, Cardiovascular Radiology and Intervention Council, and the Atherosclerotic Peripheral Vascular Disease and Quality of Care Outcomes in Research Interdisciplinary Working Groups: The American Academy of Neurology affirms the value of this guideline as an educational tool for neurologists. *Stroke* 2007;**38**:1655–1711.

152 Furlan AJ, Higashida R, Wechsler L, Gent M, Rowley H, Kase C, Pessin M, Ahuja A, Cahallan F, Clark WM, Silver F, Rivera F, for the PROACT Investigators. Intra-arterial prourokinase for acute ischemic stroke. The PROACT II study: a randomized controlled trial. *JAMA* 1999;**282**:1999.

153 Sherman DG for the STAT Writers Group. Defibrinogenation with Viprinex™ (ancrod) for the treatment of acute ischemic stroke (abstract) *Stroke* 1999;**30**:234.

154 Hickenbottom SL, Barsan WG. Acute ischemic stroke therapy. *Neurol Clin North Am* 2000;**18**(2):379–397.

23 The management of peripheral arterial disease in patients with type 2 diabetes

Sydney A. Westphal[1], Pasquale J. Palumbo[2]
[1]*Department of Medicine, Maricopa Medical Center, Phoenix, AZ, USA*
[2]*Department of Medicine, Mayo Clinic, Scottsdale, AZ, USA*

Introduction

Peripheral arterial disease (PAD) is atherosclerotic disease of the lower extremities. Occlusion of these arteries results in decreased perfusion to the legs and feet. The earliest and most frequent presenting symptom is intermittent claudication, pain in the leg muscles from inadequate blood flow with walking that is relieved with rest.[1] However, clinical presentation ranges from asymptomatic disease that is found only by objective testing to foot ulcers, rest pain and gangrene.[2] These latter manifestations are problems that increase morbidity and are associated with increased risk for lower extremity amputation. However, the major impact of PAD reaches beyond the problems occurring in the lower extremities. PAD is part of a generalized, ongoing atherogenesis that also includes the coronary and cerebral vasculature. This is why the cause of death in patients with PAD is rarely a direct result of lower extremity disease itself. Instead, typically the cause of death is a stroke or myocardial infarction.[1,2] Even those who have asymptomatic PAD have a mortality risk that exceeds that of the general population.[3,4]

PAD, as with other manifestations of atherosclerotic disease, is much more common in patients with type 2 diabetes than the general population.[5] In addition, patients with both type 2 diabetes and PAD are at even higher risk regarding both lower extremity complications and cardiovascular morbidity and mortality compared with those with PAD who do not have diabetes.[2,4]

In the management of patients with type 2 diabetes and PAD, it is important to keep in mind the systemic nature of the atherosclerosis and to take measures that will prevent the occurrence of cardiovascular events. With respect to disease in the lower extremity itself, management should focus on reducing the symptoms of claudication and preventing its progression to more serious consequences.

Because of the increasing prevalence of type 2 diabetes in the population, the burden of PAD and its complications is likely to rise unless the incidence of PAD can be reduced and its complications prevented. Therefore, it is important for physicians to be aware of what the presence of PAD foreshadows and the potential value of various options for managing these patients.

Epidemiology of PAD in type 2 diabetes and its cardiovascular impact

Having diabetes places a patient at high risk for developing PAD.[4,5] Palumbo *et al.* demonstrated a major role of diabetes and other cardiovascular risk factors in the development and progression of peripheral arterial disease.[6] The population-based Framingham Heart Study found that the risk of developing symptomatic PAD – intermittent claudication – was increased 2–3-fold in patients with diabetes compared with those without diabetes, even when controlling for age and other risk factors of PAD.[7] This study probably underestimated the risk of PAD because many people who have it are asymptomatic. The prevalence of PAD is much higher when sensitive, non-invasive testing such as the ankle brachial index (ABI) is used to determine

The Evidence Base for Diabetes Care, Second Edition, Edited by William H. Herman, Ann Louise Kinmonth, Nicholas J. Wareham and Rhys Williams.

the diagnosis of arterial insufficiency.[8–10] A population-based study of patients with type 2 diabetes showed a prevalence of PAD diagnosed with ABI of 23.5%, which was two times higher than that detected by symptoms.[11] This is similar to clinic-based studies that have reported a prevalence of PAD in type 2 diabetes of 16–22% with non-invasive testing.[10,12]

The presence of PAD by itself, independent of any association with type 2 diabetes, causes an increased risk of major cardiovascular events.[4] The combination of diabetes and PAD places these patients at especially high risk.[3] The Framingham Heart Study found that the risk of coronary heart disease, stroke and heart failure was increased 3–4-fold in women with both intermittent claudication and diabetes compared with either alone.[7] In men with both problems, the risk of stroke doubled and that of congestive heart failure tripled compared with either alone.[7]

Lower extremity problems from PAD

Claudication is the most common symptom of PAD. It restricts the patient's ability to walk and is associated with reduced overall functional ability and quality of life.[13] Longitudinal study of patients with claudication has shown that symptoms will remain stable over 4–9 years in about 75% but will progress in about 25%.[14] If disease progresses in severity to the point that arterial flow cannot meet the needs of the resting tissue, critical leg ischaemia occurs. Critical leg ischaemia is manifested by rest pain, ischaemic ulceration or gangrene.[14] In this situation, the integrity of the limb is threatened and patients are at risk for amputation.

Diabetes magnifies the likelihood of lower limb complications.[15] Type 2 diabetes increases the risk of disease progression.[6,12] Patients with both diabetes and PAD are much more prone to developing critical leg ischaemia and gangrene and to requiring lower extremity amputation.[2] Non-healing foot ulcers and their association with osteomyelitis and gangrene are a major cause of lower extremity amputation in diabetes.[5]

The increased risk of limb-related complications in diabetes is probably multifactorial. The more diffuse nature of the atherosclerosis that tends to occur in diabetes may be one factor.[3] In addition, impaired sensation from diabetic peripheral neuropathy may make the foot more susceptible to traumatic ulceration and infection.[5]

Management of the diabetic foot ulcer in the setting of PAD

PAD in patients with type 2 diabetes is a major contributor to diabetic foot ulcers. Diabetic foot ulcers, especially if they are not healing, should be evaluated for an ischaemic component.[16] This should be done with non-invasive testing such as the ABI. A patient with evidence of arterial insufficiency who has a non-healing ulcer should be referred to a vascular surgeon.[2]

Local management of lower extremity ulcers in patients with type 2 diabetes and PAD includes wound debridement and appropriate dressings. Special foot casts and boots may be helpful in off-loading weight from the affected area.[17]

It has been shown that minor trauma that resulted in ulceration and then the subsequent failure of the ulcer to heal preceded 72% of amputations in patients with diabetes who had underlying PAD.[18] This underscores the importance of paying attention to foot care in all patients with type 2 diabetes and PAD and taking measures that will prevent foot wounds from developing in the first place. Clinical practice recommendations from the American Diabetes Association (ADA) include educating patients about wearing proper shoes and socks, clipping toenails carefully, keeping feet clean and examining feet regularly.[19] Taking these simple precautions would be easier for the patient than dealing with a foot ulcer that otherwise might develop.

Risk factors associated with PAD in type 2 diabetes

The United Kingdom Prospective Diabetes Study (UKPDS) examined risk factors for the development of PAD in type 2 diabetes.[20] PAD was defined as two of the following: ABI <0.8, absence of both dorsalis pedis and posterior tibial pulses to palpation in one or both extremities or intermittent claudication. Study participants who did not have PAD at the time of diagnosis of diabetes were followed for 6 years. Independent risk factors that were identified for developing PAD were increased age, increased HbA_{1c}, elevated systolic blood pressure, low HDL, the presence of cardiovascular disease and smoking.

The coexistence of multiple risk factors increases the risk substantially.[6,21] For example, the relative risk of having PAD in a randomly selected sub-study population of the Veterans Administration-HDL Intervention Trial (VA-HIT) increased from 1.6 in someone with diabetes to 2.5 in someone with both diabetes and hypertension and to 3.9 in someone with diabetes and hypertension who smoked, compared with someone with none of these risk factors.[21] Palumbo *et al.* also reported the adverse impact of coexisting risk factors on the course of PAD.[6]

In general, important risk factors associated with increased risk for developing PAD are similar to those for developing cardiovascular disease – age, hypertension, smoking and lipid abnormalities. These, along with the duration of diabetes, have also been identified as predictors for progression in the lower extremities of PAD in type 2 diabetes.[6,12,22] Many of the risk factors that have been implicated in PAD in type 2 diabetes – smoking, glycaemic control, hypertension and dislipidaemia – are potentially modifiable.

Risk factor modification in the management of PAD of type 2 diabetes

Smoking

The UKPDS found that those with type 2 diabetes who were current smokers increased their likelihood of developing PAD 2.9-fold compared with those who were not smokers.[20] In the general population, a dose-dependent relationship has been found between smoking and severity of PAD.[23] In those with PAD, smoking is associated with disease progression and amputation.[24] In addition, observational studies have reported that the patency of lower extremity bypass grafts is worse in smokers.[25]

A dose-dependent relationship between smoking and risk for coronary heart disease was shown in women with type 2 diabetes in the Nurses' Health Study, a prospective cohort study.[26] Compared with a woman with type 2 diabetes who never smoked, the relative risk for coronary heart disease was 1.21 for a past smoker, 1.66 for someone smoking 1–14 cigarettes per day and 2.68 for someone smoking 15 or more cigarettes per day. Among the women who quit smoking, the risk continued to be high until about 10 years after quitting, when it was similar to those who had never smoked. Others have reported that smoking cessation reduces the risk of all-cause mortality in patients with diabetes but that the risk remains high for several years after quitting and is highly dependent on the duration of smoking.[27]

Because of the marked morbidity and mortality of patients with diabetes who smoke and the fact that smoking cessation has been shown to decrease coronary heart disease risk and risk for all-cause mortality, patients with type 2 diabetes and PAD need to stop smoking.

Hyperglycaemia

The UKPDS demonstrated a direct relationship between the risk of PAD and glycaemia as measured by HbA_{1c} in patients with type 2 diabetes.[20] The lower the HbA_{1c}, the lower is the risk. Each 1% decrease in HbA_{1c} was associated with a 28% decreased risk of

incident PAD, independent of other risk factors for PAD. The UKPDS also demonstrated a correlation between the incidence of cardiovascular events and glycaemic control.[28] These observations suggest that hyperglycaemia contributes to the excess risk of PAD and coronary artery disease seen in patients with type 2 diabetes compared with those without diabetes, and suggest that improved control should decrease the occurrence of PAD and cardiovascular disease. Tight control does lead to a significant reduction in microvascular complications in patients with type 2 diabetes, but this has not been matched with a comparable reduction in macrovascular endpoints.[29] Intensive glycaemic control in patients with type 2 diabetes in the UKPDS had a non-statistically significant reduction in the risk of death or amputation due to PAD. Similarly, the reduction in risk of myocardial infarction did not achieve statistical significance.[29]

There is evidence in patients with type 1 diabetes that tight glycaemic control can reduce macrovascular complications. The Diabetes Control and Complications Trial/Epidemiology of Diabetes Interventions and Complications (DCCT/EDIC) Study, a long-term observation study of the DCCT study cohort, found after a mean follow-up of 17 years, that prior intensive glycaemic control was associated with a significant 57% reduction in relative risk of non-fatal myocardial infarction, stroke or death from cardiovascular cause.[30] This raises the possibility that perhaps studies of longer duration are needed in patients with type 2 diabetes in order to see a beneficial effect of tight glycaemic control that extends to macrovascular complications.

Although hyperglycaemia is a risk factor for PAD and coronary artery disease in type 2 diabetes, treatment of hyperglycaemia alone in these patients has not been shown to prevent macrovascular disease. Nevertheless, good glycaemic control clearly does reduce the risk of microvascular complications and should be attempted at least for this reason.

Hypertension

Prospective observation data from the UKPDS identified elevated systolic blood pressure as an independent risk factor for the development of PAD in type 2 diabetes and demonstrated a direct relationship between the risk of developing PAD and systolic blood pressure over time.[20] Every 10 mmHg decrease in systolic blood pressure was associated with a 25% decrease in the risk of developing PAD and a 16% decrease in the risk of amputation or death from PAD. The lowest risk was in those with a systolic blood pressure of <120 mmHg.[31]

In the UKPDS clinical trial of tight control (mean blood pressure 144/82 mmHg) versus less tight control (mean blood pressure 154/87 mmHg), relative risk of amputation or death from PAD with tight blood pressure control was 0.51 for each, but this did not reach statistical significance ($p = 0.17$ and 0.63, respectively).[32] In addition, a non-statistically significant reduction in myocardial infarction was seen.

The Appropriate Blood Pressure Control in Diabetes (ABCD) Trial was a prospective interventional study that evaluated the effect of intensive versus moderate diastolic blood pressure reduction on complications in type 2 diabetes. *Post hoc* analysis of trial data showed that more intensive blood pressure control (mean 128/75) was more effective than moderate control (mean 137/81 mmHg) for preventing cardiovascular events in patients ($N = 53$) with type 2 diabetes and PAD.[33] The moderately well-controlled group was found to have an inverse relationship between ABI and cardiovascular events that was statistically significant. In the group with intensive blood pressure control, on the other hand, the risk of an event was not increased, even at the lowest ABI values, and was the same as in patients without PAD.[33]

Evidence for the benefit of angiotensin-converting enzyme inhibitors in PAD came from the Heart Outcome Prevention Evaluation (HOPE) Study.[34] Patients enrolled ($N = 9297$) had evidence of vascular disease or diabetes plus one other cardiovascular risk factor. Patients were randomly assigned to the angiotensin-converting enzyme inhibitor ramipril or placebo. The group treated with ramipril had a significant relative risk reduction of the composite endpoint of myocardial infarction, stroke or death from cardiovascular cause of 0.78 over 5 years. Sub-group analyses that included those with PAD ($N = 4051$) and those with diabetes ($N = 3577$) found a beneficial effect with ramipril that was similar to that for the ramipril treatment group as a whole. This benefit was felt to be independent of the small effect (a decrease of 3/2 mmHg) of ramipril on blood pressure, suggesting that the use of angiotensin-converting enzyme inhibitors in these high-risk patients may confer protection against cardiovascular events that goes beyond any effect it may have on blood pressure lowering.

The effects of treating hypertension on cardiovascular events or measures of atherosclerosis in the legs have not been directly studied in patients with both type 2 diabetes and PAD. However, the available data do support the value of tight blood pressure control in these patients in order to decrease their cardiovascular morbidity and mortality.

The use of an angiotensin-converting enzyme inhibitor or angiotensin receptor blocker is recommended by the ADA as first-line therapy in patients with diabetes needing anti-hypertension therapy.[19] Evidence from the HOPE Study actually supports the use of an angiotensin-converting enzyme inhibitor in every patient with type 2 diabetes and PAD.

Clinical trials have shown that it is not uncommon for three or four drugs to be required to reach strict blood pressure targets in patients with type 2 diabetes, so additional classes of anti-hypertensive agents will often need to be used to achieve the ADAs recommended goal of a blood pressure <130/80 mmHg.[19]

Beta-blockers have been considered to be contraindicated in patients with PAD because of concern that they will worsen it. However, a meta-analysis of 11 randomized controlled trials found that beta-blockers do not adversely affect the walking capacity or symptoms of intermittent claudication in patients with mild to moderate PAD.[35] There has also been concern that beta-blockers could blunt hypoglycaemic awareness and thus increase the risk of hypoglycaemia in patients with diabetes. However, in patients with type 2 diabetes, hypoglycaemic unawareness is uncommon and these effects have not been clinically significant.[36] Therefore, beta-blockers can be used safely in patents with PAD and type 2 diabetes.

Hyperlipidaemia

In the Heart Protection Study (HPS), patients ($N = 20\,536$) with coronary artery disease, other occlusive arterial disease or diabetes were randomly allocated to receive simvastatin or placebo.[37] After 5 years of follow-up, the group allocated to simvastatin had a significant reduction of 24% of the composite endpoint of stroke, myocardial infarction, vascular death and revascularization procedures compared with the placebo group. The reduction in event rate was similar and significant both in the subjects who had PAD and in those who had diabetes. Thus, simvastatin had a substantial benefit not only on those already known to have coronary artery disease but also in those without coronary artery disease who had PAD ($p < 0.0001$) or diabetes ($p < 0.001$). Among those with PAD allocated to simvastatin, there was a 19% reduction in risk for a major vascular event compared with those allocated to the placebo group.

In an observational study, patients ($N = 660$) with symptomatic PAD and LDL $\geq 125\,\text{mg dl}^{-1}$ were followed.[38] Those who were on a statin had a significant decrease in new coronary events compared with those who were not at a mean follow-up of 39 months.

The possibility that lipid reduction therapy has beneficial effects on the course of PAD in the legs themselves has been studied. However, many of these intervention studies excluded patients with diabetes.

In one study, patients ($N = 24$) with symptomatic PAD were randomized to 'usual care' versus diet plus cholestyramine, nicotinic acid or clofibrate.[39] After an average follow-up of 19 months, the drug-treated group was shown by arteriography measures to have had a significant reduction in the rate of progression of femoral artery atherosclerosis.

In the Cholesterol-Lowering Atherosclerosis Study (CLAS), patients ($N = 788$) with evidence of both cardiovascular disease and PAD were randomized to placebo or treatment with colestipol and niacin.[40] At 2 years, arteriograms of the femoral arteries showed that the drug treated group was doing significantly better compared with the placebo group.

In the Probucol Quantitative Regression Swedish Trial (QRST), patients ($N = 303$) were treated with diet and cholestyramine and then randomized to receive either placebo or probucol for 3 years.[41] Arteriograms showed that both groups had statistically significant evidence of improvement from baseline, but the use of probucol had no additional benefit.

The Progression on the Surgical Control of the Hyperlipidaemias (POSCH) Study was a randomized trial ($N = 838$) of diet versus diet plus partial ileal bypass surgery for the treatment of hyperlipidaemia.[42] The group treated with surgery had a significant reduction in PAD defined as developing an ABI of <0.95 (relative risk = 0.557) at 5 years of follow-up. This group also had a significant reduction in claudication or limb-threatening ischaemia (relative risk 0.656) compared with the control group. No appreciable differences in progression and regression of PAD by arteriography were seen between the two groups.

In an analysis of patients treated with simvastatin in the Scandinavian Simvastatin Survival Study, relative risk of new claudication or worsening of pre-existing claudication over mean follow-up of 5.4 years was significantly reduced by 38% compared with patients randomly assigned to the placebo group.[43]

In several randomized controlled trials of duration 6–12 months, lovastatin and simvastatin have been shown to improve pain-free walking time significantly in patients with claudication.[44–46]

In general, the authors of these studies have linked the retardation or regression of atherogenesis that was seen in the lower limbs with a reduction in cholesterol and LDL cholesterol values.

There are no data specifically evaluating the effect of lipid-lowering therapy on the course of lower extremity disease in patients with PAD and type 2 diabetes. However, primary and secondary prevention trials have proven the benefit of lipid-lowering therapy in reducing the risk of cardiovascular disease in patients with diabetes.[47–51] These benefits also appear to be tied to the lipid-lowering effects of the drugs. Taken together, the available data suggest that lipid-lowering therapy has benefit in patients with type 2 diabetes and PAD, who usually have coexisting cardiovascular disease, in decreasing cardiovascular morbidity and mortality. In studies of patients without diabetes, it does appear that lipid-lowering therapy slows the atherogenic process in the lower extremity vasculature, not just the coronary arteries, and therefore also has the effect of limiting progression of the disease in the lower extremities and improving function of the legs.

Clinical practice recommendations of the ADA advise an LDL cholesterol goal of $<100\,\mathrm{mg\,dl}^{-1}$ in patients with diabetes. For patients over the age of 40 years, they recommend statin therapy to achieve an LDL cholesterol reduction of 30–40% regardless of the baseline LDL cholesterol.[19]

Anti-platelet therapy

Randomized clinical trials have shown that anti-platelet therapy is effective in preventing occlusive vascular events in a variety of patients who are at increased cardiovascular risk.[52,53] In cardiovascular disease, anti-platelet drugs reduce the risk of non-fatal myocardial infarction, ischaemic stroke and death from vascular causes. Specific studies of anti-thrombotic prophylaxis in patients with type 2 diabetes and PAD are much less common. However, the data that are available from these studies suggest that the benefit of aspirin and other anti-platelet agents may be less in patients with diabetes. One prospective study investigated the effect of aspirin and dipyridamole in preventing disease progression and major vascular events in patients with type 2 diabetes with either recent amputation for gangrene or active gangrene. Patients were randomized to a daily aspirin and dipyridamole or placebo. Anti-platelet therapy had no significant effect on atherosclerotic vascular death or amputations.[54]

In the Early Treatment of Diabetic Retinopathy Study (ETDRS), patients with diabetes were randomized to aspirin 650 mg daily or a placebo.[55] The group treated with aspirin had a significant reduction in risk of myocardial infarction (the relative risk reduction was 0.83) but did not see a statistically significant effect on cardiovascular mortality or stroke.

In a sub-group analysis of patients with type 2 diabetes in the Primary Prevention Project (PPP) Trial, subjects randomized to 100 mg of aspirin and vitamin E daily did not do significantly better than placebo in the composite endpoint of cardiovascular death, stroke and myocardial infarction.[56]

In a meta-analysis of nine randomized trials ($N = 4961$), the odds reduction of serious vascular events (non-fatal myocardial infarction or stroke or vascular death) with anti-platelet drugs (mostly this was with aspirin) in the diabetes sub-group with or without previous vascular events was 7%, which did not reach statistical significance.[53] A meta-analysis of 42 randomized trials ($N = 9214$) of patients with PAD (i.e. intermittent claudication, those having peripheral grafting and those having peripheral angioplasty) showed that the incidence of non-fatal myocardial infarction, non-fatal stroke or vascular death was significantly decreased by 23% with anti-platelet drugs (mostly this was with aspirin).[53] These data favour the use of aspirin in patients with PAD.

Aspirin has been shown to reduce graft failure in patients who have undergone revascularization procedures. The Antiplatelet Trialists' Collaboration (ATTC) found that anti-platelet therapy (mostly this was with aspirin) significantly improved vascular patency in patients with PAD who underwent bypass surgery or peripheral angioplasty.[57]

In the Physicians' Health Study ($N = 22\,071$), a primary prevention trial, the group randomized to one aspirin every other day had a reduced need for peripheral arterial surgery compared with the placebo group.[58] This study included patients with diabetes.

Although aspirin may generally be believed to be effective in patients with type 2 diabetes and PAD, many of the studies on which this feeling is based appear to have been sub-group analysis of trials that included patients with diabetes or meta-analyses of trials including both patients with diabetes and without diabetes instead of trials carried out only in patients with diabetes. Although there are groups who clearly benefit from aspirin, such as prevention in patients without diabetes who have PAD or patients who need secondary cardiovascular prevention, the efficacy of aspirin in patients with type 2 diabetes and PAD is not as clear cut.

According to current recommendations of the ADA, all patients with type 2 diabetes who are at increased cardiovascular risk (so this should apply to patients with PAD) should take aspirin 75–162 mg day^{-1}.[19] In view of data indicating benefit in various high-risk patients who do not have diabetes and since low-dose aspirin is inexpensive and relatively safe, this recommendation is sensible, as even a potentially small benefit would be valuable for these high-risk patients.

The Clopidogrel versus Aspirin in Patients at Risk of Ischemic Events (CAPRIE) Trial compared the antiplatelet agent clopidogrel (75 mg once daily) with aspirin(325 mg once daily) in patients with recent myocardial infarction, ischaemic stroke or symptomatic PAD.[59] Clopidogrel was found to have a significant 8.7% relative risk reduction compared with aspirin for stroke, myocardial infarction or death from vascular cause. In a sub-group analysis of patients with PAD, clopidogrel was associated with a significant 23.8% relative risk reduction compared with aspirin. Based on this study, clopidogrel was approved by the FDA for the prevention of ischaemic events in patients with PAD. The CAPRIE Trial did include patients with diabetes. However, there have been no studies specifically evaluating the value of clopidogrel in patients with type 2 diabetes and PAD.

Clopidogrel is much more expensive than aspirin and therefore does have a cost disadvantage compared with aspirin. The ADA currently recommends that consideration be given to clopidogrel as adjunctive therapy in very high-risk patients with diabetes or as an alternative for patients who cannot tolerate aspirin.[19]

Exercise therapy for intermittent claudication

Prospective studies have demonstrated symptomatic benefit of formal exercise training programs in patients with claudication.[13,60] Typical benefits include improvement in walking speed and distance and overall physical function. Various types of programmes have been used, but the most successful involve a supervised exercise setting, typically modelled after cardiac rehabilitation programmes. One study evaluated the value of walking training specifically in patients with diabetes.[61] Patients with and without diabetes who had PAD and limiting intermittent claudication were enrolled in a supervised walking training programme for 6 months. Symptom-free and maximum walking distance were increased significantly in both. The relative gain in maximum walking distance was 88% greater in those with diabetes. These results suggest that walking training is at least as effective for intermittent claudication in patients with diabetes as in patients without diabetes.

The mechanism for performance improvement has been studied and does not involve changes in PAD that are measurable by ABI. Mechanisms that have been cited as possible explanations for the benefits include improvement in endothelial vasodilation function resulting in improved circulation, decreased oxygen consumption resulting in improved cardiopulmonary function and alterations in gait and walking efficiency resulting in improved walking economy.[13]

Exercise therapy is an effective treatment for intermittent claudication, the primary symptom of PAD and this has also been shown in patients with diabetes. Therefore, this is an option to offer symptomatic patients.

Pharmacological therapy for intermittent claudication

Patients with claudication may also benefit from use of pharmacological therapy. Two medications, pentoxifylline and cilostazol, have been approved by the FDA for use in the United States for intermittent claudication.

Pentoxifylline is felt to exert its effect mainly by improving deformability of erythrocytes.[62] Several meta-analyses of randomized controlled clinical trials of pentoxifylline have been published.[63–65] One of these studies concluded that the limited amount and quality of reported data precluded a reliable estimate of the drug's efficacy.[63] Two of the studies found a significant improvement in pain-free and absolute walking distances.[64,65] The most recent study reported these distances as 21 and 43.8 m, respectively, compared with placebo.[65] Thus, although some investigators have shown a measurable benefit of pentoxifylline compared with placebo, the effect may be small. In addition, none of these reports evaluated the drug specifically in patients with diabetes. Hence further study is needed to determine if pentoxifylline offers a clinically meaningful improvement and if patients with diabetes would have a similar benefit.

Cilostazol is a potent inhibitor of platelet aggregation and promotes vasodilation.[66] Randomized studies have demonstrated that cilostazol is effective in symptomatic treatment of claudication, both versus placebo and versus pentoxifylline.[67–70] In general, cilostazol improves quality of life as assessed by questionnaire and walking distance. A meta-analysis of eight randomized controlled trials of patients with claudication reported that cilostazol increased pain-free walking distance by 67% and maximum walking distance by 50%.[71] Although many of the studies of cilostazol included patients with diabetes, none specifically evaluated its efficacy in these patients. A sub-group analysis of patients with diabetes in studies in the meta-analysis showed that they also achieved increases in pain-free and maximum walking distance. Based on these studies, cilostazol would be an option to consider in patients with type 2 diabetes who need pharmacological therapy for intermittent claudication.

Surgical treatment of PAD

Indications for surgical intervention include ischaemia of the limb resulting in rest pain, ulcers or gangrene.[72,73] Disabling claudication may be considered a relative indication for invasive intervention.[13,72,73]

Bypass grafting and endovascular interventions with stenting or angioplasty are the two main techniques of revascularization. Endovascular intervention may be appropriate for focal disease, for stenosis of large, more proximal arteries and when the procedure is being done for claudication.[2] Published data on invasive vascular intervention in patients with diabetes mostly centre on outcomes with peripheral bypass surgery.

PAD in patients with diabetes is more likely to be associated with tibial and peroneal arterial disease with a sparing of the superficial femoral artery in addition to the foot arteries.[16] This allows for successful bypass to these distal vessels, restoring blood flow to the dorsalis pedis or posterior tibial artery. This below the knee bypass procedure accounts for about 75% of infra-inguinal procedures in patients with diabetes.[2]

Retrospective review of pedal artery bypass surgery has reported this to be an effective, durable option in patients with diabetes with ischaemic foot complications.[74] In addition, in retrospective reviews that compared general groups of patients undergoing peripheral bypass surgery for various reasons, patients with diabetes appeared to do as well as patients without diabetes with respect to the important outcomes of lower extremity revascularization surgery such as late mortality, graft patency and limb salvage.[75,76]

Level of evidence interpretation

Table 23.1 provides a summary of the formal levels of evidence and recommendation grades for the management of PAD in patients with diabetes.[77] Recommendation grades would be higher for most of these interventions if they were being evaluated for patients in general with PAD and not specifically for patients with diabetes and PAD. Thus, the information in this table highlights the lack of clinical trial data in patients with type 2 diabetes and PAD and shows a need for further studies in these patients. In addition, it is important to keep in mind that the recommendation grades for some of these interventions would be higher in patients with diabetes and PAD if other problems for which they are at risk, such as cardiovascular disease or microvascular disease, were being assessed.

Table 23.1 Level of evidence of management of PAD in patients with diabetes[77]

Intervention	Level of evidence	Recommendation grade
Smoking cessation	3	C
Glycaemic control	4	C
Blood pressure control	2	B
Hyperlipidaemia treatment	4	C
Anti-platelet therapy	4	C
Exercise therapy	2	B
Pentoxifylline[a]	-	D
Cilostazol	3	C
Surgery	3	C

[a]Lacked study data on patients with diabetes.

Conclusion

Type 2 diabetes is a major risk factor for PAD. The presence of PAD in these patients, in turn, portends serious cardiovascular consequences, impaired walking ability, increased risk for amputation and poorer quality of life. The most important part of managing PAD in patients with type 2 diabetes is recognizing that coronary artery disease is present in the majority of these patients and therefore taking measures that will prevent the occurrence of myocardial infarction and stroke in these patients. Because of their high cardiovascular risk, patients with type 2 diabetes should be considered candidates for secondary prevention strategies for cardiovascular disease. Proven benefits have been demonstrated from smoking cessation, tight blood pressure control and LDL cholesterol reduction. It is also possible that treatment that lowers LDL cholesterol retards and maybe even causes regression of atherogenesis in the lower extremity vasculature. Other studies provide data supporting the use of angiotensin enzyme inhibitors and the anti-platelet agents aspirin and clopidogrel in these patients.

Walking training has been shown to improve mobility in patients with diabetes and PAD. This, in turn, can improve the patient's quality of life. Cilostazol also appears to improve mobility and functional status in these patients. If peripheral bypass surgery is needed, it appears that diabetes should not be a deterrent.

Of course, the best solution would be one in which patients with type 2 diabetes do not develop PAD. Prevention measures at the primary level would be the most effective way of reducing the morbidity and mortality associated with this disease. Hyperglycaemia, hyperlipidaemia, smoking and hypertension are associated with the subsequent development of PAD in type 2 diabetes and these are all risk factors that could be modified. Minimizing these risk factors right at the start may serve to reduce the occurrence of PAD in this population. Although it seems reasonable to assume that modifying risk factors responsible for atherogenesis will result in primary prevention of PAD, the effectiveness of this approach has not yet been proven. Longitudinal studies with strict control of glucose, lipids and blood pressure at the diagnosis of type 2 diabetes are needed to see if such interventions are indeed effective. If so, this approach to managing PAD in patients with type 2 diabetes should lead to happier, healthier, longer lives for our patients.

References

1 Ouriel K. Peripheral arterial disease. *Lancet* 2001;**358**: 1257–1264.

2 American Diabetes Association. Peripheral arterial disease in people with diabetes. *Diabetes Care* 2003;**26**: 3333–3341.

3 Eberhardt RT, Coffman JD. Cardiovascular morbidity and mortality in peripheral arterial disease. *Curr Drug Targets Cardiovasc Haematol Disord* 2004;**4**:209–217.

4 Leibson CL, Ransom JE, Olson W, Zimmerman BR, O'Fallon WM, Palumbo PJ. Peripheral arterial disease, diabetes and mortality. *Diabetes Care* 2004;**27**:2843–2849.

5 Palumbo PJ, Melton LJ III. Peripheral vascular disease and diabetes. In: *Diabetes in America*, 2nd edn; NIH Publication No. 95-1468, US Government Printing Office, Washington, DC, 1995, Chapter 17.

6 Palumbo PJ, O'Fallon M, Osmundson PJ, Zimmerman BR, Langworthy AL, Kazmier FJ. Progression of peripheral occlusive arterial disease in diabetes mellitus. *Arch Intern Med* 1991;**151**:717–721.

7 Brand FN, Abbott RD, Kannel WB. Diabetes, intermittent claudication and risk of cardiovascular events: The Framingham Study. *Diabetes* 1989;**38**:504–509.

8 Osmundson PJ, O'Fallon WM, Zimmerman BR, Kazmier FJ, Langworthy AL, Palumbo PJ. Course of peripheral occlusive arterial disease in diabetes: Vascular laboratory assessment. *Diabetes Care* 1990;**13**:143–152.

9 McDermott MM, Greenland P, Liu K *et al*. The ankle brachial index is associated with leg function and physical activity: the Walking and Leg Circulation Study. *Ann Intern Med* 2002;**136**:873–883.

10 Kallio M, Forsblom C, Groop P-H *et al*. Development of new peripheral arterial occlusive disease in patients with type 2 diabetes during a mean follow-up of 11 years. *Diabetes Care* 2003;**26**:1241–1245.

11 Walters DP, Gatling W, Mullee MA, Hill RD. The prevalence, detection and epidemiological correlates of peripheral vascular disease: a comparison of diabetic and non-diabetic subjects in an English community. *Diabet Med* 1992;**9**: 710–715.

12 Beach KW, Bedford GR, Bergelin RO et al. Progression of lower-extremity arterial occlusive disease in type II diabetes mellitus. *Diabetes* 1988;**11**:464–472.

13 Stewart KJ, Hiatt WR, Regensteiner JG, Hirsch AT. Exercise training for claudication. *N Engl J Med* 2002;**347**:1941–1951.

14 Hiatt WR. Medical treatment of peripheral arterial disease and claudication. *N Engl J Med* 2001;**344**:1608–1621.

15 Humphrey LL, Palumbo PJ, Butters MA, Hallett JW Jr, Chu C-P, O'Fallon WM, Ballard DJ. The contribution of non-insulin-dependent diabetes to lower-extremity amputation in the community. *Arch Intern Med* 1994;**154**:885–892.

16 LoGerfo Coffman JD. Vascular and microvascular disease in the foot in diabetes. *N Engl J Med* 1984;**311**:1615–1619.

17 American Diabetes Association. Consensus statement. Diabetic foot wound care. *Diabetes Care* 1999;**21**:1354–1360.

18 Pecoraro RE, Reiber GE, Burgess EM. Pathways to diabetic limb amputation: basis for prevention. *Diabetes Care* 1990;**13**: 513–521.

19 American Diabetes Association. Clinical Practice Recommendations 2006. *Diabetes Care* 2006;**29**:S1–S42.

20 Adler AJ, Stevens RJ, Neil A et al. Hyperglycemia and other potentially modifiable risk factors for peripheral vascular disease in type 2 diabetes. UKPDS 59. *Diabetes Care* 2002;**25**:894–899.

21 Papademetriou V, Narayan P, Rubins H et al. Influence of risk factors on peripheral and cerebrovascular disease in men with coronary artery disease, low high-density lipoprotein cholesterol levels and desirable low-density lipoprotein cholesterol levels. *Am Heart J* 1998;**136**:734–740.

22 Bendick PJ, Glover JL, Kuebler TE, Dilley RS. Progression of atherosclerosis in diabetics. *Surgery* 1983;**93**:834–838.

23 Willigendael EM, Teijink JAW, Bartelink ML et al. Influence of smoking on incidence and prevalence of peripheral arterial disease. *J Vasc Surg* 2004;**40**:1158–1165.

24 Lassila R, Lepantalo M. *Cigarette smoking and the outcome after lower limb arterial surgery. Acta Chir Scand* 1988;**154**: 635–640.

25 Myers KA, King RB, Scott DF et al. The effect of smoking on the late patency of arterial reconstructions in the legs. *Br J Surg* 1978;**65**:267–271.

26 Wael KA-D, Manson JE, Solomon CG et al. Smoking and risk of coronary heart disease among women with type 2 diabetes mellitus. *Arch Intern Med* 2002;**162**:273–279.

27 Chaturvedi N, Stevens L, Fuller JH and The World Health Organization Multinational Study Group. Which features of smoking determine mortality risk in former cigarette smokers with diabetes? *Diabetes Care* 1997;**20**:1266–1272.

28 Stratton IM, Adler AI, Neil AW et al. Association of glycaemia with macrovascular and microvascular complications of type 2 diabetes (UKPDS 35): prospective observational study. *BMJ* 2000;**321**:405–412.

29 UK Prospective Diabetes Study (UKPDS) Group. Intensive blood glucose control with sulphonylureas or insulin compared with conventional treatment and risk of complications in patients with type 2 diabetes (UKPDS 33). *Lancet* 1998;**352**:837–853.

30 The Diabetes Control and Complications Trial/Epidemiology of Diabetes Interventions and Complications (DCCT? EDIC) Study Research Group. Intensive diabetes treatment

and cardiovascular disease in patients with type 1 diabetes. *N Engl J Med* 2005;**353**:2643–2653.

31 Adler AI, Stratton IM, Neil AW et al. Association of systolic blood pressure with macrovascular and microvascular complications of type 2 diabetes (UKPDS 36): prospective observation study. *BMJ* 2000;**321**:412–419.

32 UK Prospective Diabetes Study Group. Tight blood pressure control and risk of macrovascular and microvascular complications in type 2 diabetes: UKPDS 38. *BMJ* 1998;**317**: 703–713.

33 Mehler PS, Coll JR, Estacio R. Intensive blood pressure control reduces the risk of cardiovascular events in patients with peripheral arterial disease and type 2 diabetes. *Circulation* 2003;**107**:753–756.

34 The Heart Outcomes Prevention Evaluation Study Investigators. Effects of an angiotensin-converting-enzyme inhibitor, ramipril, on cardiovascular events in high-risk patients. *N Engl J Med* 2000;**342**:145–153.

35 Radack K, Deck C. Beta-adrenergic blocker therapy does not worsen intermittent claudication in subjects with peripheral arterial disease. *Arch Intern Med* 1991;**151**:1769–1776.

36 Lorber DL. Clinical controversies in diabetes: nonglycemic issues. *Practical Diabetology* 2002; September, pp. 22–32.

37 Heart Protection Study Collaborative Group. MRC/BHF Heart Protection Study of cholesterol lowering with simvastatin in 20536 high-risk individuals: a randomized placebo-controlled trial. *Lancet* 2002;**360**:2–3.

38 Aronow WS, Ahn C. Frequency of new coronary events in older persons with peripheral arterial disease and serum low density lipoprotein cholesterol ≥125 mg/dL treated with statins versus no lipid-lowering drug. *Am J Cardiol* 2002; **90**:789–791.

39 Duffield RGM, Miller NE, Brunt JNH et al. Treatment of hyperlipidaemia retards progression of symptomatic femoral atherosclerosis: a randomized controlled trial. *Lancet* 1983**ii**:;639–642.

40 Blankenhorn DH, Azen SP, Crawford DW et al. Effects of colestipol–niacin therapy on muan femoral atherosclerosis. *Circulation* 1991;**83**:438–447.

41 Wallidius G, Erikson U, Olsson AG et al. The effect of probucol on femoral atherosclerosis: The Probucol Quantitative Regression Swedish Trial (PQRST). *Am J Cardiol* 1994;**74**:875–883.

42 Buchwald H, Bourdages HR, Campos CT et al. Impact of cholesterol reduction on peripheral arterial disease in the Program on the Surgical Control of the Hyperlipidemias (POSCH). *Surgery* 1996;**120**:672–679.

43 Pedersen TR, Kjekshus J, Pyorala K et al. Effect of simvastatin on ischemic signs and symptoms in the Scandinavian Simvastatin Survival Study 4ˢ. *Am J Cardiol* 1998;**81**:333–335.

44 Aronow WS, Nayak D, Woodworth S, Ahn C. Effect of simvastatin versus placebo on treadmill exercise time until the onset of intermittent claudication in older patients with peripheral arterial disease at six months and at one year after treatment. *Am J Cardiol* 2003;**92**:711–712.

45 Mondillo S, Ballo P, Barbati R et al. Effects of simvastatin on walking performance and symptoms of intermittent claudication in hypercholesterolemic patients with peripheral vascular disease. *Am J Med* 2003;**114**:359–364.

46 Mohler ER, Hiatt WR, Creager MA for the Study Investigators. Cholesterol reduction with atorvastatin improves walking distance in patients with peripheral arterial disease. *Circulation* 2003;**108**:1481–1486.

47 Pyorala K, Pedersen TR, Kjekshus *et al*. Cholesterol lowering with simvastatin improves prognosis of diabetic patients with coronary heart disease: a sub-group analysis of the Scandinavian Simvastatin Survival Study 4[S]. *Diabetes Care* 1997;**20**:614–620.

48 Goldberg RB, Mellies MJ, Sacks FM *et al*. Cardiovascular events and their reduction with pravastatin in diabetic and glucose intolerant myocardial infarction survivors with average cholesterol levels: sub-group analysis in the cholesterol and recurrent events (CARE) Trial. *Circulation* 1998;**98**:2513–2519.

49 Keech A, Colquhoun D, Best J, Kirby A, Simes RJ, Hunt D, Hague W, Beller E, Arulchelvam M, Baker J, Tonkin A and the LIPID Study Group. Secondary prevention of cardiovascular events with long-term pravastatin in patients with diabetes or impaired fasting glucose results from the LIPID Trial. *Diabetes Care* 2003;**26**:2713–2721.

50 Heart Protection Study Collaborative Group. MRC/BHF Heart Protection Study of cholesterol-lowering with simvastatin in 5963 people with diabetes: a randomized placebo-controlled trial. *Lancet* 2003;**361**:2005–2016.

51 Colhoun HM, Betteridge DJ, Durrington PN *et al*. Primary prevention of cardiovascular disease with atorvastatin in type 2 diabetes in the Collaborative Atorvastatin Diabetes Study (CARDS); multicentre randomized placebo-controlled trial. *Lancet* 2004;**364**:685–696.

52 Antiplatelet Trialists' Collaboration. Collaborative overview of randomized trials of antiplatelet therapy. Prevention of death, myocardial infarction and stroke by prolonged antiplatelet therapy in various categories of patients. *BMJ* 1994;**308**:81–106.

53 Antithrombotic Trialists' Collaboration. Collaborative meta-analysis of randomized trial of antiplatelet therapy for prevention of death, myocardial infarction and stroke in high risk patients. *BMJ* 2002;**324**:71–86.

54 Colwell JA, Bingham SF, Abraira C *et al*. Veterans Administration Cooperative Study on antiplatelet agents in diabetic patients after amputation for gangrene: II. Effects of aspirin and dipyridamole on atherosclerotic vascular disease rates. *Diabetes Care* 1986;**9**:140–148.

55 ETDRS Investigators. Aspirin effects on mortality and morbidity in patients with diabetes mellitus: Early Treatment Diabetic Retinopathy Study Report 14. *JAMA* 1992;**268**: 1292–1300.

56 Sacco M, Pellegrini F, Roncaglioni MC *et al*. Primary prevention of cardiovascular events with low-dose aspirin and vitamin E in type 2 diabetic patients. *Diabetes Care* 2003;**26**: 3264–3272.

57 Antiplatelet Trialists' Collaboration. Collaborative overview of randomized trials of antiplatelet therapy. II: Maintenance of vascular graft or arterial patency by antiplatelet therapy. *BMJ* 1994;**308**:159–168.

58 Goldhaber SZ, Manson JE, Stampfer MJ *et al*. Low-dose and subsequent peripheral arterial surgery in the Physicians' Health Study. *Lancet* 1992;**340**:143–145.

59 CAPRIE Steering Committee. A randomized, blinded, trial of clopidogrel versus aspirin in patients at risk of ischaemic events (CAPRIE). *Lancet* 1996;**348**:1329–1339.

60 Gardner AW, Poehlman ET. Exercise rehabilitation programs for the treatment of claudication pain. *JAMA* 1995;**274**:975–980.

61 Ubels FL, Links TP, Sluiter WJ *et al*. Walking training for intermittent claudication in diabetes. *Diabetes Care* 1999;**22**: 198–201.

62 Samlaska CP, Winfield EA. Pentoxifylline. *J Am Acad Dermatol* 1994;**30**:603–621.

63 Radack K, Wyderski RJ. Conservative management of intermittent claudication. *Ann Intern Med* 1990;**113**:135–146.

64 Hood SC, Moher D, Barber GG. Management of intermittent claudication with pentoxifylline: meta-analysis of randomized controlled trials. *Can Med Assoc J* 1996;**155**:1053–1059.

65 Girolami B, Bernardi E, Prins MH *et al*. Treatment of intermittent claudication with physical training, smoking cessation, pentoxifylline or nafronyl. *Arch Intern Med* 1999;**159**: 337–345.

66 Okuda Y, Kimura Y, Yamashita K. Cilostazol. *Cardiovasc Drug Rev* 1993;**11**:451–465.

67 Money SR, Herd JA, Isaacsohn JL *et al*. Effect of cilostazol on walking distances in patients with intermittent claudication caused by peripheral vascular disease. *J Vasc Surg* 1998;**27**:267–275.

68 Dawson DL, Cutler BS, Meissner MH *et al*. Cilostazol has beneficial effects in treatment of intermittent claudication. *Circulation* 1998;**98**:678–686.

69 Beebe HG, Dawson DL, Cutler BS *et al*. A new pharmacological treatment for intermittent claudication: results of a randomized, multicentric trial. *Arch Intern Med* 1999;**159**: 2041–2050.

70 Dawson DL, Cutler BS, Hiatt WR *et al*. A comparison of cilostazol and pentoxifylline for treating intermittent claudication. *Am J Med* 2000;**109**:523–530.

71 Thompson PD, Zimet R, Forbes WP, Zhang P. Meta-analysis of results from eight randomized, placebo-controlled trials on the effect of cilostazol on patients with intermittent claudication. *Am J Cardiol* 2002;**90**:1314–1319.

72 Coffman JD. Intermittent claudication – be conservative. *N Engl J Med* 1991;**325**:577–578.

73 Weitz JI, Byrne J, Clagett P *et al*. Diagnosis and treatment of chronic arterial insufficiency of the lower extremities: a critical review. *Circulation* 1996;**94**:3026–3049.

74 Pomposelli FB, Kansal N, Hamdan A *et al*. A decade of experience with dorsalis pedis artery bypass: analysis of outcome in more than 1000 cases. *J Vasc Surg* 2003;**37**: 307–315.

75 Akbari C, Pomposelli FB Jr, Gibbons GW. Lower extremity revascularization in diabetes. *Arch Surg* 2000;**135**:452–456.

76 Reed AB, Conte MS, Belkin M *et al*. Usefulness of autogenous bypass grafts originating distal to the groin. *J Vasc Surg* 2002;**35**:48–55.

77 AACE Ad Hoc Task Force for Standardized Production of Clinical Practice Guidelines. American Association of Clinical Endocrinologists protocol for standardized production of clinical practice guidelines. *Endocrine Pract* 2004;**10**: 353–361.

24 Epidemiology of foot ulcers and amputations in people with diabetes: evidence for prevention

Gayle E. Reiber[1], *William R. Ledoux*[2]

[1]*VA Health Services Research and Development and VA Rehabilitation Research and Development Center for Excellence in Limb Loss Prevention and Prosthetic Engineering, VA Puget Sound, and Department of Health Services and Epidemiology, University of Washington, Seattle, WA, USA*
[2]*VA Rehabilitation Research and Development Center for Excellence in Limb Loss Prevention and Prosthetic Engineering, VA Puget Sound, and Department of Orthopaedics and Sports Medicine, University of Washington, Seattle, WA, USA*

Introduction

There are striking increases in diabetes mellitus prevalence in the United States and the rest of the world that portend future increases in serious long-term complications. In 2007, 7.8% of the United States population (24 million people) had diagnosed or undiagnosed diabetes.[1] It is estimated that global diabetes prevalence will more than double between the years 1996 and 2025 from 135 million to 300 million people.[2] Many people with diabetes develop cardiovascular disease, renal failure and lower limb complications, including foot ulcers and amputations.

The cumulative lifetime incidence of a foot ulcer is estimated at 15%.[3] Age-adjusted hospital discharge ulcer rates show the incidence of foot ulcers peaked in 1993 at 8.5 per 1000, decreased to a low of 5.8 per 1000 in 1998 and slowly increased to 6.9 per 1000 in 2003 (Figure 24.1).[4] Foot ulcers may become complicated by infection or gangrene and ultimately result in amputation. Studies report foot ulcers represent 71–84% of the amputations in persons with diabetes.[5,6]

In 2007, over 60% of non-traumatic amputations in the United States were performed in persons with diabetes.[1] Overall age-adjusted incidence of lower limb amputations decreased by over 50% in people with diabetes discharged from short-stay hospitals in the United States from a high of 8.1 per 1000 in 1996 to 3.9 per 1000 in 2005 (Table 24.1).[7]

The purpose of this chapter is to review the analytical and experimental studies concerning risk factors for ulcers and amputations in people with diabetes and to present evidence-based interventions for their prevention. In situations where multiple articles described basic, well-documented, risk factors, the earliest publications were used unless subsequent publications contributed new information. The evidence reviewed for this chapter by a professional medical records librarian was restricted to articles on human subjects that were published in English between 1986 and 2007. We performed a keyword search on 'patient education', 'self management education', 'foot examinations', 'therapeutic footwear' and 'systems of care for foot care delivery'. Evidence-based articles for 'prevention of ulcers' and 'prevention of amputations' were also searched.

The Evidence Base for Diabetes Care, Second Edition, Edited by William H. Herman, Ann Louise Kinmonth, Nicholas J. Wareham and Rhys Williams.
© 2010 John Wiley & Sons, Ltd

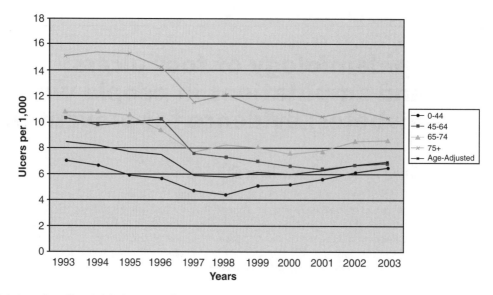

Figure 24.1 Age-adjusted hospital discharge rates for ulcers, inflammation and infection as first diagnosis per 1000 diabetic population, United States, 1993–2003

Risk factors for ulcers and amputations

Ulcers

Foot ulcer prevalence is 3.5-fold higher in people with diabetes compared with people without diabetes. The 1999–2000 NHANES United States population-based study directly observed and measured lower limb disease.[8] Study findings for adults aged ≥40 years reported the prevalence of foot ulcers in people with diabetes as 2.8%.[9,10] There is considerable global variance between published incidence and prevalence for foot ulcers. For example, among people with diabetes and foot ulcers, incidence ranges from 1.2 to 3 per 100 and prevalence from 1.18 to 11 per 100.[6,11–13] This 2.5–6-fold variation in prevalence of foot ulcers among people with diabetes is in part due to the different populations studied, methods of ascertainment and different diagnostic definitions.

Comprehensive surveillance of all outpatient foot ulcers is limited to managed care settings with sophisticated data management systems. Hospital discharge surveillance data for foot ulcers, inflammation and infection, listed as the first reason for discharge in the CDC National Hospital Discharge Survey (NHDS), shows in Figure 24.1 an age-specific decline in incident foot ulcers in short-stay hospitals between

Table 24.1 Age-adjusted hospital discharge rates for non-traumatic lower limb amputations, 1993–2005

Year	Number in thousands	Age-adjusted rate per 1000 with diabetes by level and total				
		Toe	Foot	Transtibial	Transfemoral	Total age-adjusted rate
1993	61	3.4	1.1	2.1	1.0	6.6
1994	67	3.4	1.1	2.3	1.1	6.6
1995	77	3.5	1.3	2.5	1.1	7.6
1996	82	3.6	1.5	2.4	1.2	8.1
1997	84	2.8	1.1	2.0	0.9	6.9
1998	82	2.9	1.1	2.1	1.0	6.6
1999	80	2.7	1.1	1.9	0.9	6.0
2000	81	2.8	0.9	1.9	0.8	5.6
2001	81	2.6	0.8	1.7	0.8	5.2
2002	79	2.5	0.8	1.6	0.7	4.8
2003	75	2.6	0.8	1.5	0.7	4.4
2004	71	2.4	0.7	1.4	0.7	4.1
2005	71	2.3	0.7	1.2	0.6	3.9

Source: Centers for Disease Control and Prevention, Division of Diabetes Translation.[14]

1993 and 2003.[14] Rates are generally highest in older patients, in males compared with females and in blacks compared with whites (data not shown).

Multivariate analyses were employed in several analytical studies to identify independent risk factors for diabetic foot ulcers. Table 24.2 shows that the most commonly reported factors include long duration of diabetes, neuropathy and peripheral arterial disease. Several studies also reported a significantly elevated ulcer risk associated with poor glycaemic control, foot deformity, increased plantar pressure, low high-density lipoprotein (HDL), prior foot ulcers and prior amputations.

Long duration of diabetes is a common although not uniform risk factor for foot ulcers.[11,12,15–20] The development of peripheral neuropathy, which has been associated with hyperglycaemia, was reduced by 69% in intervention patients in the Diabetes Control and Complications Trial (DCCT).[21] This trial also demonstrated that intensive treatment of hyperglycaemia over an average of 6 years reduced the risk of developing retinopathy by 76% and microalbuminuria by 34% in patients without vascular pathology at baseline.

Several of the measures used to quantify peripheral neuropathy were found to predict foot ulcers independently. Three studies found a positive relationship between insensitivity to the Semmes–Weinstein 5.07 mm (10 g) monofilament and ulcers.[16,18,20] However, the study by Abbott et al.[17] reported no relationship between the monofilament test and foot ulcers. They found that both vibration perception threshold and reflex/muscle strength score were significantly related to ulcer development. Other neuropathy risk factors significantly associated with foot ulcers included the neuropathy disability score,[12,22] absent light touch sensation[11] and impaired pain perception.[11]

High plantar pressure has also been linked to ulcer development. In a prospective study of people with diabetes attending a diabetes client foot clinic, Veves et al. used a modified neuropathic deficit score (NDS) to define neuropathy (reduced or absent reflexes and reduced or absent sensation to pain, touch and vibration) in a study of 58 neuropathic and 28 non-neuropathic subjects.[23] Plantar pressure was measured at baseline and again after an average of 35 months. Incidence of neuropathic ulcers was noted. At baseline, 53% of neuropathic and 43% of non-neuropathic patients exhibited high plantar pressure. After follow-up, 34% of neuropathic and 4% of non-neuropathic patients with high pressures developed foot ulcers. However, 55% of diabetic neuropathic patients with high foot pressures did not develop neuropathic ulcers, suggesting that high plantar pressure and insensitivity alone are not sufficient to predict ulcer development.

In a prospective study investigating the relationship between plantar pressure and ulcer development, 248 patients from three large diabetic foot centres were evaluated for peripheral neuropathy, joint mobility, peak plantar pressure and vascular status.[22] Multivariate analyses were conducted to identify ulcer risk factors. After an average of 30 months of follow-up, ulcers had developed in 29% of patients. Persons with ulcers at any site on the foot had significantly more neuropathy and significantly higher foot pressures. The increased pressure and ulcer location were not simultaneously correlated.

The association between peripheral arterial disease and foot ulcer was ascertained using several measures: (1) the ankle–arm index (AAI) (suggesting impaired large vessel perfusion), (2) low transcutaneous oxygen tension ($TcPO_2$) (indicating diminished skin oxygenation) and (3) absent peripheral pulses. In a cohort study, both AAI and $TcPO_2$ were significant ulcer predictors.[18] Absent pulses[11,12] and a history of revascularization (angioplasty or bypass surgery)[12] have also been identified as independent risk factors associated with foot ulcers.

Smoking was not found to be a statistically significant risk factor for foot ulcers in most studies.[11,12,18,22] Moss et al. reported a borderline significant finding in persons diagnosed with early onset diabetes.[15] Smoking is one of the major alterable risk factors implicated in atherosclerosis development in non-diabetic patients along with lipoprotein abnormalities and high blood pressure. These three risk factors are assumed to be similarly atherogenic in persons with diabetes.[24,25] Despite the fact that smoking has not been conclusively linked to ulcer development in persons with diabetes, it is a significant risk factor for many other adverse health outcomes.[26]

High levels of glycosylated haemoglobin (HbA_{1c}) were reported as an ulcer risk factor in only one of three studies addressing this parameter.[15,18,19] Other risk factors commonly associated with risk for ulcer include a history of ulcers and a history of amputation.[12,18]

The number of risk factors was shown to be proportional to development of foot ulcers in a case–control study of Pima Indians.[27] Persons with diabetes who had any risk factor (peripheral neuropathy, peripheral vascular disease, bony deformities and a history of foot ulcers) were 2.1 (95% CI 1.4 to 3.3) times more likely to develop an ulcer than the control subjects, persons with two risk factors were 4.5 (95% CI 2.9 to 6.9) times more likely and persons with three or four risk factors were 9.7 (95% CI 6.3 to 14.8) times more likely to develop a foot ulcer.

Table 24.2 Selected analytical studies of risk factors for diabetic foot ulcers[a]

Study Analysis	Study design Diabetes type	Long DM duration	Neuropathy (monofilament, reflex, vibration or neurological summary score)	Low AAI, TcPO$_2$ or absent pulses	High HbA$_{1c}$	Deformity	Smoking	Ulcer	Amputation
Abbott et al.[17] Cox regression	RCT Patients with VPT ≥ 25; type 1 = 255 type 2 = 780	0	0 Monofilament + VPT + Reflex	Exclusion criteria			Exclusion criteria	Exclusion criteria	Exclusion criteria
Boyko et al.[18] Cox regression	Cohort Veterans type 1 = 48 type 2 = 701	0	+ Monofilament	+ AAI + TcPO$_2$	0	+ Charcot	0	+	+
Kumar et al.[12] Logistic regression	Cross-sectional 811 type 2 from U.K. general practices	+	+ NDS	+ Absent pulses			0	0	0
LeMaster et al.[20] Intention-to-treat RR	RTC Intervention = 41 control = 38	+	[t]Monofilament [t]VPT	0				0	
Litzelman et al.[19] Generalized estimation equations	RTC 352 type 2	0	+	0	0				
Moss et al.[15] Logistic regression	Cohort 2990 patients with early and late-onset diabetes	Borderline older			+		Borderline young		+
Pham et al.[22] Multivariate analyses	Cohort type 1 = 49 type 2 = 199	Control variable	+ NDS + VPT 0 Monofilament + Monofilament	Control variable				0	
Rith-Najarian et al.[16] Chi squared	Cohort 358 type 2 Chippewa Indians	+	+ Monofilament			0			
Walters et al.[11] Logistic regression	Cohort 10 UK general practices, 1077 type 1 = 212 type 2 = 865	+	+ Absent light touch + Impaired pain perception 0 VPT	+ Absent pulses			0	+	

[a] AAI = ankle–arm index; DM = diabetes mellitus; HbA$_{1c}$ = haemoglobin A$_{1c}$; NDS = neuropathy disability score; RCT = randomized control trial; TcPO$_2$ = transcutaneous oxygen tension; VPT = vibration perception threshold; + = statistically significant finding; 0 = no statistically significant finding; t = enrolment criteria; blank cell = not studied.

Amputations

Non-traumatic lower limb amputation hospital discharge rates obtained from the US NHDS from 1993 to 2005 show important decreases in amputations. Between 1996 and 2005, there was a 50% reduction in age-adjusted amputations at both the transtibial (from 2.4 to 1.2 per 1000) and transfemoral level (from 1.2 to 0.6 per 1000). The majority of amputations were performed at the toe and foot level and demonstrate the effect of age, gender and race.[14] The highest amputation discharge rates were in patients 75 years of age or older. After controlling for age, male patients have higher hospital discharge amputation rates than females across all years. Similarly, age-standardized comparisons of blacks and whites showed uniformly higher amputation discharge rates in blacks than whites across this interval.[14]

As with ulcers, several studies employed multivariate analyses to explore the risk factors associated with amputation (Table 24.3). Rigorous analytical studies were selected for inclusion in this chapter to identify the amputation risk factors. Long-term duration of diabetes was found to be statistically significant related to amputation in five of the seven studies assessing this risk factor,[27–31] two others found no relationship[26,32] and one study included duration as a control variable.[33]

Peripheral neuropathy, diagnosed using the methods described above, was a significant independent risk factor in all of the studies measuring this variable.[27,28,30–33] Lack of protective sensation results in diminished patient awareness of painful and potentially harmful stimuli.

Peripheral arterial disease, also diagnosed with methods described previously, was found to be an independent risk factor in all of the studies making direct lower limb assessments.[27,28,31–33] Circulatory problems may also contribute to faulty wound healing.[34]

Findings implicating high blood pressure as a risk factor for lower limb amputation were inconsistent. Three studies reported systolic, diastolic or elevations of both systolic and diastolic blood pressure as independent risk factors for amputation.[26,29,30] However, none of these studies also used a direct measure of peripheral arterial disease. Aspirin use was identified as a significant protective factor decreasing amputation risk.[26]

High fasting plasma glucose or glycosylated haemoglobin was a statistically significant risk factor for amputation in most studies[26–31,33] Poor glycaemic control has been shown to increase the risk of neuropathy.[21]

A history of retinopathy was found to be a risk factor for amputation in most studies.[26–31,33] Retinopathy is thought to reflect the extent of microvascular disease and may be a proxy measure for diabetes severity.[35]

A history of ulcers was found to increase the risk of amputation in three of the four studies that examined this parameter.[26,27,32] Other significant risk factors for amputation included use of insulin,[29,32] elevated cholesterol,[29,31] the presence of urinary proteins[31] and a prior history of amputation.[33] In two studies assessing the case–control impact of prior patient education on amputation risk, findings were mixed. There was a significant protective effect in one study[33] and no significant finding in the other.[29]

Evidence-based research: interventions that prevented ulcers and amputations

Foot-related self-management education

Bloomgarden et al. randomized 749 patients requiring insulin treatment to either a special diabetes education group or to a control group.[36] While the primary study aim was a reduction in HbA$_{1c}$, a secondary aim was reduction of foot lesions. Among the 266 participants who completed the study (average 1.5-year follow-up), there were no significant differences in the frequency of foot lesions between the intervention and control groups.

Malone et al. demonstrated that a simple education programme can be used to lower the incidence of lower extremity ulcers and amputations in patients with diabetes (Table 24.4).[37] Veterans with uninfected foot ulcers were prospectively randomized into two groups: an education group (103 patients, 203 limbs) and a control group with no education (100 patients, 193 limbs). Patients from both groups received the same clinical care, except for a 1 h education class, which consisted of slides depicting infected and amputated limbs and a set of patient care instructions. Following the class, no other education was provided. Follow-up averaged 13.2 months for the education group and 9.2 months the control group. There was a significant reduction in both ulcers and amputations on comparing the education group with the control group, 7/177 amputations in the intervention group and 21/177 in the control group.

In an Australian population, Barth et al. provided 14 h of education over 3 days to 70 patients with diabetes.[38] The intervention group in this study ($n = 32$) then received an additional 9 h of content on foot care over four weekly sessions. Differences in foot care problems including foot ulcers were significantly lower in the intervention group at 1 month, but not at 3 or 6 months.

Foot examinations and physical activity

In a randomized clinical trial in Finland, groups were randomized to podiatric foot care, counselling and

Table 24.3 Selected analytical studies of risk factors for diabetic foot amputation[a]

Study Analysis	Study design Diabetes type	Long DM duration	Neuropathy (monofilament, reflex, vibration)	PAD, AAI, TcPo$_2$ or pulses	HBP	High HbA$_{1c}$	History			Pt Ed
							Smoking	Ulcer	Retinopathy	
Adler et al.[32] Survival analysis	Cohort 776 veterans type 1 = 51 type 2 = 725	0	+	+		0	0	+		
Lee et al.[29] Survival analysis	Cohort 875 type 2 Oklahoma Indians	+			+ SBP male + DBP female	+ Male	0	0	+	0
Lehto et al.[31] Univariate and multivariate regression	Cohort 1044 type 2, Finland	+	+	+	0	+	0		+	
Mayfield et al.[27] Logistic regression	Retrospective case–control 244 type 2 Pima Indians	+	+	+	0	+	0	+	+	
Moss et al.[26] Logistic regression	Cohort 2990 early and late onset, WI, US	0			+ DBP	+	+ Younger	+	+	
Nelson et al.[28] Stratified	Cohort 4399 Pima Indians, AZ, USA, type 2	+	+	+[b]	0	+	0		+	
Reiber et al.[33] Logistic regression	Prospective case–control 316 type 1 and 2 veterans	Control variable	+	+	0	+	0		+	+
Selby and Zhang[30] Logistic regression	Nested retrospective case–control type 1 = 9 type 2 = 390 29 undetermined HMO	+	+		+ SBP	+	0		+	

[a]AAI = ankle–arm index; DBP = diastolic blood pressure; DM = diabetes mellitus; HbA$_{1c}$ = haemoglobin A$_{1c}$; HBP = high blood pressure; Pt Ed = patient outpatient education; PVD = peripheral vascular disease; SBP = systolic blood pressure; TcPO$_2$ = transcutaneous oxygen tension; + = statistically significant finding; 0 = no statistically significant finding; blank cell = not studied.
[b]Medial arterial calcification.

Table 24.4 Effectiveness of foot-related self-management education and foot examinations in reducing foot ulcers and amputations

Study Analysis	Study design Diabetes type	Intervention (groups/arms/comparisons)	Prevent ulcer	Prevent LEA
Foot-related self-management education				
Bloomgarden et al.[36] Analysis of variance	RCT 266 type 1 patients	Intervention group (n = 127) received 9 education sessions and control group (n = 139) received usual care	Non-significant differences in foot lesions including ulcers	
Malone et al.[37] Chi-squared corrected for continuity	RCT 203 veterans, randomized into 2 groups Diabetes type not stated	Group 1, education (n = 90, with 177 limbs) and group 2 (n = 92, with 177 limbs), no education	Invention group had 8/177 ulcers; control group had 26/177 ulcers, p ≤ 0.005	Intervention group had 7/177 amputations; control group had 21/177 amputations, p ≤ 0.025
Barth et al.[38] Multiple linear regression	Prospective intervention Volunteers with type 2 diabetes	Intervention group (n = 38, normal plus intensive education); normal education (14 h over 3 days) plus 4 special foot care sessions over 4 weeks (additional 9 h); provided in groups of 8–10 persons. Control group (n = 32, normal education)	Reduction in foot problems at 1 month, p < 0.006, but no reduction at 6 months Foot problems included foot ulcer	
Foot examinations and activity				
Hamalainen et al.[39]	RCT Type 1 and type 2 diabetes n = 530	Intervention group (n = 267) podiatric care with counselling and primary prevention. Control group (n = 263) written instructions	Non-significant difference	Non-significant difference
Mayfield et al.[40] Logistic regression	Case–control Pima Indians 61 cases, 183 controls type 2	1166 preventive foot examinations over 3 years (foot scans, comprehensive examinations and therapeutic examination)		Benefit of 1 or more foot examinations on amputation risk OR = 0.55 (95% CI 0.2 to 1.7); foot examinations may or may not decrease LEA in Pima Indians

(continued)

Table 24.4 (Continued)

Study Analysis	Study design Diabetes type	Intervention (groups/arms/ comparisons)	Prevent ulcer	Prevent LEA
Lavery et al.[41] Kaplan–Meier survival analysis	Single (physician) blinded, multicentre, randomized trial, type 1 and type 2 diabetes n = 173	Standard therapy (n = 58) Structured foot examination (n = 56) Enhanced therapy (n = 59)	Enhanced therapy had significantly few ulcers (8.5%) than standard therapy (29.3%) or structured foot examination (30.4%)	
LeMaster et al.[20] Kaplan–Meier	Observer blinded RCT 75 type 2 4 type 1	Intervention group (n = 41), leg strengthening, balance, walking programme and follow-up calls; control, usual care	No significant difference in foot ulcer occurrence despite increased activity	

primary prevention or regular care and written foot care instruction. After a 7 year follow-up interval there were no statistically significant reductions in ulcers or amputations.[39]

The effectiveness of foot examinations in reducing the risk of diabetic amputation was studied by Mayfield *et al.* in a case–control study of 61 patients who developed ulcers and 183 controls who did not (Table 24.4).[40] Patient's preventive foot examinations over a 3 year period were classified into three groups: (1) a visual scan to check for breaks in the skin, (2) a comprehensive exam which included a visual examination plus an evaluation for bony deformity, neurological status and vascular status and (3) a therapeutic examination, conducted when a preventive procedure was performed such as callus removal. Persons requiring the fourth type of foot examination, a treatment examination for foot ulcers and lesions, were excluded from this analysis. The odds ratio (OR) of 0.55 (95% CI 0.2 to 1.7, $p = 0.31$) suggested a protective effect from preventive foot examinations yet the confidence interval included 1.

The effectiveness of using an at-home temperature monitoring device was explored by Lavery *et al.* in a physician-blinded, multicentre, randomized trial.[41] Subjects with a previous history of ulcers were randomly assigned to one of three groups: standard therapy, structured foot exams or enhanced therapy. The standard therapy included regular foot examinations, therapeutic footwear and diabetic foot education. The structured foot examination group also received training on how to use a mirror to examine their feet twice per day, whereas the enhanced therapy group was taught to use a digital infrared thermometer to measure foot temperature. If elevated temperatures were present for two consecutive days, this group was instructed to contact the research nurse. After a 15 month follow-up, 17 patients (29.3%) in the standard therapy group and 17 patients (30.4%) in the structured foot examination group developed ulcers, compared with five patients (8.5%) in the enhanced therapy group; this was over a 4-fold increase over the standard (OR 4.5, CI 1.53–13.14) and structured foot examination (OR 4.71, 95% CI 1.60 to 13.85) groups.

In a cohort study, LeMaster et al. dispelled a common misconception that physical activity in persons with peripheral neuropathy would increase the risk of foot ulcers.[42] In this observer-blinded, randomized, controlled trial, LeMaster et al. tested a lower extremity exercise and walking intervention on weight-bearing activity and foot ulcer incidence in people with diabetes and peripheral neuropathy.[20] The study findings show that there was no statistically significant increase in ulcers in the intervention group randomized to increasing daily steps, compared with the usual care group.

Therapeutic footwear

Edmonds *et al.* studied 239 ulcer patients with either ischaemic ($n = 91$) or neuropathic ($n = 148$) ulcers.[43] Subjects were either given therapeutic and custom shoes or wore their own footwear. Among the neuropathic group, 121 subjects reulcerated after an average follow-up time of 26 months. The reulceration rates were 26% among the therapeutic footwear group and 83% among those who wore their own footwear. However, these findings may have been influenced by the inclusion of subjects with severe foot deformities.

Uccioli *et al.* explored the efficacy of therapeutic shoes in preventing reulceration in people with diabetes (Table 24.5).[44] Patients ($n = 69$) with previous ulcers or those at risk for developing ulcers were alternatively allocated into two groups; Group 1 ($n = 36$) wore their ordinary, non-therapeutic shoes, whereas Group 2 ($n = 33$) wore therapeutic shoes with custom-moulded insoles. Ulcer relapses occurred in 58.3% of the group with their own shoes, but only occurred with 27.7% of the patients with therapeutic shoes. The OR was 0.26 (95% CI 0.2 to 1.54, $p = 0.009$) and indicates a protective association between the use of therapeutic shoes and ulcer development in this population.

Reiber *et al.* conducted a randomized clinical trial of 400 men and women from two Western Washington health care organizations.[45] Participants were randomized into one of three study groups. Group 1 ($n = 121$) wore study shoes and customized, medium-density cork inserts with a closed-cell Neoprene cover. Group 2 ($n = 119$) wore study shoes and non-customized medium-density polyurethane inserts with a nylon cover, and the controls in Group 3 ($n = 160$) wore their own footwear. Two-year cumulative reulceration incidence across Groups 1, 2 and 3 was low: 15, 14 and 17%, respectively. Patients in study shoes did not have a significantly lower risk of reulceration compared to controls: Group 1, risk ratio (RR) 0.88 (95% CI 0.51 to 1.52); Group 2, RR 0.85 (95% CI 0.48 to 1.48). All ulcer episodes in study shoes and 88% in non-study shoes occurred in patients with insensate feet. The authors concluded that the study shoes and custom cork or polyurethane inserts conferred no significant ulcer reduction benefit compared with control patients' footwear. This study suggested that careful attention to foot care by providers may be more important than therapeutic footwear. The study did not negate the possibility that special footwear is beneficial in patients with diabetes who do not receive such close attention to foot care by their providers.

Table 24.5 The effectiveness of therapeutic footwear in reducing foot ulcers and amputations

Study Analysis	Study design Diabetes type	Intervention (groups/arms/comparisons)	Prevent ulcer	Prevent LEA
Edmonds et al.[43] Descriptive analysis	Descriptive 148 patients with foot ulcers and sensory loss type 1 = 86 type 2 = 62	Footwear (n = 86), no footwear (n = 35) Follow up averaged 26 months	26% ulcer reduction in footwear group, 83% reulceration in own footwear group	Pre–post amputation reduction of 50% noted
Uccioli et al.[44] Chi-squared	Alternate allocation 69 diabetic patients (type 1 = 17, type 2 = 52) with previous ulcers or high risk of developing ulcers, randomized from 2 Italian teaching hospitals	Group 1 (n = 36): own, non-therapeutic shoes Group 2 (n = 33): therapeutic shoes with custom-moulded insoles 1 year follow-up	Reulceration with intervention shoes = 27.7% versus 58.3% in own footwear OR = 0.26 (95% CI 0.2 to 1.54), p = 0.009	
Reiber et al.[45] Chi-squared, Fisher's exact test	RCT 400 men and women with type 1 or 2 diabetes and a history of foot ulcers from 2 Western Washington health care organizations type 1 = 20 type 2 = 380	Group 1 = 3 pair study shoes and custom inserts Group 2 = 3 pair study shoes and prefabricated polyurethane inserts Group 3 (controls) = own footwear All participants received slippers 2 year follow-up	Ulcer rates comparing study shoes and cork inserts with controls, RR = 0.88 (95% CI 0.51 to 1.52) Ulcer rates comparing study shoes and polyurethane inserts with controls, RR = 0.85 (95% CI 0.48 to 1.48) There was no significant reduction in ulcers	

Table 24.6 The impact of changes in foot care to health care systems on ulcers and amputations in people with diabetes

Study Analysis	Study design Diabetes type	Intervention (groups/arms/ comparisons)	Prevent ulcer	Prevent LEA
Carrington et al.[53] Chi squared and t-test	Retrospective; pre/post comparison Diabetes type not stated	Intervention group: 143 with unilateral lower limb loss; foot care programme based on critical pathway plus lower limb assessment, podiatric care and education Control group: 148 with lower limb loss		15.4% amputations in intervention group, 14% in matched controls No significant difference
Dargis et al.[49] Analysis of variance	Non-randomized 2 year prospective study of patients with diabetes and prior ulcer Intervention = 56, patients control = 89 patients from other geographic areas type 1 = 31 type 2 = 114	Intervention group received multidisciplinary team foot care; control group received regular care	Significant reduction in reulceration between groups (30.4 vs 58.4%), $p < 0.001$	
Edmonds et al.[43] Descriptive analysis	Descriptive 148 patients with neuropathic foot ulcers	Average 26 months follow-up; comprehensive team foot care (inpatient and outpatient); footwear	Reulceration in 26% of patients in special shoes and 83% in own shoes	Pre–post amputation reduction of 50% noted
Larsson and Apelqvist[6] Mann–Whitney, chi-squared	Retrospective 224 126 residents of Lund or Orup Districts, Sweden, with an estimated 2.4% diabetic subjects	Multidisciplinary team to diagnose/prevent/treat diabetic foot ulcers	Not assessed	Decrease in amputations from 7.9/1000 in 1982 to 4.1/1000 in 1993

(continued)

Table 24.6 (*Continued*)

Study Analysis	Study design Diabetes type	Intervention (groups/arms/comparisons)	Prevent ulcer	Prevent LEA
Litzelman et al.[19] Chi-squared	Randomized clinical trial 352 type 2 patients in intercity clinic	Intervention group = 191, control group = 205 Patient interventions = foot care education group with education, behavioural contracting, telephone and postcard prompts Physician interventions = practice guidelines, information on amputation risk factors, foot care practice and prompts	Patients increased self-foot care behaviours Prevented minor lesions Better ulcer detection and documentation in intervention group	Intervention = 0.5%, control = 2.0%, p = 0.20
McCabe et al.[50] Chi-squared	Prospective 2001 patients Diabetes type not stated	Intervention group (n = 1000): for foot screening, examination, 128 high-risk patients in foot protection programme Control group (n = 1000): routine care, 2 year follow-up	Non-significant difference	Non-significant difference for minor amputation Significant reduction in major amputation
Patout et al.[51] Descriptive and cumulative ulcer rates	Pre–post intervention historic controls 197 patients with type 1 or 2 diabetes	Foot outcomes 1 year pre and post LEAP programme. Programme provided components included risk stratified, case managed education, foot care, foot wear Staged diabetes management	Decreased foot ulcer days, hospitalizations, emergency room visits and antibiotics for foot ulcers	Decreased lower limb amputations
Rith-Najarian et al.[52]	Cohort 639 American Indians, MN 98% type 2			Amputation reduction from 29/1000 to 21/1000 to 15/1000 (~50%)

Systems of care changes

Systems approaches have been used to improve health care outcomes in a variety of health care settings (Table 24.6).[46,47] Components for an optimal system for chronic illness care have been identified as (1) coordinated community resources and politics, (2) health care system organization, (3) patient self-management support, (4) provider decision support, (5) health system delivery design and (6) clinical information systems. The ideal foot care system would provide cost-effective care to maintain patient function and quality of life and prevent or delay the development of ulcers and amputation. Foot care systems usually involve multidisciplinary health professionals working as a team. These teams flourish with administrative support and a foot care 'champion.'

The influence of systems of care has been addressed in several historical and analytical studies. In studies published since the mid-1980s, Edmonds and colleagues designed and implemented a specialized foot clinic to manage patients with diabetes from a large referral area in South London. Over a 3 year period this multidisciplinary group demonstrated a high frequency of ulcer healing and a reduction in major amputations.[43]

A population-based retrospective study addressed the impact of a multidisciplinary programme for foot care persons with diabetes.[6] Larsson and Apelqvist[6] noted the total incidence of amputation in persons with diabetes decreased from 7.9 to 4.1 per 1000 over an 11 year interval. This success was attributed to the combination of increased availability of preventive foot care and footwear, a prompt and coordinated evaluation and follow-up of foot problems, increased use of non-invasive vascular testing, greater use of peripheral vascular procedures and strict criteria for amputation level. Falkenberg described similar successes by a multidisciplinary team also in Sweden.[48]

In Lithuania, Dargis et al. allocated 56 patients residing in one city to multidisciplinary foot care team follow-up whereas 89 patients living in 13 other geographic areas received standard care.[49] The foot care intervention included multidisciplinary foot care, footwear, foot care education and re-education on foot problems every 3 months. After 2 years of follow-up, there were significantly fewer recurrent ulcers in the intervention group than the standard treatment group (30 vs 58%).

McCabe et al. selected 2001 people with diabetes and allocated them into two groups.[50] The 1000 targeted for intervention received foot screening, which yielded 128 high-risk patients, who were then enrolled in a foot protection programme. Clinical and administrative data for the control group were used for comparison. After a 2 year follow-up, no significant differences were reported in minor amputations but a significant reduction was reported in major amputations.

Litzelman et al. targeted an intercity population of 395 patients with type 2 diabetes with a multifaceted intervention.[19] Participants received education prior to initiating a behavioural contract for self-foot care. Study staff provided support and reminders. Providers received practice guidelines, foot care flow sheets and prompts to stimulate routine foot examination and education. After a 1 year intervention, there was a statistically significant decrease in serious foot lesions between the intervention and control groups. The providers were significantly more likely to examine feet, document foot findings and refer patients for podiatric services.

Patout et al. instituted a foot care programme and followed 197 patients with diabetes for 1 year.[51] A decrease in foot ulcer days, hospitalizations and emergency room visits was observed over the year when they were in the lower extremity amputation prevention programme compared with their experience in the year prior to the programme.

Rith-Najarian et al. in Minnesota began to follow a cohort of 639 American Indians with diabetes in 1985.[52] After instituting a staged diabetes management programme that included foot evaluations and foot care, a 50% reduction in amputations was documented (from 29 to 15 per 1000).

Carrington et al. targeted patients with a prior unilateral amputation.[53] A special foot care programme was provided to 143 based on critical pathways which included physical assessment, podiatric care and education, and 148 matched controls did not receive this special programme. After a 2 year follow-up there were no significant differences in reamputation frequency between the intervention group and their matched controls.

Conclusion

In summary, prospective research on foot ulcers and amputations in persons with diabetes has identified risk factors common to both conditions: longer diabetes duration, impaired glycaemic control, peripheral neuropathy and peripheral vascular disease. Preventive intervention strategies have been explored and the most promising include patient self management education, digital infrared thermometers for high-risk individuals and alterations in systems of care. These strategies have statistically significantly reduced both ulcers and/or amputations. The effect of two additional preventative strategies, namely foot examinations and therapeutic footwear, is less conclusive, but still may be beneficial in some populations.

Acknowledgements

This research was supported by the Department of Veterans Affairs, Veterans Health Administration, Health Services Research and Development Service and Rehabilitation Research and Development Service.

References

1 CDC. *National Diabetes Fact Sheet*, p. 5 of 14; http://www.cdc.gov/diabetes/pubs/pdf/ndfs_2007.pdf. Accessed 16 December 2008.

2 King H, Aubert RE, Herman WH. Global burden of diabetes, 1995–2025: prevalence, numerical estimates and projections. *Diabetes Care* 1998;**21**:1414–1431.

3 Palumbo PJ, Melton LJ. Peripheral vascular disease and diabetes. In *Diabetes in America* (eds MI Harris, RF Hamman), NIH Publication No. 95-1468, US Government Printing Office, Washington, DC, 1985, Chapter 17.

4 CDC. *Diabetes Data and Trends: Age-Adjusted Hospital Discharge Rates for Ulcer/Inflammation/Infection (ULCER) as First-Listed Diagnosis per 1,000 Diabetic Population, United States, 1980–2003*, 2006;http://www.cdc.gov/diabetes/statistics/hosplea/diabetes_complications/fig2_ulcer.htm. Accessed 16 December 2008.

5 Pecoraro RE, Reiber GE, Burgess EM. Pathways to diabetic limb amputation: basis for prevention. *Diabetes Care* 1990;**13**:513–521.

6 Larsson J, Apelqvist J. Toward less amputations in diabetic patients: incidence, causes, cost, treatment and prevention. *Acta Ort Scand* 1995;**66**:(2):181–192.

7 CDC. *Data and Trends: Crude and Age-Adjusted Hospital Discharge Rates for Nontraumatic Lower Extremity Amputation per 1,000 Diabetic Population, United States, 1980–2005*, 2008; http://www.cdc.gov/diabetes/statistics/lea/fig3.htm. Accessed 17 December 2008.

8 Gregg EW, Sorlie P, Paulose-Ram R *et al.* Prevalence of lower-extremity disease in the U.S. adult population ≥40 years of age with and without diabetes. *Diabetes Care* 2004;**27**:(7):1591–1597.

9 CDC. History of foot ulcer among persons with diabetes – United Sates 2000–2002. *MMWR Morb Mortal Wkly Rep* 2003;**52**:(45):1098–1102.

10 CDC. *History of Foot Ulcer Among Persons with Diabetes – United States, 2000–2002*, 2005;http://www.cdc.gov/mmwr/preview/mmwrhtml/mm5245a3.htm. Accessed 31 January 2005.

11 Walters DP, Gatling W, Mullee MA, Hill RD. The distribution and severity of diabetic foot disease: a community study with comparison to a non-diabetic group. *Diabet Med* 1992;**9**: 354–358.

12 Kumar S, Ashe HA, Parnell LN *et al.* The prevalence of foot ulceration and its correlates in type 2 diabetic patients: a population-based study. *Diabet Med* 1994;**11**:(5):480–484.

13 Ramsey SD, Newton K, Blough D *et al.* Incidence, outcomes and cost of foot ulcers in patients with diabetes. *Diabetes Care* 1999;**22**:(3):382–387.

14 CDC. *Data and Trends: Age-Adjusted Hospital Discharge Rates for Non-traumatic Lower Extremity Amputation per 1,000 Diabetic Population, by Level of Amputation, United States, 1993–2005*, 2008;http://www.cdc.gov/diabetes/statistics/lealevel/fig8.htm. Accessed 16 December 2008.

15 Moss SE, Klein R, Klein BEK. The prevalence and incidence of lower extremity amputation in a diabetic population. *Arch Intern Med* 1992;**152**:(3):610–616.

16 Rith-Najarian SJ, Stolusky T, Gohdes DM. Identifying diabetic patients at high risk for lower-extremity amputation in a primary health care setting. A prospective evaluation of simple screening criteria. *Diabetes Care* 1992;**15**:(10): 1386–1389.

17 Abbott CA, Vileikyte L, Williamson S, Carrington AL, Boulton AJM. Multicenter study of the incidence of and predictive risk factors for diabetic neuropathic foot ulceration. *Diabetes Care* 1998;**21**:1071–1075.

18 Boyko EJ, Ahroni JH, Stensel V, Forsberg RC, Davignon DR, Smith DG. A prospective study of risk factors for diabetic foot ulcer. The Seattle Diabetic Foot Study. *Diabetes Care* 1999;**22**: (7):1036–1042.

19 Litzelman DK, Slemenda CW, Langefeld CD *et al.* Reduction of lower extremity clinical abnormalities in patients with non-insulin-dependent diabetes mellitus. A randomized, controlled trial. *Ann Intern Med* 1993;**119**:(1):36–41.

20 LeMaster JW, Mueller MJ, Reiber GE, Mehr DR, Madsen RW, Conn VS. Effect of weight-bearing activity on foot ulcer incidence in people with diabetic peripheral neuropathy: feet first randomized controlled trial. *Phys Ther* 2008;**88**: (11):1385–1398.

21 Diabetes Control and Complications Trial Research Group. The effect of intensive treatment of diabetes on the development and progression of long-term complications in insulin-dependent diabetes mellitus. *N Engl J Med* 1993;**329**:(14): 977–986.

22 Pham H, Armstrong DG, Harvey C, Harkless LB, Giurini JM, Veves A. Screening techniques to identify people at high risk for diabetic foot ulceration: a prospective multicenter trial. *Diabetes Care* 2000;**23**:(5):606–611.

23 Veves A, Murray HJ, Young MJ, Boulton AJM. The risk of foot ulceration in diabetic patients with high foot pressure: a prospective study. *Diabetologia* 1992;**35**:(7):660–663.

24 Gordon T, Kannel WB. The Framingham Study: predisposition to atherosclerosis in the head, heart and legs. *JAMA* 1972;**221**:661–666.

25 Kannel WB, McGee DL. Diabetes and cardiovascular disease: The Framingham Study. *JAMA* 1979;**241**:(19):2035–2038.

26 Moss SE, Klein R, Klein BE. The 14-year incidence of lower-extremity amputations in a diabetic population. The

Wisconsin Epidemiologic Study of Diabetic Retinopathy. *Diabetes Care* 1999;**22**:(6):951–959.

27 Mayfield JA, Reiber GE, Nelson RG, Greene T. A foot risk classification system to predict diabetic amputation in Pima Indians. *Diabetes Care* 1996;**19**:(7):704–709.

28 Nelson R, Gohdes D, Everhart J *et al*. Lower-extremity amputations in NIDDM: 12-yr follow-up study in Pima Indians. *Diabetes Care* 1988;**11**:8–16.

29 Lee J, Lu M, Lee V, Russel D, Bahr C, Lee E. Lower extremity amputation. Incidence, risk factors and mortality in the Oklahoma Indian Diabetes Study. *Diabetes* 1993;**42**:876–882.

30 Selby JV, Zhang D. Risk factors for lower extremity amputation in persons with diabetes. *Diabetes Care* 1995;**18**:(4): 509–516.

31 Lehto S, Pyorala K, Ronnemaa T, Laakso M. Risk factors predicting lower extremity amputations in patients with NIDDM. *Diabetes Care* 1996;**19**:(6):607–612.

32 Adler AL, Boyko EJ, Ahroni JH, Smith DG. Lower-extremity amputation in diabetes: the independent effects of peripheral vascular disease, sensory neuropathy and foot ulcers. *Diabetes Care* 1999;**22**:1029–1035.

33 Reiber GE, Pecoraro RE, Koepsell TD. Risk factors for amputation in patients with diabetes mellitus. *Ann Intern Med* 1992;**117**:(2):97–105.

34 Baranoski S, Ayello E. Wound Care Essentials: Practice Principles, 2nd edn, Lippincott Williams & Wilkins, Philadelphia, 2008.

35 Reiber GE, Smith DG, Carter J *et al*. A comparison of diabetic foot ulcer patients managed in VHA and non-VHA settings. *J Rehabil Res Dev* 2001;**38**:(3):309–317.

36 Bloomgarden ZT, Karmally W, Metzger MJ *et al*. Randomized, controlled trial of diabetic patient education: improved knowledge without improved metabolic status. *Diabetes Care* 1987;**10**:(3):263–272.

37 Malone JM, Snyder M, Anderson G, Bernhard VM, Holloway GA Jr, Bunt TJ. Prevention of amputation by diabetic education. *Am J Surg* 1989;**158**:(6):520–524.

38 Barth R, Campbell LV, Allen S, Jupp JJ, Chisholm DJ. Intensive education improves knowledge, compliance and foot problems in type 2 diabetics. *Diabet Med* 1991;**8**:111–117.

39 Hamalainen H, Ronnemaa T, Toikka T, Liukkonen I. Long-term effects of one year of intensified pediatric activities on foot-care knowledge and self-care habits in patients with diabetes. *Diabetes Educator* 1998;**24**:734–740.

40 Mayfield JA, Reiber GE, Nelson RG, Greene T. Do foot examinations reduce the risk of diabetic amputation? *J Fam Pract* 2000;**49**:(6):499–504.

41 Lavery LA, Higgins KR, Lanctot DR *et al*. Home monitoring of foot skin temperatures to prevent ulceration. *Diabetes Care* 2004;**27**:(11):2642–2647.

42 LeMaster J, Reiber GE, Smith DG, Heagerty PJ, Wallace C. Daily weight-bearing activity does not increase the risk of diabetic foot ulcers. *Med Sci Sports Exercise* 2003;**35**:(7): 1093–1099.

43 Edmonds M, Blundell M, Morris M, Thomas M, Cotton L, Watkins P. Improved survival of the diabetic foot: the role of a specialized foot clinic. *Q J Med* 1986;**60**: 763–771.

44 Uccioli L, Faglia E, Monticone G *et al*. Manufactured shoes in the prevention of diabetic foot ulcers. *Diabetes Care* 1995;**18**: (10):1376–1378.

45 Reiber GE, Smith DG, Wallace C *et al*. Effect of therapeutic footwear on foot reulceration in patients with diabetes: a randomized controlled trial. *JAMA* 2002;**287**:(19): 2552–2558.

46 Wagner EH, Austin BT, Von Korff M. Organizing care for patients with chronic illness. *Milbank Q* 1996;**74**:(4): 511–544.

47 Berwick DM. Developing and testing changes in delivery of care. *Ann Intern Med* 1998;**128**:651–656.

48 Falkenberg M. Metabolic control and amputations among diabetics in primary health care – a population-based intensified programme governed by patient education. *Scand J Clin Lab Invest* 1990;**8**:25–29.

49 Dargis V, Pantelejeva O, Jonushaite A, Vileikyte L, Boulton AJ. Benefits of a multidisciplinary approach in the management of recurrent diabetic foot ulceration in Lithuania: a prospective study. *Diabetes Care* 1999;**22**:(9):1428–1431.

50 McCabe CJ, Stevenson RC, Dolan AM. Evaluation of a diabetic foot screening and protection program. *Diabet Med* 1998;**15**:80–84.

51 Patout CA, Birke JA, Horswell R, Williams D, Cerise FP. Effectiveness of a comprehensive diabetes lower-extremity amputation prevention program in a predominantly low-income African-American population. *Diabetes Care* 2000;**23**: 1339–1342.

52 Rith-Najarian S, Branchaud C, Beaulieu O, Gohdes D, Simonson G, Mazze R. Reducing lower-extremity amputations due to diabetes. Application of the staged diabetes management approach in a primary care setting. *J Fam Pract* 1998;**47**:(2):127–132.

53 Carrington AL, Abbott CA, Griffiths J, *et al*. A foot care program for diabetic unilateral lower-limb amputees. *Diabetes Care* 2001;**24**:216–221.

Part 5: Self-management, healthcare organization and public policy

25 What is the evidence that increasing engagement of individuals in self-management improves the processes and outcomes of care?

Debra L. Roter[1], *Ann Louise Kinmonth*[2]

[1]*Department of Health Policy and Management, Johns Hopkins School of Public Health, Baltimore, MD, USA*
[2]*General Practice and Primary Care Research Unit, Department of Public Health and Primary Care, University of Cambridge, Cambridge, UK*

Introduction

Treatment decisions in the care of patients with a chronic disorder, such as diabetes, have traditionally relied upon the judgment of physicians. However, the end of the 20th and beginning of the 21st century have witnessed a shift in medical care relationships towards greater self-reliance among patients in disease management as a matter of health care policy in Europe and North America.[1]

While these policies may be in keeping with global social, economic and political pressures and perhaps moral imperatives and patient preferences, they go beyond the currently established evidence base of medicine.[2] Nevertheless, the emerging evidence shows promise with a growing number of studies indicating that collaborative decision making between a patient and physician can lead to a more active and engaged patient in the treatment process, with more effective disease management skills and, under certain circumstances, better clinical outcomes.[2–4] In addition, a range of approaches drawing on social processes, beyond the core consultation between patient and practitioner, are under development to support self-management which may contribute to the same ends.[5,6–9]

It has been argued that one factor limiting active patient engagement in the treatment process has been the narrow approach to patient behaviour implied by the term 'compliance'. Compliance has historically connoted patient deference to expert medical authority consistent with a biomedical paradigm that implicitly devalues independent patient judgment and sees failures to comply as the result of patient ignorance, incompetence, deviance or irresponsibility. In reaction to the authoritarian and directive tone of 'compliance', 'adherence' has been proposed as a less imposing alternative semantic, carrying a suggestion of active cooperation.[10] The difference in terms, however, is subtle and the change has not been widely adopted by researchers in the field.[11]

A more substantive departure from the directive terminology of compliance or adherence, more in keeping with an emphasis on patient autonomy in treatment decision making, is evident in increasing reference to patient self-care or self-management activities. Self-management approaches reflect patient judgments and values within the context of daily living and their incorporation to inform how a comprehensive treatment plan can be best agreed upon and implemented. This approach has been pioneered among patients with asthma, arthritis and diabetes, where a consideration of the broader life context within which treatment decisions must be carried out is especially relevant.[12] Consistent with this self-management perspective, the American and British Diabetes Associations now refer to diabetes education as diabetes self-management education and the American Academy of Diabetes

The Evidence Base for Diabetes Care, Second Edition, Edited by William H. Herman, Ann Louise Kinmonth, Nicholas J. Wareham and Rhys Williams.
© 2010 John Wiley & Sons, Ltd

Educators refers to diabetes education as 'an interactive, collaborative, ongoing process'.[13] This conceptual shift has been underpinned by the development of a range of programmes, to prepare patients to cope with the consequences of chronic disease and to participate as management partners with physicians and other health professionals on the one hand, and to enable health professionals to be effective teachers and health care partners with patients on the other.[14,15] Individual countries have developed their own standards for self-management education,[16–18] and international curricula have been developed[19,20]

Self-management programmes for diabetes in Europe[21] began as structured inpatient training in intensive insulin therapy and self-management and have been adapted and delivered there as outpatient courses[22] and as the DAFNE (Dose Adjustment For Normal Eating) project in the UK.[23] Although the model was originally developed for people with type 1 diabetes, it has been adapted for people with type 2 diabetes.[24–26]

The term self-management has been used in these programmes to cover a wide range of domains including, in addition to the core activity of participation in medical decisions, involvement in monitoring of symptoms and disease parameters (e.g. hypoglycaemia, blood glucose levels) in changing and monitoring health-related behaviours (medication use, diet, physical activity) and in adapting to and managing changed social and work circumstances and emotional distress.

Since semantics can have so powerful a role in shaping and focusing debate and in providing a guide to how social reality is interpreted, understood and acted upon, self-management will be used in the remainder of this chapter to reflect active patient engagement in making decisions about the management plan and adherence will be used to connote patient success in carrying out the planned treatment related behaviours and monitoring activities agreed upon.

Evidence from systematic and meta-analytic reviews of the literature

Several meta-analytic or systematic reviews of relevant diabetes-related intervention studies (or a diabetes subset of chronic disease studies) promoting self-management or adherence have been conducted over the past two decades[2,11,27–30] There is considerable agreement that intervention programmes can confer benefits on patients across a range of cognitions, behaviours and psycho-social and clinical outcomes.

For example, Norris et al.[31] evaluated 72 studies and found short-term (less than 6 months) positive effects of self-management training on knowledge, frequency and accuracy of self-monitoring blood glucose, self-reported dietary habits and glycaemic control.

Effect sizes were often largest for self-report measures, including knowledge, diet and exercise change, and smaller for more objectively measured outcomes such as increasing skills, weight change and control of blood glucose. The Brown meta-analysis[29] estimated a small effect size (as measured by a Cohen's d) for educational interventions of 0.41 for HbA_{1c} and somewhat smaller effects for other measures (Cohen's $d = 0.35$ for blood glucose and 0.27 for psychological outcomes). An exception to this pattern of results was a large knowledge effect (Cohen's $d = 1.0$) produced by the interventions. In the meta-analysis by Roter et al.[34] of compliance-specific interventions, the effect size for the subset of diabetes studies (HbA_{1c} and blood glucose) was moderate in magnitude (Cohen's $d = 0.56$). A notably stronger effect was evident for compliance indicators measured through pill count and pharmacy record review (Cohen's $d = 1.0$) and, as in the Brown study, for knowledge (Cohen's $d = 0.8$).

What approaches might be effective?

The focus of reported diabetes interventions has until recently been primarily cognitive; didactic instruction alone or in combination with behavioural training in diet, exercise and/or self-monitoring techniques, or behavioural; characterized by behaviour modification or social learning strategies. Only a few studies address techniques such as relaxation and biofeedback therapies or psychodynamic counselling; until recently, even fewer addressed patient empowerment and activation strategies. Findings demonstrate that interventions based on ideas of informed choice (actions consonant with knowledge, beliefs and values), acquiring self-management skills and including group work, the addition of audiovisual aids and use of behavioural and social learning approaches are more effective than narrowly didactic approaches.[2,14,27,31–34]

How long do effects last?

The intervention effects evident in the reviews, however, may not be long-lasting. In addition to finding similar short-term estimates as those reported by Brown, Roter and colleagues, Padgett et al.[32] calculated effect sizes over time. This analysis found that effect sizes averaging 0.36 for HbA_{1c} at 6 months following interventions fell to virtually zero (0.03) by 12 months; effects for blood glucose measures were reduced somewhat less, falling from 0.58 at 6 months to 0.20 at 12 months. Only psychological and knowledge effect sizes were maintained at moderate levels of success over time. Norris et al.'s more recent analysis similarly notes a decline in HbA_{1c} immediately following interventions.[35] That review of 31 diabetes self-management education intervention studies found an average reduction in HbA_{1c} from baseline of 76% immediately after exposure to an intervention, but substantially lower sustained reductions (26%) at later follow-up.

The interpretation of the findings from these reviews is problematic because of widespread methodological weaknesses in individual studies and the differential application of inclusion criteria for studies in the reviews. The early meta-analyses in particular had many limitations, with poor descriptions of the sample characteristics, the interventions and the underpinning theoretical models. An attempt by the UK National Health Service Centre for Reviews and Dissemination, University of York, to classify interventions by type into information and skills, cognitive-behavioural approaches and patient empowerment concluded that further research is necessary to determine whether interventions to promote self-management of any type have long term impacts.[28]

No studies have demonstrated effects on diabetes disease endpoints such as cardiovascular morbidity or mortality and economic analyses are absent or weak.

It is clear that short-term effects of interventions on HbA_{1c} are far stronger than longer term effects and all reviewers conclude that further research is necessary to determine which components of interventions to promote self-management have positive significant long-term effects and for whom.

Evidence for the role of social support, relationship and attachment

Recent attention to the role of social support and family interventions appear especially noteworthy in facilitating patient adherence to medical treatments in general.[5,27,36] Although few randomized studies are available in this area, the evidence suggests that social support, based on experiential knowledge, can provide both direct and indirect benefits to patients through the provision of informational, appraisal and emotional resources. Informational support provides advice, suggestions, alternative actions, feedback and factual information. Appraisal support includes encouraging persistence and optimism for resolving problems, affirmation of a peer's feelings and behaviours and reassurance that frustrations can be dealt with. Emotional support involves expressions of caring, empathy, encouragement and reassurance, and is generally seen to enhance self-esteem.[8] Interventions drawing on these concepts include group consultations and peer support directly or via the Internet or the telephone.[5,8]

Do group interventions work?

A Cochrane review[6] has reported the effects of group-based, patient-centred training on clinical, lifestyle and psycho-social outcomes in people with type 2 diabetes without specific consideration of the processes of social support. All trials evaluated a group-based diabetes education programme for patients alone or with friends and relations compared with routine treatment, waiting list control or no intervention. Studies were only included if the length of follow-up was 6 months or more. The size of the groups varied from 4 to 18 participants. Only 11 studies with HbA_{1c} outcomes were included, all judged by the Cochrane reviewers to have design flaws putting them at moderate to high risk of bias. They comprised 1532 participants in eight randomized controlled trials (RCTs) and three controlled trials. Age, duration of diabetes and ethnic group varied widely.

Programmes varied in duration, with the least intensive being 3 h per year for 2 years and the most intense being 52 h over 1 year. Educators were health professionals (physicians, nurses, dieticians or paramedics), except in one study where they were lay health advisors. Only five studies reported a theoretical model for the intervention; three studies drew on the Diabetes Treatment and Teaching Programme (DTTP) developed in Germany for adults with type 1 diabetes[21] and based on the concept of therapeutic patient education.[37] One study was based on patient-centred education and used an empowerment model developed by Anderson *et al.*[38] Another study drew on the psychological models of behaviour change.[39] The comparison groups received various forms of routine treatment with or without waiting list control. Meta-analysis was performed in sub-groups where heterogeneity was low. A meta-analysis comparing glycated haemoglobin levels at 12–14 months between intervention and comparison groups was possible among seven studies involving a total of 1044 participants. The pooled difference in glycated haemoglobin of 0.8% (95% CI 0.7 to 1.0; $Z = 9.63$; $p < 0.00001$) favoured the group-based diabetes education programmes. Further results favouring group-based diabetes education programmes at 12–14 months included lower body weight (1.6 kg; 95% CI 0.3 to 3.0; $p = 0.02$) and greater diabetes knowledge [standardized mean difference (SMD) 1.0; 95% CI 0.7 to 1.2; $p < 0.00001$]. There was also evidence of a reduced need for diabetes medication [odds ratio (OR) 11.8, 95% CI 5.2 to 26.9; $p < 0.00001$; relative difference = 0.2; number needed to treat = 5]. Despite limitations in quality, these data provide strong evidence that group-based training for self-management in people with type 2 diabetes can be more effective in supporting effective self-management than individual routine care alone.

Does internet peer support work?

A further Cochrane review has assessed the effects of interactive health communication applications (IHCAs) for people with chronic disease.[7] IHCAs are computer-based, usually web-based, packages for patients that combine health information with at least one of social/peer support, decision support or behaviour change support. These are innovations in health care delivery and their effects on health are uncertain. The review included 24 RCTs (3739 participants) including six among children or adults with type 1 or 2 diabetes. The review highlighted the preliminary nature of the data available. IHCAs have been developed for a range of chronic diseases across the age ranges. Conclusions regarding their effects are limited by the range of populations in the trials, the different conditions studied, the nature of the IHCAs and the differing intensity of exposure (from 20 min to many hours spread over 6–9 months). Researchers used very different outcomes and even where similar outcomes were studied, different outcome measures were used. Control groups received varied interventions. Moderate effects on knowledge and social support were found, but only small effects on clinical outcomes (SMD 0.18; 95% CI 0.01 to 0.35). It was not possible to determine the effects of IHCAs on emotional or economic outcomes or on the pathways of action of the interventions.

The Diabetes Network (D-Net) Internet-based self-management project demonstrates the potential and challenges of this approach. The project is a randomized trial evaluating the incremental effects of adding (1) tailored self-management training or (2) peer support components to a basic Internet-based, information-focused comparison intervention.[40]

It compared home access with an Internet-enabled computer system providing information and a professionally mediated e-mail diabetes peer support forum, with computer access to information only for adults with type 2 diabetes mellitus. A total of 320 adult patients managed in primary care who were relatively new to the Internet participated (mean age 59 years; SD = 9.2). The basic D-Net intervention was implemented well and improvements in behavioural, psycho-social and some clinical outcomes were found. However, there were difficulties in maintaining usage by patients over time and addition of tailored self-management or peer support components generally did not improve results significantly.

Evidence for the role of psychological and personality attributes

Other potentially important factors influencing effective self-management include a variety of psychological and personality attributes. For instance, Ciechanowski and colleagues have conducted a fascinating series of studies exploring the relationship between the psychological attributes associated with patients' interpersonal attachment style (secure, dismissing, preoccupied or fearful) and a variety of self-management behaviours relevant to diabetes.[41–43,44] Depression has also been explored as a significant risk factor for inadequate diabetes self-management.[41,45]

The influence of sociodemographic factors

In contrast to social, psychological and interpersonal factors, sociodemographic characteristics are often weak predictors of successful diabetes self-management. There is no consistent relationship between gender, education, income, intelligence, general knowledge about health and illness and adherence to medical regimes,[10] although there are some sociodemographic relationships – related to both patients and physician — with effective engagement in the communication and decision-making process.[46]

Specificity of self-management decisions

Perhaps a portion of the difficulty in the development of a demographic profile predicting individual action is the multifaceted nature of self-management decisions. Effective management of diabetes is complex; it demands not only changes in behaviours in the medical sphere through, for example, the regular taking of medications and glucose testing, but also the adoption of health lifestyle behaviours, including diet, exercise, safety precautions and other preventive self-care actions. These behaviours appear relatively independent; effective self-management in one area is not necessarily predictive of effective performance in others. Indeed, patients appear to engage in a process of decision making that often involves trading off behaviour in one sphere against others so that patients may only selectively, partially or erratically engage in medical and lifestyle activities recommended by their physician.[3]

Decisions to forgo self-management activities are much more complex and less responsive to traditional interventions than inadvertent errors attributable to forgetfulness, confusion or lack of resources. In the domain of volitional non-compliance, ambivalence plays an important challenge to successful self-management. In this context, applications from the cognitive field (techniques to test and strengthen motivations to act) and the behavioural field (support to implement chosen activities and build them into habits) may be highly relevant.[47–49]

The influence of the patient–practitioner relationship

Another area of increasing study and importance is the nature of the patient–practitioner relationship within which self-management activities are discussed and agreed upon. Patient engagement in the deliberative process is hypothesized to be the vehicle through which effective treatment plans are made and subsequently adhered to or not. Much of the supportive evidence for this contention was first synthesized in Stewart's 1995 review of analytical and randomized controlled trials of physician–patient communication,[50] in which a health-related outcome was reported. The nature and process of communication was reported to influence patient outcomes, particularly emotional distress, but also symptom resolution, functional status and physiology, including blood pressure and blood glucose. Characteristics of the consultation linked to positive health and treatment outcomes included: patients asking questions, agreeing about the nature of the problem and the need for follow-up and perceiving that a full discussion of the problem had taken place; practitioners answering patients' questions with clear information, asking questions about the patients' ideas, concerns and expectations and showing empathy.

Van Dam et al.[51] reviewed eight publications evaluating the effects of modifying provider–patient interaction and consulting style on diabetes self-care and diabetes outcomes. Patient behaviour-focused interventions, the enhancement of patient participation by assistant-guided patient preparation for visits to doctors, empowering group education and automated telephone management were all found to be more effective than focusing on provider behaviour to change health professional consulting style into a more patient-centred one.

Other recent systematic reviews have been more critical.[2,52] A systematic review of 35 randomized trials that assessed the impact on health-related outcomes of interventions to alter the interaction between patients and practitioners drew attention to the limitations in trial methodology in this field. Trials were heterogeneous in populations, settings, interventions and measures. Interventions frequently combined several poorly described elements. Explicit theoretical underpinning was rare and only one study linked intervention through process to outcome measures. Health outcomes were rarely measured objectively (six of 35) and only four trials with health outcomes met predefined quality criteria.[2]

Nevertheless, the review demonstrated that interventions frequently altered the process of interactions (significantly in 73%, 22 of 30 trials). Simple approaches to increasing the participation of patients in the clinical encounter, such as providing practitioners with a note from patients about their concerns beforehand, showed promise, as did more complex programmes providing specific information about disease and attention to emotion. However, while the interaction between patient and practitioner was amenable to change, impacts on health-related outcomes were more elusive. In more than half of the trials there were no significant positive effects on health outcomes.

A Cochrane review assessing the effects of interventions for health care providers that aimed to promote patient-centred approaches in clinical consultation supported the conclusion that they can significantly increase the patient-centredness of care, but again drew attention to the limited and mixed evidence on the effects of interventions on patients' health care behaviours or health status.[52] It included many of the same studies as Griffin et al.[2] along with controlled clinical trials, controlled before-and-after studies and interrupted time-series studies. Patient-centred care was defined as a philosophy of care that encourages (a) shared control of the consultation, decisions about interventions or management of the health problems with the patient, and/or (b) a focus in the consultation on the patient as a whole person who has individual preferences situated within social contexts (in contrast to a focus in the consultation on a body part or disease).

Patient engagement in communication during the clinic visit

The remaining sections of this chapter aim to describe patient engagement in clinical visit communication and its relationship to effective diabetes self-management and patient outcomes. Although focusing on the medical dialogue, we also appreciate the array of socio-political, individual and social factors that impact on the interpersonal relationship that underlies effective communication. These include those economic, social, cultural and political forces that define the health care system and its practitioners, in addition to factors that define family and social support, individual resilience and personality and the illness experience. Consequently, we propose a conceptual framework that provides a broad heuristic for appreciating levels of patient engagement in the communication dynamics of the clinic visit while understanding the broader context within which

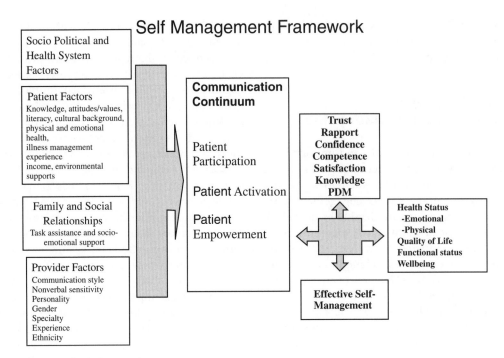

Figure 25.1 Self-management framework

self-management and health outcomes exist (see Figure 25.1).

Patient communication continuum

A point of departure for many health education interventions designed to enhance self-management is a patient engagement continuum reflected in the dialogue of the consultation. A critical reading of this literature identifies three levels of patient engagement: patient participation, patient activation and patient empowerment that can be incorporated into the self-management framework.[53,54] Key randomised control trials of patient activation/empowerment are summarised in Table 25.1 and discussed below.

Patient participation

The first level of engagement is simple participation in the medical dialogue. This can be defined as any patient or physician strategy which facilitates the inclusion of the patient's perspective or preferences into the medical plan, primarily through facilitated disclosure of their illness narrative.[3] The primary vehicle for enhanced patient participation is the use of patient-centred interviewing skills.[46] Patients may participate in the dialogue by simply telling their story. At its most basic level, feeling listened to and heard is a fundamental function of the therapeutic relationship. As expressed by George Engel in

recognizing the power for the patient in telling their story '... interpersonal engagement required in the clinical realm rests on complementary and basic human needs, especially the need to know and understand and the need to feel known and understood'.[55] The power of disclosing relevant life experiences, perspectives and preferences is not only in these being validated and the person feeling recognized and known, but also in the power of one's narrative to act as a vehicle of self-reflection.[56] Within this context, the patient is transformed from a reporter of symptoms to a 'co-investigator' of his or her health problems.[57]

The critical communication skills that facilitate active patient participation in the medical visit include those originally derived from the psychotherapy literature and applied to a functional analysis of interviewing skills: data gathering, relationship building and partnering skills.[53] At its most elementary level, patient participation in the medical visit can be seen as reactive; physicians enquire and patients respond. Data-gathering skills reflect a variety of questioning behaviours that encompass variation in both form and content. Restricted opportunities for patient participation in the visit are provided through closed-ended questions to which the patient provides direct answers. The transformation from restricted to full participation is contingent on broadening the parameters of elicitation so that patients can fully and most meaningfully tell their story. Open questions by their very nature allow more room for patient discretion in response than closed-ended questions. Questions about things patients know and care about and that are relevant to daily experience and context potentially enhance the relevance and the meaning of disclosure.

Relationship-building skills, including emotional support, empathy, reassurance and personal regard, create an atmosphere that facilitates open and sensitive disclosure by optimizing rapport and trust. Partnership skills also make it easier for a patient to tell their story by actively facilitating patient input through prompts and signals of interest, interpretations, paraphrase and requests for opinion and probes for understanding. In addition, patients may be encouraged to participate more actively in the visit by having the physician assume a less dominating relationship stance. This includes lowered verbal dominance, for example, by listening more and talking less, using head nods and eye contact and forward body lean to signal interest.

Attempting to understand the use and consequence of patient-centred skills for patient activation, Street *et al.* undertook a descriptive study of natural communication patterns in which patient participation in the medical dialogue could be linked to metabolic control.[58] For this study, following an initial educational programme, audiotape recordings were made of consultations between newly diagnosed diabetic patients and nurses during a session to review strategies for managing diabetes and progress and problems related to metabolic control. Patients of nurses with a participatory style, facilitating patient input into the medical dialogue and limiting the use of controlling communication, experienced better metabolic control than patients of 'take charge' nurses (that is, those who issued directives, recommendations and orders, interrupted the patient, disagreed with the patient or changed a patient-initiated topic).

It was suggested that a controlling communication style may inhibit patients' ability to convey the full spectrum of their concerns and communicate their illness narrative, which is to tell the story of their illness and engage in the process of reflection and understanding. This includes raising concerns of a psycho-social and emotional nature and becoming actively involved in problem solving for disease management. A controlling style may act to depersonalize both the visit and the therapeutic regimen. A somewhat similar conclusion was drawn by a group of Finnish researchers who found, in a cross-sectional study, that patient report of a positive doctor–patient relationship (for example, taking notice of the patient as an individual) correlated with tighter metabolic control.[59]

Patient activation

The second level of patient engagement is patient activation, which moves the process from one of disclosure to exploration and inquiry into the conditions and circumstances that may contribute to the medical problem or may be useful in treatment and management. The medical dialogue provides the vehicle of patient activation in agenda setting, question asking and joint problem solving. Active involvement in the dialogue transforms the patient role from reactive to proactive, with patients taking the initiative in assuring that their agenda is presented and their needs are met.

Activation interventions have generally included guides or algorithms given directly to patients by a researcher or via trained practitioners. They aim to help patients identify, phrase and rehearse questions, concerns and issues to be included in the agenda of the visit.[60] Physicians can be taught to assist patients by providing full and relevant information and counselling, by the use of partnership-building skills, including the solicitation of patient questions, expectations, preferences and probing the patient's explanatory framework, or by engaging in a process of negotiation and problem solving related to treatment and lifestyle regimens, which values individual context in addition to population-based evidence. A particularly important partnership-building behaviour is simply not to interrupt. Observational studies show that physicians frequently interrupt patients, beginning on average less than 25 s after the statement of their primary problem.[61] The interruption often leads to follow-up of the first, but not necessarily the most important, patient concern.

The first of the studies to link glycosylated haemoglobin, as a measure of diabetic control, to active patient engagement in medical visit communication was the seminal work of Greenfield *et al.*[62] They conducted an experimental intervention which was designed to improve information-seeking skills so that patients could interact more effectively, in a more participatory manner, with their physician. Patients who attended two university hospital outpatient clinics were enrolled in the study and randomly assigned to intervention or comparison groups. The first of these clinics was exclusively devoted to diabetes treatment, administered by the Endocrinology Division in a Department of Medicine, and the second was a general medical clinic.

During the 20 min immediately preceding the medical visit on two consecutive visits, patients allocated to the experimental group were approached by a clinic assistant who undertook the following to develop patient activation:

1 Reviewed the patient's medical record with the patient.

2 Acquainted the patient with how his or her disease was treated at that clinic.

3 Helped the patients identify relevant medical decisions likely to arise during the upcoming visit, with special emphasis on treatment issues that could be affected by his or her lifestyle and preferences.

4 Taught the patient simple skills designed to increase their involvement in the doctor–patient interaction. Patients were encouraged to ask questions, recognize relevant medical decisions and negotiate these decisions with physicians. Assistants also coached patients in the use of simple techniques for overcoming common barriers to discussing issues with physicians including embarrassment, fear of appearing foolish, forgetting to bring up an issue and intimidation by the physician.

The control group of patients received an 'attention control' intervention comprising 20 min of standardized educational materials on diabetes. The investigators then tape-recorded visits by both experimental and control group patients and gathered post-visit questionnaires from patients and doctors, including a mailed questionnaire 12 weeks later. The audiotapes showed that the 'activated' patients were 30% more active in the conversation with the doctor than attention-controls.

Not only did patients in the intervention group talk more with their providers, they also were more assertive, controlling the consultation more than those in the comparison group, and eliciting twice the number of factual statements from their providers, so that the talk was more explicitly related to the patient's agenda for improving their health. However, this process did not lead to any differences between groups in satisfaction or knowledge of diabetes. Activated patients were found to have lower glycosylated haemoglobin levels at follow-up than the comparison group after adjusting for baseline values. They also reported significantly fewer physical limitations in the weeks that followed the visit, including fewer days off work and less limitation on their ability to perform other important social roles.

In an exploration of the relationships between behaviour during the visit and blood glucose control, significant correlations were found between the number of conversational acts (Pearson's $r = -0.29$, p 0.001), number of controlling acts ($r = -0.38$, p 0.001), effective information elicitation ($r = -0.51$, p 0.01) and subsequent glycosylated haemoglobin. In a regression analysis of predictors of functional limitation at follow-up, four variables explained 66% of the variance: the intervention, functional limitation at follow-up and number of diabetic complications. This strongly suggests that the intervention had an effect not mediated through blood glucose or disease severity alone. The authors proposed that an increased sense of control gained from the intervention may alter the way in which individuals perceive their health status and their physical limitations.[62]

In a replication of this study in a hospital setting, Rost *et al.* attempted to specify further the intervention's effective element by distinguishing participation in decision making from increased information seeking.[63] They also explored the pathways by which the intervention might influence metabolic control and functional status. The investigators replicated the links between patient activation in information seeking and improved physical functioning at four months using a validated measure.[64] They demonstrated no significant impact of the intervention on glycosylated haemoglobin [baseline levels of 13% ($\pm$ 3.5) I and 13.5% ($\pm$ 3.6) C falling at 4 months in both groups to 11.8% ($\pm$ 3.0) and 12.4% ($\pm$ 3.3), respectively]. Among the 37 patients with audiotapes available, those in the experimental group asked significantly more questions at discharge than the control group, (a mean of eight in the experimental group compared with three in the control; $p < 0.001$, after adjustment for number of questions asked at the admission interview). Moreover, in a subsequent exploratory analysis, the perception of patients that they were successful in question asking predicted improved glycosylated haemoglobin at 4 months ($p = 0.05$).

There was greater support for the link between question asking and subsequent metabolic control than for involvement in decision making. However, patient decision making was somewhat idiosyncratically defined as the frequency of patient requests, disagreements and interruptions, rather than factors relating to, for example, choice of personally important goals and individual steps to their achievement. Pathways to improved outcomes were explored but remained unclear; there was no evidence that the functional status improvements associated with the intervention were mediated by increases in patient recall or understanding of information, satisfaction with care or the satisfaction of the treating physicians.

Patient empowerment

The final level of engagement, empowerment, is concerned with aiding the patient to take thoughtful action on their own behalf.[53] Although physicians have long recognized the importance of patients taking responsibility for behaviours affecting health, relatively little attention has been paid to the extent to which they themselves facilitate this process. A contribution in this regard has been made by the Medical Outcomes Study (MOS).[65] This prospective cohort study surveyed over 7000 patients after visits with 300 physicians to determine the extent to which the patients reported having been offered choice, control and responsibility over treatment decisions. Physician practice and patient experience in terms of shared decision making were found to vary widely. Most notably, physicians with primary care or interviewing skills training were reported to be more facilitative of active patient engagement in the decision-making process than were other physicians. Although the MOS study did not identify particular facilitative skills for participatory decision making, other observational studies have found that physicians trained in interviewing skills differed from other physicians in key ways: trained physicians were more likely to engage in discussion of psycho-social issues, be emotionally supportive, ask questions in an open manner, ask for patient opinion, be skilled in interpersonal communication, be psychologically minded and be less verbally dominant.[66–69]

In using these communication skills for empowerment, the physician's communication role is to provide an atmosphere in which confidence and competence are built, emotional support given and in which support for choice, control and responsibility for health behaviour is recognized and reinforced.

Taking an empowerment approach, Langewitz et al.[22] in Switzerland and Anderson et al.[70] in the United States designed programmes to build patients' competence and confidence to self-manage their diabetes effectively. Although not directly equivalent to one another in content, the programmes do have a common theme of promoting patient competence for decision making and treatment self-management. The Langewitz programme provided patients with more sophisticated knowledge regarding insulin requirements in relation to different glucose challenges. This went beyond conventional approaches to insulin therapy and enabled individuals to take informed control of their insulin regimen. An important element of the training programme was its focus on the importance of patient autonomy in self-management of insulin therapy. The Anderson programme also emphasized diabetes management, but included biomedical as well as psychological and social coping.

The Langewitz study investigated whether an empowering approach to insulin self-management improved the doctor-patient relationship, quality of life or metabolic control in 43 patients with longstanding type 1 diabetes (mean age 33 ± 10 years, mean duration of diabetes 15 ± 10 years).[22] A before-and-after design was used with follow-up at 1 year. Patients volunteered for the study and were younger and had more frequent severe hypoglycaemia than the clinic population as a whole. Indeed, baseline HbA_{1c} was $6.61 \pm 1.46\%$, leaving little room for improvement. However, there was a significant improvement 4 months after treatment ($6.29 \pm 1.01\%$, $p < 0.05$) but not at 1 year. Improvements were also found at 1 year in the doctor–patient relationship, patient satisfaction, depression and anxiety in general and particularly a reduction in worry about diabetes, in association with a reduction in frequency of severe hypoglycaemic attacks.

The intervention appeared to affect the doctor–patient relationship, with patients reporting a closer and more egalitarian partnership with their physicians. This finding supports the primary advantage of training identified by patients in insulin management as greater freedom to choose when to eat. Metabolic control did not deteriorate in this group, despite the patients' greater autonomy in self-care.

Anderson et al. provided a randomized evaluation of their empowerment programme, with a focus on self-efficacy and its component skills.[70] These included the ability to identify areas of satisfaction and dissatisfaction related to living with diabetes, to identify and achieve personal goals, to use problem solving to eliminate barriers to these goals, to cope with the emotional aspects of living with diabetes, to manage stress, to attain appropriate social support, to strengthen motivation to act and to make cost–benefit decisions about planned behaviours. Forty-six volunteers, mainly overweight, well-educated women, who already felt comfortable living with diabetes, were randomized to immediate programme attendance or waiting list control, after a full induction into the study design and intervention approach. Participants were asked to complete experiential worksheets, attend six sessions and participate in group discussions. At 12 weeks from baseline, the intervention group demonstrated a significantly greater improvement in glycosylated haemoglobin than the control group (intervention 11.75 ± 3.01 to $11.02 \pm 2.89\%$, control 10.82 ± 2.94 to $10.87 \pm 2.59\%$, $p = 0.05$). Self-efficacy was significantly increased among the intervention group in terms of setting goals, managing stress, obtaining social support and making self-care treatment decisions. There was also a significant reduction in perceived impact of diabetes and negative attitudes towards diabetes among the intervention group.

Two subsequent trials in the United Kingdom among individuals with type 2 diabetes, built on the earlier trials reported from the United States, using larger study populations and longer follow-up periods.[71,72] The study by Pill et al. devised an intervention for general practitioners and nurses drawing on elements of patient participation, activation and empowerment facilitation.[72] Simple visual aids were designed to assist clinicians in encouraging active patient participation. The core message was that individual patients should be encouraged to air personal concerns about their condition, to choose particular areas of lifestyle and self-management they felt most relevant for discussion, test out their readiness to change behaviour and, if appropriate, set personal goals. The intervention was provided by a multidisciplinary team at practice visits of 1 h each, continuing until practitioners felt competent to deliver the programme in consultations. Half way through the study 71% of practitioners reported using the materials frequently. However, at 2 years, fewer than 20% reported using the intervention systematically with patients. Lack of application may explain the lack of effect on glycosylated haemoglobin, measures of health status, wellbeing, satisfaction with treatment and attitudes to diabetes.

The study group was not dissimilar to those in the trials in the United States in terms of relatively poor diabetic control, and the study had greater power to detect differences. Problems with assay changes during the study may have compromised the measures of metabolic control, but the main difference between this and the trials in the United States would appear to be the attempt to deliver the programme through education of practitioners and routine practice rather than through expert coaching of patients themselves.

A similar approach was taken in the study by Kinmonth et al.,[71] but this time among patients with newly diagnosed type 2 diabetes. Nurses and GPs were trained in groups. In the first half day they were given evidence for a patient-centred approach and taught how to offer to patients a booklet, 'Diabetes in Your Hands', to encourage patients to ask questions and prepare their agenda before consultations and an insert of possible concerns for people with diabetes, including diabetic complications. Nurses attended a full day of skills training, learning to elicit and listen well to the patient agenda, negotiate behaviour change and use a framework for supporting individual choice and change, using the stages of change model[73] with a focus on identifying individual costs and benefits of choices before providing tailored lifestyle advice.[74] Patients who were seen by trained, compared with untrained, practitioners reported at 1 year better communications with their doctors (OR 2.8, 95% CI 1.8 to 4.3), greater treatment satisfaction (OR 1.6, 95% CI 1.1 to 2.5) and wellbeing [difference in means (d) 2.8, 95% CI 0.4 to 5.2]. There were no differences between groups in self-reported diet or exercise. However, body mass index was significantly higher in the intervention group (difference = 2.0, 95% CI 0.3 to 3.8) as were triglyceride concentrations ($d = 0.4 \, \text{mmol} \, l^{-1}$; 95% CI 0.07 to 0.73 mmol l^{-1}) and knowledge of critical/self-care issues was lower. HbA$_{1c}$ levels were not significantly improved in the intervention group and achieved control was good in both groups.

As in the study by Pill et al.,[72] nurses became less keen on the approach over time and were frustrated by time constraints. Patients diagnosed later in the study were less likely to recognize the materials than those diagnosed earlier. The smaller effect sizes in this study compared with those in the United States may relate to the indirect delivery of the intervention to patients via training of their practitioners. Practitioners appeared to find it easier to learn data gathering, relationship and partnering skills, rather than to integrate them with patient education and counselling, negotiation and joint problem solving.

Effective communication pathways

The communication studies described were built upon a foundation of patient–physician collaboration and partnership. However, the causal pathways linking these approaches to the improvements in process and outcomes demonstrated remain unclear.

A direct pathway explaining these results might propose that information leads to more informed, appropriate and efficacious action; a better educated patient will have the capacity to comply more fully with medical recommendations. Alternatively, one might speculate that the interventions leading to better perceived communication with practitioners and less hierarchical relationships might increase patient satisfaction and lead to higher levels of commitment to the doctor–patient relationship and subsequently to the therapeutic plan.

The very complexity of the interventions evaluated and the limits of the measures employed constrain conclusions. However, neither the Greenfield[62] nor Rost[63] studies found that activated patients scored any higher in recall or understanding of diabetes-related information and, in the Kinmonth study,[71] knowledge of self-care was greatest among patients consulting practitioners without additional training in patient-centred care.[71] Nor did patients in the intervention groups of Greenfield and Rost report greater satisfaction than those in the comparison groups despite better metabolic control or functional status. Some other mechanism must have been at work in these studies.

Patient activation may have acted as a vehicle for increased self-efficacy and 'internality training'.

Table 25.1 Randomized control trials of patient activation/empowerment

Study Country Setting Diabetes type	Randomized participants N, age, gender (M/F), baseline HbA$_{1c}$	Intervention (I) and control (C) • No. evaluated (N) • Delivery • Duration • Type	Process Measures and direction of effect*	Outcome Measures and direction (effect size)	Design issues Length of follow-up from baseline % attrition > or <30% Notes on randomization method
Greenfield,[62] 1988 USA OPD Mixed type 1, type 2 Established diabetes	N = 73 Mean age 50 years (± 14) F: 50% HbA$_{1c}$ (NR 4.0–6.8%) 10.5 ± 2.0%	— • To patients • 2 × 20 min • Patient activation pre-consultation • C:N = 26 • Attention control – standardized education	Audiotape of consultation: • Conversational acts (+) • Question asking (0) • Controlling acts (+) • Information eliciting (+) Questionnaire: • Patient satisfaction (0) • Knowledge (0)	HbA$_{1c}$ (+) (0.72) Functional status (+) Health-related quality of life (+)	12 weeks <30% Small study with short follow-up
Rost,[63] 1991 USA Hospital Mixed type 1, type 2 Established diabetes	N = 61 Mean age 40 years (± 15) F: 60% HbA$_{1c}$ (NR 4.4–6.3%) 13.2 + 3.5%	— • To patients • 3 day evaluation + educational programme • 45 min • Patient activation • 1 h • Self-administered booster, post-discharge (adapted from Greenfield) • C:N = 29 • To patients • 3 day evaluation + education programme only	Audiotape of question asking at discharge (+) Questionnaires: • Patient involvement (0) • Patient satisfaction (0) • Patient knowledge (0) • Practitioner satisfaction at discharge (0)	HbA$_{1c}$ (0) Functional status: Physical (+) Psychological (0)	16 weeks <30% Block randomization by week of admission, with allocation concealment Small study with short follow-up
Anderson,[70] 1995 USA Diabetes education centre volunteers Mixed type 1, type 2 Established diabetes	N = 46 Mean age 50 years F: 70% HbA$_{1c}$ (NR 4–8%) 11.3 ± 3%	I: N = 23 • To patients • 6 × 2 h empowerment programme over 6 weeks • C:N = 22 • Waiting list controls	Questionnaires: • Self-efficacy scales (+) • Diabetes attitudes scales (+)	HbA$_{1c}$ (+) (0.27)	12 weeks <30% Small study among motivated volunteers Randomization by patient

(continued)

431

Table 25.1 (*Continued*)

Study Country Setting Diabetes type	Randomized participants N, age, gender (M/F), baseline HbA$_{1c}$	Intervention (I) and control (C) • No. evaluated (N) • Delivery • Duration • Type	Process Measures and direction of effect*	Outcome Measures and direction (effect size)	Design issues Length of follow-up from baseline % attrition > or <30% Notes on randomization method
Pill,[72] 1998 UK General Practice Type 2 Established diabetes	N = 190 Mean age 58 years (±9.4) F: 50% HbA$_{1c}$ (NR 5.7–8%) 11.6 ± 11.2%	I: N = 77 • To practitioners • 3 + h • Patient activation skills and materials • C:N = 88 • Usual practice	Audiotapes of practitioners' competence (+) Questionnaires: • Application of intervention by practitioners: 19% at 2 years	HbA$_{1c}$ (0) (−0.17) BP (0) BMI (0) Functional status (0)	18 months <30% *Randomization by practice* (I: N = 15, C:N = 14)
Kinmonth,[71] 1998 UK General Practice Type 2 Newly diagnosed diabetes	N = 360 Mean age 57 years (range 30–71 years) F: 41% HbA$_{1c}$ NR 4.7–6.8% (at outcome) 7.1 Range 4.2–14.0%	I: N = 142 • To practitioners • 1.5 days • Patient activation skills and materials, Diabetic Association guidelines and materials • C:N = (108) • Diabetic Association guidelines + materials only	Questionnaires: • Patient ratings of communication (+) • Satisfaction with treatment (+) • Wellbeing (+) • Knowledge of self-care B (−) • Lifestyle change (0)	HbA$_{1c}$ (0) (0.05) BP (0) BMI (−) Triglyceride (−) Functional status (0)	12 months >30% *Randomization by practice* (I: N = 21, C:N = 20)

* + = sig diff in favour of intervention $p \leq 0.05$ 0 no sig diff − sig diff in favour of control group

Enhanced internal locus of control provides a plausible mechanism by which improved metabolic control and functional status are achieved. Internality may result in health benefits directly by inspiring greater patient initiative in responsible health behaviours (appointment keeping and conscientious adherence to regimes), but also indirectly as an effective coping mechanism for the anxiety and uncertainty associated with illness. Simply feeling that one's health is not beyond one's control may, itself, reduce stress and improve metabolic processes and functional status. Neither of these explanations is necessarily linked to patient satisfaction or improved understanding of the underlying mechanisms and rationale of the therapy.

The Greenfield and Anderson studies paid particular attention to the management of negative emotions about either diabetes itself or about consultations about diabetes and its care, such as fear, anxiety and embarrassment. Both demonstrated improvements in metabolic control. In the Anderson study, an emphasis on psycho-social coping was associated with increased self-efficacy in stress management and obtaining social support, plausibly mediating the improvements in attitude to diabetes, reduction in impact of the disease on life and positive metabolic outcomes.

The balance of evidence from the studies reviewed suggests that when the physician is patient-centred (and non-controlling), when patients are verbally active overall and especially in information seeking and when the patient is empowered to make treatment decisions, self-reported health and functional status and metabolic control are improved. The different findings in the Kinmonth study deserve some comment in this regard. Despite the intervention proving successful in improving patients' views of communication with their practitioners, with patients reporting greater satisfaction with treatment and wellbeing at 1 year compared with controls, their disease status was worse; with significantly greater weight gain and higher triglycerides, and their HbA$_{1c}$ was not significantly improved. The more successful interventions appeared to pay greater attention to patient education and counselling about the disease than was achieved in the Kinmonth study, drawing attention to the importance of practitioners not losing the focus on disease management while attempting to achieve the benefits of more patient-centred consulting.

There are also differences between the activation interventions in the Greenfield and Rost studies and the empowerment interventions in the Anderson and Langewitz studies that are noteworthy. Activation focuses on encouraging patients to work through

their physicians in eliciting information and establishing a partnership, whereas the empowerment programmes directly provide patients with the capacity to act independently of the physician if need be. Although both approaches may act to enhance internality (and achieve benefits described earlier), activation may put strains on the patient–physician relationship by linking patient's success at partnering to physician's receptivity. Empowerment, however, may act to 'level the playing field' to some extent by providing patients with skills in self-management, thus diminishing the usual layman–professional gap. This may in fact act to optimize patient–physician relations by equipping the patient with the wherewithal to assume a collaborative relationship.

The studies described provided the platform for the more recent pragmatic trials of self-management described earlier.[23,26,40] They point the way to further evaluations of very clearly defined interventions, integrating the well-operationalized interventions from the patient–practitioner literature with the more strongly theorised models of behavioural choice and change from psychology. The gap between the apparent efficacy of interventions aimed directly at patients to activate or empower and of those applied through practitioner training programmes, with their weak application over time, is a particular challenge.

Translating research results to clinical practice

The foundation of patient-centred skills are those core communication elements which allow the physician to partner, inform, activate and support their patients.[59] In operational terms, this means the application of critical principles of good communication.[46]

The first of these is to hear the patient's perspective. Too often treatment discussions begin and end in a focus on identifying the 'right' drug or therapy. A more fruitful search, however, might be for a better understanding of the patient. Patients often have very specific ideas regarding the cause of their medical problems and what might help. By probing the patient's perspective and determining what the patient knows, believes and expects in terms of treatment, the physician or nurse can gain insight into anxieties and motivation and possibly idiosyncratic or contradictory explanatory framework held by the patient.

Key questions that are useful for eliciting the patient's perspective include:

- 'What do you think caused it?'
- 'What do you think will help?'
- 'What do you want me to do?'

A second principle is to provide information that is useful and relevant. A consistent finding in studies of providers and patients conducted over the past 25 years has been that patients want as much information as possible from their provider. Unfortunately, the provision of information unrelated to the patients' position has not been shown to be very effective in improving processes or outcomes of care. The patient is often thought of as devoid of knowledge and experience, an empty vessel into which directives, advice and rules for living are poured. The alternative is to start where the patient is, by asking 'what do you already know about your diabetes?'.

Even well-informed patients are surprised by informational gaps they discover when attempting to articulate what they know and understand about their condition and its treatment. This process allows for a tailored approach to patient education in which new information is presented in such a way that misinformation may be corrected, informational gaps filled and an assessment of the patient's fund of knowledge made more accurate.

Before a provider can assume that a patient has integrated new information in a way that has meaning for a daily routine, specific checks for accuracy must be made. The most straightforward of these is to ask the patient directly to repeat back the information given. This again provides the opportunity to correct misinformation and misinterpretations and reinforce an accurate report.

A third principle is the need to negotiate a plan and anticipate problems. In most instances, a range of treatment goals and options is reasonable. Often, however, decisions are made unilaterally by the provider when patient input could be elicited and accommodated. To the extent that patient's preferences and concerns can be accommodated and regimens tailored, the data suggest that the likelihood of success is increased. Of course, not all aspects of the treatment regimen are open to negotiation and these must be clear. However, a surprisingly high level of control over the regimen may be afforded the patient without compromising good medicine, as demonstrated by Rost and colleagues.

Examples of negotiation include:

- 'I need to know if you can live with what we discussed?'
- 'Do you think you will have any trouble with anything we talked about – anything at all?'
- 'What do you think would work for you? Any ideas? What else could we try?'

A fourth principle is the need to offer ongoing monitoring of compliance and compliance difficulties; problems should be expected even for patients with well-established regimens. It is critical to monitor compliance at every visit; but in ways that allows a patient to admit to non-compliance without feeling a failure. Framing compliance monitoring questions in a way that allows for an acceptable negative answer, for instance 'Most people have some trouble, what kinds of problems have you been having?'. has been a successful strategy in facilitating open and honest patient disclosure of compliance problems.

This leads to the next principle: finding problems and renegotiating solutions. Once compliance difficulties are established, the problems need to be specified and addressed. Misunderstandings and misinformation can be corrected with the use of simple, direct language and written aids. Unanticipated side-effects, cost, forgetting and simple demotivation may be dealt with through problem solving and brainstorming. For instance, the following may be helpful:

- 'What is it about the diet that is most troublesome?'
- 'What do you think would work?'
- 'What one thing are you willing to try?'

Finally, the last communication principle is to provide emotional support to the patient. Although patients certainly want as much information as possible from their doctors and nurses, the evidence suggests that information is not all that patients need for effective participation in self-care. Physicians are not simply expert consultants, although they are that; the physician or nurse is also someone to whom people go when they are particularly vulnerable. It is important that they are able to respond to patient emotions and provide support, reassurance, partnership and respect to assure commitment to the therapeutic relationship and also motivation for compliance with therapeutic regimen. Phrases that may be helpful in this context include:

- 'This must be hitting you pretty hard.'
- 'Anyone would feel overwhelmed by it all at first.'
- 'I'm here to help you through; we'll work it out together.'
- 'I'm sure we'll be able to get this under control.'

Summary of the current position

While medicine has always sought to serve patients' needs, it has relied upon physicians to define those needs. The broadening definition of quality in medical care of the past decade, which includes providers' interpersonal skills, calls for systematic efforts to incorporate the patient's perspective into medical care at all levels.

Engagement of the patient as an active participant in self-management has become seen as one of the key characteristics of a whole system approach to effective diabetes care moving beyond the consultation. The rhetoric of engagement, however, still outstrips the evidence. Evidence is now strong that some patients can be engaged to participate with practitioners in the self-management of their diabetes, with important effects on both psycho-social and clinical outcomes, at least in the short term.

Exactly how to achieve this for different groups of patients, by what route and which of the many facets of patient-centred care can be cost-effectively operationalized in modern medical practice remain research questions.

Answers depend on the collection of better evidence. Improvements are needed across the board, from characterization of study populations to study designs. Process measures of participation, activation and empowerment are still needed. Outcome measures themselves should include both objective measures of disease outcomes and patient-centred measures (e.g. of functional status and quality of life). Interventions should be more carefully developed and specified to allow understanding of individual component effects and their interdependence.[75] Rigorous explanatory trials of such interventions are still needed before pragmatic studies of cost-effectiveness. To advance knowledge further, we need to replicate promising studies using rigorous methods. These studies should include explicit theoretical frameworks for interventions, designed to link effects on key characteristics of patient practitioner interaction through to effects on health outcomes. Only in this way will the field advance beyond a series of tantalizing but disconnected and unconfirmed results.

References

1 Institute of Medicine. *Crossing the Quality Chasm: a New Health System*. National Academy Press, Washington, DC, 2007.

2 Griffin SJ, Kinmonth AL, Veltman MWM, Gillard S, Grant J, Steward M. Effect on health-related outcomes of interventions to alter the interaction between patients and practitioners: a systematic review of trials. *Ann Fam Med* 2004;**2**(6): 595–608.

3 Golin CE DiMatteo MR Gelberg L. The role of patient participation in the doctor visit – implications for adherence to diabetes care. *Diabetes Care* 1996;**19**(10):1153–1164.

4 Golin CE, DiMatteo MR, Leake B, Duan N, Gelberg L. A diabetes-specific measure of patient desire to participate in medical decision making. *Diabetes Educ* 2001;**27**(6):875–886.

5 van Dam HA, van der Horst FG, Knoops L, Ryckman RM, Crebolder HFJM, van den Borne BHW. Social support in diabetes: a systematic review of controlled intervention studies. *Patient Educ Counsel* 2005;**59**(1):1–12.

6 Deakin T, McShane C, Cade JE. Williams RDRR. Group based training for self-management strategies in people with type 2 diabetes mellitus. *Cochrane Database Syst Rev* 2005;(2): CD003417.pub2.

7 Murray E, Burns J, Tai SS, Lai R, Nazareth I. Interactive health communication applications for people with chronic disease. *Cochrane Database Syst Rev* 2005 Oct 19;(4):CD004274.

8 Doull M, O'Connor AM, Robinson V, Tugwell P, Wells GA. Peer support strategies for improving the health and well-being of individuals with chronic diseases protocol. *Cochrane Database Syst Rev* (3):2005;CD005352.

9 Griffiths C, Taylor S, Feder G, Candy B, Ramsay J, Eldridge S *et al*. Self-management education by lay leaders for people with chronic conditions. *Cochrane Database Syst Rev* 2007 Oct 17(4):CD005108.

10 DiMatteo MR, DiNicola DD. *Achieving Patient Compliance: The Psychology of the Medical Practitioner's Role*. Pergamon Press, New York, 1982.

11 DiMatteo MR. Variations in patients' adherence to medical recommendations – a quantitative review of 50 years of research. *Med Care* 2004;**42**(3):200–209.

12 Holman HR, Lorig KR. Viewpoint. Patient self-management: a key to effectiveness and efficacy in care of chronic disease. *Public Health Rep* 2004;**119**(3):239–243.

13 American Assoication of Diabetes Educators. The 1999 scope of practice for diabetes educators and the standards of practice for diabetes educators. *Diabetes Educ* 2006;**23**(1):25–31.

14 Lorig KR, Holman HR. Self-management education: history, definition, outcomes and mechanisms. *Ann Behav Med* 2003; **26**(1):1–7.

15 Glasgow RE, Hiss RG, Anderson RM, Friedman NM, Hayward RA, Marrero DG *et al*. Report or the Health Care Delivery Work Gr*oup – Behavioral research related to the establishment of a chronic disease model for diabetes care. *Diabetes Care* 2001;**24**(1):124–130.

16 Mensing C, Boucher J, Cypress M, Weinger K, Mulcahy K, Barta P *et al*. National standards for diabetes self-management education. *Diabetes Care* 2003;**26**(S1):S149–S156.

17 Diabetes UK, Najib J. *Patient Education for Effective Diabetes Self-Management: Report, Recommendations and Examples of Good Practice*. Diabetes UK, London, 2002.

18 National Institute for Clinical Excellence (NICE). *Guidance on the Use of Patient-Education Models for Diabetes*. Technology Appraisal 60. National Institute for Clinical Excellence, London, 2003.

19 DECS Consultative Section on Diabetes Education. *International Curriculum for Diabetes Health Professional Education*. International Diabetes Federation, Brussels, 2002.

20 DECS Consultative Section on Diabetes Education. *International Standards for Diabetes Education*. International Diabetes Federation, Brussels, 2003.

21 Muhlhauser I, Jorgens V, Berger M, Graninger W, Gurtler W, Hornke L *et al*. Bicentric evaluation of a teaching and treatment program for type-1 (insulin-dependent) diabetic-patients – improvement of metabolic control and other

measures of diabetes care for up to 22 months. *Diabetologia* 1983;**25**(6):470–476.

22 Langewitz W, Wossmer B, Iseli J, Berger W. Psychological and metabolic improvement after an outpatient teaching program for functional intensified insulin therapy (FIT). *Diabetes Res Clin Pract* 1997;**37**(3):157–164.

23 DAFNE Study Group. Training in felxible intensive insulin management to enable dietary freedom in people with type 1 diabetes: dose adjustment for normal eating (DAFNE) randomised controlled trial. *BMJ* 2002;**325**:746–751.

24 Kronsbein P, Jorgens V, Muhlhauser I, Scholz V, Venhaus A, Berger M. Evaluation of a structured treatment and teaching programme on non-insulin-dependent diabetes. *Lancet* 1988; **ii**:1407–1411.

25 Pieber TR, Brunner GA, Schnedl WJ, Schattenberg S *et al*. Before and after evaluation of structured outpatient group education programmes for intensive insulin therapy. *Diabetes Care* 1995;**18**:625–630.

26 Davies MJ, Heller S, Skinner TC, Campbell MJ, Carey ME, Cradock S *et al*. Effectiveness of the diabetes education and self-management for ongoing and newly diagnosed (DESMOND) programme for people with newly diagnosed type 2 diabetes: cluster randomised controlled trial. *BMJ* 2008;**336**:491–495.

27 DiMatteo MR. Social support and patient adherence to medical treatment: a meta-analysis. *Health Psychol* 2004;**23**(2): 207–218.

28 NHS Centre for Reviews, Dissemination. Complications of diabetes: renal disease and promotion of self-management. *Effective Health Care* 2000;**6**(1):1–12.

29 Brown SA. Meta-analysis of diabetes patient *education research: variations in intervention effects across studies. Res Nurs Health* 1992;**15**(6):409–419.

30 Norris SL, Nichols PJ, Caspersen CJ, Glasgow RE, Engelgau MM, Jack L *et al*. Increasing diabetes self-management education in community settings – a systematic review. *Am J Prev Med* 2002;**22**(4):39–66.

31 Norris SL, Engelgau MM, Narayan KMV. Effectiveness of self-management training in type 2 diabetes – a systematic review of randomized controlled trials. *Diabetes Care* 2001; **24**(3):561–587.

32 Padgett D, Mumford E, Hynes M, Carter R. Meta-analysis of the effects of educational and psychosocial interventions on management of diabetes mellitus. *J Clin Epidemiol* 1988;**41** (10):1007–1030.

33 Brown SA. Interventions to promote diabetes self-management: state of the science. *Diabetes Educ* 1999;**25**(6):52–61.

34 Roter DL, Hall JA, Merisca R, Nordstrom B, Cretin D, Svarstad B. Effectiveness of interventions to improve patient compliance A meta-analysis. *Med Care* 1998;**36**(8): 1138–1161.

35 Norris SL, Lau J, Smith SJ, Schmid CH, Engelgau MM. Self-management education for adults with type 2 diabetes – a meta-analysis of the effect on glycemic control. *Diabetes Care* 2002;**25**(7):1159–1171.

36 Armour TA, Norris SL, Jack L, Zhang X, Fisher L. The effectiveness of family interventions in people with diabetes mellitus: a systematic review. *Diabet Med* 2005;**22**(10): 1295–1305.

37 World Health Organization. *Therapeutic Patient Education: Continuing Education Programmes for Health Care Providers in the Field of Prevention of Chronic Diseases*. World Health Organization, Geneva, 1998.

38 Anderson RM, Funnell MM, Fitzgerald JT, Marrero DG. The Diabetes Empowerment Scale – a measure of psycho-social self-efficacy. *Diabetes Care* 2000;**23**(6):739–743.

39 Rickheim PL, Flader JL, Weaver TW, Kendall DM. Assessment of group versus individual diabetes education – a randomized study. *Diabetes Care* 2002;**25**(2):269–274.

40 Glasgow RE, Boles SM, Mckay HG, Feil EG, Barrere M. The D-Net diabetes self-management program: long-term implementation, outcomes and generalization results. *Prev Med* 2003;**36**(4):410–419.

41 Ciechanowski PS, Katon WJ, Russo JE. Depression and diabetes – impact of depression symptoms on adherence, function, costs. *Arch Intern Med* 2000;**160**(21):3278–3285.

42 Ciechanowski P, Katon WJ. The interpersonal experience of health care through the eyes of patients with diabetes. *Soc Sci Med* 2006;**63**(12):3067–3079.

43 Ciechanowski P, Russo J, Katon W, Simon G, Ludman E, Von Korff M *et al*. Where is the patient? The association of psycho-social factors and missed primary care appointments in patients with diabetes. *Gen Hosp Psychiatry* 2006;**28**(1):9–17.

44 Ciechanowski P, Russo J, Katon W, Von Korff M, Ludman E, Lin E, *et al*. Influence of patient attachment style on self-care and outcomes in diabetes. *Psychosom Med* 2004;**66**(5):720–728.

45 DiMatteo MR, Lepper HS, Croghan TW. Depression is a risk factor for noncompliance with medical treatment – meta-analysis of the effects of anxiety and depression on patient adherence. *Arch Intern Med* 2000;**160**(14):2101–2107.

46 Roter DL, Hall JA. *Doctors Talking to Patients/Patients Talking to Doctor: Improving Communication in Medical Visits*. 2nd edn, Praeger, Westport, CT, 2006.

47 Glasgow RE, Hampson SE, Strycker LA, Ruggiero L. Personal-model beliefs and social-environmental barriers related to diabetes self-management. *Diabetes Care* 1997;**20**(4):556–561.

48 Bandura A. *Self-Efficacy: The Exercise of Control*. Freeman, New York, 1997.

49 Sutton S. Predicting and explaining intentions and behaviour: how well are we doing? *J Appl Soc Psychol* **28**:1998; 1317–1338.

50 Stewart MA. Effective physician–patient communication and health outcomes - a review. *Can Med Assoc J* 1995; **152**(9):1423–1433.

51 van Dam HA, van der Horst F, van den Borne B, Ryckman R, Crebolder H. Provider–patient interaction in diabetes care: effects on patient self-care and outcomes – a systematic review. *Patient Educ Counsel* 2003;**51**(1):17–28.

52 Lewin SA, Skea ZC, Entwistle V, Zwarenstein M, Dick J. Interventions for providers to promote a patient-centred approach in clinical consultations. *Cochrane Database Syst Rev* 2001;(4):CD003267.

53 Roter DL, Stashefsky-Margalit R, Rudd R. Current perspectives on patient education in the US. *Patient Educ Counsel* 2001;**44**(1):79–86.

54 Roter D. The medical visit context of treatment decision-making and the therapeutic relationship. *Health Expect* 2000; **3**(1):17–25.

55 Engel GL. How much longer must medicine's science be bound by a seventeenth century world view? In: *The Task of Medicine: Dialogue at Wickenburg*. (ed. K White), Henry J Kaiser Family Foundation, Menlo Park, CA, 1998.

56 Freire P. *Education for Critical Consciousness.* Continuum Press, New York, 1983.

57 Wallerstein N, Bernstein E. Empowerment education – Freire's ideas adapted to health education. *Health Educ Q* 1988;**15**(4):379–394.

58 Street RLJr, Piziak VK, Carpenter WS *et al.* Provider–patient communication and metabolic control. *Diabetes Care* 1993;**16**: 714–721.

59 Viinamaki H, Niskanen L, Korhonen T, Tahka V. The patient–doctor relationship and metabolic control in patients with type-1 (insulin-dependent) diabetes mellitus. *Int J Psychiatry Med* 1993;**23**(3):265–274.

60 Roter DL. Patient participation in patient–provider interaction – effects of patient question asking on quality of interaction, satisfaction and compliance. *Health Educ Monogr* 1977;**5**(4):281–315.

61 Marvel MK, Epstein RM, Flowers K, Beckman HB. Soliciting the patient's agenda – have we improved? *JAMA* 1999;**281**(3): 283–287.

62 Greenfield S, Kaplan S, Ware J. Expanding patient involvement in care – effects on blood sugar control and quality of life in diabetes. *J Gen Intern Med* 1988;**3**:448–457.

63 Rost KM, Flavin KS, Cole K, McGill JB. Change in metabolic control and functional status after hospitalization – impact of patient activation intervention in diabetic-patients. *Diabetes Care* 1991;**14**(10):881–889.

64 Jette AM, Davies AR, Cleary PD, Calkins DR, Rubenstein LV, Fink A *et al.* The functional status questionnaire – reliability and validity when used in primary care. *J Gen Intern Med* 1986;**1**(3):143–149.

65 Kaplan SH, Greenfield S, Gandek B, Rogers WH, Ware JE. Characteristics of physicians with participatory decision-making styles. *Ann Intern Med* 1996;**124**(5):497–504.

66 Levinson W, Roter D. The effects of two continuing medical education programmes on communication skills of practicing primary care physicians. *J Gen Intern Med* 1993;**8**(6): 318–324.

67 Roter DL, Hall JA, Kern DE, Barker LR, Cole KA, Roca RP. Improving physicians' interviewing skills and reducing patients emotional distress – a randomized clinical-trial. *Arch Intern Med* 1995;**155**(17):1877–1884.

68 Roter DL, Larson S, Shinitzky H, Chernoff R, Serwint JR Adamo G *et al.* Use of an innovative video feedback technique to enhance communication skills training. *Med Educ* 2004;**38**(2):145–157.

69 Kern DE, Grayson M, Barker LR, Roca RP, Cole KA, Roter D *et al.* Residency training in interviewing skills and the psychosocial domain of medical practice. *J Gen Intern Med* 1989; **4**(5):421–431.

70 Anderson RM, Funnell MM, Butler PM, Arnold MS, Fitzgerald JT, Feste CC. Patient empowerment – results of a randomized controlled trial. *Diabetes Care* **18**:(7):1995; 943–949.

71 Kinmonth AL, Woodcock A, Griffin S, Spiegal N, Campbell MJ. Randomised controlled trial of patient centred care of diabetes in general practice: impact on current wellbeing and future disease risk. *BMJ* 1998;**317**(7167):1202–1208.

72 Pill R, Stott N, Rollinick SRRM. A randomised controlled trial of an intervention designed to improve the care given in general practice to Type II diabetic patients: patient outcomes and professional ability to change behaviour. *Fam Pract* 1998;**15**:229–235.

73 Prochaska JO, DiClemente CC. *The Transtheoretical Approach: Crossing Traditional Boundaries of Therapy.* Dow Jones-Irwin, Homewood, IL, 1984.

74 Kinmonth AL, Spiegal N, Woodcock A. Developing a training programme in patient-centred consulting for evaluation in a randomised controlled trial; diabetes care from diagnosis in British primary care. *Patient Educ Counsel* 1996;**29**(1): 75–86.

75 Campbell NC, Murray E, Darbyshire J, Emery J, Farmer A, Griffiths F, *et al.* Designing and evaluating complex interventions to improve health care. *BMJ* 2007;**334**(7591): 455–459.

26 Delivering care to the population

Rhys Williams[1], Ann John[1], Ambady Ramachandran[2], Chamukuttan Snehalatha[2]

[1]School of Medicine, Swansea University, Swansea, UK
[2]India Diabetes Research Foundation and Dr A Ramachandran's Diabetes Hospitals Egmore, Chennai, India

Introduction

This chapter considers the literature on methods of delivering diabetes care to populations. It draws upon analyses and recommendations contained in published reviews. It takes a global view of health care delivery, considering the impact of the increasing incidence and prevalence of diabetes on both developing and developed countries and the central need for primary care based strategies for the prevention and management of chronic disease.

We consider three important reviews which deal with interventions to improve the management of diabetes in primary care, outpatient and community settings,[1] a meta-analysis of randomized controlled trials of general practice diabetes care[2] and a review of shared (hospital and primary care) largely focused on the United Kingdom.[3] From these, a synthesis is provided of existing knowledge on the most effective means of delivering diabetes care to populations and recommendations are made for future studies in this area. These reviews deal almost exclusively with studies from developed countries. The needs of people with chronic conditions are now being addressed on a global scale,[4] and it has been pointed out that, for chronic non-communicable conditions in general, including diabetes, 'many health care providers are ill-equipped to manage [them] effectively and many governments cannot cope with the escalating disease burden and costs'.[5]

A recent report[6] from the Economist Intelligence Unit (sponsored by a major insulin-producing company) has estimated the economic impacts of diabetes in developed and developing countries. These data and others compiled from a similar standpoint have been critiqued in some detail elsewhere.[7] They relate to five countries – China, Denmark, India, the United Kingdom and the United States – and include estimates of costs in two important categories – direct health care costs and costs associated with lost production resulting from diabetes and its complications.

In the face of a rising prevalence of diabetes in almost every country [as clearly indicated by data from the International Diabetes Federation (IDF)[8]], direct health care costs of diabetes, as calculated by the Economist Intelligence Unit in 2007,[7] stand at 14.2% of total health care expenditure for China, 2.5% for Denmark, 4.5% for India, 3.5% for the United Kingdom and 6.0% for the United States. In all of these countries, productivity losses are considerable. In China, they are estimated to equal health care costs and in India they exceed health care costs.

The recent report of the World Health Organization (WHO) on the implementation of its global strategy on the prevention and control of non-communicable diseases[9] (adopted by the World Health Assembly in May 2008) recognizes the need for 'strengthening health care for people with non-communicable diseases by developing evidence-based norms, standards and guidelines for cost-effective interventions and by reorienting health systems to respond to the need for effective management of diseases of a chronic nature'. In terms of national policies and plans to enable this to occur, one of its proposals for action by member states is that the training of health professionals should be significantly improved 'with a special focus on primary care'.[9]

The Evidence Base for Diabetes Care, Second Edition, Edited by William H. Herman, Ann Louise Kinmonth, Nicholas J. Wareham and Rhys Williams.

Primary care – strengths and weaknesses

The ideal primary care service offers 'first contact, continuous, comprehensive and coordinated care to individuals and populations [ideally] undifferentiated by gender, disease, organ system or social status'.[10] Primary care has long been perceived to be the rational core of an efficient, equitable and effective health service in both developed and developing nations.[11]

Many features of primary care are particularly suited to meet the clinical needs of people with diabetes. For example, in systems such as that in the UK and many Western European nations, primary care provides open access, free at the point of delivery and a generalist approach well suited to initial diagnosis over a whole range of conditions. It also has, at its heart, a preventive approach depending on the infrastructure to enable maintenance of registers of people with long-term conditions and periodic recall and review organized on a population basis. In the UK this has recently been enshrined in the terms and conditions of general practitioners. They now work within a voluntary Quality and Outcomes Framework which includes financial incentives for achievement of specified goals in diabetes surveillance and intensification of treatment. In the ideal situation, primary care is local and convenient, provides 24 hour cover and takes a holistic approach, with the primary care team aware of and sensitive to family circumstances and effects.

This encouraging picture is balanced, however, by certain obstacles to the delivery of effective primary care. These include the need for the care team to be alert to non-specific presentations which may be missed in a complex clinical situation. More complex diagnostic and investigative needs may be best met by the specialist team in a hospital setting with extensive diagnostic and therapeutic back-up. Also, many of the advantages listed in the previous paragraph rely on *well-organized* primary care. Without appropriate infrastructure and organization, patients' needs will remain unidentified and the individuals may be lost to surveillance, particularly as many in the early stages of type 2 diabetes do not feel ill. When more specialized skills are needed for surveillance, and consequential action, these may be lacking or may have deteriorated with infrequent use. Examples within the field of diabetes care are fundoscopy skills and the knowledge and confidence to make changes in treatment, such as the intensification of treatment or cardiovascular risk reduction or initiation of insulin therapy. Lack of sufficient time to devote to individual patients and to continuing education for primary care professionals can lead to less effective care and professional and patient discontent.

One of the most important functions of general practitioners is as coordinators of continuous and comprehensive care. In this role, they are well suited to offer, or to ensure referral to, a structured programme of clinical surveillance based on registers, recall and regular review and to call on the wide range of generalist and specialist agencies available in the community or hospital sectors to support the diabetes patient in self-care.

A number of characteristics of the nature and current epidemiology of diabetes and the evolution of health care systems have contributed to a recent increase in the involvement of primary care. Among these is the recognition that effective clinical surveillance leading to near-normal control of blood glucose, blood pressure and other cardiovascular risk factors are associated with better outcomes and that continuing patient education, self-care and family support are likely to enhance such control. Diabetes epidemiology is changing such that incidence rates and prevalence are rising, especially in children and some minority groups. These changes, coupled with severe pressures on resources, are leading to overcrowded hospital clinics, some of which are, in any case, difficult for patients to access. These difficulties in access will be particularly severe in scattered rural communities, in countries without affordable transport systems and for people who are economically disadvantaged or disabled in some way.

Patient preferences also have an influence, with some, although by no means all, favouring the convenience and familiarity of their local primary care setting as opposed to the less comforting atmosphere of the hospital, especially when self-care is going well. In addition to this, depending on the means by which health care is funded in different countries, patients may be unable to afford hospital treatment even if they can physically access it. For a variety of reasons, many of them also economic, policy makers have lately favoured devolution of care away from secondary to primary care with chronic disease management schemes and financial incentives to widen the role of primary care teams in this area of practice.

Recognition of the widening role of the general practitioner in diabetes care has occurred in parallel with the developing role of the practice nurse and community diabetes specialist nurse, podiatrist, dietician and ophthalmic optician. Where these specialist skills are available in the community, they can be brought together into a community-based team joined, in some instances, by hospital-based physicians, clinical biochemists and other specialists on an 'outreach' basis. The current concept of the 'extended or integrated diabetes team' embraces professionals based in either primary care, secondary care or both in conjunction with the patient and their family.

The nature of currently available evidence

Randomized trials of health care delivery are uncommon, largely because the interventions being evaluated are usually complex. In his systematic review, published in 1998,[2] Griffin set out to identify and evaluate all published randomized trials of hospital versus general practice care for people with diabetes, to compare the effectiveness of general practice and hospital care through the use of meta-analysis of the identified trials and to explore variations in the findings of the individual trials. He identified only a few trials which met the inclusion criteria.

Details of the search strategies used can be found in the original publication. In brief, the medical subject heading 'diabetes' was combined with a number of others (e.g. 'family practitioner', 'family medicine', 'primary care') to identify all relevant studies in all languages. A wide range of databases was used (EMBASE, CRIB, Dissertation Abstracts, the UK National Research Register, MEDLINE, CINAHL, PsycLIT and Healthstar). These automated searches were combined with manual searches for further trial references. Studies were included in which people with diabetes (type 1 or type 2) were randomly allocated to hospital or general practice or 'shared care' for routine review and surveillance for complications, regardless of the quality of allocation concealment or choice of outcome measures.

The combined searches identified over 1200 studies but only five publications[12–16] describing six studies (Table 26.1) met the inclusion criteria. These were based in the United Kingdom (four trials) or Australia. All six trials employed satisfactory randomization of individual subjects. However, they were of short duration, only one lasting more than 2 years. One of these trials was published almost 25 years ago. The most recent of them was published in 1994.

On aggregate, 1058 people seen in hospital diabetes clinics were eligible and agreeable to randomization to continuing hospital outpatient review or follow-up in the community, either by their family doctor alone or as part of a shared care scheme. The organization of care for the hospital outpatient group was not clearly defined, although the descriptions appear to be broadly similar. All the general practitioners were provided with educational sessions or protocols before the trials. However, the support for care in general practice changed over time.

The two studies published in the 1980s evaluated basic general practice care. Two of the more recent studies included computer prompting systems. The publication by Hoskins et al.[15] compared both basic and prompted general practice care with hospital care and was therefore included as two separate studies.

The outcome measures used included process measures (primary care follow-up appointments and reviews, hospital consultations and admissions); morbidity measures (symptoms, weight, blood pressure, blood glucose, HbA_1, etc.), patient satisfaction and diabetes knowledge and mortality (in all studies except those of Hoskins et al.). The latter study alone included measures of cost.

There was heterogeneity between these trials. In the shared care schemes featuring more intensive support by means of computerized prompting systems, there was no difference in mortality between those patients randomized to hospital and those randomized to hospital follow-up. Those randomized to primary care tended to have lower values of HbA_1 [a weighted difference in means of -0.28%, 95% confidence interval (CI) -0.59 to 0.03]. Losses to follow-up were significantly less in the case of prompted general practitioner care (odds ratio 0.37, 95% CI 0.22 to 0.61). Patients randomized to primary care with less well-developed support tended to have worse outcomes than those allocated to hospital follow-up in the same study (Figures 26.1 and 26.2).

Hence these results supported the provision of 'regular prompted recall and review of selected people with diabetes by willing general practitioners'. These were a small number of trials, however, carried out in only two developed countries with comparatively similar systems of health care delivery.

Since the publication of that review, another randomized controlled trial, based in Denmark,[17] has been published. In this study, 311 general practitioners, in 474 general practices, took part in a 6 year study which included regular patient follow-up and individual goal setting supported by the prompting of doctors, clinical guidelines, feedback and continuing medical education. The results included significantly lower (at the $p < 0.001$ level) median plasma glucose levels in the intervention group than in the comparison group (7.9 versus 8.7 mmol l^{-1}), lower median glycated haemoglobin levels (8.5 versus 9.0%) and lower median systolic blood pressures (145 versus 150 mmHg). The doctors in the intervention group 'arranged more follow-up consultations, referred fewer patients to [hospital] diabetes clinics and set more optimistic goals'.

The trial, although well conducted and exceeding the follow up period of all of the six trials analysed by Griffin in 1998, does not allow a judgement to be made as to whether the interventions studied could be introduced throughout primary care in Denmark. The patients selected for the study were a representative sample of patients with diabetes attending these

Table 26.1 Characteristics of trials of general practice versus hospital care for diabetes (cited in Griffin[2]). Reproduced with permission from BMJ Group

Study	Setting	Follow-up (years)	Method of random allocation	Exclusion criteria	N	Type of diabetes	Mean duration of diabetes Mean age (years)[a]	Intervention	Main outcome measures
Porter 1982[12]	Fife, Scotland	2	Opaque sealed envelopes, independently prepared using random number tables	Insulin treatment	197	Type 2 diabetes from hospital clinic	Not stated	• Routine GP care • Diabetes team meetings • Record card • Recall system for those GPs without one	Symptoms, limb function, fundi, weight, blood pressure, blood glucose, urinalysis, costs, mortality
Hayes and Harries 1984[13]	Cardiff, Wales	5	Independently prepared (MRC) sealed envelopes	Diabetic complications Serious medical problems	200	Type 2 diabetes from hospital clinic	7 GP 59.7 H 58.4	• Routine GP care	Follow-up: reviews and blood tests, HbA₁, hospital admissions, mortality
Hurwitz et al. 1993[14]	London, England	2	Random number tables	Diabetic complications Serious medical problems	181	Type 2 diabetes from hospital clinic	GP 62.0 H 63.1	• Prompted GP care • GP education sessions • Structured review form • Fundoscopy by optometrists • Central computerized recall • Patient and GP prompts	Follow up: reviews and blood test, weight, blood pressure, HbA₁, consultation rates, hospital admission, satisfaction, mortality
Hoskins et al. 1993[15]	Sydney, Australia	1	A number (1 to 3) was drawn from a bag by an independent person	Diabetic complications Serious medical problems	134	Type 1 and type 2 diabetes newly referred to hospital clinic	3 GP 54 H 52	• Prompted GP care • Individual management protocols sent to patient and GP • Central liaison nurse prompting patient and GP	Follow up: reviews and blood tests, weight, blood pressure, HbA₁, costs
Hoskins et al. 1993[15]	Sydney, Australia	1	A number (1 to 3) was drawn from a bag by an independent person	Diabetic complications Serious medical problems	134	Type 1 and type 2 diabetes newly referred to hospital clinic	3 GP 54 H 52	• Routine GP care	Follow up: reviews and blood tests, weight, blood pressure, HbA₁, costs

(continued)

Table 26.1 (Continued)

Study	Setting	Follow-up (years)	Method of random allocation	Exclusion criteria	N	Type of diabetes	Mean duration of diabetes Mean age (years)[a]	Intervention	Main outcome measures
DiCE 1994[16]	Grampian, Scotland	2	Opaque sealed envelopes, independently prepared using random number tables	Age <18 years Planning pregnancy Serious medical problems	274	Type 1 and type 2 diabetes	9 GP 58.1 H 59.6	• Prompted GP care • Hospital annual review • Guideline and structure review form • Central computerized recall • Patient and GP prompts	Follow: reviews and blood tests, blood pressure, body mass index, creatinine, HbA_1, costs, knowledge, psychological tests, mortality

[a]MRC = Medical Research Council; GP = patients randomized to general practice care.; H = patients randomized to hospital care.

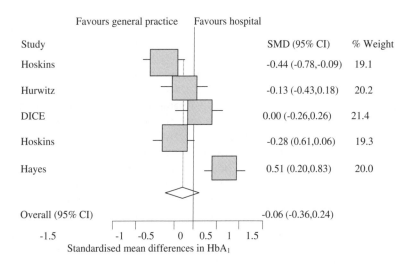

Figure 26.1 Standardized mean differences in HbA₁ (%). Reproduced from[2] with permission of BMJ Group

practices, but the practices were not representative of those in Denmark. To what extent these encouraging outcomes can be achieved by less well-motivated practices, particularly when such practices are faced with the combination of a rising prevalence of diabetes and limited resources, is not known. More recently,[18] a publication by some of the same authors suggested that improvement in HbA$_{1c}$ following the introduction of 'structured personal diabetes care' is found in women but not in men. Again, the extent to which this finding can be generalized outside this particular trial is uncertain. Mean HbA$_{1c}$ was lower in men provided with structured care than in men provided with routine care (8.5% compared with 8.9%), a difference which was not statistically significant ($p = 0.052$).

A review by Renders *et al.*[1] was conducted within the Effective Practice and Organization of Care (EPOC) review group of the Cochrane Collaboration. The EPOC search strategy was combined with free-text words and keywords regarding 'diabetes' and 'primary care' or 'community care' or 'outpatient care'. The databases searched were MEDLINE (1966 to 2000), EMBASE (1980 to 2000), CINAHL (1982 to 2000), the EPOC trials register (1999) and the Cochrane Clinical Trials' Register (1999).

The details of the study selection methods are included in the original review. In summary, they were studies aimed at evaluating the effectiveness of interventions *directed at health care professionals* who care for patients with type 1 or type 2 diabetes in primary care, outpatient or community settings and which fulfilled certain EPOC quality criteria. In order to be included, the studies must have used a 'reliable, objective, predetermined measure of the process of health care or patient outcomes'.

The review included 48 publications describing 41 studies. Of these, 27 were randomized controlled trials (RCTs), 12 were 'before-and-after' studies and two were interrupted time series.

All of the studies included were regarded as having methodological limitations. Only six of the RCTs were

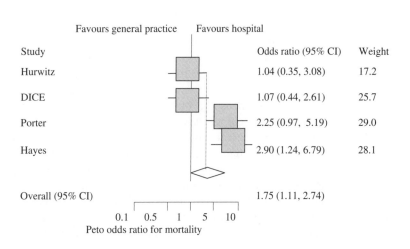

Figure 26.2 Peto odds ratios for mortality in general practice and hospital care. Reproduced from[2] with permission of BMJ Group

regarded as having adequate methods for the concealment of allocation. Contamination of the comparison groups was likely in the 15 studies in which patients or health care professionals were randomized within a clinic or practice. In a further two studies, it was likely that the comparison group also received the intervention (in that, for one of these, both intervention and control clinics were staffed by the same personnel, and in the other, a crossover design was used). Other methodological limitations were observed, such as lack of comparability of intervention and comparison groups, inadequate 'blinding' in the assessment of outcomes, less than satisfactory follow-up of patient outcomes, failure to provide 'intention-to-treat analysis' or the lack of a priori statistical power calculations.

From the detailed results of this review, a number of important conclusions were drawn. First, although complex professional interventions often improved the process of care, the effects on health-related outcomes was unclear, as these were rarely assessed. Significant improvement in patient outcome was reported in only one study. Second (and echoing the earlier results of the Griffin review), process improvements were also observed in studies of organizational interventions which included structured and regular review. A small beneficial effect in glycaemic control was observed in studies in which a nurse or pharmacist assumed part of the physician's role. Third, in studies which combined professional and organizational interventions, computer-assisted recall and reminder systems, in combinations with professional interventions, were associated with improvements in process measures. The involvement of nurses and the inclusion of patient education were associated with positive effects on patient outcomes. Overall, despite the methodological flaws and inconsistencies which this review described, it seems clear that combinations of professional interventions, organizational interventions, nurse involvement and the incorporation of patient education often *do* make a positive difference in the process of care and *can* make a positive difference in the outcome of care. The review also makes the point that diabetes care is a good model for the care of many chronic diseases.

Chronic conditions, such as diabetes, contribute around two-thirds of the global burden of disease worldwide.[5] This burden impacts on society, health care systems and individuals and families, often those who can least afford to bear the direct health care costs and resulting losses of income. As a result, there has been much interest in chronic disease management programmes as a means of improving the quality and efficiency of care for patients with chronic illness, thereby reducing their direct and indirect costs. Epping-Jordan et al. defined chronic disease management as a population-based approach to health care that identifies patients at risk, intervenes with specific programmes of care and measures outcomes.[5] Weingarten et al. systematically reviewed, from 1987 to 2001, the published evidence regarding the characteristics and effectiveness of disease management programmes.[19] They included 102 articles evaluating 118 disease management programmes. The study showed that many different interventions were effective; provider education, reminders and feedback led to improved adherence to practice care guidelines and improved disease control. Patient education, reminders and patient financial incentives also led to improved disease control. However, no study directly compared different interventions and most chronic disease management programmes used two or more interventions. The study concluded that currently it is difficult to define the most effective strategies for disease management programmes since the wide variety of interventions used can give limited practical guidance for programme development. Further study is needed in this area to assess the effectiveness of different strategies in specific situations.

The burden of diabetes as a chronic illness will fall heavily on low-income countries which also suffer substantial burdens from communicable disease and the long-term health effects of physical injuries (for example, those sustained in traffic accidents and resulting from wars and humanitarian disasters). If diabetes care is to be a model for the effective delivery of care to populations, then the knowledge base for practice and policy needs to be widened to include countries and health systems that are not represented in the available studies and reviews. Some of their conclusions will be applicable to other countries, many will not be.

Currently, evidence on delivering diabetes care in low-income countries is sparse. There is a need to develop sustainable interventions in line with the aims of the WHO.[9] Beyond health promotion programmes and community-based education, these countries will need support to develop their own infrastructure and expertise in this area. Additionally, the prevention and control of diabetes at a population level will have to extend beyond bio-medical and lifestyle approaches to addressing wider political, economic and social environments. For example, policies encouraging cash cropping of tobacco or coffee will need to be balanced with consideration of local nutritional needs. This requires a broad, multidisciplinary approach to delivering diabetes care to the populations of developing countries.

The developing country perspective

It is clear, from the developing epidemiology and health economics of diabetes, that the future holds many challenges for the delivery of care to populations. While evidence is accumulating to inform decisions in developed countries, the requirement now is for such evidence also to be obtained, analysed and acted upon in developing countries where the burden of diabetes and its complications will fall most significantly, on individuals, families and society, in the decades to come.

According to the predictions made by the IDF[20] and also by the WHO,[21] 70% of the expected increase in the diabetic population will occur in the developing world and, more importantly, it will affect people aged under 65 years who are in the economically productive stages of their life and crucial to the economic wellbeing of society. India is the country with the highest number of people currently affected by the disorder and is likely to remain so for some time, with a projected number of 71 million by 2025.[20] In China, where diabetes was relatively uncommon a few decades ago, it is already become a major health concern, with an estimated 21 million cases in 2000. Increasing urbanization and increasing prevalence of obesity contribute greatly to the increase in diabetes and, indirectly, to the related complications.[21]

Developing countries face a dual burden from communicable and non-communicable diseases (NCDs). The main challenges in delivering care are the inadequate facilities to cope with the increasing burden and the often inappropriate government budget allocations to health care.[22] These lead to severe economic burdens on the patient, his or her family, society and the government and are a major public health challenge. With the availability of effective treatments, ideally it is possible to achieve good metabolic control and thus reduce or prevent diabetic complications. However, the quality of diabetes care remains suboptimal in a large number of developing countries, including India.[23]

Health care systems in most developing countries are equipped to manage acute illness and have limitations in managing chronic disorders such as diabetes. Chronic disease management needs a team approach, which is frequently lacking. In addition, because of the relatively asymptomatic nature of diabetes, it is often considered to be a less serious disorder until a patient presents with complications.

India, a typical example of a rapidly progressing economy with multiple health care challenges, faces several limitations in the effective management of diabetes. Health care in India is provided by the central or state government hospitals, at district municipal and tertiary teaching hospital levels or through private general practitioners, specialists in their clinics or hospitals or by large corporate hospitals. Great disparity occurs between these centres in the quality, amenities and cost of care, depending on the training and interest in diabetes of the treating doctors. Except in government institutions, which provide free or subsidized consultation and treatment, the patient has to pay heavily 'out of pocket' for investigations and treatment. Due to the pressing needs for taking care of acute diseases, limited resources and infrastructure exist for chronic disorders such as diabetes. As a consequence, the quality of care suffers badly.

There is a wide disparity in the health care facilities available in rural and urban areas of India. The Government of India has built up an extensive infrastructure of rural health services based on primary health centres and subcentres. However, these often have inadequate facilities in terms of staff, equipment, laboratory facilities and essential drugs. Even in the private sector, no uniform standard is maintained. Facilities for patient education and awareness programmes are limited. The problem is aggravated by the prevailing disparities among patients in literacy, health consciousness and purchasing power, which determine their health-seeking behaviour.

In developing countries, the lower socio-economic stratum of society has a lower prevalence of diabetes because of the associated adherence to traditional lifestyles.[24] This is in contrast to the developed world, where prevalence is higher among the lower socioeconomic groups. However, complications are proportionally more frequent among the poorer members of society because of neglected diabetes management,[24] as a result of lack of awareness[25] about the disease and also due to economic constraints.[26,27] This scenario is similar in most developing countries.[28,29] Care of type 1 diabetes and other insulin-requiring patients is beset with multiple problems resulting from lack of sufficient insulin and other supplies and non-availability of trained health care personnel.[28]

The studies in developing countries that indicate that treatment of people with diabetes is far from optimal[30–32] include the Diabetes Care Asia project, which analysed data from a large patient pool from multiple centres and which showed that in India,[31] Singapore[33] and Taiwan[34] between 30 and 50% of the diabetic population had poor glycaemic and lipid control.

Many socio-economic factors and issues related to health care delivery impact the outcome of diabetes and consequently the costs. A major problem lies in the lack of a support system and non-availability of trained paramedical personnel, including nurse educators, podiatrists and dieticians. The entire responsibility for caring for these patients usually falls on the physicians. Moreover, many patients are unwilling to pay for these additional support services, thereby hindering their development of knowledge about the condition and endangering its management. Lack of medical reimbursement also is a barrier to quality care, because most patients of low socio-economic status cannot afford the costs of tests or treatment.

Nearly 70% of patients are diagnosed by non-specialists who may be ill-trained and poorly informed about diabetes.[31] They are unable to devote time to diabetes due to their busy practice. However, unfortunately, it is this group of doctors who are the prime link in early detection, diagnosis and guidance of the patients. Most physicians are trained to provide acute care, where effort and success are easily measurable and are linked to a sense of achievement and power. Physicians make decisions for the patients and many have concerns about their patients' apprehensions and capability for self-care.[35]

The treatment of acute illness is also economically more rewarding and private hospitals are interested and equipped for it. Patients belonging to middle and upper socio-economic groups with sufficient financial resources are good clients of corporate hospitals as they spend money on acute care and in treatments such as coronary bypass surgery. On the other hand they are not properly equipped for chronic care of disorders such as diabetes, partly because the long-term care of diabetes is not financially rewarding. A patient who is aware of the disorder and is motivated to participate in the daily management regimen has a better prognosis[36] and the physician has to be the guide for this.

In the absence of a comprehensive social security system, the burden of treating illness falls on the patient and their family. Diabetes-related complications account for 60% of diabetes health care costs and about 80–90% of indirect costs. Although the amounts spent by the upper and the lower socio-economic group families are similar, the percentage of the income spent is higher among the latter, owing to their lower income.[37] This percentage is increasing with time.[38] Health insurance is not yet popular. Employee state insurance benefits, although available, do not appear to be utilized fully.

The burden of health care in India can be judged from the fact that the *per capita* expenditure on health care in India is only 6.4% of the average world spending, whereas India accounts for 23.5% of world disability-adjusted life years (DALYs) lost due to diabetes.[39] Higher family income increases the likelihood of appropriate care provided to the patient, and this is likely to lead to the lowest risk of complications.

Studies show that type 2 diabetes starts early in Indians and more than half of the cases are diagnosed opportunistically, mostly by general practitioners.[30,31,40] The availability of specialists in cities prompts patients to consult them. However, even among the urban populations, many patients use alternative medicines for diabetes. This is similar to the situation in many African countries, where health care is delivered largely by traditional healers, particularly in rural areas.[28]

The availability of medical facilities and public awareness about the disease varies between Indian states. Despite the availability of specialized treatments, more than 50% of patients show poor glycaemic control and only a few undergo tests for complications, even in the cities. Similar observations have been made in Singapore[33] and Taiwan.[34] Hypertension and dyslipidaemia are common in all areas irrespective of the level of urbanization. These problems are, however, not confined to developing countries, since glycaemic and lipid control in Indian studies are comparable to the data from the United Kingdom.[40]

Good glycaemic control and the effective management of hypertension and dyslipidaemia in diabetes have multiple benefits, the most important of which is the prevention or delay of diabetic complications. However, there is a pressing need for primary prevention of diabetes in developing countries, which face multiple problems related to the increase in prevalence of diabetes, inadequate facilities to provide adequate health care to all the patients, the high cost of treating diabetes and its complication and the sub-optimal control of diabetes. It has been shown that moderate lifestyle modifications or the use of metformin in small doses prevents or delays the progression of IGT to diabetes in the Asian Indian population and that both interventions are cost effective.[41] These approaches may be useful in other developing countries also.

Several programmes have been initiated by the IDF, WHO, the World Bank and the World Diabetes Foundation (WDF) to create awareness of the consequences of non-communicable diseases (NCDs) in developing countries. These have subsequently led to the launch of national diabetes control programmes. For primary and secondary prevention of NCDs, including diabetes, cardiovascular disease and stroke, countries such as China, India, Bangladesh, Pakistan, Sri Lanka, Costa Rica, El Salvador, Malaysia, several countries in Africa and the Western Pacific (IDF) Region have given priority to the implementation of these strategies and have laid down guidelines for the effective management of these disorders.[42]

Based on the guidance, support and recommendations by an expert committee, the government of India

Table 26.2 Factors that will have impact on the delivery of diabetes care in developing and developed nations

1. Early diagnosis of diabetes
2. Early institution of appropriate interventions
3. Creation of awareness about diabetes and its complications among the public
4. National capacity building to improve the skills of intervention among doctors and paramedical personnel at different levels of healthcare system throughout the country
5. Patient education and empowerment to manage diabetes
6. A network system where by expert opinion and improved up-to-date facilities for treatment are available to the needy
7. Involvement of the government and steps to improve knowledge and facilities for diagnosis and treatment of diabetes even at the primary health centre level
8. Availability of medicines to the patients in the low socio-economic strata at a subsidised cost
9. A social support system or insurance programmes to support diabetic patients

and the Indian Council of Medical Research have laid down guidelines for minimum standards of care, prevention, disease prevalence surveys and for human resources development.[43] The pilot phase of the National Programme for Prevention and Control of Diabetes, cardiovascular disease and stroke has been launched by the Ministry of Health and Family Welfare,[44] the financial outlay for which is approximately US$1.3 million, undertaken in six districts and in six states, which in due course will grow into a larger project with allocation of a higher budget. Based on the deliberations of this expert committee, Table 26.2 shows the factors that will improve the management of diabetes in India and in other developing countries and also in those in a more advanced state of development.

References

1 Renders CM, Valk GD, Griffin SJ, Wagner EH, van Eijk JTM, Assundelft WJJ. Interventions to improve the management of diabetes mellitus in primary care, outpatient and community settings: a systematic review. *Cochrane Database Syst Rev* 2001; (1):CD001481.
2 Griffin S. Diabetes care in general practice: meta-analysis of randomized control trials. *BMJ* 1998;**317**:390–395.
3 Griffin SJ, Kinmonth AL. The management of diabetes by general practitioners and shared care. In: *Textbook of Diabetes*, 2nd edn, Vol 2 (eds J Pickup, G Williams,), Blackwell Science, Oxford, 1997, pp. 80.1–80.2.
4 Wagner EH. Meeting the needs of chronically ill people. *BMJ* 2001;**323**:945–946.
5 Epping-Jordan J, Bengoa R, Kawar R, Sabate E. The challenge of chronic conditions: WHO responds. *BMJ* 2001;**323**:947–948.
6 Economist Intelligence Unit. *The Silent Epidemic. An Economic Study of Diabetes in Developed and Developing Countries.* Sponsored by Novo Nordisk, The Economist, London, 2007.
7 Williams R, Songer TJ, Economic costs. In: *The Epidemiology of Diabetes Mellitus*, 2nd edn (eds J-M Ekoé, M Rewers, R Williams, P Zimmet), John Wiley & Sons, Ltd, Chichester, 2008.
8 Gan D, (ed.). *Diabetes Atlas*, 3rd edn, International Diabetes Federation, Brussels, 2006.
9 World Health Organization. *Prevention and Control of Non-communicable Diseases: Implementation of the Global Strategy*, World Health Organization, Geneva, 2008.
10 Starfield B, Fox R. Primary care tomorrow. *Lancet* 1994;**344**:1129–1133.
11 World Health Organization, Regional Office for Europe. *Alma Ata Declaration*. World Health Organization, Copenhagen, 1978.
12 Porter AMD. Organisation of diabetic care. *BMJ* 1982;**285**:1121–1124.
13 Hayes TM, Harries J. Randomised controlled trial of routine hospital clinic care versus routine general practice care for type II diabetes. *BMJ* 1984;**289**:728–730.
14 Hurwitz B, Goodman C, Yudkin J. Prompting the clinical care of non-insulin dependent (type II) diabetic patients in an inner city area: one model of community care. *BMJ* 1993;**206**:5624–5630.
15 Hoskins PL, Fowler PM, Constantino M, Forest J, Yue DK, Turtle JR. Sharing the care of diabetic patients between hospital and general practitioners: does it work?. *Diab. Med.* 1993;**10**:81–86.
16 Diabetes Integrated Care Evaluation (DICE) Team. Integrated care for diabetes: clinical, psychosocial and economic evaluation. *BMJ* 1994;**308**:1208–1212.
17 de Fine Olivarius N, Beck-Nielsen H, Andreasen AH, Harder M, Pedersen P. Randomised controlled trial of structured personal care of type 2 diabetes mellitus. *BMJ* 2001;**323**:970–975.
18 Nielsen ABS, de Fine Olivarius N, Gannik D, Hindsberger C, Hollnagel H. Structured personal care in primary health care affects only women's HbA$_{1c}$. *Diabetes Care* 2006;**29**:963–969.
19 Weingarten SR, Henning JM, Badamgarav E. Review: most disease management programmes for providers and patients lead to improvements in care. *Evidence Based Med* 2003;**8**:64.
20 Sicree R, Shaw J, Zimmet P. Diabetes and impaired glucose tolerance. In: *Diabetes Atlas* 3rd edn (ed. D Gan), International Diabetes Federation, Brussels, 2006, pp. 15–103.
21 World Health Organization. Diabetes cases could double in developing countries in next 30 years; http://www.who.int/mediacentre/news/releases/2003/pr86/en/index.html (accessed 10 February 2008).
22 Colagiuri R, Colagiuri S, Yach D, Pramming S. The answer to diabetes prevention: science, surgery, service delivery or social policy? *Am J Public Health* 2006;**96**:1562–1569.
23 Engelgau MM, Narayan KMV. Translation research for improving diabetes care: a perspective for India. *Int. J Diab Dev Countries* 2004;**24**:7–10.

24 Ramachandran A, Snehalatha C, Vijay V, King H. Impact of poverty on the prevalence of diabetes and its complications in Urban Southern India. *Diabet Med* 2002;**19**:130–135.

25 Murugesan N, Snehalatha C, Shobhana R, Roglic G, Ramachandran A. Awareness about diabetes and its complications in the general and diabetic population in a city in southern India. *Diabetes Res Clin Pract* 2007;**77**:433–437.

26 Herman WH, Eastman RC. The effects of treatment on the direct costs of diabetes. *Diabetes Care* 1998;**21**:(Suppl 3): C19–C24.

27 Rayappa PH, Raju KNM, Kapur A, Bjork S, Sylvist C, Dilip-Kumar KM. Economic costs of diabetes. The Bangalore urban district diabetes study. *Int J Diab Dev Countries* 1999;**19**:87–96.

28 Beran D, Yudkin JS, Courten MD. Access to care for patients with insulin-requiring diabetes in developing countries. Case studies of Mozambique and Zambia. *Diabetes Care* 2005;**28**:2136–2140.

29 Ei-Shazly M, Abdel-Fattah M, Zaki A, Bedwani R, Assad S, Tognoni G, Nicolucci A. Health care for diabetic patients in developing countries a case from Egypt. *Public Health* 2000;**114**:276–281.

30 Ramachandran A, Mary S, Sathish CK, Selvam S, Catherin Seeli A, Muruganandam M, Yamuna A, Murugesan N, Snehalatha C. Population based study of quality of diabetes care in southern India. *JAPI* 2008;**56**:513–516.

31 Raheja BS, Kapur A, Bhoraskar A *et al.* Diabetes Care Asia–India Study: diabetes care in India – current status. *J Assoc Physicians India* 2001;**49**:717–722.

32 Nagpal J, Bhartia A. Quality of diabetes care in the middle- and high-income group populace. *Diabetes Care* 2006;**29**: 2341–2348.

33 Lee WRW, Lim HS, Thai AC, Chew WLS, Emmanuel S, Goh LG, Lau HC, Lee HC, Soon PC, Tambyah JA, Tam YT, Jorgensen LN, Chua A, Yeo JP. A window on the current status of diabetes mellitus in Singapore – the Diabetes Care Singapore 1998 study. *Singapore Med J* 2001;**42**:501–507.

34 Chuang LM, Tsai ST, Huang BY, Tai TY. The current state of diabetes management in Taiwan. *Diabetes Res Clin Pract* 2001;**54**(Suppl 1): S55–S65.

35 Hunt LM, Valenzuela MA, Pugh JA. NIDDM patients' fears and hopes about insulin therapy. *Diabetes Care* 1997;**20**:292–298.

36 Herman WH. Diabetes epidemiology: guiding clinical and public health practice (The Kelly West Award Lecture 2006). *Diabetes Care* 2007;**30**:1912–1919.

37 Shobana R, Rama Rao P, Lavanya A, Williams R, Vijay V, Ramachandran A. Expenditure on health care incurred by diabetic subjects in a developing country – a study from southern India. *Diabetes Res Clin Pract* 2000;**48**:37–42.

38 Ramachandran A, Ramachandran S, Snethalatha C, Augustine C, Murgesan M, Viswanathan V, Kapur A, Williams R. Increasing expenditure on health care incurred by diabetic subjects in a developing country. *Diabetes Care* 2007;**30**:252–256.

39 Kapur A. Economic analysis of diabetes care. *Indian J Med Res* 2007;**125**:473–482.

40 Hippisley-Cox J, O'Hanlon S, Coupland C. Association of deprivation, ethnicity and sex with quality indicators for diabetes: population based survey of 53,000 patients in primary care. *BMJ* 2004;**329**:1267–1269.

41 Ramachandran A, Snehalatha C, Yamuna A, Mary S, Ping Z. Cost-effectiveness of the interventions in the primary prevention of diabetes among Asian Indians: within-trial results of the Indian Diabetes Prevention Programme (IDPP). *Diabetes Care* 2007;**30**:2548–2552.

42 Willett WC, Jeffrey P, Koplan JP, Nugent R, Dusenbury C, Puska P, Gaziano TA. Prevention of chronic disease by means of diet and lifestyle changes. In: *Disease Control Priorities in Developing Countries*, 2nd edn (eds DT Jamison, JG Breman, AR Measham, *et al.*), Oxford University Press, New York, 2006, Chapter 44, pp. 833–850.

43 Association of Physicians of India. API–ICP Guidelines for Diabetes, 2nd edn, 2007. *J Assoc Physicians India* 2007;**55**: www.japi.org.

44 A new initiative for a healthy nation: 'National programme for prevention and control of diabetes, cardiovascular and stroke (NPDCS)'; http://mohfw.nic.in/for%20websitediabetes.htm (accessed 11 March 2008).

27 Cost-effectiveness of interventions for the prevention and control of diabetes

Rui Li, Ping Zhang

Centers for Disease Control and Prevention, Atlanta, GA, USA

Public health and clinical decisions related to patient care, including diabetes care, have traditionally been based on projected medical outcomes; new treatments have usually been adopted if the health benefits to patients receiving them exceed any harm the treatments may cause. However, after several decades of rising health care costs, cost has become an increasingly important factor in the decision to implement a public health or clinical intervention. From 1961 to 2006, health care spending in the United States grew at an average annual rate of 9.9% or about 2.5% faster than the gross domestic product (GDP). United States health care costs as a percentage of GDP increased from 7.2% in 1965 to more than 16% in 2006. Health care expenditures reached $2.6 trillion or $7110 per person in 2006 and are projected to reach more than $4 trillion or $12 782 per person by 2016.[1] The estimated direct medical costs of diabetes care in the United States increased from $92 billion in 2002[2] to $116 billion in 2007.[3]

The rapid rate of growth in United States health care expenditures has raised both public and private decision makers' concerns about the United States health care system's financial sustainability. The federal government is particularly concerned about the longer term affordability of the publicly financed Medicare and Medicaid programmes. Private employers are concerned about their long-term ability to pay increasing premiums to provide health insurance coverage for employees, and also about the impact of medical costs on the competitiveness of their products in both the domestic and international markets. Now, many believe that, in deciding whether to cover a particular treatment, employers and other health care payers are justified in asking whether the net benefits of the treatment are worth its costs.

Costs are already a consideration in the establishment of public health priorities or recommendations for clinical practices in much of the world. Britain's National Institute for Health and Clinical Excellence (NICE) has formally incorporated both the cost and the effectiveness of a drug into its decision-making process concerning drug coverage. In Australia and in Ontario, Canada, drug costs are integrated into reimbursement decision-making. In the United States, however, the cost of medical services and drugs is not formally considered in national health care decisions such as decisions about Medicare reimbursement policy. However, the cost of intervention is beginning to play a greater role in some public heath and clinical decisions. For example, managed care health plans have begun considering an intervention's cost in addition to evidence about its effectiveness in their service and drug coverage decisions;[4] many federal agencies, including the Centers for Disease Control and Prevention (CDC), the Agency for Health Research and Quality and the Department of Defense, have considered the cost of interventions in their health policy and drug formulary decisions.[5] Independent scientific panels, such as the United States Task Force on Preventive Services, have also formally integrated the cost consequence of health interventions in their recommendations.

In this chapter, we describe the economic framework used to determine whether an intervention is worth its cost, describe how such a framework

The Evidence Base for Diabetes Care, Second Edition, Edited by William H. Herman, Ann Louise Kinmonth, Nicholas J. Wareham and Rhys Williams.
© 2010 John Wiley & Sons, Ltd

informs and guides public health and clinical decision-making and present the results of a systematic review of current evidence concerning the cost-effectiveness of interventions used for the prevention and control of diabetes.

Cost-effectiveness analysis

What is cost-effectiveness analysis?

Cost-effectiveness analysis is an analytical tool in which the costs and positive effects of an intervention and those of an alternative are calculated and presented as a ratio of incremental cost to incremental effectiveness.[6] Thus the cost-effectiveness ratio (CER) of intervention A compared with intervention B, is calculated as

$$CER = \text{incremental cost/incremental effectiveness}$$

where incremental cost = cost of intervention B — cost of intervention A and incremental outcome = health outcome of intervention B — health outcome of intervention A.

When the health outcome of an intervention is measured in physiological units, such as number of diabetes cases prevented or delayed or number of life-years gained (LYGs), the analysis is called a cost-effectiveness analysis; when the health outcome is measured by a quality of life-adjusted measure, such as quality-adjusted life-year (QALY), the analysis is called a cost–utility analysis; and when the health outcome is quantified in monetary terms, the analysis is called a cost–benefit analysis. Because of the difficulties in converting health outcomes into a monetary value, cost-effectiveness analyses and/or cost–utility analyses are more common than cost–benefit analyses.

How can cost-effectiveness analysis be used for health care decision-making?

Figure 27.1 illustrates how cost-effectiveness analysis can be used to guide decisions concerning the allocation of health care resources.[7] In a comparison of intervention A with intervention B, four cost and effectiveness scenarios are possible. Scenario 1, better outcome at lower cost, is the most desirable, but is probably the least frequently achieved. Scenario 2, better outcome at higher cost, may be acceptable, depending on how much the patient's outcome is improved and the increase in cost at which this is achieved. Scenario 3, worse outcome at higher cost, is the least desirable. Scenario 4, worse outcome at lower cost, may be acceptable when resources are limited and the amount of benefit being forgone is comparatively small.

The better outcome at higher cost (scenario 2) quadrant shown in Figure 27.1 is divided into two zones of cost acceptability by a line representing society's willingness to pay (WTP) to achieve the benefits of an intervention. Thus a CER above the WTP line indicates that society does not consider an intervention to be an acceptable use of scarce resources and a CER below the line indicates that society does consider the intervention to be an acceptable use of resources.

Current evidence on the cost-effectiveness of diabetes interventions

Systematic review to compile cost-effectiveness data

We searched MEDLINE, EMBASE, CINAHL, PsycINFO, Soc Abs, Web of Science and Cochrane databases in accordance with a systematic review protocol developed by the Cochrane Collaboration.[8] We sought cost-effectiveness, cost–utility and

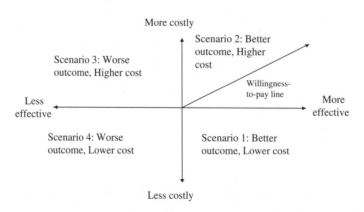

Figure 27.1 A framework for using cost-effectiveness analysis results in allocating health care resources

cost–benefit analyses of interventions related to the prevention and control of diabetes and its complications that were published from January 1985 to August 2005. We excluded review articles, commentaries and letters, published abstracts only, dissertations and cost of illness studies. We also excluded those studies with poor quality, which we assessed using the *BMJ* authors' guidelines[9] for economic studies. We also excluded studies from developing countries because of lack of availability and poor quality of the studies. Because of differences in health care financing system, health insurance coverage in particular, between the United States and other developed countries, we reported the cost-effectiveness of United States diabetes interventions separately from that of interventions in other developed countries (primarily western Europe, Canada and Australia).

We grouped interventions into the following five categories: (1) interventions to prevent type 2 diabetes among people at high risk for the condition; (2) interventions to screen for undiagnosed diabetes including GDM; (3) interventions to prevent diabetes-related complications among people with diabetes; (4) interventions to screen and provide early treatment for diabetes-related complications; and (5) interventions to treat diabetes-related complications.

All CERs are expressed in 2005 United States dollars per life-year or quality-adjusted life-year gained.

Interventions to prevent diabetes among people with impaired glucose tolerance

People with impaired glucose tolerance (IGT) have a higher risk of developing type 2 diabetes than those without. This risk can be reduced significantly by lifestyle modifications, such as eating a healthier diet and exercising more frequently or by pharmacological interventions. Two large randomized clinical trials[10,11] showed that improved diet and increased exercise reduced the risk of diabetes among people with IGT by 42–58% over periods of 3–6 years. The United States Diabetes Prevention Program (DPP) showed that, at the end of a 2.8 year trial period, metformin had reduced the relative risk for diabetes among people with IGT compared with those left untreated by 31%.[12]

Lifestyle interventions

United states

Three major studies[13,14,15] based on the DPP estimated the cost-effectiveness of intensive lifestyle modifications involving dietary improvements and increased physical activity in preventing type 2 diabetes among

people with IGT. Within the trial period, the CER for the intensive lifestyle intervention compared with the standard lifestyle recommendation was $19 000 per case prevented or $30 288 per additional QALY gained from the health system perspective and $32 156 per case prevented or $67 720 per additional QALY gained from the societal perspective.[13]

Because the health benefit of the intensive lifestyle modification will extend beyond the clinical trial period, possibly over a lifetime, Herman *et al.*[14] and Eddy *et al.*[15] estimated the cost effectiveness of the intensive lifestyle modification over a lifetime using a disease progression simulation model. Herman *et al.* estimated that the intensive lifestyle intervention would likely reduce the lifetime risk of developing type 2 diabetes by 20% among people with IGT and Eddy *et al.* estimated that it would reduce their lifetime risk by 11%. Herman *et al.* estimated that the lifetime CER of the intensive lifestyle intervention was $1400 per additional QALY gained (health system perspective) and $10 855 per additional QALY gained (societal perspective), relative to the standard lifestyle recommendation. Eddy *et al.* estimated that the CER of the intensive lifestyle intervention compared with dietary advice was $78 000 per additional QALY gained (societal perspective). The difference in the CERs in the two studies may be due to different assumptions about intervention effectiveness and different model structures. Eddy *et al.* also estimated that the CER of the intensive lifestyle intervention compared with standard lifestyle recommendations was $177 329 per additional QALY gained from the perspective of a 100 000-person health plan

The three studies[13–15] also estimated the cost-effectiveness of the intensive lifestyle intervention if it were conducted in a group setting instead of one-on-one as it was in the intervention trial. The DPP Research Group[13] estimated that the CER of the intervention in a group setting of 10 people would be $11 138 per additional QALY gained from a health care system perspective and $36 024 per additional QALY gained from a societal perspective over a 3 year period. The intervention was cost saving in the study by Herman *et al.*[14] or $14 880 per additional QALY gained over the lifetime (societal perspective) in the study by Eddy *et al.*[15] Eddy *et al.* estimated that the CER of the intervention in a group setting would be $33 480 per additional QALY gained from a health plan perspective.

Other developed countries

Segal *et al.*[16] and Palmer *et al.*[17] estimated the cost-effectiveness of lifestyle interventions in France, Germany, Switzerland, the United Kingdom and Australia; and Caro *et al.*[18] estimated the cost-effectiveness of lifestyle interventions in France, Germany,

Switzerland, the United Kingdom and Canada. Palmer *et al.* and Caro *et al.* used data on the effectiveness of the interventions from the DPP, while Segal at al used effectiveness data from other previously published studies. From a health system perspective, intensive lifestyle interventions among people with IGT were found to be cost saving in all countries except Canada (where Caro *et al.* found the CER to be $600 per additional LYG) and the United Kingdom (where Palmer *et al.* found the CER to be $7600 per additional LYG or $8,552 per additional QALY gained).

In Australia, Segal *et al.* found that group behavioural modification in the workplace for men and a community-supported media campaign were both cost saving when compared with standard lifestyle recommendation and that general practitioner advice on healthy lifestyle cost $964–2340 per additional LYG. Compared with standard care for women with IGT or normal glucose tolerance (NGT), they found that intensive dietary and behavioural modification cost $1239 per additional LYG for women with IGT only and $2340 per additional LYG for women with IGT or NGT.

Pharmaceutical interventions

United states
Three studies[13–15] used results from the DPP trial and computer simulation models to estimate the cost effectiveness of metformin in preventing type 2 diabetes among people with IGT. The DPP trial[13] showed that metformin reduced users' risk of developing diabetes by 31% at the end of the 2.8 year trial period; Herman *et al.*[14] estimated that metformin would reduce users' lifetime diabetes risk by 5.5% and Eddy *et al.*[15] estimated that it would reduce their lifetime risk by 8%. Within the clinical trial period, the CER for metformin use was $38 859 per case of diabetes prevented and $123 350 per additional QALY gained from a health system perspective and $42 780 per case of diabetes prevented and $122 805 per additional QALY gained from a societal perspective.[13] Over a lifetime, metformin was estimated to cost $38 700 per additional QALY gained from a health system perspective[14] and from $37 022 to $44 084 per additional QALY gained from a societal perspective.[14,15] If the generic form of the drug was used, metformin was estimated to cost $56 814 per additional QALY gained within the DPP trial period,[13] $2176 per additional QALY gained over a lifetime from a health system perspective[14] and $1800 per additional QALY gained over a lifetime from a societal perspective.[15]

Other developed countries
In studies that estimated the cost-effectiveness of metformin in Australia, Germany, Switzerland and England[17] and in Canada,[18] metformin treatment was found to be cost saving in terms of QALYs gained or LYGs over 10 years or a lifetime in all countries except England, where it was estimated to cost $6500 per LYG. In addition, acarbose treatment was found to be cost saving in terms of QALYs gained and LYGs over a 10 year period for people with IGT in Canada.[18] In Sweden, acarbose was estimated to cost $8351 per case of diabetes prevented over a 3.3 year trial period when used among people at high risk for type 2 diabetes and to be cost saving when used among people at high risk both for type 2 diabetes and for CHD.[19]

Summary
Three United States studies[13–15] showed that, over the long-term, an intensive lifestyle intervention in a group setting among people with IGT cost less than $20 000 per additional QALY gained from both a health system and a societal perspective. In other developed countries, an intensive lifestyle intervention cost less than $10 000 per LYG or additional QALY gained.

Three United States studies and two studies in other developed countries (all rated as being excellent in quality) used DPP clinical trial data to estimate the cost-effectiveness of metformin treatment for people with IGT. The three United States studies showed that, over the long term, metformin cost less than $50 000 per additional QALY gained and the two studies in other developed countries showed that it cost less than $10 000 per additional QALY gained.

Screening for undiagnosed type 2 diabetes or gestational diabetes (GDM)

Type 2 diabetes is often not detected until microvascular complications and the development of risk factors for macrovascular complications have already occurred. Although the health benefits of early detection and treatment of type 2 diabetes have not been established directly by randomized clinical trials there is a good reason to believe that early treatment can slow the progression of the disease and prevent or delay diabetes-related complications.[20]

GDM increases women's risk for macrosomia, spontaneous abortions and the later development of type 2 diabetes. Identifying women with GDM and managing their disease appropriately during pregnancy can reduce the number of pregnancy-related hospitalizations and improve birth outcomes. Although most United States obstetricians screen for GDM, we found no randomized clinical trials on the effectiveness of GDM screening.

We also found no studies of the long-term cost-effectiveness of screening for undiagnosed diabetes in developed countries other than the United States. We found five United States studies and one study in Germany that compared the cost-effectiveness of different methods of screening for type 2 or gestational diabetes.

United States

Two studies[20,21] estimated the cost-effectiveness of one-time screening for type 2 diabetes compared with no screening among United States adults who had a physician visit in the previous year (opportunistic screening). Both studies used comprehensive diabetes disease simulation models and one of them[21] also evaluated the cost-effectiveness of opportunistic screening in a United States subpopulation group at high risk for both diabetes and hypertension. The CER of screening per additional QALY gained ranged from $82 707 to more than $100 000 in the study by the CDC Study Group[20] and from $48 146 to $126 238 in the study by Hoerger et al.,[21] depending on the age group involved. However, the estimated cost of targeted screening among people with hypertension was only $42 985 to $64 531 per additional QALY gained.[21] In addition, the estimated cost-effectiveness of screening among population groups at high risk for undiagnosed diabetes was much lower, for example, less than $2000 per additional QALY gained among African Americans aged 25–54 years.[20]

One of these studies showed that the CERs of screening were lower among younger people,[20] whereas the other showed that they were lower among older people.[21] This difference in the relationship between age and the cost-effectiveness of screening may reflect differences in the models used or in assumptions concerning the intensity of glycaemic and hypertension control that those with positive screening results would receive. For example, Hoerger et al.[21] assumed that participants identified as having diabetes would receive intensive glycaemic control and that those identified as hypertensive would receive intensive hypertension control, whereas the authors of the other study[20] assumed that participants found to have diabetes would receive standard glycaemic control.

Zhang et al.[22] estimated the effectiveness and cost-effectiveness of five screening strategies per case of pre-diabetes (either impaired glucose tolerance or impaired fasting glucose) or previously undiagnosed diabetes identified: (1) giving a 2 h oral glucose tolerance test (OGTT) to the entire study population; (2) giving a fasting plasma glucose (FPG) test to the entire study population and giving an OGTT only to those who test positive; (3) giving an HbA$_{1c}$ screening test to the entire study population and giving an OGTT only to those who test positive; (4) giving a capillary blood glucose (CBG) screening test to the entire study population and giving an OGTT only to those who test positive; and (5) using a type 2 diabetes risk assessment questionnaire to identify people to be given an OGTT. They estimated that the cost per case identified ranged from $176 to $236 from a single-payer perspective, that testing everyone with the OGTT was the most effective strategy (i.e. identified the most cases), but that either using the CBG test or using the risk assessment questionnaire were the least costly strategies. Hence the best strategy for a diabetes screening programme will depend on the extent to which the goal of the programme is to identify as many diabetes cases as possible or to identify cases at the lowest cost per case.

In a later study, Zhang et al.[23] estimated the most cost-effective cutoff points for three screening tests for undiagnosed diabetes and pre-diabetes: the FPG test, the HbA$_{1c}$ test and the CBG test. From a single-payer perspective, they estimated that the most efficient cutoff points were 100 mg dl^{-1} (5.5 mmol/L) for the fasting plasma glucose test ($141 per case identified), 5.0% for the HbA$_{1c}$ test ($190 per case identified) and 100 mg dl^{-1} (5.5 mmol/L) for the random capillary blood glucose test ($155 per case identified). However, if the purpose of screening was to detect undiagnosed diabetes alone, the most efficient cutoff points were 110 mg dl^{-1} (6.1 mmol/L) for the fasting plasma glucose test ($689 per case identified), 5.7% for the HbA$_{1c}$ test ($732 per case identified) and 120 mg dl^{-1} (6.7 mmol/L) for the random capillary blood glucose test ($486 per case identified). In short, they found that a lower cutoff value should be used when screening for pre-diabetes and undiagnosed diabetes together than when screening for undiagnosed diabetes alone.

Johnson et al.[24] estimated the cost per case of diabetes detected using random plasma glucose (RPG) screening with three different cutoff points (100, 130 and 160 mg dl^{-1}) (5.5, 7.2, 8.9 mmol/L) and at three different screening intervals (1, 3 and 5 years) among Americans aged 45–74 years. All study participants with positive screening results were given a diagnostic fasting plasma glucose test or an oral glucose tolerance test. From a societal perspective, over 15 years, they estimated that RPG screening with a cutoff point of 130 mg dl^{-1} (7.2 mmol/L) conducted every 3 years would have the optimal combination of sensitivity and specificity and that the cost per type 2 diabetes case identified with this strategy was $275 for opportunistic screening and $1745 for population screening.

Nicholson et al.[25] used a simulation model to study the short-term cost-effectiveness of three screening methods to detect GDM in the United States: (1) a 75 g glucose tolerance test (GTT); (2) an initial 50 g glucose challenge test, followed by a 100 g GTT for those testing positive on the initial test (sequential methods); and (3) a 100 g GTT. Maternal outcomes considered were hypertensive disease, polyhydramnios, Caesarean delivery and delivery complications. Neonatal outcomes considered were mild hypoglycaemia, macrosomia, respiratory distress syndrome, shoulder dystocia, moderate morbidity and severe morbidity or death. Costs were screening costs, short-term costs for maternal and infant care and the costs of lost productivity, including lost wages. From a societal perspective, they estimated that use of the challenge test in conjunction with a 100 g GTT was most cost-effective ($35 218 per additional QALY gained among mothers and $8977 per additional QALY gained among infants compared with the second most cost-effective strategy, sequential methods). The 75 g GTT method was the least effective and most costly. All of the screening methods yielded better outcome and less cost compared with no screening.

Kim et al.[26] simulated several strategies for type 2 diabetes screening among women with histories of GDM: a fasting plasma glucose (FPG) test, a 2 h oral glucose tolerance test (OGTT) and an HbA_{1c} test. Screening intervals were annually, every 2 years and every 3 years. From a health system perspective, over a period of 12 years, they estimated that the OGTT had the lowest cost per diabetes case detected and that less frequent testing led to lower costs per case detected. Screening for undiagnosed diabetes every 3 years with the OGTT had the lowest CER: $373 per case detected.

Other developed countries

Icks et al.[27] compared the cost-effectiveness of different screening methods for detecting undiagnosed type 2 diabetes among Germans aged 55–74 years. They evaluated the cost-effectiveness of (1) the fasting glucose test (FGT) only, (2) the FGT plus the OGTT if FGT results were positive (FGT + OGTT), (3) the OGTT only and (4) the HbA_{1c} test plus the OGTT if HbA_{1c} results were >5.6% (HbA_{1c} + OGTT). They found that the FGT alone detected the highest proportion of previously undiagnosed diabetes cases, followed in order by FGT + OGTT, OGTT and HbA_{1c} + OGTT. They also evaluated the cost per case of diabetes detected from a health system perspective over a 1 year period. They found that all the screening methods were more effective and less costly in population screening than in targeted screening of people who were obese, had a family history of diabetes or had hypertension or a high cholesterol level. Under the scenario of population screening for diabetes, OGTT alone was more cost-effective than IFG alone and IFG + OGTT. HbA_{1c} + OGTT cost $921 per additional case of diabetes detected when compared with OGTT alone.

Summary

United States studies have shown that screening for undiagnosed type 2 diabetes among all adults was less cost-effective than targeted screening among those with risk factors for diabetes. However, we found little evidence from other developed countries concerning the cost-effectiveness of mass or targeted diabetes screening. Screening for GDM, when compared with no screening, may be cost saving. Four studies estimated the most cost-effective diabetes screening methods or the most cost-effective cutoff points to use in various biological screening tests for diabetes. Most of the CERs were less than $1000 per case identified. In the United States, the CBG test and the risk assessment questionnaire were the most efficient diabetes screening methods in terms of the cost per case of pre-diabetes or previously undiagnosed diabetes that they identified. The most efficient cutoff points in screening for either pre-diabetes or diabetes were 100 mg dl^{-1} (5.5 mmol/L) on the FPG test, 5.0% on the HbA_{1c} test and 100 mg dl^{-1} (5.5 mmol/L) on the CBG test. However, the most efficient cutoff point were higher (110 mg dl^{-1} (6.1 mmol/L) on the FPG test, 5.7% on the HbA_{1c} test and 120 mg dl^{-1} (6.7 mmol/L) on the CBG test) in screening for diabetes alone. For women with a history of GDM, screening for undiagnosed diabetes every 3 years with the OGTT was the most cost-effective strategy. In Germany, OGTT screening only for people with HbA_{1c} levels 5.6% or higher was the most cost-effective strategy. However, the German analysis was based on data from population studies and the outcomes were neither LYGs nor QALYs gained.

Interventions for glucose management

A number of studies have examined the effectiveness of intensive glycaemic control interventions in slowing the progression of diabetes and reducing the occurrence of diabetes complications. Such interventions include intensive lifestyle modification, the use of insulin alone, the use of anti-diabetic medications such as sulfonylureas and metformin, either alone or in combination with insulin, diabetes education programmes and disease management programmes. However, intensive glycaemic control interventions may increase diabetes patients' risk for hypoglycaemic events, including neurogenic symptoms such as palpitations, tremor, hunger and sweating, in addition to more severe consequences such as seizure, coma and even death.

United States

The Diabetes Control and Complications Trial (DCCT) Research Group[28] evaluated the cost-effectiveness of intensive insulin therapy among type 1 diabetes patients on the basis of results from the DCCT trial. The goal of the intensive insulin therapy was to lower patients' HbA$_{1c}$ level from around 9% to a level that was as close as possible to that of people without diabetes. Compared with conventional glycaemic control, the intensive insulin therapy cost $43 851 per additional LYG or $30 580 per additional QALY gained.

We identified three studies that evaluated the cost-effectiveness of intensive glycaemic control interventions for type 2 diabetes patients. In a 1997 study, Eastman et al.[29] estimated the cost-effectiveness of a comprehensive treatment to lower HbA$_{1c}$ levels from an average of 10% to near 7% among people with newly diagnosed type 2 diabetes compared with 'standard care' with insulin or oral diabetes drugs They estimated that the comprehensive treatment cost $25 337 per additional QALY gained. However, the efficacy of intensive glycaemic control was based on the DCCT for persons with type 1 diabetes.

Eddy et al.[15] used a simulation to evaluate the cost-effectiveness of intensive glucose management with the intensive lifestyle modification used in the DPP to maintain patients' HbA$_{1c}$ level below 7%. They simulated both health and cost consequences assuming that type 2 diabetes patients received the intervention as soon as they developed the disease and additional treatments as recommended by the American Diabetes Association (ADA) if the lifestyle modification failed to bring their HbA$_{1c}$ level below 7% and that the comparison group received only standard dietary recommendations plus the intensive treatment recommended by ADA if their HbA$_{1c}$ level exceeded 7%. They estimated that the intensive lifestyle intervention would cost $30 367 per additional QALY gained from a health system perspective.

In 2002, the CDC Diabetes Cost-Effectiveness Study Group[30] evaluated the cost-effectiveness of an intensive glucose control intervention in which sulfonylurea or insulin treatment was used to keep patients' fasting plasma glucose levels below 108 mg dl^{-1}. The comparative intervention was conventional therapy with diet alone or a combination of diet and drug treatment if hyperglycaemic symptoms were present. The study group assumed that this conventional therapy would produce an average HbA$_{1c}$ level of 7.9% as it did in the United Kingdom Prospective Diabetes Study (UKPDS). They estimated that among Americans aged 25 years or older with newly diagnosed type 2 diabetes, the intensive intervention would cost $57 110 per additional QALY gained. However, the CER estimates varied substantially by age, from less than $25 000 for diabetes patients aged 25–44, to $100 000 for those aged 55–64, to $2.9 million for those aged 85–94 years.

Other developed countries

Three studies estimated the cost-effectiveness of intensive glucose control for type 1 diabetes patients in England. One study compared a structured treatment and teaching program (STTP) for diabetes self-management plus usual care with usual care alone, one compared a continuous subcutaneous insulin intervention with multiple daily insulin injections[31] and one compared insulin detemir-based basal/bolus therapy with protamine hagendorm human insulin-based basal/bolus therapy.[32] From a health system perspective, STTP was found to be cost saving and the other two interventions cost less than $20 000 per additional QALY gained. However, the data from all three studies were based on results of single small-scale clinical trials.

Eight studies evaluated the cost-effectiveness of intensive glucose control among type 2 diabetes patients or a mix of type 1 and type 2 diabetes patients in UK[33,34,36] Canada,[35] Sweden,[37] Japan,[38] Australia[39] and Germany.[40] Three studies were based on data from the UKPDS.[33,34,36] One was based on other clinical trial data,[38] two were based on data from a literature review[36,40] and two were based on data from trials conducted before UKPDS.[37,39] These studies evaluated the cost-effectiveness of intensive glycaemic management with insulin, sulfonylureas or metformin compared with conventional glycaemic management (usually defined as diet control)[33,34,36] or conventional insulin therapy;[38,37] of pioglitazone as a second-line anti-diabetic medication compared with metformin, acarbose or sulfonylurea;[40] of pioglitazone as a first-line anti-diabetic medication compared with metformin or diet and exercise;[35] and of a community-pharmacist-initiated disease-management service (defined as one initial and six follow-up visits in 9 months) compared with standard anti-diabetic care.[39] Compared with conventional anti-diabetic treatment, intensive glycaemic control treatment with insulin, sulfonylureas or metformin was either cost saving[33,34,38] or cost less than $20 000 per additional LYG or QALY gained [33,36,37] from a health system's perspective. Although one study[37] estimated that intensive glycaemic control through insulin–glucose infusion followed by subcutaneous insulin would cost $20 444 per additional LYG and $29 161 per additional QALY gained (societal perspective) when compared with standard anti-diabetic therapy using anti-diabetics and subcutaneous insulin, that study included the added cost of intensive treatment over the increased projected lifespan of those given the treatment, a cost excluded in the other referenced studies. If this cost was excluded, the CERs would decrease to $1210 per additional LYG or $1815 per additional QALY gained.

In Germany, the use of pioglitazone as a second-line anti-diabetic drug following the failure of sulfonylureas was estimated to cost $23 694 per additional LYG when compared with metformin and $11 606 per additional LYG when compared with acarbose (both from a health system perspective). When compared with sulfonylureas or acarbose as a second-line anti-diabetic drug following the failure of metformin, pioglitazone as a second-line drug cost $57 163 per additional LYG and $16 063 per additional LYG, respectively.[40] If pioglitazone was used as a first-line anti-diabetic drug, the therapy cost $35 670 compared with glyburide, $45 240 compared with metformin or $23 490 compared with diet and exercise as a first-line anti-diabetic therapy in terms of per additional LYG in Canada.[35] In Australia, Taylor et al.[39] reported that, compared with standard care, community pharmacists disease management cost $2041 for each 1% reduction in mean HbA$_{1c}$ level.

Summary

In the United States, intensive insulin therapy among type 1 diabetes patients was estimated to cost less than $50 000 per additional QALY gained on the basis of data collected in the DCCT, a multi-centre, randomized clinical trial. Among type 2 diabetes patients, intensive glycaemic control in conjunction with sulfonylurea or insulin treatment was estimated to cost between $50 000 and $60 000 per additional QALY gained overall, but to be more cost-effective for younger patients. Intensive lifestyle modification or comprehensive anti-diabetic therapy to achieve an HbA$_{1c}$ level of less than 7% among people with newly diagnosed diabetes was estimated to cost about $30 000 per additional QALY gained. All of these estimates were from high-quality economic studies based on data from large multi-centre randomized clinical trials.

In other developed countries, the estimated CERs for glycaemic control interventions were lower than those in the United States. All CERs for interventions among type 1 diabetes patients were under $20 000 per additional QALY gained; however, the interventions were diverse and cost-effectiveness data were based on small-scale clinical trials. For type 2 diabetes patients, intensive glycaemic control using insulin, sulfonylureas or metformin to reduce HbA$_{1c}$ levels to less than 7% were also estimated to cost less than $20 000 per additional LYG or QALY gained and those estimates were based on high-quality data from randomized clinical trials such as the UKPDS. In Germany, use of pioglitazone as a second-line anti-diabetic drug was found to cost less than $50 000 per additional LYG when compared with glyburide, metformin or diet and exercise, and in Canada it was found to cost between $25 000 and $60 000 per additional LYG as a first-line anti-diabetic drug when

compared with metformin or acarbose. In all studies that assessed the cost-effectiveness of intensive glycaemic management by patients' age, its cost-effectiveness was negatively associated with age.

Interventions for blood pressure control

Among people with type 2 diabetes, hypertension is associated with an increased risk of macrovascular complications. Studies have shown that ACE (angiotensin-converting enzyme) inhibitors or beta-blockers are effective in reducing blood pressure and thus in reducing the incidence of stroke and myocardial infarction among people with type 2 diabetes. Data on the effectiveness of hypertension control among type 2 diabetes patients are mainly from the UKPDS.[12]

United States

Two United States studies estimated the cost-effectiveness of tight blood pressure (BP) control to reduce the incidence of macrovascular complications among type 2 diabetes patients with hypertension but no history of cardiovascular heart disease or end-stage renal disease (ESRD). One analysis of ACE inhibitor treatment showed that the average BP of treated patients was 144/82 mmHg and the average BP of those who received 'standard care' was 154/86 mmHg as in the UKPDS.[30] The other study[43] was a systematic review and meta-analysis of data from clinical trials and tight BP control (defined as a diastolic blood pressure of less than 85 mmHg instead of 9 mmHg). Both studies found that tight hypertension control was cost saving.

Other developing countries

Four studies, all conducted in UK, estimated the cost-effectiveness of interventions to control high BP.[43–47] Three of these studies were based on the results from the UKPDS, which compared tight BP control with ACE inhibitors with standard BP control.[44,45,47] In the UKPDS, the goal was to achieve a BP of less than 150/85 mmHg, whereas the goal of standard blood control was to achieve a BP of less than 180/105 mmHg. Tight BP control was found to be cost saving in two studies[44,45] and to cost $210 per additional QALY gained in the other.[36]

Mason et al.[46] evaluated the cost-effectiveness of implementing a BP control programme in routine clinical practice in England. This programme included a 45 min consultation session at a specialist nurse-led clinic plus follow-up clinic visits for lifestyle and hypertension medication review, in addition to the usual care. The treatment goal was a BP of 130/85 mmHg. The comparison group received the usual BP treatment delivered in hospitals or by primary care providers in England. The comprehensive BP control programme was estimated to cost $4382 per additional QALY gained when compared with the usual treatment. In another study, Gray et al.[47] used UKPDS data to show that use of the beta-blocker atenolol to treat hypertension was cost saving compared with the use of ACE inhibitors such as captopril.

Summary

Several well-conducted economic studies based on data from the UKPDS, a large, multi-centre, randomized clinical trial and simulation model showed that intensive BP control with ACE inhibitors was cost saving or had very low CERs. A translational intervention in which the ACE inhibitor intervention used in the UKPDS trial was adopted by specialist nurse-led clinics also was estimated to have a low CER; however, this estimate was based on data from a small-scale clinical trial.

Interventions for cholesterol control

People with diabetes are at substantially higher risk of cardiovascular disease than those without, even if they are not hypertensive.[48] Several large prospective randomized controlled clinical trials such as the Scandinavian Simvastatin Survival Study (4S)[49] have shown that statin treatment is clinically effective in improving lipid values among patients with dyslipidaemia. Evidence that lipid control reduces patients' risk for cardiovascular disease is stronger among those with a history of coronary heart disease (CHD) than among those without.

United States

Two studies estimated the cost-effectiveness of HMG-CoA reductase inhibitors such as simvastatin or pravastatin compared with placebos among diabetes patients with dyslipidaemia.[30,49] One study was based on 4S data[49] and the other was based on data from the West of Scotland Coronary Prevention Study.[30] In the study based on 4S data, Herman et al.[49] estimated that simvastatin treatment for secondary prevention of CVD was cost saving compared with treatment with a placebo. In the second study, the CDC Diabetes Cost-Effectiveness Study Group estimated that the CER of pravastatin for primary prevention of CVD among people with newly diagnosed diabetes was $71 607 per additional QALY gained compared with no drug treatment.[30]

Other developed countries

The cost-effectiveness of lipid control was evaluated in three studies using data from 11 European countries and Canada.[46,50,51] Two studies used data from the 4S study,[50,51] one used data from the Cholesterol and Recruitment Events (CARE) trial[51] and one used data from the Specialist Nurse-Led Clinics to Improve Hyperlipidaemia in Diabetes (SPLINT) trial and the Heart Protection Study (HPS).[46]

For diabetes patients with a CHD history, Jonsson et al.[50] reported that the CERs of simvastatin treatment in the 11 European countries varied from cost saving to $8663 per additional LYG, depending on the country in which the treatment occurred; the median CER of simvastatin treatment was $2622 per additional LYG. Grover et al.[51] reported that in Canada, among men with an average pretreatment LDL of 5.46 mmol l^{-1}, the CER of simvastatin treatment ranged from $5640 per additional LYG among 60-year-olds to $11 280 per additional LYG among 40-year-olds and that results were similar among Canadian women with cardiovascular disease.[51]

Among Canadian men with diabetes but no cardiovascular disease and an average pretreatment LDL level of 5.46 mmol l^{-1}, Grover et al.[51] reported that CERs of simvastatin treatment per additional YLG ranged from $5640 among 60-year-olds to $14 100 among 70-year-olds and that among women free of cardiovascular disease, they ranged from $14 100 among 60-year-olds to $25 380 among 70-year-olds. The relationship between the cost-effectiveness of simvastatin treatment and age was a 'U' shape (high for the young and old, low for those in the middle). Similarly, for diabetes patients with nearly 'normal' lipid levels (3.5 mmol l^{-1}) and no cardiovascular disease, CERs of simvastatin treatment ranged from $9870 to $21 150 per additional LYG among men and from $33 840 to $56 400 per additional LYG among women.

Mason et al.[46] estimated that a policy of using specialist nurse-led clinics in England to treat and control hyperlipidaemia among diabetes patients with a total cholesterol level ≥5.0 mmol l^{-1} would cost $21 745 per additional QALY gained.

Summary

A United States study based on 4S trial data indicated that simvastatin was cost saving when used for secondary CVD prevention.[49] Another study based on a randomized clinical trial[30] reported that pravastatin for primary prevention of CVD cost more than $50 000 per additional QALY gained.

Two studies based on data from Europe and Canada reported that pharmaceutical cholesterol control generally cost less than $25 000 per additional LYG for both primary and secondary prevention of CVD among diabetes patients except among women with near to normal LDL levels, for whom such treatment was estimated to cost $30 000 to $60 000 per additional LYG. However, the use of cholesterol control drugs for primary CVD prevention among diabetes patients was not as cost-effective as their use for secondary CVD prevention. Most of the studies discussed in this section used efficacy data extrapolated from the 4S trial, which included only patients with a history of CVD. In addition, the use of cholesterol control drugs was more cost-effective among men than among women, independent of country setting.

Drug therapy for weight loss

Obesity is common among type 2 diabetes patients.[52] Treating obesity may enhance hypoglycaemic treatment and contribute to the reduction of long-term microvascular and macrovascular complications through better glycaemic control.[53] One pharmacological treatment option to help patients with type 2 diabetes lose weight, orlistat, has also been shown to reduce their risk for cardiovascular risk factors such as high HbA_{1c} and LDL-cholesterol levels and hypertension.[54] However, the trials used to assess orlistat's effectiveness were of poor quality and had high drop-out rates. Two studies[55,56] analysed the cost-effectiveness of orlistat.

United states

In a meta-analysis of data from several clinical trials, Maetzel et al.[55] estimated the cost-effectiveness of orlistat treatment among overweight or obese patients with type 2 diabetes but without pre-existing complications. They compared treatment with orlistat in conjunction with the standard regimen of anti-diabetic drugs and weight management through diet and exercise with the standard regimen alone. From a payer's perspective, they estimated that orlistat would cost $9826 per additional vascular-event-free LYG under the assumption that the effect of orlistat would persist for 3 years after the treatment stopped, and $27 817 per additional event-free LYG under the assumption that its effect would persist for 1 year in a sensitivity analyses.

Other developed countries

In Belgium, Lamotte et al.[56] estimated the cost-effectiveness of orlistat treatment plus usual diabetes care treatment with usual treatment alone (from the patient's perspective) They estimated that adding orlistat treatment cost $23 783 per additional LYG among obese diabetes patients without arterial hypertension or hypercholesterolemia, $8792 per additional LYG among those with hypercholesterolemia alone and $4120 per additional LYG among those with both hypercholesterolemia and arterial hypertension.

Summary

Estimates from two studies of excellent quality based on data from clinical trials indicated that orlistat

would cost less than $28 000 per event-free LYG or per additional LYG However, the quality of the several trials from which these studies drew their data is problematic.

Interventions to prevent or delay diabetic retinopathy

Diabetic retinopathy causes macular oedema and is the leading cause of new cases of blindness. Because clinical trials have demonstrated that timely laser photocoagulation treatment substantially reduces the likelihood of blindness among patients with diabetic retinopathy,[57,58] screening for diabetic retinopathy and providing early treatment for people who need it may be effective in preventing diabetes eye complications and blindness. The cost-effectiveness of screening for diabetic retinopathy has been evaluated both in the United States and in other developed countries.

United States

Using a disease simulation model, Javitt and Aiello[59] evaluated the cost-effectiveness of universal screening for eye disease among type 1 diabetes patients (screening conducted annually for patients with no retinopathy and every 6 months for those with a history of retinopathy) compared with such screening among only 60% of diabetes patients. They estimated that universal screening and treatment would cost $2814 per additional QALY gained from a health system perspective.

Three studies[59,60,61] estimated the cost-effectiveness of screening for diabetic retinopathy among type 2 diabetes patients in the United States. Javitt et al.[60] conducted an analysis from the federal government's perspective in which both the decrease in disability payments and the increase in income taxes attributable to increased income among diabetes patients who would otherwise have become blind were considered as benefits. The study showed that universal screening of diabetes patients every 2, 3 or 4 years, with more frequent follow-up screenings for those with background diabetic retinopathy, were all cost saving compared with screening 60% of all diabetes patients with the same intervals. For patients with no or mild background retinopathy, screening every 2 years was slightly cost saving relative to annual screening. Once patients developed moderate non-proliferative or more advanced retinopathy, savings in sight-years were sensitive to the screening interval: screening every 6 months saved more sight-years than screening annually and screening annually saved more sight-years than screening every 2 years. However, this study reported no incremental CERs between screening methods with different intervals.

In a later study, Javitt and Aiello[59] evaluated the cost-effectiveness of screening for eye diseases among type 2 diabetes patients from a health system perspective. They assumed that the intervention evaluated would result in annual screenings for all diabetes patients with retinopathy and screening every 6 months for patients with background retinopathy and that all other parameters were the same as in their previous study.[60] From a health system's perspective, they estimated that annual ophthalmologic screening for diabetes patients and treating those found to have diabetic retinopathy would cost $4494 per additional QALY gained among insulin-treated patients and $8112 per additional QALY gained among non-insulin-treated patients.

Vijan et al.[61] evaluated the cost-effectiveness of screening for eye diseases at various frequencies by age group and HbA$_{1c}$ level among United States diabetes patients aged 40 years or older. Interventions were screening for retinopathy every 5, 3 or 2 years or annually among patients without retinopathy, with subsequent annual screening among patients with background retinopathy. From the health system perspective, compared with no screening, they estimated that screening every 5, 3 and 2 years and annually for eye diseases cost $21 637, $24 838, $28 230 and $36 410, respectively, per additional QALY gained. Unlike the results of the two studies by Javitt's group,[59,60] the results of this study showed that screening less frequently had better CERs than screening more frequently. For example, compared with screening every 5 years, screening every 3 years cost $38 867 per additional QALY gained and compared with screening every 2 years, screening annually cost $138,548 per additional QALY gained. However, screening annually may be more cost-effective than screening less frequently for diabetes patients at high risk for retinopathy. For example, for a hypothetical 45-year-old person with an HbA$_{1c}$ level of 11%, the CER of screening every year compared with screening every other year was $37 216 per additional QALY gained.

To explore this difference, Vijan et al.[61] conducted sensitivity analyses using the cost of blindness and utility scores used in the study by Javitt et al.[60] and found that doing so had little effect on their estimates.

Shama et al.[62] analysed the cost-effectiveness of early vitrectomy compared with deferral vitrectomy for the management of vitreous eye haemorrhage secondary to diabetic retinopathy. The study population was a hypothetical group of patients assumed to have characteristics similar to those of participants in the Diabetic Retinopathy Vitrectomy Study trial. Early vitrectomy was the dominant strategy in all analyses. From the payer's perspective, they estimated that, over lifetime, the use of early vitrectomy rather than deferral vitrectomy would cost $2461 per additional QALY gained.

Other developed countries

Polak et al.[63] compared the cost-effectiveness of different intervals of eye disease screening with no screening among diabetes patients who received minimal glycaemic control in The Netherlands. The screening intervals evaluated were every 8, 4 or 2 years or annually among patients who had not developed retinopathy and double or quadruple these frequencies among patients had developed background retinopathy or retinopathy. For patients with type 1 diabetes, the CERs ranged from $1346 to $2563 per sight-year gained. For patients with type 2 diabetes, the CERs ranged from $6000 to $30 000 per sight-year gained depending on screening interval and age, except that screening every 8 years beginning at age 65 years was estimated to be cost saving. For all other scenarios considered, age was negatively associated with the estimated cost-effectiveness of screening and screening every 8 years was much less cost-effective than the other shorter screening intervals. For example, at age 35 years, screening every 8 years cost about $30 000 per additional sight-year gained and more frequent screening cost $6500 to $9000 per additional sight-year gained; at age 50 years, screening every 8 years cost $80 000 per additional sight-year gained and more frequent screening cost $9500 to $10 000 per additional sight-year gained.

Two studies assessed the cost-effectiveness of alternative screening methods to detect diabetic retinopathy, such as using ophthalmoscopy to detect the condition in patients with type I or type II diabetes.[64,65] In one study, James et al.[64] evaluated a newly introduced systematic screening programme in which ophthalmoscopies were performed in a mobile screening unit (camera) in inner-city general practices and at dedicated hospital assessment clinics in Liverpool, England. The screening involved three-field, non-stereoscopic photography using mydriasis, 35 mm transparencies and validated grading. The comparison group received pre-existing opportunistic screening. Members of the comparison groups received a direct ophthalmoscopy performed by general practitioners, optometrists or diabetologists without specialized systematic training. From the health system's perspective, the systematic screening programme had a CER of $39 per additional diabetic retinopathy case identified. In the other study, Maberley et al.[65] assessed the cost-effectiveness of photographic screening of diabetes patients in James Bay, a remote area of Northern Ontario, Canada. They compared using a portable digital camera with the existing screening practice every 6 months and with no screening. Because the digital images could be produced instantaneously, patients' diabetic retinopathy status could be assessed immediately at a remote reading centre. Maberley et al. estimated that the retinal camera screening programme and follow-up care would cost $13 445 per additional QALY gained or $3496 per additional year of vision gained and that the retina specialist programme would cost $33 165 per additional QALY gained or $8784 per additional sight-year gained (both compared with no screening). The retinal camera screening programme was cost saving compared with the retina specialist programme.[65]

Using a simulation model, Davies et al.[66] assessed the cost-effectiveness of various diabetic retinopathy screening methods (mydriatic or non-mydriatic, ophthalmoscopy or photograph) and screening intervals (12 to 24 months and 6 to 12 months) among English diabetes patients. They found that annual screening with a mobile camera with 6 month follow-up screening after the detection of background retinopathy was the most cost-effective method. Among type 1 and type 2 diabetes patients combined, they estimated that this screening scheme cost $2330 per additional sight-year gained compared with no screening ($1147 among type 1 patients and $2746 among type 2 patients).

Summary

One United States study and two studies in Europe showed that the cost of annual diabetic retinopathy screening and treatment from a health system perspective was less than $3000 per additional QALY gained among type 1 diabetes patients and $8000 to $40 000 per additional QALY gained among type 2 diabetes patients when compared with no screening. Estimates of the most cost-effective screening interval differed, although they generally indicated that annual eye screening may be more cost-effective than screening every other year in high-risk subpopulations, such as patients with poor glycaemic control. Two non-United States studies showed that annual screening for diabetic retinopathy among type 2 diabetes patients without background retinopathy cost less than $20 000 per additional sight-year gained compared with no screening. Mobile digital camera screening was estimated to be more cost-effective than other eye screening methods in studies in England and Canada. However, both estimates were based on data from local studies and might not be generalizable to other locations. In addition, for treatment of eye haemorrhage secondary to diabetic retinopathy, early vitrectomy was estimated to cost less than $5000 per additional QALY gained when compared with deferral vitrectomy.

Interventions to prevent or delay diabetic neuropathy

Lower extremity amputation (LEA) is a serious and costly complication of diabetes. Foot ulcers precede 80% of LEAs. Preventing the development of foot ulcers in patients with diabetes can reduce the frequency of LEAs by 50–85%.[67] Interventions used to prevent or delay diabetic neuropathy include intensive glycaemic control (IGC), comprehensive foot care programmes, treatment with becaplermin gel (a biotechnology product containing recombinant human platelet-derived growth factor) and treatment with apligraf (a bio-engineered skin substitute) plus good wound care.

United States

We found no United States studies that evaluated the cost-effectiveness of interventions to prevent or delay the development of diabetic neuropathy.

Other developed countries

We found six European studies that evaluated the cost-effectiveness of interventions to prevent or delay the development of diabetic neuropathy. Tennvall and Apelqvist[67] estimated the cost-effectiveness of a comprehensive foot care programme for patients at three levels of risks for diabetic neuropathy (high, medium and low) in Sweden. Following international recommendations for foot care of diabetes patients, the programme included annual foot examinations, appropriate footwear, appropriate treatment for non-ulcerative pathology and patient education. The high-risk group consisted of patients with a previous foot ulcer or amputation; the moderate-risk group consisted of those with neuropathy and/or peripheral vascular disease and those with foot deformity; and the low-risk group consisted of those without specific risk factors. Compared with Sweden's existing prevention programme, the comprehensive foot care programme was cost saving for the high-risk group at all ages; the CERs ranged from cost saving to $6000 per additional QALY gained for the moderate-risk group; and the intervention cost more than $100 000 per additional QALY gained for the low-risk group.

Ortegon et al.[68] evaluated the cost-effectiveness of three Netherlands foot care programmes for patients with newly diagnosed type 2 diabetes whose initial mean age was 61 years: (1) optimal foot care (OFC), which included professional protective foot care, education of patients and staff, regular foot inspections, identification of high-risk patients and treatment of non-ulcerative lesions; (2) intensive glycaemic control (IGC); and (3) a combination of OFC and IGC. Compared with standard diabetes care, they estimated that OFC would cost $15 690 per additional QALY gained under the assumption that OFC would reduce the number of foot lesions by 90%, and cost $283,929 per additional QALY gained under the assumption that it would reduce the number of foot lesions by 10%. IGC cost $41 354 per additional QALY gained. Applying both interventions (optimal foot care and intensive glycaemic control) cost $10 139 per additional QALY gained under the assumption of 90% foot lesion reduction and $31 677 per additional QALY gained under the assumption of 10% foot lesion reduction.

Three studies estimated the cost-effectiveness of becaplermin gel for wound care. Compared with good wound care alone, becaplermin gel plus good wound care was found to be cost saving in England,[69,70] Switzland,[70] Sweden[71] and France[70] and found to cost $25 per each additional ulcer-free month gained in Sweden.[70] Using apligraf in addition to good wound care was also estimated to be cost saving compared with good wound care alone.[72]

Summary

In Europe, optimal foot ulcer prevention was estimated to be cost saving or to have very low CERs among diabetes patients at high or moderate risk for foot ulcers but less cost-effective among those at low risk. Estimates of the cost-effectiveness of optimal foot care ranged from $15 000 to more than $200,000 per additional QALY gained. The use of medications such as becaplermin and apligraf for wound care were estimated to be cost saving.

Interventions to prevent or delay diabetic nephropathy

Diabetes is a leading cause of end-stage renal disease (ESRD). ESRD can be prevented or delayed by screening diabetes patients for microalbuminuria and treating those who screen positive with ACE inhibitors or other angiotensin receptor antagonists, which have blood pressure-independent reno-protective effects. The cost-effectiveness of such screening and targeted treatment and of providing everyone with newly diagnosed diabetes with ACE inhibitors has been evaluated for both type 1 and type 2 diabetes patients.

United States

Dong et al.[73] examined the cost-effectiveness of treating all type 1 diabetes patients with ACE inhibitors beginning 1 year after diagnosis (the 'treating-all' strategy) compared with annual screening for microalbuminuria and targeted treatment for those who screen positive. Data on treatment effectiveness and disease progression were based on DCCT results.

They estimated that the overall cost-effectiveness of the 'treating-all' strategy was $35 014 per additional QALY gained but that the strategy was more cost-effective among patients with a high baseline HbA$_{1c}$ level. For example, they estimated that strategy would cost less than $25 000 per additional QALY gained among patients with a baseline HbA$_{1c}$ of 9% but $42 533–50,993 per additional QALY gained among those with a baseline HbA$_{1c}$ of 7% at different ages.

Herman et al.[74] evaluated the within-trial cost-effectiveness of losartan after 3.5 years of follow-up based on the Reduction of End Points in Type 2 Diabetes With the Angiotensin II Antagonist Losartan (RENAAL) study. Compared with standard treatment that did not include ACE inhibitors or angiotensin II receptor agonists, losartan treatment reduced the incidence of ESRD and was estimated to be cost saving.

Palmer et al.[75] evaluated the cost-effectiveness of two treatment schemes (early irbesartan treatment for patients with microalbuminuria and late irbesartan treatment for patients who have developed advanced overt nephropathy). In both evaluations, the comparison treatment was given only to patients with overt nephropathy and consisted of the standard anti-hypertension drug treatment, which did not include ACE inhibitors, other angiotension-2 receptor antagonists or dihydropyridine calcium channel blockers. The assumed effectiveness of the intervention was based on Irbesartan In Diabetic Nephropathy (IDNT) results. Both treatment schemes were found to be cost saving compared with standard care and early irbesartan treatment was found to be cost saving compared with late irbesartan treatment.

Golan et al.[76] compared the cost-effectiveness of three ACE inhibitor treatment strategies among patients aged 50 years or older with newly diagnosed type 2 diabetes: 'treat all,' 'screen for microalbuminuria' and 'screen for gross proteinuria'. With the 'treat all' strategy, all patients received ACE inhibitor therapy at the time of their diagnosis With the other two strategies, patients were treated only if their screening test results were positive. From a health system perspective, the 'treat all' and 'screen for microalbuminuria' strategies were estimated to be cost-saving compared with the 'screen for gross proteinuria' strategy, and compared with the 'screen for microalbuminuria' strategy, the 'treat all' approach was estimated cost $9975 per additional QALY gained.

Rosen et al.[77] estimated the cost-effectiveness of Medicare fully covering the cost of ACE inhibitors for all the Medicare beneficiaries with diabetes and found such coverage to be cost saving compared both with no coverage and with the current Medicare Modernization Act coverage from both Medicare and societal perspectives.

Other developed countries

Two studies evaluated the cost-effectiveness of ACE inhibitor treatment of type 1 diabetes patients compared with their treatment with other antihypertensive medication, one in England[78] and one in Italy;[79] both studies were based on data from the Diabetic Nephropathy Collaborative Study (DNCS). They reported cost savings in terms of LYGs or months of dialysis-free life gained.

Borch-Johnsen et al.[80] reported that, in Germany, annual screening for microalbuminuria among diabetes patients 5 years after the onset of diabetes and treating those who tested positive with anti-hypertension medication was cost-saving compared with not treating patients with anti-hypertension medication until ESRD. The study was based on data from a Danish cohort study conducted in the1980s. However, 'treat at ESRD', the comparison practice, is not part of current clinical guidelines for the prevention of diabetic nephropathy, calling into question the applicability of this analysis.

In Canada, Kiberd and Jindal[81] used DNCS data to evaluate the cost-effectiveness of screening patients who had type 1 diabetes for more than 5 years for microalbuminuria and treating those who tested positive with ACE inhibitors compared with treating such patients only after they develop hypertension or macro-proteinuria. They estimated that early screening and targeted treatment would cost $55 498 per additional QALY gained compared with treatment only after patients develop macroalbuminuria or hypertension.

In Canada, Clarke et al.[82] found that publicly funding ACE inhibitors for type 1 diabetes patients with microproteinuria was cost saving compared with not funding this treatment.

Four studies in Europe[83–86] estimated the cost-effectiveness of losartan or irbesartan in preventing diabetic nephropathy among type 2 diabetes patients. Szucs et al.[83] and Souchet et al.[84] used data from the RENAAL study to estimate the cost-effectiveness of losartan compared with standard hypertension treatment and in two studies, Palmer et al.[85,86] used IDNT data to estimate the cost-effectiveness of irbesartan compared with standard hypertension treatment. The results of these studies showed that adding either losartan or irbesartan to conventional antihypertensive therapies (any antihypertensive medications except for a ACE inhibitor or another angiotensin II receptor blocker) was cost saving.

Summary

One United States study showed that treating all patients with newly diagnosed type 1 diabetes with ACE inhibitors cost less than $40 000 per additional QALY gained compared with screening for microalbuminuria and treating only those who tested positive. For patients with inadequate glycaemic control, the CER of the screening was less than $25 000 per additional QALY gained, and for patients with type 2 diabetes, the CERs were much lower. Compared with screening for proteinuria and treating patients who test positive with either ACE inhibitors or irbesartan, screening patients for microalbuminuria and providing similar treatment for those who test positive was cost saving. Treating all patients with newly diagnosed type 2 diabetes with ACE inhibitors was estimated to cost $10 000 per additional QALY gained compared with treating only patients who screen positive for microalbuminuria.

In other developed countries, screening type 1 diabetes patients for microalbuminuria and treating those who test positive with ACE inhibitors was estimated to cost around $55 000 per additional QALY gained compared with providing ACE inhibitor treatment to all patients with hypertension or macroproteinuria. Among type 1 diabetes patients, ACE inhibitor treatment was found to be cost saving compared with treatment with other anti-hypertensive medications. Among type 2 diabetes patients, treatment with losartan and with irbesartan were both cost saving in terms of preventing diabetic nephropathy.

Two well-conducted studies in the United States and Canada also showed that public insurance payment for ACE inhibitors for diabetes patients was cost saving compared with having patients pay for the medications out of their own pockets.

Multi-component interventions

The only two cost-effectiveness studies of multi-component interventions for diabetes that we found were conducted in Switzerland. In one, Palmer et al.[87] estimated the cost-effectiveness of various combinations of the following four interventions for type 1 diabetes patients: conventional insulin therapy (C); intensive insulin therapy (I); annual screening for proliferative retinopathy and treatment with laser photocoagulation if proliferative retinopathy was detected (EYE); and annual screening for microalbuminuria with urine test strips and treatment with captopril if microalbuminuria was detected (ACE). From a Swiss health insurance payer's perspective, they estimated that, compared with C alone, C + EYE, C + ACE and C + EYE + ACE were all cost saving and that I cost $14 291, I + EYE cost $15 135, I + ACE cost $11 716 and I + EYE + ACE cost $12 321 per additional LYG.

In the other study, Gozzoli et al.[88] used a computer simulation model to evaluate the cost-effectiveness of several combinations of the following treatments: a standard treatment and educational programme; nephropathy screening with ensuing ACE inhibitor therapy; retinopathy screening with ensuing laser therapy; and a single comprehensive multi-factorial intervention, which included an educational programme, screening for nephropathy and retinopathy and control of cardiovascular risk factors, early diagnosis and treatment of complications; and health education. The comparison group received standard anti-diabetic treatment alone (57% of the patients were treated with insulin, 35% with oral anti-diabetic agents and 8% with diet treatment alone). Combined treatments (standard care plus education; standard care plus education plus nephropathy screening and treatment; standard care plus education plus retinopathy screening and treatment; and standard care plus education plus retinopathy screening and treatment plus nephropathy screening and treatment) were evaluated from the Swiss health insurance payer's perspective. All combinations were found to be cost saving compared with standard care.

Summary

In Switzerland, multi-component interventions to optimize diabetes management were found to be either cost saving or very cost-effective.

Classifying the results of cost-effectiveness analyses for use in formulating public health and clinical recommendations

There is no consensus concerning the criteria to use in classifying the results of cost-effectiveness analyses of diabetes interventions. We divided interventions into eight cost-effectiveness categories according to their estimated cost-effectiveness (cost saving, cost-effective, marginally cost-effective or not cost-effective) and the quality of the evidence upon which these estimates were based (strong or weak). We also created a ninth category to describe interventions about which cost-effectiveness estimates were inconsistent (Table 27.1).

We considered evidence for a cost-effectiveness assessment to be strong if it met either of two multi-part criteria: Criterion 1 – the cost effectiveness of the intervention was evaluated by at least two studies AND these studies were rated as 'good' or 'excellent' in quality AND the effectiveness of the interventions were based on good quality randomized clinical trials or good diabetes disease simulation models

Table 27.1 Classification of Diabetes prevention and control interventions by estimated cost-effectiveness and strength of evidence for estimates

Strong evidence	Weak evidence	Cost-effectiveness uncertain
I. Cost-saving	V. Cost-saving	IX. Contradictory conclusions
II. Cost-effective ($0–25 000 per QALY gained or LYG)	VI. Cost-effective ($0–25000 per QALY gained or LYG)	
III. Marginally cost-effective ($25 000–100 000 per QALY gained or LYG)	VII. Marginally cost-effective ($25 000–100 000 per QALY gained or LYG)	
IV. Not cost-effective (>$100 000 per QALY gained or LYG)	VIII. Not cost-effective (>$100 000 per QALY gained or LYG)	

that were validated AND the studies produced similar CERs; Criterion 2 – only one study evaluated the cost-effectiveness of the intervention AND the study was rated as 'excellent' in quality AND the estimation of the effectiveness of the intervention was based on data from well-known randomized clinical trials such as the DCCT, the UKPDS and the 4S studies.

We considered evidence for a cost-effectiveness assessment to be weak if only one study evaluated the cost-effectiveness of the intervention AND/OR the estimate of an intervention's effectiveness was based on epidemiological data or data from trials that were small or not randomized, was simulated by diabetes disease models that were not validated or was assessed by studies rated as 'fair' in quality.

Table 27.2 summarizes the interventions for which evidence was strong enough for us to reach a conclusion concerning their cost-effectiveness. United States interventions for which we found strong evidence that they were cost saving or cost-effective included generic metformin treatment for primary prevention of type 2 diabetes, ACE inhibitors and beta-blockers for intensive hypertension control among type 2 diabetes patients, intensive group lifestyle interventions for preventing type 2 diabetes among persons with IGT and annual diabetic retinopathy screening among type 1 diabetes patients. These interventions should be adopted because they have been shown to be effective and to make efficient

Table 27.2 Estimated cost-effectiveness of diabetes interventions in the United States and other developed countries for which cost-effectiveness evidence was strong, 1985–2005

Cost-effectiveness	Interventions	
	United States	**Other developed countries**
I. Cost saving	• ACE inhibitors or beta-blocker treatment for intensive hypertension control among type 2 diabetes patients • Screening for and treating microalbuminuria with ACE inhibitors or irbesartan for type 2 diabetes compared with screening for and treating proteinuria	• ACE inhibitors or beta-blocker treatment for intensive hypertension control among type 2 diabetes patients[a] • Treatment with ACE inhibitors, losartan and irbesartan for preventing nephropathy among type 2 diabetes patients • Becaplermin treatment for foot ulcer for type 1 or type 2 diabetes patients
II. Cost-effective: less than $25 000 per additional QALY gained or LYG	• Generic metformin for preventing type 2 diabetes among persons with IGT • Intensive group lifestyle intervention for preventing type 2 diabetes among persons with IGT • Intensive glycaemic control targeting at fast plasma glucose concentration less than 108 mg dl^{-1} (6.0 mmol/L) among type 2 diabetes patients aged 25–44 years • Simvastatin for preventing CVD among type 2 diabetes patients with dyslipidaemia and CHD history • Screening for diabetic retinopathy in persons with type 1 diabetes • ACE inhibitor for preventing ESRD among type 1 diabetes patients with an HbA$_{1c}$ level of 9% or more	• Metformin for preventing type 2 diabetes • Intensive group lifestyle intervention for preventing type 2 diabetes • Intensive glycaemic control using insulin, sulfonylureas or metformin targeting an HbA$_{1c}$ level of less that 7% among type 2 diabetes patients • Simvastatin treatment for preventing CVD among type 2 diabetes patients with dyslipidaemia and CHD history
III. Marginally cost-effective: $25 000–100 000 per additional QALY gained or LYG	• Non-generic metformin for preventing type 2 diabetes among persons with IGT • Intensive insulin therapy among with type 1 diabetes patients • ACE inhibitor treatment for all newly diagnosed type 1 diabetes compared with screening for and treating microalbuminuria • Annual screening for diabetic retinopathy and ensuing laser treatment compared with no screening in persons with type 2 diabetes • Intensive glycaemic control targeting a fasting plasma glucose concentration less than 108 mg dl^{-1} (6.0 mmol/L) using sulfonylureas or insulin for type 2 diabetes patients aged 45–54 years	
IV. Not cost-effective: more than $100 000 per additional QALY gained or LYG	• Intensive glycaemic control targeting a fasting plasma glucose concentration less than 108 mg dl^{-1} (6.0 mmol/L) using sulfonylureas or insulin for type 2 diabetes patients aged 55 years and older • Universal screening for undiagnosed type 2 diabetes (2 based on modelling)	

[a] ACE inhibitors for intensive hypertension control among persons with type 2 diabetes were reported cost saving in most of the studies and very cost-effective in one study.

use of resources. Interventions that had strong evidence and were marginally cost-effective were brand-name metformin for preventing diabetes among people with IGT, intensive glycaemic control to reduce diabetes patients' HbA$_{1c}$ levels to 7%, intensive glycaemic control to reduce fasting plasma glucose levels of type 2 diabetes patients aged 45–54 years to 108 mg dl^{-1} (6.0 mmol/L) annual diabetic retinopathy screening and ensuing treatment for type 2 diabetes patients and ACE inhibitor treatment to prevent ESRD for everyone with newly diagnosed type 1 diabetes. We recommend that these interventions be adopted only if additional justification for their use is provided, particularly if they cost more than $50 000 per additional QALY gained or LYG.

Only universal screening for undiagnosed type 2 diabetes and intensive glycaemic control designed to reduce plasma glucose levels to 108 mg dl^{-1} (6.0 mmol/L) in type 2 diabetes patients aged 55 years or older were classified as having strong evidence and not being cost-effective. Unless further studies show different results or demonstrate some as yet undetected deficiency in the previous studies, these ratings indicate that universal screening for undiagnosed type 2 diabetes in the general population and intensive glycaemic control among older diabetes patients are suboptimal uses of resources.

In other developed countries, analyses of three interventions had strong evidence and indicated the interventions were cost saving: ACE inhibitors for intensive hypertension control among type 2 diabetes patients; ACE inhibitors, losartan and irbesartan treatment for preventing nephropathy among type 2 diabetes patients; and becaplermin treatment for foot ulcers among type 1 or type 2 diabetes patients. Analyses of four interventions had strong evidence indicated the interventions were cost-effective: metformin and intensive group lifestyle intervention for preventing type 2 diabetes among people at high risk for the condition; intensive glycaemic control among type 2 diabetes patients with the goal of achieving an HbA$_{1c}$ level of 7% or less; and simvastatin treatment for secondary prevention of CVD among type 2 diabetes patients with dyslipidaemia. We recommend all these interventions for adoption in Europe and Canada.

Table 27.3 summarizes the interventions for which cost-effectiveness evidence was weak. United States interventions in this group included orlistat therapy for weight loss; cholesterol control using pravastatin for primary CVD prevention; and the most cost-effective screening strategies for gestational diabetes. In other developed countries, the interventions in this category included acarbose treatment for

Table 27.3 Estimated cost-effectiveness of diabetes interventions in the United States and other developed countries for which cost-effectiveness evidence was weak or contradictory, 1985–2005

Cost-effectiveness	Interventions	
	United States	**Other developed countries**
V. Cost saving	• Early vitrectomy for managing various eye haemorrhage secondary to diabetic retinopathy compared with deferral vitrectomy for type 2 diabetes patients • Screening for gestational diabetes during pregnancy compared with no screening • Sequential screening strategy compared with 75 g glucose tolerance test for gestational diabetes during pregnancy • Government paying for ACE inhibitors for all Medicare beneficiaries with diabetes	• Acarbose for preventing type 2 diabetes • Intensive glycaemic control among type 1 diabetes patients • Intensive hypertension control using atenolol compared with captopril among persons with type 2 diabetes and hypertension • Optimal foot ulcer prevention for persons with previous foot ulcer or amputation for foot ulcer • Apligraf for treating foot ulcer • Canadian provincial government paying for ACE inhibitors for persons with type 1 diabetes and overt nephropathy • Conventional insulin therapy, plus screening for and treating retinopathy and screening for and treating microalbuminuria compared with conventional insulin therapy alone for type 1 diabetes patients

(continued)

Table 27.3 (*Continued*)

Cost-effectiveness	Interventions	
	United States	**Other developed countries**
VI. Cost-effective: less than $25 000 per additional QALY gained or LYG	• Target screening for undiagnosed type 2 diabetes among African Americans aged 25–54 years • Orlistat for losing weight for obese type 2 diabetes patients • Early vitrectomy for managing various eye haemorrhages compared with late vitrectomy	• Educational programme, plus screening for and treating retinopathy and screening for and treating microalbuminuria compared with standard anti-diabetic care for type 2 diabetes patients • Intensive hypertension control for patients with type 2 diabetes by specialist-led clinics • Orlistat for losing weight for obese type 2 diabetes patients • Simvastatin for preventing CVD among type 2 diabetes patients with dyslipidaemia but without CHD history • Annual retinopathy screening among type 2 diabetes patients with poor glycaemic control (HbA$_{1c}$ of 10%) • Annual eye retinopathy screening among type 1 diabetes patients • Retinal camera screening for eye diseases compared with retina-specialist programme in remote areas • Intensive insulin therapy, plus screening for and treating retinopathy and screening for and treating microalbuminuria compared with conventional insulin therapy alone for type 1 diabetes • Optimal foot care for preventing foot ulcer among persons with neuropathy and peripheral vascular disease • Good wound care plus standard anti-diabetic care for treating foot ulcer compared with standard care alone
VII. Marginally cost-effective: $25 000 to $100,000 per additional QALY or LY gained	• Annual eye screening for and treating retinopathy for type 2 diabetes patients with poor glycaemic control or in younger age group or with insulin-treated diabetes compared with screening every other year • Target screening for undiagnosed type 2 diabetes among persons with hypertension • Cholesterol control using pravastatin for primary preventing CVD	• Pioglitazone as a first-line anti-diabetic drug compared with glyburide, metformin or diet and exercise • Screening for and treating microalbuminuria with ACE inhibitors for type 1 diabetes patients compared with ACE inhibitor treatment in patients with hypertension, macroproteinuria or both
VIII. Not cost-effective: more than $100,000 per additional QALY or LY gained		• Optimal foot care for preventing foot ulcer among persons with diabetes with low risk for foot ulcer
IX. Contradictory evidence	• Relative cost-effectiveness of screening for undiagnosed type 2 diabetes between age groups • Optimal frequency of screening for and treating retinopathy among type 2 diabetes patients	

preventing type 2 diabetes; screening for and treating diabetic retinopathy; orlistat treatment for weight loss; primary CVD prevention using simvastatin; foot ulcer prevention and control; GDM prevention; and multiple component interventions. The difference between the United States and other developed countries is mainly attributable to unequal numbers of the cost-effectiveness studies and type of interventions conducted in the two regions.

Most interventions in this group with weak evidence were estimated to cost less than $50 000 per additional QALY gained and we classified more than half of the them as having weak evidence of being cost saving or very cost-effective. We classified only a few interventions, such as optimal foot ulcer prevention for diabetes patients at low risk for foot ulcers, as having weak evidence and of being not cost-effective.

We could not draw a conclusion concerning the cost-effectiveness of a few interventions because different studies produced conflicting results. We found great uncertainty, for example, concerning the most cost-effectiveness age parameters to set in screening people for undiagnosed type 2 diabetes and the most cost-effective intervals to use in screening for retinopathy among type 2 diabetes patients.

Estimates of the cost-effectiveness of screening for micro-albuminuria or proteinuria as a means of preventing ESRD among type 1 diabetes patients in other developed countries were based on data from small-scale clinical trials conducted in the1990s before the DCCT results were published. Thus new studies that apply the DCCT results in the European setting would provide more reliable results.

Many cost-effectiveness studies evaluated a single intervention that targeted only one component of diabetes treatment. However, many patients probably receive multi-component diabetes treatment. More studies are needed to estimate the cost-effectiveness of the multi-component interventions, particularly in the United States.

We found only three studies that evaluated the cost-effectiveness of population-level or diabetes interventions in real-world settings, such as policy changes or the implementation of interventions in clinical settings: specialist nurse-led clinics offering intensive hypertension and cholesterol control to diabetes patients in England, the United States Medicare programme paying for ACE inhibitor treatment for Medicare recipients with diabetes and provincial governments paying for ACE inhibitors for diabetes patients in Canada. Population-level translational interventions, particularly policy changes, could substantially improve the health of diabetes patients in a country or region. More efforts are needed to evaluate the cost-effectiveness of population-level interventions.

Results from cost-effectiveness studies of diabetes interventions should be used cautiously in making public health and clinical decisions. Such studies provide very limited information concerning the distribution of benefits and costs of an intervention, and who pays for and who benefits from any intervention are an important aspect of public health and clinical policy decisions. A cost-effective intervention could, for example, apply to the entire population or only to those at high risk; interventions that benefit different groups differentially can raise issues of equity.

Although estimates derived from cost-effectiveness analyses can be an important source of advice to inform the judgement of officials making public policy and clinical decisions, they cannot provide definitive answers concerning whether a particular intervention should be adopted. Answering such questions also requires willingness-to-pay information, which is not obtainable from a cost-effectiveness analysis.

Cost-effectiveness estimates should be considered as one factor in the multi-factoral process of judging whether a particular intervention should be adopted. Other factors that need to be considered include the treatment preferences and values of patients, society and other stakeholders. Judgments about these preferences – acceptability, feasibility and strategic planning – also should contribute substantially to the decision-making process concerning whether an intervention should be adopted.

References

1 Centers for Medicare, Medicaid Services, Office of the Actuary, National Health Statistics Group; http://www.cms.hhs.gov/NationalHealthExpendData (accessed 31 October 2007).

2 American Diabetes Association. Economic cost of diabetes in the US in 2002. *Diabetes Care* 2003;**26**:917–932.

3 American Diabetes Association. Economic cost of diabetes in the US in 2007. *Diabetes Care* 2008;**31**:596–615.

4 Neumann P. The arrival of economic evidence in managed care formulary decisions: the unsolicited request process. *Med Care* 2005;**43**(7)(Suppl II):27–32.

5 Bryan L. What will it take to make cost-effectiveness analysis acceptable in the United States? *Med Care* 2005;**43**(7 Suppl II): 44–48.

6 Gold MR, Siegel JE, Russell LB, Weinstein MC. *Cost-Effectiveness in Health and Medicine*. Oxford University Press, New York, 1996.

7 Laupacis A, Feeny D, Detsky A, Tugwell PX. How attractive does a new technology have to warrant adoption and utilization? Tentative guideline for using clinical and economic evaluations. *CMAJ* 1992;**146**:473–481.

8 Clarke M, Oxman AD. *Cochrane Reviewers Handbook (Updated October 2001)* Update Software, Oxford, 2001.

9 Drummond MF. Guidelines for authors and peer reviewers of economic submissions to the BMJ. *BMJ* 1996;**313**:275–283.

10 Knowler WC, Barrett-Connor E, Fowler SE, Hamman RF, Lachin JM, Walker EA *et al.* Reduction in the incidence of type 2 diabetes with lifestyle intervention or metformin. *N Engl J Med* 2002;**346**:393–403.

11 Tuomilehto J, Lindstrom J, Eriksson JG, Valle TT, Hamalainen H, Ilanne-Parikka P *et al.* Prevention of type 2 diabetes mellitus by changes in lifestyle among subjects with impaired glucose tolerance. *N Engl J Med* 2001;**344**:1343–1350.

12 Wylie-Rosett J, Herman WH, Goldberg RB. Lifestyle intervention to prevent diabetes: intensive and cost effective. *Curr Opin Lipidol* 2006;**17**:37–44.

13 The Diabetes Prevention Program Research Group. Within-trial cost-effectiveness of lifestyle intervention or metformin for the primary prevention of type 2 diabetes. *Diabetes Care* 2003;**26**:2518–2523.

14 Herman WH, Hoerger TJ, Brandle M, Hicks K, Sorensen S, Zhang P, Hamman RF, Ackermann RT, Engelgau MM. Ratner RE, and the Diabetes Prevention Program Research Group. The cost-effectiveness of lifestyle modification or metformin in preventing type 2 diabetes in adults with impaired glucose tolerance. *Ann Intern Med* 2005;**142**: 323–332.

15 Eddy DM, Schlessinger L, Kahn R. Clinical outcomes and cost-effectiveness of strategies for managing people at high risk for diabetes. *Ann Intern Med* 2005;**143**:251–264.

16 Segal L, Dalton AC, Richardson J. Cost-effectiveness of the primary prevention of non-insulin dependent diabetes mellitus. *Health Promotion Int* 1998;**13**:197–209.

17 Palmer AJ, Roze S, Valentine WJ, Spinas GA, Shaw JE, Zimmet PZ. Intensive lifestyle changes or metformin in patients with impaired glucose tolerance: modeling the long-term health economic implications of the diabetes prevention program in Australia, France, Germany, Switzerland and the United Kingdom. *Clin Ther* 2004;**26**:304–321.

18 Caro JJ, Getsios D, Caro I, Klittich WS, O'Brien JA. Economic evaluation of therapeutic interventions to prevent Type 2 diabetes in Canada. *Diabet Med* 2004;**21**:1229–1236.

19 Quilici S, Chancellor J, Maclaine G, McGuire A, Andersson D, Chiasson JL. Cost-effectiveness of acarbose for the management of impaired glucose tolerance in Sweden. *Int J Clin Pract* 2005;**59**:1143–1152.

20 CDC Diabetes Cost-Effectiveness Study Group. The cost-effectiveness of screening for type 2 diabetes. *JAMA* 1998; **280**:1757–1763.

21 Hoerger TJ, Harris R, Hicks KA, Donahue K, Sorensen S, Engelgau M. Screening for type 2 diabetes mellitus: a cost-effectiveness analysis. *Ann Intern Med* 2004;**140**:689–699.

22 Zhang P, Engelgau MM, Valdez R, Benjamin SM, Cadwell B, Venkat Narayan KM. Costs of screening for pre-diabetes among U.S. adults: a comparison of different screening strategies. *Diabetes Care* 2003;**26**:2536–2542.

23 Zhang P, Engelgau MM, Valdez R, Benjamin SM, Cadwell B, Narayan KMV. Efficient cutoff points for three screening tests for detecting undiagnosed diabetes and pre-diabetes: an economic analysis. *Diabetes Care* 2005;**28**:1321–1325.

24 Johnson SL, Tabaei BP, Herman WH. The efficacy and cost of alternative strategies for systematic screening for type 2 diabetes in the US population 45–74 years of age. *Diabetes Care* 2005;**28**:307–311.

25 Nicholson WK, Fleisher LA, Fox HE, Powe NR. Screening for gestational diabetes mellitus: a decision and cost-effectiveness analysis of four screening strategies. *Diabetes Care* 2005; **28**:1482–1484.

26 Kim C, Herman WH, Vijan S. Efficacy and cost of postpartum screening strategies for diabetes among women with histories of gestational diabetes mellitus. *Diabetes Care* 2007;**30**: 1102–1106.

27 Icks A, Rathmann W, Haastert B, John J, Lowel H, Holle R, Giani G. Cost-effectiveness of type 2 diabetes screening: results from recently published studies. *Gesundheitswesen* 2005;**67**:S167–S171.

28 The DCCT Research Group. Lifetime benefits and costs of intensive therapy as practiced in the diabetes control and complications trial. *JAMA* 1996;**276**:1409–1415.

29 Eastman RC, Javitt JC, Herman WH, Dasbach EJ, Zbrozek AS, Dong F, Manninen D, Garfield SA, Copley-Merriman C, Maier W, Eastman JF, Kotsanos J, Cowie CC, Harris M. Model of complications of NIDDM. I. Model construction and assumptions. *Diabetes Care* 1997; **20**:725–734.

30 CDC Diabetes Cost-effectiveness Group. Cost-effectiveness of intensive glycemic control, intensified hypertension control and serum cholesterol level reduction for type 2 diabetes. *JAMA* 2002;**287**:2542–2551.

31 Starostina EG, Antsiferov M, Galstyan GR, Trautner C, Jorgens V, Bott U, Muhlhauser I, Berger M, Dedov II. Effectiveness and cost–benefit analysis of intensive treatment and teaching programmes for type 1 (insulin-dependent) diabetes mellitus in Moscow – blood glucose versus urine glucose self-monitoring. *Diabetologia* 1994;**37**:170–176.

32 Palmer AJ, Roze S, Valentine WJ, Smith I, Wittrup-Jensen KU. Cost-effectiveness of detemir-based basal/bolus therapy versus NPH-based basal/bolus therapy for type 1 diabetes in a UK setting: an economic analysis based on meta-analysis results of four clinical trials. *Curr Med Res Opin* 2004;**20**: 1729–1746.

33 Gray A, Raikou M, McGuire A, *et al.* Cost effectiveness of an intensive blood glucose control policy in patients with type 2 diabetes: economic analysis alongside randomized controlled trial (UKPDS 41). United Kingdom Prospective Diabetes Study Group. *BMJ* 2000;**320**:1373–1378.

34 Clarke PM, Gray AM, Briggs A, Stevens RJ, Matthews DR, Holman RR. Cost–utility analyses of intensive blood glucose and tight blood pressure control in type 2 diabetes (UKPDS 72). *Diabetologia* 2005;**48**:868–877.

35 Coyle D, Palmer AJ, Tam R. Economic evaluation of pioglitazone hydrochloride in the management of type 2 diabetes mellitus in Canada. *Pharmacoeconomics* 2002;**20**(Suppl 1): 31–42.

36 Clarke P, Gray A, Adler A, Stevens R, Raikou M, Cull C, Stratton I, Holman R, and the UKPDS Group. United Kingdom Prospective Diabetes Study: cost-effectiveness analysis of intensive blood-glucose control with metformin in overweight patients with type II diabetes (UKPDS No. 51). *Diabetologia* 2001;**44**:298–304.

37 Almbrand B, Johannesson M, Sjostrand B, Malmberg K, Ryden L. Cost-effectiveness of intense insulin treatment after acute myocardial infarction in patients with diabetes mellitus; results from the DIGAMI study. *Eur Heart J* 2000;**21**(9): 733–739.

38 Wake N, Hisashige A, Katayama T *et al*. Cost-effectiveness of intensive insulin therapy for type 2 diabetes: a 10-year follow-up of the Kumamoto study. *Diabetes Res Clin Pract* 2000;**48**:201–210.

39 Taylor SJ, Milanova T, Hourihan F, Krass I, Coleman C, Armour CL. A cost-effectiveness analysis of a community pharmacist-initiated disease state management service for type 2 diabetes mellitus. *Int J Pharmacy Pract* 2005;**13**:33–40.

40 Neeser K, Lubben G, Siebert U, Schramm W. Cost effectiveness of combination therapy with pioglitazone for type 2 diabetes mellitus from a German statutory healthcare perspective. *Pharmacoeconomics* 2004;**22**:321–341.

41 Heart Outcomes Prevention Evaluation Study Investigators. Effects of ramipril on cardiovascular and microvascular outcomes in people with diabetes mellitus: results of the HOPE study and MICRO-HOPE substudy. *Lancet* 2000;**355**: 253–258.

42 UKPDS Group. Tight blood pressure control and risk of macro-vascular and microvascular complications in type 2 diabetes: UKPDS 38. UK Prospective Diabetes Study Group. *BMJ* 1998;**317**:703–713.

43 Elliott, WJ, Weir DR, Black HR, Irving, BH. Cost-effectiveness of the lower treatment goal (of JNC VI) for diabetic hypertensive patients. *Arch Intern Med* 2000;**160**(9):1277–1283.

44 UK Prospective Diabetes Study Group. Cost effectiveness analysis of improved blood pressure control in hypertensive patients with type 2 diabetes: UKPDS 40. *BMJ* 1998;**317**: 720–726.

45 Gray A, Raikou M, McGuire A *et al*. Cost effectiveness of an intensive blood glucose control policy in patients with type 2 diabetes: economic analysis alongside randomized controlled trial (UKPDS 41). United Kingdom Prospective Diabetes Study Group. *BMJ* 2000;**320**:1373–1378.

46 Mason JM Freemantle N, Gibson JM, New JP. Specialist nurse-led clinics to improve control of hypertension and hyperlipidemia in diabetes: economic analysis of the SPLINT trial., *Diabetes Care* 2005;**28**:40–46.

47 Gray A, Clarke P, Raikou M *et al*. An economic evaluation of atenolol vs. captopril in patients with Type 2 diabetes (UKPDS 54). *Diabet Med* 2001;**18**:438–444.

48 Kannel WB, McGee, DL. Diabetes and glucose tolerance as risk factors for cardiovascular disease: the Framingham Study. *Diabetes Care* 1979;**2**:120–126.

49 Herman WH, Alexander CM, Cook, JR *et al*. Effect of simvastatin treatment on cardiovascular resource utilization in impaired fasting glucose and diabetes: findings from the Scandinavian Simvastatin Survival Study. *Diabetes Care* 1999;**22**:1771–1778.

50 Jonsson B, Cook JR, Pedersen TR. The cost-effectiveness of lipid lowering in patients with diabetes: results from the 4S trial. *Diabetologia* 1999;**42**:1293–1301.

51 Grover SA, Coupal L, Zowall H, Dorais M. Cost-effectiveness of treating hyperlipidemia in the presence of diabetes: who should be treated? *Circulation* 2000;**102**:722–727.

52 Wolf AM, Colditz GA. Current estimates of the economic cost of obesity in the United States. *Obesity Res* 1998;**6**:97–106.

53 Hollander PA, Elbein SC, Hirsch IB, Kelley D, McGill J, Taylor T, Weiss SR, Crockett SE, Kaplan RA, Comstock J, Lucas CP, Lodewick PA, Canovatchel W, Chung J, Hauptman J. Role of orlistat in the treatment of obese patients with type 2 diabetes: a 1-year randomized double-blind study. *Diabetes Care* 1998;**21**:1288–1294.

54 Heymsfield SB, Segal KR, Hauptman J, Lucas CP, Boldrin MN, Rissanen A, Wilding JPH, Sjostrom L. Effects of weight loss with orlistat on glucose tolerance and progression to type 2 diabetes in obese adults. *Arch Intern Med* 2000;**160**: 1321–1326.

55 Maetzel A, Ruof J, Covington M, Wolf A. Economic evaluation of orlistat in overweight and obese patients with type 2 diabetes mellitus. *Pharmacoeconomics* 2003;**21**:501–512.

56 Lamotte M, Annemans L, Lefever A, Nechelput M, Masure J. A health economic model to assess the long-term effects and cost-effectiveness of orlistat in obese type 2 diabetic patients. *Diabetes Care* 2002;**25**:303–308.

57 The Diabetic Retinopathy Study Research Group. Photocoagulation treatment of proliferative diabetic retinopathy: clinical application of Diabetic Retinopathy Study (DRS) findings. DRS report number 8. *Ophthalmology* 1981;**88**:583–600.

58 Early Treatment Diabetic Retinopahty Study Research Group Photocoagulation for diabetic macular edema: Early Treatment Diabetic Retinopathy Study report number 1. *Arch Ophthalmol* 1985;**103**:1796–1806.

59 Javitt JC, Aiello, LP. Cost-effectiveness of detecting and treating diabetic retinopathy. *Ann Intern Med* 1996;**124**:164–169.

60 Javitt JC, Aiello LP, Chiang Y, Ferris FL III, Canner JK, Greenfield S. Preventive eye care in people with diabetes is cost-saving to the federal government. Implications for health-care reform. *Diabetes Care* 1994;**17**:909–917.

61 Vijan S, Hofer TP, Hayward RA. Cost–utility analysis of screening intervals for diabetic retinopathy in patients with type 2 diabetes mellitus. *JAMA* 2000;**283**:889–896.

62 Sharma S, Hollands H, Brown GC, Brown MM, Shah GK, Sharma SM. The cost-effectiveness of early vitrectomy for the treatment of vitreous hemorrhage in diabetic retinopathy. *Curr Opin Ophthalmol* 2001;**12**:230–234.

63 Polak BC, Crijns H, Casparie AF, Niessen LW. Cost-effectiveness of glycemic control and ophthalmological care in diabetic retinopathy. *Health Policy* 2003;**64**:89–97.

64 James M, Turner DA, Broadbent DM, Vora J, Harding SP. Cost effectiveness analysis of screening for sight threatening diabetic eye disease [published erratum appears in *BMJ* 2000; **321** (7258): 424]. *BMJ* 2000;**320**:1627–1631.

65 Maberley D, Walker H, Koushik A, Cruess A. Screening for diabetic retinopathy in James Bay, Ontario: a cost-effectiveness analysis. *CMAJ* 2003;**168**:160–164.

66 Davies R, Roderick P, Canning C, Brailsford S. The evaluation of screening policies for diabetic retinopathy using simulation. *Diabet. Med* 2002;**19**:762–770.

67 Tennvall GR, Apelqvist J. Prevention of diabetes-related foot ulcers and amputations: a cost–utility analysis based on Markov model simulations. *Diabetologia* 2001;**44**:2077–2087.

68 Ortegon MM, Redekop WK, Niessen LW. Cost-effectiveness of prevention and treatment of the diabetic foot: a Markov analysis. *Diabetes Care* 2004;**27**:901–907.

69 Ghatnekar O, Persson U, Willis M, Wright T, Odegaard K. The cost-effectiveness in the UK of treating diabetic lower extremity ulcers with becaplermin gel. *J Drug Assess* 2000;**3**: 243–251.

70 Ghatnekar O, Persson U, Willis M, Odegaard K. Cost effectiveness of becaplermin in the treatment of diabetic foot

ulcers in four European countries. *Pharmacoeconomics* 2001;**19**:767–778.

71 Persson U, Willis M, Odegaard K, Apelqvist J. The cost-effectiveness of treating diabetic lower extremity ulcers with becaplermin (Regranex): a core model with an application using Swedish cost data. *Value in Health* 2000;**3**:S39–S46.

72 Redekop WK, McDonnell J, Verboom P, Lovas K, Kalo Z. The cost effectiveness of apligraf treatment of diabetic foot ulcers. *Pharmacoeconomics* 2003;**21**:1171–1183.

73 Dong FB, Sorensen SW, Manninen DL *et al.* Cost effectiveness of ACE inhibitor treatment for patients with type 1 diabetes mellitus. *Pharmacoeconomics* 2004;**22**:1015–1027.

74 Herman WH, Shahinfar S, Carides GW, Dasbach EJ, Gerth WC, Alexander CM, Cook JR, Keane WF, Brenner BM. for the RENAAL Investigators. Losartan reduces the costs associated with diabetic end-stage renal disease: The RENAAL Study Economic Evaluation. *Diabetes Care* 2003;**26**:683–687.

75 Palmer AJ, Annemans L, Roze S *et al.* Cost-effectiveness of early irbesartan treatment versus control (standard antihypertensive medications excluding ACE inhibitors, other angiotensin-2 receptor antagonists and dihydropyridine calcium channel blockers) or late irbesartan treatment in patients with type 2 diabetes, hypertension and renal disease. *Diabetes Care* 2004;**27**:1897–1903.

76 Golan L, Birkmeyer JD, Welch HG. The cost-effectiveness of treating all patients with type 2 diabetes with angiotensin-converting enzyme inhibitors. *Ann Intern Med* 1999;**131**:660–667.

77 Rosen AB, Hamel MB, Weinstein MC, Cutler DM, Fendrick AM, Vijan S. Cost-effectiveness of full Medicare coverage of angiotensin-converting enzyme inhibitors for beneficiaries with diabetes. *Ann Intern Med* 2005;**143**:89–99.

78 Hendry BM, Viberti GC, Hummel S, Bagust A, Piercey J. Modeling and costing the consequences of using an ACE inhibitor to slow the progression of renal failure in type 1 diabetic patients. *Q J Med* 1997;**90**:277–282.

79 Garattini L, Brunetti M, Salvioni F, Barosi M. Economic evaluation of ACE inhibitor treatment of nephropathy in patients with insulin-dependent diabetes mellitus in Italy. *Pharmacoeconomics* 1997;**12**:67–75.

80 Borch-Johnsen K, Wenzel H, Viberti GC, Mogensen CE. Is screening and intervention for microalbuminuria worthwhile in patients with insulin dependent diabetes? [published erratum appears in *BMJ*. 1993; **307**: (6903): 543]. *BMJ* 1993;**306**:1722–1725.

81 Kiberd BA, Jindal KK. Screening to prevent renal failure in insulin dependent diabetic patients: an economic evaluation. *BMJ* 1995;**311**:1595–1599.

82 Clark WF, Churchill DN, Forwell L, Macdonald G, Foster S. To pay or not to pay? A decision and cost–utility analysis of angiotensin-converting-enzyme inhibitor therapy for diabetic nephropathy [published erratum appears in *CMAJ* 2000; **162** (7): 973]. *CMAJ* 2000;**162**(2):195–198.

83 Szucs TD, Sandoz MS, Keusch GW. The cost-effectiveness of losartan in type 2 diabetics with nephropathy in Switzerland – an analysis of the RENAAL study. *Swiss Med Wkly* 2004;**134**:440–447.

84 Souchet T, Durand ZI, Hannedouche T, Rodier M, Gaugris S, Passa P. An economic evaluation of losartan therapy in type 2 diabetic patients with nephropathy: an analysis of the RENAAL study adapted to France. *Diabetes Metab* 2003; **29**:29–35.

85 Palmer AJ, Annemans L, Roze S, Lamotte M, Rodby RA, Cordonnier DJ. An economic evaluation of irbesartan in the treatment of patients with type 2 diabetes, hypertension and nephropathy: cost-effectiveness of Irbesartan in Diabetic Nephropathy Trial (IDNT) in the Belgian and French settings. *Nephrol Dial Transplant* 2003; **18**:2059–2066.

86 Palmer AJ, Annemans L, Roze S, Lamotte M, Rodby RA, Bilous RW. An economic evaluation of the Irbesartan in Diabetic Nephropathy Trial (IDNT) in a UK setting. *J Hum Hypertens* 2004;**18**:733–738.

87 Palmer AJ, Weiss C, Sendi PP *et al.* The cost-effectiveness of different management strategies for type I diabetes: a Swiss perspective. *Diabetologia* 2000;**43**:13–26.

88 Gozzoli V, Palmer AJ, Brandt A, Spinas GA. Economic and clinical impact of alternative disease management strategies for secondary prevention in type 2 diabetes in the Swiss setting. *Swiss Med Wkly* 2001;**131**:303–310.

28 The role of public policy

Julia Critchley, Nigel Unwin

Institute of Health and Society, Newcastle University, Newcastle upon Tyne, UK

Healthy public policy – introduction

Policy can be defined as 'a course or principle of action adopted or proposed by a government, party, business or individual'[1] and public policy as policy formulated at any level of government.[2,3] The concept of 'healthy public policy' highlights the fact that all areas of government activity can impact upon the health of individuals and populations. It has been used to argue that at the very least the health impact of all public policies should be explicitly considered and that such considerations should influence whether policies are adopted and how they are implemented. For example, the Ottawa Charter of the World Health Organization emphasizes that health should be on the policy agenda in all areas of government and that governments should be held to account for the health consequences of their policies.[4,5] In simple terms, healthy public policies are those which improve the conditions under which people live and have a demonstrable net benefit for health.[2]

Public policy has played, and continues to play, a central role in improving public health. A few examples from the older industrialized countries of the world in which public policy has played a key role include: food hygiene; the provision of clean water and safe disposal of sewerage; safety at work; road safety; cleaner air; tobacco control; and vaccination programmes for major infectious diseases. It is now widely accepted that well-directed public policies, across several sectors, are needed to address the obesity epidemic. The rationale for this is succinctly put in this quotation from a World Health Organization report:[6] 'what has been demonstrated ... is that approaches that are firmly based on the principle of personal education and behaviour change are unli-

kely to succeed in an environment in which there are plentiful inducements to engage in opposing behaviours ... It would therefore seem appropriate to devote resources to programmes which focus on reducing the exposure of the population to obesity promoting agents by addressing the environmental factors such as transportation, urban design, advertising and food pricing'.

It is plausible that it is only through addressing the broader environmental factors that influence physical activity and diet[7,8] that real progress towards the primary prevention of type 2 diabetes will be made. Attempting to modify such environmental factors is firmly within the remit of healthy public policy.

Well-intended public policies in other fields can, of course, have perverse effects on health (e.g. road building, promotion of small businesses selling fast foods). It is therefore important to consider explicitly the health impacts of all public policies [health impact assessment (HIA)] and not just those directly concerned with health. Recent UK government publications, such as the Wanless report[9] and the Department of Health white paper 'Choosing Health: Making Healthier Choices Easier,'[10] have highlighted the need to consider health impacts of 'non-health' interventions and policies and embed HIA into policy.

The policy-making process

A simple and idealized schema of the policy making process is shown in Figure 28.1.[11] Although policy making in the real world is almost always more iterative and complicated than this figure suggests, it provides a useful way of considering the main

The Evidence Base for Diabetes Care, Second Edition, Edited by William H. Herman, Ann Louise Kinmonth, Nicholas J. Wareham and Rhys Williams.
© 2010 John Wiley & Sons, Ltd

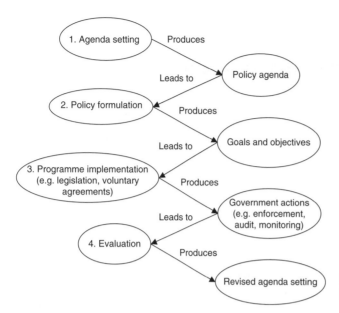

Figure 28.1 The policy making progress (based on Anderson and Hussey[11])

elements in the process. The first main element is agenda setting, which is the process of government deciding which issues it will address and towards what broad goals. The second element is the policy formulation stage, which involves deciding on the aims and objectives towards addressing the broad goals on the policy agenda. The third element is the actions taken to meet the aims and objectives, that is, the implementation of the policy. The fourth and final element in this schema is evaluation of policy, which should then feed back into the agenda-setting process.

Public policy making is first and foremost a political process. Considerations of public opinion, media attention, lobbying from interest groups, party politics, the funding of political parties, financial power of certain industries and so on, all play a role in setting the policy agenda and in how that agenda is acted on. Evidence on what is good for public health is but one factor in the policy making process. How to ensure that it is one of the more important factors that policy makers consider is beyond the scope of this chapter. However, it is a crucial issue for anyone interested in promoting healthy public policy.[12]

Policy levers for promoting health

Policy levers (or policy instruments) refer to the broad types of interventions that are available to implement public policy. The World Health Organization, in its report 'Preventing Chronic Diseases: a Vital Investment',[13] identifies six main categories of policy levers. These are shown and described in Box 28.1. These categories are not discrete entities. For example, legislative measures might be used in approaches to

health financing and improving the built environment and advocacy initiatives and community mobilization often go hand in hand.

BOX 28.1 Types of 'levers' for healthy public policy.[13]

- **Health financing**
  At its most basic level, this includes ensuring that the annual health budget has a line item for diabetes prevention and control. More sophisticated approaches might include the use of specific tax revenues (e.g. on tobacco, alcohol or certain food items) to fund preventive activities.[14]

- **Legislation and regulation**
  This has played a key role in tobacco control, including banning advertising, forbidding sales to minors and banning smoking in public places. Its potential to modify food consumption and promote physical activity seems great but is largely untested.[3,15]

- **Improving the built environment**
  This refers to changing the built environment in order to promote physical activity. It includes the provision of cycle ways and walk ways, changes in the lay out of residential and shopping areas and changes in the interior design of workplaces and public buildings.[16]

- **Advocacy initiatives**
  This refers to the systematic engagement of opinion leaders in order to help change and lead public opinion on the need for preventive action. Advocacy initiatives are considered an essential adjunct to the other policy levers, most of which require substantial public support if they are to be politically possible.[17]

- **Community mobilization**
  This refers to the active engagement of organizations and individuals in preventive activities. Examples include schemes to engage local employers in the promotion of physical activity amongst their employees

---

and school-based programmes to promote healthier diets amongst their pupils.[18]
- **Health services organization and delivery**
This refers to policy that is designed to coordinate and direct the provision of health services towards the goal of improved prevention and control for diabetes. An example is the design and implementation of a National Service Framework for diabetes in England.[19]

Evidence for public policy

Scope of review

In this review, we focus on those policy levers for promoting health which influence risks outside of the health sector. Issues to do with health care organization, delivery and content (interventions largely affecting patients or individuals) are covered elsewhere in this volume. As we are considering interventions outside of the health sector, the target of these interventions is generally whole populations or specific groups in the population, rather than individuals.

In public health terms, we are interested in public policy that will shift the distribution of major risk factors or behaviours for type 2 diabetes and the complications of diabetes (particularly cardiovascular disease) towards healthier levels.[20] As has been reviewed in Chapter 5, well-designed randomized controlled trials have shown that a package of measures that includes increased physical activity, reductions in the caloric density and improvements in the composition of diets can reduce or delay the incidence of type 2 diabetes in those at high risk. The epidemiological evidence is strong enough to suggest that similar measures amongst those at lower risk would also contribute to reducing the incidence of type 2 diabetes.

In people with diabetes (as reviewed in Chapter 7), increased levels of physical activity, improved diets, lower levels of obesity and avoidance of smoking are all desirable for the prevention of both macrovascular and microvascular complications. The effectiveness of different interventions to reduce tobacco use is not covered here (except where it forms part of a multi- risk factor reduction strategy), as it has been the subject of numerous reviews and discussion papers.[21–28]

Hence in this review, we focus on the evidence for public policy measures to increase physical activity, improve diets and reduce obesity that are relevant to areas outside the health sector. We use as our framework the policy levers described by the World Health Organization and shown in Box 28.1, focusing on community mobilization and advocacy, legislation and regulation and changing the built environment.

Types of evidence for healthy public policy

In evidence-based medicine, systematic reviews of randomized controlled trials (RCTs) are widely regarded as the best possible evidence for decision making. This is because RCTs are less prone to bias (particularly selection bias) and confounding than other study designs.[29,30] Typically in clinical guidelines, a hierarchy of evidence approach is used with systematic reviews of RCTs at the top, representing the strongest possible evidence for any particular intervention. These are followed by single large and preferably multi-centre RCTs, then single-centre RCTs, then observational studies (cohort and case–control studies in that order), case reports and finally expert opinion.[31] However, when it comes to public health initiatives and especially public policy-based initiatives, RCTs are not always feasible or available to guide decision making and the 'hierarchy' approach can therefore be problematic.[32,33] In many instances, it may not be possible to randomize whole communities to receive or not receive an intervention. Examples include community health promotion projects to prevent coronary heart disease, such as the North Karelia project in Finland,[34] or interventions to modify the built environment (e.g. more cycling or walking paths) to promote physical activity.[35] The 'hierarchy' approach is also based around being able to identify a study design and place it appropriately in the hierarchy, thus equating study design with the quality or strength of evidence.[36] In practice, this can be more difficult to achieve with public health interventions, as the criteria designed for classifying studies of clinical evidence may not readily apply to studies of public health interventions.[37] The actual quality or reliability of a study may be related as much to the appropriateness and quality of implementation of the intervention, as to the design per se.[33,36,38] Inclusion of results from various types of studies, apart from RCTs, is therefore essential when assessing the evidence for making healthy public policy.[38]

Another difficulty is that it is not always clear which sectors of the population benefit the most. There are concerns that the most socially and economically disadvantaged in the community, likely to be at higher diabetes risk, may be less likely to respond to advocacy interventions.[39] Few community or advocacy interventions have been able to assess benefits by socioeconomic group.[40,41] However, further evidence on how to target those most at risk would be informative.

In public health terms, what constitutes evidence itself is rarely explicitly defined in most discussions – for some this may be RCTs only, but for others expert opinion or recommendations may be included.[33] Evidence-based public health has recently been defined as 'public health endeavour in which there is an informed, explicit and judicious use of evidence that has been derived from any of a variety of science and social science research and evaluation methods',[42] which highlights the need for an explicit consideration of the types of evidence relevant to public health and a framework for interpreting and applying that evidence. In this chapter, we include evidence from any type of experimental or observational study design, highlighting systematic reviews of experimental studies or observational studies with a plausible comparison group, particularly where individual studies are consistent.

We describe the evidence as 'good evidence' if there is at least one systematic review of five or more other studies which consistently find evidence of benefit; 'some evidence' if there are five or more studies showing benefits, but effect sizes are small or follow-up short; 'limited' if there is no comprehensive review and less than five studies; 'no supporting evidence' if there is evidence from several well-designed studies that the intervention is not effective; and 'not yet evaluated' if no studies have considered the health effects of a policy initiative.

Table 28.1 is not a comprehensive listing of the effectiveness of every possible public health policy

Table 28.1 Examples of policy interventions which may be effective in reducing type 2 diabetes risk with notes on design and strength of evidence base (see text)

Risk factor(s)	Intervention	Nature of evidence (design)	Strength of evidence
Advocacy and community mobilization			
Physical activity	Community-wide campaigns to promote physical activity, including mass media interventions with support of self-help groups, counselling, risk factor screening and education and environmental or policy changes. Many of the studies aimed to reduce cardiovascular disease risk	Systematic review of mainly before-and-after studies, some with control areas, half from US and remainder from other developed countries. Task Force on Community Preventive Services;[43] http://www.thecommunityguide.org/pa/pa-int-comm-campaigns.pdf	Good evidence of effect; 10 studies reviewed were all effective, although relative contributions of individual components not clear. Outcomes measured in original studies included % active at some level, activity levels and estimated energy expenditure. Median physical activity changes across studies included a 5% increase in proportion of people active and a 16% increase in energy expenditure. Results were similar in different urban and rural environments and in different ethnic and socio-economic groups
Physical activity	Mass media campaigns to promote physical activity. Campaign used a variety of media (TV, newspapers) to provide information on health benefits of physical activity and promote moderate intensity activities (such as walking)	3 year prospective longitudinal survey using a multi-stage, cluster random probability design to select participants. Participants were a representative sample of 3189 adults aged 16–74 years. Survey evaluated the UK media campaign 'Active for Life'[44]	No supporting evidence – no increases in physical activity levels, either overall or in any sub-groups
Physical activity	Interventions to promote walking, including brief interventions with individuals or households, group-based approaches, use of pedometers, community-level approaches, active commuting, school travel and financial incentives/motives.	Systematic review of 19 randomized and 29 non-randomized studies; all these were before-and-after or with some control group, area or population[41]	Some evidence – the most successful studies increased walking by 30–60 min per week on average in the short term among targeted groups. The most convincing evidence was from individual/household studies, but this partly reflects the studies undertaken

(continued)

Table 28.1 (*Continued*)

Risk factor(s)	Intervention	Nature of evidence (design)	Strength of evidence
Multiple risk factors (focus mainly on CHD prevention)	Community cardiovascular primary prevention programmes, which use multi-factorial intervention strategies to promote healthy eating, weight control, physical activity and reductions in tobacco consumption	Evaluations of programmes and systematic reviews of programmes comparing intervention with control communities. Examples of projects include North Karelia,[34] Stanford Five-Cities,[45] Minnesota,[46] Pawtucket Heart Health Program,[48] Heart Beat Wales[49]	Some evidence of small but potentially important declines in risk factors in some communities. For example, a joint analysis of three US community trials (Stanford Five-City, Minnesota and Pawtucket) showed small reductions in risk in men and women of all ages, but none were statistically significant.[50] The reason for this was the very small differences observed between intervention and control cities, rather than sample size limitations. The analysis highlights the difficulties in maintaining suitable control communities for evaluation, as beneficial effects were found in many control cities
Obesity	Worksite interventions for obesity aimed at diet, physical activity and cognitive change (including nutrition education, prescriptions for exercise, training in behavioural techniques, self-help materials, group exercise sessions)	Systematic review of 7 studies. All studies had before-and-after measurements or control groups. Effectiveness defined as an average weight loss of at least 4 lb (1.8 kg), 6 months or longer after start of intervention[51]	Some evidence that worksite interventions using a combination of strategies were effective [average weight loss 4–26 lb (1.8–11.8 kg)], but those based on single interventions (e.g. diet, physical activity) were not effective. Studies with longer term follow-up (>6 months) were less effective, suggesting that benefits may not be maintained
Obesity	School-based programmes for obesity. Most interventions targeted both physical activity and nutrition behaviour, although there were some interventions that focused on only one dimension such as TV watching or restricting drinking of carbonated drinks or increasing physical education time in the school. Most of the interventions were based on some behavioural theory and the most popular theory was social cognitive theory. Most focused on individual level behaviour change approaches and evaluated short-term changes right after the intervention	Review of 11 such interventions between 1999 and 2004, all from USA and UK.[18] Most were evaluated in RCTs, but some used pre–post designs, non-randomized controls groups or were observational in design. Outcomes measured were highly variable, including BMI, % overweight or obese, triceps skinfold thickness, waist circumference, fruit/vegetable intake, physical activity, TV viewing in hours per week, length of PE activities at school, percentage fat in food, stages of change for physical activity	Some evidence of modest changes in behaviour and mixed results with indicators of obesity. Typically, in successful programmes, BMI was reduced by around 0.3 kg m^{-2}. Some studies reported improvements in fruit and vegetable intake or modest increases in physical activity levels. Some showed improvements in knowledge, attitudes or stages of change for physical activity
Nutrition/diet	School-based programmes to improve nutritional status of children and adolescents. These	Systematic review of 41 studies.[52] Wide variations in activities, length of study, age of population and	Some evidence. Reported changes (improvements in intake of fruit and vegetables,

(continued)

Table 28.1 (*Continued*)

Risk factor(s)	Intervention	Nature of evidence (design)	Strength of evidence
	include educational components (e.g. classroom instruction by teachers, integrating nutrition education across curricula, peer training), environmental components (e.g. improving school menus) and other components (such as physical activity, family education and involvement, community involvement)	length of follow-up. Study outcomes were self-reported changes in dietary intake (fruit and vegetables, fat, saturated fats), which may be prone to reporting bias	fats, saturated fats) were in the desired direction, but small and questionable due to potential biases
Physical activity	Increasing physical activity in schools (increasing lengths of time in PE classes or amount of time children are active during PE classes)	13 studies with comparison groups (who mostly receive standard health and PE curriculum)[53]	Good evidence – interventions effective increasing length of time physically active and aerobic capacity (by a median of 8.4%, IQR 3.1–9.0%)
Environment			
Physical activity	Point of decision prompts to increase physical activity (e.g. signs or posters promoting stair use, rather than taking the lift or escalator)	Systematic review of 6 studies, mostly before-and-after designs;[54] http://www.thecommunityguide.org/pa/pa-int-decision-prompts.pdf; also review for NICE[16]	Some evidence. One review of 6 studies estimated a net 54% increase in stair use[54] but another found they mostly had only a short-term effect, with one study reporting a 29% increase in stair use at 6 months.[16] No controlled trials are available and most studies only measured short-term effects. It is also unclear whether those who respond are physically active
Physical activity – promoting walking or cycling as alternatives to using cars for commuting	Interventions at the level of individual commuters to encourage them to shift to walking, cycling or public transport, instead of car use	Systematic review of 22 observational and experimental studies (some controlled studies, some before-and-after studies.[35] Main outcomes were % change in trips by different modes of transport and time spent walking	Some evidence that behaviour change programmes targeted at motivated volunteers can slightly increase trips by walking, cycling or public transport (by about 5% in one study). Single studies found small effects from commuter subsidies and new railway stations. No evidence that engineering (improved bicycle lanes) or publicity campaigns were effective
Physical activity	Development of new cycle and walking paths (with support from local promotional campaigns) can encourage use	Systematic review for NICE including 2 before-and-after studies, one cross-sectional study, from USA and Australia, which evaluated new cycle or walking paths[16]	Limited evidence. Use of paths appeared to be increased by support with local promotional campaigns and is associated with proximity and safety concerns. Few well-designed studies available and results should be viewed with caution. Unclear if paths attract 'new exercisers' or only those already active

(continued)

Table 28.1 (*Continued*)

Risk factor(s)	Intervention	Nature of evidence (design)	Strength of evidence
Physical activity	Traffic calming studies in many countries have shown reductions in traffic speed and accidents. They may also have the potential to increase physical activity through improving road safety and the general environment, to promote cycling and walking	Before-and-after study[55]	Limited evidence. One small before-and-after study found modest improvements in walking (20% increase), cycling (4%) increase and allowing children to play outdoors, walk or cycle. However, the study was small with low response rates and a high potential for selection bias
Legislation, regulation and voluntary agreements			
Diet	Economic or agricultural subsidies and policies which promote consumption of healthy food stuffs such as fruit and vegetables and discourage consumption of less healthy foodstuffs such as hydrogenated fat	Observational (generally before-and-after) studies in individual countries/communities	Reasonable evidence from large-scale studies of individual policy change such as Poland, Finland, Singapore. In Poland, subsidies for dairy and animal fats were abolished, followed by a rapid fall in CHD mortality.[56] In Finland, agricultural policies were altered to favour berry farming over dairy farming, contributing to falls in cholesterol levels[57]
Diet (specifically lipid levels)	Modifying the food supply to promote the consumption of foods promoting cardiovascular health, e.g. eliminating the partial hydrogenation of vegetable oils, which destroys essential omega-3 fatty acids and creates trans-fatty acids	Observational (generally before-and-after) studies in individual countries/communities	Reasonable evidence from large-scale studies of individual policy change. Examples include Mauritius, where saturated palm oils were replaced by unsaturated soybean oils for use in cooking in 1987. Total cholesterol levels fell by about 0.8 mmol l^{-1} between 1987 and 1992.[58] Reductions in salt consumption would also be beneficial,[59] but examples of successful legislation and manufacturing are not available
Diet	Legislation and regulation in schools. These include regulations to improve nutrition in schools including nutritional standards for school meals, restricting competitive food sales (e.g. vending machines) and 'closed-campus' policies keeping children at school during lunch hours	Little evidence available[60]	Not yet evaluated
Diet	Taxes on 'junk foods'	A number of US states have tried to tax foods that are not nutritious (e.g. sweets, soft drinks)[60]	Not yet evaluated. No direct evidence that taxes on foods will affect diet or obesity, but there is evidence to suggest an effect is plausible. Econometric models have linked food prices with consumption and cigarette taxes with patterns of use. The possible effect size is unclear

(continued)

Table 28.1 (*Continued*)

Risk factor(s)	Intervention	Nature of evidence (design)	Strength of evidence
Diet	Voluntary agreements with industry (e.g. to reduce salt in processed foods or limit advertising of unhealthy foods to children or for improved food labelling)	Limited evidence. Select UK Committee on Health has favoured voluntary agreements over legislation on the grounds that this would lead to faster implementation[61]	Not yet evaluated. Different models of policy development have been compared to restrict TV advertising to children.[60] There are concerns that voluntary agreements may not be powerful enough to achieve any real public health benefits and need continual monitoring. A recent example is the 'traffic light' scheme recommended by the National Consumer Council for nutrient profiling by food.[62] Some supermarkets are implementing this scheme, but other major UK retailers are developing competing schemes, which have not been tested with consumers
Physical activity	'Zoning' laws to limit prevalence of fast foods, expand recreational opportunities and encourage healthier lifestyles[63]	Little or no evidence, although some areas have zoning restrictions on fast food outlets including wholesale prohibitions, limited bans on fast food chains and quotas on the number of restaurants[63]	Not yet evaluated

intervention, but aims to provide an indication of the types of policy interventions which might be possible and the evidence for the effectiveness of these interventions within this framework. It is categorized first by the type of policy measure or lever (advocacy and community mobilization, changes to the environment, legislation, regulations, including voluntary regulation through voluntary agreements), and second by the diabetes risk factor it aims to intervene on. However, it should be recognized that interventions are likely to be more effective if they act on several policy levers and risk factors simultaneously – see, for example, physical activity promotion interventions in Table 28.1.[43] Following the table, we discuss some of the difficulties with evaluating healthy public policy initiatives and summarize the evidence for different types of policy measures and interventions. Finally, we identify the main policy areas already shown to be effective and potentially beneficial policies where evidence is currently lacking and further research required.

The limited evidence base

There is, in general, far less evidence available for the effectiveness (or lack of effectiveness) of different public health interventions than for clinical treatments.[9] This is partly because these are much more difficult to evaluate, as the interventions are often not amenable to randomization[32] (a recent example of this might be legislation to prevent smoking in public places). In other cases, controlled trials are possible, but tend to be expensive and difficult to carry out (this includes many environmental or community interventions, such as traffic calming measures, ideally requiring evaluation through cluster RCTs). Even where controlled trials are possible, there can still be problems in maintaining a control group which is not exposed to the intervention. It is not always feasible to randomize whole communities, and even if this is possible, the intervention may be rolled out to control areas before there is time for its full effects to become apparent.[64] Many community interventions have shown diffusion or contamination of the intervention from the 'active' area to the 'control' area, diluting its apparent impact.[65] Changes to public health policies cannot take place in a social vacuum and it is therefore almost impossible to prevent such 'diffusion' from occurring. The effectiveness of some well-known community health promotion projects is much disputed (e.g. the coronary heart disease prevention programme which commenced in North Karelia, Finland[34]), mainly due to difficulties in allocating large areas to an intervention, selecting appropriate control groups and avoiding contamination with the intervention in control group areas.[57]

Limitations in design are not the only difficulty with public health policy research. If a public health policy or programme does not show a beneficial effect, it can be difficult to distinguish whether the programme itself was flawed, whether the programme was not properly implemented or whether the outcome measures to evaluate the programme were not sensitive or accurate enough to show an effect.[36] High-quality process evaluation of interventions is therefore important to determine the quality of implementation of any programme (particularly delivery and take-up of the programme), in addition to outcome evaluation.[44,66] Moreover, in some studies outcome measures can be limited to self-reported changes in lifestyle behaviours, such as diet, smoking or physical activity, which can be subject to bias.[67–70] More objective measurements, such as accelerometry (for physical activity), urinary cotinine (for smoking) or plasma vitamin levels (for self-reported fruit and vegetable intake) would be ideal, but are often not practical or cost-effective in large-scale community surveys. If objective measurements of outcomes are not possible, measurement tools should be validated as far as possible (e.g. physical activity questionnaires should be validated against accelerometers or heart rate monitors).

Rigorous evaluations of public health interventions are often very expensive for all these reasons, but funding for public health research has in general been more limited than that available for biomedical or clinical research.[9] Much basic biomedical science is funded by the pharmaceutical sector and, at least in the United Kingdom, government funding has tended in the past to favour basic sciences over more applied public health interventions or implementation research. Further, public policies addressing health are often introduced for political reasons, when policy makers feel under pressure to respond to real or perceived public health problems, often raised by powerful groups in society.[71] Increasingly, this includes pressure from powerful patient groups, sometimes supported by the pharmaceutical sector.[72] In-

terventions introduced in this way may or may not be effective, but the political context and time pressures under which they are implemented makes rigorous evaluation less likely to occur.

Effectiveness of public health interventions

Advocacy and community health mobilization

In practice, it is difficult to distinguish advocacy levers from community mobilization levers, as many interventions directed at local 'communities' contain elements of both. In general, community health promotion interventions have been subject to more evaluation than other types of public health policy initiatives (see Table 28.1), partly because they tend to be easier to carry out and evaluate than other types. Interventions generally target whole communities, sometimes defined geographically and sometimes socially (such as workplaces or schools, often termed a 'settings' approach[73]). Typically, such studies show small to modest benefits, at least in the short term, for example, increases in physical activity[43] or in consumption of fruit and vegetables.[52] These could potentially be important if they were maintained, but evidence over the longer term is usually lacking. There are few reports of beneficial changes in obesity or overweight, which have been maintained over the longer term, from such interventions. One national programme, based in schools in Singapore, has shown modest reductions in before-and-after surveys of obesity among school children (a reduction in prevalence of obesity from 16.6 to 14.6% between 1999 and 2000 for 11–12-year-olds and from 15.5 to 13.1% for 15–16-year-olds).[74] The programme included both a general intervention (improving food standards in schools, nutrition education) and targeted a programme for students who were overweight. This included special exercise programmes and assessment and management at a health centre where appropriate.[74] Other school-based programmes have shown some modest improvements in diet and physical activity,[18] but these are generally self-reported and their interpretation is equivocal.[52]

The most effective interventions seem to be those which use a variety of media and messages to target different groups.[43] More intense interventions also tend to be more effective, particularly if they target several policy levers simultaneously – an example is the North Karelia community cardiovascular health promotion programme, which included advocacy and community mobilization (awareness raising, media campaigns, competitions to lower community cholesterol levels and financial incentives (to change types of farming).[34] However, even here, the longer term effectiveness of most interventions has seldom been evaluated.

Most community-based advocacy interventions have focused on 'the demand' side (providing information and encouragement to make healthier choices), but the supply side, largely supermarkets in most Western countries, is very influential in shaping our diets. Collaborative interventions with supermarkets may have value in improving diets. For example, a recent RCT evaluated an intervention which prompted Internet shoppers to swap food items they chose with lower fat alternatives.[75] In a short-term evaluation (4 months), this seemed to be effective in reducing the saturated fat content of foods chosen (by 0.66%), although we do not know whether the lower fat alternatives were actually eaten or by which members of the family unit. More generally, supermarkets could play a major role in promoting the consumption of healthier foods through a variety of initiatives, including store design and layout and location, (e.g. placing low-fat foods at eye level, ensuring equivalent prices for different foodstuffs in high- and low-income areas), pricing policies and promotions which incentivize the selection of healthy foods, including fresh fruit and vegetables. However, it is unclear to what extent supermarkets will be prepared to cooperate with initiatives to promote healthier eating at the possible expense of their business plans.

Changing the built environment

Interventions which attempt to change the environment (e.g. to promote cycling and walking for transport, instead of car use) should have an enormous potential for preventing and controlling diabetes, because they can become a part of routine daily life (i.e. through walking to work or to the shops). It has been suggested that such 'active commuting' could play a major role in promoting physical activity and preventing diabetes.[76,77] However, relatively few studies have tried to evaluate the benefits of such schemes and the evidence for benefits is equivocal at best. This is partly because the appropriate behavioural outcome measures (e.g. physical activity) have not always been measured.[32] For example, many studies have attempted to evaluate the effectiveness of traffic calming measures in built-up areas (such as road humps, chicanes or lower speed limits). Such interventions may have considerable potential for promoting active commuting (by improving the safety or perceived safety of roads for cyclists and pedestrians, thereby encouraging use[55]). However, often the only

health outcomes measured have been accidents or injuries.[78] In most places, the built environment has been under the control of town and country planners, rather than public health experts, which may explain some of the lack of health outcomes evaluated. Changes to the built environment could have other benefits for preventing diabetes and complications of diabetes, in addition to promoting physical activity. In particular, changes to the environment which promote higher consumption of fruit and vegetables (such as local markets or allotments for growing vegetables) could be beneficial, but the health benefits of these have rarely been evaluated. The creation of new green spaces (parks, safe cycling and walking routes) could also be beneficial, but again evidence is lacking.[16]

Considering the dearth of evidence, it is essential that any future environmental change interventions should include a careful evaluation of their health impacts. This should cover not only changes in total physical activity levels among the local community, but also consideration of who benefits from these schemes (the 'target group'). In particular, it is important to assess whether traffic calming and new cycle/walking routes encourage any increases in physical activity among those who are currently sedentary or whether they are largely used by people who are already physically active. The greatest health gain and impact on diabetes is likely to come from projects which encourage inactive people to take any additional activity, rather than from promoting activity levels among those who are already active or diverting them into different activities.[20,79]

Legislation and regulations

Types of legal changes
Some of the most important public health improvements over the past 50 years or so (such as reduced rates of smoking, seatbelt legislation, improvements in health and safety at work), have come from changes in the law.[60] In general, these take three forms – new legislation (such as nutritional standards for school dinners), increases in regulatory enforcements (e.g. school district policies banning sugary drinks from school vending machines) or litigation (e.g. legal action against local authorities or school boards which permit school to accept money from soft drink companies in return for vending rights).[60] Litigation has been of critical importance in tobacco control,[80] but there are few successful examples of litigation against the food industry, although high-profile cases such as the suit against McDonald's brought by obese children in

New York may have contributed to decisions made by some food companies to provide healthier products.[60] For further details of the arguments for and against specific legal interventions (such as disclosure, surveillance, taxation and prohibition), the reader is directed to Gostin's recent review article.[63]

Country-level changes in legislation and food Subsidies

There are many examples of changes in legislation or regulations which may contribute to healthier diets. Rigorous evaluation of legislative changes is not always possible, but in some cases the dietary changes (shown from representative before-and-after surveys and using biochemical measurements such as cholesterol levels, as well as self-reported behaviour change) have been so rapid and substantial that it is reasonable to attribute the benefits to changes in legislation. There is, for example, some reasonable evidence that legislative changes can be highly effective in improving diets at the country level, particularly the types of fats consumed, (mostly from before-and-after studies, often using routine or cross-sectional data), although successful examples are limited. Possible legislation could involve abolishing unhelpful subsidies (e.g. for animal fats), and also promoting consumption of healthier food stuffs. At the national level, the example of Poland is often cited. Mortality from coronary heart disease was increasing rapidly in Poland in the 1980s. However, with the fall of communism, subsidies for dairy and animal fats were abolished, followed by a very rapid change in the ratio of saturated to unsaturated fats consumed and fall in CHD mortality.[56,81] The fall observed may not be entirely due to the change in fat consumption, as other favourable dietary changes also occurred around this time, such as some increase in imports of fruits. However, most observers agree that the legislative change was likely to have been the most important factor changing dietary behaviour and thus reducing CHD mortality in Poland (and CHD mortality in Poland fell earlier than in other similar Eastern European countries[82]). Another country where legislative change appears to have had substantial dietary benefits is Mauritius. Here, saturated palm oil for cooking was replaced with unsaturated soybean oil towards the end of the 1980s. Total cholesterol levels fell substantially in the population following this change.[58] More recently (2003), Denmark became the first country to set an upper limit of trans-fatty acids in food and New York City is introducing a ban or upper limit of artificial trans-fatty acids in all food service establishments and restaurants, respectively.[63] Any future evaluations of the health impacts of these limits would be highly valuable.

In addition to legislation, financial incentives and subsidies can be used to improve diets at national levels. In Finland, dairy farmers were provided with financial incentives and support to alter production from dairy to berries. Cholesterol levels and CHD mortality have fallen substantially in Finland, although it is difficult to attribute this to changes in farming or any one intervention solely, as a large-scale community health promotion intervention was implemented in North Karelia from the late 1970s and rolled out to the rest of Finland soon after.[34,83] Legislation to reduce the salt content in processed foods is likely to be effective in reducing salt content in diets, as approximately 80% of salt in our diets is estimated to come from processed foods, rather than salt added during cooking or at the table.[59] Consequently, this may reduce blood pressure levels, although the magnitude of the reduction which can be achieved is currently unclear and a matter of debate.[84–87] We are not aware of any wide-scale evaluation of legislative, regulatory or voluntary agreements to reduce the amount of salt in processed foods, although there are many reports suggesting the food industry is taking some steps to reduce salt in such foods[88]

Legislation or voluntary agreements with the food and advertising industries

A current area of controversy and debate surrounds the role of the food and advertising industries and how they are regulated. To date, much health promotion research has focused on educating people to improve their food choices. However, major suppliers such as supermarkets play a critical role in determining food consumption. Legislation or voluntary agreements with supermarkets to improve labelling of 'healthful' foods is another under-evaluated intervention.[62] In the United Kingdom, recent voluntary agreement with major supermarkets has resulted in new labelling systems, but the systems introduced differ between supermarkets (some use coloured 'traffic lights', endorsed by the Food Standards Authority,[89] but others are using 'guideline daily amounts'), and the latter has been criticized for being over-complicated and potentially misleading.[90] The National Heart Forum report suggests that the traffic light system is easier for the consumer to understand quickly,[90] but further work may be needed to establish the extent to which improved labelling can be effective in changing diet.[63]

TV advertising to children

Obesity in children has increased dramatically in many countries over the past few decades and children are particularly vulnerable to targeting by the food industry.[91] Banning advertising of cigarettes is thought to have played an important role in reducing cigarette smoking in many Western countries, particularly among young people.[3] Younger children are considered incapable of understanding or critically appraising the marketing content of adverts,[91] or of understanding the potential long-term implications of poor dietary choices. Children are also important in determining the food choices of the whole family through 'pester power'.[92] Recent reviews have highlighted the impact of advertising on food choice[93] and the contribution of children's TV advertising to rising rates of obesity. For these reasons, children are often deemed worthy of regulatory protection from food industry marketing campaigns.

Regulatory agreements have taken varying formats in different countries.[60] Sweden has prohibited outright advertising to children (defined as those aged <12 years) since 1991. The French government has recently banned advertising to children and introduced legal measures to require food advertisers to display health warnings on advertisements for high-sugar and high-salt foods. Other countries such as Ireland are introducing new statutory codes which cover a range of measures, including not using celebrities, sports stars or cartoon characters to promote food or drink (unless part of public health campaigns), not encouraging consumption of fast or snack foods as the main part of the diet and placing advertised foodstuffs in the context of a balanced diet. The most common form of regulation in many countries including the United States and United Kingdom is to rely largely on voluntary agreements or codes of practice, although this is under review in the United Kingdom, and in the United States the Institute of Medicine has recently recommended restrictions on advertising if the food industries do not voluntarily shift emphasis from unhealthy foodstuffs. In the United Kingdom, there has been lobbying for a ban on television advertising of 'junk foods' aimed at young children before the 'watershed' (9 pm), and although this has not yet been successful, a total ban on all advertising of junk foods around all children's programming, on all children's channels was phased in during 2007.

Most examples of legislative or regulatory agreements with food and advertising industries are confined to developed countries, although the recent WHO Global Strategy for Diet, Physical Activity and Health also sets out provisions for marketing, advertising and sponsorship and encourages governments to work with consumer groups and industry to develop appropriate approaches to deal with these issues.[94] With increases in satellite TV, it is increasingly argued that agreement on such issues is needed at a global or at least regional level; banning advertising in one country will not prevent children from viewing advertisements made for TV elsewhere.[91] A global agreement and legislation to improve diets, similar to the Framework Convention on Tobacco Control,[95] which countries sign up to and ratify, may be more effective in improving diet than piecemeal country-wide legislation and regulations. Well-designed, qualitative and quantitative evaluations should accompany any future restrictions on advertising.

Legislation and regulations to promote physical activity

Evidence of any legislative changes which have resulted in an increase in physical activity are currently lacking. Legislation which makes it more difficult to drive into city centres (e.g. congestion charging, higher parking fees and dedicated lanes for public transport) may be able to increase physical activity levels. Congestion charging in Central London is thought to have greatly reduced the number of cars coming into the centre. It may be expected that this has resulted in increases in physical activity, but little data or evidence for this are currently available.[96] A health impact assessment of the congestion charge is under way, but this appears to focus on air quality, rather than changes in physical activity.[97] There is some evidence of an increase in the number of cyclists in London (a 100% increase in journeys by bicycle from 2000 to 2005,[98] including a 20% rise in cyclists entering the congestion zone during charging hours[99]). This may not be due solely to congestion charging, as cycling was already increasing before the charge was implemented, but the rate of increase accelerated following the introduction of charging.[100] Further research is required to identify whether such schemes encourage 'new exercisers' (who have most to gain in public health terms) or whether they largely promote increases in cycling amongst those who are already physically active. Future schemes to reduce congestion in cities should be carefully designed to promote and evaluate changes in population levels of physical activity before and after the legislation is introduced.

Healthy public policies: a global perspective

Almost all public policy intervention studies relevant to the prevention of type 2 diabetes come from a limited number of Western countries, mainly the United States, Australia, the United Kingdom or Western Europe. With burgeoning epidemics of chronic diseases, including diabetes, in many low- and middle-income countries, there is an urgent need for evaluation and widespread dissemination of public health policies in these countries. Although evidence from Western nations provides a useful guide, it cannot be assumed that interventions developed in the West can be uncritically applied to low- and middle-income countries. For example, there is some evidence that prompts to use the stairs instead of lifts or escalators may be effective in promoting physical activity in Western populations.[16] A recent evaluation of a 'point of decision' prompt to use the stairs at the mid-level escalators in Hong Kong found no effect of the intervention, although some increases in walking up the escalators was observed.[101] Baseline levels of stair walking were also much lower than in Western studies.[101] The authors pointed out that such interventions have rarely been evaluated outside of an English language community and careful consideration will be needed to translate such interventions to communities which are culturally and linguistically very different from those for which they were originally designed.[101] The recent WHO Global Strategy for Diet, Physical Activity and Health is one of the first international public health strategies to put forward an agenda for healthy public health policy in low- and middle-income countries.[94] Internationally, it is likely that a global agreement (e.g. around obesity reduction or improving diet), similar to the Framework Convention on Tobacco Control,[95] may provide the best opportunity for implementing policies to prevent diabetes in low- and middle-income countries

Healthy public policy: the example of international tobacco control

Public policy for tobacco control is far more developed, compared with that to improve diets or physical activity, and is a good example of what can be achieved with focused multi-sectorial and appropriately financed interventions. Tobacco control interventions have been extensively studied in a variety of settings[15,25,26,102,103] and there are examples of successful policy levers covering advocacy/community, environment and legislation.[104] Information on the adverse health effects of tobacco has been widely available and disseminated since the 1960s,[105,106] and in many Western countries cigarette smoking started to decline (particularly in men) from around the 1970s onwards.[107–110] In most countries, legislation includes banning the sale of cigarettes to minors and in many banning advertising and sponsorship. Many countries have recently started to implement widespread bans on smoking in almost all public places. The WHO Framework Convention on Tobacco Control (FCTC) has been an influential piece of international public health policy, explicitly recognizing that globalization has facilitated the spread of the tobacco epidemic through a complex mix of factors that transcend national borders. This means that countries cannot regulate tobacco solely through domestic legislation. The FCTC is a binding international legal instrument which establishes broad commitments and a general system of governance. As of February 2007, 168 countries have signed the treaty and over 140 ratified.[95] Once signed and ratified, the treaty requires countries to implement a wide range of tobacco control initiatives, such as imposing restrictions on tobacco advertising, sponsorship and promotion, establishing new packaging and labelling of tobacco products, establishing clean indoor air controls and strengthening legislation to clamp down on tobacco smuggling.[95]

Another example of a successful tobacco control programme is that of California, where independent evaluation of the California Tobacco Control Program (CTCP) showed that per capita consumption fell by 57% in California in the 1990s, compared with 27% for the rest of the United States over the same time period.[80] The programme was established in 1989, after state legislation that increased the tax on tobacco products and earmarked the new revenues for tobacco control, medical care and research activities.[14] The CTCP is a comprehensive programme involving multiple, coordinated tobacco control strategies that aim to reduce tobacco use at the population level, largely through changing community norms regarding the acceptability of tobacco use. The goal of the programme is to alter the social–political environment in which tobacco initiation and cessation occur and one of the primary mechanisms used to attain this goal is the passage and enforcement of local and state policies.[14] The CTCP had three main components. The first is a media campaign, which disseminated hard-hitting anti-tobacco messages through television, radio, print media and outdoor advertising. The second programme component consists of local tobacco control initiatives, policy development and public education programmes implemented by county health departments and community-based organizations. The third component comprises school-based tobacco prevention programmes, activities and policies. Smoking prevalence has fallen to around 16% of adults in California, compared with about 21% in the United States generally. California has also been a leader in developing comprehensive restrictions on smoking in public places and protecting the population from passive smoking.[14,45,80]

Tobacco control initiatives also provide us with many good lessons on how legislative changes (such as the banning of smoking in public places) have been successfully achieved. It is often assumed by public health activists that senior policy markers are the most important group to target to achieve change. However, ASH Scotland points out that a critical factor in the recent English legislation has been the frequent canvassing and harnessing of public opinion; once it was shown in repeated surveys that public opinion largely favoured bans on smoking in public places, this was perceived as a 'vote-winner' and political opinion followed. Both the general public and media engaged in the debate openly and over a long period of time.[17] Voluntary health organizations lobbied together for comprehensive legislation and were able to expose the tobacco industry influences and strategies. Advances in scientific knowledge and research technologies have contributed; although the potential adverse medical effects of passive smoking have been known for some time, it has often been assumed that the doses received are low and unimportant for most people. Improved methods of measuring indoor air quality and lung function have shown that the health impacts of passive smoking are more immediate and greater than previously thought.[111,112] Most critically, ASH was able to promote smoke-free successes in other countries and clearly summarize both the scientific and medical evidence on passive smoking.[17]

Summary: evidence for the effectiveness of public policies to prevent type 2 diabetes

In summary, there is relatively little good evidence for the effectiveness of many public policy measures which should prevent diabetes through improvements to diet and physical activity. There are successful examples of community mobilization and advocacy policies, but interventions need to be high profile and sustained to have significant effects on risk factors. The cost-effectiveness of such interventions is also generally uncertain. They are also more likely to be successful if combined with supportive environmental changes and/or financial incentives and legislation. Policies to change the built environment should offer increased opportunities for physical activity, but there is a dearth of evidence in this area. Legislative or regulatory agreements may also have the scope to achieve larger improvements in diabetes risk factors at a population level, but have rarely been studied, particularly in low- and middle-income settings. There are, however a number of examples of regulatory changes or financial incentives improving diet at a country level. Much can be learnt from the experience of tobacco control, particularly the importance of garnering support from general populations

before lobbying for legislative change. Evidence for the ability of such policy measures to improve physical activity is almost completely absent. The WHO Global Strategy on Diet and Physical Activity has recently published a set of indicators which can be used to monitor strategy implementation and could be combined with country level research to obtain further evidence of the effectiveness of a range of policy measures in different settings.

Summary: what works?

Interventions for which there is good evidence of effectiveness:

• Sustained multi-media multiple risk factor interventions to improve diet and physical activity, if supported by community and legislative, regulatory or financial incentives.

Interventions for which there is some evidence of effectiveness:

• Legislation to remove subsidies on potentially harmful foods or to promote the consumption of healthier options.

Interventions requiring further research:

• The impact of changes to the built environment (such as new parks, walking or cycle routes and traffic calming schemes) on physical activity.

• The impact of legislation or financial incentives (e.g. congestion charging, increases in car parking fees) on physical activity.

• Legislation or regulations banning advertising of junk foods to children.

• Interventions with suppliers (food industry and supermarkets) to improve labelling and promote healthier food choices.

References

1 Oxford University Press. *Oxford English Dictionary Online* [online], 2006; http://dictionary.oed.com/ (accessed: 1 February 2007).
2 Milio N. Glossary: healthy public policy. *J Epidemiol Community Health* 2001;**55**(9):622–623.
3 Pierce JP, Gilpin E, Burns DM, Whalen E, Rosbrook B, Shopland D, Johnson M. Does tobacco advertising target young people to start smoking? Evidence from California. *JAMA* 1991;**266**(22):3154–3158.
4 World Health Organization. *Ottawa Charter for Health Promotion*, World Health Organization, Geneva, 1986.
5 Nutbeam D. Developing healthy public policy. In: *Oxford Handbook of Public Health Practice* (eds D Pencheon, C Guest, D Melzer, J Muir Grey), Oxford University Press, Oxford, 2006, Chapter 4.2.

6 World Health Organization. *Obesity: Preventing and Managing the Global Epidemic – Report of a WHO Consultation on Obesity*, World Health Organization, Geneva, 1998.

7 Egger G, Swinburn B. An ecological approach to the obesity pandemic. *BMJ* 1997;**315**:477–480.

8 Jain A. Treating obesity in individuals and populations. *BMJ* 2005;**331**(7529):1387–1390.

9 Wanless D. *Securing Good Health for the Whole Population: Final Report [The Wanless Report]*, HM Treasury, London, 2004.

10 Department of Health. *Choosing Health: Making Healthier Choices Easier*. The Stationery Office, Norwich, 2004.

11 Anderson G, Sotir Hussey P. Influencing government policy: a framework. In: *Oxford Handbook of Public Health Practice* (eds D Pencheon, C Guest, D Melzer, J Muir Grey), Oxford University Press, Oxford, 2006, Chapter 4.1.

12 Chapman S. Advocacy for public health: a primer. *J Epidemiol Community Health* 2004;**58**(5):361–365.

13 World Health Organization. *Preventing Chronic Diseases: a Vital Investment: WHO Global Report*, World Health Organization, Geneva, 2005.

14 Rohrbach L, Howard-Pitney B, Unger J, Dent C, Howard K, Cruz T, Ribisl K, Norman G, Fishbein H, Johnson C. Independent evaluation of the California Tobacco Control Program: relationships between program exposure and outcomes, 1996–1998. *Am J Public Health* 2002;**92**(6): 975–983.

15 Callinan JE, Clarke A, Doherty K, Kelleher C. Smoking bans for reducing smoking prevalence and tobacco consumption (Protocol). *Cochrane Database Syst Rev* 2006;(2): CD005992.

16 Foster C, Hillsdon M, Cavill N, Bull F, Buxton K, Crombie H. *Interventions that Use the Environment to Encourage Physical Activity. Evidence Review*, HDA Publications, London, 2006; http://www.nice.org.uk/page.aspx?o=366133.

17 Scotland ASH. *The Unwelcome Guest: How Scotland Invited the Tobacco Industry to Smoke Outside*, 2005; http://www.ashscotland.org.uk/ash/files/The%20Unwelcome%20Guest.pdf (accessed 24 July 2009).

18 Sharma M. School-based interventions for childhood and adolescent obesity. *Obesity Rev* 2006;**7**:261–269.

19 Department of Health. *Diabetes National Service Frameworks* [Online], 2007; http://www.dh.gov.uk/en/Policyandguidance/Healthandsocialcaretopics/Diabetes/index.htm.

20 Rose G. Sick individuals and sick populations. *Int J Epidemiol* 1985;**14**(1):32–38.

21 Hopkins DP, Briss PA, Ricard CJ, Husten CG, Carande-Kulis VG, Fielding JE, Alao MO, McKenna JW, Sharp DJ, Harris JR *et al.* Reviews of evidence regarding interventions to reduce tobacco use and exposure to environmental tobacco smoke. *Am J Prev Med* 2001;**20**(2 Suppl): 16–66.

22 Lancaster T, Stead L, Silagy C, Sowden A. Regular review: effectiveness of interventions to help people stop smoking: findings from the Cochrane Library. *BMJ* 2000;**321** (7257):355–358.

23 Sowden A, Arblaster L. Mass media interventions for preventing smoking in young people. *Cochrane Database Syst Rev* 1998;(4):CD001006.

24 Sowden A, Stead L. Community interventions for preventing smoking in young people. *Cochrane Database Syst Rev.* 2003;(1):CD001291.

25 Secker-Walker R, Gnich W, Platt S, Lancaster T. Community interventions for reducing smoking among adults. *Cochrane Database Syst Rev* 2002;(2):CD001745.

26 Bala M, Strzeszynski L, Hey K. Mass media interventions for smoking cessation in adults (Protocol). *Cochrane Database Syst Rev* 2004;(2):CD004704.

27 Hey K, Perera R. Quit and win contests for smoking cessation. *Cochrane Database Syst Rev.* 2005;(2):CD004986.

28 Thomas R, Perera R. School-based programmes for preventing smoking. *Cochrane Database Syst Rev.* 2006;(3): CD001293.

29 Juni P, Altman D, Egger M. Systematic reviews in health care: assessing the quality of controlled clinical trials. *BMJ* 2001;**323**(7303):42–46.

30 Deeks J, Dinnes J, DAmico R, Sowden A, Sakarovitch C, Song F, Petticrew M, Altman D. Evaluating non-randomised intervention studies. *Health Technol Assess* 2003;**7**(27):173.

31 Sackett D, Rosenberg W, Gray J, Haynes R, Richardson W. Evidence based medicine: what it is and what it isn't. *BMJ* 1996;**312**:71–72.

32 Petticrew M. Why certain systematic reviews reach uncertain conclusions. *BMJ* 2003;**326**(7392):756–758.

33 Petticrew M, Roberts H. Evidence, hierarchies and typologies: horses for courses. *J Epidemiol Community Health* 2003;**57**(7):527–529.

34 Puska P, Tuomilehto J, Nissinen A, Vartiainen E. *The North Karelia Project. 20 Year Results and Experiences*, National Public Health Institute, KTL, Helsinki, 1995.

35 Ogilvie D, Egan M, Hamilton V, Petticrew M. Promoting walking and cycling as an alternative to using cars: systematic review. *BMJ* 2004;**329**(7469):763.

36 Rychetnik L, Frommer M, Hawe P, Shiell A. Criteria for evaluating evidence on public health interventions. *J Epidemiol Community Health* 2002;**56**(2):119–127.

37 Thomson H, Hoskins R, Petticrew M, Ogilvie D, Craig N, Quinn T, Lindsay G. Evaluating the health effects of social interventions. *BMJ* 2004;**328**(7434):282–285.

38 Glasziou P, Vandenbroucke J, Chalmers I. Assessing the quality of research. *BMJ* 2004;**328**(7430):39–41.

39 White M, Adams J, Heywood P. How and why do interventions that increase health overall widen inequalities within populations? In: *From Equity to Health: International and Interdisciplinary Perspectives on the Link between Social Inequality and Human Health* (ed. S Babones), Johns Hopkins Press, Baltimore, 2007.

40 Weinehall L, Hellsten G, Boman K, Hallmans G, Asplund K, Wall S. Can a sustainable community intervention reduce the health gap? – 10-year evaluation of a Swedish community intervention program for the prevention of cardiovascular disease. *Scand J Public Health* 2001;Suppl;56: 59–68.

41 Ogilvie D, Foster CE, Rothnie H, Cavill N, Hamilton V, Fitzsimons CF, Mutrie N, on behalf of the Scottish Physical Activity Research C. Interventions to promote walking: systematic review. *BMJ* 2007;**334**(7605):1204.

42 Rychetnik L, Hawe P, Waters E, Barratt A, Frommer M. A glossary for evidence based public health. *J Epidemiol Community Health* 2004;**58**(7):538–545.

43 Task Force on Community Preventive Services. *Community-wide Campaigns are Recommended to Promote Physical Activity*, 2005; http://www.thecommunityguide.org/pa/pa-int-comm-campaigns.pdf (accessed 25 October 2006).

44 Hillsdon M, Cavill N, Nanchahal K, Diamond A, White IR. National level promotion of physical activity: results from Englands ACTIVE for LIFE campaign. *J Epidemiol Community Health* 2001;**55**(10):755–761.

45 Fortmann SP, Varady AN. Effects of a community-wide health education program on cardiovascular disease morbidity and mortality: the Stanford Five-City Project. *Am J Epidemiol* 2000;**152**(4):316–323.

46 Luepker RV, Rastam L, Hannan PJ, Murray DM, Gray C, Baker WL, Crow R, Jacobs D-RJ Pirie PL, Mascioli SR, Mittelmark MB, Blackburn H. Community education for cardiovascular disease prevention. Morbidity and mortality results from the Minnesota Heart Health Program. *Am J Epidemiol* 1996;**144**(4):351–362.

47 Luepker RV, Raczynski JM, Osganian S, Goldberg RJ, Finnegan JR, Hedges JR, Goff DC, Eisenberg MS, Zapka JG, Feldman HA, Labarthe DR, McGovern PG, Cornell CE, Proschan MA, Simons-Morton DG. Effect of a community intervention on patient delay and emergency medical service use in acute coronary heart disease: The Rapid Early Action for Coronary Treatment (REACT) Trial. *JAMA* 2000;**284**(1):60–67.

48 Eaton CB, Lapane KL, Garber CE, Gans KM, Lasater TM, Carleton RA. Effects of a community-based intervention on physical activity: the Pawtucket Heart Health Program. *Am J Public Health* 1999;**89**(11):1741–1744.

49 Tudor-Smith C, Nutbeam D, Moore L, Catford J. Effects of the Heartbeat Wales programme over five years on behavioural risks for cardiovascular disease: quasi-experimental comparison of results from Wales and a matched reference area. *BMJ* 1998;**316**(7134):818–822.

50 Winkleby MA, Feldman HA, Murray DM. Joint analysis of three U.S. community intervention trials for reduction of cardiovascular disease risk. *J Clin.Epidemiol* 1997; **50**(6):645–658.

51 Guide to Community Preventive Services. *Worksite Programs Combining Nutrition and Physical Activity are Recommended to Control Overweight or Obesity*, 2005; http://www.thecommunityguide.org/obese/obese-int-worksite.pdf (accessed: 23 February 2007).

52 Guide to Community Preventive Services. *More Evidence is Needed to Determine the Effectiveness of School-based Programs to Improve the Nutritional Status of Children and Adolescents*, 2005; http://www.thecommunityguide.org/nutrition/nutr-int-schools.pdf (accessed 16 July 2007).

53 Task Force on Community Preventive Services. Increasing physical activity. A report on recommendations of the Task Force on Community Preventive Services. *MMWR* 2001;**50** (RR18):1–16.

54 Task Force on Community Preventive Services. *Point of Decision Prompts that Encourage People to Use the Stairs are Recommended to Promote Physical Activity*, 2005;

http://www.thecommunityguide.org/pa/pa-int-decision-prompts.pdf (accessed 25 October 2006).

55 Morrison DS, Thomson H, Petticrew M. Evaluation of the health effects of a neighbourhood traffic calming scheme. *J Epidemiol Community Health* 2004;**58**(10):837–840.

56 Zatonski WA, Willett W. Changes in dietary fat and declining coronary heart disease in Poland: population based study. *BMJ* 2005;**331**(7510):187–188.

57 Capewell S, McEwen J, Dunbar J, Puska P. Effects of the Heartbeat Wales programme: programme that originated in Finland should be adopted. *BMJ* 1999;**318**:1072–1073.

58 Uusitalo U, Feskens E. JM, Tuomilehto J, Dowse G, Haw U, Fareed D, Hemraj F, Gareeboo H, Alberti KGMM, Zimmet P. Fall in total cholesterol concentration over five years in association with changes in fatty acid composition of cooking oil in Mauritius: cross sectional survey. *BMJ* 1996;**313** (7064):1044–1046.

59 Murray CJL, Lauer JA, Hutubessy RCW, Niessen L, Tomijima N, Rodgers A, Lawes CMM, Evans DB. Effectiveness and costs of interventions to lower systolic blood pressure and cholesterol: a global and regional analysis on reduction of cardiovascular-disease risk. *Lancet* 2003;**361**(9359): 717–725.

60 Mello MM, Studdert DM, Brennan TA. Obesity – the new frontier of public health law. *N Engl J Med* 2006; **354**(24):2601–2610.

61 House of Commons. *Select Committee on Health. Third Report*, London, 2004; http://www.publications.parliament.uk/pa/cm200304/cmselect/cmhealth/23/2307.htm.

62 National Consumer Council. *Traffic Lights for Food? How Nutrient Profiling Can Help Make Healthy Choices Become Easy Choices*, 2004; http://www.ncc.org.uk/food/traffic_lights_for_food.pdf (accessed 27 February 2007).

63 Gostin L. Law as a tool to facilitate healthier lifestyles and prevent obesity. *JAMA* 2007;**297**(1):87–90.

64 Lawlor DA, Ness AR, Cope AM, Davis A, Insall P, Riddoch C. The challenges of evaluating environmental interventions to increase population levels of physical activity: the case of the UK National Cycle Network. *J Epidemiol Community Health* 2003;**57**(2):96–101.

65 Nutbeam D, Smith C, Murphy S, Catford J. Maintaining evaluation designs in long term community based health promotion programmes: Heartbeat Wales case study. *J Epidemiol Community Health* 1993;**47**:127–133.

66 Moffatt S, Mackintosh J, White M, Howel D, Sandell A. The acceptability and impact of a randomised controlled trial of welfare rights advice accessed via primary health care: qualitative study. *BMC Public Health* 2006;**6** (1):163.

67 Woodward M, Tunstall PH. Biochemical evidence of persistent heavy smoking after a coronary diagnosis despite self-reported reduction: analysis from the Scottish Heart Health Study. *Eur Heart J* 1992;**13**(2):160–165.

68 Wilson PWF, Paffenbarger RSJ, Morris JN, Havlik RJ, Assessment methods for physical activity and physical fitness in population studies: report of a NHLBI workshop. *Am Heart J* 1986;**111**:1177–1192.

69 Johansson L, Solvoll K, Bjorneboe GE, Drevon CA. Under- and overreporting of energy intake related to weight status

and lifestyle in a nationwide sample. *Am J Clin Nutr* 1998;**68**(2):266–274.

70 Barth J, Critchley J, Bengel J. Efficacy of psychosocial interventions for smoking cessation in patients with coronary heart disease: a systematic review and meta-analysis. *Ann Behav Med* 2006;**32**(1):10–20

71 Petticrew M, Whitehead M, Macintyre SJ, Graham H, Egan M. Evidence for public health policy on inequalities: 1: the reality according to policymakers. *J Epidemiol Community Health* 2004;**58**(10):811–816.

72 Herxheimer A. Relationships between the pharmaceutical industry and patients organisations. *BMJ* 2003;**326**: 1208–1210.

73 Dooris M. Healthy settings: challenges to generating evidence of effectiveness. *Health Promotion Int* 2006;**21**(1):55–65.

74 Toh CM, Cutter J, Chew SK. School based intervention has reduced obesity in Singapore. *BMJ* 2002;**324**(7334):427.

75 Huang A, Barzi F, Huxley R, Denyer G, Rohrlach B, Jayne K, Neal B. The effects on saturated fat purchases of providing Internet shoppers with purchase-specific dietary advice: a randomised trial. *PLoS Clin Trials* 2006;**1**(5):e22.

76 Mutrie N, Carney C, Blamey A, Crawford F, Aitchison T, Whitelaw A. 'Walk in to Work Out': a randomised controlled trial of a self help intervention to promote active commuting. *J Epidemiol Community Health* 2002;**56**(6): 407–412.

77 Ogilvie D, Egan M, Hamilton V, Petticrew M. Systematic reviews of health effects of social interventions: 2. Best available evidence: how low should you go? *J Epidemiol Community Health* 2005;**59**(10):886–892.

78 Bunn F, Collier T, Frost C, Ker K, Roberts I, Wentz R. Traffic calming for the prevention of road traffic injuries: systematic review and meta-analysis. *Inj Prev* 2003; **9**(3):200–204.

79 Naidoo B, Thorogood M, McPherson K, Gunning-Schepers LJ. Modelling the effects of increased physical activity on coronary heart disease in England and Wales. *J Epidemiol Community Health* 1997;**51**(2):144–150.

80 Gilpin E, Emery S, Farkas A, Distefan J, White M, Pierce J. *The California Tobacco Control Program: a Decade of Progress Results from the California Tobacco Surveys 1990–1998*, University of California, San Diego, 2001.

81 Zatonski W, McMichael A, Powles J. Ecological study of reasons for sharp decline in mortality from ischaemic heart disease in Poland since 1991. *BMJ* 1998;**316**:1047–1051.

82 Kesteloot H, Sans S, Kromhout D. Dynamics of cardiovascular and all-cause mortality in Western and Eastern Europe between 1970 and 2000. *Eur Heart J* 2006;**27**(1): 107–113.

83 Jousilahti P, Vartiainen E, Tuomilehto J, Puska P. Twenty-year dynamics of serum cholesterol levels in the middle-aged population of eastern Finland. *Ann Intern Med* 1996;**125**(9):713–722.

84 Ebrahim S, Davey-Smith GD. Lowering blood pressure: a systematic review of sustained effects of non-pharmacological interventions. *J Public Health* 1998;**20**(4):441–448.

85 He F, MacGregor G. Effect of modest salt reduction on blood pressure: a meta-analysis of randomized trials. Implications for public health. *J Hum Hypertens* 2002;**16**(11):761–770.

86 He F, MacGregor G. Effect of longer-term modest salt reduction on blood pressure. *Cochrane Database Syst Rev.* 2004;(1):CD004937.

87 He F, MacGregor G. Importance of salt in determining blood pressure in children: meta-analysis of controlled trials. *Hypertension* 2006;**48**(5):861–869.

88 Food Safety of Ireland. *Salt and Health*, 2006; http://www.fsai.ie/industry/salt/salt2.asp (accessed: 23 February 2007).

89 Krebs J. Whats on the label? *Science* 2004;**306**(5699):1101.

90 Lobstein T, Landon J, Lincoln P. *Misconceptions and Misinformation: the Problems with Guideline Daily Amounts (GDAs)*, National Heart Forum, London, 2007.

91 Caraher M, Landon J, Dalmeny K. Television advertising and children: lessons from policy development. *Public Health Nutr* 2006;**9**:596–605.

92 Wilson G, Wood K. The influence of children on parental purchases during supermarket shopping. *Int J Consumer Studies* 2004;**28**(4):329–336.

93 Hastings G, Stead M, McDermott L, Forsyth A, MacKintosh A, Rayner M, Godfrey C, Caraher M, Angus K. *Review of Research on the Effects of Food Promotion to Children*, Food Standards Agency, London, 2003.

94 World Health Organization. *Global Strategy on Diet Physical Activity and Health*, 2004; http://www.who.int/gb/ebwha/pdf_files/WHA57/A57_R17-en.pdf (accessed 23 February 2007).

95 World Health Organization. *WHO Framework Convention on Tobacco Control*, 2003; http://www.who.int/tobacco/framework/WHO_FCTC_english.pdf (accessed 27/February 2007).

96 Davis A, Cavill N, Rutter H, Crombie H. *Transport and Health*. Health Development Agency, London, 2007.

97 Kell F. *Congestion Charge Reducing Congested Chests? – King's Team Monitoring the Health Effects of Congestion Charging*, (Press Release), Environmental Research Group, King's College London, London, 2005.

98 Sport England. *The London Plan for Sport and Physical Activity. Working for an Active and Successful sporting Capital. 2004–2008*. Sport England, London, 2004.

99 Transport for London *Congestion Charging. Monitoring. Impacts Monitoring First Annual Report*, Transport for London, London, 2003.

100 Walters R, Boltong A, Mindell J. *Proposed Western Extension of the Central London Congestion Charging Scheme. Health Impact Assessment Report*, London Health Observatory, London, 2005.

101 Eves F, Masters R. An uphill struggle: effects of a point-of-choice stair climbing intervention in a non-English speaking population. *Int J Epidemiol* 2006;**35**(5): 1286–1290.

102 Lancaster T, Stead LF. Physician advice for smoking cessation. *Cochrane Database Syst Rev.* 2004;(4):CD000165.

103 Hajek P, Stead LF, West R, Jarvis M, Lancaster T. Relapse prevention interventions for smoking cessation. *Cochrane Database Syst Rev.* 2005;(1):CD003999.

104 Townsend J. Policies to halve smoking deaths. *Addiction* 1993;**88**(1):37–46.

105 Doll R, Hill A. Mortality of British doctors in relation to smoking: observations on coronary thrombosis. *Natl Cancer Inst Monogr* 1966;**19**:205–268.

106 Doll R, Peto R. Mortality in relation to smoking: 20 years observations on male British doctors. *Br Med J* 1976ii;(6051):1525–1536.

107 Peto R, Lopez AD, Boreham J, Thun M, Heath C, Doll R. Mortality from smoking worldwide. *Br Medl Bull* 1996;**52** (1):12–21.

108 Capewell S, Morrison CE, McMurray JJ. Contribution of modern cardiovascular treatment and risk factor changes to the decline in coronary heart disease mortality in Scotland between 1975 and 1994. *Heart* 1999;**81**(4):380–386.

109 Vartiainen E, Puska P, Pekkanen J, Tuomilehto J, Jousilahti P. Changes in risk factors explain changes in mortality from ischaemic heart disease in Finland. *BMJ* 1994;**309**(6946): 23–27.

110 Sigfusson N, Sigvaldson H, Steingrimsdottir L, Gudmundsdottir II, Stefansdottir I, Thorsteinsson Y, Sigurdsson G. Decline in ischaemic heart disease in Iceland and change in risk factor levels. *BMJ* 1991;**302**:1371–1375.

111 Tulunay OE, Hecht SS, Carmella SG, Zhang Y, Lemmonds C, Murphy S, Hatsukami DK. Urinary metabolites of a tobacco-specific lung carcinogen in nonsmoking hospitality workers. *Cancer Epidemiol Biomarkers Prev* 2005;**14**(5): 1283–1286.

112 Johnsson T, Tuomi T, Hyvärinen M, Svinhufvud J, Rothberg M, Reijula K. Occupational exposure of non-smoking restaurant personnel to environmental tobacco smoke in Finland. *Am J Ind Med* 2003;**43**(5):523–531.

Index

The Evidence Base for Diabetes Care, Second Edition, Edited by William H. Herman, Ann Louise Kinmonth, Nicholas J. Wareham and Rhys Williams.
© 2010 John Wiley & Sons, Ltd

This index was prepared by Neil Manley.